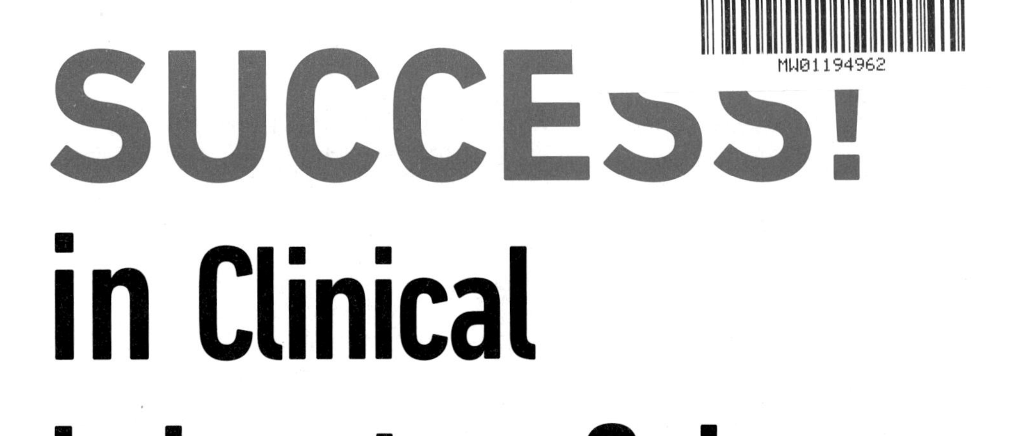

SUCCESS! in Clinical Laboratory Science

FIFTH EDITION

Donald C. Lehman, EdD, MLS(ASCP)^{CM}, SM(NRCM)
Professor
Department of Medical and Molecular Sciences
College of Health Sciences
University of Delaware

Janelle M. Chiasera, PhD, MT(ASCP)
Senior Executive Associate Dean and Professor
School of Health Professions
The University of Alabama at Birmingham

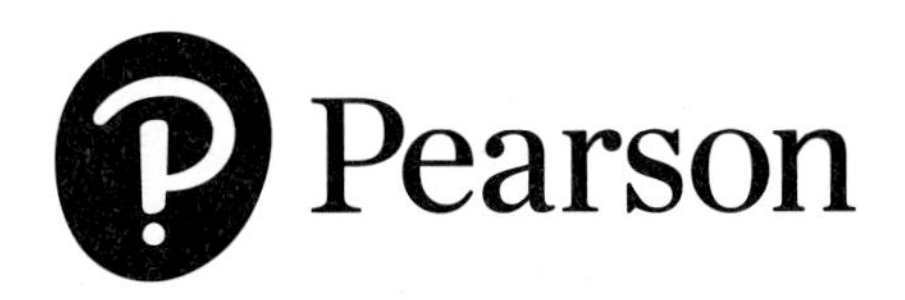

Pearson

SVP, Product Management: Adam Jaworski
Director Product Management - Health Sciences: Katrin Beacom
Content Manager - Health Professions & Nursing: Kevin Wilson
Portfolio Management Assistant: Cara Schaurer
Associate Sponsoring Editor: Zoya Zaman
Product Marketing Manager: Rachele Strober
Field Marketing Manager: Brittany Hammond
Vice President, Digital Studio and Content Production: Paul DeLuca
Director, Digital Studio and Content Production: Brian Hyland
Managing Producer: Jennifer Sargunar
Content Producer (Team Lead): Faraz Sharique Ali
Content Producer: Neha Sharma
Project Manager, Global R&P: Anjali Singh
DGM, Global R&P: Tanvi Bhatia
Operations Specialist: Maura Zaldivar-Garcia
Cover Design: SPi Global
Cover Photo: Xubingruo/E+/Getty Images
Full-Service Project Management and Composition: Ashwina Ragounath, Integra Software Services Pvt. Ltd.
Printer/Binder: LSC Communications
Cover Printer: LSC Communications
Text Font: Garamond LT Std

Library of Congress Cataloging-in-Publication Data

Names: Lehman, Donald C., author | Chiasera, Janelle M., author
Title: Success! in clinical laboratory science / Donald C. Lehman, EdD, MT(ASCP), SM(NRM), Associate Professor, Department of Medical Technology, College of Health Sciences, University of Delaware.
Other titles: Prentice Hall health's Q and A review of medical technology/clinical laboratory science.
Description: Fifth edition. | Hoboken, New Jersey: Pearson, [2020] | Includes index.
Identifiers: LCCN 2019002761 | ISBN 9780134989181 | ISBN 013498918X
Subjects: LCSH: Medical laboratory technology—Examinations, questions, etc. | Diagnosis, Laboratory—Examinations, questions, etc.
Classification: LCC RB38.25.M42 2020 | DDC 616.07/5076—dc23
LC record available at https://lccn.loc.gov/2019002761

1 2019

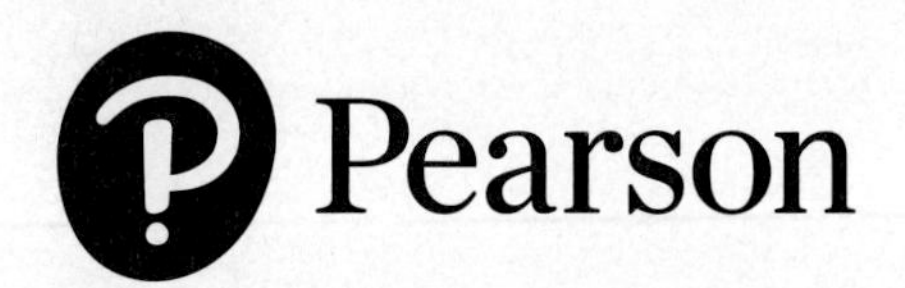

ISBN 10: 0-13-498918-X
ISBN 13: 978-0-13-498918-1

WE DEDICATE THIS BOOK

To my wife, Terri, whose love, support, and encouragement
helped make this book possible.

Donald C. Lehman

and

To my parents, John and Arleen, for their unwavering support,
love, and encouragement; and to my husband, John,
who is my best friend, my greatest support,
my biggest comfort, and my strongest motivation.

Janelle M. Chiasera

and

To all the clinical laboratory professionals who contribute their expertise daily
as members of the healthcare team and to all current clinical
laboratory science students and those who will follow.

Contents

Preface

SUCCESS! in Clinical Laboratory Science: Complete Review, Fifth Edition, is designed as an all-in-one summary and review of the major clinical laboratory science content areas generally taught in an academic program. It is designed to help examination candidates prepare for national certification or state licensure examinations. It is also a resource for practicing clinical laboratory scientists wanting a "refresher." Students enrolled in clinical laboratory science programs can use the text to prepare for undergraduate examinations. The excellent reception received by the first four editions of the book spurred the writing of this fifth edition. Educators and students alike have commented that the strengths of the book are concise summaries of important information and the paragraph explanations that accompany each answer to the review questions. The explanations help readers of the book augment their knowledge or clear up misunderstandings.

In the fifth edition, we continued the concise outline of each content area that began in the fourth edition. The outlines are not intended to replace discipline-specific textbooks, but the outlines will provide a quick review of important material.

Color plates of 58 full-color pictures are included to provide the user with an experience in answering questions based on a color photograph. Additionally, a 200-question self-assessment test and a 100-question self-assessment test on the Student Resource Website are included as mechanisms for final evaluation of one's knowledge, thus allowing for the identification of one's strengths and weaknesses while there is still time to improve.

The book contains more than 2000 multiple choice questions that cover all the areas commonly tested on national certification and state licensure examinations. The questions are based on current clinical laboratory practice, and case study questions are incorporated to hone problem-solving and critical thinking skills. The paragraph rationales expand upon the correct answer, and matching puzzles on the Student Resource Website provide an alternate means to assess recall knowledge. Overall, this book provides the essential components needed in an effective clinical laboratory science examination review book. We hope that you find this book and the accompanying Student Resource Website useful, and we wish you success in your academic studies, with the certification examination, and with your career as a clinical laboratory professional.

New to the fifth edition:

- We expanded the content on molecular biology and added more review questions.
- Information was added on matrix assisted-laser desorption/ionization time of flight for the identification of microorganisms.
- The section on antimicrobial testing was expanded to include detecting extended-spectrum beta-lactamases and carbapenemases.
- New medications used in hemostasis treatments were added.
- Celiac disease, pathology and diagnosis, was added to the immunology chapter.
- Revisions were made to many of the multiple-choice questions and answer explanations.
- Several color images were updated.

STUDENT RESOURCES

To access the material on student resources that accompany this book, visit www.pearsonhighered.com/healthprofessionsresources. Click on view all resources and select Clinical Lab Science from the choice of disciplines. Find this book and you will find the complimentary study materials.

Acknowledgments

This book is the end product of the labor and dedication of a number of outstanding professionals. The editors would like to acknowledge these individuals for their invaluable assistance in completing this project. The editors greatly appreciate the efforts of the contributing authors who worked so diligently to produce quality materials. A note of recognition and appreciation is extended to Karen A. Keller, Mary Ann McLane, and Linda Sykora, who allowed use of their color slides in the fourth edition, many of which were maintained in the fifth edition. We want to thank Linda Smith who contributed new images for the fifth edition. In addition, we extend a special acknowledgment to Elmer W. Koneman, MD, Professor Emeritus, University of Colorado School of Medicine and Medical Laboratory Director, Summit Medical Center, Frisco, CO for use of color slides from his private collection.

Certifying Agencies

Information pertaining to certification examinations, education and training requirements, and application forms may be obtained by contacting the certifying agency of your choice. The following is a list of the certification agencies that service clinical laboratory professionals.

American Society for Clinical Pathology Board of Certification (ASCP/BOC)
33 West Monroe Street, Suite 1600
Chicago, IL 60603
312-541-4999
E-mail: bor@ascp.org
Web site: http://www.ascp.org

American Medical Technologists (AMT)
10700 West Higgins Road, Suite 150
Rosemont, IL 60018
847-823-5169 or 800-275-1268
E-mail: MT-MLT@amt1.com
Web site: http://www.americanmedtech.org/

American Association of Bioanalysts (AAB)
906 Olive Street, Suite 1200
St. Louis, MO 63101-1434
314-241-1445
E-mail: aab@aab.org
Web site: http://www.aab.org

Contributors

Charity Accurso, PhD, MLS(ASCP)[CM]
Associate Professor
Director, Medical Laboratory Science Program
Department Head, Clinical and Health Information Sciences
College of Allied Health Sciences
University of Cincinnati
Cincinnati, Ohio

Leslie Allshouse
Senior Instructor and
Medical Laboratory Science Program Director
University of Delaware
Newark, Delaware

Lela Buckingham, PhD, retired
Assistant Professor
Department of Laboratory Science
Rush University
Chicago, Illinois

Sabrina Bryant, PhD
Assistant Professor
Department of Medical Laboratory Science
University of Southern Mississippi
Hattiesburg, Mississippi

Janelle Chiasera, PhD
Professor and
Chair, Department of Clinical and Diagnostic Sciences
Senior Executive Associate Dean, School of Health Professions
University of Alabama at Birmingham
Birmingham, Alabama

Floyd Josephat, EdD, MT(ASCP)
Associate Professor and
Program Director, Clinical Laboratory Sciences
Program Director, Clinical Pathologist Assistant
Department of Clinical and Diagnostic Sciences
University of Alabama at Birmingham
Birmingham, Alabama

Don Lehman, EdD MLS(ASCP)[CM], SM(NRCM)
Professor and
Director Medical Diagnostic Program
Department of Medical and Molecular Sciences
University of Delaware
Newark, Delaware

Dave McGlassen, MS, MLS, retired
Wilford Hall Medical Center
59th Clinical Research Division (Laboratory)
Joint Base San Antonio
Lackland, Texas

Mary Ann McLane, PhD, MLS(ASCP)^{CM}
Professor Emeritus
Department of Medical and Molecular Sciences
University of Delaware
Newark, Delaware

Ana Oliveira, DPH
Assistant Professor
Department of Clinical and Diagnostic Sciences
University of Alabama at Birmingham
Birmingham, Alabama

Linda Smith, PhD, MLS(ASCP)^{CM}, BB^{CM}
Professor
Department of Health Sciences
University of Texas Health Science Center
San Antonio, Texas

Cheryl Katz, MS, MT(ASCP), SH, CLS(NCA)
Vice President Pathology and Laboratory Sciences
Christiana Healthcare System
Newark, Delaware

Brian Singh, BS, MLS
Clinical Laboratory Section Supervisor
Children's Hospital of Philadelphia
Philadelphia, Pennsylvania

Reviewers

Stacy Askvig, MS MT(ASCP)
University of North Dakota
Minot, Newark, Delaware

Tracy Buch, MA RT(R)(M)
Southeast Community College
Lincoln, Nebraska

Kathryn Dugan, MEd, MT(ASCP)
Auburn University at Montgomery
Montgomery, Alabama

Liz Johnson, MLS ASCP, CLS NCA, MT AMT
University of New Mexico
Albuquerque, New Mexico

Timothy Maze
Lander University
Greenwood, South Carolina

Catherine Moran Robinson, BSc, MSc, MEd, MT(ASCP); MLT (CSMLS)
New Brunswick Community College
Saint John, New Brunswick
Canada

Jo Ellen Russell, MT(ASCP), RHIT, RMA(AMT)
Panola College
Carthage, Texas

Matthew Schoell, MLS (ASCP)CM
Nazareth College
Rochester, New York

Tyra Stalling, CLS (ASCP)
Dalton State College
Dalton, Georgia

Lorraine Torres, Ed.D, MT(ASCP)
The University of Texas at El Paso
El Paso, Texas

Joan Young, MHA, MT(ASCP)
Southwest Wisconsin Technical College
Fennimore, Wisconsin

Introduction

If you are currently preparing for a Clinical Laboratory Science/Medical Laboratory Science certification or licensure examination, or if you are a practicing clinical laboratory professional who wants to "brush up" on clinical laboratory information, then this is the review book for you. ***SUCCESS! in Clinical Laboratory Science: Complete Review, Fifth Edition*** is a comprehensive text containing content outlines and more than 2000 questions with paragraph explanations accompanying each answer. Unique to this book is an outline of each content area that concisely summarizes important information. The question and rationale format not only tests your knowledge of the subject matter but also facilitates additional learning. Color plates of 58 full-color pictures are included to help you prepare for national examinations in as realistic a manner as possible. There is a 200-question self-assessment test and a 100-question self-assessment test on the Student Resource Website. Both assessments will assist you in determining your mastery of the material while allowing computer practice for certification examinations.

ORGANIZATION

The book is organized into 17 chapters corresponding to the areas tested on clinical laboratory science/medical laboratory science certification examinations with Chapter 17 being a review exam. The chapters are as follows:

1. Clinical Chemistry
2. Hematology
3. Hemostasis
4. Immunology and Serology
5. Immunohematology
6. Bacteriology

7. Mycology
8. Parasitology
9. Virology
10. Molecular Diagnostics
11. Urinalysis and Body Fluids
12. Laboratory Calculations
13. General Laboratory Principles, Quality Assessment, and Safety
14. Laboratory Management
15. Medical Laboratory Education and Research
16. Computers and Laboratory Information Systems
17. Self-Assessment Test

The chapters are organized into an outline, review questions, and answers with paragraph explanations. A list of references is located at the end of each chapter for further review. The last chapter is a 200-question self-assessment test that should be used to determine overall competency upon completion of the previous chapters. To further synthesize important material, case studies in clinical chemistry, hematology, immunology and serology, immunohematology, and microbiology are included. The Student Resource Website has three types of assessment tools including a 100-question self-assessment test to assist you in preparing for computerized national examinations. In addition, matching puzzles are available to help you to review major points associated with each content area.

QUESTIONS

The style of the questions used adheres to that prevalent in most certification examinations. Each chapter contains questions in a multiple-choice format with a single answer. In some cases, a group of two or more questions may be based on a case study or other clinical situation. Questions are divided among three levels of difficulty: Level 1 questions test recall of information, level 2 questions test understanding of information and application to new situations, and level 3 questions test problem-solving ability. Each of the multiple-choice questions is followed by four choices, with only one of the choices being completely correct. Although some choices may be partially correct, remember that there can only be one best answer.

HOW TO USE THIS BOOK

The best way to use ***SUCCESS! in Clinical Laboratory Science: Complete Review, Fifth Edition*** is to first read through the outline. If you find that some of the material is not fresh in your memory, go to a textbook or recent class notes to review the area in more detail. Then work through short sections of the questions at a time, reading each question carefully, and recording an answer for each. Next, consult and read the correct answers. It is important to read the paragraph explanations for both those questions answered correctly as well as for those missed, because very often additional information will be presented that will reinforce or clarify knowledge already present. If you answer a question incorrectly, it would be wise to consult the references listed at the end of the chapter.

Lastly, you should take the 200-question self-assessment test as if it was the actual examination. Find a quiet place, free of interruptions and distractions, and allow yourself 3 hours and 30 minutes to complete the self-assessment test. Record your answers; then check the answer key. Review topic areas that seemed difficult. As final preparation, take 2 hours to complete the 100-question computerized test on the Student Resource Website. These tests will give you a more realistic evaluation of your knowledge and your ability to function within a time constraint. It is important that you are comfortable taking a test that is computerized, because the certifying agencies now use either computer-administered or computer-adaptive testing. So be sure to practice on the computer using the Student Resource Website. By the time you have worked through the outlines, the questions and rationales, the two self-assessment tests, case studies, and the matching puzzles, you will have gained a solid base of knowledge.

For students of clinical laboratory science/medical laboratory science and clinical laboratory practitioners, this book has been designed to summarize important information, to test your knowledge, and to explain unfamiliar information through use of the paragraph explanations that accompany each question. Working through the entire book will make you aware of the clinical areas in which you are strong or weak. This review will help you gauge your study time before taking any national certification or state licensure examination. Remember, there is no substitute for knowing the material.

TEST-TAKING TIPS

In addition to studying and reviewing the subject matter, you should also consider the following points:

1. Contact the Sponsoring Agency
   Check the Website of the sponsoring agency that administers the examination and review the general information about the test, including
   - The outline of the test content areas
   - The test question format
   - If it is computer administered or computer adaptive
   - The time allowed to complete the test and the number of test questions to expect
   - The scoring policy

   Note: Because certification examination requirements vary, it is important to read thoroughly all directions published by the sponsoring agency and to read carefully the directions presented on the day of the examination. After completing the computerized examinations, most agencies permit you to return to previously answered questions and entered responses can be changed. In some cases the sponsoring agency allows you to skip a question and return to it at the end of the exam, whereas other agencies require that you select an answer before being allowed to move to the next question. So know the rules! Checking your answers is a very important part of taking a certification exam. During the exam, check the computer screen after an answer is entered to verify that the answer appears as it was entered.

2. Prepare before Examination Day
   - Study thoroughly prior to taking the exam. Set up a study schedule that allows sufficient time for review of each area. Treat studying like a job.
   - Use this review book to help you to identify your strengths and weaknesses, to sharpen your test-taking skills, and to be more successful with multiple choice examinations.
   - Know the locations of the test center and the parking facilities. If the area is unfamiliar to you, a visit to the site a week before the exam may help to prevent unnecessary anxiety on the morning of the test.
   - Check your calculator (if one is allowed) for proper function and worn batteries. Some agencies allow a nonprogrammable calculator to be used during the exam.
   - Get plenty of rest. Do not cram. A good night's sleep will prove to be more valuable than cramming the night before the exam.
3. On the Examination Day
   - Eat a good breakfast.
   - Take two types of identification with you—your photo identification and another form of identification, with both illustrating your current name and signature, as these are generally required—and your admission letter (if required by the agency).
   - Take a nonprogrammable calculator (if one is allowed) to the test center. Most test centers do not permit any paper, pencils, or study materials in the testing area. In addition, electronic devices such as cell phones, etc. are not permitted in the test center.
   - Allow sufficient time to get to the test center without rushing. Most agencies require that you be at the test center 30 minutes before the start of the exam.
   - Wear a wristwatch in order to budget your time properly.
   - Read the directions thoroughly and carefully. Know what the directions are saying.
   - Read each question carefully. Be sure to answer the question asked. Do not look for hidden meanings.
   - Take particular note of qualifying words such as "least," "not," "only," "best," and "most."
   - Rapidly scan each choice to familiarize yourself with the possible responses.
   - Reread each choice carefully, eliminating choices that are obviously incorrect.
   - Select the one best answer.
   - Enter the correct response in accordance with the directions of the test center.

- Budget your time. If the test has, for example, 100 questions and 2 hours and 30 minutes are allowed for completion, you have approximately 1 minute and 30 seconds for each question.
- Above all, don't panic! If you "draw a blank" on a particular question or set of questions, skip it and go on unless the directions indicate that all questions must be answered when presented. At the end of the exam, if you are permitted, return to review your answers or to complete any skipped questions. Stay calm and do your best.

KEYS TO SUCCESS ACROSS THE BOARDS

Study, review, and practice.
Keep a positive, confident attitude.
Follow all directions on the examination.
Do your best.

Good luck!

CHAPTER

1 Clinical Chemistry

contents

Note: *The reference ranges used throughout the book are meant to function as guides to understand and relate to the analytes; each laboratory facility will have established its own reference ranges based on the laboratory's specific instrumentation, methods, population, and so on.*

I. INSTRUMENTATION AND ANALYTICAL PRINCIPLES

A. Spectrophotometry General Information

1. **Electromagnetic radiation** has wave-like and particle-like properties.
   a. **Radiant energy** is characterized as a spectrum from short wavelength to long wavelength: cosmic, gamma rays, X-rays, ultraviolet, visible, infrared, microwaves, and radiowaves.
   b. **Wavelength (λ)** is the distance traveled by one complete wave cycle (distance between two successive crests) measured in **nanometers (nm).**
   c. The **shorter the wavelength**, the **greater the energy** contained in the light, and the greater the number of photons.
   d. Light is classified according to its wavelength: **Ultraviolet (UV) light** has very short wavelengths and **infrared (IR) light** has very long wavelengths. When all **visible wavelengths** of light (400–700 nm) are combined, white light results.
      1) Visible color: wavelength of light transmitted (not absorbed) by an object
2. Particles of light are called **photons.** When an atom absorbs a photon, the atom becomes **excited** in one of three ways: An electron is moved to a higher energy level, the mode of the covalent bond vibration is changed, or the rotation around its covalent bond is changed.
   a. When energy is absorbed as a photon, an **electron** is moved to a higher energy level where it is **unstable.**
      1) An excited electron is not stable and will **return to ground state.**
      2) An electron will **emit** energy in the form of **light** (radiant energy) of a characteristic wavelength.
      3) Absorption or emission of energy forms a **line spectrum** that is characteristic of a molecule and can help identify a molecule.

B. Spectrophotometer

1. In order to determine the concentration of a light-absorbing analyte in solution, a **spectrophotometer measures light transmitted** by that analyte in solution. Such an analyte may absorb, transmit, and reflect light to varying degrees, but always of a characteristic nature for the analyte.
2. **Components of a spectrophotometer**
   a. Power supply
   b. Light source
   c. Entrance slit
   d. Monochromator
   e. Exit slit
   f. Cuvet/sample cell
   g. Photodetector
   h. Readout device

3. The **light source** or **exciter lamp** produces an intense, reproducible, and constant beam of light. A variety of light sources exist to measure within the visible and ultraviolet regions as described further.
   a. Incandescent lamps
      1) **Tungsten (incandescent tungsten or tungsten-iodide):** Most common, used in visible and near-infrared regions. Approximately 15% of radiant energy falls within the visible region, the rest falls in the near-infrared region; therefore, a heat absorbing filter is placed between the lamp and the sample to absorb the infrared radiation. NOTE: This lamp does not provide sufficient energy for measurements in the UV region.
      2) **Deuterium:** Used in the ultraviolet region; provides continuous emission down to 165 nm
      3) **Mercury arc (low, medium, and high pressure):** Used in the ultraviolet region; low-pressure mercury arc lamps (not practical for absorbance measurements) emit sharp ultraviolet and visible line spectra; medium- to high-pressure lamps emit continuum from ultraviolet to the mid-visible region.
      4) **Xenon arc:** Used in the ultraviolet region; provide continuous spectra
   b. **Lasers (light amplification by stimulated emission of radiation):** Lasers produce extremely intense, focused, and nearly nondivergent beam of light.
   c. **Important:** When a lamp is changed in the spectrophotometer, the instrument must be recalibrated because changing the light source changes the angle of the light striking the monochromator.
4. The **monochromator** is a device used to isolate radiant energy of wider wavelengths to a mechanically selected narrow band of desirable wavelengths of light, in other words, it is a wavelength isolator. When a monochromator is set to a particular wavelength, light with a Gaussian distribution of wavelengths emerges from the exit slit. This information can be used to describe **bandpass.** The bandpass, or spectral bandwidth, is defined as the width of the band of light at one-half the peak maximum. The bandpass describes the purity of light emitted from the monochromator, which is a reflection of the resolution capabilities of the instrument. For example, if a spectrophotometer is set to read at 550 nm, light with a Gaussian distribution of wavelengths between 540 and 560 nm emerges from the exit slit. Bandpass may be determined by locating one-half the maximum intensity of light (50%) on the *y*-axis and dropping two vertical lines down to the *x*-axis from these midpoints, 545 and 555 nm. The distance between these two points (545–555) is equal to the bandpass, in other words, 10 nm. See Figure 1–1■. Types of monochromators are described further.
   a. **Filters**
      1) **Glass filters** are used in **photometers;** simple and inexpensive; isolate a relatively wide band of radiant energy and therefore have low transmittance of the selected wavelength; considered less precise.
      2) **Interference filters:** Produce monochromatic light using constructive interference of waves using two pieces of glass; can be constructed to yield a very narrow range of wavelengths with good efficiency.

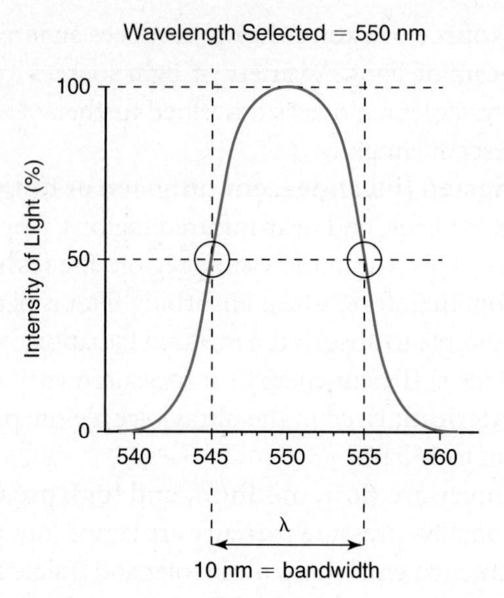

FIGURE 1–1 ■ Determining spectral bandwidth.

b. **Diffraction gratings** are the most commonly used monochromators in **spectrophotometers;** consist of a flat glass plate coated with a thin layer of aluminum-copper alloy with rulings of many parallel grooves into the coating. The more rulings, the better the grating, for example, better diffraction gratings contain 1000–2000 lines/mm.

c. **Prisms:** Used in **spectrophotometers;** separate light through refraction with shorter wavelengths that are bent (refracted) more than longer wavelengths as they pass through the prism.

1) **Wavelength selection:** Entrance slit allows lamp light to enter; slit is fixed in position and size. Monochromator disperses the light into wavelengths. Exit slit selects the bandpass of the monochromator that allows light of the selected wavelength to pass through the cuvet onto the detector.

5. **Photodetectors:** A **detector converts** the **electromagnetic radiation** (light energy) transmitted by a solution **into an electrical signal.** The more light transmitted, the more energy, and the greater the electrical signal that is measured.
6. **Readout devices:** Electrical energy from a detector is displayed on some type of digital display or readout system. The readout system may be a chart recorder or a computer printout.

C. Atomic Absorption Spectrophotometry

1. **Principle: Ground-state atoms absorb light at defined wavelengths.**

a. **Line spectrum** refers to the wavelengths at which an atom absorbs light; each metal exhibits a specific line spectrum.

b. The sample is **atomized in a flame** where the atoms of the metal to be quantified are dissociated from its chemical bonds and placed at ground state.

Once in this state, it is at a low-energy level and is now capable of absorbing light corresponding to its own line spectrum.

c. Then a beam of light from a **hollow-cathode lamp** (HCL) is passed through a chopper to the flame.

d. The **ground-state atoms** in the flame **absorb** the same wavelengths of **light** from the HCL as the atoms emit when excited.

e. The **light not absorbed** by the atoms is **measured as a decrease in light intensity by the detector.** The detector (photomultiplier tube) will selectively read the pulsed light from the chopper that passes through the flame and will not detect any light emitted by the excited atoms when they return to ground state.

f. The difference in the amount of light leaving the HCL and the amount of light measured by the detector is **indirectly proportional to the concentration** of the metal analyte in the sample.

2. **Components**

Hollow-cathode lamp → chopper → burner head for flame →
monochromator → detector → readout device

3. **Hollow-cathode lamp (HCL)**

a. HCL contains an anode, a cylindrical cathode made of metal being analyzed, and an inert gas such as helium or argon.

b. **Principle:** Applied voltage causes ionization of the gas, and these excited ions are attracted to the cathode, where they collide with the metal coating on the cathode, knocking off atoms, and causing atomic electrons to become excited. When the electrons of the metal atoms from the cathode return to ground state, the characteristic light energy of that metal is emitted.

c. Vaporized metal atoms from the sample can be found in the flame. The flame serves as the sample cuvet in this instrument.

d. The light produced in the HCL passes through a chopper and then to the flame, and the light is absorbed by the metal in the sample. The light not absorbed will be read by the photomultiplier tube.

e. A **flameless system** employs a carbon rod (graphite furnace), tantalum, or platinum to hold the sample in a chamber. The temperature is raised to vaporize the sample being analyzed. The atomized sample then absorbs the light energy from the HCL. This technique is more sensitive than the flame method.

D. Nephelometry

1. **Definition:** Nephelometry is the **measurement of light scattered** by a particulate solution. Generally, scattered light is measured at an angle to the incident light when small particles are involved; for large molecules, forward light scatter can be measured. The **amount of scatter is directly proportional** to the number and size of particles present in the solution.

2. The **sensitivity of nephelometry** depends on the absence of background scatter from scratched cuvets and particulate matter in reagents.

E. Turbidimetry

1. **Definition:** Turbidimetry **measures light blocked** as a decrease in the light transmitted through the solution; dependent on particle size and concentration.
2. **Turbidimetry uses a spectrophotometer** for measurement, and it is limited by the photometric accuracy and sensitivity of the instrument.

F. Molecular Emission Spectroscopy

1. Types of **luminescence** where **excitation requires absorption of radiant energy**
   a. **Fluorescence** is a process where atoms absorb energy at a particular wavelength (excitation), electrons are raised to higher-energy orbitals, and the electrons release energy as they return to ground state by emitting light energy of a longer wavelength and lower energy than the exciting wavelength. The emitted light has a very short lifetime.
      1) **Fluorometry:** Frequently UV light is used for excitation and is passed through a primary filter for proper wavelength selection for the analyte being measured. The excitation light is absorbed by the atoms of the analyte in solution, which causes the electrons to move to higher-energy orbitals. Upon return to ground state, light is emitted from the fluorescing analyte and that light passes through a secondary filter. The secondary filter and the detector are placed at a right angle to the light source to prevent incident light from being measured by the detector. Whereas fluorometers use filters, spectrofluorometers use prisms or diffraction gratings as monochromators.
      2) **Advantages:** Fluorometry is about 1000 times more **sensitive** than absorption techniques and has increased **specificity** because optimal wavelengths are chosen both for absorption (excitation) and for monitoring emitted fluorescence.
      3) **Limitations:** It changes from the established protocol that affect pH, temperature, and solvent quality; self-absorption; quenching.

   b. **Phosphorescence** is the emission of light produced by certain substances after they absorb energy. It is similar to fluorescence except that the time delay is longer (greater than 10^{-4} seconds) between absorption of radiant energy and release of energy as photons of light.
2. Types of **luminescence** where excitation does **not** require **absorption of radiant energy**
   a. **Chemiluminescence** is the process where the **chemical energy** of a reaction produces excited atoms, and upon electron return to ground state, photons of light are emitted.

b. **Bioluminescence** is the process where an **enzyme-catalyzed** chemical reaction produces light emission. For example, this may occur in the presence of the enzyme luciferase because of oxidation of the substrate luciferin.
   1) **Luminometer** is a generic term for the type of instrument that is used to measure chemiluminescence and bioluminescence.

G. Chromatography

1. **Chromatography** is a technique where solutes in a sample are separated for identification based on **physical differences** that allow their differential distribution between a mobile phase and a stationary phase.
   a. **Mobile phase:** Phase that passes through the column; may be an inert gas or a liquid
   b. **Stationary phase:** Phase bound to the column therefore, it does not pass through the column; may be silica gel bound to the surface of a glass plate or plastic sheet; may be silica or a polymer that is coated or bonded within a column

H. Thin-Layer Chromatography (TLC)

1. TLC is a type of planar chromatography. The **stationary phase** may be silica gel that is coated onto a solid surface such as a glass plate or plastic sheet. The **mobile phase** is a solvent, where solvent polarity should be just enough to achieve clear separation of the solutes in the sample. TLC is a technique used clinically for **urine drug screening.**
2. **The mobile phase moves through the stationary phase by absorption and capillary action.** The solute components move at different rates because of solubility in the mobile phase and electrostatic forces of the stationary phase that retard solute movement. These two phases work together to provide **solute resolution and separation.**
   a. Solute will stay with the **solvent front** if solvent is too polar for the solute.
   b. Solute will remain at **origin** if solvent is insufficiently polar.
3. Basic steps in performing TLC include sample extraction using a liquid-liquid or column technique; concentration of the extracted sample; sample application by spotting onto the silica gel plate; development of the solute in the sample using the stationary and mobile phases; solute detection using chromogenic sprays, UV light, fluorescence, and heat; and interpretation of chromatographic results utilizing R_f values of solutes in comparison to aqueous standards.
4. **R_f values** are affected by chamber saturation, temperature, humidity, and composition of the solvent.

I. Gas-Liquid Chromatography (GLC)

1. **Gas-liquid chromatograph** components include a carrier gas with a flow-control device to regulate the gas flow, a heated injector, chromatographic column to separate the solutes, heated column oven, detector, and computer to process data and control the operation of the system.

2. **Gas-liquid chromatography** is a technique used to **separate volatile solutes.**
   a. The sample is injected into the injector component of the instrument where the **sample is vaporized** because the injector is maintained approximately 50°C higher than the column temperature.
   b. An **inert carrier gas (mobile phase)** carries the vaporized sample into the column. Carrier gases commonly used include hydrogen, helium, nitrogen, and argon. The **carrier gas flow rate is critical** to maintaining column efficiency and reproducibility of elution times.
   c. The types of **columns (stationary phase)** used are designated as packed or capillary. When the volatile solutes carried by the gas over the stationary phase of the column are eluted, the column effluent is introduced to the detector. The solutes are introduced to the detector in the order that each was eluted.
   d. The **detector** produces a signal for identification and quantification of the solutes. Commonly used detectors include flame ionization, thermal conductivity, electron capture, and mass spectrometer.
   e. Separation of solutes is a function of the relative differences between the vapor pressure of the solutes and the interactions of the solutes with the stationary column. The **more volatile** a solute, **the faster it will elute** from the column; the **less interaction** of the solute **with the column**, the **faster it will elute.**
   f. **Identification** of a solute is based on its **retention time** and **quantification** is based on **peak size** where the amount of solute present is proportional to the size of the peak (area or height of the sample peak is compared to known standards).

J. High-Performance Liquid Chromatography (HPLC)

1. **High-performance liquid chromatograph** components include solvent reservoir(s), one or more pumps to propel the solvent(s), injector, chromatographic column, detector, and computer to process data and control the operation of the system.
2. HPLC is a type of liquid chromatography where the **mobile phase** is a **liquid** that is passed over the **stationary phase** of the **column.** The separation of solutes in a sample is governed by the selective distribution of the solutes between the mobile and stationary phases.
   a. **Solvents** commonly used for the **mobile phase** include acetonitrile, methanol, ethanol, isopropanol, and water.
      1) **Isocratic elution:** Strength of solvent **remains constant** during separation.
      2) **Gradient elution:** Strength of solvent **continually increases** (%/min) during separation.
   b. **Stationary phase** is an **organic material covalently bonded to silica** that may be polar or nonpolar in composition.
      1) **Normal-phase** liquid chromatography: Polar stationary phase and nonpolar mobile phase
      2) **Reversed-phase** liquid chromatography: Nonpolar stationary phase and polar mobile phase

3. The **solvent-delivery system** utilizes a solvent reservoir from which the pump can push the mobile phase through the column. The sample is introduced through a loop injector. A precolumn and guard column function to maintain the integrity of the column and are positioned prior to the sample reaching the main column. The column, which functions as the stationary phase, generally operates at room temperature. The effluent from the column passes to a detector system. The solutes are introduced to the detector in the order that each was eluted.
4. The **detector** produces a signal for identification and quantification of the solutes. Commonly used detectors include spectrophotometer, photodiode array, fluorometer, electrochemical, and mass spectrometer.

K. Mass Spectrometry

1. A **mass spectrometer** is an instrument that uses the principle of **charged particles moving through a magnetic or electric field**, with **ions** being **separated** from other charged particles **according to their mass-to-charge ratios.** In this system, electrons bombard a sample, ionizing the compound into **fragment ions**, which are separated by their mass-to-charge ratios. The **mass spectrum** produced is unique for a compound **(identification)**, and the **number of ions** produced relates proportionally to **concentration** (quantification).
2. **Mass spectrometry** is a high-quality technique for identifying drugs or drug metabolites, amino acid composition of proteins, and steroids. In addition, mass spectrometry has applications in the field of proteomics. The **eluate gas from a gas chromatograph** may be introduced into a mass spectrometer that functions as the detector system, or the **liquid eluate** may be introduced **from** a high-performance liquid chromatograph.
3. **Instrumentation**
   a. **Mass spectrometer** components include ion source, vacuum system, analyzer, detector, and computer.
   b. **Ion source:** Samples enter the ion source and are bombarded by the ionization beam. When the sample is in gas form and introduced from a gas chromatograph, the ion source may be electron or chemical ionization. Other types, such as electrospray ionization and sonic spray ionization, may be used when a high-performance liquid chromatograph is used in conjunction with a mass spectrometer.
   c. **Vacuum system:** Prevents the collision of ions with other molecules when electronic or magnetic separation is occurring.
   d. **Analyzer:** Beam-type and trapping-type
      1) **Beam-type** is a destructive process, where ions pass through the analyzer one time and then strike the detector.
      2) **Quadrupole** is a beam-type analyzer, where mass-to-charge ratios are scanned during a prescribed time period to form a mass spectrum.

e. **Detector** usually detects ions using electron multipliers, such as discrete dynode and continuous dynode electron multipliers.
f. **Computer and software** convert the detector's signal to a digital form. Sample **identification** is achieved because each compound produces a **unique spectrum**, which is analyzed by a database for matching to a computerized reference library.

4. To further improve selectivity and sensitivity, a system known as **tandem mass spectrometers** can be employed, where a gas chromatograph or a high-performance liquid chromatograph is connected to **two** mass spectrometers (GC/MS/MS) or (HPLC/MS/MS). In these systems, ions of a specific mass-to-charge ratio are allowed to continue to the **second mass spectrometer**, where **additional fragmentation** occurs and final analysis is done.

L. Polarography

1. **Polarography** employs an **electrochemical cell.**
   a. Gradually increasing the voltage applied between two electrodes of the cell in contact with a solution containing the analyte
   b. Current measured; voltage change versus current plotted to produce a polarogram
   c. Voltage at which sharp rise in current occurs characteristic of the electrochemical reaction involved
   d. Amount of increase in current (i.e., the wave height) proportional to the concentration of analyte
2. **Anodic stripping voltammetry** is based on polarography.
   a. Negative potential applied to one of the electrodes
   b. Trace metal ions in the solution reduced and **plated onto anodic electrode;** preconcentrating step
   c. Plated electrode used as anode in polarographic cell; **metal stripped off anode**
   d. Current flow during stripping provides polarogram that **identifies** and **quantifies** the analyte being measured (trace metals)
   e. Used to assay heavy metals such as **lead in blood**

M. Potentiometry

1. **Potentiometry** is a technique used to determine the concentration of a substance in solution employing an **electrochemical cell** that consists of two half-cells, where the potential difference between an indicator electrode and a reference electrode is measured.
   a. Half-cell, also called an electrode, composed of single metallic conductor surrounded by solution of electrolyte
   b. Two different half-cells are connected to make a complete circuit; current flows because of potential difference between two electrodes (reference and indicator electrodes)

c. Salt bridge connection between two metallic conductors and between two electrolyte solutions
d. Comparison made between the voltage of one half-cell connected to another half-cell
e. Half-cell potentials compared to potential generated by standard (reference) electrode; desirable to use one half-cell (reference electrode) with known and constant potential, not sensitive to composition of material to be analyzed
f. Universally accepted standard (reference) half-cells; standard hydrogen electrode, arbitrarily assigned a potential E° of 0.000 volt
g. Calomel electrode, consisting of mercury covered by a layer of mercurous chloride in contact with saturated solution of potassium chloride; silver-silver chloride (Ag/AgCl) electrode; common type of reference electrode; consists of a silver wire coated with silver chloride dipped in a solution containing silver
h. Other half-cell **(indicator electrode)** selected on basis of change in its potential with change in concentration of analyte to be measured. Types of indicator electrodes include, glass, solid state, ion-exchange, gas, and polymer

2. A **pH/blood gas analyzer** employs a pH-sensitive glass electrode for measuring blood pH, and it employs PCO_2 and PO_2 electrodes for measuring gases in blood. For measuring pH, the **pH electrode** is a functioning **glass electrode** that is dependent on properties of pH-sensitive glass.
   a. Glass electrode made by sealing thin piece of pH-sensitive glass at the end of glass tubing and filling tube with solution of hydrochloric acid saturated with silver chloride
   b. Glass electrode constructed from specially formulated glasses consisting of a melt of silicon dioxide with added oxides of various metals; membrane thickness ranged from 10 to 100 μm; glass membranes have been made with selectivity for H^+, Na^+, K^+, Li^+, Rb^+, Cs^+, Ag^+, Tl^+, and NH_4^+
   c. Silver wire immersed in tube's solution with one end extending outside the tube for external connection; silver-silver chloride reference electrode sealed within tube with pH-sensitive glass tip
   d. pH-sensitive glass must be saturated with water. Surface of the glass develops a hydrated lattice, allowing exchange of alkaline metal ions in the lattice for hydrogen ions in the test solution. A potential is created between the inside and the outside of the electrode, and that potential is measured.
   e. Glass electrode calibrated by comparison with two primary standard buffers of known pH
   f. Because pH readings are temperature sensitive, the calibration must be carried out at a constant temperature of 37°C.

3. In a pH/blood gas analyzer, the **PCO_2 electrode** for measuring the **partial pressure of carbon dioxide (PCO_2)** in blood is actually a pH electrode immersed in a bicarbonate solution.
   a. The bicarbonate solution is separated from the sample by a membrane that is permeable to gaseous CO_2 but not to ionized substances such as H^+ ions.

b. When CO_2 from the sample diffuses across the membrane, it dissolves, forming carbonic acid and thus lowering the pH.
c. The pH is inversely proportional to the log of the PCO_2. Hence, the scale of the meter can be calibrated directly in terms of PCO_2.

4. The **ion-exchange electrode** is a type of potentiometric **ion-selective electrode.**
   a. Consists of liquid ion-exchange membrane made of inert solvent and ion-selective neutral carrier material
   b. Collodion membrane may be used to separate membrane solution from sample solution.
   c. **K^+ analysis:** Antibiotic **valinomycin**, because of its ability to bind K^+, used as a neutral carrier for K^+-selective membrane
   d. **NH_4^+ analysis:** Antibiotics **nonactin** and **monactin** used in combination as neutral carrier for NH_4^+-selective membrane
5. **Sodium analysis:** Ion-selective electrodes based on principle of potentiometry
   a. Utilize **glass membrane electrodes** with selective capability
   b. Constructed from glass that consists of silicon dioxide, sodium oxide, and aluminum oxide

N. Amperometry: Electrochemical technique that measures the amount of current produced through the oxidation or reduction of the substance to be measured at an electrode held at a fixed potential

1. In a pH/blood gas analyzer, the electrode for measuring the **partial pressure of oxygen (PO_2)** in the blood is an electrochemical cell consisting of a platinum cathode and a Ag/AgCl anode connected to an external voltage source. The cathode potential is adjusted to -0.65 V.
2. The cathode and anode are immersed in the buffer. A polypropylene membrane selectively permeable to gases separates the electrode and buffer from the blood sample.
3. When there is no oxygen diffusing into the buffer, there is practically no current flowing between the cathode and the anode because they are polarized.
4. When oxygen diffuses into the buffer from a sample, it is reduced at the platinum cathode.
5. The electrons necessary for this reduction are produced at the anode. Hence a current flows; the current is directly proportional to the PO_2 in the sample. For every molecule reduced at the cathode, four electrons of current will flow.

O. Coulometry

1. A **chloride coulometer** employs a coulometric system based on Faraday's law, which states that in an electrochemical system, the **number of equivalent weights of a reactant oxidized or reduced is directly proportional to the quantity of electricity used in the reaction.** The quantity of electricity is measured in coulombs. The coulomb is the unit of electrical quantity; 1 coulomb of electricity flowing per minute constitutes a current of 1 ampere.

2. If the current is constant, the number of equivalent weights of reactant oxidized or reduced **depends only on the duration of the current.**
3. In the chloride coulometer, the electrochemical reaction is the generation of Ag^+ ions by the passage of a direct current across a pair of silver electrodes immersed in a conducting solution containing the sample to be assayed for chloride. As the Ag^+ ions are generated, they are immediately removed from solution by combining with chloride to form insoluble silver chloride. When all the chloride is precipitated, **further generation of Ag^+ ions** causes an **increase in conductivity** of the solution.
4. The **endpoint** of the titration is indicated by the **increase in conductivity** of the solution. **Amperometry** is used to **measure the increase in conductivity.**

P. Electrophoresis

1. Used clinically to separate and identify proteins, including serum, urine and cerebrospinal fluid (CSF) proteins, lipoproteins, isoenzymes, and so on.
2. **Electrophoresis** is defined as the **movement of charged molecules** in a liquid medium when an electric field is applied.
3. **Zone electrophoresis** is defined as the movement of charged molecules in a porous supporting medium where the **molecules separate as distinct zones.**
4. **Support medium** provides a matrix that allows molecules to separate (e.g., agarose gel, starch gel, polyacrylamide gel, and cellulose acetate membranes).
5. Movement of charged particles through a medium depends on the nature of the particle, including net charge, size and shape, the character of the buffer and supporting medium, temperature, and the intensity of the electric field.
   a. Nature of the charged particle: **Proteins are amphoteric** and may be charged positively or negatively depending on the pH of the buffer solution.
   b. The pH at which negative and positive charges are equal on a protein is the **protein's isoelectric point.**
6. **Buffer solutions of pH 8.6** are generally used for serum protein electrophoresis. Using agarose gel or cellulose acetate at this alkaline pH, **serum proteins** take on a **net negative charge** and will migrate toward the **anode (+)**. Albumin migrates the fastest toward the anode and the gamma-globulins remain closer to the cathode (−).
7. **Visualizing the separated analyte:** Following electrophoresis, treat the support medium with colorimetric stains or fluorescent chemicals. **Amido black B, Ponceau S, and Coomassie brilliant blue stains** are used for visualizing **serum proteins.** Silver nitrate is used for CSF proteins, fat red 7B and oil red O are used for lipoproteins, and nitrotetrazolium blue is used for lactate dehydrogenase isoenzymes.
8. Detection and quantification of the separated protein are accomplished using a **densitometer.**

9. Commonly encountered problems in electrophoresis
   a. **Holes in staining pattern:** Analyte present in too high a concentration
   b. **Very slow migration:** Voltage too low
   c. **Sample precipitates in support:** pH too high or low; excessive heat production
10. **Isoelectric focusing** is a type of zone electrophoresis in which protein separation is based on the **isoelectric point (pI)** of the proteins. This method utilizes polyacrylamide or agarose gel containing a pH gradient formed by ampholytes in the medium. When exposed to an electric field, the ampholytes migrate based on their pI to their respective positions in the gradient. In turn, the serum proteins will migrate in the gel to the position where the gel's pH equals the pI of the respective protein.
11. **Capillary electrophoresis** is based on **electroosmotic flow** (EOF). When an electric field is applied, the flow of liquid is in the direction of the cathode. Thus, EOF regulates the speed at which solutes move through the capillary.

Q. Hemoglobin Electrophoresis

1. **Hemoglobin:** Tetramer composed of **four globin chains**, four heme groups, and four iron atoms
   a. **Hemoglobin A_1:** Two alpha chains and **two beta chains**
   b. **Hemoglobin A_2:** Two alpha chains and **two delta chains**
   c. **Hemoglobin F:** Two alpha chains and **two gamma chains**
2. A number of hemoglobinopathies exist where a **substitution** of one amino acid on either the alpha chain or the beta chain causes the formation of an abnormal hemoglobin molecule.
   a. **Hemoglobin S:** Substitution of valine for glutamic acid in position 6 of the beta chain.
   b. **Hemoglobin C:** Substitution of lysine for glutamic acid in position 6 of the beta chain.
3. Although hemoglobin differentiation is best achieved by use of electrophoresis, hemoglobin F may be differentiated from the majority of human hemoglobins because of its alkali resistance.
4. At **pH 8.6**, hemoglobins have a net negative charge and migrate from the point of application toward the anode. Using **cellulose acetate:**
   a. Hemoglobin A_1 moves the fastest toward the anode, followed by hemoglobin F and hemoglobins S, G, and D, which migrate with the same mobility.
   b. Hemoglobins A_2, C, O, and E have the same electrophoretic mobility and migrate slightly slower than hemoglobins S, G, and D.
5. At **pH 6.2 on agar gel**, hemoglobins exhibit different electrophoretic mobilities in comparison with hemoglobins electrophoresed at pH 8.6 on cellulose acetate.
   a. Order of migration, from the most anodal hemoglobin to the most cathodal hemoglobin, is hemoglobins C and S; followed by hemoglobins A_1, A_2, D, E, and G, which migrate as a group with the same mobility; followed by hemoglobin F.
   b. The different migration patterns seen with cellulose acetate at pH 8.6 and agar gel at pH 6.2 are useful in differentiating hemoglobins that migrate with the same electrophoretic mobility.

R. Automation Parameters/Terminology

1. **Centrifugal analysis:** Centrifugal force moves samples and reagents into cuvet areas for simultaneous analysis.
2. **Discrete analysis:** Each sample reaction is compartmentalized. This may relate to an analyzer designed to assay only one analyte (e.g., glucose) or an analyzer capable of performing multiple tests where the sample and reagents are in a separate cuvet/reaction vessel for each test.
3. **Random access:** Able to perform individual test or panel, and allows for stat samples to be added to the run ahead of other specimens
4. **Batch analysis:** Samples processed as a group
5. **Stand-alone:** Instrument from a single discipline with automated capability
6. **Automated stand-alone:** Instrument from a single discipline with additional internal automated capability (e.g., autorepeat and autodilute)
7. **Modular workcell:** At least two instruments from a single discipline with one controller
8. **Multiple platform:** Instrument able to perform tests from at least two disciplines
9. **Integrated modular system:** At least two analytical modules supported by one sample and reagent processing and delivery system
10. **Pneumatic tube system:** Transports specimens quickly from one location to another
11. **Throughput:** Maximum number of tests generated per hour
12. **Turnaround:** Amount of time to generate one result
13. **Bar coding:** Mechanism for patient/sample identification; used for reagent identification by an instrument
14. **Dead volume:** Amount of serum that cannot be aspirated
15. **Carry-over:** The contamination of a sample by a previously aspirated sample
16. **Reflex testing:** Use of preliminary test results to determine if additional tests should be ordered or canceled on a particular specimen; performed manually or automated
17. **Total laboratory automation:** Automated systems exist for laboratories where samples are received, centrifuged, distributed to particular instruments using a conveyor system, and loaded into the analyzer without operator assistance. This kind of automation is seen in large medical center laboratories and commercial laboratories where the volume of testing is high.

S. Principles of Automation

1. Automated instruments use robotics and fluidics to replicate manual tasks.
2. **Specimen handling:** Some instruments have **level-sensing probes** that detect the amount of serum or plasma in the tube. Some systems have a reading device that **allows bar-coded sample tubes** to be loaded onto the instrument. Although not as common, other instruments require the operator to **manually enter** the position of the patient sample.

3. **Reagents**
   a. **Dry reagents** can be packaged as **lyophilized powder** or **tablet form** that must be reconstituted with a buffer or reagent-grade water. Reconstituting of reagents may need to be done manually and then the reagents placed on an analyzer for use, or reconstituting the reagents may be part of the total automation process as employed by the Dimension® analyzer.
   b. **Dry reagents** can be spread over a support material and assembled into a **single-use slide.** This technique is employed by the Vitros® analyzer.
   c. **Liquid reagents** are pipetted by the instrument and mixed with the sample.
4. **Testing phase**
   a. Mixing of sample and reagents occurs in a vessel called a **cuvet.** Some instruments have permanent, nondisposable cuvets made of quartz glass. Other cuvets are made of plastic and are disposable.
   b. **Reaction temperatures and times** vary for each analyte. The most common reaction temperatures are 37°C and 30°C.
   c. **Kinetic assays:** Determination of sample concentration is based on **change in absorbance** over time.
   d. **Endpoint/colorimetric assays:** Incubated for a specific time, absorbance determined, absorbance related to calibrators for calculation of sample concentration
   e. A spectrophotometer is built within the system to read absorbances for kinetic and colorimetric assays. These systems may use a diffraction grating or a series of high-quality filters. Some automated analyzers incorporate fluorometry or nephelometry.
5. **Data management**
   a. The **computer module** of most automated instruments has a data management system that allows analysis of quality control (QC) materials and assessment of patient values (e.g., delta check) before releasing patient results.
   b. Instruments/laboratory information systems (LISs) also archive patient results and QC values. These archived results are stored by the laboratory for various lengths of time.

T. Point-of-Care Testing (POCT)

1. **Definition:** Defined as performing diagnostic tests outside the main laboratory and at or near patient care areas.
2. **Applications:** POCT is designed to provide immediate laboratory test results for immediate patient assessment and determination of appropriate treatment. POCT may be used in neonatal intensive care, coronary care, intensive care, or the emergency department.
3. **Operators:** Only waived laboratory tests can be performed using point-of-care instruments. Clinical laboratory technicians and clinical laboratory scientists must operate instruments that perform complex or high-complexity laboratory tests.

4. **Point-of-care (POC) instrument evaluations:** All POC instruments must be evaluated in accordance with the Clinical Laboratory Improvement Amendments of 1988 (CLIA '88). The values obtained from POC instruments must correlate with values obtained from larger laboratory instruments. Linearity testing, calculation of control ranges, correlations of sample data, and reference range validations/verifications must be done for each instrument.
5. **Training:** All POC instrument operators must be trained and training must be documented.
6. **Quality control:** All effective quality control systems must be set up for each POC instrument. The program must use appropriate standards and controls, statistical analyses, and a proficiency testing system. This information must be documented.

U. Immunochemical Techniques

1. **Immunoassays** encompass a number of immunochemical techniques used to detect an extremely small amount of analyte (functions as antigen) by reacting it with an antibody (functions as reagent) to form an **antigen-antibody complex.** The signal measured has a relationship to the **label** used, and the label may be attached to either a reagent antigen or a reagent antibody.
   a. **Detection limits:** Immunochemical techniques detect very small amounts of substances. Monoclonal antibodies increase the specificity of the procedure.
   b. **Polyclonal antiserum:** Antibodies produced in an animal from many cell clones in response to an immunogen; heterogeneous mixture of antibodies
   c. **Monoclonal antiserum:** Antibodies produced from a single clone or plasma cell line; homogeneous antibodies
   d. **Used to quantify:** Hormones, tumor markers, drugs, and other analytes present in small concentrations
2. **Methods**
   a. **Competitive-binding immunoassays** are based on the **competition between an unlabeled antigen** (sample analyte) and a **labeled antigen** for an antibody. In this type of assay, the unlabeled antigen (sample analyte) is an unknown concentration and varies from sample to sample, whereas the labeled antigen concentration and the antibody concentration are constant for a particular method.
      1) As the assay proceeds, there will be some free labeled antigen remaining that does not bind to antibody.
      2) The concentration of the antibody binding sites is limited with respect to total antigens (unlabeled and labeled) present, which leads to less-labeled antigen bound to antibody when sample analyte concentration is high.

3) It is then necessary to measure either the free labeled antigen or the labeled antigen-antibody complex and relate it to the concentration of analyte in the sample. Depending on the method, it may be necessary to separate the free labeled antigen from the labeled antigen-antibody complex.
   a) **Heterogeneous** assays require that free labeled antigen be physically removed from the labeled antigen bound to antibody. Radioimmunoassay (RIA), enzyme-linked immunosorbent assay (ELISA), and immunoradiometric assay (IRMA) are examples of this technique.
   b) **Homogeneous** assays do **not** require physical removal of free labeled antigen from bound-labeled antigen.
4) The **original labels** used for immunoassays were **radioactive isotopes** (e.g., I^{125}); thus the term **radioimmunoassay.** Most immunoassays in use today use nonradioactive labels. **Enzyme** (e.g., alkaline phosphatase), **fluorophore** (e.g., fluorescein), and **chemiluminescent** (e.g., acridinium ester) **labels** are commonly used for immunoassays.

b. **Enzyme multiplied immunoassay technique (EMIT)** is a **homogeneous** immunoassay where the **sample** analyte (functions as **unlabeled antigen**) competes with the **enzyme-labeled antigen** for the binding sites on the antibody. The more analyte (unlabeled antigen) present in the mixture, the less binding of enzyme-labeled antigen to the antibody. The unbound enzyme-labeled antigen will react with substrate because the enzyme is in a conformational arrangement that allows for substrate to bind at the active site of the enzyme. The product formed is read spectrophotometrically. The more product formed, the greater the concentration of analyte in the sample.

c. **Fluorescent polarization immunoassay (FPIA)** is based on measuring the degree to which fluorescence intensity is greater in one plane than in another **(polarized versus depolarized).** FPIA is based on the amount of polarized fluorescent light detected when the fluorophore label is excited with polarized light.

1) FPIA is a **homogeneous** technique where the **sample** analyte (functions as **unlabeled antigen**) competes with the **fluorophore-labeled antigen** for the binding sites on the antibody. The more analyte (unlabeled antigen) present in the mixture, the less binding of fluorophore-labeled antigen to the antibody.
2) The **free fluorophore-labeled antigen** has **rapid** rotation and emits **depolarized light.** The **fluorophore-labeled antigen-antibody complex** rotates more **slowly;** light is in the vertical plane **(polarized light)** and is detected as **fluorescence polarization.**
3) The greater the concentration of analyte in the sample, the less binding between antibody and fluorophore-labeled antigen (bound complex emits polarized light), the greater the amount of free fluorophore-labeled antigen (emits depolarized light), and thus the lesser amount of polarization sensed

by the detector. The amount of **analyte** in the sample is **inversely proportional** to the amount of fluorescence polarization. That is, the greater the concentration of analyte, the less the amount of polarized light detected.

4) It is used to measure hormones, drugs, and fetal pulmonary surfactant to assess fetal lung maturity.

d. **Chemiluminescent immunoassay** is a technique between antigen and antibody that employs a chemiluminescent indicator molecule such as isoluminol and acridinium ester as labels for antibodies and haptens. In the presence of hydrogen peroxide and a catalyst, isoluminol is oxidized, producing light emission at 425 nm. In such an assay, the chemiluminescent signal is proportional to the concentration of analyte in the serum sample.

e. **Luminescent oxygen channeling immunoassay (LOCI™)** is a homogeneous technique that is an adaptation of the chemiluminescent immunoassay.

1) Antigen (from serum sample) links to two antibody-coated particles. The first is an antibody-coated sensitizer particle containing a photosensitive dye (singlet oxygen source), and the second is an antibody-coated particle (singlet oxygen receptor) containing a precursor chemiluminescent compound and a fluorophore.

2) Irradiation of the immunocomplex produces singlet oxygen at the surface of the sensitizer particle that diffuses to the second particle being held in close proximity.

3) Singlet oxygen reacts with the precursor chemiluminescent compound to form a chemiluminescent product that decays and emits light. This light energy is accepted by a fluorophore, which results in light emission of a longer wavelength.

4) In this assay, the chemiluminescent signal is enhanced by the resulting fluorescent signal, which is proportional to the concentration of analyte in the serum sample.

f. **Electrochemiluminescence immunoassay** uses an indicator label such as **ruthenium** in sandwich and competitive immunoassays. Following a wash procedure to remove unbound label, label bound to magnetic beads at an electrode surface undergoes an electrochemiluminescent reaction with the resulting light emission measured by a photomultiplier tube.

II. PROTEINS AND TUMOR MARKERS

A. Characteristics of Proteins

1. Proteins are macromolecules made of **amino acids**, with each amino acid being linked to another via a **peptide bond.**

a. **Peptide bond** is formed when the **carboxyl** (−COOH) group of one amino acid links to the **amino** ($-NH_2$) group of another amino acid with the loss of a water molecule.

b. **N-terminal:** End of protein structure with a free amino group

c. **C-terminal:** End of protein structure with a free carboxyl group
d. **Nitrogen content:** Proteins consist of 16% nitrogen, which differentiates proteins from carbohydrates and lipids.

2. Protein structure
    a. **Primary structure:** The amino acids are linked to each other through covalent peptide bonding in a specific sequence to form a polypeptide chain.
    b. **Secondary structure:** The polypeptide chain winds to form alpha helixes and beta sheets through the formation of hydrogen bonds between CO and NH groups of the peptide bonds.
    c. **Tertiary structure:** The coiled polypeptide chain folds upon itself to form a three-dimensional structure through the interactions of the *R* groups of the amino acids. Such interactions include the formation of disulfide linkages, hydrogen bonds, hydrophobic interactions, and van der Waals forces.
    d. **Quaternary structure:** Two or more folded polypeptide chains bind to each other through hydrogen bonds and electrostatic interactions to form a functional protein.

B. Classification of Proteins

1. **Simple proteins:** Polypeptides composed of only amino acids
    a. **Globular proteins:** Symmetrical, compactly folded polypeptide chains (e.g., albumin)
    b. **Fibrous proteins:** Elongated, asymmetrical polypeptide chains (e.g., troponin and collagen)
2. **Conjugated proteins:** Composed of protein (apoprotein) and nonprotein (prosthetic group) components; **prosthetic groups** are commonly metal, lipid, and carbohydrate in nature
    a. **Metalloproteins:** Protein with a metal prosthetic group (e.g., ceruloplasmin)
    b. **Lipoproteins:** Protein with a lipid prosthetic group (e.g., cholesterol, triglyceride)
    c. **Glycoproteins:** Protein with 10–40% carbohydrates attached (e.g., haptoglobin)
    d. **Mucoproteins:** Protein with $>$40% carbohydrates attached (e.g., mucin)
    e. **Nucleoproteins:** Protein with DNA or RNA nucleic acids attached (e.g., chromatin)

C. Protein Functions

1. **Energy production:** Proteins can be broken down into amino acids that can be used in the citric acid cycle to produce energy.
2. **Water distribution:** Proteins maintain the colloidal osmotic pressure between different body compartments.
3. **Buffer:** The ionizable *R* groups of the individual amino acids of a protein provide buffering capacity by binding or releasing H^+ ions as needed.

4. **Transporter:** Binding of proteins to hormones, free hemoglobin, lipids, drugs, calcium, unconjugated bilirubin, and so on, allows movement of these and other molecules in the circulation.
5. **Antibodies:** Defined as proteins that protect the body against "foreign" invaders
6. **Cellular proteins:** These function as receptors for hormones so that the hormonal message can activate cellular components; some hormones are protein in nature [e.g., adrenocorticotropic hormone (ACTH), follicle-stimulating hormone (FSH), luteinizing hormone (LH), and thyroid-stimulating hormone (TSH)].
7. **Structural proteins:** Collagen is the fibrous component that maintains the structure of body parts such as skin, bone, cartilage, and blood vessels.
8. **Enzymes:** Catalysts that accelerate chemical reactions

D. Plasma Total Protein

1. **Regulation**
   a. The **liver synthesizes** most of the **plasma proteins. Plasma cells synthesize** the **immunoglobulins.**
      1) Proteins are synthesized from amino acids, with one amino acid linked to another through the formation of a peptide bond.
      2) When proteins **degrade**, their constituent amino acids undergo **deamination** with the **formation of ammonia**, which is **converted to urea** for excretion in the urine. The liver and kidneys play a key role in the process of amino acid deamination as they are responsible for riding the body of potentially toxic levels of ammonia.

   b. Some **cytokines** released at the site of injury or inflammation cause the **liver** to **increase synthesis** of the **acute-phase reactant proteins.** This is a nonspecific response to inflammation that may be caused by autoimmune disorders or infections, as well as a nonspecific response to tissue injury from tumors, myocardial infarctions, trauma, or surgical procedures. On the other hand, some proteins will decrease in concentration and are referred to as **negative acute-phase proteins**, including prealbumin (transthyretin), albumin, and transferrin.
   c. Immunoglobulins are humoral antibodies produced in response to foreign antigens for the purpose of destroying them.
   d. **Reference ranges:** Total protein 6.5–8.3 g/dL; albumin 3.5–5.0 g/dL
2. In general, changes in total protein concentration are associated with:
   a. **Hypoproteinemia** caused by urinary loss, gastrointestinal tract inflammation, liver disorders, malnutrition, inherited immunodeficiency disorders, and extensive burns
   b. **Hyperproteinemia** caused by dehydration, increased protein production associated with monoclonal and polyclonal gammopathies, and chronic inflammatory diseases associated with paraprotein production

E. Clinical Significance of the Major Proteins

1. **Prealbumin** (also termed transthyretin): Act as indicator of nutritional status and is one of the proteins that transports thyroid hormones.
   a. **Decreased** in liver disorders, inflammation, malignancy, and poor nutrition
   b. **Increased** in steroid therapy, chronic renal failure, and alcoholism
2. **Albumin** is synthesized in the liver and has the **highest concentration of all plasma proteins.** Albumin is a nonspecific binder of many analytes **for transport** in blood, including unconjugated bilirubin, steroids, and ions such as calcium and magnesium, fatty acids, and drugs, and it significantly contributes to plasma **osmotic pressure.**
   a. **Decreased** in liver disorders because of decreased production, gastrointestinal disease associated with malabsorption, muscle-wasting diseases, severe burns caused by loss, renal disease caused by loss (nephrotic syndrome, glomerulonephritis), starvation, and malnutrition
   b. **Increased** in dehydration (relative increase)
3. **α_1-Antitrypsin** is an acute-phase reactant and a protease inhibitor that neutralizes trypsin-type enzymes that can damage structural proteins.
   a. **Decreased** in emphysema-associated pulmonary disease and severe juvenile hepatic disorders that may result in cirrhosis
   b. **Increased** in inflammatory disorders
4. **α_1-Fetoprotein (AFP)** is synthesized during gestation in the yolk sac and liver of the fetus, peaking at 13 weeks and declining at 34 weeks. Normally, adult levels are very low.
   a. **Maternal serum AFP** is measured between 15 and 20 weeks of gestation and is reported as **multiples of the median** (MoM).
      1) **Increased** AFP level in maternal serum: neural tube defects, spina bifida, and fetal distress
      2) **Decreased** AFP level in maternal serum: Down syndrome, trisomy 18
   b. **In adults, increased** levels of AFP can be indicative of hepatocellular carcinoma and gonadal tumors.
5. **α_1-Acid glycoprotein (orosomucoid):** Acute-phase reactant; binds to basic drugs
   a. **Increased** in inflammatory disorders such as rheumatoid arthritis, pneumonia, and conditions associated with cell proliferation
   b. **Decreased** in nephrotic syndrome
6. **Haptoglobin:** α_2-globulin that binds free hemoglobin and is an acute-phase reactant
   a. **Increased** in inflammatory conditions, burns, trauma
   b. **Decreased** in intravascular hemolysis because of formation of a haptoglobin-hemoglobin complex for removal by the liver
7. **Ceruloplasmin** is an acute-phase reactant that is an α_2-globulin, **copper-containing protein** with enzymatic activity. Approximately 90% of serum copper is bound in ceruloplasmin.
   a. **Increased** in pregnancy, inflammatory disorders, malignancies, and with intake of oral estrogen and oral contraceptives
   b. **Decreased** in **Wilson disease**, malnutrition, malabsorption, and severe liver disease

8. **α_2-Macroglobulin:** It is a proteolytic enzyme inhibitor that inhibits thrombin, trypsin, and pepsin.
   a. **Increased** in nephrotic syndrome, contraceptive use, pregnancy, and estrogen therapy
   b. **Decreased** slightly in acute inflammatory disorders and prostatic cancer; decreased markedly in acute pancreatitis
9. **Transferrin:** β-globulin that **transports iron**
   a. **Decreased** in infections, liver disease, and nephrotic syndrome
   b. **Increased** in iron-deficiency anemia and pregnancy
10. **C-reactive protein (CRP):** β-globulin that is an acute-phase reactant
    a. Increased in tissue necrosis, rheumatic fever, infections, myocardial infarction, rheumatoid arthritis, and gout
    b. The American Heart Association (AHA) and the Centers for Disease Control (CDC) have defined risk groups for future coronary events according to hs-CRP levels. <1.0 mg/L = low risk, 1.0–3.0 mg/L = average risk, and >3.0 mg/L = high risk.
11. **Immunoglobulins:** Antibodies
    a. Five major classes: IgA, IgD, IgE, IgG, and IgM
       1) Synthesized in **plasma cells** as an immune response
       2) One of the immunoglobulins will be increased in a **monoclonal gammopathy** (e.g., **multiple myeloma**). Such disorders are generally associated with an increase in IgG, IgA, or IgM; seldom is the increase associated with IgD or IgE.
    b. **IgG** can cross the placenta.
       1) **Increased** in liver disorders, infections, and collagen disease
       2) **Decreased** in the presence of increased susceptibility to infection and when a monoclonal gammopathy is associated with an increase in another immunoglobulin
    c. **IgA** levels increase after birth.
       1) **Increased** in liver disorders, infections, and autoimmune diseases
       2) **Decreased** in inhibited protein synthesis and hereditary immune disorders
    d. **IgM** cannot cross the placenta; it is made by the fetus.
       1) **Increased** in various bacterial, viral, and fungal infections and **Waldenström macroglobulinemia**
       2) **Decreased** in renal diseases associated with protein loss and immunodeficiency disorders
    e. **IgD** is increased in liver disorders, infections, and connective tissue disorders.
    f. **IgE** is increased in allergies, asthma, and hay fever, and during parasitic infections.
12. **Fibronectin:** Fetal fibronectin is used to **predict risk of premature birth.** It is a normal constituent in the placenta and amniotic fluid. In cases of stress, infection, or hemorrhage these can cause leakage of fibronectin into the cervicovaginal secretions, increased fibronectin is suggestive of risk for premature birth.

F. Methodology for Serum Total Protein, Albumin, and Protein Fractionation

1. **Refractometry** is based on the change in velocity of light (light is bent) as light passes through the boundary between air and water, which function as two transparent layers. In protein analysis, the light is bent and such change is proportional to the concentration of the solutes (proteins) present in the water (serum).
2. The **biuret method** is based on cupric ions complexing with peptide bonds in an alkaline medium to produce a purple-colored complex. The amount of purple complex produced is directly proportional to the number of peptide bonds present and reflects protein concentration.
3. **Dye binding** techniques allow proteins to bind to a dye, forming a protein-dye complex that results in a shift of the maximum absorbance of the dye (e.g., **Coomassie brilliant blue**). The increase in absorbance is directly proportional to protein concentration.
4. The **Kjeldahl** technique for the determination of total protein is too cumbersome for use in routine testing. It is considered the **reference method** of choice to validate materials used with the biuret method. The Kjeldahl technique is based on the quantification of the nitrogen content of protein.
5. **Electrophoresis**
   a. **Serum protein electrophoresis:** Serum is applied at the cathode region of an agarose gel or cellulose acetate plate saturated with a buffer of pH 8.6. At a pH of 8.6, serum proteins have a **net negative charge** and migrate toward the **anode**, with **albumin traveling the farthest**, followed by α_1-globulins, α_2-globulins, β-globulins, and γ-globulins. The proteins are fixed in the medium, stained, and then quantified using a densitometer.
   b. **High-resolution protein electrophoresis** is a modified technique that uses agarose gel, a higher voltage, a cooling system, and a more concentrated buffer to separate proteins into as many as 12 zones.
   c. **Isoelectric focusing** is a type of zone electrophoresis in which protein separation is based on the **isoelectric point (pI)** of the proteins.
6. **Immunochemical methods**
   a. Homogeneous and heterogeneous immunoassays
   b. Immunonephelometry
   c. Immunoelectrophoresis
   d. Radial immunodiffusion (RID)
   e. Electroimmunodiffusion
   f. Immunofixation
7. **Test methodology for albumin: Dye binding** techniques using **bromcresol green** and **bromcresol purple** dyes allow albumin to be positively charged for binding to the anionic dye, forming an albumin-dye complex that results in a shift of the maximum absorbance of the dye. The increase in absorbance is directly proportional to the albumin concentration.

8. **Test methodology for globulins:** The direct measurement of total globulins is not generally performed. The concentration of the globulins is determined by calculation. **Globulins = Total Protein − Albumin**

G. Proteins in Other Body Fluids
   1. **Urinary proteins: Quantification** performed on 24-hour urine specimens
      a. **Test methods:** Sulfosalicylic acid, trichloroacetic acid, benzethonium chloride (turbidimetric), and Coomassie brilliant blue (spectrophotometric)
      b. **Reference range urine total protein:** 1–14 mg/dL; <100 mg/day
      c. Clinical significance of proteinuria
         1) **Increased** protein in urine may result from tubular or glomerular dysfunction, multiple myeloma, Waldenström macroglobulinemia, and nephrotic syndrome.
         2) **Bence Jones protein** may be found in urine of patients with multiple myeloma.
         3) Glomerular membrane can be damaged in diabetes, amyloidosis, and collagen diseases.
         4) Glomerular dysfunction can be detected in its early stages by measuring albumin in urine. **Albuminuria** is a condition where the quantity of albumin in the urine is greater than normal, yet it is not able to be detected by the urine dipstick method. The presence of albuminuria in a diabetic individual is a concern because it **generally precedes nephropathy.**
            a) **Methods** for quantification: Enzyme immunoassays and immunonephelometric assays
            b) **Reference range for urine albumin:** <30 mg/day
   2. **Cerebrospinal fluid (CSF) proteins**
      a. CSF is an **ultrafiltrate of plasma** formed in the ventricles of the brain.
      b. **Test methods** include sulfosalicylic acid, trichloroacetic acid, benzethonium chloride, and Coomassie brilliant blue.
      c. **Reference range:** 15–45 mg/dL
      d. **Clinical significance**
         1) **Increased** in viral, bacterial, and fungal meningitis, traumatic tap (bloody), multiple sclerosis, herniated disk, and cerebral infarction
         2) **Decreased** in hyperthyroidism and with central nervous system leakage of CSF

H. Tumor Marker Utilization
   1. In general, tumor markers used today are **not very useful in diagnosis**, but they are **useful** in tumor staging, monitoring therapeutic responses, predicting patient outcomes, and detecting cancer recurrence. **Ideal characteristics** for tumor markers include:
      a. Measured easily
      b. High analytical sensitivity of assay method
      c. High analytical specificity of assay method
      d. Cost-effective
      e. Test results contribute to patient care and outcome

2. **Prostate-specific antigen (PSA)**
   a. **Function**
      1) Produced by epithelial cells of the **prostate gland** and secreted into seminal plasma
      2) Glycoprotein protease that functions in liquefaction of seminal coagulum
   b. **Forms of PSA found in blood**
      1) **Enveloped** by protease inhibitor, α_2-macroglobulin; **lacks** immunoreactivity
      2) **Complexed** to another protease inhibitor, α_1-antichymotrypsin; **immunologically detectable**
      3) **Free PSA**, not complexed to protease inhibitor; **immunologically detectable**
      4) **Total PSA** assays measure complexed and free PSA forms, as both are immunologically detectable.
   c. **Specificity**
      1) PSA is a tissue-specific marker but **not** tumor specific.
      2) Small amounts present in serum normally
      3) Lacks specificity because serum level of PSA is increased in benign prostate hypertrophy as well as in adenocarcinoma of the prostate
   d. **Prostate cancer detection**
      1) Early-detection guidelines endorse lower cutoff of **PSA up to 2.5 ng/mL.**
      2) PSA >2.5 ng/mL perform biopsy
      3) **PSA velocity** is measurement of the **rate of change per year.**
         a) Biopsy recommended when PSA rises more than 0.75 ng/mL/year even when PSA is <2.5 ng/mL
      4) **Free PSA:** Men with **prostate cancer** tend to have **lower % free PSA** (free PSA/total PSA) than men with benign disease. Lower % free PSA is associated with a higher risk of prostate cancer.
      5) PSA is used to monitor therapeutic response and to follow radical prostatectomy.
   e. Methods used to measure serum levels of PSA include fluorescence immunoassay, enzyme immunoassay, and chemiluminescence immunoassay.
3. α_1**-Fetoprotein (AFP)**
   a. Oncofetal glycoprotein antigen
      1) Synthesized in liver, yolk sac, and gastrointestinal (GI) tract of **fetus**
      2) Fetal serum AFP peaks at 12–15 weeks of gestation with levels of 2–3 mg/mL.
      3) At birth, levels fall to 50 μg/mL, and at 2 years of age only trace amounts are present.
      4) **Adult levels <20 ng/mL**
   b. **Clinical significance**
      1) **Increased** levels of AFP in adults are associated with hepatocellular carcinoma, testicular and ovarian teratocarcinomas, pancreatic carcinoma, and gastric and colonic carcinomas.

2) **Increased** levels of AFP in adults are also seen in **nonmalignant** disorders, including viral hepatitis and chronic active hepatitis.
3) It is useful in monitoring therapeutic response of cancer patients to treatment protocols.
4) In **pregnancy, increased** maternal serum levels are associated with **spina bifida, neural tube defects**, and **fetal distress. Decreased** levels of maternal serum AFP are associated with increased incidence of **Down syndrome.**

c. Enzyme immunoassay methods are used for measurement.

4. **Carcinoembryonic antigen (CEA)**
   a. Oncofetal glycoprotein antigen
   b. Normally found in epithelial cells of the **fetal** GI tract
   c. **Clinical significance in adults**
      1) **Increased** levels of CEA are associated with adenocarcinoma of digestive tract and colorectal carcinoma.
      2) Elevations are seen in other malignancies and noncancerous disorders.
      3) These are useful in monitoring therapeutic response of cancer patients to treatment protocols.
   d. Enzyme immunoassay methods are used for measurement.
5. **Human chorionic gonadotropin (hCG)**
   a. hCG is a glycoprotein composed of α- and β-subunits. The **β-subunit is unique** and not common to other hormones; α-subunit is common to other hormones.
   b. Normally secreted by the trophoblast cells of the placenta.
   c. **Increased** secretion is associated with **trophoblastic tumors,** choriocarcinoma, nonseminomatous testicular tumors, and ovarian tumors.
   d. It is useful for monitoring the progress of patients.
   e. Immunoassay measurement is made of **β-hCG**.
6. **CA 15-3**
   a. Mucin glycoprotein antigen
   b. It is useful for monitoring therapeutic response and for detecting recurrence of **breast cancer** in patients previously treated.
   c. Elevated levels are observed in nonmalignant diseases such as chronic hepatitis, tuberculosis, and systemic lupus erythematosus.
   d. Immunoassay methods are used for measurement.
7. **CA 125**
   a. Mucin glycoprotein antigen
   b. Marker for **ovarian** and endometrial cancer
   c. It is useful for monitoring the progress of patients.
   d. Immunoassay methods are used for measurement.
8. **CA 19-9**
   a. Glycolipid blood group antigen-related marker; sialylated derivative of the Lewis blood group system, known as Le^{xa}

b. Marker for **pancreatic, colorectal**, lung, and gastric carcinomas
c. It is useful for monitoring the progress of patients.
d. Immunoassay methods are used for measurement.

III. NONPROTEIN NITROGENOUS COMPOUNDS

A. Urea

1. **Regulation:** Urea is the **major nitrogen-containing compound** in the blood. It results from protein catabolism and is synthesized in the liver from the deamination of amino acids. Urea is **excreted by the kidneys.**
2. **Clinical significance:** Abnormal serum urea levels may be due to prerenal, renal, or postrenal disorders.
   a. **Increased serum urea:** Renal failure, glomerular nephritis, urinary tract obstruction, congestive heart failure, dehydration, and increased protein catabolism
   b. **Decreased serum urea:** Severe liver disease, vomiting, diarrhea, and malnutrition
3. Blood urea nitrogen (BUN) is an older term still in use, and the terminology was based on previous methodology where nitrogen was measured. To convert BUN to urea: BUN $\times$ 2.14 =Urea.
4. **Test methodology**
   a. **Kinetic method: Urease/GLDH coupled enzymatic method**

$$\text{Urea} + H_2O \xrightarrow{\text{Urease}} 2NH_4^+ + CO_3^{2-}$$

$$NH_4^+ + \alpha\text{-ketoglutaric acid} + \text{NADH} \xrightarrow{\text{GLDH}} \text{NAD}^+ + \text{Glutamic acid}$$

   b. **Chemical method**

$$\text{Diacetyl monoxime} + H_2O \longrightarrow \text{diacetyl} + \text{hydroxylamine}$$

$$\text{Diacetyl} + \text{urea (acid medium)} \longrightarrow \text{diazine derivative (yellow)}$$

5. **Reference range:** 6–20 mg/dL

B. Creatinine

1. **Regulation:** Creatinine is a waste product of muscle contraction that is formed from phosphocreatine, a high-energy compound. Creatinine levels are **regulated by kidney excretion.** Measurements of creatinine in serum and urine (creatinine clearance) are used to assess the glomerular filtration rate (GFR). Creatinine levels are not changed by diet or rate of urine flow. Creatinine is not reabsorbed by renal tubules.
2. **Clinical significance**
   a. **Increased serum creatinine:** Renal disease, renal failure
3. **Test methodology**
   a. **Jaffe method**

$$\text{Creatinine} + \text{picric acid (alkaline solution)} \rightarrow \text{creatinine picrate (red tautomer)}$$

b. **Enzymatic method: Creatininase (creatinine amidohydrolase)**

$$\text{Creatinine} + H_2O \xrightarrow{\text{creatinine amidohydrolase}} \text{Creatine}$$

$$\text{Creatine} + H_2O \xrightarrow{\text{creatinase}} \text{sarcosine} + \text{urea}$$

$$\text{Sarcosine} + O_2 + H_2O \xrightarrow{\text{sarcosine oxidase}} \text{glycine} + \text{formaldehyde} + H_2O_2$$

$$H_2O_2 + \text{indicator (reduced)} \xrightarrow{\text{peroxidase}} \text{indicator (oxidized)} + 2H_2O$$

4. **Reference ranges:** Male, 0.9–1.3 mg/dL; female, 0.6–1.1 mg/dL
5. **Creatinine clearance** is used to **assess** the **GFR.** Testing requires a plasma sample and a 24-hour urine collection.
   a. **P:** plasma creatinine mg/dL, **U:** urine creatinine mg/dL, **V:** urine flow in mL/min, and **SA:** body surface area; 1.73 m^2 = average body surface area
   b. **Creatinine clearance formula:**

$$\text{CrCl (mL/min)} = \frac{U \times V}{P} \times \frac{1.73\ m^2}{SA}$$

   c. **Reference ranges:** Differ according to age and sex; values decrease with age
   Creatinine clearance (males): 105 ± 20 mL/min/1.73 m^2
   Creatinine clearance (females): 95 ± 20 mL/min/1.73 m^2
   d. **Estimated glomerular filtration rate (eGFR)** uses a **serum creatinine** or **serum cystatin C** in conjunction with multiple equations including, CKD-EPI creatinine equation (2009), CKD-EPI creatinine-cystatin equation (2012), CKD-EPI cystatin C equation (2012), and the **MDRD** (Modification of Diet in Renal Disease) equation. The National Kidney Foundation recommends using the CKD-EPI Creatinine equation (2009) to estimate GFR.
      1) CKD-EPI creatinine equation (2009) is expressed as a single equation:

$$eGFR = 141 \times \min(SCr/\kappa, 1)\alpha \times \max(SCr/\kappa, 1) - 1.209 \times 0.993Age \times 1.018\ [\text{if female}] \times 1.159\ [\text{if African American}]$$

      2) Recommended method for estimating GFR in adults; designed for use with laboratory creatinine values that are standardized to IDMS; estimates GFR from serum creatinine, age, sex, and ethnicity; more accurate than the MDRD Study equation, particularly in people with higher levels of GFR; based on the same four variables as the MDRD Study equation, but uses a two-slope "spline" to model the relationship between estimated GFR and serum creatinine, and a different relationship for age, sex, and ethnicity.

      Some clinical laboratories are still reporting GFR estimates using the MDRD study equation. The National Kidney Foundation has recommended that clinical laboratories should begin using the CKD-EPI equation to report estimated GFR in adults.
      3) Results only reported as a number if <60 mL/min/1.73 m^2

C. Uric Acid

1. **Regulation:** Uric acid, the major waste product of purine (adenosine and guanine) catabolism, is synthesized in the liver. Uric acid **elimination** from the blood is **regulated by the kidneys** through glomerular filtration, and some uric acid is excreted through the GI tract.
2. **Clinical significance**
   a. **Increased serum uric acid:** Gout, renal disorders, treatment of myeloproliferative disorders, lead poisoning, lactic acidosis, toxemia of pregnancy, and Lesch-Nyhan syndrome
   b. **Decreased serum uric acid:** Severe liver disease as a secondary disorder, tubular reabsorption disorders, and drug induced
3. **Test methodology**
   a. **Chemical method**

$$\text{Uric acid} + \text{phosphotungstic acid} + O_2 \rightarrow \text{allantoin} + CO_2 + \text{tungsten blue}$$

   b. **Enzymatic uricase method:** Decrease in absorbance monitored at 293 nm

$$\text{Urate} + O_2 \xrightarrow{\text{uricase}} \text{allantoin} + H_2O_2 + CO_2$$

$$2H_2O_2 + \text{phenol} + \text{4-aminophenazone} \xrightarrow{\text{peroxidase}} \text{quinine-monoimine dye} + 2H_2O$$

4. **Reference ranges:** Male, 3.5–7.2 mg/dL; female, 2.6–6.0 mg/dL

D. Ammonia

1. **Regulation**
   a. Ammonia produced from **deamination of amino acids**.
   b. Hepatocytes convert ammonia **to urea** for excretion.
   c. With severe liver cell malfunction, blood levels of ammonia **increase**.
   d. Ammonia is neurotoxic.
2. **Type of specimen and storage**
   a. Venous blood free of hemolysis; **place on ice immediately**
   b. Blood collected in ethylenediaminetetra-acetic acid (EDTA) may be used.
   c. Centrifuge sample within 20 minutes of collection and remove plasma.
   d. Plasma stable up to 3½ hours in ice bath; stable several days frozen
3. **Clinical significance:** Increased plasma ammonia levels seen in hepatic failure and Reye syndrome
4. **Test methodology**

$$NH_4^+ + \alpha\text{-ketoglutaric acid} + \text{NADH} \xrightarrow{\text{GLDH}} \text{NAD}^+ + \text{glutamic acid}$$

5. **Interferences**
   a. Incorrect handling of blood sample
   b. Ammonia contamination
6. **Reference range:** 11–32 μmol/L

IV. CARBOHYDRATES

A. Glucose Metabolism

1. During a fast, the blood glucose level is kept constant by mobilizing the **glycogen** stores in the liver.
2. During long fasts, **gluconeogenesis** is required to maintain blood glucose levels because glycogen stores are used up in about 24–48 hours.
3. An individual with a **fasting blood glucose level >100 mg/dL** is referred to as **hyperglycemic.** An individual with a **fasting blood glucose level <50 mg/dL** is referred to as **hypoglycemic.**

B. Hormones Affecting Blood Glucose Levels

1. **Insulin:** Produced by the beta cells of the pancreatic islets of Langerhans; promotes the entry of glucose into liver, muscle, and adipose tissue to be stored as glycogen and fat; inhibits the release of glucose from the liver, resulting in a decreased glucose level
2. **Somatostatin:** Synthesized by delta cells of the pancreatic islets of Langerhans; inhibits secretion of insulin, glucagon, and growth hormone, resulting in an increase in plasma glucose level
3. **Growth hormone** and adrenocorticotropic hormone (**ACTH**): Hormones secreted by the anterior pituitary that raise blood glucose levels
4. **Cortisol:** Secreted by the adrenal glands; stimulates glycogenolysis, lipolysis, and gluconeogenesis
5. **Epinephrine** is secreted by the medulla of the adrenal glands. It stimulates glycogenolysis and lipolysis; it inhibits secretion of insulin. Physical or emotional stress causes increased secretion of epinephrine and an immediate increase in blood glucose levels.
6. **Glucagon:** Secreted by the α cells of the pancreatic islets of Langerhans; increases blood glucose by stimulating glycogenolysis and gluconeogenesis
7. **Thyroxine:** Secreted by the thyroid gland; stimulates glycogenolysis and gluconeogenesis; increases glucose absorption from the intestines

C. Renal Threshold for Glucose

1. Glucose is filtered by the glomeruli, reabsorbed by the tubules, and normally **not** present in urine. If the blood glucose level is elevated, glucose appears in the urine, a condition known as **glucosuria.**
2. An individual's **renal threshold** for glucose varies between **160 and 180 mg/dL.** When blood glucose reaches this level or exceeds it, the renal tubular transport mechanism becomes saturated, which causes glucose to be excreted into the urine.

D. Abnormal Carbohydrate Metabolism

1. **Classification of diabetes mellitus**
   a. **Type 1 diabetes mellitus**
      1) This has been characterized by **insulinopenia**, a deficiency of insulin.
      2) Individuals require **treatment with insulin** to sustain life.
      3) Most individuals exhibit it as an autoimmune disorder where β cells of the islets of Langerhans are destroyed by the body.

4) Peak incidence is in childhood and adolescence, but it may occur at any age.
5) Primary symptoms include polyuria, polydipsia, and weight loss.
6) **Ketosis-prone:** It can produce excess ketones, resulting in diabetic ketoacidosis; this is a result of the breakdown of fatty acids for energy.

b. **Type 2 diabetes mellitus**
1) This is characterized by defect in insulin secretion, insulin action, and cellular resistance to insulin.
2) Individuals are **not dependent on treatment with insulin.** Individuals generally respond to dietary intervention and oral hypoglycemic agents, but some may require insulin therapy.
3) It is associated with obesity and sedentary lifestyle; symptoms include polyuria, polydipsia, and weight loss.
4) Although associated with individuals over the age of 40, type 2 diabetes mellitus is becoming a significant problem in children and adolescents.
5) **Nonketosis-prone:** Without exogenous insulin or oral hypoglycemic medication, these individuals will have an elevated glucose but will not go into diabetic ketoacidosis.

c. **Gestational diabetes mellitus (GDM)**
1) GDM is the onset of diabetes mellitus during **pregnancy**.
2) After childbirth, the individual generally returns to normal metabolism. However, there is an increased chance that type 2 diabetes mellitus may develop later in life.

2. **Inherited disorders of carbohydrate metabolism**

a. **Glycogen storage diseases**, of which there are 10 types, are inherited diseases involving the deficiency of particular enzymes; these deficiencies cause defects in the normal metabolism of glycogen.
1) **von Gierke, type I:** Glucose-6-phosphatase deficiency
2) **Pompe, type II:** α-1,4-glucosidase deficiency
3) **Cori, type III:** Amylo-1,6-glucosidase deficiency

b. **Galactosemia**
1) This is characterized by a deficiency or absence of galactokinase, galactose 1-phosphate uridyl transferase, or uridyl diphosphate glucose-4-epimerase; the enzyme defect prevents metabolism of galactose. Galactose is found in milk as a component of lactose, with galactosemia generally identified in infants.
2) Most commonly, **galactose 1-phosphate uridyl transferase** is deficient, which leads to excessive galactose in blood and excretion in urine.

E. Laboratory Diagnosis

1. **Normal** fasting plasma glucose (FPG) $<$**100 mg/dL**
2. **Impaired fasting glucose (IFG)** is defined as a fasting plasma glucose level that **ranges between 100 and 125 mg/dL.**
3. **Provisional diagnosis of diabetes mellitus** is made when **FPG $\geq$126 mg/dL.** The diagnosis **must be confirmed** by one of the three methods described in the following outline section.

4. **Diagnosis of diabetes mellitus**
   a. A plasma glucose analysis that yields **any one** of the following results is **diagnostic for the presence of diabetes mellitus**, provided that unequivocal hyperglycemia is apparent. If unequivocal hyperglycemia is not apparent, the **glucose result must be confirmed** by repeat analysis on a subsequent day using any one of the following three methods. However, the American Diabetes Association does **not** recommend the oral glucose tolerance test (OGTT) for routine clinical use.
      1) An individual expressing physical symptoms and a **casual plasma glucose level of ≥200 mg/dL**
      2) **Fasting plasma glucose** level that is **≥126 mg/dL** (fasting defined as no caloric intake for minimum of 8 hours)
      3) Plasma glucose level of **≥200 mg/dL at 2-hour point** of an **OGTT** as described by the World Health Organization (WHO)
      4) A1c ≥ 6.5%; performed with a method traceable to the DCCT
   b. **Gestational diabetes mellitus (GDM)**
      1) A woman at **high risk** for GDM should have an **initial screening early** in the pregnancy. If she is not found to have GDM during the initial screening, the woman should be **retested at 24–28 weeks** of gestation. For women of **average risk**, testing should be performed at 24–28 weeks of gestation.
         a) Screening and diagnosis of GDM
         b) One-step approach: 75-g OGTT with plasma glucose measurement at fasting, 1 and 2 hours, at 24–28 weeks of gestation in women not previously diagnosed with overt diabetes.
         c) The OGTT should be performed in the morning after an overnight fast of at least 8 hours.
         d) The diagnosis of GDM is made when any of the following plasma glucose values are met or exceeded:
            - Fasting: 92 mg/dL (5.1 mmol/L)
            - 1 hour: 180 mg/dL (10.0 mmol/L)
            - 2 hours: 153 mg/dL (8.5 mmol/L)
         e) Two-step approach: 50-g (nonfasting) screen followed by a 100-g OGTT for those who screen positive
            Step 1: Perform a 50-g GLT (nonfasting), with plasma glucose measurement at 1 hour, at 24–28 weeks of gestation in women not previously diagnosed with overt diabetes; plasma glucose level measured 1 hour after the load; glucose ≥130 mg/dL, 135 mg/dL, or 140 mg/dL, proceed to Step 2.
            Step 2: 100-g OGTT performed when the patient is fasting; glucose measured at fasting, 1, 2, and 3 hours postload.

            The diagnosis of GDM is made if at least two* of the following four plasma glucose levels (measured fasting and 1, 2, and 3 hours during OGTT) are met or exceeded

	Carpenter-Coustan	OR	NDDG
Fasting	95 mg/dL		105 mg/dL
1 hour	180 mg/dL		190 mg/dL
2 hours	155 mg/dL		165 mg/dL
3 hours	140 mg/dL		145 mg/dL

5. **Oral glucose tolerance test** based on the criteria published by the World Health Organization (WHO). NOTE: American Diabetes Association does **not** recommend the OGTT for routine clinical use.
   a. Timed measurements of plasma glucose before and after ingesting a specific amount of glucose
   b. **Patient preparation:** It includes unrestricted carbohydrate-rich diet for 3 days before the test with physical activity, restrict medication on the test day, 12-hour fast required, no smoking.
   c. Adult patient ingests 75 g of glucose in 300–400 mL of water and children 1.75 g/kg up to 75 g of glucose. For assessment of GDM, 50, 75, or 100 g of glucose may be used (see previous description for details).
   d. Plasma glucose specimen is collected fasting at 10 minutes before glucose load and at 120 minutes after ingestion of glucose. Urine glucose may be measured.
   e. **Interpretation of OGTT results** is based on the criteria published by the WHO.
      1) **Impaired fasting glucose (IFG)** is diagnosed when fasting plasma glucose ranges between 110 and 125 mg/dL.
      2) The following two criteria must be met for diagnosis of **impaired glucose tolerance (IGT):** Fasting plasma glucose level must be ≤126 mg/dL and the 2-hour plasma glucose level of the OGTT must fall between 140 and 199 mg/dL.
      3) **Diabetes mellitus** is diagnosed when the fasting plasma glucose level is ≥126 mg/dL or the 2-hour glucose is ≥200 mg/dL.
6. **Glycated/glycosylated hemoglobin**
   a. Hemoglobin A is composed of three forms, HbA_{1a}, HbA_{1b}, and HbA_{1c}, which are referred to as **glycated** or **glycosylated hemoglobin.** $\mathbf{HbA_{1c}}$ represents the **main form.**
   b. Glycated hemoglobin is formed from the **nonenzymatic, irreversible attachment of glucose** to hemoglobin A_1.
   c. Measurement of glycated hemoglobin **reflects blood glucose levels for the past 2–3 months.** It is useful in monitoring effectiveness of treatment and compliance of diabetic individual to treatment protocol.
   d. **Measured** by affinity chromatography, ion-exchange chromatography, and high-performance liquid chromatography
   e. **Specimen collection:** Nonfasting blood drawn in EDTA tubes
   f. **Reference range:** 4–6% HbA_{1c}; effective treatment range <7% HbA_{1c}

7. **Fructosamine**
   a. Ketoamine linkage forms between glucose and protein, mainly represented by albumin.
   b. **Clinical significance:** Measurement of fructosamine **reflects blood glucose levels for 2–3 weeks** before sampling.
   c. **Measured** by spectrophotometric/colorimetric methods, affinity chromatography, and high-performance liquid chromatography
   d. **Reference range:** 205–285 μmol/L
8. Measurement of albumin excretion is useful for patients with **renal complications of diabetes mellitus.** Performed on random urines, microalbumin analysis always requires the simultaneous analysis of creatinine, and it is reported as an albumin/creatinine ratio. Abnormal values **(albuminuria)** will be ≥**30 mg albumin/g creatinine.**

F. Measurement of Plasma Glucose

1. **Glucose oxidase method**

$$\beta\text{-D-Glucose} + H_2O + O_2 \xrightarrow{\text{glucose oxidase}} \text{gluconic acid} + H_2O_2$$

$$H_2O_2 + \text{reduced chromogen} \xrightarrow{\text{peroxidase}} \text{oxidized chromogen (colored)} + H_2O$$

2. **Hexokinase method**

$$\text{Glucose} + \text{ATP} \xrightarrow[\text{Mg}^{2+}]{\text{hexokinase}} \text{glucose-6-phosphate} + \text{ADP}$$

$$\text{Glucose-6-phosphate} + \text{NADP}^+ \xrightarrow[\text{dehydrogenase}]{\text{glucose-6-phosphate}} \text{6-phosphogluconate} + \text{NADPH} + H^+$$

3. **Clinical significance:** An increase in the blood glucose level is the hallmark of diabetes mellitus, but it can also be indicative of other hormonal disorders such as Cushing disease.
4. **Reference range:** Adult fasting, 74–99 mg/dL

G. Lactate

1. The normal end-product of glucose metabolism is pyruvate; however, lactate is produced under conditions of oxygen deficit (anaerobic metabolism). The production and accumulation of lactate in the blood and its measurement aid in assessing the degree of oxygen deprivation that is occurring. Change in the blood lactate level precedes a change in blood pH. Lactate is metabolized by the liver via gluconeogenesis.
2. **Test methodology**

$$\text{Lactate} + O_2 \xrightarrow{\text{lactate oxidase}} \text{pyruvate} + H_2O_2$$

$$H_2O_2 + \text{reduced chromogen} \xrightarrow{\text{peroxidase}} \text{oxidized chromogen (colored)} + H_2O$$

3. **Clinical significance: Type A lactic acidosis** is caused by depressed oxygen levels that may occur in acute myocardial infarction, congestive heart failure,

shock, pulmonary edema, and so on. **Type B lactic acidosis** is caused by metabolic processes that may occur in diabetes mellitus, renal disorders, liver disease, ingestion of toxins (salicylate overdose and excess ethanol), and so on.

4. **Special specimen handling** is required and includes the following: Avoid using a tourniquet because venous stasis will falsely raise blood lactate levels; place the specimen on ice and immediately transport to the laboratory; centrifuge the specimen and remove the plasma (additives NaF and $K_2C_2O_4$) as soon as possible.
5. **Reference range (venous):** 0.5–1.3 mmol/L

V. LIPIDS AND LIPOPROTEINS

A. Lipid Structure

1. **Fatty acids** exist as short, medium, and long chains of molecules that are major constituents of triglycerides and phospholipids. Minimal amounts of fatty acids are bound to albumin and circulate free (unesterified) in plasma.
2. **Triglyceride**
   a. Triglyceride is formed from one glycerol molecule with three fatty acid molecules attached via ester bonds.
   b. Triglycerides comprise 95% of all fats stored in adipose tissue.
   c. Triglycerides are **transported** through the body by **chylomicrons** and **VLDL** (very-low-density lipoprotein).
   d. Metabolism involves releasing the fatty acids to the cells for energy, then recycling the glycerol into triglyceride.
   e. Lipase, lipoprotein lipase, epinephrine, and cortisol breakdown triglycerides.
3. **Cholesterol**
   a. It is unsaturated steroid alcohol; exists in the **esterified** form, where a fatty acid forms an ester bond at carbon-3, and the **free** (unesterified) form.
   b. Act as **a precursor for synthesis** of bile acids, steroid hormones, and vitamin D.
   c. Low-density lipoprotein (LDL) is the primary carrier of cholesterol.
4. **Phospholipid**
   a. Composed of one glycerol molecule and two fatty acid molecules attached via ester bonds
   b. Found on the surface of lipid layers, they are major constituents of cell membranes and outer shells of lipoprotein molecules.

B. Classification of Lipoproteins

1. **Lipoproteins** are molecules that combine water-insoluble dietary lipids and water-soluble proteins (apolipoproteins) so that lipids can be transported throughout the body. Micelles are spherical and have an inner core of neutral fat.
2. **Chylomicrons** are the largest lipoproteins and have the lowest density. They are formed in the intestines and transport **triglycerides** after a meal, giving serum a turbid appearance. Because of their low density, chylomicrons will float to the top and form a creamy layer when plasma is stored overnight. **Chylomicrons** are composed of **86% triglyceride**, 5% cholesterol, 7% phospholipid, and

2% apolipoprotein. Chylomicrons have apoproteins **B-48**, mainly, and lesser amounts of A-I, C-I, C-II, and C-III on their surface. In **normal lipid metabolism**, chylomicrons enter the circulation and are metabolized to remnant particles for uptake and further modification by the liver.

3. **Very-low-density lipoprotein** carries endogenous **triglycerides** synthesized in the liver. **VLDL** molecules are composed of **55% triglycerides**, 19% cholesterol, 18% phospholipid, and 8% apolipoprotein and have apolipoproteins B-**100**, mainly, and C-I, C-II, C-III, and E on their surface. In **normal lipid metabolism,** VLDLs are secreted into the blood by the liver for metabolism in peripheral tissues.
4. **Intermediate-density lipoprotein** (IDL) is a transitional form, as it is **formed from VLDL** and then further **modified** in the liver **to LDL.** IDLs carry endogenous triglycerides and cholesterol esters. IDL molecules are composed of 23% triglycerides, 38% cholesterol, 19% phospholipid, and 19% apolipoprotein and have apolipoproteins **B-100**, mainly, and some E on their surface.
5. **Low-density lipoprotein** is the body's **major cholesterol carrier** and transports a large amount of endogenous cholesterol. Known as **bad cholesterol,** LDL is easily taken up by cells, so elevated levels are associated with increased risk for atherosclerosis. **LDLs** are composed of **50% cholesterol,** 22% phospholipids, 6% triglycerides, and 22% protein and have apoprotein **B-100** on their surface. In **normal lipid metabolism,** this lipoprotein brings cholesterol to peripheral cells for membrane synthesis and formation of adrenal and reproductive hormones.
6. **High-density lipoprotein** (HDL) is also known as **good cholesterol. HDL** is synthesized in the intestine and liver cells. **HDL** molecules are recycled chylomicron and VLDL molecules. **HDL** is composed of **50% protein,** 28% phospholipids, 19% cholesterol, and 3% triglycerides. HDL has apoproteins **A-I**, mainly, and A-II on its surface. In **normal lipid metabolism,** HDL removes excess cholesterol from peripheral tissues and transports it to other catabolic sites. This function has an **antiatherogenic effect.**
7. **Lp(a)** is composed primarily of cholesterol esters, phospholipids, and **apolipoprotein (a)** and B-100. **Elevated** levels of Lp(a) are associated with **increased risk for coronary heart disease**, myocardial infarction, and cerebrovascular disease.

C. Clinical Significance

1. Abnormal lipid metabolism can be due to genetic defects or it can be acquired. Abnormal lipid metabolism is associated with risk of coronary heart disease and other disorders.
2. The National Cholesterol Education Program established the Adult Treatment Panel III Classification (ATP III), which sets cutoff values for cholesterol and triglyceride levels based on a 9- to 12-hour fast. See Tables 1–1■–1–4■.

TABLE 1–1 TOTAL CHOLESTEROL REFERENCE RANGE

	Desirable	Borderline High	High
Total Cholesterol (mg/dL)	<200	200–239	≥240

TABLE 1–2 HDL CHOLESTEROL REFERENCE RANGE

	Protective against Heart Disease	The Higher, the Better	Major Risk Factor for Heart Disease
HDL Cholesterol (mg/dL)	≥60	40–59	<40

TABLE 1–3 LDL CHOLESTEROL REFERENCE RANGE

	Optimal	Near Optimal	Borderline High	High	Very High
LDL Cholesterol (mg/dL)	<100	100–129	130–159	160–189	≥190

TABLE 1–4 TRIGLYCERIDE REFERENCE RANGE

	Normal	Borderline High	High	Very High
Triglyceride (mg/dL)	<150	150–199	200–499	≥500

NOTE: In 2013, the ACC/AHA released updated guidelines for the treatment of blood cholesterol to reduce atherosclerotic cardiovascular risk in adults. This report, loosely known as the adult treatment panel IV, puts statins as the linchpin for management of those with high blood cholesterol. The guidelines recommend people be put into one of four statin benefit group as described further.

1. Patients with any form of clinical ASCVD
2. Patients with primary LDL-C levels of 190 mg/dL or greater
3. Patients with diabetes mellitus, 40–75 years of age, with LDL-C levels of 70–189 mg/dL
4. Patients without diabetes, 40–75 years of age, with an estimated 10-year ASCVD risk ≥ 7.5%

Risk assessment for 10-year and lifetime risk is recommended using an updated ASCVD risk calculator: http://my.americanheart.org/cvriskcalculator

The updated guidelines did not find evidence to support the use of specific LDL-C or HDL-C target levels. The expert panel stated that using LDL-C targets could lead to undertreating with evidence-based statin therapy or overtreating with nonstatin drugs that have not been shown to reduce ASCVD events in RCTs.

3. **Hyperlipoproteinemias** have been classified using the Fredrickson-Levy classification system, which is not commonly used today. However, some of the

abnormal lipid types are still referenced in the literature and for that reason are included here.

a. **Type I hyperlipoproteinemia (Hyperchylomicronemia): Elevated chylomicrons**
   1) Serum appearance: Creamy layer of chylomicrons over clear serum
   2) Total cholesterol: Normal to moderately elevated
   3) Triglyceride: Extremely elevated
   4) Apo B-48 increased, Apo A-IV increased
b. **Type IIa hyperlipoproteinemia (Hyperbetalipoproteinemia): Increased LDL**
   1) Serum appearance: Clear
   2) Total cholesterol: Generally elevated
   3) Triglyceride: Normal
   4) Apo-B 100 increased
c. **Type IIb hyperlipoproteinemia (Hyperbetalipoproteinemia):: Increased LDL and VLDL**
   1) Serum appearance: Clear or slightly turbid
   2) Total cholesterol: Elevated
   3) Triglyceride: Elevated
   4) Apo B-100 increased
d. **Type III hyperlipoproteinemia (Dysbetalipoproteinemia): Increased IDL**
   1) Serum appearance: Creamy layer sometimes present over a turbid layer
   2) Total cholesterol: Elevated
   3) Triglyceride: Elevated
   4) Apo E-II increased, Apo E-III decreased, and Apo E-IV decreased
e. **Type IV hyperlipoproteinemia (Hyperprebetalipoproteinemia): Increased VLDL**
   1) Serum appearance: Turbid
   2) Total cholesterol: Normal to slightly elevated
   3) Triglyceride: Moderately to severely elevated
   4) Apo C-II either increased or decreased, and Apo B-100 increased
f. **Type V hyperlipoproteinemia (Mixed Hyperlipoproteinemia): Increased VLDL with increased chylomicrons**
   1) Serum appearance: Turbid with creamy layer
   2) Total cholesterol: Slightly to moderately elevated
   3) Triglyceride: Severely elevated
   4) Apo C-II increased or decreased, Apo B-48 increased, and Apo B-100 increased

4. The most common familial form is **familial combined hyperlipidemia (FCHL).** FCHL is characterized by increased plasma levels of total and LDL cholesterol (type IIa), or triglyceride (type IV), or a combination of both (type IIb). Also, Apo B-100 is increased. The level of HDL cholesterol may be decreased.
5. **Hyperapobetalipoproteinemia** is associated with VLDL and Apo B-100 overproduction in the liver. It is characterized by normal or moderate elevation of LDL cholesterol with an elevated Apo B-100. Total cholesterol and triglyceride are generally elevated but may be normal. HDL cholesterol and Apo A-I levels are decreased.

6. **Familial hypertriglyceridemia** is characterized by a moderate elevation of triglyceride with excess production of VLDL. Both triglyceride and cholesterol are present in higher concentrations than normal in VLDL. LDL cholesterol and Apo B-100 are within their reference ranges. HDL cholesterol is decreased.
7. **Type V hyperlipoproteinemia** is characterized by increased VLDL and chylomicrons.
8. **Familial hypercholesterolemia** is characterized by increased LDL cholesterol. The plasma triglyceride level may be normal or slightly increased, and the plasma HDL cholesterol level is slightly decreased.
9. **Secondary lipoproteinemia:** Many conditions cause lipoproteins to be abnormally metabolized. Some of those conditions include diabetes mellitus, hypothyroidism, obesity, pregnancy, nephrotic syndrome, pancreatitis, alcoholism, and myxedema.
10. **Hypolipoproteinemias**
    a. **Abetalipoproteinemia:** Total cholesterol level very low, triglyceride level nearly undetectable, LDL and Apo B-100 absent
    b. **Hypobetalipoproteinemia:** Unable to synthesize Apo B-100 and Apo B-48, low total cholesterol level and normal to low triglyceride level
    c. **Hypoalphalipoproteinemia:** Severely elevated triglyceride level and low HDL level
    d. **Tangier disease:** HDL absent, Apo A-I and Apo A-II very low levels, LDL low, total cholesterol level low, triglyceride level normal to slightly increased

D. Cholesterol Test Methodology

1. **Elevated** cholesterol concentrations have been linked to atherosclerosis, coronary artery disease, and increased risk for myocardial infarction.
2. **Decreased** cholesterol levels are present in various forms of liver disease, most notably alcoholic cirrhosis.
3. **Enzymatic methodology**

$$\text{Cholesteryl ester} + H_2O \xrightarrow{\text{cholesteryl esterase}} \text{cholesterol} + \text{fatty acid}$$

$$\text{Cholesterol} + O_2 \xrightarrow{\text{cholesterol oxiudase}} \text{cholestenone} + H_2O_2$$

$$H_2O_2 + \text{phenol} + \text{4-aminoantipyrine} \xrightarrow{\text{peroxidase}} \text{quinoneimine dye} + 2H_2O$$

E. HDL Cholesterol Test Methodology

1. **HDL decreases the atherosclerotic process.** Increased HDL cholesterol is associated with **decreased risk** of coronary artery disease, and decreased HDL cholesterol is associated with **increased risk** of coronary artery disease.
2. **Test methodology**
    a. **Precipitate LDL and VLDL** cholesterol with dextran sulfate-magnesium chloride or heparin sulfate-manganese chloride, then **assay the supernatant** for cholesterol using an enzymatic technique. **Cholesterol present is HDL.**

b. **Homogeneous assay** uses an antibody to Apo B-100 to bind LDL and VLDL. An enzymatic cholesterol analysis can then be performed with only HDL cholesterol able to react.

F. LDL Cholesterol Test Methodology

1. **LDL** is directly **associated with atherosclerosis and coronary heart disease.**
2. **Test methodology:** LDL cholesterol may be **calculated or measured directly.**
   a. **Friedewald formula** (indirect, not valid for triglycerides over 400 mg/dL):

$$\text{LDL-Cholesterol} = \text{Total Cholesterol} - (\text{HDL-C} + \text{TG}/5)$$

   b. **Homogeneous** assay uses detergents to block HDL and VLDL from reacting with the dye to form a colored chromogen product. An enzymatic cholesterol analysis is performed with only LDL cholesterol able to react.

G. Triglyceride Test Methodology

1. **Elevated** triglyceride levels may be seen in Fredrickson types I, IIb, IV, and V hyperlipoproteinemias, pancreatitis, alcoholism, obesity, hypothyroidism, nephrotic syndrome, and storage diseases (Gaucher, Niemann-Pick).
2. **Enzymatic methodology**

$$\text{Triglyceride} + 3\,H_2O \xrightarrow{\text{lipase}} \text{glycerol} + 3 \text{ fatty acids}$$

$$\text{Glycerol} + \text{ATP} \xrightarrow{\text{Glycerol Kinase}} \text{Glycerol 3 phosphate} + \text{ADP}$$

$$\text{ADP} + \text{phosphoenolpyruvate} \xrightarrow{\text{Pyruvate kinase}} \text{ATP} + \text{Pyruvate}$$

$$\text{Pyruvate} + \text{NAHD} + H^+ \xrightarrow{\text{Lactate Dehydrogenase}} \text{Lactate} + \text{NAD}^+$$

H. Apo A-1, Apo B, and Lp(a)

1. **Clinical significance**
   a. **Apo A-1** is the major protein found in HDL. It activates lecithin-cholesterol acyltransferase (LCAT) and removes free cholesterol from extrahepatic tissues. Thus, it is considered **antiatherogenic.**
   b. **Apo B-100** is the major protein found in LDL. It is **associated with increased risk of coronary artery disease.**
   c. **Lp(a)** is an independent risk factor associated with impaired plasminogen activation and thus decreased fibrinolysis. A high level suggests **increased risk for coronary heart disease and stroke.**
2. **Test methodology**
   a. Apo-A, Apo-B, and Lp(a) are measured by immunochemical methods such as immunoturbidimetric and immunonephelometric.
3. **Reference ranges**
   a. **Apo-A:** 120–160 mg/dL
   b. **Apo-B:** <120 mg/dL
   c. **Lp(a):** <30 mg/dL

VI. ENZYMES AND CARDIAC ASSESSMENT

A. General Properties

1. **Definition: Enzymes** are **proteins** that function as **biological catalysts** and are neither consumed nor permanently altered during a chemical reaction. They appear in the serum in increased amounts after cellular injury or tissue damage.
2. **Isoenzyme:** These are **different forms** of the same enzyme capable of the **same catalytic function** in the body. Isoenzymes may be differentiated based on electrophoretic mobility and resistance to heat denaturation.
3. **Cofactor:** A nonprotein compound that may be required for enzyme activity
4. **Activators:** Inorganic cofactors needed for enzymatic activity, such as Mg^{2+}, Zn^{2+}, or Cl^{-}
5. **Coenzyme:** Organic cofactor, such as NAD^{+} (nicotinamide adenine dinucleotide)
6. **Prosthetic group:** Organic cofactor tightly bound to the enzyme
7. **Active site:** Location on an enzyme where the three-dimensional arrangement of amino acid residues allows binding of substrate
8. **Denaturation:** Causes change in enzyme structure that results in loss of activity; may be caused by elevated temperature, extreme change in pH, and certain chemicals

B. Enzyme Kinetics

1. **Activation energy** is the energy required to raise all molecules to the transition state in a chemical reaction so that products may be formed.
2. **Enzymes** increase the rate of chemical reactions by lowering the activation energy required by substrate to react and form the product.

C. Factors That Influence Enzyme Reactions

1. **Substrate concentration**
   a. **Substrate** binds to free enzyme **at low substrate concentration**. As long as the enzyme exceeds the amount of substrate, the reaction rate increases as more substrate is added. The rate of the reaction is directly proportional to substrate concentration **(first-order kinetics)**.
   b. When the **substrate concentration is high** enough to bind with all available enzyme, the **reaction velocity is at its maximum**. As product is formed, the enzyme becomes available to react with additional substrate **(zero-order kinetics)**. When excess substrate is present, the rate of the reaction depends only on the concentration of enzyme.
2. **Enzyme concentration:** The reaction velocity is proportional to the enzyme concentration, provided that substrate concentration exceeds enzyme concentration.
3. **pH:** It is important that pH be controlled, because extreme pHs can denature an enzyme or change its ionic state and, possibly, the reactivity of the active site. Most enzymes of physiological interest function at pH 7.0–8.0.
4. **Temperature:** An increase in temperature will increase the rate of a chemical reaction. In general, the rate of an enzymatic reaction will double with each 10°C increase in temperature, until the rise in temperature causes the enzyme to

denature. Enzymes have an optimal reaction temperature, which is usually 37°C. Denaturation generally occurs at 40–50°C.

5. **Inhibitors**
   a. It is a substance that **interferes** with an enzyme-catalyzed reaction.
   b. **Competitive inhibitor** competes with substrate for the active site. This inhibition is reversible.
   c. **Noncompetitive inhibitor** binds with the enzyme at a site different from the active site and prevents the enzyme-catalyzed reaction from taking place. This inhibition may be reversible or irreversible. It may be irreversible if the active site is affected.
   d. **Uncompetitive inhibitor** binds to the enzyme-substrate complex so that increasing the concentration of substrate leads to the formation of more enzyme-substrate complexes and more inhibition.

D. Measuring Enzyme Activity

1. Enzyme reactions are performed in **zero-order kinetics**, with substrate in excess.
2. It is extremely important in enzyme reactions that the pH and temperature **remain constant**, and that additives (e.g., cofactors, coenzymes, and activators) are present in sufficient amounts.
3. There are **two methods** used to measure enzyme reactions: endpoint and kinetic.
   a. **Endpoint:** This type of reaction combines reactants, stops the reaction at a fixed time (e.g., 20 minutes), and then measures the product formed. Activity of the enzyme is based on the final absorbance reading.
   b. **Kinetic:** This type of reaction combines reactants, then measures the change in absorbance at specific time intervals (e.g., 60 seconds) over a specific time period. Activity of the enzyme is based on the change in absorbance over time.

E. Calculation of Enzyme Activity

1. Enzymes are reported in **activity units** because they are measured based on their activity instead of their concentration.
2. **International unit (IU or U)** is the quantity of enzyme that catalyzes the reaction of one micromole of substrate per minute under specified conditions, including temperature, pH, substrates, and activators. Results are generally reported as IU/L, U/L, or mU/mL.

F. Specific Enzymes of Clinical Interest

1. In general, each enzyme of clinical significance is found in **many tissues** of the body, and in healthy individuals, these enzymes exhibit **very low levels in serum.** In certain disease states or with cell injury, these **intracellular enzymes** are **released into the blood** and are indicative of the **presence of a pathological condition.** Quantification of enzyme levels in serum is useful in determining the presence of disease. Based on the individual's physical symptoms, several enzymes may be chosen for analysis to determine if a pattern develops that aids in identifying the tissue source of the enzyme elevation in the serum.

2. **Lactate dehydrogenase (LD)**
   a. **Tissue location**
      1) **Highest concentrations:** Liver, heart, skeletal muscle, kidney, erythrocytes, with lesser amounts in many other tissues
      2) **LD isoenzymes**
         a) LD isoenzymes consist of **four subunits** (polypeptide chains) derived from two types of polypeptides designated **M** (muscle/liver) and **H** (heart).
         b) Each LD isoenzyme is a tetramer with five isoenzyme types: LD-1 through LD-5. LD-1 and LD-2 are associated with acute myocardial infarction (AMI) and erythrocyte destruction. LD-3 is associated with pulmonary disorders, pancreatitis, and lymphocytosis. LD-4 and LD-5 are associated with liver and skeletal muscle disorders.
   b. **Clinical significance**
      1) Level of LD is **elevated** in cardiac disorders (acute myocardial infarction), hepatic diseases (viral hepatitis, cirrhosis, infectious mononucleosis), skeletal muscle diseases, hemolytic and hematologic disorders (pernicious anemia exhibits extreme elevation of LD), and neoplastic disorders (acute lymphoblastic leukemia)
      2) In **AMI**, LD levels rise within 8–12 hours, peak at 24–48 hours, and return to normal in 7–10 days. Although LD and LD isoenzymes are **not used to diagnose AMI**, knowledge of their pattern may be **useful when assessing concurrent liver damage**.
   c. **Test methodology**

$$\text{Lactate} + \text{NAD}^+ \xrightarrow{\text{LD(pH 8.3–8.9)}} \text{pyruvate} + \text{NADH} + \text{H+}$$

   Optimal pH for the forward reaction is 8.3–8.9
      1) **Sources of error:** Hemolysis; LD-4 and LD-5 labile at 4°C
      2) **Reference range:** 100–225 U/L at 37°C
3. **Creatine kinase (CK) and CK isoenzymes**
   a. **Tissue location**
      1) **Highest concentrations:** Skeletal muscle, heart muscle, and brain tissue
      2) **CK isoenzymes**
         a) CK isoenzymes consist of **two subunits: M** for muscle and **B** for brain.
         b) Each CK isoenzyme is a dimer with three possible types: **CK-MM** (or CK-3), **CK-MB** (or CK-2), and **CK-BB** (or CK-1).
         c) In serum, healthy individuals have **CK-MM** as the **major isoenzyme** and a small amount of **CK-MB** (less than 6% of total CK), whereas **CK-BB** is **not normally detectable.**
         d) **CK-MB** increases are associated with heart muscle damage, and elevations are indicative of AMI when used in conjunction with other markers, such as troponin. However, CK-MB also increases in other disorders, such as skeletal muscle damage. **CK-MM** increases are

associated with skeletal muscle and heart muscle disorders. **CK-BB** is elevated in central nervous system disorders and tumors of various organs, including the prostate gland.

b. **Clinical significance**
   1) Elevations of **total CK** in serum are associated with cardiac disorders, such as AMI, and skeletal muscle disorders, such as muscular dystrophy. Occasionally, elevations are due to disorders of the central nervous system, including seizures and cerebral vascular accidents.
   2) **CK-MB** values **greater than 6%** of total CK are **suggestive of AMI.** When AMI is suspected, **troponin** is assayed in conjunction with CK-MB, and sometimes **myoglobin** is assayed. **Following AMI, CK-MB levels rise within 4–6 hours, peak at 12–24 hours, and return to normal within 2–3 days.**
c. **Test methodology**
   1) **CK isoenzymes** are measured by electrophoresis, ion-exchange chromatography, and several types of immunoassays. Immunoassays that measure **enzyme mass** are more sensitive than activity-based assays.
   2) **Methodology**

$$\text{Creatine phosphate} + \text{ADP} \xrightarrow[\text{Mg}^{2+}]{\text{creatine kinase}} \text{creatine} + \text{ATP}$$

$$\text{ATP} + \text{glucose} \xrightarrow{\text{hexokinase}} \text{ADP} + \text{glucose-6-phosphate}$$

$$\text{Glucose-6-phosphate} + \text{NADP}^{+} \xrightarrow{\text{G6PD}} \text{6-phosphogluconate} + \text{NADPH} + \text{H}^{+}$$

      a) **Sources of error:** Moderate hemolysis
      b) **Reference ranges:**
      Total CK: male, 15–160 U/L; female, 15–130 U/L at 37°C
      CK-MB: <6% of total CK; mass assay 0–5 ng/mL

4. **Aspartate aminotransferase (AST)**
   a. **Tissue location:** Highest concentrations in heart, liver, and skeletal muscle, with lesser amounts in kidney and other tissues, including erythrocytes
   b. **Clinical significance**
      1) **AST** is used to evaluate **hepatocellular disorders** (up to 100 times upper reference limit in viral hepatitis, up to 20 times upper reference limit in infectious mononucleosis, and up to four times upper reference limit in cirrhosis), skeletal muscle disorders (up to eight times upper reference limit), and pulmonary emboli (up to three times upper reference limit) and acute pancreatitis.
      2) In **AMI, AST rises** within 6–8 hours, peaks at 18–24 hours, and returns to normal within 4–5 days. **AST** is **not used to diagnose AMI**, but awareness of the AST pattern may be **useful when ruling out other disorders, including concurrent liver damage.**

c. **Test methodology**

$$\text{Aspartate} + \alpha\text{-ketoglutarate} \xrightarrow{\text{AST (p-5'-p)}} \text{oxaloacetate} + \text{glutamate}$$

$$\text{Oxaloacetate} + \text{NADH} + \text{H}^+ \xrightarrow{\text{malate dehydrogenas}} \text{malate} + \text{NAD}^+$$

1) **Sources of error:** Hemolysis
2) **Reference range:** 5–30 U/L at 37°C

5. **Alanine aminotransferase (ALT)**

a. **Tissue location:** Highest concentrations in liver, with lesser amounts in other tissues, including kidneys and erythrocytes

b. **Clinical significance:** Hepatocellular disorders (hepatitis, cirrhosis) exhibit higher ALT levels than intra- or extrahepatic obstruction. **ALT** is **more specific for liver disease** than AST. ALT, in conjunction with an elevated AST, is used to assess liver involvement with diagnosis of an AMI. ALT does not exhibit a significant increase in muscular dystrophy, and it is not affected in cases of pulmonary emboli or acute pancreatitis.

c. **Test methodology**

$$\text{Alanine} + \alpha\text{-ketoglutarate} \xrightarrow{\text{ALT (p-5'-p)}} \text{pyruvate} + \text{glutamate}$$

$$\text{Pyruvate} + \text{NADH} + \text{H}^+ \xrightarrow{\text{LD}} \text{lactate} + \text{NAD}^+$$

1) **Sources of error:** Slight hemolysis does not interfere.
2) **Reference range:** 6–37 U/L at 37°C

6. **Alkaline phosphatase (ALP)**

a. **Tissue location:** Highest concentrations are found in liver, bone, intestines, spleen, kidney, and placenta. ALP is found on cell surfaces, in sinusoidal and bile canalicular membranes in the liver, and in bone osteoblasts. In normal adult serum, ALP is mainly of liver origin, with a small amount from bone.

b. **Clinical significance**

1) **Increased** serum ALP levels are seen in hepatobiliary disease and bone disorders (with osteoblastic involvement). In hepatobiliary disorders, the increased levels are due to **obstructive disease**, and the **ALP** levels are **increased more significantly than ALT and AST.**
   a) **In biliary tract obstruction**, synthesis of ALP is induced by cholestasis, which causes serum ALP levels to rise 3–10 times the upper reference limit. The elevation is usually greater in cases of extrahepatic obstruction in contrast to intrahepatic obstruction.
   b) In hepatitis and cirrhosis, which are classified as hepatocellular conditions, ALP rises up to three times the upper reference limit.
   c) Highest elevations of ALP are seen in Paget disease.
   d) ALP levels increase with healing bone fractures.
2) **Decreased serum** ALP levels are seen in **hypophosphatasia** because of lack of ALP bone isoenzyme. This disorder is characterized by insufficient bone calcification.

3) ALP levels are **normally higher in children** than adults because of bone growth.
4) ALP levels are **normally higher in** women during **pregnancy** because the placenta is a source of ALP.

c. **Test methodology**

$$\underset{\text{(colorless)}}{p\text{-Nitrophenylphosphate}} + H_2O \xrightarrow{\text{ALP (pH 10.2)}} \underset{\text{(yellow)}}{p\text{-nitrophenol}} + \text{phosphate ion}$$

1) **Sources of error:** Hemolysis
2) **Reference ranges:**
   Adults: 50–115 U/L at 37°C
   Children aged 4–15 years: 54–369 U/L at 37°C

7. **Acid phosphatase (ACP)**

a. **Tissue location:** Highest concentration in **prostate gland**, with lesser amounts in bone (osteoclasts), liver, spleen, erythrocytes, and platelets

b. **Clinical significance**

1) **Increased** in prostate cancer, benign prostatic hypertrophy, bone disease, Paget disease, breast cancer with bone metastases, Gaucher disease, platelet damage, and idiopathic thrombocytopenic purpura
2) ACP is **useful in forensic cases** involving rape because vaginal washings containing seminal fluid would exhibit ACP activity.

c. **Test methodology**

$$p\text{-Nitrophenylphosphate} \xrightarrow{\text{ACP(pH 4.9)}} p\text{-nitrophenol} + \text{NaOH} \xrightarrow{\text{(pH 11.0)}} \text{quinoid form (410 nm)}$$

Prostatic ACP = Total ACP − ACP after tartrate inhibition

1) **Sources of error:** Hemolysis; loss of activity in 1–2 hours at room temperature
2) **Reference ranges:**
   Total ACP: male 2.5–11.7 U/L; female 0.3–9.2 U/L at 37°C
   Prostatic ACP: male 0.2–5.0 U/L; female 0.0–0.8 U/L at 37°C

8. **Gamma-glutamyltransferase (GGT)**

a. **Tissue location:** GGT is found in liver (canaliculi of hepatic cells and epithelial cells lining biliary ductules), kidneys, pancreas, intestine, and many other tissues. GGT is **not** found in skeletal muscle tissue or bone.

b. **Clinical significance**

1) **Increased** levels in all **hepatobiliary** diseases, with levels increasing to two to five times the upper reference limit (e.g., viral hepatitis, alcoholic cirrhosis); very sensitive indicator for these conditions
2) Higher levels observed in **intra- and posthepatic biliary tract obstruction**, with levels increasing to 5–30 times the upper reference limit; increases before and remains elevated longer than ALP, AST, and ALT

3) GGT activity **induced by drugs** (e.g., phenobarbital and phenytoin) and by alcohol consumption
4) GGT levels are **normal in** the presence of **bone disease** and during **pregnancy** in contrast to alkaline phosphatase, where levels would be elevated.

c. **Test methodology:** Selected method of American Association for Clinical Chemistry

$$(\gamma\text{-L-Glutamyl})\text{-4-nitroanilide} \xrightarrow{\text{GGT}} \text{2-nitroaniline (405 nm)}$$

1) **Sources of error:** Hemolysis does not interfere.
2) **Reference ranges:** Male, up to 55 U/L; female, up to 38 U/L at 37°C

9. **Amylase (AMS)**

a. **Tissue location:** Found in pancreas, salivary glands, small intestine, fallopian tubes, and other tissues

b. **Clinical significance**

1) **Increased** serum levels in **acute pancreatitis** occur in 2–12 hours after the onset of pain, with peak values in 24 hours, and return to normal in 3–4 days.
2) **Increased:** Mumps, perforated peptic ulcer, intestinal obstruction, cholecystitis, ruptured ectopic pregnancy, mesenteric infarction, and acute appendicitis

c. **Test methodology**

1) **Amyloclastic:** Measures decrease in starch substrate
2) **Saccharogenic:** Measures formation of the product produced from starch (maltose)
3) **Chromogenic:** Measures the formation of soluble starch fragments coupled with a chromogenic dye
4) **Enzymatic:** Defined substrate used in coupled-enzymatic reactions
   a) **Sources of error:** In hyperlipidemia, triglycerides suppress AMS activity; morphine and other opiates falsely elevate AMS levels
   b) **Reference range:** 28–100 U/L at 37°C

10. **Lipase (LPS)**

a. **Tissue location:** Found in pancreas, with lesser amounts in gastric mucosa, intestinal mucosa, and adipose tissue

b. **Clinical significance:**

1) **Increased** serum levels in **acute pancreatitis** occur in 4–8 hours after the onset of pain, with peak values in 24 hours, and return to normal in 8–14 days.
2) **Increased:** Perforated peptic ulcer, duodenal ulcers, intestinal obstruction, and cholecystitis

c. **Test methodology**

$$\text{Oleic acid emulsion (0.8\%)} + H_2O \xrightarrow{\text{LPS}} \text{fatty acids}$$
(measure decreased turbidity)

1) **Sources of error:** Hemolysis because hemoglobin inhibits LPS activity
2) **Reference range:** Up to 38 U/L at 37°C

11. **Cholinesterase**
    a. Two related enzymes: **Acetylcholinesterase (AChE)/true cholinesterase** and **acylcholine acylhydrolase (PChE)/pseudocholinesterase**
    b. **Tissue location**
        1) **True cholinesterase** found in **red blood cells**, lungs, spleen, nerve endings, and gray matter of brain
        2) **Pseudocholinesterase** found in liver, pancreas, heart, white matter of brain, and **serum**
    c. **Clinical significance**
        1) **Pseudocholinesterase** found in serum in decreased amount in hepatocellular disease due to decreased synthesis, e.g., hepatitis, cirrhosis
        2) Decreased PChE occurs in **insecticide poisonings.**
        3) PChE testing identifies individuals with atypical forms who are **at risk** of prolonged response to muscle relaxants used in surgery.
    d. **Test methodology**

$$\text{Propionylthiocholine} + H_2O \xrightarrow{\text{CHS}} \text{Propionate} + \text{Thiocholine}$$

$$\text{Thiocholine} + \text{DTNB (5,5'-dithiobis(2-nitrobenzoic acid)} \longrightarrow \text{Yellow Compound}$$

        1) **Reference ranges (PChE serum):** Male, 40–78 U/L; female, 33–76 U/L at 37°C

12. **Glucose-6-phosphate dehydrogenase (G6PD)**
    a. **Tissue location:** Found in **erythrocytes**, adrenal glands, thymus, lymph nodes, and spleen
    b. **Clinical significance**
        1) **Decreased:** Primary importance of **G6PD** is in cases of **deficiency**, inherited as a sex-linked trait (X-chromosome). In G6DP deficiency, a drug-induced hemolytic anemia occurs when an individual is administered antimalarial drugs or primaquine. Hemolysis may also be caused by infections and after ingestion of fava beans.
        2) **Increased:** Megaloblastic anemias and AMI
    c. **Test methodology**

$$\text{Glucose-6-phosphate} + \text{NADP}^+ \xrightarrow{\text{G6PD}} \text{6-hogluconate} + \text{NADPH} + H^+$$

        1) **G6PD deficiency** requires the analysis of a **red blood cell hemolysate**.
        2) Analysis of **G6PD elevations** requires a **serum** sample.
        3) **Reference range (RBC):** 8–14 U/g Hgb

G. Cardiac Profile

1. Upon arrival to the emergency department, a cardiac profile would be ordered to establish **baseline values**. Then the cardiac profile would be ordered for several samplings in **3- to 8-hour intervals** over a 12- to 24-hour period.

Frequently blood is drawn every 3 hours for analysis during the first 12-hour period. Laboratory testing used to assess AMI includes **cardiac troponin T or I, CK-MB, and sometimes myoglobin**. In many institutions, once the cardiac troponin appears elevated, additional sampling and testing is halted and the elevated cardiac troponin is considered diagnostic for AMI.

2. **Troponin**
   a. **Tissue location:** Troponins T, I, and C form a complex of three proteins that bind to filaments of skeletal muscle and cardiac muscle to regulate muscle contraction.
   b. **Clinical significance**
      1) **cTnT or cTnI** (cardiac troponin T or cardiac troponin I) is used as an **AMI indicator** because of specificity and early rise in serum concentration following AMI.
      2) **In cases of AMI, cTnT** increases in 3–4 hours following infarction, peaks in 10–24 hours, and returns to normal in 10–14 days. **cTnI** increases in 3–6 hours following infarction, peaks in 14–20 hours, and returns to normal in 5–10 days.
   c. **Test methodology**
      1) Quantified by immunoassay: Fourth generation assay example. NOTE: Fifth generation troponin assays became available for use in the United States in 2018. The fifth generation assays are referred to as high-sensitivity troponin assays. The fifth generation assays appear to allow for more rapid detection of cardiomyocyte necrosis and at an earlier time point. Serum or plasma is mixed with biotinylated monoclonal anti-cTnT antibody and monoclonal anti-cTnT antibody labeled with a ruthenium complex; antibody-antigen-labeled-antibody sandwich binds to the solid phase via interaction with biotin and streptavidin, and microparticles are magnetically captured onto an electrode; application of a voltage emits chemiluminescence, which is measured by a photomultiplier and is proportional to cTnT in the sample.
      2) **Reference ranges:** cTnT < 0.03 ng/mL; cTnI < 0.40 ng/mL (Values vary considerably among laboratories and are dependent on the methodology employed. The new fifth generation assays will report troponins to the whole number with different units)

3. **Myoglobin**
   a. **Tissue location:** Found in skeletal and cardiac muscles
   b. **Clinical significance**
      1) **Increased** in skeletal muscle injuries, muscular dystrophy, and AMI
      2) Myoglobin is released early **in cases of AMI**, rising in 1–3 hours and peaking in 5–12 hours, and returns to normal in 18–30 hours. However, it is **not tissue specific**. It is better used as a negative predictor in the first 2–4 hours following chest pain.

c. **Test methodology**
   1) Quantified by immunoassay: preferred method uses a two-site sandwich technique
   2) **Reference ranges:** Male, 30–90 ng/mL; female, <50 ng/mL

4. **Creatine kinase and CK-MB** previously discussed in section VI. ENZYMES AND CARDIAC ASSESSMENT, pages 43–44.

H. Natriuretic Peptides: Polypeptide Hormones

1. **Tissue location and function**
   a. Three forms: ANP, CNP, and BNP
   b. Although effects are minimal, they function to **promote excretion of sodium and water** by increasing the glomerular filtration rate and decreasing the tubular reabsorption of sodium by the kidneys.
   c. **B-type (brain) natriuretic peptide (BNP)** is synthesized in and secreted from myocardial ventricles in response to ventricular volume expansion and pressure overload. BNP causes dilation of blood vessels and promotes sodium and water loss, thus reducing fluid load on the heart to improve cardiac function.
2. **Clinical significance:** BNP **increased** in **congestive heart failure** (CHF)
3. **Test methodology**
   a. BNP quantified by immunoassays
   b. **Reference range:** BNP <100 pg/mL
4. **ProBNP** assay measures N-terminal proBNP **(NT-proBNP)**, which is released when BNP is cleaved from precursor proBNP.
   a. NT-proBNP has a longer half-life than BNP.
   b. Measurement of NT-proBNP shows no interference from nesiritide (human recombinant BNP) administration to treat CHF.
   c. NT-proBNP is measured by electrochemiluminescence.

I. High-Sensitivity CRP (hs-CRP)

1. **C-reactive protein (CRP):** β-globulin that is an acute-phase reactant
2. **High-sensitivity CRP** refers to the sensitivity of the assay to determine low levels in serum.
3. **Clinical significance:** Used as a **predictor for cardiovascular risk;** increased levels seen in inflammation, infection, stress, trauma, and AMI
4. **Test methodology**
   a. Quantified by immunoassay; hs-CRP detection limit 0.05 mg/L
   b. **Reference ranges:** Males, 0.3–8.6 mg/L; females, 0.2–9.1 mg/L
   c. **Cardiovascular risk classification:**

      Low risk < 1.0 mg/L; average risk 1.0–3.0 mg/L; high risk > 3.0 mg/L

J. Homocysteine

1. **Clinical significance:** Elevated levels cause damage to arterial walls that precedes formation of plaques. It is an indicator of arterial inflammation.
2. **Test methodology**
   a. Immunoassay, fluorometric, and chromatographic
   b. **Reference range:** 5–15 μmol/L

VII. LIVER FUNCTION AND PORPHYRIN FORMATION

A. Liver Function: Synthesis, Excretory, and Detoxification

1. **Synthesis:** Liver synthesizes proteins, coagulation factors, ammonia, carbohydrates, fat, ketones, vitamin A, enzymes, and so on
2. **Bilirubin:** Principal pigment in bile that is derived from hemoglobin breakdown
   a. Bilirubin is produced in the reticuloendothelial system from the breakdown of hemoglobin from senescent red blood cells (RBCs). **Bilirubin** forms a **complex with albumin** for transport to the liver. In this form, bilirubin is **unconjugated** and **not** water soluble.
   b. **Bilirubin** is **conjugated** in the hepatocyte endoplasmic reticulum **with glucuronic acid to form bilirubin diglucuronide** (conjugated bilirubin). The reaction is catalyzed by **uridine diphosphate (UDP) glycuronyltransferase.** Conjugated bilirubin is **water soluble.** Conjugated bilirubin is excreted into the bile for storage in the gallbladder, secreted into the duodenum in response to gallbladder stimulation, and reduced by anaerobic bacteria in the intestine to **urobilinogen.** Some intestinal urobilinogen is reabsorbed; a portion returns to the liver and some enters the circulation for excretion in the urine, whereas the remaining portion in the intestines is oxidized by anaerobic bacteria for excretion in the stool as **urobilin.** Urobilin is an **orange-brown pigment** that gives stool its characteristic color.
   c. **Jaundice (icterus)** is a yellow discoloration that occurs when the bilirubin concentration in the blood rises **(>2–3 mg/dL)** and the bilirubin is deposited in the skin and sclera of the eyes.
   d. **Kernicterus:** Elevated bilirubin deposits in **brain tissue of infants**, affecting the central nervous system and resulting in intellectual disability.
3. **Liver secretes bile** to assist in digestion. Bile salts are composed of cholic acid and chenodeoxycholic acid conjugated with glycine or taurine. **Bile** is **stored** in the **gallbladder.**
4. **Detoxification and drug metabolism:** The **liver** is the primary site in the body for synthesis of waste products (e.g., urea), conjugation of hormones and bilirubin to water-soluble forms, and conversion of drugs to metabolites for excretion in urine or stool.

B. Classification of Causes of Jaundice

1. **Prehepatic jaundice occurs** when there is **excessive erythrocyte destruction**, as seen in hemolytic anemias, spherocytosis, toxic conditions, hemolytic disease

of the newborn caused by Rh or ABO incompatibility, and so on. In these cases, the rate of hemolysis exceeds the liver's ability to take up the bilirubin for conjugation. Prehepatic jaundice is characterized by an **increased level of unconjugated bilirubin** in the serum.

2. **Hepatic jaundice** occurs when the **liver cells malfunction** and cannot take up, conjugate, or secrete bilirubin.
   a. **Gilbert syndrome:** Defect in the ability of hepatocytes to take up bilirubin; due to **transport problem** of bilirubin from the sinusoidal membrane to the microsomal region; characterized by **mild increase** in serum level of **unconjugated bilirubin** (1.5–3.0 mg/dL)
   b. **Crigler-Najjar disease:** Partial or complete deficiency of **UDP-glycuronyltransferase**; little, if any, conjugated bilirubin formed, which causes **increased** serum level of **unconjugated bilirubin** (moderate to extremely elevated)
   c. **Dubin-Johnson syndrome:** Defective liver cell excretion of bilirubin due to **impaired transport in the hepatocyte** of conjugated bilirubin from microsomal region to the bile canaliculi; characterized by **increased** serum level of **conjugated bilirubin** with mild increase in unconjugated bilirubin
   d. **Neonatal physiological jaundice:** Level of **UDP-glycuronyltransferase** is **low at birth**; takes several days for the liver to synthesize an adequate amount of the enzyme to catalyze bilirubin conjugation; causes **increased** serum level of **unconjugated bilirubin**
   e. **Intrahepatic cholestasis:** May be caused by hepatocyte injury such as cirrhosis, bile duct injury such as Rotor syndrome, or neoplasms
3. **Posthepatic jaundice** occurs when an **obstruction blocks the flow of bile into the intestines.** This is referred to as **extrahepatic cholestasis** and may be caused by gallstones obstructing the common bile duct, neoplasms such as carcinoma of the ampulla of Vater or carcinoma of the pancreas, and inflammatory conditions such as acute cholangitis or acute pancreatitis. Posthepatic jaundice is characterized by a **significantly increased** level of **conjugated bilirubin** in serum, increased level of unconjugated bilirubin in serum, increased conjugated bilirubin in the urine, decreased urine and fecal urobilinogen, and **stool** that appears **pale in color.**

C. Other Disorders of the Liver

1. **Cirrhosis:** Result of **chronic scarring** of liver tissue turning it into nodules; may be caused by excessive alcohol ingestion over a long period of time, hemochromatosis, complication of hepatitis
2. **Tumors**
   a. **Hepatocellular carcinoma or hepatoma:** Primary cancer of the liver
   b. **Metastatic liver tumors:** Arise from other cancerous tissue where the primary site was of lung, pancreas, gastrointestinal tract, or ovary origin

3. **Reye syndrome**
   a. **Cause is unknown**, but the **symptoms include** encephalopathy, neurologic abnormalities including seizures or coma, and abnormal liver function tests due to hepatic destruction.
   b. It occurs mainly in children, usually after a viral infection (varicella or influenza) and aspirin therapy.
4. **Drug-related disorders:** Drugs, including phenothiazines, antibiotics, antineoplastic drugs, and anti-inflammatory drugs such as acetaminophen, may cause liver damage.
5. Acute and chronic **hepatitis**

D. Serum Enzymes Used to Assess Liver Function

1. Markers for **hepatocellular necrosis**
   a. **ALT:** Most specific for hepatocyte injury
   b. **AST:** Less specific than ALT; significant presence in other tissues
   c. **LD:** Least specific; significant presence in other tissues
2. Markers that reflect **cholestasis**
   a. **Alkaline phosphatase**
   b. **Gamma-glutamyl transferase**
3. Other tests to assess liver disorders
   a. Total bilirubin, direct bilirubin (conjugated), and indirect bilirubin (unconjugated)
   b. Albumin
   c. Ammonia
   d. AFP

E. Test Methodology for Bilirubin

1. **Jendrassik-Grof total bilirubin test**

Bilirubin + sodium acetate + caffeine-sodium benzoate + diazotized sulfanilic acid
→ purple azobilirubin + alkaline tartrate → green-blue azobilirubin (600 nm)

2. **Direct spectrophotometric:** For newborns, bilirubin concentration is read directly by spectrophotometry and concentration is proportional to absorbance at 455 nm.
3. **Sources of error:** Hemolysis, lipemia; avoid exposure to sunlight and fluorescent lighting
4. **Reference ranges**
   Infants: Total bilirubin 2–6 mg/dL (0–1 day, full term)
   Adults: Total bilirubin 0.2–1.0 mg/dL
   Indirect bilirubin 0.2–0.8 mg/dL
   Direct bilirubin 0.0–0.2 mg/dL

TABLE 1–5 CAUSES OF JAUNDICE

	Reference Range	Hemolytic Jaundice	Intrahepatic Early Hepatitis	Extrahepatic Obstructive
Serum Conj. Bilirubin	0.0–0.2 mg/dL	Normal or sl. ↑	↑	↑↑
Serum Unconj. Bilirubin	0.2–0.8 mg/dL	↑	↑↑	↑
Feces Urobilinogen	75–400 EU/d or (+2)	↑(+4)	↓(+1)	↓ or Neg
Urine Urobilinogen	0.5–4.0 EU/d or (+1)	↑(+4)	↑	↓ or Neg
Urine Bilirubin	Negative (Neg)	Neg	↑	↑

F. Test Methodology for Urobilinogen

1. Urobilinogen is the collective term for stercobilinogen, mesobilinogen, and urobilinogen.
2. **Urine urobilinogen assay**

   urobilinogen + *p*-dimethyl aminobenzaldehyde → red colored complex

3. **Sources of error:** Oxidation will occur if urine is allowed to stand; other compounds react, such as porphobilinogen
4. **Clinical significance (see Table 1–5■)**
   a. In **posthepatic obstruction, urobilinogen** formation is **decreased** because of impaired bilirubin excretion into the intestines. This is evidenced by a clay-colored (partial biliary obstruction) or chalky white stool (complete biliary obstruction).
   b. **Increased** urine urobilinogen is associated with hemolytic disease and hepatocellular disease, such as hepatitis.
5. **Reference range urine urobilinogen:** 0.1–1.0 Ehrlich units/2 hours

G. Porphyrin Formation

1. Heme is derived from a series of biochemical reactions that begin with the formation of aminolevulinic acid (ALA) from succinyl coenzyme A and glycine. Through a second condensation reaction, two molecules of ALA condense and cyclize to form porphobilinogen (PBG). Because porphobilinogen is a monopyrrole, four molecules of porphobilinogen condense and cyclize to form the various porphyrinogens. Specific enzymes catalyze the formation of **uroporphyrinogen, coproporphyrinogen, protoporphyrinogen**, and protoporphyrin IX. Protoporphyrinogen IX is the immediate precursor of protoporphyrin IX.
   a. **Deficiency** of any of the specific **enzymes** that catalyze the formation of the porphyrinogens results in **excess formation** of the corresponding **porphyrin**. The enzyme deficiencies may be inherited or acquired.
   b. Protoporphyrin IX chelates iron to form heme.
2. The **porphyrins** that are of clinical significance include **uroporphyrin, coproporphyrin**, and **protoporphyrin**. Types of **porphyrias** include:
   a. Plumboporphyria
   b. Acute intermittent porphyria

c. Congenital erythropoietic porphyria
d. Porphyria cutanea tarda
e. Hepatoerythropoietic porphyria
f. Hereditary coproporphyria
g. Variegate porphyria
h. Erythropoietic porphyria

3. General characteristics of the porphyrias
   a. Overproduction or accumulation of porphyrins and precursors, such as porphobilinogen, in the **bone marrow** is termed **erythropoietic porphyrias** and in the **liver** it is termed **hepatic porphyrias**.
   b. Excess of early precursors, such as ALA and PBG, causes **neuropsychiatric** symptoms, including abdominal pain, vomiting, constipation, tachycardia, hypertension, and psychiatric symptoms.
   c. Excess of later intermediates, uroporphyrins, coproporphyrins, and protoporphyrins, causes **cutaneous** symptoms including photosensitivity, blisters, excess facial hair, and hyperpigmentation. Photosensitivity results from the deposition of porphyrins in the skin.
   d. Excess of early precursors and later intermediates causes **neurocutaneous** symptoms.
4. **Methods:** For measurement of aminolevulinic acid, porphobilinogen, uroporphyrin, and coproporphyrin, a 24-hour urine specimen should be collected.
   a. Refrigerate urine during collection; store in brown bottle to protect light-sensitive compounds.
   b. Porphobilinogen more stable under alkaline conditions and aminolevulinic acid more stable under acid conditions; sodium bicarbonate used as a compromise to maintain the pH near 7.
   c. **Watson-Schwartz test** employs ***p*-dimethylaminobenzaldehyde** reagent (also known as Ehrlich's aldehyde reagent) to form a red condensation product with **porphobilinogen.**
   d. Porphyrin compounds may be detected in acid solution by irradiating the solution with long-wave ultraviolet light, which causes the **porphyrins** to **fluoresce.** The intense orange-red fluorescence of the porphyrins is due to the conjugated unsaturation of the tetrapyrrole ring structure.
   e. Porphyrins may be differentiated and quantified using HPLC with a fluorescence detector system.

VIII. ELECTROLYTES AND OSMOLALITY

A. Osmolality

1. **Colligative properties** refer to the properties of a solution that are influenced by the number of molecules in solution, but not their individual composition. There are four types of colligative properties: **boiling point, freezing point, osmotic pressure**, and **vapor pressure.**

2. **Osmolality**
   a. **Osmolality** is the measure of the number of dissolved particles in solution expressed as **osmoles per kilogram of water.** Serum osmolality is expressed as **milliosmoles/kg**; the reference range for serum is 275–295 mOsm/kg.
   b. Osmolality is **regulated by** the **hypothalamus** through the sensation of thirst and the signaling to secrete antidiuretic hormone (ADH). When the osmolality of the blood is increased, two processes occur:
      1) Consuming more water will decrease the osmolality.
      2) Posterior pituitary secretion of ADH will cause renal reabsorption of water and decrease the osmolality.
   c. **Osmometry:** Method used to measure all particles (molecules and ions) in solution; measure of osmolality
   d. Two formulas used to **calculate estimated osmolality:**

$$\mathbf{1.86Na + glucose/18 + BUN/2.8 + 9 = mOsm/kg}$$

$$\mathbf{2(Na) + glucose/20 + BUN/3 = mOsm/kg}$$

      1) In healthy individuals, the **calculated osmolality** equals the **measured osmolality**.
      2) The **osmolal gap** represents the difference between the measured and calculated osmolality. The osmolal gap **should be <15.** An **osmolal gap can exist** for a variety of reasons, including excess production of β-hydroxybutyrate, ingestion of toxins such as ethylene glycol, or ingestion of an excessive amount of alcohol.
3. **Measuring osmolality**
   a. Measuring **serum** and **urine osmolality** is useful in assessing electrolyte disorders and acid-base status. Major molecules measured by serum osmolality include **sodium, chloride, glucose,** and **urea.**
   b. **Freezing point depression osmometry:** Particles in solution cause the freezing point of pure water to be decreased, with the decrease in temperature being directly proportional to the total number of particles present.
   c. **Vapor pressure depression osmometry:** Water evaporation is decreased when solute is present in water, which is indicated by an inverse relationship between the osmolality of the solution (amount of particles present) and the vapor pressure.

B. Electrolytes: Sodium, Potassium, Chloride, and Total Carbon Dioxide
   1. **Electrolytes:** Charged ions found in intracellular fluid, extracellular fluid, and interstitial fluid
      a. **Cations** are **positively** charged ions. The **major cations** in the body are sodium, potassium, calcium, and magnesium.
      b. **Anions** are **negatively** charged ions. The **major anions** in the body are chloride, bicarbonate, phosphate, sulfate, organic acids, and protein.

c. Clinically, when electrolytes are ordered on an individual, the **term** "electrolytes" is understood to mean the **measurement of serum sodium, potassium, chloride,** and **total carbon dioxide** (bicarbonate). The serum concentration of these four electrolytes is quantified using **ion-selective electrodes (ISEs).**

2. **Sodium (Na^+)**
   a. **Major cation of extracellular fluid**
   b. **Reference range:** 136–145 mmol/L
   c. Changes in sodium result in changes in plasma volume.
   d. **Largest** constituent of plasma osmolality
   e. Sodium is excreted in the urine when the renal threshold for serum sodium exceeds 110–130 mmol/L.
   f. **Clinical significance**
      1) **Hyponatremia** occurs when serum sodium level is <135 mmol/L.
         a) **Depletional hyponatremia** can be due to diuretics, hypoaldosteronism (Addison disease), diarrhea or vomiting, and severe burns or trauma.
         b) **Dilutional hyponatremia** can be due to overhydration, syndrome of inappropriate antidiuretic hormone (SIADH), congestive heart failure, cirrhosis, and nephrotic syndrome.
      2) **Hypernatremia** occurs when serum sodium level is >150 mmol/L.
         a) Usually occurs when water is lost as through diarrhea, excessive sweating, or diabetes insipidus, and when sodium is retained as through acute ingestion, hyperaldosteronism, or infusion of hypertonic solutions during dialysis

3. **Potassium (K^+)**
   a. **Major intracellular cation**
   b. **Reference range:** 3.4–5.0 mmol/L
   c. Because the concentration of potassium in red blood cells is higher than in serum, any level of hemolysis will falsely increase serum potassium results.
   d. **Clinical significance**
      1) **Hypokalemia** occurs when serum potassium level is <3.0 mmol/L.
         a) Results from decreased dietary intake, hyperaldosteronism, diuretics, vomiting, diarrhea, laxative abuse, and excess insulin which causes increased cellular uptake of potassium
      2) **Hyperkalemia** occurs when serum potassium level is >5.0 mmol/L.
         a) Results from increased intake, renal failure, hypoaldosteronism, metabolic acidosis, increased red blood cell lysis, leukemia, and chemotherapy

4. **Chloride (Cl^-)**
   a. **Major anion of extracellular fluid**
   b. **Reference range:** 98–107 mmol/L
   c. Chloride levels change proportionally with sodium.
   d. **Clinical significance**
      1) **Hypochloremia** occurs when serum chloride level is <98 mmol/L.
         a) Results from excessive vomiting, use of diuretics, burns, and aldosterone deficiency

2) **Hyperchloremia** occurs when serum chloride level is >107 mmol/L.
   a) Results from prolonged diarrhea, renal tubular disease, dehydration, and excess loss of bicarbonate

5. **Bicarbonate (HCO_3^-)**
   a. **Second largest anion fraction of extracellular fluid**
   b. **Reference range:** 22–29 mmol/L
   c. Clinically, the concentration of total carbon dioxide ($ctCO_2$) is measured because it is difficult to measure HCO_3^-. $ctCO_2$ is comprised primarily of HCO_3^- along with smaller amounts of H_2CO_3 (carbonic acid), carbamino-bound CO_2, and dissolved CO_2. HCO_3^- accounts for approximately 90% of measured $ctCO_2$.
   d. Bicarbonate is able to buffer excess H^+, making bicarbonate an important buffer system of blood.
   e. **Clinical significance**
      1) **Decreased $ctCO_2$** associated with metabolic acidosis, diabetic ketoacidosis, and salicylate toxicity
      2) **Increased $ctCO_2$** associated with metabolic alkalosis, emphysema, and severe vomiting

6. **Anion gap:** This is a mathematical formula used to demonstrate electroneutrality of body fluids. It represents the difference between cations and anions that are not actually measured analytically when serum "electrolytes" are quantified. The unmeasured cations include calcium and magnesium, whereas the unmeasured anions include phosphate, sulfate, organic acids, and protein.
   a. Two **calculation methods are** commonly used:

$$Na^+ - (Cl^- + HCO_3^-) = \text{anion gap}$$

expected anion gap: 7–16 mmol/L

$$(Na^+ + K^+) - (Cl^- + HCO_3^-) = \text{anion gap}$$

expected anion gap: 10–20 mmol/L

   b. **Increased anion gap** can be caused by uremia, lactic acidosis, ketoacidosis, hypernatremia, and ingestion of methanol, ethylene glycol, or salicylate. It is also used as an assessment of instrument errors.
   c. **Decreased anion gap** can be caused by hypoalbuminemia and hypercalcemia.

C. Calcium

1. **Calcium** exists in plasma in three forms: 50% **free (ionized)**, 40% **bound to protein**, and 10% **bound to anions.** It is the **free form** of calcium that is **biologically active.**
2. Decreased free (ionized) calcium levels cause muscle spasms or uncontrolled muscle contractions called **tetany.**

3. **Regulation: Serum calcium** is controlled by parathyroid hormone, vitamin D, and calcitonin.
   a. **Parathyroid hormone (PTH)**
      1) A **decrease** in free (ionized) calcium **stimulates** the release of PTH by the parathyroid gland, and a **rise** in free calcium **terminates** PTH release.
      2) In bone, PTH **activates osteoclasts** to breakdown bone with the release of calcium.
      3) In the kidneys, PTH **increases tubular reabsorption** of calcium and **stimulates hydroxylation of vitamin D** to the active form.
   b. **Vitamin D (cholecalciferol)**
      1) Obtained by diet or exposure to sunlight
      2) Initially, vitamin D is transported to the liver, where it is hydroxylated but still inactive. Then the hydroxylated form is transported to the kidneys, where it is **converted to 1,25-dihydroxycholecalciferol**, the **active form** of the vitamin.
      3) **Calcium absorption** in the intestines is enhanced by vitamin D. In addition, PTH increases tubular reabsorption of calcium in the kidneys.
   c. **Calcitonin**
      1) Calcitonin is released by the parafollicular cells of the thyroid gland when serum calcium level increases.
      2) It **inhibits vitamin D and parathyroid hormone** activity, thus decreasing serum calcium.
      3) Medullary carcinoma of the thyroid gland is a neoplasm of the parafollicular cells, resulting in elevated serum levels of calcitonin.
4. **Clinical significance**
   a. **Hypercalcemia** is caused by primary hyperparathyroidism, other endocrine disorders such as hypothyroidism and acute adrenal insufficiency, malignancy involving bone, and renal failure.
   b. **Hypocalcemia** is caused by hypoparathyroidism, hypoalbuminemia, chronic renal failure, magnesium deficiency, and vitamin D deficiency.
5. **Methods, interferences, and reference range**
   a. **Methods used to measure total serum calcium:** Spectrophotometric (ortho-cresolphthalein complexone, arsenazo III dye), ISE (ion-specific electrode), and atomic absorption (reference method)
      1) Spectrophotometric methods use metallochromic indicators that bind calcium causing a color change. These methods are easily automated.
      2) With ISE analysis, the specimen must be acidified to convert protein-bound and complexed calcium to the free form in order to measure total calcium.
   b. **Measure free (ionized) serum calcium:** Ion-specific electrode measures free form. Measurement is temperature sensitive, and generally analysis is performed at 37°C.
   c. **Sources of error:** Cannot use oxalate, citrate, or EDTA anticoagulants; interferences for spectrophotometric methods include hemolysis, icterus,

and lipemia; interferences for ion-specific electrode methods include protein buildup on electrode and change in blood pH *in vitro* before analysis

d. **Reference ranges**
Total calcium (adults): 8.6–10.3 mg/dL
Free calcium (adults): 4.6–5.3 mg/dL

D. Phosphorus

1. **Regulation**
   a. **Phosphate** in the blood is absorbed from dietary sources, released from cells, or released from bone. Regulation occurs by reabsorption or excretion by the **kidneys.**
   b. Most important regulatory hormone is **PTH**, which increases renal excretion of phosphate.
   c. **Vitamin D** regulates phosphate by causing intestinal absorption and renal reabsorption.
2. **Clinical significance**
   a. **Hyperphosphatemia** is caused by renal failure, hypoparathyroidism, neoplastic diseases, lymphoblastic leukemia, and intense exercise.
   b. **Hypophosphatemia** is caused by diabetic ketoacidosis, hyperparathyroidism, asthma, alcoholism, and malabsorption syndrome.
3. **Methods, interferences, and reference range**
   a. Ammonium molybdate + phosphate ions $\longrightarrow$ phosphomolybdate complex (colorless) read at 340 nm
   b. When aminonaphtholsulfonic acid is used to reduce the complex, a colored product is formed and read at 600–700 nm.

   $$\text{Phosphomolybdenum} \xrightarrow{+\text{electrons}} \text{molybdenum blue}$$

   c. **Sources of error:** Hemolysis, lipemia, icterus; cannot use oxalate, citrate, or EDTA anticoagulants
   d. **Reference range (adults):** 2.5–4.5 mg/dL

E. Magnesium

1. **Magnesium** exists in plasma in three forms: 55% **free (ionized)**, 30% **bound to protein**, and 15% **complexed.** It is the **free form** of magnesium that is **biologically active**.
2. Regulation
   a. The magnesium level is regulated by the **kidneys** through reabsorption and excretion.
   b. **PTH enhances** reabsorption by the kidneys and intestinal absorption.
3. **Clinical significance**
   a. **Hypermagnesemia** is caused by renal failure and excess antacids.
   b. **Hypomagnesemia** is caused by gastrointestinal disorders; renal diseases; hyperparathyroidism (hypercalcemia); drugs (e.g., diuretic therapy, cardiac

glycosides, cisplatin, cyclosporine); diabetes mellitus with glycosuria; and alcoholism due to dietary deficiency.

4. **Methods, interferences, and reference range**
   a. **Methods used to measure total serum magnesium:** Calmagite, methylthymol blue, and atomic absorption spectrophotometry (reference method)
   b. **Measure free (ionized) serum magnesium:** Ion-selective electrode
   c. **Sources of error:** Hemolysis; cannot use oxalate, citrate, or EDTA anticoagulants
   d. **Reference range (adults):** 1.7–2.4 mg/dL

F. Serum Iron and Total Iron-Binding Capacity

1. **Iron** is found in several locations in the body, including: component of hemoglobin and myoglobin, stored form **(ferritin and hemosiderin)**, tissue compartment (component of enzymes and coenzymes), and labile pool. Iron is transported in the blood by **transferrin.**
   a. **Serum iron** exhibits **diurnal variation,** with values being highest in the morning.
   b. **Transferrin** is **increased** in iron-deficiency disorders, and it is **decreased** in conditions of iron overload, hemochromatosis, and severe infections. Transferrin is measured directly by immunochemical methods. **Transferrin** has a **reference range** of 200–360 mg/dL.
   c. **Ferritin reflects iron stores.** Ferritin **decreases early** in iron-deficiency disorders, making it a sensitive, early indicator of disease. It is **increased** in conditions of iron overload, hemochromatosis, and severe infections. Ferritin is an acute-phase protein measured directly by immunochemical methods. **Ferritin reference ranges** are 20–250 ng/mL for males and 10–120 ng/mL for females.
2. **Clinical significance (see Table 1–6■)**
   a. **Decreased serum iron** is associated with iron-deficiency anemia, malnutrition, blood loss, and chronic infection.
   b. **Increased serum iron** is associated with iron overdose, sideroblastic anemia, viral hepatitis, and hemochromatosis.

TABLE 1–6 DISEASE STATES RELATED TO IRON METABOLISM

Test	Iron Deficiency	Malnutrition	Iron Overdose	Hemochromatosis
Serum Iron	Decreased	Decreased	Increased	Increased
% Saturation	Decreased	Varies	Increased	Increased
TIBC (indirect transferrin)	Increased	Decreased	Decreased	Decreased

3. **Test methodology**
   a. **Total iron content (serum iron):** Measures serum **Fe^{3+}** bound to transferrin. An acid solution is used to release Fe^{3+} from transferrin, Fe^{3+} is reduced to Fe^{2+} by a reducing agent, Fe^{2+} is complexed with a chromogen reagent such as bathophenanthroline or ferrozine.
   b. **Total iron-binding capacity (TIBC):** Measures the quantity of iron bound to transferrin **if all** the **binding sites** on transferrin were **occupied** (i.e., saturated with iron). Fe^{3+} is added to serum to saturate transferrin. $MgCO_3$ is added to remove unbound Fe^{3+}. The mixture is centrifuged and the supernatant is used in the serum iron procedure.
   c. **Percent transferrin saturation:** This is a calculated value that represents the amount of iron that transferrin is **capable** of binding.

   Calculate using serum iron and TIBC:

$$\textbf{\% transferrin saturation} = \textbf{serum iron } (\mu\textbf{g/dL}) \div \textbf{TIBC } (\mu\textbf{g/dL}) \times 100\%$$

4. **Reference ranges**
   Serum iron: 45–160 μg/dL
   TIBC: 250–425 μg/dL
   % Saturation: 15–55

IX. ACID-BASE METABOLISM

A. Major Buffer Systems

1. **Buffer:** System that can resist change in pH; composed of a weak acid or a weak base and its corresponding salt
2. Four buffer systems of clinical importance exist in whole blood:
   a. The **bicarbonate-carbonic acid buffer system** uses HCO_3^- and H_2CO_3 to minimize pH changes in plasma and erythrocytes. It is the most important buffer system in plasma.
   b. The **protein buffer system** uses plasma proteins to minimize pH changes in the blood.
   c. The **phosphate buffer system** uses HPO_4^{2-} and $H_2PO_4^-$ to minimize pH changes in plasma and erythrocytes.
   d. The **hemoglobin buffer system** uses the hemoglobin in red blood cells to minimize pH changes in the blood. It is the most important intracellular buffer.

B. Definitions

1. **Respiration:** It is a process to supply cells with oxygen for metabolic processes and remove the carbon dioxide produced during metabolism.
2. **Partial pressure:** In a mixture of gases, partial pressure is the amount of pressure contributed by each gas to the total pressure exerted by the mixture.
3. **Acidemia** occurs when arterial blood $pH < 7.35$.
4. **Alkalemia** occurs when arterial blood $pH > 7.45$.
5. **Hypercapnia** is increased blood PCO_2.

6. **Hypocapnia** is decreased blood PCO_2.
7. **Partial pressure of carbon dioxide (PCO_2):** Measured in blood as mm Hg
8. **Concentration of dissolved carbon dioxide ($cdCO_2$):** Includes undissociated carbonic acid (H_2CO_3) and carbon dioxide dissolved in blood **(represented by PCO_2)**
9. **Concentration of total carbon dioxide ($ctCO_2$):** Includes bicarbonate (primary component), carbamino-bound CO_2, carbonic acid, and dissolved carbon dioxide

C. Acid-Base Balance

1. The **pH of plasma** is a function of two independent variables: the **partial pressure of carbon dioxide (PCO_2)**, which is regulated by the **lungs** or (respiratory mechanism), and the concentration of **bicarbonate** (HCO_3^-), which is regulated by the **kidneys** (renal mechanism).
2. Carbon dioxide is transported as bicarbonate, carbamino compound (bound to serum proteins and hemoglobin), and dissolved carbon dioxide. Even though these forms transport the carbon dioxide, they also serve as buffers to maintain blood pH. Carbon dioxide, pH, and PCO_2 are related according to the **Henderson-Hasselbalch equation:**

$$\mathrm{pH} = \mathrm{pK}' + \log \frac{[\mathrm{HCO_3}]}{[\mathrm{H_2CO_3}]}$$

$$\mathrm{pH} = 6.1 + \log \frac{c\mathrm{HCO_3^-}}{c\mathrm{dCO_2}}$$

$$\boldsymbol{c\mathrm{dCO_2} = P\mathrm{CO_2} \times \alpha \text{ (solubility coefficient of } \mathrm{CO_2})}$$

$$\textbf{where } \alpha = \textbf{0.03 mmol/L per mm Hg}$$

The average normal ratio of $cHCO_3^-$ to $cdCO_2$ is **20:1.** So any change in the bicarbonate concentration or the dissolved carbon dioxide concentration (includes H_2CO_3) would result in a change in blood pH. Because laboratories measure the concentration of total carbon dioxide ($ctCO_2$), this value is substituted for $cHCO_3^-$ in the equation. If $ctCO_2 = 24$ mmol/L and $PCO_2 = 40$ mm Hg, then

$$\mathrm{PH} = 6.1 + \log \frac{(\mathrm{HCO_3})}{\mathrm{PCO_2}(\alpha)}$$

$$\mathrm{pH} = 6.1 + \log \frac{[24 \text{ mmol/L}]}{[40 \text{ mm Hg} \times 0.03 \text{ mmol/L/mm Hg}]}$$

$$\mathrm{pH} = 6.1 + \log \frac{[24]}{[1.2]}$$

$$\mathrm{pH} = 6.1 + \log \frac{[20]}{[1]}$$

$$\mathrm{pH} = 6.1 + 1.3 = 7.4$$

3. **Reference ranges for arterial blood gas analysis**

   pH: 7.35–7.45

   ***c*tCO_2:** 22–26 mmol/L

   ***P*CO_2:** 35–45 mm Hg

D. Acid-Base Disorders
   1. Acid-base disorders are classified as metabolic acidosis, metabolic alkalosis, respiratory acidosis, and respiratory alkalosis.
      a. **Metabolic** acid-base disorders primarily involve **bicarbonate concentration.**
      b. **Respiratory** acid-base disorders primarily involve **dissolved carbon dioxide concentration.**
   2. **Metabolic acidosis (nonrespiratory): Primary bicarbonate deficit**
      a. In **metabolic acidosis**, the **bicarbonate concentration decreases**, causing a decrease in the 20:1 ratio between $cHCO_3^-$ and $cdCO_2$, which results in a decrease in the blood pH.
      b. **Metabolic acidosis** may be **caused by** organic acid production or when ingestion exceeds the excretion rate. Disorders include diabetic ketoacidosis due to the production of acetoacetic acid and β-hydroxybutyric acid; lactic acidosis due to the production of lactic acid; poisonings such as salicylate, ethylene glycol, and methyl alcohol; reduced acid excretion due to renal failure or tubular acidosis; and loss of bicarbonate due to diarrhea or excessive renal excretion.
      c. **Laboratory findings in metabolic acidosis**
         1) $ctCO_2$ decreased
         2) PCO_2 normal
         3) pH decreased
      d. **Respiratory compensatory mechanism:** A decreased pH triggers **hyperventilation** that **lowers PCO_2** and results in an increase in pH. This increases the ratio between $cHCO_3^-$ and $cdCO_2$ to 20:1, which increases the blood pH.
      e. **Laboratory findings in compensation**
         1) $ctCO_2$ decreased
         2) PCO_2 decreased
         3) pH normal
   3. **Metabolic (nonrespiratory) alkalosis: Primary bicarbonate excess**
      a. In **metabolic alkalosis**, the **bicarbonate concentration increases**, causing an increase in the 20:1 ratio between $cHCO_3^-$ and $cdCO_2$, which results in an increase in the blood pH.
      b. **Metabolic alkalosis** may be **caused by** ingestion of excess base, decreased elimination of base, or loss of acidic fluids. Disorders include ingestion of excess alkali (antacids); intravenous administration of bicarbonate; renal bicarbonate retention; prolonged diuretic use; loss of hydrochloric acid

from the stomach after vomiting, intestinal obstruction, or gastric suction; glucocorticoid excess as in Cushing syndrome; and mineralocorticoid excess as in hyperaldosteronism.

c. **Laboratory findings in metabolic alkalosis**
   1) $ctCO_2$ increased
   2) PCO_2 normal
   3) pH increased

d. **Respiratory compensation mechanism:** The pH increase slows breathing **(hypoventilation)**, thus **increasing the amount of CO_2 retained** by the lungs. This increased CO_2 retention causes an increase in H_2CO_3, which results in more dissolved CO_2 in the blood. The carbonic acid lowers the pH. This decreases the ratio between $cHCO_3^-$ and $cdCO_2$ to 20:1, which decreases the blood pH.

e. **Laboratory findings in compensation**
   1) $ctCO_2$ increased
   2) PCO_2 increased
   3) pH normal

4. **Respiratory acidosis: Primary $cdCO_2$ excess expressed as increase in PCO_2 (hypercapnia)**

a. Inability of a person to exhale CO_2 through the lungs **(hypoventilation)** causes an **increase of PCO_2.** The increased PCO_2 causes an increase in the concentration of dissolved carbon dioxide, which forms carbonic acid in the blood. This decreases the 20:1 ratio between $cHCO_3^-$ and $cdCO_2$, which decreases the blood pH.

b. **Respiratory acidosis** may be **caused by** chronic obstructive pulmonary disease, such as chronic bronchitis and emphysema, ingestion of narcotics and barbiturates, and severe infections of the central nervous system such as meningitis.

c. **Laboratory findings in respiratory acidosis**
   1) $ctCO_2$ normal
   2) PCO_2 increased
   3) pH decreased

d. **Renal compensatory mechanism:** The **kidneys** increase sodium-hydrogen exchange, ammonia formation, and bicarbonate retention. The **increased bicarbonate** concentration aids the return of the 20:1 ratio, which raises the blood pH.

e. **Laboratory findings in compensation**
   1) $ctCO_2$ increased
   2) PCO_2 increased
   3) pH normal

5. **Respiratory alkalosis: Primary cdCO_2 deficit expressed as decrease in PCO_2 (hypocapnia)**
   a. **Decreased PCO_2** results from an accelerated rate or depth of respiration, or a combination of both. Excessive exhalation of carbon dioxide **(hyperventilation) reduces the PCO_2,** causing a decrease in the concentration of dissolved carbon dioxide, which forms less carbonic acid in the blood (i.e., less hydrogen ions). This increases the 20:1 ratio between $cHCO_3^-$ and cdCO_2, which increases the blood pH.
   b. **Respiratory alkalosis** may be **caused by** hypoxia, anxiety, nervousness, excessive crying, pulmonary embolism, pneumonia, congestive heart failure, salicylate overdose, and so on.
   c. **Laboratory findings in respiratory alkalosis**
      1) ctCO_2 normal
      2) PCO_2 decreased
      3) pH increased
   d. The **renal compensatory mechanism** corrects respiratory alkalosis by **excreting bicarbonate.**
   e. **Laboratory findings in compensation**
      1) ctCO_2 decreased
      2) PCO_2 decreased
      3) pH normal

E. Oxygen Metabolism
   1. **Oxygen** is **transported bound to hemoglobin** present in red blood cells and in a **physically dissolved** state.
      a. Three factors control oxygen transport: the PO_2, free diffusion of oxygen across the alveolar membrane, and affinity of hemoglobin for oxygen.
      b. Release of oxygen to the tissues is **facilitated by** an increase in H^+ concentration and PCO_2 levels at the tissue level.
      c. Under normal circumstances, the saturation of hemoglobin with oxygen is 95%. When the PO_2 is >110 mm Hg, greater than 98% of hemoglobin binds to oxygen.
      d. When a person's oxygen saturation falls below 95%, either the individual is not getting enough oxygen or does not have enough functional hemoglobin available to transport the oxygen.
      e. The amount of functional hemoglobin available in the blood can be altered due to decreased red blood cells or presence of nonfunctional hemoglobin (e.g., carboxyhemoglobin or cyanmethemoglobin).
   2. **Clinical significance of PO_2 levels in blood**
      a. Increased values (>95%) are observed with supplemental oxygen.
      b. **Hypoxemia:** Causes include decreased pulmonary diffusion, decreased alveolar spaces due to resection or compression, and poor ventilation/perfusion (due to obstructed airways—asthma, bronchitis, emphysema, foreign body, and secretions).

X. ENDOCRINOLOGY

A. Hormones

1. **Hormones** are chemical compounds secreted into the blood that affect target tissues generally at a site distant from original production.
2. **General function**
   a. **Multiple hormones** can **affect one physiological function** (e.g., carbohydrate metabolism under the control of insulin, glucagon, growth hormone, cortisol, and epinephrine).
   b. A **Single hormone** can **affect several organs** to produce different physiological effects (e.g., cortisol).
3. Three classes of hormones: **steroids, proteins** (peptides or glycoproteins), and **amines**
   a. **Steroid hormones**
      1) Synthesized by **adrenal glands, gonads, and placenta**
      2) Synthesized from **cholesterol** as needed, not stored, **lipid-soluble**
      3) **Need a carrier protein** to circulate in the blood
      4) Clinically significant hormones include **cortisol, aldosterone, testosterone, estrogen**, and **progesterone.**
      5) **Mechanism of action: Free hormone** is transported across cell membrane to interact with **intracellular receptor forming a complex**; complex binds to chromatin, producing mRNA; mRNA initiates production of proteins that carry out the function attributed to the specific hormone.
      6) Hormone synthesis is regulated through **negative feedback** by another hormone (e.g., **cortisol/ACTH**).
   b. **Protein hormones**
      1) Synthesized by **anterior pituitary, placenta, pancreas, and parathyroid glands**
      2) Synthesized, then stored in the cell as secretory granules until needed
      3) Do **not** need carrier proteins to enter blood; **water soluble**
      4) Clinically significant hormones include **follicle-stimulating hormone** (FSH), **luteinizing hormone** (LH), **thyroid-stimulating hormone** (TSH), **human chorionic gonadotrophin** (hCG), **insulin, glucagon, parathyroid hormone, growth hormone**, and **prolactin.**
         a) Glycoprotein hormones, **FSH, LH, TSH,** and **hCG,** composed of alpha and beta chains; alpha chains identical and **beta** chains **unique** for each hormone
         b) Peptide hormones synthesized as prohormone, cleaved to produce circulating hormone (e.g., insulin)
      5) **Mechanism of action:** Protein hormones interact with a **cell membrane receptor.** This activates a second messenger system and then cellular action.

6) Hormone synthesis is regulated through **change in analyte concentration** in serum (e.g., **insulin/glucose**) and **negative feedback** by another hormone (e.g., **testosterone/FSH**).

c. Amine hormones
1) Synthesized by **thyroid and adrenal glands**
2) Synthesized from **amino acids**
3) **Some** amine hormones **require a carrier protein** and others do not.
4) Clinically significant hormones include **epinephrine, norepinephrine, thyroxine**, and **triiodothyronine.**
5) **Mechanism of action: Epinephrine and norepinephrine** do not bind to carrier proteins and interact with the **receptor site on the cell membrane. Thyroxine and triiodothyronine** circulate bound to carrier proteins, with the **free hormone** being transported across the cell membrane to interact with the **intracellular receptor**.
6) Hormone synthesis is regulated by **nerve stimulation, another hormone** (e.g., thyroxine/TSH), and **negative feedback**.

4. Methods for quantifying hormones need to be **sensitive** because of the extremely low levels of hormones in circulation. Some of the more commonly used methods include enzyme-multiplied immunoassay technique (EMIT), fluorescent immunoassay (FIA), fluorescent polarization immunoassay (FPIA), chemiluminescent immunoassay (CLIA), electrochemiluminescence immunoassay (Electro CLIA), and high-performance liquid chromatography (HPLC).

B. Hypothalamus: Overview and Clinical Significance

1. Hormones produced by the hypothalamus and their function:
   a. **Corticotropin-releasing hormone** (CRH): Stimulates secretion of adrenocorticotropic hormone (ACTH)
   b. **Gonadotropin-releasing hormone** (GnRH): Stimulates secretion of follicle-stimulating hormone (FSH) and luteinizing hormone (LH)
   c. **Growth hormone-releasing hormone** (GHRH): Stimulates secretion of growth hormone (GH)
   d. **Thyrotropin-releasing hormone** (TRH): Stimulates secretion of thyroid-stimulating hormone (TSH) and prolactin
   e. **Dopamine:** Inhibits prolactin release
   f. **Somatostatin:** Inhibits secretion of TSH and GH
2. **Supraoptic and paraventricular nuclei** of the **hypothalamus** produce **antidiuretic hormone** (ADH), also known as vasopressin, and **oxytocin**. These hormones are transported to the **posterior pituitary for storage.**
3. **Diseases:** Tumors, inflammatory or degenerative processes, and congenital disorders

C. Anterior Pituitary: Overview and Clinical Significance

1. Hormones secreted by the anterior pituitary include **ACTH, LH, FSH, TSH, GH, and prolactin.**
2. **Adrenocorticotropic hormone**
   a. Corticotropin-releasing hormone stimulates secretion of ACTH, which in turn stimulates synthesis of cortisol.
   b. **Increased cortisol** levels turn off secretion of ACTH and CRH.
   c. **Decreased cortisol** levels stimulate secretion of ACTH through negative feedback, which promotes cortisol synthesis.
   d. ACTH and cortisol exhibit **diurnal variation**, with **highest levels** in the **morning** and lowest levels in late afternoon to early evening.
3. **Growth hormone** (also known as somatotropin)
   a. Hypothalamus controls the release of growth hormone from the anterior pituitary with growth hormone-releasing hormone, which is stimulatory, and somatostatin, which is inhibitory.
   b. Direct effect on metabolism in numerous tissues: Antagonistic effect to insulin in relationship to glucose metabolism, stimulates gluconeogenesis in the liver, stimulates lipolysis, and promotes protein synthesis
   c. **Reference range:** Basal level 2–5 ng/mL
   d. **Clinical significance**
      1) **Increased levels** in childhood result in pituitary **gigantism** and in adulthood in **acromegaly** (enlarged feet, hands, and facial bones, impaired glucose tolerance, hypertension). Acromegaly is generally caused by a growth hormone-secreting pituitary tumor.
      2) **Decreased levels**
         a) Adults: Caused by pituitary adenomas or irradiation
         b) Children: May be familial or caused by a tumor, craniopharyngioma; results in **pituitary dwarfism**
4. **Prolactin:** Secreted by pituitary lactotroph cells and released upon stimulation from TRH; dopamine inhibits release
   a. **Function:** Initiates and maintains lactation; effects reproduction through ovarian and testicular steroidogenesis; affects the immune system
   b. **Reference ranges:** Male: 3.0–14.7 ng/mL; female: 3.8–23.0 ng/mL
   c. **Clinical significance**
      1) **Increased prolactin levels** may be caused by pituitary adenomas that produce prolactin, trauma, inflammation, chronic renal failure, and as a side effect of the administration of certain drugs (e.g., tricyclic antidepressants, phenothiazines, and reserpine). Hyperprolactinemia results in hypogonadism.
      2) **Decreased prolactin** levels may be caused by a tumor that compresses or replaces normal pituitary tissue. This is seen in panhypopituitarism, where there is loss of all anterior pituitary function.

5. **Follicle-stimulating hormone** will be discussed under "Ovaries: Overview and Clinical Significance" and "Testes: Overview and Clinical Significance."
6. **Luteinizing hormone** will be discussed under "Ovaries: Overview and Clinical Significance" and "Testes: Overview and Clinical Significance."
7. **Thyroid-stimulating hormone** will be discussed under "Thyroid: Overview and Clinical Significance."

D. Posterior Pituitary: Overview and Clinical Significance

1. **Posterior pituitary (neurohypophyseal system): Antidiuretic hormone (ADH), also known as vasopressin, and oxytocin** are hormones released by the posterior pituitary, but they are synthesized in the hypothalamus, where they form secretory granules for transport down the nerve axons to the posterior pituitary for storage. Upon stimulation, the hormones are secreted by the posterior pituitary.
2. **Antidiuretic hormone**
   a. **Function:** ADH controls water homeostasis by affecting the permeability of the collecting tubules of the kidney and enhancing water resorption, which makes the urine more concentrated and the blood more dilute. The osmolality of plasma has a regulatory effect on secretion of ADH. In addition, ADH raises blood pressure by stimulating musculature of arterioles and capillaries, affects uterine contraction, and promotes intestinal muscle contraction.
   b. **Clinical significance**
      1) **Increased ADH level** (hyperfunction): The **syndrome of inappropriate ADH secretion (SIADH)** occurs when there is uncontrolled secretion of ADH without any known stimulus for such release. In this syndrome, ADH is released even though the blood volume is normal or increased and plasma osmolality is low. This disorder may be caused by ectopic tumor production of ADH as in small cell carcinoma of the lung, central nervous system (CNS) disease, pulmonary disease, or as a side effect of administration of certain drugs.
      2) **Decreased ADH level** (hypofunction): Results in **polyuria**, causing **diabetes insipidus** and polydipsia
3. **Oxytocin**
   a. **Function:** Uterine stretch receptors stimulate the release of oxytocin, which in turn stimulates uterine contractions during childbirth. The action of suckling stimulates tactile receptors that promote the secretion of oxytocin, which causes ejection of breast milk.
   b. Although oxytocin is present in males, its function is unknown.

E. Adrenal Glands: Overview and Clinical Significance

1. **Adrenal glands:** Located above each kidney
   a. **Adrenal cortex (produces steroid hormones):** Outer portion of the gland, composed of three layers
      1) **Zona glomerulosa**, outermost layer, secretes **mineralocorticoids,** with **aldosterone** being the major hormone.

2) **Zona fasciculata,** second layer, secretes **glucocorticoids,** with **cortisol** being the major hormone.
3) **Zona reticularis,** third layer, secretes **sex hormones, principally the androgens**. Excessive production of androgens causes virilization.

b. **Adrenal medulla (produces amine hormones):** Inner portion of the gland
1) **Epinephrine** and **norepinephrine** are secreted and are known collectively as **catecholamines.**

2. **Steroid hormones** secreted by the adrenal glands are divided into three groups:
a. **Mineralocorticoids:** Regulate salt balance
b. **Glucocorticoids:** Assist with carbohydrate metabolism
c. **Androgens:** Required for sexual function (contribution from the adrenal glands is minimal as compared to the gonads)

3. **Aldosterone** controls the retention of Na^+, Cl^-, and H_2O, the excretion of K^+ and H^+ and, therefore, the amount of fluid in the body.
a. Aldosterone production is controlled by the **renin-angiotensin system** of the kidney. When the juxtaglomerular apparatus of the kidney detects low serum sodium or pressure changes in the blood perfusing the kidneys, due to decreased blood pressure or blood volume, **renin** is **produced**. Renin is a protein that acts on angiotensinogen to produce angiotensin I, which is acted on by angiotensin-converting enzyme to catalyze the formation of angiotensin II. **Angiotensin II** stimulates the **secretion of aldosterone** and is a **potent vasoconstrictor**.
b. **Function** of aldosterone is to **increase salt and water conservation** through renal tubular retention of Na^+ and Cl^- and H_2O secondarily and to promote excretion of K^+ and H^+.
1) Overall effect is vasoconstriction, which increases blood pressure (BP), and Na^+ retention, which promotes increase in blood volume (BV).
2) Increase in BP and BV suppresses secretion of renin and, thus, the synthesis of aldosterone.

c. **Reference ranges:** Adult supine, 3–16 ng/dL; adult upright, 7–30 ng/dL; blood levels of aldosterone are higher in the morning
d. **Clinical significance**
1) **Hyperaldosteronism**
a) **Primary hyperaldosteronism:** Adrenal diseases such as an aldosterone-secreting adrenal adenoma (Conn syndrome), aldosterone-secreting adrenal carcinoma, or hyperplasia of adrenal cortex
b) **Secondary hyperaldosteronism:** Renin-angiotensin system disorder due to excess production of renin, malignant hypertension, or a renin-secreting renal tumor

2) **Hypoaldosteronism**
a) Atrophy of adrenal glands

b) Symptoms of **Addison disease:** Atrophy of adrenal glands with depressed production of aldosterone and the glucocorticoids
   i. Hypoadrenalism causes decreased secretion of aldosterone and cortisol, increased ACTH, increased β-MSH, decreased blood glucose; decreased Na^+ and Cl^-, and increased K^+.
   ii. Pigmentation of the skin, muscle weakness, weight loss, decreased blood pressure, nausea, and diarrhea

c) **Congenital deficiency of 21-hydroxylase enzyme**

4. Cortisol
   a. **Physiological effects of cortisol include** anti-insulin effects on carbohydrates that result in increased blood glucose levels, increased gluconeogenesis, increased lipolysis, increased protein catabolism, decreased protein synthesis, decreased antibody formation, and suppressed inflammatory response. Cortisol is high levels can result in mineralocorticoid effects so you can see glucose and electrolyte changes simultaneously.
   b. **Regulation of cortisol:** The hypothalamus secretes corticotropin-releasing hormone and the anterior pituitary secretes adrenocorticotropic hormone, which controls cortisol production via a feedback loop.
      1) Low levels of plasma cortisol promote ACTH release.
      2) Elevated levels of plasma cortisol inhibit ACTH release.
   c. **Reference ranges total cortisol:** 8 A.M., 5–23 μg/dL; 4 P.M., 3–16 μg/dL; cortisol and ACTH exhibit **diurnal variation**
   d. Clinical significance
      1) **Hypercortisolism**
         a) **Two types of hypercortisolism:** 1) **ACTH-dependent** and 2) **ACTH-independent**
            i. ACTH-dependent hypercortisolism is due to excess ACTH from one of the following, pituitary disease (Cushing's disease), Ectopic ACTH production, or Ectopic CRH production. Excess ACTH drive the hypercortisolism.
            ii. **ACTH-independent hypercortisolism is due to excess cortisol from one of the following: adrenal adenoma, adrenal carcinoma, nodular adrenal hyperplasia, or exogenous administration of glucocorticoids. Excess cortisol drives the hypercortisolism.**
            iii. **The term Cushing's disease is used when the source of the ACTH is the pituitary gland, all others are labeled as Cushing's syndrome.**
            iv. **Cushing's disease is the most common cause of hypercortisolism, accounting for 70% of all cases.**
         b) **Symptoms of Cushing syndrome**
            i. Increased serum cortisol; cortisol lacks diurnal variation; and hyperglycemia
            ii. When adrenal gland secretes excess cortisol, the ACTH will be decreased.

iii. Weight gain in the face (moon face) and abdomen, buffalo hump back, thinning of skin, easy bruising, hypertension, muscle wasting, decreased immune response, and hyperpigmentation (if ACTH-dependent)

c) **Diagnosis: Three-step process**

i. Rule out exogenous cortisol use (oral, topical, injected, and inhaled).

ii. Establish hypercotisolism using any one of the following tests.

a. Urine free cortisol (UFC), 24-hour urine, positive on two separate occasions. A cortisol level three times above the normal is suggestive of hypercortisolism. NOTE: Fluid intake greater than 5 L/day and urine volume greater than 3 L/day can cause false positive results; depression on alcohol intake can influence results as pseudo-Cushing's.

b. Midnight salivary cortisol positive on two occasions

c. Dexamethasone suppression test, 1 mg dexamethasone taken at 11 P.M. followed by an 8 A.M. cortisol. 0800 cortisol $< 1.8 \mu g/dL$

iii. Differentiate the cause of hypercortisolism by performing the following tests

a. Plasma ACTH at 0800: Value $> 15 \mu g/dL$ consider ACTH-dependent causes of hypercortisolism; value $< 5 \mu g/dL$ consider ACTH-independent cause of hypercortisolism. NOTE: Strict guidelines for collection of ACTH must be adhered to.

b. Inferior pertrosal sinus sampling (IPSS): Gold standard test for determining the source of ACTH production; test yields a ratio of inferior pertrosal sinus ACTH to peripheral ACTH; ratios $> 3:1$ are suggestive of pituitary production of ACTH (Cushing's syndrome)

2) **Hypocortisolism**

a) **Primary hypocortisolism:** Atrophy of adrenal gland, autoimmune disease, tuberculosis, and prolonged high-dosage cortisol therapy

b) **Secondary hypocortisolism:** Pituitary hypofunction

5. **Adrenal medulla: Inner portion**

a. Catecholamines synthesized from **tyrosine** by chromaffin cells of the adrenal medulla, brain, and sympathetic neurons

b. **Catecholamines** include the hormones **epinephrine, norepinephrine,** and **dopamine.**

c. **Function**

1) **Epinephrine:** Mobilizes energy stores by converting glycogen to glucose, which allows the voluntary muscles to have greater work output; released in response to low blood pressure, hypoxia, cold exposure, muscle exertion, and pain

2) **Norepinephrine:** Functions as a neurotransmitter affecting the vascular smooth muscle and heart; released primarily by the postganglionic sympathetic nerves

3) **Dopamine:** Functions as a neurotransmitter in the brain affecting the vascular system

d. Epinephrine and norepinephrine are **metabolized into metanephrine** and **normetanephrine** and then to final end-product **vanillylmandelic acid** (VMA). Some metanephrine and normetanephrine along with the end-product VMA are excreted in the urine.

e. Increased levels of epinephrine and norepinephrine are associated with **pheochromocytoma** (rare chatacholamine producing tumor); tumors arising from the adrenal medulla are referred to as pheochromocytomas and those arising from the sympathetic ganglia are referred to as paraganglioma (extra-adrenal pheochromocytoma)

1) Classic triad of symptoms: Palpitations, sweating, and headaches; less commonly seen symptoms include weight loss, dizziness, hyperglycemia, hypotension, and symptoms of a panic attack.

2) Diagnosis: Initial testing involves measuring **plasma metanephrines (metanephrine** and **normetanephrine)** or 24-hour urine fractionated metanepherines and catecholamines

a) Fluorometric methods or HPLC methods used for quantifying plasma epinephrine and norepinephrine

b) Colorimetric/spectrophotometric method used for quantifying VMA

f. **Neuroblastoma** is a **malignant tumor** of the adrenal medulla that occurs in **children.** This tumor produces epinephrine and norepinephrine along with dopamine. The end-product of dopamine metabolism is homovanillic acid (HVA).

1) Characterized by increase in HVA and VMA urinary excretion

2) May be quantified using HPLC, gas chromatographic, and spectrophotometric methods

F. Ovaries: Overview and Clinical Significance

1. Ovaries are part of the **hypothalamic-pituitary-gonadal axis.**

a. The anterior pituitary secretes **follicle-stimulating hormone**, which stimulates growth of the **ovarian follicles** and **increases** the **plasma estrogen level.** FSH is under the control of gonadotropin-releasing hormone.

b. The anterior pituitary secretes **luteinizing hormone**, which stimulates production of **progesterone at ovulation.** LH is under the control of GnRH.

c. Estrogens and progesterone exert **negative feedback** to the hypothalamus and pituitary, which controls FSH and LH synthesis.

d. Abnormal synthesis of estrogens may be caused by the ovaries (primary disorder) or as a secondary disorder due to a primary disorder of the pituitary or hypothalamus.

2. **Estrogens and progesterone** are the principal **female sex hormones.**
   a. **Estrogens** are secreted by the ovarian follicles and by the placenta in pregnancy (and to a much lesser extent by the adrenal glands and testes).
      1) There are three primary estrogens: **estradiol-17β, estrone,** and **estradiol.**
      2) **Estradiol** is the **principal estrogen** synthesized by the ovaries.
   b. **Progesterone** is secreted by the ovarian follicles, mainly the corpus luteum following ovulation, and by the placenta in pregnancy.
   c. **Function: Estrogen** promotes development and maintains the female reproductive system, including the uterus, fallopian tubes, and vagina. It is responsible for development and maintenance of secondary female sex characteristics (e.g., breast development, maturation of external genitalia, fat deposition, and termination of bone growth). **Progesterone** is secreted by the corpus luteum following ovulation, and in pregnancy progesterone is secreted by the placenta to maintain the uterus.
   d. Hormone changes in the **menstrual cycle**
      1) In the first-half of the menstrual cycle, **FSH** promotes growth of ovarian follicles and an increase in estrogen (low in first 7 days of cycle).
      2) **Estrogen peaks at midcycle**, causing a decrease in FSH but promoting the **LH surge** at midcycle.
      3) **LH triggers ovulation,** which is followed by a decrease in estrogen and LH levels.
      4) The **follicle becomes** the **corpus luteum**, which **produces estrogen** and **progesterone.**
      5) **Lack of fertilization** (thus absence of human chorionic gonadotropin) causes the **corpus luteum** to **degenerate** along with decrease in the estrogen and progesterone levels. **Progesterone falls** to the initial low level of the follicular phase about 24 hours prior to onset of menstruation.
      6) Menstruation results, and then the cycle begins again.
      7) Menstrual cycle
         a) **Follicular phase** (first-half): Characterized by **estrogen** stimulating growth of the uterine lining; progesterone levels are low
         b) **Luteal phase** (second-half): Characterized by **progesterone** promoting endometrium tissue to accept the fertilized ovum; progesterone measurements clinically useful to confirm ovulation
   e. **Clinical significance**
      1) **Hyperestrinism in females:**
         a) **Precocious puberty:** Ovarian tumor, hypothalamic tumor, and adrenal tumors (rare); may be difficult to determine
         b) **Infertility and irregular menses:** Polycystic ovaries, estrogen-producing ovarian tumors, and disorders of the hypothalamus or pituitary
         c) **Postmenopausal bleeding:** Cervical or endometrial carcinoma, estrogen-producing ovarian tumors, and exogenous estrogen consumption

2) **Hyperestrinism in males** results in testicular atrophy and enlargement of the breasts.
3) **Hypoestrinism**
   a) **Ovarian insufficiency** can be primary or secondary to disorders of the hypothalamus or pituitary.
   b) **Delayed puberty:** Primary amenorrhea due to lack of ovarian function or secondary to disorders of the hypothalamus or pituitary
   c) **Amenorrhea** occurs at menopause, with radiation or chemotherapy, severe stress, intense athletic training, and excessive weight loss.
   d) **Turner syndrome** is a genetic defect in females where there is partial or complete loss of one of the two X chromosomes, resulting in nonfunctional ovaries. Exogenous estrogen can be administered to develop secondary sex characteristics.
4) **Hyperprogesteronemia:** Prevents menstrual cycle from occurring
5) **Hypoprogesteronemia:** Causes infertility, abortion of fetus

3. Estrogens in pregnancy
   a. **Placenta** is the main source of estrogen synthesis during pregnancy, making primarily **estriol.**
   b. Placenta requires a precursor compound that can **only** be made by the **fetal adrenal glands**, the **hydroxylated form of DHEAS** (16α-OH dehydroepiandrosteronesulfate); placenta **lacks** the enzyme 16α-hydroxylase.
   c. Use **maternal estriol** blood level/urine excretion to **assess fetoplacental status.**
4. **Triple screen** consists of **α_1-fetoprotein** (AFP), **unconjugated estriol** (uE3), and **human chorionic gonadotropin** (hCG).
   a. Maternal blood sample collected at 15–20 weeks gestation
   b. Triple screen helps to **estimate risk of Down syndrome.** Following pattern is suggestive of increased risk:
      1) **Decreased AFP** (made by fetal liver; found in maternal blood)
      2) **Decreased uE3** (made by joint effort of fetus and mother)
      3) **Increased hCG** (made by placenta)
      4) Interpretation utilizes **MoMs: Multiples of the median**
      5) Definitive testing would follow: Amniocentesis and chromosome analysis
5. **Quadruple (Quad) screen** includes the analytes of the triple test **plus inhibin A**, a polypeptide hormone. **Inhibin A** would be **increased** in Down syndrome. In pregnancy, inhibin A is produced by the fetoplacental unit; function is to inhibit production of FSH.

G. Placenta: Overview and Clinical Significance

1. Placenta synthesizes and secretes **estrogens, progesterone, human chorionic gonadotropin**, and **human placental lactogen.**

2. **Human chorionic gonadotropin** prolongs the viability of the corpus luteum, which synthesizes progesterone and estrogens in early pregnancy until the placenta can assume the function. hCG levels are highest in the first trimester.
   a. **hCG qualitative** measurement used to **detect pregnancy.** Utilize monoclonal antibody to detect hCG in 1–2 days following fertilization.
   b. hCG quantitative measurement
      1) **Increased hCG:** Hydatidiform mole, choriocarcinoma, and preeclamptic toxemia
      2) **Decreased hCG:** Threatened abortion, ectopic pregnancy
      3) hCG is used to monitor success of surgery and chemotherapy.
3. **Human placental lactogen** (HPL) functions with hCG to produce estrogen and progesterone during pregnancy. HPL level rises throughout gestation and reaches its highest level near term.
   a. HPL reflects integrity of placental function, so serial analysis may be helpful in high-risk pregnancies.
   b. **Decreased HPL** suggestive of placental malfunction and **potential fetal distress.**

H. Testes: Overview and Clinical Significance
1. Testes are part of the **hypothalamic-pituitary-gonadal axis.**
   a. The anterior pituitary secretes **follicle-stimulating hormone**, which stimulates **spermatogenesis.** FSH is under the control of GnRH.
   b. The anterior pituitary secretes **luteinizing hormone,** which stimulates production of **testosterone.** LH is under the control of GnRH.
   c. Through **negative feedback** to the hypothalamus, increased levels of testosterone shut off FSH and LH synthesis.
   d. Abnormal synthesis of testosterone may be caused by the testes (primary disorder) or as a secondary disorder due to a primary disorder of the pituitary or hypothalamus.
2. **Testosterone** is the principal **male sex hormone** and is secreted by the testes (and to a much lesser extent by the adrenal glands and ovaries).
   a. **Function: Testosterone** promotes development and maintains the **male reproductive system.** It is responsible for development and maintenance of secondary male sex characteristics (e.g., facial and body hair, muscle development).
   b. **Clinical significance**
      1) **Hyperandrogenemia:** In adult males, there are no observable symptoms. In prepubertal males, precocious puberty occurs (may be caused by hypothalamic tumors, congenital adrenal hyperplasia, testicular tumor). In female children, development of male secondary sex characteristics/virilization occurs (increased androgen production by ovaries or adrenals as androgens are estrogen precursors in females).
         a) **Congenital adrenal hyperplasia** (CAH) is caused by an enzyme defect of **21-hydroxylase,** which prevents cortisol production and results in accumulation of cortisol precursors, including 17-α-hydroxyprogesterone

(17-OHP). CAH is characterized by **increased** blood levels of **17-OHP** and ACTH and decreased cortisol.

1) **Hypoandrogenemia:** In adult males, impotence and loss of secondary sex characteristics occurs; in prepubertal males, delayed puberty results.
   a) **Primary hypoandrogenemia:** Causes include infections, tumors, congenital disorders (Klinefelter syndrome)
      i) **Klinefelter syndrome:** Male possesses an extra X chromosome (XXY). Characteristics include tall with long extremities, small testes, gynecomastia, infertility, and low IQ.
   b) **Secondary hypoandrogenemia:** Causes include primary hypofunction disorders of the pituitary or hypothalamus, which in turn cause decreased synthesis of LH and FSH

I. Thyroid Gland: Overview and Clinical Significance

1. **Thyroid gland** located in trachea-larynx area; composed of two lobes that consist of two types of cells
   a. **Follicular cells** are single layer of epithelial cells arranged spherically to create a follicle.
      1) **Make and secrete thyroid hormones**
         a) $\mathbf{T_4}$, L-thyroxine
         b) $\mathbf{T_3}$, L-triiodothyronine
         c) $\mathbf{rT_3}$, reverse T_3 biologically inactive
      2) Hormones **stored** in lumina of follicle (colloid)
   b. **Parafollicular cells** secrete **calcitonin**, which is involved with calcium regulation.
2. **Function:** Thyroid hormones aid in regulation of several metabolic functions, including rate of O_2 consumption and heat production, growth, sexual maturity, and protein and carbohydrate metabolism.
3. **Hypothalamic-pituitary-thyroid axis**
   a. **Thyrotropin-releasing hormone** (TRH) is released by hypothalamus and stimulates anterior pituitary to secrete thyroid-stimulating hormone.
   b. **TSH** is a polypeptide hormone that originates in the anterior pituitary gland. TSH regulates synthesis and release of the thyroid hormones.
   c. Secretion of TSH is **regulated** by TRH, somatostatin, free T_3 (FT_3), and free T_4 (FT_4).
      1) **Somatostatin** functions as an inhibitory factor.
      2) FT_3 and FT_4 stimulate hypothalamus to secrete somatostatin.
      3) FT_3 and FT_4 exert negative feedback to the anterior pituitary to inhibit TSH secretion.
   d. It is estimated that 40% of secreted $\mathbf{T_4}$ undergoes enzymatic **monodeiodination** in tissues to **produce** $\mathbf{T_3}$ and approximately 45% is converted to $\mathbf{rT_3}$, which is **biologically inactive.**
      1) **Thyroid hormones** circulate in blood **bound** to **thyroxine-binding globulin (TBG)**, thyroxine-binding prealbumin, and thyroxine-binding albumin.

2) **TBG** is the principal carrier protein.
3) The **free hormones**, FT_3 and FT_4, are **physiologically active.**
4) $\mathbf{T_3}$ is four to five times **more metabolically potent** in the tissues than T_4.

4. **Thyroid antibodies:** Appear with some autoimmune thyroid diseases but they are not specific
   a. **Thyroid-stimulating immunoglobulins** (TSI) are classified as **thyrotropin-receptor antibodies** (TRAbs). They **bind to TSH receptor sites** and activate thyroid epithelial cells.
   b. **Thyroid antimicrosomal antibodies** (TMAbs) cause tissue destruction, and analysis is generally directed to measurement of **antithyroid peroxidase antibodies** (TPOAbs). TPOAbs are detected in Hashimoto thyroiditis and in Graves' disease.
   c. **Antithyroglobulin antibodies** (TgAbs) do not cause damage to the gland.
5. **Clinical significance (see Table 1–7■)**
   a. **Hypothyroidism** characterized by enlarged thyroid gland (goiter), impaired speech and memory, fatigue, weight gain, personality changes, cold intolerance, increased serum cholesterol and LDL, and so on.
      1) In **primary hypothyroidism**, total T_3 (TT_3), total T_4 (TT_4), FT_3, and FT_4 are decreased in the serum; TSH is increased in the serum.
      2) **Myxedema:** Advanced form of hypothyroidism
      3) **Congenital hypothyroidism/cretinism:** If untreated in first 3 months of life, irreversible neurological and mental deficiency occurs; newborn screening is required in the United States.
      4) **Hashimoto disease:** Most common cause of primary hypothyroidism; chronic autoimmune thyroiditis; TPOAb, TMAb, and TgAb present
      5) **Hypothyroidism may be secondary or tertiary** to lack of TSH (pituitary disorder) or lack of TRH (hypothalamus disorder), respectively.
      6) Due to the sensitivity of the TSH assay, hypothyroidism may be "overt" or "subclinical"; in subclinical hypothyroidism thyroid hormones are in the normal range and TSH is abnormally high.

TABLE 1–7 DISORDERS RELATED TO THE THYROID GLAND

Clinical Condition	TT_4	TT_3	FT_4	TSH
Primary Hypothyroidism	↓	↓	↓	↑
Secondary Hypothyroidism	↓	↓	↓	↓
Primary Hyperthyroidism	↑	↑	↑	↓
Secondary Hyperthyroidism	↑	↑	↑	↑
Primary Increase TBG	↑	↑	N	N
Primary Decrease TBG	↓	↓	N	N
↑ = Increased; ↓ = Decreased; N = Normal (within reference range)				

b. **Hyperthyroidism** is characterized by weight and muscle loss, fatigue, heat intolerance, nervousness, and exophthalmos.
   1) In **primary hyperthyroidism**, total T_3, total T_4, FT_3, and FT_4 are increased in the serum; TSH is decreased in the serum.
   2) **Thyrotoxicosis:** Increased serum levels of thyroid hormones
   3) **Thyroid storm:** Life-threatening complication of uncontrolled thyrotoxicosis
   4) **Graves' disease:** Most common cause of thyrotoxicosis; exhibits diffuse toxic goiter; autoimmune disorder with TRAb and TSI present
   5) **Hyperthyroidism may be secondary or tertiary** to increased levels of TSH (pituitary disorder) or increased levels of TRH (hypothalamus disorder), respectively.
   6) Due to the sensitivity of the TSH assay, hyperthyroidism may be "overt" or "subclinical"; in subclinical hyperthyroidism thyroid hormones are in the normal range and TSH is abnormally low

6. Methods of measurement for **total thyroid hormone** and **TSH** include competitive immunoassays, enzyme immunoassays, and chemiluminescence immunoassays; **direct measurement of free thyroid hormones** includes direct equilibrium dialysis and ultrafiltration methods, whereas **indirect methods for estimating free thyroid hormones** include two-step microparticle capture immunoassays and one-step immunochemiluminometric assays.
7. With availability of **highly sensitive TSH assays**, TSH testing is used to **screen for thyroid disorders** and to follow success of treatment protocols. TSH reflects the physiological action of the thyroid hormones at the level of one of its target tissues, the pituitary gland. The secretion of TSH by the pituitary gland is very sensitive to changes and reflective of such changes in thyroid hormone concentration in the blood. Most TSH immunometric assays are third-generation assays, which display functional sensitivity between 0.01 and 0.02 mU/L and can be used to not only diagnose hypothyroidism and hyperthyroidism but also assess severity of hyperthyroidism.
8. Nonthyroidal illness (Euthyroid Sick syndrome) is a condition where you will see abnormal thyroid function tests in clinically euthyroid patients with nonthyroidal systemic illness. Nonthyroidal illness associated with abnormal thyroid function tests include, fasting, starvation, severe trauma, myocardial infarction, chronic kidney disease, diabetic ketoacidosis, cirrhosis, and sepsis.
   Diagnosis of nonthyroidal illness involves ruling out hypothyroidism through TSH results. In nonthyroidal illness the TSH will be low, normal, or only slightly elevated (not as elevated as you would see in hypothyroidism).
9. An electrochemiluminescence immunoassay can be used for the **T uptake (TU)** test, which measures the **unsaturated serum binding capacity of TBG**; or, rephrased, TU measures available binding sites on TBG. **Thyroid hormone binding ratio (THBR)** expresses a ratio of T uptake in a patient's serum with a normal or reference serum.

a. There is an **inverse** relationship between **THBR** levels and the **concentration of TBG.** When the serum concentration of TBG is increased (as in euthyroid primary increase in TBG), THBR is decreased.
b. The **free T_4 index (FT_4I)** is an indirect estimation of the free T_4 concentration in serum adjusted for any interference that may be caused by an abnormality in the binding proteins.

$$\textbf{Free } T_4 \textbf{ index } (FT_4I) = \textbf{Total } T_4 \times \textbf{THBR}$$

J. Parathyroid Glands: Overview and Clinical Significance
1. **Four parathyroid glands** are located bilaterally on or near the thyroid gland capsule. Parathyroid glands are composed of chief cells and oxyphil cells. Chief cells synthesize, store, and secrete **parathyroid hormone** (PTH).
   a. PTH is synthesized as a **preprohormone.**
   b. **Amino N-terminal third is biologically active.**
   c. In the blood, intact PTH has half-life of **<5 minutes.**
2. **Function: PTH** aids in the **regulation of calcium** and **phosphate**, having direct action on bone and kidney and indirect action on the intestines through vitamin D. PTH increases the serum calcium level by increasing calcium resorption from bone, increasing calcium reabsorption in the renal tubules, and increasing intestinal absorption of calcium by stimulating production of vitamin D.
   a. In **kidneys, PTH increases calcium reabsorption** in the distal tubule and decreases reabsorption of phosphate in the proximal tubule, resulting in phosphaturia.
   b. In **intestines, PTH promotes absorption of calcium** and phosphate by stimulating increased production of **$1{,}25(OH)_2D$.**
   c. In **bone**, PTH stimulates **bone resorption** (alters osteoclasts) **or bone formation** (alters osteoblasts); elevated PTH increases bone resorption.
   d. Combined effects cause
      1) **Serum:** Calcium increased, phosphate reduced
      2) **Urine:** Phosphate increased, calcium increased due to larger filtered load overriding increased tubular reabsorption
   e. **Increase in serum-free calcium reduces secretion of PTH** through negative feedback, conversely decrease in serum-free calcium stimulates secretion of PTH.
3. PTH quantified in plasma (EDTA preferred—stabilizes PTH) by measuring different forms of the hormone: **intact PTH, N-terminal PTH, mid-molecule PTH, and C-terminal PTH**.
   a. Electrochemiluminescence immunoassay (ECLIA)
   b. Measures **intact PTH** using a sandwich technique
   c. Reference range: 15–65 pg/mL
4. Measurement of PTH **during surgery for adenoma resection of the parathyroid glands** assists the surgeon in determining completeness of the resection

based on the rapid fall of PTH. Need preincision baseline sample as surgery starts, second baseline sample following exposure of the gland, and postexcision sample drawn 10 minutes following gland removal. At 10 minutes postexcision, the PTH level should fall to 50% or less of the preincision value or the value at the time of gland resection. If the PTH remains increased and such a decrease does not occur or if the PTH rises again after what initially appeared to be a decrease, multigland disease or ectopic production needs to be investigated.

5. **Clinical significance**
   a. **Hyperparathyroidism**
      1) **Primary hyperparathyroidism** (results in increased blood calcium) may be caused by parathyroid adenoma (tumor), parathyroid carcinoma, or hyperplasia.
      2) **Secondary hyperparathyroidism** may be caused by vitamin D deficiency (presents with low blood calcium levels) or chronic renal failure.
   b. **Hypoparathyroidism** (results in decreased calcium and increased phosphate blood levels) may be caused by osteomalacia, autoimmune disease, inborn errors of metabolism, or unintentional removal during thyroid surgery.

K. Gastrointestinal Hormones: Overview and Clinical Significance

1. **Gastrin** is secreted by the stomach in response to the vagus and food entering the stomach. Maximum secretion occurs in the stomach at pH 5–7.
   a. **Function:** Gastrin stimulates secretion of gastric HCl and pancreatic enzymes.
   b. **Acidification** of the antrum of the stomach causes a **decrease in gastrin secretion.**
   c. **Zollinger-Ellison syndrome:** An **elevated gastrin** level accompanied by gastric hyperacidity; caused by gastrinomas, duodenal, or pancreatic endocrine tumors that secrete gastrin
2. **Serotonin** is synthesized from **tryptophan** and secreted by the enterochromaffin cells in the gastrointestinal tract.
   a. **Function:** Serotonin is a smooth muscle stimulant and vasoconstrictor that is transported by platelets.
   b. Liver **metabolizes serotonin to 5-hydroxyindole acetic acid** (5-HIAA).
      1) **Metastatic carcinoid tumors** occur in the appendix, ileum, or rectum.
      2) Produce excessive amount of **serotonin** and its metabolite **5-HIAA**, which is measured in urine.

L. Pancreas: Overview and Clinical Significance

1. **Pancreas** has both endocrine and exocrine functions
   a. **Endocrine function:** Islets of Langerhans secrete insulin, glucagon, gastrin, and somatostatin into the blood; secretions flow directly to the blood stream
   b. **Exocrine function:** Digestive fluid containing bicarbonate and digestive enzymes is made in the acinar cells and secreted into the duodenum. Digestive enzymes include lipase, amylase, trypsin, chymotrypsin, elastase, collagenase,

leucine aminopeptidase, and nucleases; secretions flow through pancreatic ducts

1) **Secretion** of the digestive fluid is regulated by the vagus nerve and the endocrine hormones cholecystokinin and secretin.

2. **Insulin** is synthesized in the islets of Langerhans by the β-cells and secreted into the blood when the blood glucose level is elevated.
   a. **Insulin lowers blood glucose** by binding to cell membrane receptors, which increases membrane permeability in the liver, muscle, and adipose tissue. Insulin affects glucose metabolism by promoting glycogenesis and lipogenesis while inhibiting glycogenolysis.
   b. Insulin is **inhibited** by epinephrine and norepinephrine release and certain drugs (e.g., thiazide, dilantin, and diazoxide).
   c. **Clinical significance**
      1) **Hyperinsulinemia:** May be caused by insulinomas (insulin-producing tumors of the β-cells of the pancreas [also known as spontaneous hyperinsulinemia]) or are a result of overtreatment with pharmacological insulin (factitious hyperinsuliemia); both result in hypoglycemia; differentiation between factitious and spontaneous hyperinsulemia can be done through the measurement of C-Peptide; with spontaneous hyperinsulinemia C-peptide is increased.
      2) **Hypoinsulinemia:** Lack of insulin or ineffective insulin, which results in diabetes mellitus; diagnosed through the presence of Whipple's Triad Whipple's Triad involves:
         1) Symptoms of hypoglycemia (behavioral changes, fatigue, seizures, altered consciousness, palpitations, tremors, anxiety, sweating, hunger, and altered sensations)
         2) Low plasma glucose by an accurate method
         3) Relief of the symptoms when the plasma glucose level is raised

3. **Glucagon** is synthesized in the islets of Langerhans by the α-cells and secreted into the blood when the blood glucose level is low. Glucagon increases blood glucose by promoting glycogenolysis in the liver and gluconeogenesis.
   a. The secretion of glucagon is promoted by exercise, stress, and amino acids.
   b. Secretion is **inhibited** by insulin.
   c. **Clinical significance**
      1) **Hyperglucagonemia** is associated with glucagon-secreting tumors of the pancreas (glucagonomas). These tumors are malignant and have usually metastasized by the time they are diagnosed.

XI. THERAPEUTIC DRUG MONITORING

A. Therapeutic Drug Monitoring (TDM): It entails the analysis, interpretation, and evaluation of drug concentration in serum, plasma, or whole blood samples.

1. **Purpose:** TDM is employed to establish maximum benefits with minimal toxic effects for drugs whose correlation with dosage, effect, or toxicity is not clear.

2. **Common routes of drug administration:** Oral, IV (intravenous), IM (intramuscular), and SC (subcutaneous)
3. **Therapeutic range:** Drug concentration that produces benefits

B. Drug Absorption and Distribution

1. Most drugs are **absorbed** from the **GI tract** in a consistent manner in healthy individuals.
2. **Liquids are absorbed more quickly** than tablets and capsules.
3. **First-pass metabolism:** All drugs absorbed from the GI tract must go through the liver before entering the general circulation.
4. **Most drugs circulate** in the blood **bound to plasma proteins.** A number of disorders may affect drug-protein binding, including kidney disease, hepatic disease, malnutrition, and inflammatory processes. In addition, drugs compete with other ingested drugs, as well as endogenous molecules such as the steroids and bilirubin, for protein binding sites.
   a. **Acidic drugs** primarily bind to **albumin.**
   b. **Basic drugs** primarily bind to **α_1-acid glycoprotein** (AAG).
   c. Some drugs **bind to both** albumin and AAG.
5. Only **free drugs** can **interact with target sites and produce a response.** Thus, the quantity of free drug correlates the best with monitoring therapeutic and toxic effects. Most TDM assays **quantify total drug** concentration rather than free drug.
6. **Measuring the free drug level** may be warranted for highly protein bound drugs or when clinical response is not consistent with the total drug level.
7. In general, drugs are **eliminated** from the circulation through **hepatic metabolic processes and renal filtration**. In the liver, drugs are chemically altered to metabolites, and they are conjugated to make them water soluble. Conjugated drugs can be eliminated through the urine or the bile.
8. Drugs are usually **administered in a scheduled manner** with multiple doses administered over a period of time. This manner of drug administration produces high (**peak** drug level) and low (**trough** drug level) variations in drug concentration. The aim is to keep the trough level from dropping below a concentration of **therapeutic benefit** and to keep the peak concentration from rising to the **toxic level.** Approximately **five to seven doses** of a drug are required to achieve a **steady state** where peak and trough levels can be assessed.

C. Sample Collection and Measurement

1. **Timing of blood sample collection is critical in TDM.**
2. When the **trough level** is required, the blood sample should be drawn immediately **before next dose** is administered.

3. Sample collection for **peak levels**
   a. Drawing blood sample **1 hour after oral administration** is the rule of thumb. However, collection time varies and is drug specific; variations in peak levels occur due to different absorption, metabolic, and excretion rates for individual drugs.
   b. Draw blood sample 0.5 hour after completion of IV administration.
4. Most drugs can be quantified using immunoassay techniques or chromatography (e.g., GC and HPLC).

D. Cardioactive Drugs

1. **Digoxin**
   a. **Function:** Cardiac glycoside used to treat **congestive heart failure**
   b. **Mechanism of action:** Digoxin inhibits membrane Na^+-K^+-ATPase, causing decrease in intracellular K^+ and increase in intracellular Ca^{2+} in cardiac myocytes; increased Ca^{2+} improves contraction of cardiac muscle. Electrolytes need to be monitored because digoxin function is enhanced by a low serum K^+ level.
   c. **Metabolism:** Digoxin levels need to be monitored to ensure blood concentrations are therapeutic because absorption of the drug is variable. Although the blood level **peaks in 2–3 hours** following oral ingestion, **tissue uptake** of digoxin is **slow**, making it necessary to monitor serum 8 hours after an oral dose, which correlates better with the tissue level.
   d. **Therapeutic range:** 0.8–2.0 ng/mL
2. **Lidocaine**
   a. **Function: Antiarrhythmic** drug used to treat ventricular arrhythmia and prevent ventricular fibrillation
   b. **Metabolism:** Lidocaine is usually given by **continuous IV administration** after a loading bolus, and it is primarily metabolized by the liver to the metabolic by-product monoethylglycinexylidide (MEGX). Although **MEGX** does not contribute to therapeutic effect, it does **enhance toxicity.** Hence the **need to measure both lidocaine and MEGX**; some immunoassays are able to quantify both. Oral administration is contraindicated, because lidocaine would be removed from the circulation during the first pass through the liver.
   c. **Therapeutic range:** 1.5–4.0 μg/mL
   d. **Toxicity:** Individuals with blood levels of 4–8 μg/mL exhibit CNS depression and >8 μg/mL exhibit seizures and severe hypotension.
3. **Quinidine**
   a. **Function: Antiarrhythmic** drug used to treat cardiac arrhythmia
   b. **Metabolism:** Quinidine may be administered orally as the sulfate or gluconate form, and it is primarily metabolized by the liver. **Quinidine sulfate** is absorbed more quickly than the gluconate form, with **peak** plasma levels occurring **2 hours** after oral ingestion. In contrast, **peak** plasma levels of **quinidine gluconate** occur in **4–5 hours**.
   c. Usually, the **trough level** is monitored to ensure achievement of therapeutic levels. In the case of quinidine gluconate administration, sample collection is

performed 1 hour following the last ingested dose for trough determination because of its slow absorption rate.

d. **Therapeutic range:** 2–5 μg/mL

4. **Procainamide**

a. **Function: Antiarrhythmic** drug used to treat cardiac arrhythmia

b. **Metabolism:** Procainamide is administered orally, with elimination dependent on it being metabolized by the liver and filtered by the kidney. Procainamide is **metabolized to *N*-acetylprocainamide (NAPA)**, which exhibits a similar physiological effect as the parent drug. Thus, it is necessary to **quantify both** procainamide and NAPA when assessing serum concentration. **Peak plasma levels** occur approximately 1 hour after ingestion.

c. **Therapeutic range:** 4–8 μg/mL

E. Antibiotic Drugs

1. **Aminoglycosides**

a. **Function:** It is used to **treat infections** caused by **gram-negative** bacteria; include gentamicin, tobramycin, kanamycin, and amikacin.

b. **Metabolism:** The aminoglycosides are administered IV or IM because gastrointestinal absorption is poor. Elimination is via kidney filtration.

c. It is associated with nephrotoxicity and ototoxicity.

2. **Vancomycin**

a. **Function:** It is used to **treat infections** caused by **gram-positive** bacteria.

b. **Metabolism:** Vancomycin is administered by IV because of poor gastrointestinal absorption.

c. It may be associated with nephrotoxicity, ototoxicity, and "red-man syndrome" (erythemic flushing of extremities).

F. Antiepileptic Drugs

1. **Phenobarbital**

a. **Function:** Slow-acting barbiturate used to **control seizures**

b. **Metabolism:** Phenobarbital is administered orally with a **peak** plasma level occurring at **10 hours** following ingestion. It is characterized by slow absorption and a long half-life. Elimination is dependent on it being metabolized by the liver and filtered by the kidney.

c. **Primidone** is the **inactive form** of phenobarbital, and this proform is administered when rapid absorption is indicated. **Primidone** is quickly **converted** to phenobarbital. When primidone is administered, both compounds need to be quantified.

d. **Toxicity** effects are drowsiness, depression, fatigue, and altered mental ability.

e. **Therapeutic range:** 15–40 μg/mL

2. **Phenytoin** (diphenylhydantoin)

a. **Function:** Used to **control seizures** and to keep the brain from swelling and injuring tissue during brain traumas

b. **Metabolism:** Phenytoin, administered orally with slow GI absorption, has low solubility in aqueous solutions; thus it is 90–95% protein bound in the circulation. The small free component of this drug is physiologically active. Drug elimination is controlled by liver metabolism. For **trough** levels, the sample is **drawn before the next dose** is ingested. For **peak** levels when toxicity is a concern, the sample is **drawn 4–5 hours after the last dose.**
c. Toxicity characterized by seizures.
d. **Therapeutic range:** Total serum level 10–20 μg/mL; free serum level 1–2 μg/mL
e. **Fosphenytoin: IM** injectable proform of the drug

3. **Valproic acid**
   a. **Function:** Used to **control seizures**
   b. **Metabolism:** Administered orally, 93% protein bound in the circulation, and metabolized by the liver for elimination
   c. **Therapeutic range:** 50–100 μg/mL
4. **Carbamazepine**
   a. **Function:** Used to **control seizures**
   b. **Metabolism:** Administered orally, 70–80% protein bound in the circulation, and metabolized by the liver for elimination
   c. **Therapeutic range:** 4–12 μg/mL

G. Antipsychotic Drugs

1. **Lithium**
   a. **Function:** Used to treat **manic depression**
   b. **Metabolism:** Administered orally as lithium carbonate, does not bind to plasma proteins in the circulation, **peak** plasma levels occur **2–4 hours** after oral ingestion, and filtered by the kidney for elimination
   c. **Therapeutic range:** 1.0–1.2 mmol/L
2. **Tricyclic antidepressants** (TCAs)
   a. **Function:** TCAs include amitriptyline, imipramine, and doxepin, which may be used in cases of depression, insomnia, extreme apathy, and loss of libido.
   b. **Metabolism:** TCAs are administered orally, but GI absorption is slow. This results in **peak** concentrations occurring **2–12 hours after ingestion.** TCAs are metabolized by the liver for elimination. Amitriptyline and imipramine are metabolized to the **active metabolites nortriptyline and desipramine**, respectively.
   c. **Therapeutic range:** Amitriptyline 120–150 ng/mL; imipramine 150–300 ng/mL; nortriptyline 50–150 ng/mL; and desipramine 150–300 ng/mL

H. Bronchodilator Drugs

1. **Theophylline**
   a. **Function:** Used to treat **asthma** and other chronic obstructive pulmonary disorders (COPDs)

b. **Metabolism:** Administered orally, with elimination dependent on it being metabolized by the liver and filtered by the kidney
c. **Therapeutic range:** 10–20 µg/mL

I. Immunosuppressive Drugs

1. **Cyclosporine**
   a. **Function:** It is used to **suppress transplant rejections** and **graft-versus-host disease.**
   b. **Metabolism:** Cyclosporine is administered orally with **peak** levels reached in **4–6 hours**; elimination dependent on it being metabolized by the liver.
   c. **Therapeutic range:** Specimen of choice is **whole blood.** Therapeutic ranges vary with organ transplanted; liver, pancreas, and heart require 200–350 ng/mL, and renal transplants require 100–300 ng/mL.
2. **Tacrolimus** (Prograf)
   a. **Function:** Used to **suppress transplant rejections** and **graft-versus-host disease** (potency far exceeds cyclosporine by a factor of 100)
   b. **Metabolism:** Administered orally, with elimination dependent on it being metabolized by the liver
   c. **Therapeutic range:** 10–15 ng/mL, with therapeutic ranges varying with organ transplanted; specimen of choice, **whole blood**
3. **Sirolimus** (Rapamune)
   a. **Function:** Used to **suppress transplant rejections** and **graft-versus-host disease**
   b. **Metabolism:** Administered orally with peak levels reached in about 2 hours; elimination dependent on it being metabolized by the liver
   c. **Therapeutic range:** 4–12 ng/mL with therapeutic ranges varying with organ transplanted; specimen of choice **whole blood**

J. Antineoplastic Drugs

1. **Methotrexate**
   a. **Function:** Methotrexate is used to **destroy neoplastic cells.** Although methotrexate inhibits the synthesis of DNA in all cells, its action is based on the principle that neoplastic cells contain a greater amount of DNA because of their rapid rate of division as compared to normal cells. Thus, neoplastic cells are more susceptible to the loss of DNA.
   b. **Metabolism:** May be administered IV; filtered by the kidney for elimination
   c. **Leucovorin rescue** refers to the administration of leucovorin to offset the effect of methotrexate in an attempt to prevent cytotoxicity of normal cells. Leucovorin dosage is based on the amount of methotrexate in the circulation.
   d. **Therapeutic monitoring:** High-dose therapy generally exceeds 50 mg/m^2, and serum levels vary with the time interval following dosage. Serum levels of methotrexate are monitored at 24, 48, and 72 hours after drug administration.

XII. TOXICOLOGY

A. Elements of Toxicology

1. **Toxicology:** The **study** of poisonous substances
2. **Exposure to toxins:** May be due to suicide attempt, accidental exposure, or occupational exposure
3. **Routes of exposure:** Ingestion, inhalation, and transdermal absorption
4. **Toxic response:** The amount of damage done to an organism when the substance is administered at less than the lethal dose
5. **Acute toxicity:** A one-time exposure of short duration to an agent that immediately causes a toxic response
6. **Chronic toxicity:** Multiple exposures for extended time periods to an agent at a dosage that will not cause an acute response

B. Analysis of Toxic Agents

1. **Screening test:** Performed first and usually of a qualitative nature; may lack specificity
2. **Confirmatory test:** Usually quantitative with good specificity and sensitivity (e.g., gas chromatography and immunoassays)

C. Analysis of Specific Substances

1. **Alcohols:** Volatile organic substances
   a. Types of alcohols
      1) **Ethanol:** Chronic exposure is associated with toxic hepatitis and cirrhosis.
      2) **Methanol:** Ingestion is related to severe acidosis, blindness, and even death due to methanol conversion to formaldehyde, which is metabolized to formic acid.
      3) **Isopropanol:** Ingestion produces severe, acute symptoms, similar to ethanol intoxication, that persist for a long period of time because isopropanol is metabolized to acetone, which has a long half-life.
      4) **Ethylene glycol** (found in antifreeze): Ingestion produces severe metabolic acidosis and renal tubular damage.

   b. **Analysis for ethanol:** Enzymatic and gas-liquid chromatography
      1) Ethanol + $NAD^+ \xrightarrow{ADH}$ acetaldehyde + NADH
      2) Gas-liquid chromatography (GLC) is the reference method. GLC can differentiate among the various types of alcohols and quantify them.
2. **Carbon monoxide**
   a. Toxic because it **binds very tightly to hemoglobin** and does not allow oxygen to attach to the hemoglobin; forms carboxyhemoglobin
   b. Produces **hypoxia** in brain and heart
   c. Whole blood is required for analysis.
   d. **Analysis:** Gas-liquid chromatography is the reference method.

3. **Cyanide**
   a. **Supertoxic** substance with exposure occurring through various routes, including oral ingestion, inhalation, or transdermal absorption
   b. Used in insecticide and rodenticide products
   c. Cyanide **binds** to heme iron and mitochondrial cytochrome oxidase.
   d. **Analysis:** Ion-selective electrode
4. **Metals**
   a. **Arsenic**
      1) **Binds to thiol groups** in proteins; ionized arsenic excreted in urine
      2) **Specimens:** Blood and urine used to assess short-term exposure; hair and fingernails used to assess long-term exposure
      3) **Analysis:** Atomic absorption spectrophotometry
   b. **Lead**
      1) **Lead binds to proteins** and it inhibits many enzymes; it also inhibits heme synthesis. Toxicity may occur when lead is ingested, inhaled, or contacted dermally.
      2) Lead **interferes** in heme biosynthesis at several stages, the last of these being the incorporation of **iron** into the tetrapyrrole ring. This alteration results in the formation and accumulation of **zinc protoporphyrin (ZPP)**, with zinc replacing the iron in the tetrapyrrole ring.
      3) **Lead poisoning** in children is generally associated with the ingestion of lead-laden paint chips. Laboratory results indicate:
         a) **Basophilic stippling** of RBCs
         b) Increased urinary excretion of **aminolevulinic acid** and **coproporphyrins**
      4) **Acceptable blood lead level:** <5 μg/dL in young children
      5) **Lead analysis: Whole blood** specimen required; methods include spectrophotometric dithizone, atomic absorption spectrophotometry and anodic stripping voltammetry
   c. **Mercury**
      1) **Binds to proteins** and inhibits many enzymes
      2) **Analysis:** Atomic absorption spectrophotometry and anodic stripping voltammetry
5. **Pesticides**
   a. Include insecticides and herbicides that may contaminate food or be inhaled, absorbed through the skin, and ingested via hand-to-mouth contact
   b. Organophosphate and carbamate insecticides **inhibit acetyl cholinesterase.**
   c. **Analysis:** Assess enzyme activity of erythrocyte acetylcholinesterase or serum pseudocholinesterase.
6. **Therapeutic drugs commonly abused**
   a. **Salicylate** (aspirin)
      1) **Function:** Used as an analgesic, antipyretic, and anti-inflammatory
      2) **Metabolism:** Administered orally

3) **Toxic effects at high dosages:** Causes mixed acid-base imbalance seen as metabolic acidosis and respiratory alkalosis (respiratory center stimulant), ketone body formation, excess formation of lactate
4) **Analysis:** Ferric nitrate method with colored product read spectrophotometrically; gas or liquid chromatography

b. **Acetaminophen** (Tylenol)
1) **Function:** Used as an analgesic
2) **Metabolism:** Administered orally, with elimination dependent on it being metabolized by the liver
3) **Toxic effect at high dosages:** Liver toxicity
4) **Analysis:** Immunoassays and high-performance liquid chromatography

7. **Drugs of abuse**

a. **Amphetamine and methamphetamine**
1) **Function:** Used to treat narcolepsy and disorders that affect ability to focus; stimulants, provide sense of mental and physical well-being
2) **Analysis:** Immunoassays and gas or liquid chromatography

b. **Anabolic steroids**
1) **Function:** Used to increase muscle mass and athletic performance
2) **Analysis:** Gas or liquid chromatography

c. **Cannabinoids**
1) **Function:** It is hallucinogenic, provide a feeling of mental well-being and euphoria, impair mental function and short-term memory.
2) **Marijuana: Tetrahydrocannabinol (THC)** primary cannabinoid component; THC half-life in blood is one day following single use and 3–5 days following chronic use.
3) **Metabolism:** THC distributes in lipophilic tissue such as the brain and adipose tissue. Elimination is dependent on THC being metabolized by the liver to 11-nor-Δ-tetrahydrocannabinol-9-carboxylic acid (THC-COOH) with this metabolic product filtered by the kidney. **THC-COOH** (major urinary metabolite) is detectable in urine for 3–5 days following single use and for as long as 4 weeks following chronic use.
4) **Analysis:** Immunoassays and gas chromatography/mass spectrometry

d. **Cocaine**
1) **Function:** Used as a local anesthetic and at higher levels functions as a CNS stimulant
2) **Metabolism:** Half-life 0.5–1 hour, with elimination dependent on liver metabolism; **benzoylecgonine** (half-life 4–7 hours) **primary metabolite** and filtered by the kidney
3) **Benzoylecgonine** is detectable in urine for 3 days following single use and for as long as 20 days following chronic use.
4) **Analysis:** Immunoassays and gas chromatography/mass spectrometry

e. **Opiates**
   1) Types of opiates
      a) **Naturally occurring:** Opium, morphine, and codeine
      b) **Chemically modified:** Heroin, dilaudid, and oxycodone
      c) **Synthetic:** Demerol, methadone, darvon, talwin, and fentanyl
   2) **Function:** Narcotics used for their analgesic, sedative, and anesthetic properties
   3) **Metabolism:** Respiratory center depressant causing respiratory acidosis
   4) **Analysis:** Immunoassays and gas chromatography/mass spectrometry

f. **Phencyclidine** (PCP)
   1) **Function:** Produces stimulant, depressant, anesthetic, and hallucinogenic effects
   2) **Metabolism:** Distributes in lipophilic tissue such as the brain and adipose tissue; elimination dependent on it being metabolized by the liver, with 10–15% of the parent compound filtered by the kidney; detectable in urine for as long as 7–30 days following chronic use
   3) **Analysis:** Immunoassays and gas chromatography/mass spectrometry

g. **Tranquilizers**
   1) Types of tranquilizers
      a) **Barbiturates:** Phenobarbital (long acting), amobarbital (intermediate acting), and secobarbital and pentobarbital (short acting)
      b) **Benzodiazepines:** Diazepam (valium), chlordiazepoxide (librium), and lorazepam (ativan)
   2) **Function:** Sedative hypnotics that produce depression of the CNS
   3) **Metabolism:** Respiratory center depressants causing respiratory acidosis
   4) **Analysis:** Immunoassays and gas-liquid chromatography

XIII. VITAMINS

A. Solubility

1. **Fat-soluble** vitamins include A, D, E, and K.
2. **Water-soluble** vitamins include C, ascorbic acid; B_1, thiamin; B_2, riboflavin; B_6, pyridoxine; B_{12}, cobalamin; niacin, nicotinic acid; pantothenic acid; biotin; and folate, folic acid.

B. Metabolism

1. Fat-soluble vitamins **stored in liver or adipose tissue**; may accumulate to toxic levels
2. Water-soluble vitamins **easily excreted in urine**; generally do not accumulate to toxic levels

C. Clinical Significance of Vitamins

1. **Vitamin A deficiency:** Drying, degeneration, and increased risk of infection in conjunctiva, cornea, skin, and mucous membranes; night blindness
2. **Vitamin D deficiency:** Rickets, osteomalacia, and osteoporosis

3. **Vitamin E deficiency:** Hemolytic disease of premature neonates
4. **Vitamin K deficiency:** Hemorrhage
5. **Vitamin C deficiency:** Scurvy, necrosis of gums, and emotional disturbances
6. **Vitamin B_1 deficiency:** Beriberi
7. **Vitamin B_2 deficiency:** Cheilosis, angular stomatitis, glossitis, seborrheic dermatitis, and ocular disturbances
8. **Vitamin B_6 deficiency:** Eczema, seborrheic dermatitis, cheilosis, glossitis, angular stomatitis, mental depression, and anemia
9. **Vitamin B_{12} deficiency:** Hematologic effects, including macrocytic anemia, and neurologic effects, including peripheral nerve degeneration
10. **Niacin deficiency:** Pellagra
11. **Pantothenic acid deficiency:** Metabolism affected; causes nausea, vomiting, muscular weakness, and malaise
12. **Biotin deficiency:** Cutaneous, ophthalmic, and neurologic symptoms
13. **Folate deficiency:** Megaloblastic anemia, anorexia, glossitis, nausea, hepatosplenomegaly, and hyperpigmentation of skin

D. Methods for Quantification

1. A number of methods exist for quantifying vitamins, including fluorometric assays, HPLC, liquid chromatography-tandem mass spectrometry, competitive protein-binding assays, immunoassays, bioassays, microbiological assays, enzyme activation tests, spectrophotometric, electrochemical, and RIA.

REFERENCES

Bishop, M. L., Fody, E. P., and Schoeff, L. (Eds.) (2018). *Clinical Chemistry Principles, Techniques, and Correlations,* 8th ed. Philadelphia: Wolters Kluwer.

Burtis, C. A., and Bruns, D. E. (Eds.) (2015). *Tietz Fundamentals of Clinical Chemistry and Molecular Diagnostics,* 7th ed. Philadelphia: Saunders.

Haven, M. C., Tetrault, G. A., and Schenken, J. R. (Eds.) (1995). *Laboratory Instrumentation,* 4th ed. New York: Van Nostrand Reinhold.

Kaplan, L. A., and Pesce, A. J. (Eds.) (2010). *Clinical Chemistry Theory, Analysis, Correlation,* 5th ed. St. Louis: Mosby.

Westgard, J. O., Quam, E., and Barry, T. (Eds.) (1998). *Basic QC Practices.* Madison, WI: WesTgard® Quality Corporation.

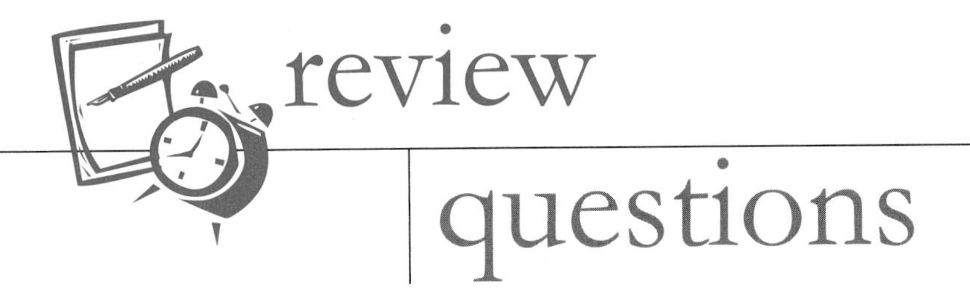

review questions

INSTRUCTIONS Each of the questions or incomplete statements that follow is comprised of four suggested responses. Select the *best* answer or completion statement in each case.

Instrumentation and Analytical Principles

1. Which of the following lamps provides a continuous spectrum of radiant energy in the visible, near IR, and near UV regions of the spectrum?
   A. Tungsten-filament
   B. Hydrogen
   C. Deuterium
   D. Mercury vapor
2. Which of the following isolates light within a narrow region of the spectrum?
   A. Photomultiplier tube
   B. Monochromator
   C. Photovoltaic cell
   D. Detector
3. Which of the following represents a feature unique to the hollow cathode lamp?
   A. It emits wavelengths of light in the UV region.
   B. It is lined with the element of interest.
   C. It cannot be used with a chopper.
   D. It serves to amplifies the initial signal received.
4. Which of the following best describes a monochromator?
   A. A device used to isolate a specified range of wavelengths
   B. A device used to amplify signals from a photoemissive device
   C. A device used to decrease interference from light scatter
   D. A device used to UV from visible wavelengths of light
5. Which type of photodetector employs a linear arrangement that allows it to respond to a specific wavelength resulting in complete UV/visible spectrum analysis?
   A. Photomultiplier tube
   B. Phototube
   C. Barrier layer cell
   D. Photodiode array

6. When performing spectrophotometer quality assurance checks, what is the holmium oxide glass filter used to assess?
   A. Linearity
   B. Stray light
   C. Absorbance accuracy
   D. Wavelength accuracy

7. In spectrophotometric analysis, what is the purpose of the reagent blank?
   A. Correct for interfering chromogens
   B. Correct for lipemia
   C. Correct for protein
   D. Correct for color contribution of the reagents

8. In fluorescent polarization assays:
   A. Fluorescent tagged Ag/Ab complexes rotate out of orientation resulting in an increase in intensity of polarized light.
   B. Fluorescent tagged antibody complexes absorb light at one wavelength and re-emit light at a longer wavelength of lower energy.
   C. Fluorescent tagged Ag/Ab complexes rotate rapidly emitting light in different planes leading to a decrease in polarized light.
   D. Fluorescent tagged Ag/Ab complexes maintain orientation and result in an increase in intensity of polarized light.

9. The bandpass of a spectrophotometer is 10 nm. If an instrument is set at 540 nm, the wavelengths of light that are permitted to impinge on the sample will be within what wavelength range?
   A. 530–540 nm
   B. 530–550 nm
   C. 535–545 nm
   D. 540–550 nm

10. Which of the following formula is an expression of the Beer-Lambert law that is routinely applied to spectrophotometric analysis?
    A. $A_u \times \frac{C_s}{A_s} = C_u$
    B. $C_u \times \frac{C_s}{A_s} = A_u$
    C. $A_s \times \frac{C_s}{C_u} = A_u$
    D. $A = 2 - \log \%T$

11. In spectrophotometry, which of the following is a mathematical expression of the relationship between absorbance and transmittance?
    A. $A = abc$
    B. $\frac{A_u}{C_u} = \frac{A_s}{C_s}$
    C. $A = 2 - \log \%T$
    D. $A = \log \%T$

12. Which of the following techniques measures light scattered and has a light source placed at 90 degrees from the incident light?
    A. Chemiluminescence
    B. Atomic absorption spectrophotometery
    C. Nephelometry
    D. Turbidity

13. Which of the following may be associated with reflectance spectrophotometry as it relates to the dry reagent slide technique?
    A. Light projected to the slide at 180-degree angle
    B. Dye concentration directly proportional to reflectance
    C. Unabsorbed, reflected light detected by photodetector
    D. Reflectance values are linearly proportional to transmission values

14. Fluorometers are designed so that the path of the exciting light is at a right angle to the path of the emitted light. What is the purpose of this design?
    A. Prevent loss of emitted light
    B. Prevent loss of the excitation light
    C. Focus emitted and excitation light upon the detector
    D. Prevent excitation light from reaching the detector
15. Which of the following represents a primary advantage of performing fluorometric over absorption spectroscopic methods of analysis?
    A. Increased specificity and increased sensitivity
    B. Increased specificity and decreased sensitivity
    C. Purity of reagents used not as critical
    D. Ease of performing assays
16. Which of the following may be associated with fluorescence polarization?
    A. Plane-polarized light is used for sample excitation.
    B. Small molecular complexes show a greater amount of polarization.
    C. It is a heterogeneous technique employed in fluorophore-ligand immunoassays.
    D. Polarized light detected is directly proportional to concentration of ligand in sample.
17. Which of the following may be associated with bioluminescence?
    A. Light emission produced due to enzymatic oxidation of a substrate
    B. Less sensitive than direct fluorescent assays
    C. Electron excitation caused by radiant energy
    D. Employs a radioactive label
18. Nephelometry is based on the measurement of light that is
    A. Absorbed by particles in suspension
    B. Scattered by particles in suspension
    C. Produced by fluorescence
    D. Produced by excitation of ground-state atoms
19. Which of the following instruments is used in the clinical laboratory or in reference laboratories to detect beta and gamma emissions?
    A. Fluorometer
    B. Nephelometer
    C. Scintillation counter
    D. Spectrophotometer
20. Which of the following best describes chemiluminescence?
    A. Electron excitation caused by radiant energy
    B. Enzymatic oxidation of a substrate produces light emission
    C. Chemical energy excites electrons that emit light upon return to ground state
    D. Employs a fluorescent label that produces light
21. In assaying an analyte with a single-beam atomic absorption spectrophotometer, what is the instrument actually measuring?
    A. Intensity of light emitted by the analyte on its return to the ground state
    B. Intensity of light that the analyte absorbs from the hollow-cathode lamp
    C. Intensity of light that the analyte absorbs from the flame
    D. Intensity of the beam from the hollow-cathode lamp after it has passed through the analyte-containing flame

22. What is the function of the flame in atomic absorption spectroscopy?
    A. Absorb the energy emitted from the metal analyte in returning to ground state
    B. Supply the thermal energy needed to excite the metal analyte
    C. Bring the metal analyte to its ground state
    D. Supply the light that is absorbed by the metal analyte
23. Most atomic absorption spectrophotometers incorporate a beam chopper and a tuned amplifier. The purpose of these components is to avoid errors that would be caused by
    A. Variations in flame temperature
    B. Deterioration of the hollow-cathode lamp
    C. Stray light from the hollow-cathode lamp
    D. Measurement of light emitted by the analyte
24. In potentiometry, which of the following is considered a reference electrode?
    A. Hydrogen electrode
    B. Calcium electrode
    C. Potassium electrode
    D. Copper electrode
25. In an electrolytic cell, which of the following is the half-cell where reduction takes place?
    A. Anode
    B. Cathode
    C. Combination electrode
    D. Electrode response
26. Mercury covered by a layer of mercurous chloride in contact with saturated potassium chloride solution is a description of which of the following types of electrodes?
    A. Sodium
    B. Calomel
    C. Calcium
    D. Silver/silver chloride
27. When a pH-sensitive glass electrode is not actively in use, in what type of solution should it be kept?
    A. Tap water
    B. Physiologic saline solution
    C. The medium recommended by the manufacturer
    D. A buffer solution of alkaline pH
28. When measuring K^+ with an ion-selective electrode by means of a liquid ion-exchange membrane, what antibiotic will be incorporated into the membrane?
    A. Monactin
    B. Nonactin
    C. Streptomycin
    D. Valinomycin
29. Which of the following techniques measures an excitation event caused by a chemical or electrochemical reaction?
    A. Atomic absorption
    B. Chemiluminescence
    C. Nephelometry
    D. Turbidometry
30. What are the principles of operation for a chloride analyzer that generates silver ions as part of its reaction mechanism?
    A. Potentiometry and amperometry
    B. Amperometry and polarography
    C. Coulometry and potentiometry
    D. Amperometry and coulometry
31. When quantifying glucose using an amperometric glucose electrode system, which of the following is *not* a component of the system?
    A. Product oxidation produces a current
    B. Hydrogen peroxide formed
    C. Hexokinase reacts with glucose
    D. Platinum electrode

32. To calibrate the pH electrode in a pH/blood gas analyzer, it is necessary that
    A. The barometric pressure be known and used for adjustments
    B. Calibrating gases of known high and low concentrations be used
    C. The calibration be performed at room temperature
    D. Two buffer solutions of known pH be used

33. The measurement of CO_2 in blood by means of a PCO_2 electrode is dependent on the
    A. Passage of H^+ ions through the membrane that separates the sample and the electrode
    B. Change in pH because of increased carbonic acid in the electrolyte surrounding the electrodes
    C. Movement of bicarbonate across the membrane that separates the sample and the electrode
    D. Linear relationship between PCO_2 in the sample and measured pH

34. The measurement of oxygen in blood by means of a PO_2 electrode involves which of the following?
    A. Wheatstone bridge arrangement of resistive elements sensitive to oxygen concentration
    B. Direct relationship between amount of oxygen in the sample and amount of current flowing in the measuring system
    C. Change in current resulting from an increase of free silver ions in solution
    D. Glass electrode sensitive to H^+ ions

35. Which of the following blood gas parameters are measured directly by the blood gas analyzer electrochemically as opposed to being calculated by the instrument?
    A. pH, HCO_3^-, total CO_2
    B. PCO_2, HCO_3^-, PO_2
    C. pH, PCO_2, PO_2
    D. PO_2, HCO_3^-, total CO_2

36. What indicator electrode uses a membrane made of dioxides that combine with and result in an ion exchange with the analyte of interest in a patient sample?
    A. Glass
    B. Liquid
    C. Silver-silver chloride
    D. Calomel

37. Which of the following methods allows for the separation of charged particles based on their rates of migration in an electric field?
    A. Rheophoresis
    B. Electrophoresis
    C. Electroendosmosis
    D. Ion exchange

38. Which of the following techniques is based on electro-osmotic flow?
    A. Capillary electrophoresis
    B. Zone electrophoresis
    C. Iontophoresis
    D. Isoelectric focusing

39. In isoelectric focusing electrophoresis, ampholytes create a pH gradient where:
    A. The higher pH gradient is toward the anode.
    B. The higher pH gradient is toward the cathode.
    C. The higher pH gradient is toward the middle of the gel.
    D. The higher pH gradient is found at the extreme ends of the gel.

40. In serum protein electrophoresis, when a buffer solution of pH 8.6 is used, which of the following characterizes the proteins?
    A. Exhibit net negative charge
    B. Exhibit net positive charge
    C. Exhibit charge neutrality
    D. Migrate toward the cathode

41. Which of the following characteristics will a protein have at its isoelectric point?
    A. Net negative charge
    B. Net positive charge
    C. Net zero charge
    D. Mobility

42. What dye may be used for staining protein bands following electrophoresis?
    A. Fat red 7B
    B. Sudan black B
    C. Ponceau S
    D. Oil red O

43. When electrophoresis is performed, holes appear in the staining pattern, giving the stained protein band a doughnut-like appearance. What is the probable cause of this problem?
    A. Protein denatured and will not stain properly.
    B. Ionic strength of the buffer was too high.
    C. Protein reached its isoelectric point and precipitated out.
    D. Protein concentration was too high.

44. What is the purpose of using ampholytes in isoelectric focusing?
    A. Maintain the polyacrylamide gel in a solid state
    B. Maintain the protein sample in a charged state
    C. Maintain the pH of the buffer solution
    D. Establish a pH gradient in the gel

45. After performing protein electrophoresis, you notice a band between the beta and gamma zones. This band most likely represents:
    A. Prealbumin
    B. Fibrinogen
    C. C-reactive protein
    D. Alpha 1 antitrypsin

46. Which of the following techniques uses boronate groups attached to resin to separate proteins
    A. Gel filtration
    B. Affinity chromatography
    C. Cation exchange
    D. Anion exchange

47. Which of the following is an electrophoretic technique employing a pH gradient that separates molecules with similar isoelectric points?
    A. Zone electrophoresis
    B. High-resolution electrophoresis
    C. Isoelectric focusing
    D. Immunoelectrophoresis

48. Given the following information on a particular compound that has been visualized by means of thin-layer chromatography, calculate the R_f of the compound.

    Distance from origin to spot center = 48 mm

    Distance from spot center to solvent front = 93 mm

    Distance from origin to solvent front = 141 mm

    A. 0.29
    B. 0.34
    C. 0.52
    D. 0.66

49. To achieve the best levels of sensitivity and specificity, to what type of detector system could a gas chromatograph be coupled?
    A. UV spectrophotometer
    B. Bichromatic spectrophotometer
    C. Mass spectrometer
    D. Fluorescence detector

50. Which of the following instruments has a sample-introduction system, solvent-delivery system, column, and detector as components?
    A. Atomic absorption spectrometer
    B. Mass spectrometer
    C. High-performance liquid chromatograph
    D. Nephelometer

51. Which type of elution technique may be used in high-performance liquid chromatography?
    A. Amphoteric
    B. Isoelectric
    C. Gradient
    D. Ion exchange

52. Which of the following statements best describes discrete analysis?
    A. Each sample-reagent mixture is handled separately in its own reaction vessel.
    B. Samples are analyzed in a flowing stream of reagent.
    C. Analyzer must be dedicated to measurement of only one analyte.
    D. It does not have random access capability.

53. Which of the following chromatography systems may be described as having a stationary phase that is liquid absorbed on particles packed in a column and a liquid moving phase that is pumped through a column?
    A. Thin-layer
    B. High-performance liquid
    C. Ion-exchange
    D. Gas-liquid

54. Which of the following chromatography systems is characterized by a stationary phase of silica gel on a piece of glass and a moving phase of liquid?
    A. Thin-layer
    B. Ion-exchange
    C. Gas-liquid
    D. Partition

55. What is the x-axis of a mass spectrum?
    A. Mass
    B. Mass/energy
    C. Mass/charge
    D. Charge

56. Ion-exchange chromatography separates solutes in a sample based on the
    A. Solubility of the solutes
    B. Sign and magnitude of the ionic charge
    C. Adsorption ability of the solutes
    D. Molecular size

57. Which parameter is used in mass spectrometry to identify a compound?
    A. Ion mass-to-charge ratio
    B. Molecular size
    C. Absorption spectrum
    D. Retention time

58. Which chromatography system is commonly used in conjunction with mass spectrometry?
    A. High-performance liquid
    B. Ion-exchange
    C. Partition
    D. Gas-liquid

59. Which of the following may be a sampling source of error for an automated instrument?
    A. Short sample
    B. Air bubble in bottom of sample cup
    C. Fibrin clot in sample probe
    D. All the above

60. Checking instrument calibration, temperature accuracy, and electronic parameters are part of
    A. Preventive maintenance
    B. Quality control
    C. Function verification
    D. Precision verification

61. For which of the following laboratory instruments should preventive maintenance procedures be performed and recorded?
    A. Analytical balance
    B. Centrifuge
    C. Chemistry analyzer
    D. All the above

62. In the Clark electrode, for every molecule of oxygen reduced at the cathode, how many electrons of current flow?
    A. 1
    B. 2
    C. 4
    D. 8

63. Which globin chains compose hemoglobin A_1?
    A. Two alpha chains and two beta chains
    B. Two alpha chains and two delta chains
    C. Two alpha chains and two gamma chains
    D. Two beta chains and two delta chains

64. Which hemoglobin may be differentiated from other hemoglobins on the basis of its resistance to denature in alkaline solution?
    A. A_1
    B. A_2
    C. C
    D. F

65. Hemoglobin S is an abnormal hemoglobin that is characterized by a substitution of which amino acid?
    A. Valine for glutamic acid in position 6 on the beta chain
    B. Valine for glutamic acid in position 6 on the alpha chain
    C. Lysine for glutamic acid in position 6 on the beta chain
    D. Lysine for glutamic acid in position 6 on the alpha chain

66. When performing electrophoresis at pH 8.6, which hemoglobin molecule migrates the fastest on cellulose acetate toward the anode?
    A. A_1
    B. A_2
    C. F
    D. S

67. Because of similar electrophoretic mobilities, several hemoglobins cannot be differentiated on cellulose acetate medium. Electrophoresis of hemoglobins at pH 6.2 on agar gel may be useful in differentiating which hemoglobins?
    A. A_1 from A_2
    B. A_1 from D
    C. A_1 from E
    D. C from A_2

68. In addition to performing hemoglobin electrophoresis, a solubility test may be performed to detect the presence of what hemoglobin?
    A. A_1
    B. C
    C. F
    D. S

69. Which of the following statements correctly describes zero-order kinetics
    A. Substrate is in excess and the rate of reaction is driven by the temperature of the test system.
    B. Enzyme is in excess and the rate of reaction is dependent on the time of the assay.
    C. Substrate is in excess, time and temperature are constant and the rate of reaction is dependent on the enzyme concentration.
    D. Enzyme is in excess, time and temperature are constant and the rate of reaction is dependent on the enzyme concentration.

70. Which of the following is a homogeneous immunoassay where separation of the bound from the free labeled species is *not* required?
    A. Radioimmunoassay
    B. Enzyme-linked immunosorbent assay
    C. Immunoradiometric assay
    D. Enzyme-multiplied immunoassay technique

71. Which of the following is immobilized on the microtiter well in a sandwich ELISA?
    A. Capture antibody
    B. Detection antibody
    C. The sample
    D. The secondary antibody conjugated to an enzyme

72. Which of the following is *not* associated with the enzyme-multiplied immunoassay technique (EMIT)?
    A. Is a homogeneous enzyme immunoassay
    B. Determines antigen concentration
    C. Employs a labeled reactant
    D. Enzyme reacts with drug in serum sample

73. When using EMIT, the enzyme is coupled to
    A. Antibody
    B. Antigen
    C. Substrate
    D. Coenzyme

74. The enzyme activity measured in the EMIT is the result of the reaction between the substrate and coenzyme with
    A. Free antibody
    B. Free unlabeled antigen
    C. Free labeled antigen
    D. Labeled antigen-antibody complexes

75. Singlet oxygen reacting with a precursor chemiluminescent compound to form a decay product whose light energizes a fluorophore best describes
    A. Fluorescent polarization immunoassay
    B. Enzyme-multiplied immunoassay technique
    C. Electrochemiluminescence immunoassay
    D. Luminescent oxygen channeling immunoassay

76. Which of the following stimulates the production of singlet oxygen at the surface of the sensitizer particle in a luminescent oxygen channeling immunoassay?
    A. Radiant energy
    B. Heat energy
    C. Enzymatic reaction
    D. Fluorescent irradiation

Proteins and Tumor Markers

77. Proteins, carbohydrates, and lipids are the three major biochemical compounds of human metabolism. What is the element that distinguishes proteins from carbohydrate and lipid compounds?
    A. Carbon
    B. Hydrogen
    C. Oxygen
    D. Nitrogen

78. Proteins may become denatured when subjected to mechanical agitation, heat, or extreme chemical treatment. How are proteins affected by denaturation?
    A. Alteration in primary structure
    B. Alteration in secondary structure
    C. Alteration in tertiary structure
    D. Increase in solubility

79. What is the basis for the Kjeldahl technique for the determination of serum total protein?
    A. Quantification of peptide bonds
    B. Determination of the refractive index of proteins
    C. Ultraviolet light absorption by aromatic rings at 280 nm
    D. Quantification of the nitrogen content of protein

80. When quantifying serum total proteins, upon what is the intensity of the color produced in the biuret reaction dependent?
A. Molecular weight of the protein
B. Acidity of the medium
C. Number of peptide bonds
D. Nitrogen content of the protein

81. Which of the following reagents can be used to measure protein in cerebrospinal fluid?
A. Biuret
B. Coomassie brilliant blue
C. Ponceau S
D. Bromcresol green

82. The tumor marker that is used to monitor reoccurrence of testicular cancer and used to screen for neural tube defects during pregnancy is:
A. Alpha-fetoprotein
B. Carcinoembryonic antigen
C. Human chorionic gonadotropin
D. Norepinephrine

83. Which term describes a congenital disorder that is characterized by a split in the albumin band when serum is subjected to electrophoresis?
A. Analbuminemia
B. Anodic albuminemia
C. Prealbuminemia
D. Bisalbuminemia

84. In what condition would an increased level of serum albumin be expected?
A. Malnutrition
B. Acute inflammation
C. Dehydration
D. Renal disease

85. Identification of which of the following is useful in early stages of glomerular dysfunction?
A. Albuminuria
B. Ketonuria
C. Hematuria
D. Urinary light chains

86. Which of the following is a low-weight protein that is found on the cell surfaces of nucleated cells?
A. C-reactive protein
B. β_2-Microglobulin
C. Ceruloplasmin
D. α_2-Macroglobulin

87. Which glycoprotein binds with hemoglobin to facilitate the removal of hemoglobin by the reticuloendothelial system?
A. Haptoglobin
B. Ceruloplasmin
C. α_1-Antitrypsin
D. Fibrinogen

88. In a healthy individual, which protein fraction has the greatest concentration in serum?
A. Alpha$_1$-globulin
B. Beta-globulin
C. Gamma-globulin
D. Albumin

89. Which of the following is an anionic dye that binds selectively with albumin?
A. Amido black
B. Ponceau S
C. Bromcresol green
D. Coomassie brilliant blue

90. Which total protein method requires copper sulfate, potassium iodide in sodium hydroxide, and potassium sodium tartrate in its reagent system?
A. Kjeldahl
B. Biuret
C. Folin-Ciocalteu
D. Ultraviolet absorption

91. Which of the following plasma proteins is produced by plasma cells?
A. Albumin
B. Haptoglobin
C. Fibrinogen
D. IgG

92. There are five immunoglobulin classes: IgG, IgA, IgM, IgD, and IgE. With which globulin fraction do these immunoglobulins migrate electrophoretically?
 A. Alpha_1-globulins
 B. Alpha_2-globulins
 C. Beta_1-globulins
 D. Gamma-globulins

93. Of the five immunoglobulin classes, IgG is the most structurally simple, consisting of how many light chains/heavy chains, respectively?
 A. 5/2
 B. 1/1
 C. 2/5
 D. 2/2

94. Which immunoglobulin class, characterized by its possession of a secretory component, is found in saliva, tears, and body secretions?
 A. IgA
 B. IgD
 C. IgG
 D. IgM

95. Which immunoglobulin class is able to cross the placenta from the mother to the fetus?
 A. IgA
 B. IgD
 C. IgE
 D. IgG

96. Which of the following is an acute-phase reactant protein able to inhibit enzymatic proteolysis and having the highest concentration of any of the plasma proteolytic inhibitors?
 A. C-reactive protein
 B. Haptoglobin
 C. α_2-Macroglobulin
 D. α_1-Antitrypsin

97. Which of the following is a copper transport protein that migrates as an alpha_2-globulin?
 A. Ceruloplasmin
 B. Haptoglobin
 C. Transferrin
 D. Fibrinogen

98. Which of the following proteins is normally produced by the fetus but is found in increased amounts in the amniotic fluid in cases of spina bifida?
 A. α_1-Antitrypsin
 B. α_1-Acid glycoprotein
 C. α_1-Fetoprotein
 D. α_2-Macroglobulin

99. The physician is concerned that a pregnant patient may be at risk for delivering prematurely. What would be the best biochemical marker to measure to assess premature delivery?
 A. Inhibin A
 B. α_1-Fetoprotein
 C. Fetal fibronectin
 D. Human chorionic gonadotropin

100. Bence Jones proteinuria is a condition characterized by the urinary excretion of what type of light chain?
 A. Kappa light chains
 B. Lambda light chains
 C. Both kappa and lambda light chains
 D. Either kappa or lambda light chains

101. Which of the following conditions presents as a beta-gamma bridge on protein electrophoresis
 A. Cirrhosis
 B. Alpha 1 antitrypsin deficiency
 C. Inflammation
 D. Bisalbuminemia

102. What technique is used to quantify specific immunoglobulin classes?
   A. Immunonephelometry
   B. Serum protein electrophoresis
   C. Isoelectric focusing
   D. Immunoelectrophoresis

103. Portal cirrhosis is a chronic disease of the liver. As observed on an electrophoretic serum protein pattern, what is a predominant characteristic of this disease?
   A. Monoclonal band in the gamma-globulin region
   B. Polyclonal band in the gamma-globulin region
   C. Bridging effect between the beta- and gamma-globulin bands
   D. Increase in the alpha$_2$-globulin band

104. The abnormal metabolism of several of the amino acids has been linked with disorders classified as inborn errors of metabolism. What technique is used to differentiate among several different amino acids?
   A. Electrophoresis
   B. Microbiological analysis
   C. Enzyme immunoassay
   D. Chromatography

105. Serum protein electrophoresis is routinely performed on the serum obtained from a clotted blood specimen. If a plasma specimen is substituted for serum, how will the electrophoresis be affected?
   A. Electrophoresis cannot be performed because the anticoagulant will retard the mobilities of the protein fractions.
   B. Electrophoresis cannot be performed because the anticoagulant will cause migration of the protein fractions in the direction of the cathode.
   C. Electrophoresis will show an extra fraction in the beta-gamma region.
   D. Electrophoresis will show an extra fraction in the prealbumin area.

106. In serum protein electrophoresis, when a barbital buffer of pH 8.6 is employed, what protein fraction will migrate the fastest toward the anode?
   A. Albumin
   B. Alpha$_1$-globulin
   C. Beta-globulin
   D. Gamma-globulin

107. During the second trimester of pregnancy, it is expected that levels of this analyte will decrease?
   A. Unconjugated estriol
   B. AFP
   C. Inhibin A
   D. hCG

108. A male patient, 48 years old, mentions during his annual physical that he has been having difficulty urinating. The physician performs a rectal examination, and he orders a total prostate-specific antigen (PSA) and free PSA. The patient has the tests done the following week, and the total PSA result is 3.1 ng/mL and the free PSA is 0.3 ng/mL. What do these results suggest?
   A. Both are normal, no disease present
   B. Benign prostatic hypertrophy
   C. Increased risk of prostate cancer
   D. Free PSA is low and does not correlate with total PSA.

109. Which of the following is *not* associated with carcinoembryonic antigen?
   A. Increased levels seen with malignancies of the lungs
   B. Quantified by using capillary electrophoresis
   C. Used to monitor treatment of colon cancer
   D. Glycoprotein in nature

110. In cases of hepatoma, which protein not normally found in adult serum is synthesized by liver cells?
A. α_1-Acid glycoprotein
B. α_1-Fetoprotein
C. α_2-Macroglobulin
D. Carcinoembryonic antigen

111. The value for PSA below which the presence of prostate cancer is considered unlikely is:
A. 2.5 ng/mL
B. 4.0 ng/mL
C. ng/mL
D. ng/mL

112. Which of the following is an oncofetal antigen that is elevated in nonmucinous epithelial ovarian cancer?
A. CA 549
B. CA 125
C. CA 19-9
D. CA 15-3

113. Which of the following is a sialylated Lewis blood group antigen associated with colorectal carcinoma?
A. CA 19-9
B. CA 15-3
C. CA 549
D. CEA

114. Which of the following conditions will lead to a false positive PSA?
A. Acute myocardial infarction
B. Renal failure
C. Digital rectal exam
D. Testicular cancer

115. Which of the following PSA values warrants a biopsy
A. PSA = 5.2 ng/mL
B. PSA velocity = 0.25 ng/mL/year
C. Free PSA = increased
D. Digital rectal exam = smooth nodules

116. Although serum elevations are not generally seen in early stages, which of the following tumor markers are elevated in more advanced stages of breast cancer?
A. CEA and AFP
B. AFP and CA 125
C. PSA and CA 15-3
D. CA 15-3 and CA 549

Nonprotein Nitrogenous Compounds

117. What is the compound that comprises the majority of the nonprotein-nitrogen fractions in serum?
A. Uric acid
B. Creatinine
C. Ammonia
D. Urea

118. To convert from mg/dL of blood urea nitrogen (BUN) to mmol/L of urea, you would?
A. Multiply BUN by 1.03
B. Divide BUN by 1.03
C. Multiply BUN by 2.14
D. Divide BUN by 2.14

119. In the urea method, the enzymatic action of urease is inhibited when blood for analysis is drawn in a tube containing what anticoagulant?
A. Sodium heparin
B. Sodium fluoride
C. Sodium oxalate
D. Ethylenediaminetetra-acetic acid

120. In the most frequently used enzymatic method to measure urea, what is the enzyme that is used?
A. Uricase
B. Lipase
C. Peroxidase
D. Urease

121. What endogenous substance may cause a positive interference in the urease/glutamate dehydrogenase assay?
  A. Ammonia
  B. Creatinine
  C. Glucose
  D. Cholesterol

122. Which of the following methods utilizes urease and glutamate dehydrogenase for the quantification of serum urea?
  A. Berthelot
  B. Coupled enzymatic
  C. Conductimetric
  D. Indicator dye

123. In the Berthelot reaction, what contaminant will cause the urea level to be falsely elevated?
  A. Sodium fluoride
  B. Protein
  C. Ammonia
  D. Bacteria

124. To maintain acid-base balance, it is necessary that the blood ammonia level be kept within narrow limits. This is accomplished primarily by which of the following?
  A. Synthesis of urea from ammonia
  B. Synthesis of glutamine from ammonia
  C. Excretion of ammonia in the bile
  D. Excretion of ammonia in the stools

125. When a blood ammonia determination is performed, the blood specimen must be treated in a manner that will ensure that
  A. The deamination process continues *in vitro.*
  B. Glutamine formation *in vitro* is avoided.
  C. The transamination process continues *in vitro.*
  D. Ammonia formation *in vitro* is avoided.

126. The preferred method for measurement of plasma ammonia uses which of the following enzymes?
  A. GLDH
  B. Peroxidase
  C. Urease
  D. Lipase

127. Which of the following statements can be associated with the enzymatic assay of ammonia?
  A. Increase in absorbance monitored at 340 nm
  B. Nicotinamide-adenine dinucleotide (NAD^+) required as a cofactor
  C. Ammonium ion isolated from specimen before the enzymatic step
  D. Reaction catalyzed by glutamate dehydrogenase

128. Which of the following disorders is *not* associated with an elevated blood ammonia level?
  A. Reye syndrome
  B. Renal failure
  C. Chronic liver failure
  D. Diabetes mellitus

129. An increased serum level of which of the following analytes is most commonly associated with decreased glomerular filtration?
  A. Creatinine
  B. Uric acid
  C. Urea
  D. Ammonia

130. A serum creatinine was found to be 6.0 mg/dL. Which of the following urea nitrogen serum results would support a renal pathological condition?
  A. 6 mg/dL
  B. 20 mg/dL
  C. 35 mg/dL
  D. 70 mg/dL

131. Which of the following sets of data most closely approximates the results you would see from a person suffering from prerenal azotemia?
   A. BUN 78 mg/dL; creatinine 4.1 mg/dL
   B. BUN 62 mg/dL; creatinine 2.6 mg/dL
   C. BUN 14 mg/dL; creatinine 0.8 mg/dL
   D. BUN 29 mg/dL; creatinine 1.1 mg/dL

132. The red-colored complex developed in the jaffe method to determine creatinine measurements is a result of the complexing of creatinine with:
   A. Alkaline picrate
   B. Diacetyl monoxide
   C. Sulfuric acid
   D. Sodium hydroxide
   E. Sodium nitroprusside

133. Which of the following is added to the Jaffe creatinine measurement to control for interfering substances
   A. Peroxidase
   B. Heparin
   C. Ascorbate
   D. Fuller's earth

134. The creatinine clearance test is routinely used to assess the glomerular filtration rate. Given the following information for an average-size adult, calculate a creatinine clearance.
   Urine creatinine—120 mg/dL
   Plasma creatinine—1.2 mg/dL
   Urine volume for 24 hours—1520 mL
   A. 11 mL/min
   B. 63 mL/min
   C. 95 mL/min
   D. 106 mL/min

135. When it is not possible to perform a creatinine assay on a fresh urine specimen, to what pH level should the urine be adjusted?
   A. 3.0
   B. 5.0
   C. 7.0
   D. 9.0

136. What compound normally found in urine may be used to assess the completeness of a 24-hour urine collection?
   A. Urea
   B. Uric acid
   C. Creatine
   D. Creatinine

137. Which of the following analytes is used to calculate an eGFR?
   A. Urine creatinine
   B. Microalbumin
   C. Cystatin C
   D. Uric acid

138. An endogenous substance assayed to assess the glomerular filtration rate may be described as being filtered by the glomeruli, not reabsorbed by the tubules, and only secreted by the tubules when plasma levels become elevated. What is this frequently assayed substance?
   A. Inulin
   B. Uric acid
   C. Creatinine
   D. Urea

139. What is the end-product of purine catabolism in humans?
   A. Urea
   B. Uric acid
   C. Allantoin
   D. Ammonia

140. When mixed with phosphotungstic acid, what compound causes the reduction of the former to a tungsten blue complex?
   A. Urea
   B. Ammonia
   C. Creatinine
   D. Uric acid

141. In the ultraviolet procedure for quantifying uric acid, what does the reaction between uric acid and uricase cause?
   A. Production of reduced nicotinamide-adenine dinucleotide (NADH)
   B. The formation of allantoin
   C. An increase in absorbance
   D. A reduction of phosphotungstic acid

142. Which of the following disorders is best characterized by laboratory findings that include increased serum levels of inorganic phosphorus, magnesium, potassium, uric acid, urea, and creatinine and decreased serum calcium and erythropoietin levels?
   A. Chronic renal failure
   B. Renal tubular disease
   C. Nephrotic syndrome
   D. Acute glomerulonephritis

143. In gout, what analyte deposits in joints and other body tissues?
   A. Calcium
   B. Creatinine
   C. Urea
   D. Uric acid

144. During chemotherapy for leukemia, which of the following analytes would most likely be elevated in the blood?
   A. Uric acid
   B. Urea
   C. Creatinine
   D. Ammonia

Carbohydrates

145. What does hydrolysis of sucrose yield?
   A. Glucose only
   B. Galactose and glucose
   C. Maltose and glucose
   D. Fructose and glucose

146. In what form is glucose stored in muscle and liver?
   A. Glycogen
   B. Maltose
   C. Lactose
   D. Starch

147. The following results are from a 21-year-old patient with a back injury who appears otherwise healthy:

Analyte	Result
Whole blood glucose	84 mg/dL
Serum glucose	98 mg/dL
CSF glucose	50 mg/dL

The best interpretation of these results is that:
   A. The whole blood and serum values are expected but the CSF value is elevated.
   B. The whole blood glucose value should be higher than the serum value.
   C. All values are consistent with a healthy individual.
   D. The serum and whole blood values should be identical.

148. You report an A1c value of 9% on a patient. The corresponding estimated average glucose (eAG) is:
   A. 126 mg/dL
   B. 212 mg/dL
   C. 240 mg/dL
   D. Not enough data were provided

149. What is the glucose concentration in fasting whole blood?
   A. Less than the concentration in plasma or serum
   B. Greater than the concentration in plasma or serum
   C. Equal to the concentration in plasma or serum
   D. Meaningless because it is not stable

150. Of the following blood glucose levels, which would you expect to result in glucose in the urine?
   A. 50 mg/dL
   B. 120 mg/dL
   C. 150 mg/dL
   D. 225 mg/dL

151. Which test may be performed to assess the average plasma glucose level that an individual maintained during a previous 2- to 3-month period?
   A. Plasma glucose
   B. Two-hour postprandial glucose
   C. Oral glucose tolerance
   D. Glycated hemoglobin

152. The physician determined that the patient needed an oral glucose tolerance test (OGTT) to assist in diagnosis. The patient had blood drawn for the OGTT, and the following serum glucose results were obtained. These results are indicative of what state?

   Fasting serum glucose 124 mg/dL
   2-hour postload serum glucose 227 mg/dL

   A. Normal
   B. Diabetes mellitus
   C. Addison disease
   D. Hyperinsulinism

153. A 30-year-old pregnant woman has a gestational diabetes mellitus screening test performed at 26 weeks of gestation. Her physician chooses to order a 50-g oral glucose load. Her serum glucose level is 150 mg/dL at 1 hour. What should occur next?
   A. This confirms diabetes mellitus; give insulin.
   B. This confirms diabetes mellitus; dietary intake of carbohydrates should be lessened.
   C. This is suspicious of diabetes mellitus; an oral glucose tolerance test should be performed.
   D. This is an expected glucose level in a pregnant woman.

154. A sample of blood is collected for glucose in a sodium fluoride tube before the patient has had breakfast. The physician calls 2 hours later and requests that determination of blood urea nitrogen (BUN) be performed on the same sample rather than obtaining another specimen. The automated analyzer in your laboratory utilizes the urease method to quantify BUN. What should you tell the physician?
   A. Will gladly do the test if sufficient specimen remains
   B. Could do the test using a micro method
   C. Can do the BUN determination on the automated analyzer
   D. Cannot perform the procedure

155. Which of the following is associated with type 1 diabetes mellitus?
   A. Insulin sensitivity
   B. Hyperosmolar hyperglycemic state (HHS)
   C. Ketone production
   D. Central obesity

156. Which of the following sugars may be used directly by your body for energy?
   A. Galactose
   B. Fructose
   C. Lactose
   D. Glucose
   E. All of the above

157. Which of the following statements may be associated with the activity of insulin?
   A. Increases blood glucose levels
   B. Decreases glucose uptake by muscle and fat cells
   C. Stimulates release of hepatic glucose into the blood
   D. Stimulates glycogenesis in the liver

158. A patient presents to the ER in a hypoglycemic episode. Significant data are found below:

Analyte	Result
Glucose	35 mg/dL
Insulin	>20 μU/mL
C-Peptide	Negative

The most likely explanation for the hypoglycemia is:
A. The presence of an insulinoma (insulin producing tumor)
*B. Too much pharmacological insulin
C. Oversecretion of glucagon
D. Oversecretion of epinephrine

159. Which of the following statements applies to the preferred use of plasma or serum, rather than whole blood, for glucose determination?
A. Glucose is more stable in separated plasma or serum.
B. Specificity for glucose is higher with most methods when plasma or serum is used.
C. It is convenient to use serum or plasma with automated instruments because whole blood requires mixing immediately before sampling.
D. All the above

160. Which of the following analytes would *not* commonly be measured when monitoring complications of diabetes mellitus?
A. Serum urea nitrogen
B. Urinary albumin
C. Serum creatinine
D. Serum bilirubin

161. Ingestion of which of the following drugs may cause hypoglycemia?
A. Ethanol
B. Propranolol
C. Salicylate
D. All the above

162. Which of the following is the cutpoint for the use of a fasting plasma glucose in diagnosing diabetes mellitus?
A. 99 mg/dL
B. 126 mg/dL
C. 140 mg/dL
D. 200 mg/dL

163. Which glucose method can employ a polarographic oxygen electrode?
A. Hexokinase
B. Glucose oxidase
C. Glucose dehydrogenase
D. *o*-Toluidine

164. Which glucose method catalyzes the phosphorylation of glucose by adenosine triphosphate, forming glucose-6-phosphate and adenosine diphosphate with the absorbance of the NADPH product read at 340 nm?
A. *o*-Toluidine
B. Glucose oxidase
C. Hexokinase
D. Glucose dehydrogenase

165. Which of the following is *not* a reagent required in an enzymatic serum glucose method?
A. NAD^+
B. Glucose oxidase
C. Peroxidase
D. Reduced chromogen

166. A person who has a 2-hour oral glucose tolerance test result of 173 mg/dL would be classified in which of the following categories?
A. Impaired fasting glucose
*B. Impaired glucose tolerance
C. Normal glucose tolerance
D. Gestational diabetes

167. Which glucose method is considered to be the reference method?
A. Glucose oxidase
B. *o*-Toluidine
C. Hexokinase
D. Glucose dehydrogenase

168. An individual has a plasma glucose level of 110 mg/dL. What would be the approximate glucose concentration in this patient's cerebrospinal fluid?
A. 33 mg/dL
B. 55 mg/dL
C. 66 mg/dL
D. 110 mg/dL

169. What is the reference interval for fasting serum glucose in an adult expressed in SI units (International System of Units)?
A. 1.7–3.3 mmol/L
B. 3.3–5.6 mmol/L
C. 4.1–5.5 mmol/L
D. 6.7–8.3 mmol/L

170. At what level should a 52-year-old male diagnosed with type 2 diabetes mellitus maintain his hemoglobin A_{1c}?
A. ≤3%
B. ≤7%
C. ≤9%
D. ≤11%

171. The following results are from a 21-year-old patient with a back injury who appears otherwise healthy:

Analyte	Result
Whole blood glucose	84 mg/dL
Serum glucose	98 mg/dL
CSF glucose	50 mg/dL

The best interpretation of these results is that:
A. The whole blood and serum values are expected but the CSF value is elevated.
B. The whole blood glucose value should be higher than the serum value.
C. All values are consistent with a normal healthy individual.
D. The serum and whole blood values should be identical.

172. What effect if any would be expected when the secretion of epinephrine is stimulated by physical or emotional stress?
A. Decreased blood glucose level
B. Increased blood glucose level
C. Increased glycogen storage
D. No effect on blood glucose or glycogen levels

173. What would an individual with Cushing syndrome tend to exhibit?
A. Hyperglycemia
B. Hypoglycemia
C. Normal blood glucose level
D. Decreased 2-hour postprandial glucose

174. As part of a routine physical, a fasting plasma glucose is performed on a 45-year-old male and the test result is 105 mg/dL. How should this individual be classified?
A. Normal for his age
B. Impaired fasting glucose
C. Type 1 diabetes mellitus
D. Type 2 diabetes mellitus

175. A cerebrospinal fluid specimen is sent to the lab at 9:00 P.M. for glucose analysis. The specimen is cloudy and appears to contain red blood cells. Which of the following statements is *true?*
A. Glucose testing cannot be performed on the specimen.
B. Specimen should be centrifuged and glucose assayed immediately.
C. Specimen can be refrigerated as received and glucose assayed the next day.
D. Specimen can be frozen as received and glucose assayed the next day.

176. A patient has a urine uric acid level of 1575 mg/day. What effect will this have on the measured urine glucose level when the glucose oxidase/peroxidase method is employed?
   A. Urine glucose level will be falsely low.
   B. Urine glucose level will be falsely high.
   C. Urine glucose level will be accurate.
   D. Urine glucose level will exceed the linearity of the method.

177. Laboratory tests are performed on a postmenopausal, 57-year-old female as part of an annual physical examination. The patient's casual plasma glucose is 220 mg/dL, and the glycated hemoglobin (Hb A_{1c}) is 11%. Based on this information, how should the patient be classified?
   A. Normal glucose tolerance
   B. Impaired glucose tolerance
   C. Gestational diabetes mellitus
   D. Type 2 diabetes mellitus

178. Which of the following is characterized by a deficiency of glucose-6-phosphatase resulting in hepatomegaly, lactic acidosis, and severe fasting hypoglycemia?
   A. Type I—von Gierke disease
   B. Type II—Pompe disease
   C. Type III—Cori disease
   D. Type IV—Andersen disease

Lipids and Lipoproteins

179. Bile acids that are synthesized in the liver are derived from what substance?
   A. Bilirubin
   B. Fatty acid
   C. Cholesterol
   D. Triglyceride

180. The turbid, or milky, appearance of serum after fat ingestion is termed postprandial lipemia, which is caused by the presence of what substance?
   A. Bilirubin
   B. Cholesterol
   C. Chylomicron
   D. Phospholipid

181. Cholesterol ester is formed through the esterification of the alcohol cholesterol with what substance?
   A. Protein
   B. Triglyceride
   C. Fatty acid
   D. Digitonin

182. Which of the following tests would most likely be included in a routine lipid profile?
   A. Total cholesterol, triglyceride, fatty acid, chylomicron
   B. Total cholesterol, triglyceride, HDL cholesterol, phospholipid
   C. Triglyceride, HDL cholesterol, LDL cholesterol, chylomicron
   D. Total cholesterol, triglyceride, HDL cholesterol, LDL cholesterol

183. To produce reliable results, when should blood specimens for lipid studies be drawn?
   A. Immediately after eating
   B. Anytime during the day
   C. In the fasting state, approximately 2–4 hours after eating
   D. In the fasting state, approximately 9–12 hours after eating

184. Which of the following lipid tests is *least* affected by the fasting status of the patient?
   A. Cholesterol
   B. Triglyceride
   C. Fatty acid
   D. Lipoprotein

185. What compound is a crucial intermediary in the metabolism of triglyceride to form energy?
    A. Bile
    B. Acetyl-coenzyme A
    C. Acetoacetate
    D. Pyruvate

186. The kinetic methods for quantifying serum triglyceride employ enzymatic hydrolysis. The hydrolysis of triglyceride may be accomplished by what enzyme?
    A. Amylase
    B. Leucine aminopeptidase
    C. Lactate dehydrogenase
    D. Lipase

187. Enzymatic methods for the determination of total cholesterol in serum utilize a cholesterol oxidase-peroxidase method. In this method, cholesterol oxidase reacts specifically with what?
    A. Free cholesterol and cholesteryl ester
    B. Free cholesterol and fatty acid
    C. Free cholesterol only
    D. Cholesteryl ester only

188. Exogenous triglycerides are transported in the plasma in what form?
    A. Phospholipids
    B. Cholesteryl esters
    C. Chylomicrons
    D. Free fatty acids

189. Ketone bodies are formed because of an excessive breakdown of fatty acids. Of the following metabolites, which may be classified as a ketone body?
    A. Pyruvic acid
    B. β-Hydroxybutyric acid
    C. Lactic acid
    D. Oxaloacetic acid

190. The following laboratory data are received after performing a lipid profile. These data are most closely associated with which of the following lipoprotein electrophoresis patterns?

    Standing plasma test = fat layer; clear plasma
    Total Cholesterol = 202 mg/dL
    Triglycerides = 329 mg/dL
    HDL = 36 mg/dL

    A. Increase in chylomicrons
    B. Increase in beta lipoprotein
    C. Increase in prebeta lipoprotein
    D. Increase in beta and prebeta lipoprotein with bridging

191. Each lipoprotein fraction is composed of varying amounts of lipid and protein components. The beta-lipoprotein fraction consists primarily of which lipid?
    A. Fatty acid
    B. Cholesterol
    C. Phospholipid
    D. Triglyceride

192. What substance is the precursor to all steroid hormones?
    A. Fatty acid
    B. Cholesterol
    C. Triglyceride
    D. Phospholipid

193. The term "lipid storage diseases" is used to denote a group of lipid disorders, the majority of which are inherited as autosomal recessive mutations. What is the cause of these diseases?
    A. Excessive dietary fat ingestion
    B. Excessive synthesis of chylomicrons
    C. A specific enzyme deficiency or nonfunctional enzyme form
    D. An inability of adipose tissue to store lipid materials

194. Several malabsorption problems are characterized by a condition known as steatorrhea. Steatorrhea is caused by an abnormal accumulation of what substance in the feces?
    A. Proteins
    B. Lipids
    C. Carbohydrates
    D. Vitamins

195. Which of the following lipoprotein profiles would be indicative of the laboratory presentation of Tangier disease?
    A. Increased VLDL, increased LDL, increased HDL
    B. Absent VLDL, increased LDL, normal HDL
    C. Normal VLDL, absent LDL, normal HDL
    D. Normal VLDL, normal LDL, absent HDL

196. The quantification of the high-density lipoprotein cholesterol level is thought to be significant in the risk assessment of what disease?
    A. Pancreatitis
    B. Cirrhosis
    C. Coronary artery disease
    D. Hyperlipidemia

197. Upon standing at 24 hours a serum sample appears cloudy with a creamy layer. This is most likely due to elevations in which lipoprotein fraction(s)?
    A. Chylomicrons
    B. VLDL and Chylomicrons
    C. LDL and chylomicrons
    D. HDL and LDL

198. The VLDL fraction primarily transports what substance?
    A. Cholesterol
    B. Chylomicron
    C. Triglyceride
    D. Phospholipid

199. A 54-year-old male, with a history of type 2 diabetes mellitus for the past 8 years, is seen by his family physician. The patient indicates that during the past week he had experienced what he described as feeling lightheaded and faint. He also indicated that he became out of breath and had experienced mild chest pain when doing heavy yard work, but the chest pain subsided when he sat down and rested. The physician performed an ECG immediately, which was normal, and he ordered blood tests. The patient fasted overnight and had blood drawn the next morning. The laboratory test values follow:

Test	Patient's Values	Reference Ranges
Glucose, fasting	175 mg/dL	74–99 mg/dL
Hemoglobin A_{1c}	8.1%	4–6%
Total cholesterol	272 mg/dL	<200 mg/dL
HDL cholesterol	30 mg/dL	>40 mg/dL
LDL cholesterol	102 mg/dL	<130 mg/dL
Triglyceride	250 mg/dL	<150 mg/dL
hs-CRP	6.2 mg/L	0.3–8.6 mg/L, <1.0 mg/L low risk

Based on the patient's test results, history, and symptoms, which of the laboratory values in the chart above does *not* support the patient's diagnosis?
    A. LDL cholesterol
    B. HDL cholesterol
    C. Hemoglobin A_{1c}
    D. hs-CRP

200. Name a commonly used precipitating reagent to separate HDL cholesterol from other lipoprotein cholesterol fractions.
    A. Zinc sulfate
    B. Trichloroacetic acid
    C. Heparin-manganese
    D. Isopropanol

201. What is the principle of the "direct" or "homogeneous" HDL cholesterol automated method, which requires no intervention by the laboratorian? The direct HDL method
   A. Quantifies only the cholesterol in HDL, whereas the precipitation HDL method quantifies the entire lipoprotein
   B. Utilizes polymers and detergents that make the HDL cholesterol soluble while keeping the other lipoproteins insoluble
   C. Uses a nonenzymatic method to measure cholesterol, whereas the other methods use enzymes to measure cholesterol
   D. Uses a column chromatography step to separate HDL from the other lipoproteins, whereas the other methods use a precipitation step

202. Which of the following results would be the most consistent with high risk for coronary heart disease?
   A. 20 mg/dL HDL cholesterol and 250 mg/dL total cholesterol
   B. 45 mg/dL HDL cholesterol and 210 mg/dL total cholesterol
   C. 50 mg/dL HDL cholesterol and 180 mg/dL total cholesterol
   D. 55 mg/dL HDL cholesterol and 170 mg/dL total cholesterol

203. A patient's total cholesterol is 300 mg/dL, his HDL cholesterol is 50 mg/dL, and his triglyceride is 200 mg/dL. What is this patient's calculated LDL cholesterol?
   A. 200
   B. 210
   C. 290
   D. 350

204. A patient's total cholesterol/HDL cholesterol ratio is 10.0. What level of risk for coronary heart disease does this result indicate?
   A. No risk
   B. Half average risk
   C. Average risk
   D. Twice average risk

205. Which of the following techniques can be used to quantify apolipoproteins?
   A. Spectrophotometric endpoint
   B. Ion-selective electrode
   C. Immunonephelometric assay
   D. Refractometry

206. Which of the following may be described as a variant form of LDL, associated with increased risk of atherosclerotic cardiovascular disease?
   A. Lp(a)
   B. HDL
   C. Apo A-I
   D. Apo A-II

207. In what way is the "normal" population reference interval for total cholesterol in America different from that of other clinical chemistry parameters (i.e., protein, sodium, BUN, creatinine, etc.)?
   A. Established units for total cholesterol are mg/dL; no other chemistry test has these units.
   B. Reference interval is artificially set to reflect good health even though Americans as a group have "normally" higher total cholesterol levels.
   C. Total cholesterol reference interval must be interpreted in line with triglyceride, phospholipid, and sphingolipid values.
   D. Total cholesterol reference interval is based on a manual procedure, whereas all other chemistry parameters are based on automated procedures.

208. Your lab routinely uses a precipitation method to separate HDL cholesterol. You receive a slightly lipemic specimen for HDL cholesterol. The total cholesterol and triglyceride for the specimen were 450 and 520 mg/dL, respectively. After adding the precipitating reagents and centrifuging, you notice that the supernatant still looks slightly cloudy. What is your next course of action in analyzing this specimen?
    A. Perform the HDL cholesterol test; there is nothing wrong with this specimen
    B. Take off the supernatant and recentrifuge
    C. Take off the supernatant and add another portion of the precipitating reagent to it and recentrifuge
    D. Send specimen to a lab that offers other techniques to separate more effectively the HDL cholesterol

209. A 46-year-old known alcoholic with liver damage is brought into the emergency department unconscious. In what way would you expect his plasma lipid values to be affected?
    A. Increased total cholesterol, triglyceride, LDL, and VLDL
    B. Increased total cholesterol and triglyceride, decreased LDL and VLDL
    C. Decreased total cholesterol, triglyceride, LDL, and VLDL
    D. Normal lipid metabolism, unaffected by the alcoholism

210. A healthy, active 10-year-old boy with no prior history of illness comes to the lab after school for a routine chemistry screen in order to meet requirements for summer camp. After centrifugation, the serum looks cloudy. The specimen had the following results: blood glucose = 135 mg/dL, total cholesterol = 195 mg/dL, and triglyceride = 185 mg/dL. What would be the most probable explanation for these findings? The boy
    A. Is at risk for coronary artery disease.
    B. Has type 1 diabetes mellitus that is undiagnosed.
    C. Has an inherited genetic disease causing a lipid imbalance.
    D. Was most likely not fasting when the specimen was drawn.

211. A mother brings her obese, 4-year-old child who is a known type 1 diabetic to the laboratory for a blood workup. She states that the boy has been fasting for the past 12 hours. After centrifugation the tech notes that the serum looks turbid. The specimen had the following results: blood glucose = 150 mg/dL, total cholesterol = 250 mg/dL, HDL cholesterol = 32 mg/dL, and triglyceride = 395 mg/dL. What best explains these findings? The boy
    A. Is at low risk for coronary artery disease.
    B. Is a good candidate for a 3-hour oral glucose tolerance test.
    C. Has secondary hyperlipidemia due to the diabetes.
    D. Was not fasting when the specimen was drawn.

Enzymes and Cardiac Assessment

212. A convenient method for assaying enzyme activity is based on measuring the conversion between the oxidized and reduced forms of nicotinamide adenine dinucleotide (NAD/NADH). Which form of nicotinamide adenine dinucleotide is correctly paired with its maximum absorption?
    A. Oxidized, 550 nm
    B. Oxidized, 340 nm
    C. Reduced, 265 nm
    D. Reduced, 340 nm

213. In the assay of an enzyme, zero-order kinetics are best described by which of the following statements?
   A. Enzyme is present in excess; rate of reaction is variable with time and dependent only on the concentration of the enzyme in the system.
   B. Substrate is present in excess; rate of reaction is constant with time and dependent only on the concentration of enzyme in the system.
   C. Substrate is present in excess; rate of reaction is constant with enzyme concentration and dependent only on the time in which the reaction is run.
   D. Enzyme is present in excess; rate of reaction is independent of both time and concentration of the enzyme in the system.

214. Which type of enzyme inhibitor binds to the active site and is considered to be a reversible inhibitor?
   A. Competitive
   B. Noncompetitive
   C. Uncompetitive
   D. Allosteric

215. When measuring enzyme activity, if the instrument is operating 5°C lower than the temperature prescribed for the method, how will the results be affected?
   A. Lower than expected
   B. Higher than expected
   C. Varied, showing no particular pattern
   D. All will be clinically abnormal

216. Given the following information for a rate reaction, calculate the activity of a serum specimen for alanine aminotransferase in international units per liter (IU/L).

Time	Absorbance	
1 min	1.104	Specimen volume = 20 μL
2 min	1.025	Reagent volume = 3.0 mL
3 min	0.950	Molar absorptivity for NADH at 340 nm = 6.22×10^3 L/mol·cm
4 min	0.873	Light path = 1 cm

   A. 186
   B. 198
   C. 1857
   D. 1869

217. The properties of enzymes are correctly described by which of the following statements?
   A. Enzymes are stable proteins.
   B. Enzymes are protein catalysts of biological origin.
   C. Enzymes affect the rate of a chemical reaction by raising the activation energy needed for the reaction to take place.
   D. Enzyme activity is not altered by heat denaturation.

218. Which of the following is a *true* statement concerning serum enzymes?
   A. The presence of hemolyzed red cells is of no significance for an accurate assay of most serum enzymes.
   B. Serum asparate transaminase (AST), but not serum lactate dehydrogenase (LD), is usually elevated in acute myocardial infarction.
   C. Increased serum alkaline phosphatase may be found in bone disease.
   D. Aspartate transaminase was formerly known as glutamate pyruvate transaminase.

219. Enzymes that catalyze the transfer of groups between compounds are classified as belonging to which enzyme class?
    A. Hydrolases
    B. Lyases
    C. Oxidoreductases
    D. Transferases

220. Which of the following pH values drives the conversion of pyruvate to lactacte in the presence of lactate dehydrogenase?
    A. 6.5
    B. 8.5
    C. 9.5
    D. 7.3

221. To what class of enzymes does lactate dehydrogenase belong?
    A. Isomerases
    B. Ligases
    C. Oxidoreductases
    D. Transferases

222. Which of the following enzymes catalyzes the transfer of amino groups causing the interconversion of amino acids and α-oxoacids?
    A. Amylase
    B. Aspartate transaminase
    C. Alkaline phosphatase
    D. Lactate dehydrogenase

223. What abbreviation has been used in the past to designate alanine aminotransferase?
    A. AST
    B. AAT
    C. GOT
    D. GPT

224. When measuring CK-MB, which of the following would provide the most sensitive method?
    A. Electrophoretic
    B. Colorimetric
    C. Kinetic
    D. Mass immunoassay

225. Which of the following enzyme activities can be determined by using a dilute olive oil emulsion substrate, whose hydrolyzed product is monitored as a decrease in turbidity or light scatter?
    A. AST
    B. ALT
    C. GGT
    D. Lipase

226. Which test, if elevated, would provide information about risk for developing coronary artery disease?
    A. Troponin
    B. CK-MB
    C. hs-CRP
    D. Myoglobin

227. Lactate dehydrogenase (LD) catalyzes the following reaction:

    $$\text{Lactate} + \text{NAD}^+ \xrightleftharpoons{\text{LD}} \text{pyruvate} + \text{NADH}$$

    As the reaction is written, which of the following techniques can be used to assess LD activity?
    A. Measure the colorimetric product pyruvate
    B. Measure the colorimetric product NADH
    C. Measure the increase in absorbance at 340 nm as NADH is produced
    D. Measure the decrease in absorbance at 340 nm as NADH is produced

228. Liver function (hepatocellular) is best assessed by which of the following parameters?
    A. AST and ALT levels
    B. Amylase and Lipase levels
    C. BUN and creatinine levels
    D. ALP and GGT levels

229. Hemolysis effects creatine kinase assays because:
   A. There is an increased amount of creatine kinase in the RBC.
   B. There is an increased amount of ATP in the RBC.
   C. There is an increased amount of adenylate kinase in the RBC.
   D. There is an increased amount of NADH in the RBC.
   E. There is an increased amount of potassium in the RBC.

230. One international unit of enzyme activity is the amount of enzyme that under specified reaction conditions of substrate concentration, pH, and temperature, causes utilization of substrate at the rate of:
   A. 1 mole/min
   B. 1 millimole/min
   C. 1 micromole/min
   D. 1 nanomole/min

231. Which enzyme is measured by methodologies that use small oligosaccharides and 4-nitrophenyl-glycoside for substrates?
   A. Lipase
   B. Amylase
   C. Creatine kinase
   D. Cholinesterase

232. Which statement concerning gamma-glutamyltransferase is *false?*
   A. Present in almost all cells of the body
   B. Elevated in liver and some pancreatic diseases
   C. Elevated in chronic alcoholism
   D. Elevated in bone disease

233. Which of the following statements correctly describes alkaline phosphatase?
   A. Decreased in Paget disease
   B. Decreased in third trimester of a normal pregnancy
   C. Increased in obstructive jaundice
   D. Primarily found in cardiac muscle

234. What is the typical time course for plasma troponin I and T following acute myocardial infarction?
   A. Rise in 4–6 hours, peaks 12–24 hours, returns to normal in 1 week
   B. Rise in 4–6 hours, peaks at 12–24 hours, and returns to normal in 3 days
   C. Rise in 1–2 hours, peaks at 36 hours, and returns to normal in 72 hours
   D. Rise in 8–10 hours, peaks at 12–24 hours, and returns to normal in 3 days

235. In acute pancreatitis, a significant increase in which serum enzyme would be expected diagnostically?
   A. Creatine kinase
   B. Amylase
   C. Alkaline phosphatase
   D. Aspartate aminotransferase

236. For assessing carcinoma of the prostate, quantification of PSA has virtually replaced the measurement of which of the following enzymes?
   A. Alkaline phosphatase
   B. Acid phosphatase
   C. Alanine aminotransferase
   D. Trypsin

237. Which of the following biomarkers is the first to elevate after an acute myocardial infarction?
   A. CK
   B. CK-MB
   C. AST
   D. Myoglobin
   E. Troponin I

238. Which of the following disorders is *not* characterized by an elevated serum myoglobin?
   A. Renal failure
   B. Vigorous exercise
   C. Acute myocardial infarction
   D. Hepatitis

239. Upon stimulation of skeletal muscles, calcium is immediately made available for binding to:
A. Troponin I
B. Troponin T
C. Troponin C
D. Tropomyosin

240. Which of the following biomarkers is currently recommended at the preferred maker for acute myocardial infarction?
A. CK-MB
B. LD
C. Troponin
D. Myoglobin

241. A physician orders several laboratory tests on a 55-year-old male patient who is complaining of pain, stiffness, fatigue, and headaches. Based on the following serum test results, what is the most likely diagnosis?
Alkaline phosphatase—significantly increased
Gamma-glutamyltransferase—normal
A. Biliary obstruction
B. Cirrhosis
C. Hepatitis
D. Osteitis deformans

242. A 53-year-old female presents with fatigue, pruritus, and an enlarged, nontender liver. The physician orders a series of blood tests. Based on the following serum test results, what is the most likely diagnosis?
Alkaline phosphatase—markedly elevated
Alanine aminotransferase—slightly elevated
Lactate dehydrogenase—slightly elevated
Gamma-glutamyltransferase—markedly elevated
Total bilirubin—slightly elevated
A. Alcoholic cirrhosis
B. Infectious mononucleosis
C. Intrahepatic cholestasis
D. Viral hepatitis

243. A 42-year-old male presents with anorexia, nausea, fever, and icterus of the skin and mucous membranes. He noticed that his urine had appeared dark for the past several days. The physician orders a series of biochemical tests. Based on the following test results, what is the most likely diagnosis?
Serum alkaline phosphatase—slightly elevated
Serum alanine aminotransferase—markedly elevated
Serum aspartate aminotransferase—markedly elevated
Serum gamma-glutamyltransferase—slightly elevated
Serum total bilirubin—moderately elevated
Urine bilirubin—positive
Fecal urobilinogen—decreased
A. Acute hepatitis
B. Alcoholic cirrhosis
C. Metastatic carcinoma of the pancreas
D. Obstructive jaundice

244. To aid in the diagnosis of skeletal muscle disease, which of the following serum enzyme measurements would be of most use?
A. Creatine kinase
B. Alkaline phosphatase
C. Aspartate aminotransferase
D. Alanine aminotransferase

245. When an AMI occurs, in what order (list first to last) will the enzymes aspartate aminotransferase (AST), creatine kinase (CK), and lactate dehydrogenase (LD) become elevated in the serum?
A. AST, LD, CK
B. CK, LD, AST
C. CK, AST, LD
D. LD, CK, AST

246. Which of the following represents the sample collection times for cTn according to the Third Universal definition of Acute Myocardial Infarction?
   A. At presentation, 6–9 hours after admission, and 12–24 hours if prior results are negative
   B. At presentation and 12–24 hours after admission
   C. At presentation, 3 hours after admission, and 6 hours if prior results are negative
   D. At presentation AMD 1–2 hours after admission

247. If elevated, which laboratory test would support a diagnosis of congestive heart failure?
   A. Homocysteine
   B. Troponin
   C. Albumin cobalt binding
   D. B-type natriuretic peptide

248. A 4-year-old male child is brought to the pediatrician because the parents are concerned about the child's frequent falling, which results in bruising. The parents indicate that the child has difficulty running, walking, standing up, climbing stairs, and even sitting up straight. The child also appears somewhat weak. Which of the following results is *not* consistent with the most likely diagnosis?
   A. Moderately elevated AST
   B. Moderately elevated ALP
   C. Moderately elevated LD
   D. Markedly elevated CK

249. A 68-year-old male in an unconscious state is transported to the emergency department after being involved in a one-car crash, where he drove off the road and hit a tree. Because he was alone at the time and there was no apparent cause for the accident, it is assumed that he blacked out, which caused him to lose control of the car. He was not wearing a seat belt and has a broken leg, multiple contusions, and cuts. Blood samples were drawn upon arrival to the ED and in 3-hour intervals for 12 hours; all control values were within acceptable range. Selected test results follow:

Test	Initial Values	3 Hours	9 Hours	Reference Ranges
Myoglobin	57 ng/mL	140 ng/mL	281 ng/mL	30–90 ng/mL
Total CK	112 U/L	170 U/L	390 U/L	15–160 U/L
CK-MB	3 ng/mL	6 ng/mL	8 ng/mL	0–5 ng/mL
Troponin I	0.10 ng/mL	0.12 ng/mL	0.11 ng/mL	<0.40 ng/mL

What do these test results suggest?
   A. The man had a myocardial infarction, which caused the accident.
   B. The elevated results are from the skeletal muscle injuries sustained in the car crash.
   C. The elevated results are a combination of the car crash injuries and a myocardial infarction.
   D. The elevated total CK and CK-MB results indicate that the man had a stroke.

250. If elevated, which of the following is associated with increased risk for coronary heart disease?
   A. Homocysteine
   B. Vitamin B_6
   C. Myoglobin
   D. pro-BNP

251. Which statement best describes the clinical use of measuring NT-proBNP?
A. Used to assess risk of coronary heart disease
B. Used to assess risk of angina
C. Used to assess individuals treated with nesiritide
D. Used to assess individuals treated with vitamin B

252. A 10-year-old girl presents with varicella. The child has been experiencing fever, nausea, vomiting, lethargy, and disorientation. A diagnosis of Reye syndrome is determined. Which of the following laboratory results is *not* consistent with the diagnosis?
A. Elevated serum AST
B. Elevated serum ALT
C. Elevated plasma ammonia
D. Elevated serum bilirubin

253. Which of the following enzymes is measured using a chromolytic technique using the substrate 4,6-ethylidene(G1)-p-nitrophenyl(G7)-α-D-maltohepataoside at 30 degrees C?
A. Alkaline phosphatase
B. Amylase
C. Lipase
D. Trypsin

254. Which of the following is *not* characteristic of cystic fibrosis?
A. Decreased bicarbonate concentration in duodenal fluid
B. Decreased lipase activity in duodenal fluid
C. Decreased amylase activity in duodenal fluid
D. Increased trypsin in feces

Liver Function and Porphyrin Formation

255. Which compounds originally condense to form aminolevulinic acid?
A. Oxoglutarate and aspartate
B. Isocitrate and coenzyme II
C. Oxalacetate and malate
D. Succinyl coenzyme A and glycine

256. What compound chelates iron and is the immediate precursor of heme formation?
A. Porphobilinogen
B. Protoporphyrinogen IX
C. Uroporphyrinogen III
D. Protoporphyrin IX

257. Which of the following is a qualitative screening test for porphobilinogen that may be performed to aid in the diagnosis of the porphyrias?
A. Caraway test
B. Gutman test
C. Jendrassik-Grof test
D. Watson-Schwartz test

258. What compound may be detected by observing its orange-red fluorescence in acid solution?
A. Porphobilinogen
B. Uroporphyrinogen
C. Aminolevulinic acid
D. Coproporphyrin

259. The laboratory receives a request that assays for urinary aminolevulinic acid, porphobilinogen, uroporphyrin, and coproporphyrin are to be performed on a patient. Which of the following will *not* contribute to the integrity of the sample when these assays are performed on the same urine specimen?
A. Refrigeration
B. Addition of hydrochloric acid
C. 24-hour urine collection
D. Use of a brown bottle

260. What is the immediate precursor of bilirubin formation?
   A. Mesobilirubinogen
   B. Verdohemoglobin
   C. Urobilinogen
   D. Biliverdin

261. To quantify serum bilirubin levels, it is necessary that bilirubin couples with diazotized sulfanilic acid to form what complex?
   A. Verdobilirubin
   B. Azobilirubin
   C. Azobilirubinogen
   D. Bilirubin glucuronide

262. What enzyme catalyzes the conjugation of bilirubin?
   A. Leucine aminopeptidase
   B. Glucose-6-phosphate dehydrogenase
   C. Uridine diphosphate glucuronyltransferase
   D. Carbamoyl phosphate synthetase

263. What breakdown product of bilirubin metabolism is produced in the colon from the oxidation of urobilinogen by microorganisms?
   A. Porphobilinogen
   B. Urobilin
   C. Stercobilinogen
   D. Protoporphyrin

264. Which of the following functions as a transport protein for bilirubin in the blood?
   A. Albumin
   B. $Alpha_1$-globulin
   C. Beta-globulin
   D. Gamma-globulin

265. What term is used to describe the accumulation of bilirubin in the skin?
   A. Jaundice
   B. Hemolysis
   C. Cholestasis
   D. Kernicterus

266. In the condition kernicterus, the abnormal accumulation of bilirubin occurs in what tissue?
   A. Brain
   B. Liver
   C. Kidney
   D. Blood

267. As a reduction product of bilirubin catabolism, this compound is partially reabsorbed from the intestine through the portal circulation for reexcretion by the liver. What is this compound?
   A. Verdohemoglobin
   B. Urobilinogen
   C. Urobilin
   D. Biliverdin

268. Laboratory findings can be useful in following the progression of chronic hepatitis to cirrhosis. As this occurs, the platelet count will _____, the prothrombin time will _____, albumin will _____, and ALP will ________.
   A. Decrease, increase, decrease, increase
   B. Decrease, decrease, increase, increase
   C. Increase, decrease, increase, decrease
   D. Increase, increase, decrease, decrease

269. Which bilirubin fraction is unconjugated and covalently bound to albumin?
   A. Alpha
   B. Beta
   C. Delta
   D. Gamma

270. As the red blood cells disintegrate, hemoglobin is released and converted to the pigment bilirubin. Which organ is primarily responsible for this function?
   A. Spleen
   B. Kidneys
   C. Intestines
   D. Liver

271. Which of the following methods is *not* used for the quantification of serum bilirubin?
    A. Bilirubinometer
    B. Jendrassik and Grof
    C. Zimmerman
    D. Bilirubin oxidase

272. In which of the following conditions does no activity of glucuronyl transferase result in increased unconjugated bilirubin, kernicterus in neonates, and eventual death within 18 months?
    A. Gilbert's disease
    B. Dubin-Johnson syndrome
    C. Crigler-Najjar syndrome
    D. Physiological jaundice of the newborn

273. Which of the following reagent systems contains the components sulfanilic acid, hydrochloric acid, and sodium nitrite?
    A. Jaffe
    B. Zimmerman
    C. Diazo
    D. Lowry

274. Indirect-reacting bilirubin may be quantified by reacting it initially in which reagent?
    A. Dilute hydrochloric acid
    B. Dilute sulfuric acid
    C. Caffeine-sodium benzoate
    D. Sodium hydroxide

275. Which of the following methods employs a reaction where bilirubin is oxidized to colorless biliverdin?
    A. Bilirubinometer
    B. Bilirubin oxidase
    C. High-performance liquid chromatography
    D. Jendrassik-Grof

276. What collective term encompasses the reduction products stercobilinogen, urobilinogen, and mesobilirubinogen?
    A. Urobilinogen
    B. Mesobilirubinogen
    C. Urobilin
    D. Bilirubin

277. What condition is characterized by an elevation of total bilirubin primarily due to an increase in the conjugated bilirubin fraction?
    A. Hemolytic jaundice
    B. Neonatal jaundice
    C. Crigler-Najjar syndrome
    D. Obstructive jaundice

278. Which of the following is characteristic of hemolytic jaundice?
    A. Unconjugated serum bilirubin level increased
    B. Urinary bilirubin level increased
    C. Urinary urobilinogen level decreased
    D. Fecal urobilin level decreased

279. What may be the cause of neonatal physiological jaundice of the hepatic type?
    A. Hemolytic episode caused by an ABO incompatibility
    B. Stricture of the common bile duct
    C. Hemolytic episode caused by an Rh incompatibility
    D. Deficiency in the bilirubin conjugation enzyme system

280. Choose the diagnosis most consistent with the following laboratory findings:
    Serum: Total bilirubin 5.8 mg/dL
    Direct bilirubin 0.1 mg/dL
    Indirect bilirubin 5.7 mg/dL
    A. Physiologic jaundice of the newborn
    B. Posthepatic bile obstruction
    C. Dubin-Johnson syndrome
    D. Rotor's syndrome

281. Which of the following characterizes hepatic dysfunction in the early stage of viral hepatitis?
   A. Elevation in urobilinogen and urobilin excretion in the feces
   B. Elevation in the serum unconjugated bilirubin fraction
   C. Depression in the serum conjugated bilirubin fraction
   D. Depression in urinary urobilinogen excretion

282. Which of the following characterizes Crigler-Najjar syndrome?
   A. Inability to transport bilirubin from the sinusoidal membrane to the micro somal region
   B. Deficiency of the enzyme system required for conjugation of bilirubin
   C. Inability to transport bilirubin glucuronides to the bile canaliculi
   D. Severe liver cell damage accompanied by necrosis

283. Which of the following disorders is characterized by an inability to transport bilirubin from the sinusoidal membrane into the hepatocyte?
   A. Carcinoma of the common bile duct
   B. Crigler-Najjar syndrome
   C. Dubin-Johnson syndrome
   D. Gilbert syndrome

284. In which of the following states would you see an elevation in total bilirubin and conjugated bilirubin only?
   A. Biliary obstruction
   B. Hemolysis
   C. Neonatal jaundice
   D. Gilbert's disease

285. A healthy 28-year-old female sees her physician for a routine examination and has receives a "relatively" clean bill of health except for the results below.

   Total bilirubin 2.8 mg/dL
   Direct bilirubin 0.1 mg/dL
   Indirect bilirubin 2.7 mg/dL

   What do these results most likely indicate?
   A. Normal bilirubin metabolism
   B. Extrahepatic obstruction
   C. Dubin-Johnson syndrome
   D. Gilbert's disease

286. Which of the following disorders can be classified as a form of prehepatic jaundice?
   A. Acute hemolytic anemia
   B. Cirrhosis
   C. Dubin-Johnson syndrome
   D. Neoplasm of common bile duct

287. The following laboratory results are determined on a patient with a suggested diagnosis of biliary obstruction:

   Serum total bilirubin—increased
   Serum conjugated bilirubin—normal
   Urine bilirubin—increased
   Fecal urobilin—decreased

   Which laboratory result is the *least* consistent with such a diagnosis?
   A. Serum total bilirubin
   B. Serum conjugated bilirubin
   C. Urine bilirubin
   D. Fecal urobilin

288. A 42-year-old woman is admitted to the hospital with complaints of abdominal pain and inability to eat, which have gotten worse during the past several weeks. Although the pain had been uncomfortable, what alarmed her was noticing a slight yellow color in her eyes. Blood was drawn and the test results follow: total bilirubin 3.9 mg/dL, direct bilirubin 2.7 mg/dL, AST slightly elevated (three times the upper limit of the reference range), ALT slightly elevated (three times the upper limit of the reference range), alkaline phosphatase markedly elevated (six times the upper limit of the reference range), and urine urobilinogen decreased. What diagnosis do these test results support?
A. Viral hepatitis
B. Cirrhosis
C. Exposure to toxic chemicals
D. Biliary obstruction

289. Which of the following results is *least* consistent with a diagnosis of viral hepatitis?
A. Serum total bilirubin 7.5 mg/dL, direct bilirubin 5.5 mg/dL, indirect bilirubin 2.0 mg/dL
B. Urine urobilinogen increased
C. AST increased 10 times the upper limit of the reference range
D. ALT increased 13 times the upper limit of the reference range

Electrolytes and Osmolality

290. What is the normal renal threshold of sodium (measured in millimoles per liter)?
A. 80–85
B. 90–110
C. 110–130
D. 135–148

291. Of the total serum osmolality, sodium, chloride, and bicarbonate ions normally contribute approximately what percent?
A. 8
B. 45
C. 75
D. 92

292. The presence of only slightly visible hemolysis will significantly increase the serum level of which of the following electrolytes?
A. Sodium
B. Potassium
C. Chloride
D. Bicarbonate

293. Insulin release will stimulate the cellular uptake of which of the following electrolytes?
A. Sodium
B. Potassium
C. Chloride
D. Bicarbonate

294. Hyponatremia may be caused by depletional and dilutional causes. Which of the following is a dilutional cause of hyponatremia?
A. Renal loss
B. Skin damage
C. Syndrome of inappropriate ADH secretion (SIADH)
D. Acute myocardial infraction

295. Which of the following is a spectrophotometric method for quantifying serum chloride?
A. Ferric perchlorate
B. Ammonium molybdate
C. Bathophenanthroline
D. Cresolphthalein complexone

296. Which of the following values is the threshold critical value (alert or action level) for low plasma potassium?
   A. 1.5 mmol/L
   B. 2.0 mmol/L
   C. 2.5 mmol/L
   D. 3.5 mmol/L

297. Which of the following describes the correct meaning of anion gap = 15 mmol/L?
   A. There is a 15 mmol/L gap between the major measured cations and major measured anions.
   B. There is a 15 mmol/L gap between the major physiologically active cations and major physiologically active measured anions.
   C. There are 15 mmol/L more cations than anions in the plasma.
   D. There are 15 mmol/L more anions than cations in the plasma.

298. A patient presents with Addison disease. Serum sodium and potassium analyses are performed. What would the results reveal?
   A. Normal sodium, low potassium levels
   B. Low sodium, low potassium levels
   C. Low sodium, high potassium levels
   D. High sodium, low potassium levels

299. Primary aldosteronism results from a tumor of the adrenal cortex. How would the extracellular fluid be affected?
   A. Normal sodium, decreased potassium levels
   B. Decreased sodium, decreased potassium levels
   C. Decreased sodium, increased potassium levels
   D. Increased sodium, decreased potassium levels

300. Which of the following electrolytes is likely to be found decreased in metabolic alkalosis?
   A. Sodium
   B. Potassium
   C. Chloride
   D. Bicarbonate

301. Of the total serum calcium, free ionized calcium normally represents approximately what percent?
   A. 10
   B. 40
   C. 50
   D. 90

302. Measuring the tubular reabsorption of phosphate is useful in diagnosing diseases that affect which of the following organs?
   A. Liver
   B. Adrenal gland
   C. Thyroid gland
   D. Parathyroid gland

303. Acute metabolic acidosis resulting from acid with an associated anion promotes an increase in the plasma level of which electrolyte?
   A. Sodium
   B. Potassium
   C. Chloride
   D. Bicarbonate

304. Which of the following is an effect of increased parathyroid hormone secretion?
   A. Decreased blood calcium levels
   B. Increased renal reabsorption of phosphate
   C. Decreased bone resorption
   D. Increased intestinal absorption of calcium

305. The following laboratory results are obtained on a 60-year-old woman who is complaining of anorexia, constipation, abdominal pain, nausea, and vomiting:

     Ionized serum calcium—elevated
     Serum inorganic phosphate—decreased
     Urine calcium—elevated
     Urine phosphate—elevated

     What do these results suggest?
     A. Primary hyperparathyroidism
     B. Vitamin D deficiency
     C. Hypoparathyroidism
     D. Paget disease

306. Secondary hyperparathyroidism is often the result of
     A. Vitamin C deficiency
     B. Liver disease
     C. Renal disease
     D. Thyroid disease

307. Which of the following reagents is used to determine the concentration of serum inorganic phosphate?
     A. Ehrlich's reagent
     B. Ammonium molybdate
     C. 8-Hydroxyquinoline
     D. Bathophenanthroline

308. Which of the following reagents is used in a colorimetric method to quantify the concentration of serum calcium?
     A. Cresolphthalein complexone
     B. Lanthanum
     C. Malachite green
     D. Amino-naphthol-sulfonic acid

309. Which of the following has an effect on plasma calcium levels?
     A. Sodium
     B. Inorganic phosphate
     C. Potassium
     D. Iron

310. A patient's serum inorganic phosphate level is found to be elevated but the physician cannot determine a physiological basis for this abnormal result. What could possibly have caused an erroneous result to be reported?
     A. Patient not fasting when blood was drawn
     B. Specimen was hemolyzed
     C. Effect of diurnal variation
     D. Patient receiving intravenous glucose therapy

311. To what metal does ceruloplasmin firmly bind?
     A. Chromium
     B. Copper
     C. Zinc
     D. Iron

312. In iron-deficiency anemia, what would be the expected percent saturation of transferrin with iron?
     A. Less than 15
     B. Between 30 and 40
     C. Between 40 and 50
     D. Greater than 55

313. What is the primary storage form of iron?
     A. Apotransferrin
     B. Myoglobin
     C. Ferritin
     D. Hemosiderin

314. A serum ferritin level may not be a useful indicator of iron-deficiency anemia in patients with what type of disorder?
     A. Chronic infection
     B. Malignancy
     C. Viral hepatitis
     D. All the above

315. The first reaction step in the colorimetric measurement of serum iron involves which of the following steps?
   A. The reaction of iron with a ligand
   B. The reaction of iron with a reducing substance
   C. The reaction of bound iron with a releasing substance
   D. The reaction of iron with transferrin

316. In what disorder would an increased percent saturation of transferrin be expected?
   A. Hemochromatosis
   B. Iron-deficiency anemia
   C. Myocardial infarction
   D. Malignancy

317. Which of the following disorders is best characterized by these laboratory results?
   Serum iron—decreased
   Total iron-binding capacity—increased
   Transferrin saturation—decreased
   Serum ferritin—decreased
   Free erythrocyte protoporphyrin—increased
   A. Anemia of chronic disease
   B. Thalassemia
   C. Iron-deficiency anemia
   D. Hemochromatosis

318. A patient has the following results:
   Analyte ________ Patient values
   Serum Iron 250 μg/dL
   TIBC 350 μg/dL
   The results most likely indicate:
   A. Normal iron status
   B. Iron deficiency anemia
   C. Chronic disease
   D. Iron hemochromatosis

319. Which of the following constituents normally present in serum must be chemically eliminated so that it will not interfere with the measurement of serum magnesium?
   A. Calcium
   B. Chloride
   C. Iron
   D. Potassium

320. In the collection of plasma specimens for lactate determinations, which of the following anticoagulants would be more appropriate?
   A. Sodium heparin
   B. Sodium citrate
   C. EDTA
   D. Oxalate plus fluoride

321. Which of the following disorders is characterized by increased production of chloride in sweat?
   A. Multiple myeloma
   B. Hypoparathyroidism
   C. Cystic fibrosis
   D. Wilson disease

322. Which form of iron is the only form that will react with the ligand in the serum iron methodology?
   A. Albumin bound iron
   B. Ferrous
   C. Ferric
   D. Transferrin bound iron

323. Which of the following describes the basis for the freezing point osmometer?
   A. The freezing point depression is directly proportional to the amount of solvent present.
   B. The freezing point depression varies as the logarithm of the concentration of solute.
   C. The freezing point is raised by an amount that is inversely proportional to the concentration of dissolved particles in the solution.
   D. The freezing point is lowered by an amount that is directly proportional to the concentration of dissolved particles in the solution.

324. Given the following information, calculate the plasma osmolality in milliosmoles per kilogram: sodium—142 mmol/L; glucose—130 mg/dL; and urea nitrogen—18 mg/dL.
A. 290
B. 291
C. 295
D. 298

325. Which of the following may be associated with the colloid osmotic pressure (COP) osmometer?
A. Utilizes a cooling bath set at –7°C
B. Measures total serum osmolality
C. Negative pressure on reference (saline) side equivalent to COP of sample
D. Measures contribution of electrolytes to osmolality

Acid-Base Metabolism

326. Which is the most predominant buffer system in the body?
A. Bicarbonate/carbonic acid
B. Acetate/acetic acid
C. Phosphate/phosphorous acid
D. Hemoglobin

327. The measurement of the pressure of dissolved CO_2 (PCO_2) in the blood is most closely associated with the concentration of what substance?
A. pH
B. Bicarbonate (HCO_3^-)
C. Carbonic acid (H_2CO_3)
D. PO_2

328. What is the term that describes the sum of carbonic acid and bicarbonate in plasma?
A. Total CO_2
B. Standard bicarbonate
C. Buffer base
D. Base excess

329. To maintain a pH of 7.4 in plasma, it is necessary to maintain a
A. 10:1 ratio of bicarbonate to carbonic acid.
B. 20:1 ratio of bicarbonate to carbonic acid.
C. 1:20 ratio of bicarbonate to carbonic acid.
D. 20:1 ratio of carbonic acid to bicarbonate.

330. In the plasma, an excess in the concentration of bicarbonate without a change in PCO_2 from normal will result in what physiological state?
A. Respiratory acidosis
B. Respiratory alkalosis
C. Metabolic acidosis
D. Metabolic alkalosis

331. Which of the following characterizes respiratory acidosis?
A. Excess of bicarbonate
B. Deficit of bicarbonate
C. Excess of dissolved carbon dioxide (PCO_2)
D. Deficit of dissolved carbon dioxide (PCO_2)

332. What is the specimen of choice for analysis of acid-base disturbances involving pulmonary dysfunction in an adult?
A. Venous blood
B. Arterial blood
C. Capillary blood
D. Urine

333. What is the anticoagulant of choice for blood gas analysis?
A. EDTA
B. Heparin
C. Sodium fluoride
D. Citrate

334. If a blood gas specimen is left exposed to air, which of the following changes will occur?
   A. PO_2 and pH increase; PCO_2 decreases
   B. PO_2 and pH decrease; PCO_2 increases
   C. PO_2 increases; pH and PCO_2 decrease
   D. PO_2 decreases; pH and PCO_2 increase

335. How would blood gas parameters change if a sealed specimen is left at room temperature for 2 or more hours?
   A. PO_2 increases, PCO_2 increases, pH increases
   B. PO_2 decreases, PCO_2 decreases, pH decreases
   C. PO_2 decreases, PCO_2 increases, pH decreases
   D. PO_2 increases, PCO_2 increases, pH decreases

336. The bicarbonate ion concentration may be calculated from the total CO_2 and PCO_2 blood levels by using which of the following formulas?
   A. $0.03 \times (PCO_2 - \text{total } CO_2)$
   B. $(\text{total } CO_2 + 0.03) \times PCO_2$
   C. $0.03 \times (\text{total } CO_2 - PO_2)$
   D. $\text{total } CO_2 - (0.03 \times PCO_2)$

337. In order to maintain electrical neutrality in the red blood cell, bicarbonate leaves the red blood cell and enters the plasma through an exchange mechanism with what electrolyte?
   A. Sodium
   B. Potassium
   C. Chloride
   D. Phosphate

338. In acute diabetic ketoacidosis, which of the following laboratory findings would be expected?
   A. Fasting blood glucose elevated, pH elevated, ketone bodies present
   B. Fasting blood glucose elevated, pH low, ketone bodies present
   C. Fasting blood glucose elevated, pH normal, ketone bodies absent
   D. Fasting blood glucose decreased, pH low, ketone bodies absent

339. Which of the following is a cause of metabolic alkalosis?
   A. Late stage of salicylate poisoning
   B. Uncontrolled diabetes mellitus
   C. Renal failure
   D. Excessive vomiting

340. Which of the following statements is *true* about partially compensated respiratory alkalosis?
   A. PCO_2 is higher than normal.
   B. HCO_3^- is higher than normal.
   C. More CO_2 is eliminated through the lungs by hyperventilation.
   D. Renal reabsorption of HCO_3^- is decreased.

341. Which is a compensatory mechanism in respiratory acidosis?
   A. Hypoventilation
   B. Decreased reabsorption of bicarbonate by the kidneys
   C. Increased Na^+/H^+ exchange by the kidneys
   D. Decreased ammonia formation by the kidneys

342. Which of the following will cause a shift of the oxygen dissociation curve to the right, resulting in a decreased affinity of hemoglobin for O_2?
   A. Low plasma pH level
   B. Low PCO_2 level
   C. Low concentration of 2,3-bisphosphoglycerate
   D. Low temperature

343. Which of the following statements about carbonic anhydrase (CA) is *true?*
   A. Catalyzes conversion of CO_2 and H_2O to $HHCO_3$ in red blood cells
   B. Causes shift to the left in oxygen dissociation curve
   C. Catalyzes formation of H_2CO_3 from CO_2 and H_2O in the tissues
   D. Inactive in renal tubular cells

344. Which of the following statements best describes "base excess"?
   A. Primarily refers to carbonic acid concentration
   B. Positive values reflect metabolic alkalosis
   C. Created through metabolism of carbohydrates
   D. Negative values represent a respiratory imbalance

345. Given the following information, calculate the blood pH.
   $PCO_2 = 44$ mm Hg
   Total $CO_2 = 29$ mmol/L
   A. 6.28
   B. 6.76
   C. 7.42
   D. 7.44

346. A 75-year-old woman comes to her physician complaining of abdominal pain. She says she has had a sore stomach for the last 3 weeks and has been taking increasing doses of antacid pills to control it. Now she is taking a box of pills a day. Blood gases are drawn with the following results: pH = 7.49, $PCO_2 = 59$ mm Hg, $HCO_3^- =$ 34 mmol/L. What do these data indicate?
   A. Metabolic alkalosis, partially compensated
   B. Respiratory acidosis, uncompensated
   C. A dual problem of acidosis
   D. An error in one of the blood gas measurements

347. A 24-year-old drug abuser is brought into the emergency department unconscious. He has shallow breaths, looks pale, and is "clammy." Blood gases show the following results: pH = 7.29, $PCO_2 = 50$ mm Hg, $HCO_3^- = 25$ mmol/L. What condition is indicated by these results?
   A. Metabolic alkalosis, partially compensated
   B. Respiratory acidosis, uncompensated
   C. A dual problem of acidosis
   D. An error in one of the blood gas measurements

348. Blood gases are drawn on a 68-year-old asthmatic who was recently admitted for treatment of a kidney infection. Blood gas results are as follows: pH = 7.25, $PCO_2 =$ 56 mm Hg, $HCO_3^- = 16$ mmol/L. What condition is indicated by these results?
   A. Metabolic alkalosis, partially compensated
   B. Respiratory acidosis, uncompensated
   C. A dual problem of acidosis
   D. An error in one of the blood gas measurements

349. A mother brings her daughter, a 22-year-old medical technology student, to her physician. The patient is hyperventilating and has glossy eyes. The mother explains that her daughter is scheduled to take her final course exam the next morning. The patient had been running around frantically all day in a worried state and then started to breathe heavily. Blood gases are drawn in the office with the following results: pH = 7.58, PCO_2 = 55 mm Hg, $HCO_3^- = 18$ mmol/L. What do these data indicate?
   A. Metabolic alkalosis, partially compensated
   B. Respiratory acidosis, uncompensated
   C. A dual problem of acidosis
   D. An error in one of the blood gas measurements

Endocrinology

350. Secretion of hormones by the anterior pituitary may be controlled by the circulating levels of hormones from the respective target gland, as well as hormones secreted by what organ?
    A. Posterior lobe of the pituitary gland
    B. Intermediate lobe of the pituitary gland
    C. Hypothalamus
    D. Adrenal medulla

351. An elevated level of which of the following hormones will inhibit pituitary secretion of adrenocorticotropic hormone (ACTH)?
    A. Aldosterone
    B. Cortisol
    C. 17β-Estradiol
    D. Progesterone

352. Which of the following is the major mineralocorticoid?
    A. Aldosterone
    B. Cortisol
    C. Corticosterone
    D. Testosterone

353. Plasma renin activity (PRA) measurements are usually made by measuring which of the following using immunoassay?
    A. Angiotensinogen
    B. Angiotensin I
    C. Angiotensin II
    D. Angiotensin-converting enzyme

354. What effect would a low-salt diet, upright position, and diuretics have on the following test results?
    A. Renin ↑, aldosterone ↑, hypernatremia, hypokalemia
    B. Renin ↑, aldosterone ↓, hypernatremia, hypokalemia
    C. Renin ↓, aldosterone ↓, hyponatremia, hyperkalemia
    D. Renin ↓, aldosterone ↑, hyponatremia, hyperkalemia

355. As a screening test for Cushing syndrome, the physician wishes to see whether a patient exhibits normal diurnal rhythm in his or her cortisol secretion. At what time should the specimens be drawn for plasma cortisol determination?
    A. 6 A.M., 2 P.M.
    B. 8 A.M., 4 P.M.
    C. 12 noon, 6 P.M.
    D. 12 noon, 12 midnight

356. A patient is suspected of having Addison disease. His symptoms are weakness, fatigue, loss of weight, skin pigmentation, and hypoglycemia. His laboratory tests show low serum sodium and chloride, elevated serum potassium, and elevated urine sodium and chloride levels. The serum cortisol level is decreased and the plasma ACTH is increased. To make a definitive diagnosis, the physician orders an ACTH stimulation test, and serum cortisol levels are measured. If the patient has primary hypoadrenocortical function (Addison disease), what would be the expected level of serum cortisol following stimulation? If the patient has hypopituitarism and secondary hypoadrenocortical function, what would be the expected level of serum cortisol following stimulation?
    A. Increase from baseline; decrease from baseline
    B. Decrease from baseline; increase from baseline
    C. Slight increase from baseline; no change from baseline
    D. No change from baseline; slight increase from baseline

357. What does the concentration of urinary free cortisol mainly reflect?
    A. Total serum cortisol
    B. Conjugated cortisol
    C. Unbound serum cortisol
    D. Protein-bound serum cortisol

358. A 30-year-old woman is admitted to the hospital. She has truncal obesity, buffalo humpback, moon face, purple striae, hypertension, hyperglycemia, increased facial hair, acne, and amenorrhea. The physician orders endocrine testing. The results are as follows:

Test	Result
Urine Free Cortisol	78 μg/dL
Salivary Cortisol	1.3 μg/dL
Plasma ACTH	3.6 μg/dL

What is the most probable diagnosis?
A. Pituitary adenoma
B. Ectopic ACTH lung cancer
C. Adrenal adenoma
D. Addison disease

359. Which of the following is the most common cause of the adrenogenital syndrome called congenital adrenal hyperplasia, and which test is used for its diagnosis?
A. 17α-Hydroxylase deficiency; progesterone assay
B. 21-Hydroxylase deficiency; 17α -hydroxyprogesterone assay
C. 3β-Hydroxysteroid dehydrogenaseisomerase deficiency; 17α-hydroxypregnenolone assay
D. 11β-Hydroxylase deficiency; 11-deoxycortisol assay

360. Which of the following is the most potent androgen?
A. Androstenedione
B. Dehydroepiandrosterone
C. Androsterone
D. Testosterone

361. Stimulation of the pituitary to produce gonadotropins is regulated by the release of __________ from the hypothalamus.
A. FSH
B. LH
C. GnRH
D. None of the above

362. Which of the following is the most potent estrogen and is considered to be the true ovarian hormone?
A. Estriol (E_3)
B. Estrone (E_1)
C. 17β-Estradiol (E_2)
D. 16α-Hydroxyestrone

363. During pregnancy in the second trimester, human chorionic gonadotropin (hCG) levels __________ and progesterone and estriol levels __________.
A. Increase, increase
B. Increase, decrease
C. Decrease, increase
D. Decrease, decrease

364. Which of the following is *not* quantified in the triple test for Down syndrome?
A. α_1-Fetoprotein
B. Unconjugated estriol
C. Progesterone
D. Human chorionic gonadotropin

365. Because of infertility problems, a physician would like to determine when a woman ovulates. The physician orders serial assays of plasma progesterone. From these assays, how can the physician recognize when ovulation occurs?
A. After ovulation, progesterone rapidly increases
B. After ovulation, progesterone rapidly decreases
C. Right before ovulation, progesterone rapidly increases
D. There is a gradual, steady increase in progesterone throughout the menstrual cycle.

366. The placenta secretes numerous hormones both protein and steroid. Which of the following hormones is not secreted by the placenta?
A. Human chorionic gonadotropin (hCG)
B. Estrogen
C. Human placental lactogen (HPL)
D. Luteinizing hormone (LH)

367. During pregnancy, estriol is synthesized in the placenta from _________ formed in the _________.
A. Estradiol, mother
B. Estradiol, fetus
C. 16α-Hydroxy-DHEA-S, mother
D. 16α-Hydroxy-DHEA-S, fetus

368. What percentage decrease in plasma or urinary estriol, in comparison with the previous day's level, is considered significant during pregnancy?
A. 5
B. 10
C. 25
D. 40

369. Which of the following basic reproductive cells is responsible for maturation of sperm?
A. Leydig cells
B. Theca cells
C. Granulosa cells
D. Sertoli cells

370. When do the highest levels of gonadotropins occur?
A. During the follicular phase of the menstrual cycle
B. During the luteal phase of the menstrual cycle
C. At the midpoint of the menstrual cycle
D. Several days prior to ovulation

371. What would be an example of ectopic hormone production?
A. Prolactin production by pituitary tumors
B. Calcitonin production by thyroid tumors
C. Growth hormone production by lung tumors
D. Cortisol production by adrenal tumors

372. Which of the following hormones initiates its response by diffusing through the cell membrane and binding to cytoplasmic receptors?
A. Estradiol
B. Epinephrine
C. Growth hormone
D. Follicle-stimulating hormone

373. The adrenal medulla secretes which of the following in the greatest quantity?
A. Metanephrine
B. Norepinephrine
C. Epinephrine
D. Dopamine

374. In a patient who is suspected of having pheochromocytoma, measurement of which of the following would be most useful?
A. Metanephrine
B. Homovanillic acid
C. 5-Hydroxyindoleacetic acid
D. Homogentisic acid

375. Diabetes insipidus is associated with depressed secretion of which of the following hormones?
A. Prolactin
B. Antidiuretic hormone
C. Growth hormone
D. Oxytocin

376. A 4-year-old girl presents with a palpable abdominal mass, pallor, and petechiae. Based on family history, clinical findings, and the patient's physical examination, neuroblastoma is suspected. Which of the following does *not* support such a diagnosis?
A. Increased blood dopamine levels
B. Increased blood epinephrine levels
C. Increased urinary homovanillic acid
D. Decreased urinary vanillylmandelic acid

377. Of which of the following is 5-hydroxy indoleacetic acid (5-HIAA) the primary metabolite?
A. Epinephrine
B. Norepinephrine
C. Serotonin
D. Prolactin

378. Which of the following functions as an inhibiting factor for somatotropin release?
A. Gonadotropin-releasing hormone
B. Growth hormone-releasing hormone
C. Somatomedin
D. Somatostatin

379. Which of the following hormones is used to determine the cause of infertility, to track ovulation, and increases in concentration if fertilization of the egg occurs?
A. Progesterone
B. Testosterone
C. FSH
D. LH

380. The secretion of which of the following is controlled by growth hormone?
A. Growth hormone-releasing hormone
B. Corticotropin-releasing hormone
C. Somatomedin
D. Somatostatin

381. Which of the following would be elevated in the blood in medullary carcinoma of the thyroid?
A. Calcitonin
B. Thyroxine
C. Catecholamines
D. Secretin

382. What is the predominant form of thyroid hormone in the circulation?
A. Thyroxine
B. Triiodothyronine
C. Diiodotyrosine
D. Monoiodotyrosine

383. Once synthesized, the thyroid hormones are stored as a component of thyroglobulin in what area of the thyroid gland?
A. Epithelial cell wall of the follicle
B. Colloid in the follicle
C. Isthmus of the thyroid gland
D. Extracellular space of the thyroid gland

384. How is the majority of reverse T_3 (rT_3) made?
A. Peripheral deiodination of T_4
B. Peripheral deiodination of T_3
C. From T_3 in the thyroid gland
D. From thyroglobulin in the thyroid gland

385. Which of the following is an autoantibody that binds to TSH receptor sites on thyroid cell membranes, preventing thyroid-stimulating hormone from binding?
A. Antithyroglobulin antibodies
B. Thyroid antimicrosomal antibodies
C. Thyrotropin-receptor antibodies
D. Antithyroid peroxidase antibodies

386. In a patient with suspected primary hyperthyroidism associated with Graves disease, one would expect the following laboratory serum results: free thyroxine (FT_4) ________, thyroid hormone binding ratio (THBR) ________, and thyroid-stimulating hormone (TSH) ________.
A. Increased, decreased, increased
B. Increased, decreased, decreased
C. Increased, increased, decreased
D. Decreased, decreased, increased

387. In a patient suspected of having primary myxedema, one would expect the following serum results: free thyroxine (FT_4) ________, thyroid hormone binding ratio (THBR) ________, and thyroid-stimulating hormone (TSH) ________.
A. Decreased, increased, decreased
B. Increased, increased, decreased
C. Decreased, decreased, increased
D. Increased, decreased, increased

388. Thyroid-releasing hormone (TRH) is given to a patient. Serum thyroid-stimulating hormone (TSH) levels are taken before and after the injection, and the values are the same—low. This patient probably has which of the following disorders?
   A. Primary hypothyroidism
   B. Secondary hypothyroidism
   C. Tertiary hypothyroidism
   D. Iodine deficiency

389. The presence of a very high titer for antithyroglobulin antibodies and the detection of antithyroid peroxidase antibodies is highly suggestive of what disorder?
   A. Pernicious anemia
   B. Hashimoto thyroiditis
   C. Multinodular goiter
   D. Thyroid adenoma

390. What is the major carrier protein of the thyroid hormones in the blood?
   A. Albumin
   B. Thyroxine-binding globulin
   C. Thyroxine-binding prealbumin
   D. Thyroglobulin

391. Why are the total thyroxine (T_4) levels increased in pregnant women and women who take oral contraceptives?
   A. Inappropriate iodine metabolism
   B. Changes in tissue use
   C. Changes in concentration of thyroxine-binding globulin (TBG)
   D. Changes in thyroglobulin synthesis

392. Which of the following is the Hollander insulin test used to confirm?
   A. Hyperglycemia
   B. Vagotomy
   C. Pancreatectomy
   D. Insulinoma

393. Zollinger-Ellison syndrome is characterized by an elevated blood level of which of the following?
   A. Trypsin
   B. Pepsin
   C. Gastrin
   D. Cholecystokinin-pancreozymin

394. When performing parathyroid surgery for adenoma resection, parathyroid hormone is quantified at three points relative to the surgical procedure: baseline prior to incision, second baseline with gland exposure, and third sample at postexcision. Which of the following is *not* correct in assessing the PTH values?
   A. The second baseline value should be higher than the first baseline.
   B. The first baseline value should be the highest value of the three samples.
   C. The postexcision value should be at least 50% of or lower than the second baseline.
   D. The lack of decrease in the PTH value postexcision indicates possible multigland disease.

Therapeutic Drug Monitoring and Toxicology

395. Levels of 8–9% carboxyhemoglobin saturation of whole blood are commonly found in which of the following situations?
   A. Fatal carbon monoxide poisoning
   B. Acute carbon monoxide poisoning
   C. Nonsmoking residents of rural areas
   D. People who smoke cigarettes and cigars

396. Which of the following methods would yield reliable quantification of ethanol in the presence of isopropanol?
   A. Reaction with permanganate and chromotropic acid
   B. Conway diffusion followed by dichromate reaction
   C. Alcohol dehydrogenase reaction
   D. Gas-liquid chromatography

397. Which of the following tests would be particularly useful in determining isopropanol exposure?
A. Serum osmolality and urine acetone
B. Urine osmolality and serum osmolality
C. Urine acetone and urine osmolality
D. Serum sodium and serum acetone

398. A nurse calls the laboratory for a peak drug level on a patient already on oral digoxin for the past 2 weeks. The half-life of digoxin is 5 hours. When should the peak blood level of digoxin be drawn?
A. 15–30 minutes after the next dose
B. 1–2 hours after the next dose
C. Immediately before the next dose
D. 25 hours after the next dose

399. Heroin is synthesized from what drug?
A. Diazepam
B. Morphine
C. Ecgonine
D. Chlorpromazine

400. After absorption, codeine is rapidly metabolized to what compound?
A. Phencyclidine
B. Morphine
C. Methadone
D. Propoxyphene

401. THC (Δ^9-tetrahydrocannabinol) is the principal active component of what drug?
A. Benzodiazepine
B. Marijuana
C. Morphine
D. Codeine

402. Identification of the urinary metabolite benzoylecgonine would be useful in determining exposure to which of the following drugs?
A. Codeine
B. Cocaine
C. Amphetamine
D. Propoxyphene

403. Of the following specimens, which would be appropriate for determining exposure to lead?
A. EDTA plasma
B. Serum
C. Whole blood
D. Cerebrospinal fluid

404. Free erythrocyte protoporphyrin (FEP) levels are useful as a screening method for exposure to which of the following metals?
A. Zinc
B. Lead
C. Iron
D. Mercury

405. Anticoagulated whole blood is the preferred specimen in determining exposure to what compound?
A. Methanol
B. Mercury
C. Acetaminophen
D. Carbon monoxide

406. What is the approximate number of half-life periods required for a serum drug concentration to reach 97–99% of the steady state?
A. 1–3
B. 2–4
C. 5–7
D. 7–9

407. For what colorimetric determination is the Trinder reaction widely used?
A. Acetaminophen
B. Propoxyphene
C. Salicylate
D. Barbiturate

408. Acetaminophen is particularly toxic to what organ?
A. Heart
B. Kidney
C. Spleen
D. Liver

409. Which of the following is an example of a long-acting barbiturate?
   A. Phenobarbital
   B. Amobarbital
   C. Secobarbital
   D. Pentobarbital

410. Increased trough levels of aminoglycosides in the serum are often associated with toxic effects to which organ?
   A. Heart
   B. Kidney
   C. Pancreas
   D. Liver

411. Which of the following is an example of an antiarrhythmic drug that has a metabolite with the same action?
   A. Quinidine
   B. Digoxin
   C. Procainamide
   D. Nortriptyline

412. In what form must a drug be in order to elicit a pharmacologic response?
   A. Free
   B. Bound to albumin
   C. Bound to globulins
   D. Bound to fatty acids

413. A patient receiving phenytoin for epilepsy develops acute glomerulonephritis. What change, if any, would be expected in the patient's circulating drug level?
   A. Decrease in free drug
   B. Increase in free drug
   C. Increase in protein-bound drug
   D. No change in circulating drug level

414. Free drug levels can generally be determined by analyzing what body fluid?
   A. Whole blood
   B. Ultrafiltrate of plasma
   C. Urine
   D. Protein-free filtrate of plasma

415. Which of the following drugs is used as an immunosuppressant in organ transplantation, especially in liver transplants?
   A. Methotrexate
   B. Amiodarone
   C. Tacrolimus
   D. Paroxetine

416. Which of the following is a commonly encountered xanthine that could potentially interfere with the determination of theophylline?
   A. Nicotine
   B. Caffeine
   C. Amphetamine
   D. Procainamide

417. What is the major active metabolite of the anticonvulsant drug primidone?
   A. Phenytoin
   B. Acetazolamide
   C. NAPA
   D. Phenobarbital

418. Nortriptyline is the active metabolite of which of the following drugs?
   A. Amitriptyline
   B. Desipramine
   C. Imipramine
   D. Doxepin

419. Which of the following is used in the treatment of manic depression?
   A. Potassium
   B. Lithium
   C. Calcium
   D. Chloride

420. When is a blood sample for determination of the trough level of a drug appropriately drawn?
   A. During the absorption phase of the drug
   B. During the distribution phase of the drug
   C. Shortly before drug administration
   D. Two hours after drug administration

421. In regard to drug distribution patterns, which of the following statements is *false?*
A. Drug metabolism is slower in newborns than adults.
B. Drug metabolism is more rapid for 6-year-old children than for adults.
C. Renal clearance of drugs is faster in newborns than adults.
D. Drug metabolism often changes during pubescence.

422. Which of the following serum components is able to alter the free drug level in plasma?
A. Creatinine
B. Urea
C. Albumin
D. Calcium

423. Which of the following is an example of a phenothiazine drug?
A. Cyclosporine
B. Theophylline
C. Phenytoin
D. Chlorpromazine

424. What is the recommended name for diphenylhydantoin?
A. Phenytoin
B. Nalorphine
C. Primidone
D. Carbamazepine

425. Which of the following classes of compounds has a sedative effect and as such is used to treat anxiety?
A. Amphetamines
B. Opiates
C. Cannabinoids
D. Benzodiazepines

426. What is the active metabolite of the antiarrhythmic drug procainamide?
A. Pronestyl
B. Disopyramide
C. PEMA
D. NAPA

427. Which of the following drugs is used as a bronchodilator?
A. Theophylline
B. Phenytoin
C. Amikacin
D. Clozapine

Vitamins

428. Which of the following techniques is more commonly used to measure vitamins?
A. High-performance liquid chromatography
B. Spectrophotometry
C. Nephelometry
D. Microbiological

429. In the United States, most cases of scurvy occur in children between the ages of 7 months to 2 years. Scurvy is a disease caused by a deficiency in which of the following?
A. Vitamin A
B. Vitamin C
C. Vitamin D
D. Vitamin K

430. The term "lipid" encompasses a wide variety of compounds characterized as being insoluble in water but soluble in nonpolar solvents. Which of the following vitamins is *not* classified as fat soluble?
A. Vitamin A
B. Vitamin C
C. Vitamin D
D. Vitamin E

431. Measuring which of the following compounds is useful in the diagnosis of steatorrhea?
A. Vitamin B_{12}
B. Vitamin C
C. Carotenoids
D. Folic acid

432. Which of the following is another name for vitamin B_{12}?
   A. Retinol
   B. Pyridoxine
   C. Cyanocobalamin
   D. Riboflavin

433. Which of the following represents the preferred sample collection for the analysis of vitamin B_{12}?
   A. Nonfasting sample collected in EDTA
   B. Fasting sample collected in EDTA
   C. Fasting sample collected in heparin
   D. Nonfasting sample collected in heparin

434. Which of the following tissues is important in vitamin D metabolism?
   A. Skin
   B. Spleen
   C. Pancreas
   D. Thyroid

435. A deficiency in which of the following leads to increased clotting time and may result in hemorrhagic disease in infancy?
   A. Riboflavin
   B. Pyridoxine
   C. Tocopherols
   D. Menaquinone

436. Which vitamin is a constituent of two redox coenzymes?
   A. Vitamin A
   B. Vitamin B_2
   C. Vitamin B_6
   D. Vitamin C

437. Which disorder is associated with thiamin deficiency?
   A. Beriberi
   B. Pellagra
   C. Rickets
   D. Dermatitis

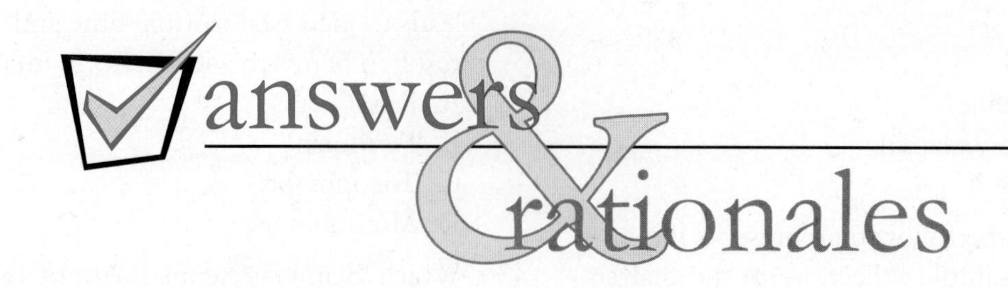

Instrumentation and Analytical Principles

1.

A. A tungsten-filament lamp is the most common light source for photometry in the visible region. It provides a continuous spectrum (360–800 nm) from the near infrared (IR) through the visible to the near ultraviolet (UV) region. Most of the radiant energy is in the near IR. Only about 15% is in the visible region—the region usually used. Because of the large emission in the near IR, tungsten lamps generate a significant amount of heat. Hydrogen and deuterium lamps are used for work in the 200–375 nm range. The mercury vapor lamp does not provide a continuous spectrum, emitting radiation at specific wavelengths.

2.

B. Photometric methods are based on the use of Beer's law, which is applicable only for monochromatic light. A monochromator is a device for selecting a narrow band of wavelengths from a continuous spectrum. The three kinds of monochromators are filters, prisms, and diffraction gratings.

3.

B. The unique feature of a hollow cathode lamp used in atomic absorption spectroscopy is that it, unlike others, is lined with the element of interest. The hollow cathode lamp contains traces of a particular element to be analyzed. Heat from the lamp causes the element to emit light of energies that are characteristic of the element. If the sample contains this element, these energies will be strongly absorbed because the same orbital energy levels are involved.

4.

A. A monochromator is a device used in spectroscopy to isolate specified wavelengths of light to impinge on the sample of interest.

5.

D. Photodiode array detectors are designed with 256–2048 photodiodes that are arranged in a linear fashion. This arrangement allows each photodiode to respond to a specific wavelength that results in a continuous UV/visible spectrum. Resolution is generally 1–2 nm.

6.

D. Wavelength calibration of a spectrophotometer is performed to verify that the radiant energy emitted from the monochromator through the exit slit is the same as the wavelength selector indicates. The glass filters holmium oxide, used in the UV and visible ranges, and didymium, used in the visible and near IR regions, are employed to check wavelength accuracy. Solutions of stable chromogens such as nickel sulfate may be used. Source lamps may be replaced with mercury-vapor or deuterium lamps. These lamps have strong emission lines and provide the most accurate method of wavelength calibration.

7.

D. The reagent blank contains the same reagents as those used for assaying the specimen. By adjusting the spectrophotometer to 100%*T* (or 0 absorbance) with the reagent blank, the instrument automatically subtracts the color contributed by the reagents from each succeeding reading of specimens, controls, and standards. This technique is used both in manual procedures and automated instruments. Because the reagent blank does not contain sample, there is no correction for interfering chromogens or lipemia.

8.

D. Fluorescent polarization immunoassay is a technique where the polarization of the fluorescence from a fluorescein-antigen conjugate is determined by its rate of rotation during the lifetime of the excited state in solution. A small, rapidly rotating fluorescein-antigen conjugate has a low degree of polarization; however, binding to a large antibody molecule slows the rate of rotation and increases the degree of polarization.

9.

C. The bandpass or bandwidth is the range of wavelengths that are passed by a monochromator. In the example given, the bandpass will permit a 10-nm range of wavelengths to pass through the monochromator and impinge on the sample solution in the cuvet. Thus, 540 ± 5 nm (10-nm bandpass) will be equivalent to a wavelength range of 535–545 nm.

10.

A. When the absorbance of a sample in solution varies directly with the concentration of the sample, Beer's law is followed. In turn, when the absorbance increases exponentially with an increase in the light path, the Lambert law is followed. Incorporation of these two laws may be stated as $A = abc$, where A = absorbance, a = absorptivity of the substance being measured, b = light path in cm, and c = concentration of the measured substance. When the Beer-Lambert law is applied to spectrophotometric analyses of standards and unknown samples that are being measured, the following equation is derived: $A_u \times C_s/A_s = C_u$, where A_u = absorbance of unknown, C_u = concentration of unknown, A_s = absorbance of standard, and A_u = absorbance of unknown. This formula is applied to assays that exhibit linear relationships between changes in absorbance with changes in concentration to calculate the concentration of the unknown sample.

11.

C. In spectrophotometry, molecules in solution will cause incident light to be absorbed while the remaining light energy will be transmitted. Absorbance is the term used to describe the monochromatic light that is absorbed by the sample, and transmittance describes the light that passes through the sample. The mathematical relationship between absorbance and transmittance is expressed by $A = 2 - \log\%T$.

12.

C. Nephelometry, by definition, is a technique that measure light scattered by particles in suspension with a detector at an angle to the incident light (Often 45 or 90 degrees).

13.

C. In the dry reagent slide technique, as light from a radiant energy source passes through an interference filter, it is projected to the slide at a 45-degree angle. The light then follows a path through the clear support material and reagent layer and hits a white spreading layer; the unabsorbed light is then reflected back through the reagent and support layers. This reflected light impinges on the photodetector, which is positioned at a 90-degree angle to the slide. Because reflectance values are neither linearly proportional to transmission values nor consequently to dye concentration, the microcomputer utilizes an algorithm as a linearizing transformation of reflectance values to transmission values so that concentration may be calculated.

14.

D. In a fluorometer, light from the excitation lamp travels in a straight line, whereas the fluorescent light is radiated in all directions. If the detector for the emitted fluorescent light is placed at a right angle to the path of the excitation light, the excitation light will not fall on the detector. In addition, baffles can be placed around the cuvet to avoid reflection of the exciting light from the surface of the cuvet to the detector. The right-angle configuration does not prevent loss of the exciting or the emitted light.

15.

A. Fluorescence occurs when a molecule absorbs light of a particular wavelength and is thereby stimulated to emit light of a longer wavelength. The emitted light has a characteristic spectrum, the emission spectrum, that is unique for each fluorescing molecule. Hence, fluorometric methods are extremely sensitive and highly specific. Because of this extreme sensitivity, reagents used must be of a higher degree of purity than is required for spectroscopy, because even slight traces of impurities may fluoresce.

16.

A. Instrumentation employing fluorescence polarization is used for such testing as therapeutic drug levels and fetal lung maturity analysis. In these immunologic assays, plane-polarized light excites fluorophors in the sample cuvet. The free fluorophore-labeled ligands rotate freely because of their small size and primarily emit depolarized light. The labeled ligand-antibody complexes rotate more slowly because of their large size and emit polarized fluorescent light. Because of the differences in emitted light, it is not necessary to separate free from bound fluorophore-labeled ligands, allowing for use of the homogeneous assay technique. The emitted fluorescence intensity is measured by a polarization analyzer in the vertical plane, followed by its 90-degree movement for measurement in the horizontal plane. The amount of polarized light detected is inversely proportional to the concentration of ligand in the serum sample.

17.

A. Bioluminescence is a type of chemiluminescence in which the excitation energy is supplied by an enzymatic chemical reaction rather than by radiant energy, as in fluorescence and phosphorescence. Bioluminescence assays may employ such systems as NADH:FMN oxidoreductase-bacterial luciferase or adenosine triphosphate-firefly luciferase. Bioluminescence assays are nonradioactive, having sensitivity levels in the attomole (10^{-18}) to zeptomole (10^{-21}) ranges, which makes them more sensitive than direct fluorescence assays. Bioluminescence has been applied in the development of immunoassays.

18.

B. Nephelometry is the measurement of the amount of light scattered by particles in suspension. The amount of light scattered depends on the size and shape of the particles and on the wavelength of the incident light. Ultraviolet light should not be used because it might produce some fluorescence, which would lead to erroneously high results.

19.

C. Radionuclides are quantified by measuring the amount of energy that they emit. This can be in the form of alpha emission ${}^{4}_{2}He^{2+}$, beta emission (electrons ejected from the nucleus of a radioisotope during radioactive decay), or gamma emission (electromagnetic radiation emitted during radioactive decay). Beta and gamma emissions can be detected by scintillation counters. The sensing element of a scintillation counter is a fluor, a substance capable of converting radiation energy to light energy. The light energy is converted to electrical energy and amplified by a photomultiplier tube. A fluor commonly employed in solid scintillation counters is a large crystal of sodium iodide containing a small amount of thallium as an activator; it is used for gamma counting. Beta emission is counted by liquid scintillation counters using fluors dissolved in organic solvents. Alpha emission has very low penetrating power and is not measured in the clinical laboratory. Although radioimmunoassay (RIA) is no longer used for routine analyses and has been replaced by nonradioactive immunoassays, it is still used in a limited manner in some clinical reference laboratories and in research settings.

20.

C. Chemiluminescence is a type of luminescence where excitation does not require absorption of radiant energy. Chemiluminescence is the process where the chemical energy of a reaction produces excited atoms, and upon electron return to ground state photons of light are emitted. Chemiluminescence has been applied in the development of immunoassays and has ultrasensitivity in the attomole (10^{-18}) to zeptomole (10^{-21}) ranges.

21.

D. Atomic absorption spectrophotometry (AAS) is based on the principle that atoms in a basic ground state are capable of absorbing energy in the form of light at a specific wavelength. In a single-beam AAS, the amount of light that the analyte absorbs from the hollow-cathode lamp is what we wish to know. However, what is actually measured is the intensity of the beam after it has passed through the flame. This measurement is made with and without sample in the flame. In this way, the instrument calculates the amount of light absorbed because of the presence of the analyte in the flame. Because most samples usually have the analyte in the form of a compound or an ion, the analyte must first be converted to nonionized atoms. This is achieved by heating in a flame. About 99% of the atoms of analyte in the flame are in the ground state and, therefore, are capable of absorbing energy at the appropriate wavelength. Hence, light absorbed is essentially proportional to the concentration of the analyte. The light source in AAS is a hollow-cathode lamp in which the cathode contains the element that is to be measured.

22.

C. The basis of AAS is the measurement of light, at a specific wavelength, that is absorbed by an element whose atoms are in a ground state. The flame in AAS serves two functions—to accept the sample, thus serving as a cuvet, and to supply heat for converting the element, which is usually present in the sample in molecular form, into its atomic form at ground-state energy level. The hollow-cathode lamp supplies the emission line of light required for the analysis. The metal element of interest is coated on the cathode of the lamp. When the inert gas, either argon or neon, becomes ionized, it is drawn toward the cathode. The impact excites the metal element coated on the cathode, resulting in the emission of spectral lines specific for the element. This light emission is then absorbed by the metal element in the sample. A flameless AAS employs a carbon rod (graphite furnace), tantalum, or platinum to hold the sample in a chamber. The temperature is raised to vaporize the sample being analyzed. The atomized sample then absorbs the light energy from the hollow-cathode lamp. This technique is more sensitive than the flame method.

23.

D. A beam chopper is a device for interrupting a beam of light so that a pulsed beam is produced. In an atomic absorption spectrophotometer, if the light entering the flame from the hollow-cathode lamp is pulsed, then the light leaving the flame will consist of unabsorbed pulsed light and unpulsed light from the flame and from a small amount of emission by excited atoms of the analyte. The detector has an amplifier that is tuned to recognize and amplify only the pulsed signal. Thus errors caused by light from the flame and light emitted by the analyte are avoided. However, the beam chopper and tuned amplifier do not compensate for errors introduced by variations in flame temperature or deterioration of the hollow-cathode lamp. AAS may be used to measure such analytes as lead, zinc, copper, aluminum, magnesium, calcium, and lithium.

24.

A. A half-cell, also called an electrode, is composed of a single metallic conductor surrounded by a solution of electrolyte. An electrochemical cell consists of two half-cells. If two different kinds of half-cells are connected in such a way as to make a complete circuit, a current will flow because of the potential difference between the two electrodes. The connection must be between the two metallic conductors and also between the two electrolyte solutions, usually by means of a salt bridge. In the analytical technique of potentiometry, a comparison is made between the voltage of one half-cell connected to another half-cell. It is customary that all half-cell potentials be compared to the potential generated by a standard electrode. The universally accepted standard half-cell with which all other half-cells are compared is the standard hydrogen electrode, arbitrarily assigned a potential E° of 0.000 volt.

25.

B. Oxidation involves the loss of electrons, and reduction the gain of electrons. In an electrolytic cell composed of two different half-cells—for example, zinc in zinc sulfate and copper in copper sulfate—electrons will flow from the anode to the cathode. Thus reduction takes place at the cathode, whereas oxidation occurs at the anode. "Combination electrode" refers to the combining of indicator and reference electrodes into a single unit. "Electrode response" refers to the ability of an ion-selective electrode to respond to a change in concentration of the ion being measured by exhibiting a change in potential.

26.

B. In practical applications of potentiometry, it is desirable to use one half-cell with a known and constant potential that is not sensitive to the composition of the material to be analyzed. This is called the reference electrode. One type of reference electrode is the calomel electrode, which consists of mercury covered by a layer of mercurous chloride in contact with a saturated solution of potassium chloride. The other half-cell, called the indicator electrode, is selected on the basis of the change in its potential with change in the concentration of the analyte of interest. The silver-silver chloride electrode is a commonly used type of reference electrode. The sodium and calcium electrodes are types of ion-selective electrodes.

27.

C. For optimum performance, pH-sensitive glass electrodes that are not actively in use should be kept immersed in an aqueous medium. Because the exact composition of the pH-sensitive glass varies from one manufacturer to another, the glass electrode should be maintained in the medium recommended by the manufacturer. Usual media are deionized water, dilute HCl, and buffer with a pH near the pH of the solution to be measured. The functioning of a glass electrode depends on the properties of the pH-sensitive glass. A typical glass electrode is made by sealing a thin piece of pH-sensitive glass at the end of a piece of glass tubing and filling the tube with a solution of hydrochloric acid saturated with silver chloride. A silver wire is immersed in the solution in the tube, with one end extending outside the tube for external connection. This is essentially a silver/silver chloride reference electrode sealed within the tube with the pH-sensitive glass tip. This pH-sensitive glass functions appropriately only when it is saturated with water. Then each surface of the glass develops a hydrated lattice, where exchange of alkaline metal ions in the lattice for hydrogen ions in the test solution can occur.

28.

D. The ion-exchange electrode is a type of potentiometric, ion-selective electrode that consists of a liquid ion-exchange membrane that is made of an inert solvent and an ion-selective neutral carrier material. A collodion membrane may be used to separate the membrane solution from the sample solution being analyzed. Because of its ability to bind K^+, the antibiotic valinomycin is used as the neutral carrier for the K^+-selective membrane. The antibiotics nonactin and monactin are used in combination as the neutral carrier for the NH_4^+-selective membrane. A special formulation is used to make a selective glass membrane for the measurement of sodium.

29.

B. Chemiluminescence involves the oxidation of an organic compound by an oxidant. When that happens light is emitted from the excited product formed in the oxidation reaction.

30.

D. A chloride coulometer employs a coulometric system based on Faraday's law, which states that in an electrochemical system, the number of equivalent weights of a reactant oxidized or reduced is directly proportional to the quantity of electricity used in the reaction. The quantity of electricity is measured in coulombs. The coulomb is the unit of electrical quantity; 1 coulomb of electricity flowing per minute constitutes a current of 1 ampere. Thus, if the current is constant, the number of equivalent weights of reactant oxidized or reduced depends only on the duration of the current. In the chloride coulometer, the electrochemical reaction is the generation of Ag^+ ions by the passage of a direct current across a pair of silver electrodes immersed in a conducting solution containing the sample to be assayed for chloride. As the Ag^+ ions are generated, they are immediately removed from solution by combining with chloride to form insoluble silver chloride. When all the chloride is precipitated, further generation of Ag^+ ions causes an increase in conductivity of the solution. Thus the instrument provides an electrometric titration, in which the titrant is Ag^+ ions and the endpoint of the titration is indicated by the increase in conductivity of the solution. Amperometry is used to measure the increase in conductivity. The amperometric circuit includes a second pair of silver electrodes that are immersed in the solution. They are provided with a small, steady, and constant voltage. The appearance of free Ag^+ ions in the solution generates a sharp increase in conductivity, which, in turn, causes a sudden rise in the current between the electrodes in the amperometric circuit. This increase in current activates a relay that stops the further generation of Ag^+ ions and also stops an automatic timer placed in the circuit to measure the total duration of current in the coulometric circuit. Although this system is no longer used for routine analysis of serum, it is still employed for sweat chloride analysis.

31.

C. In an amperometric glucose electrode system, glucose oxidase reacts with glucose to produce hydrogen peroxide and gluconic acid. The platinum electrode that operates at a positive potential oxidizes the hydrogen peroxide to oxygen. The oxidation of hydrogen peroxide produces a current that is directly proportional to the glucose level in the sample.

32.

D. A pH/blood gas analyzer contains a pH-sensitive glass electrode, a PCO_2 electrode, and a PO_2 electrode. The glass electrode is calibrated by comparison with two primary standard buffers of known pH. Because pH readings are temperature sensitive, the calibration must be carried out at a constant temperature of 37°C. pH readings are not appreciably sensitive to changes in barometric pressure. Note that if the PCO_2 and PO_2 electrodes were also to be calibrated, then it would be essential to know the barometric pressure, because that affects the PCO_2 and PO_2 calibrating gases.

33.

B. In a blood gas analyzer, the PCO_2 electrode is actually a pH electrode immersed in a bicarbonate solution. The bicarbonate solution is separated from the sample by a membrane that is permeable to gaseous CO_2 but not to ionized substances such as H^+ ions. When CO_2 from the sample diffuses across the membrane, it dissolves, forming carbonic acid and thus lowering the pH. The pH is inversely proportional to the log of the PCO_2. Hence the scale of the meter can be calibrated directly in terms of PCO_2. It should be noted that whereas pH refers to the negative logarithm of the H^+ ion concentration, PCO_2 refers to the partial pressure of CO_2.

34.

B. In a blood gas analyzer, the electrode for measuring the partial pressure of oxygen (PO_2) in the blood is an electrochemical cell consisting of a platinum cathode and a Ag/AgCl anode connected to an external voltage source. The cathode and anode are immersed in buffer. A polypropylene membrane selectively permeable to gases separates the buffer from the blood sample. When there is no oxygen diffusing into the buffer, there is practically no current flowing between the cathode and the anode because they are polarized. When oxygen diffuses into the buffer from a sample, it is reduced at the cathode. The electrons necessary for this reduction are produced at the anode. Hence a current flows; the current is directly proportional to the PO_2 in the sample.

35.

C. pH, PCO_2, and PO_2 are measured directly from the specimen by utilizing electrodes. The pH and PCO_2 electrodes are potentiometric where the voltage produced across a semipermeable membrane to hydrogen ions or CO_2 gas is proportional to the "activity" of those ions in the patient's sample. Activity is measured in voltage whose value can be presented in terms of concentration. PO_2 is measured similarly, but using an amperometric electrode. For PO_2 a small charge is put on a cathode, and electrons are drawn off the cathode in proportion to the oxygen present. The O_2 becomes part of the circuit. The amount of electrons drawn is proportional to the amount of oxygen present. Bicarbonate and other parameters, such as base excess, are calculated by the instrument using pH and PCO_2 values and the Henderson/Hasselbalch equation.

36.

A. The are multiple types of indicator electrodes used in ion selective technology including glass, liquid, solid-state, gas sensing, and enzyme. The glass electrode contains a glass tip that contains oxides that create an ion exchange with the analyte of interest. An example of a glass electrode is the pH electrode.

37.

B. Electrophoresis is a method of separating charged particles by their rates of migration in an electric field. An electrophoretic chamber consists of two electrodes, two reservoirs to hold buffer, a means of supporting a strip in the chamber so that the ends are dipping into the reservoirs, and a means of applying an electric current to the strip. The whole chamber is sealed to make it vapor-proof.

38.

A. Capillary electrophoresis is based on electro-osmotic flow (EOF). When an electric field is applied, the flow of liquid is in the direction of the cathode. Thus, EOF regulates the speed at which solutes move through the capillary. Cations migrate the fastest, because EOF and electrophoretic attraction are in the direction of the cathode.

39.

B. In isoelectric focusing a homogeneous mixture of carrier ampholytes with a pH range from 3 to 10 are added to the system with the patient sample. When current is applied to the system, the ampholytes rapidly migrate to the pH zones where net charge is zero. The ampholytes line up from lowest (at the anode) to highest pH (cathode).

40.

A. Buffer solutions of pH 8.6 are commonly used for serum protein electrophoresis. At this alkaline pH, the serum proteins have a net negative charge. Therefore, the negatively charged serum proteins migrate toward the anode. This is true for all the proteins except the gamma-globulins, which tend to show the phenomenon of endosmosis.

41.

C. Proteins are dipolar or zwitterion compounds because they contain amino acids that exhibit both negative and positive charges. The isoelectric point (pI) of a protein refers to the pH at which the number of positive charges on the protein molecule equals the number of negative charges, causing the protein to have a net charge of zero. Because the protein exhibits electrical neutrality at its isoelectric point, it is unable to migrate in an electrical field.

42.

C. Amido black 10B, Coomassie brilliant blue, and Ponceau S are dyes that are used to stain serum proteins after electrophoresis. Once the serum protein bands are stained, they may be quantified by scanning the support media at the appropriate wavelength with a densitometer. Oil red O and fat red 7B are dyes that are used to stain lipoproteins following electrophoresis.

43.

D. In electrophoresis, each band in the stained protein pattern should be uniformly colored; that is, no holes should appear within an individual band. Such a doughnut-like appearance occurs when the protein is present in too high a concentration, thus exceeding the complexing ability of the stain. To overcome this problem, dilute elevated specimens before rerunning the electrophoresis.

44.

D. Ampholytes are mixtures of polyanions and polycations used to establish a pH gradient within the gel media in isoelectric focusing. When an electrical field is applied to the gel, ampholytes seek their own isoelectric point where they become stationary, establishing a pH gradient. Similarly, proteins will migrate within the gel-gradient until they reach the pH of their isoelectric point, thus becoming stationary or focused. This system is most useful in separating proteins that have close isoelectric points.

45.

B. Serum protein electrophoresis at pH 8.5 results in a net negative charge on proteins and their subsequent movement toward the anode. This movement results in the production of five bands (zones) known as albumin, alpha1, alpha 2, beta, and gamma. Serum proteins will migrates into these five zones. Occasionally, you will see a band between the beta and gamma regions that often represents fibrinogen from an anticoagulated sample.

46.

B. Affinity chromatography is the type of chromatography that uses boronate groups attached to the resin on a chromatography column to measure glycated hemoglobin. The interaction of glycated hemoglobin and the boronate groups results in the retainment of glycated hemoglobin on the column.

47.

C. Protein molecules can exist as anions, cations, or zwitterions, depending on the pH of the solution in which they are placed. The pH at which they exist in the form of zwitterions and hence have no net charge is called the isoelectric point. The principle of isoelectric focusing is based on the ability to separate proteins because of differences in their isoelectric points. Aliphatic polyamino polycarboxylic acids, known as ampholytes, are used to produce the pH gradient.

48.

B. In thin-layer chromatography (TLC), the R_f (retention factor) describes the distance traveled by the solute (compound of interest) in relation to the distance traveled by the solvent (mobile phase). Measurements of the TLC plate are made from the origin or point of sample application to the center of the developed spot and from the origin to the solvent front. An R_f may be calculated by means of the following formula:

$$R_f = \frac{\text{Distance from origin to spot center}}{\text{Distance from origin to solvent front}}$$

$$R_f = \frac{48 \text{ mm}}{141 \text{ mm}} = 0.34$$

The R_f of the compound of interest, along with chromogenic spray characteristics, may then be compared with standards for identification of the unknown compound.

49.

C. The column and carrier gas flow rate used in gas-liquid chromatography are important aspects of the separation and resolving power of the system. When the column eluent is introduced into a mass spectrometer, additional information pertaining to elemental composition, position of functional groups, and molecular weight may be determined for the purpose of identifying compounds (e.g., drugs in biological samples). Mass spectrometers consist of a vacuum system, ion source, mass filter, and detector.

50.

C. High-performance liquid chromatography (HPLC) systems are composed of four basic units: sample-introduction system, solvent-delivery system, column, and detector. The sample-introduction system is generally a fixed-loop injection valve, which allows the sample to be injected into a stainless steel external loop for flushing onto the column by the solvent. The solvent-delivery system may be composed of one or two pumps for the purpose of forcing the mobile phase and sample through the column. Photometric, fluorometric, and electrochemical detectors are available for monitoring the eluate as it emerges from the column.

51.

C. In HPLC, the technique used for the mobile phase may be isocratic or gradient elution. With isocratic elution the strength of the solvent remains constant during the separation. With gradient elution the strength of the solvent is continually increased (percent per minute) during the separation process. The gradient elution technique is sometimes employed to improve HPLC resolution and sensitivity.

52.

A. Discrete analyzers are designed so that each specimen-reagent mixture is analyzed separately in its own vessel. Although a discrete analyzer may be designed to measure only one analyte, most discrete analyzers are very versatile and are able to run multiple tests on each sample. Some discrete analyzers also have random access capability that allows STAT samples to be accessed easily.

53.

B. High-performance liquid chromatography is also called high-pressure liquid chromatography. It is a form of column chromatography in which a liquid moving phase is actively pumped through the column, thus speeding the separation process considerably. HPLC is used in therapeutic drug monitoring and in assaying vitamin and hormone concentrations.

54.

A. Chromatography provides a variety of means of separating mixtures of substances on the basis of their physicochemical properties, primarily their solubility in a variety of solvents. Chromatographic methods always involve a stationary phase and a mobile phase. The sample containing the substances to be separated is carried in the mobile phase; the mobile phase passes over the stationary phase at different rates depending on their relative solubilities in the two phases. The amount of separation depends on (1) the rate of diffusion, (2) the solubility of the substances being separated, and (3) the nature of the solvent. In TLC, the stationary phase is a thin layer of some sorbent such as silica gel uniformly spread on a piece of glass or plastic.

55.

C. A mass spectrum is an intensity vs. mass/charge ratio plot representing an analysis. The *x*-axis is the mass/charge ratio.

56.

B. Ion-exchange chromatography uses synthetic ion-exchange resins. They may be cation- or anion-exchange resins. They can be used in either a column or a thin layer. Separation of mixtures of substances by ion-exchange chromatography depends primarily on the sign and the ionic charge density of the substances being separated.

57.

A. Mass spectrometry identifies a compound based on the principle of charged particles moving through a magnetic or electric field, with ions being separated from other charged particles according to their mass-to-charge ratios. The mass spectrum produced is unique for a particular compound. It also identifies the positioning of functional groups of the compound. Mass spectrometry is useful in the clinical laboratory for drug identification.

58.

D. Mass spectrometry is used in the clinical laboratory in conjunction with gas or liquid chromatography (GC-MS). In gas chromatography a compound is identified by its retention time. If two compounds have very similar retention times, the compound may be misidentified. Gas chromatography complements mass spectrometry in that the eluted peak is subjected to mass spectrometric analysis for molecular weight determination. Use of the two systems in tandem allows for more accurate identification of compounds.

59.

D. With automated instruments, the quality of the specimen and its handling are critical to producing accurate test results. Sampling errors can occur that cause falsely low results to be generated. These errors include short sampling, air pocket in the bottom of the sample cup, and fibrin clots in the sample probe.

60.

C. As part of a good quality assurance program, a laboratory should perform function verification, performance verification, and preventive maintenance for all instrument systems. Function verification is the monitoring of specific instrument functions and the correcting of these functions when necessary to assure reliable operation. Function verification includes monitoring temperature, setting electronic parameters, calibrating instruments, and analyzing quality control data. It is important that performance of these activities be properly documented.

61.

D. It is imperative that preventive maintenance procedures be performed and the results recorded for all laboratory instrumentation. This includes maintenance of analytical balances, refrigerators, freezers, centrifuges, ovens, water baths, heating blocks, thermometers, pipetters, dilutors, automated analyzers, and all other laboratory equipment used for analyzing specimens. Preventive maintenance is performed at scheduled times such as per shift, daily, weekly, monthly, or yearly.

62.

C. The Clark electrode (also know as a PO_2 electrode) uses amperometry as its electrochemical technique. This electrochemical cell contains a platinum cathode and a silver/silver chloride anode in a buffer with potassium chloride. The cathode is adjusted to −0.65 V. When oxygen is present in a sample, it diffuses across the gas permeable membrane to the cathode where it is reduced causing a current to flow. With each molecule of oxygen that is reduced at the cathode, it causes four electrons of current to flow.

63.

A. Hemoglobin is a tetramer composed of four globin chains, four heme groups, and four iron atoms. In adult hemoglobin, or hemoglobin A_1, there are two alpha chains and two beta chains. Hemoglobin A_2, which comprises less than 4% of the normal adult hemoglobin, is composed of two alpha chains and two delta chains. Hemoglobin F, or fetal hemoglobin, is composed of two alpha chains and two gamma chains.

64.

D. Although hemoglobin differentiation is best achieved by use of electrophoresis, hemoglobin F may be differentiated from the majority of human hemoglobins because of its alkali resistance. Hemoglobin F is able to resist denaturation and remain soluble when added to an alkaline solution. In contrast to hemoglobin F, most hemoglobins will denature in alkaline solution and precipitate on the addition of ammonium sulfate. After one year of age, the normal concentration of hemoglobin F is less than 1% of the total hemoglobin. However, hemoglobin F may be present in elevated concentrations in disorders that include thalassemia, sickle cell disease, and aplastic anemia.

65.

A. A number of hemoglobinopathies exist where a substitution of one amino acid on either the alpha chain or the beta chain causes the formation of an abnormal hemoglobin molecule. Hemoglobin S is an abnormal hemoglobin that is characterized by the substitution of valine for glutamic acid in position 6 of the beta chain. Hemoglobin C is an abnormal hemoglobin in which lysine replaces glutamic acid in position 6 of the beta chain. The structural changes that are seen in hemoglobins S and C disorders are inherited as autosomal recessive traits.

66.

A. At pH 8.6, hemoglobins have a net negative charge and migrate from the point of application toward the anode. When hemoglobin electrophoresis is performed on cellulose acetate at pH 8.6, hemoglobin A migrates the fastest toward the anode, followed respectively by hemoglobins F and S. Hemoglobins A_2 and C have the same electrophoretic mobility and migrate slightly slower than hemoglobin S. Because hemoglobins A_2 and C exhibit nearly the same mobility, they cannot be differentiated on cellulose acetate.

67.

D. At pH 6.2 on agar gel, hemoglobins exhibit different electrophoretic mobilities in comparison with hemoglobins electrophoresed at pH 8.6 on cellulose acetate. The order of migration of hemoglobins on cellulose acetate, proceeding from the most anodal hemoglobin to the most cathodal hemoglobin, is respectively A_1 and F, followed by G, D, and S, which migrate with the same mobility, followed by the group A_2, C, O, and E, which migrate the most slowly with the same mobility. This migration pattern is in contrast to agar gel electrophoresis at pH 6.2 in which the order of migration, from the most anodal hemoglobin to the most cathodal hemoglobin, is, respectively, C and S, followed by hemoglobins A_1, A_2, D, E, and G, which migrate as a group with the same mobility, followed by F. The different migration patterns seen with these two media systems are useful in differentiating hemoglobins that migrate with the same electrophoretic mobility. In the case of hemoglobins A_2 and C, which migrate with the same mobility on cellulose acetate, it is not possible to discern which hemoglobin is present in a particular blood specimen. By electrophoresing this specimen on agar gel at pH 6.2, hemoglobin A_2 may be differentiated from hemoglobin C because hemoglobin A_2 exhibits mobility similar to that of hemoglobin A_1, whereas hemoglobin C migrates alone closest to the anode.

68.

D. Although hemoglobin electrophoresis is the recommended method for hemoglobin identification, solubility testing may be warranted for large-scale screening for hemoglobin S. Solubility testing is possible because the solubility properties of most hemoglobins differ enough from those of hemoglobin S. In this method, sodium hydrosulfite acts as a reducing agent to deoxygenate hemoglobin. In the presence of hemoglobin S, the concentrated phosphate buffer test solution will become turbid because deoxygenated hemoglobin S is insoluble in the buffer solution. Hemoglobins A_1, C, D, and F, when present, will remain soluble in the phosphate buffer solution and show no visible signs of turbidity. Therefore, the detection of turbidity is associated with the presence of hemoglobin S.

69.

C. Zero-order kinetics refers to chemical reactions whose rate of the reaction does not depend on the reactant concentration. Enzyme assays in chemistry are built for zero-order kinetics where the substrate is in excess, time and temperature are constant, and the only item driving the rate of reaction is the enzyme in the patient sample.

70.

D. Enzyme-multiplied immunoassay technique (EMIT) is an example of a homogeneous immunoassay technique. A homogeneous assay is one in which separation of the bound and free fraction is unnecessary. The antigen is labeled with an enzyme and competes with the unknown antigen for binding sites on the antibody. The enzyme-labeled antigen that remains in the free fraction is enzymatically active. Therefore, the free labeled antigen can be determined by its action on a substrate in the presence of bound-labeled fraction. This type of assay is used commonly on automated instruments. The other techniques mentioned in the question, RIA, ELISA, and IRMA, are termed heterogeneous immunoassays because they require the physical separation of the bound from the free fraction before actual measurement.

71.

A. An ELISA is a sensitive and robust method which measures the antigen concentration in an unknown sample. The antigen of interest is quantified between two layers of antibodies: the capture and the detection antibody. The capture antibody is attached to a solid support (usually a polystyrene microtiter plate) and it is attracted to an antigen of interest.

72.

D. EMIT employs a homogeneous enzyme immunoassay method. This means that physical separation of the free labeled antigen from the antibody-bound-labeled antigen is not necessary for measurement. This is possible because only the free labeled antigen remains active. In the EMIT system the antigen is labeled with an enzyme (e.g., glucose-6-phosphate dehydrogenase). Determination of the drug concentration in the serum sample is made when the free enzyme-labeled drug reacts with substrate and coenzyme, resulting in an absorbance change that is measured spectrophotometrically. The drug in the serum sample is the unlabeled antigen in the assay, and it competes with the labeled drug for the binding sites on the antibody.

73.

B. The components needed in EMIT include the free unlabeled drug (unlabeled antigen) in the serum specimen, antibody specific to the drug being quantified, enzyme-labeled drug (labeled antigen), and substrate and coenzyme specific for the enzyme. In this method, the enzyme is coupled to the drug, producing an enzyme-labeled drug also referred to as an enzyme-labeled antigen. This enzyme-labeled complex competes with free unlabeled drug in the serum sample for the binding sites on the antibody. EMIT therapeutic drug monitoring assays are available for a variety of drugs that are included in the categories of antimicrobial, antiepileptic, antiasthmatic, cardioactive, and antineoplastic drugs. The EMIT system is not limited only to drug assays but is also available for hormone testing.

74.

C. In the EMIT assay, antibody specific to the drug being quantified is added to the serum sample that contains the drug. Substrate and coenzyme specific for the enzyme label being used are added. Finally, the enzyme-labeled drug (free labeled antigen) is added to the mixture. The drug in the serum sample and the enzyme-labeled drug compete for the binding sites on the antibody. The binding of the enzyme-labeled drug to the antibody causes a steric alteration that results in decreased enzyme activity. This steric change prevents the substrate from reacting at the active site of the enzyme, leaving only the free enzyme-labeled drug able to react with the substrate and coenzyme. The resulting enzyme activity, measured at 340 nm, is directly proportional to the concentration of the drug in the serum sample. The greater the amount of enzyme activity measured, the greater is the concentration of free enzyme-labeled drug and, therefore, the greater is the concentration of drug in the serum sample.

75.

D. Luminescent oxygen channeling immunoassay (LOCI™) is a homogeneous technique that is an adaptation of the chemiluminescent immunoassay. Singlet oxygen reacts with the precursor chemiluminescent compound to form a chemiluminescent product that decays and emits light. This light energy is accepted by a fluorophore, which results in light emission of a longer wavelength. In this assay, the chemiluminescent signal is enhanced by the resulting fluorescent signal which is proportional to the concentration of analyte in the serum sample.

76.

A. In a luminescent oxygen channeling immunoassay the antigen links to two antibody-coated particles. The first is an antibody-coated sensitizer particle containing a photosensitive dye (singlet oxygen source), and the second is an antibody-coated particle (singlet oxygen receptor) containing a precursor chemiluminescent compound and a fluorophore. Radiant energy is used to irradiate the immunocomplex, which stimulates the production of singlet oxygen at the surface of the sensitizer particle. The singlet oxygen diffuses to the second particle being held in close proximity.

Proteins and Tumor Markers

77.

D. The three major biochemical compounds that exert primary roles in human intermediary metabolism are proteins, carbohydrates, and lipids. The presence of nitrogen in all protein compounds distinguishes proteins from carbohydrates and lipids. Protein compounds contain approximately 16% nitrogen. Although there are only 20 common α-amino acids that are found in all proteins and a total of 40 known amino acids, a protein compound may contain from 50 to thousands of amino acids. The uniqueness of any protein is dictated by the number, type, and sequencing of the α-amino acids that compose it. The α-amino acids are linked to each other through peptide bonds. A peptide bond is formed through the linkage of the amino group of one amino acid to the carboxyl group of another amino acid.

78.

C. A variety of external factors, such as mechanical agitation, application of heat, and extreme chemical treatment with acids or salts, may cause the denaturation of proteins. When proteins are denatured, they undergo a change in their tertiary structure. *Tertiary structure* describes the appearance of the protein in its folded, globular form. When the covalent, hydrogen, or disulfide bonds are broken, the protein loses its shape as its polypeptide chain unfolds. With the loss of this tertiary structure, there is also a loss in some of the characteristic properties of the protein. In general, proteins will become less soluble, and enzymes will lose catalytic activity. Denaturation by use of chemicals has been a useful laboratory tool. The mixing of serum proteins with sulfosalicylic acid or trichloroacetic acid causes the precipitation of both the albumin and globulin fractions. When albumin is placed in water, dilute salt solutions, or moderately concentrated salt solutions, it remains soluble. However, the globulins are insoluble in water but soluble in weak salt solutions. Both the albumins and globulins are insoluble in concentrated salt solutions. *Primary structure* refers to the joining of the amino acids through peptide bonds to form polypeptide chains. *Secondary structure* refers to the twisting of more than one polypeptide chain into coils or helices.

79.

D. Although the Kjeldahl technique for the determination of protein nitrogen is too cumbersome for use in routine testing, it is considered to be the reference method of choice to validate materials used with the biuret method. The Kjeldahl technique is based on the quantification of the nitrogen content of protein. It is estimated that the average nitrogen content of protein is 16% of the total weight. In the Kjeldahl technique, protein undergoes a digestion process with sulfuric acid through which the nitrogen content of the protein is converted to ammonium ion. The ammonium ion in turn may be reacted with Nessler's reagent, forming a colored product that is read spectrophotometrically, or the ammonium ion may undergo distillation, liberating ammonia that is titrated.

80.

C. A commonly used method to quantify serum total proteins is the biuret procedure. The biuret reaction is based on the complexing of cupric ions in an alkaline solution with the peptide linkages of protein molecules. Because the amino acids of all proteins are joined together by peptide bonds, this method provides an accurate quantification of the total protein content of serum. The greater the amount of protein in a specimen, the greater will be the number of available peptide bonds for reaction and the more intense the colored reaction will be. In the biuret reaction, the intensity of the reddish violet color produced is proportional to the number of peptide bonds present. Generally, one cupric ion complexes with four to six peptide linkages. However, a colored product may be formed when the cupric ion links through coordinate bonds with at least two peptide linkages, with the smallest compound able to react being the tripeptide. Therefore, not only will proteins contribute to the formation of the colored product, but so, too, will any tripeptides and polypeptides present in a serum sample.

81.

B. The concentration of total protein in cerebrospinal fluid (CSF) is 15–45 mg/dL. Such a low level of protein requires a method with sufficient sensitivity such as Coomassie brilliant blue. Turbidimetric methods can also be used to quantify protein in CSF. Neither biuret nor Ponceau S has the sensitivity needed, and bromcresol green measures only albumin and does not react with the globulins.

82.

D. CSF, an ultrafiltrate of blood plasma, is made in the choroid plexus of the ventricles of the brain. Protein quantification is among the tests generally ordered on CSF; other tests include glucose, culture and sensitivity, and differential cell count. The reference range for CSF protein is 15–45 mg/dL. CSF protein may be quantified using turbidimetric (e.g., sulfosalicylic acid and benzethonium chloride) or dye-binding methods (e.g., Coomassie brilliant blue). Elevated levels of CSF protein are found in such disorders as bacterial, viral, and fungal meningitis; multiple sclerosis; neoplasm; disk herniation; and cerebral infarction. Low levels of CSF protein are found in hyperthyroidism and in CSF leakage from the central nervous system.

83.

D. Bisalbuminemia is a congenital disorder that does not exhibit any clinical manifestations. The only sign of this disorder is the splitting of albumin into two distinct bands when serum is subjected to electrophoresis. The extra albumin band may occur either anodically or cathodically to the normal albumin band depending on its speed of migration. The intensity of the two bands when quantified by densitometry may show that the two forms are of equal concentration. In a less common variation the abnormal albumin band may represent only 10–15% of the total albumin concentration.

84.

C. There are no physiological diseases that cause increased production of albumin by the liver. Elevated serum albumin is only associated with dehydration. It is a relative increase that will return to normal when fluids are administered to alleviate the dehydration. Disorders such as malnutrition, acute inflammation, and renal disease are characterized by decreased serum albumin levels.

85.

A. In renal disease, glomerular or tubular malfunction results in proteinuria. In early stages of glomerular dysfunction, small quantities of albumin will appear in the urine. Because the concentration is so low, urine dipstick assays are unable to detect the presence of such a small quantity of albumin; hence the term "albuminuria." Annual testing of diabetic individuals for albuminuria is recommended, because identification of these low levels of albumin that precede nephropathy would allow for clinical intervention to control blood glucose levels and blood pressure. The reference interval for urinary albumin is less than 30 mg/day. Albuminuria may be quantified using immunonephelometry and enzyme immunoassay.

86.

B. β_2-Microglobulin is a single polypeptide chain that is the light chain component of human leukocyte antigens (HLAs). It is found on the surface of nucleated cells and is notably present on lymphocytes. Increased plasma levels of β_2-microglobulin are associated with renal failure, lymphocytosis, rheumatoid arthritis, and systemic lupus erythematosus.

87.

A. Haptoglobin is a glycoprotein produced mainly by the liver that migrates electrophoretically as an alpha$_2$-globulin. Increased serum concentrations of haptoglobin are seen in inflammatory conditions and tissue necrosis, whereas decreased levels are seen in hemolytic situations in which there is extensive red blood cell destruction. In the latter situation, haptoglobin binds with free hemoglobin to form a stable complex that may then be removed by the reticuloendothelial system. Because of the size of the haptoglobin-hemoglobin complex, urinary excretion of hemoglobin by the kidney is avoided, thereby preventing the loss of iron by the kidney.

88.

D. The serum proteins are divided into five principal fractions based on their electrophoretic mobilities. The five fractions are albumin, alpha$_1$-globulin, alpha$_2$-globulin, beta-globulin, and gamma-globulin. Albumin constitutes the largest individual fraction of the serum proteins. The reference concentration of albumin in serum ranges between 3.5 and 5.0 g/dL, and the total globulin concentration is between 2.3 and 3.5 g/dL.

89.

C. Bromcresol green (BCG) and bromcresol purple (BCP) are anionic dyes that bind selectively with albumin without preliminary extraction of the globulins. The nature of the dyes is such that the color of the free dye is different from the color of the albumin-dye complex so that the color change is directly proportional to the concentration of albumin in the specimen. Although amido black, Ponceau S, and Coomassie brilliant blue are able to bind albumin, they also react with the globulins, thus prohibiting their use in a direct procedure for quantification of serum albumin.

90.

B. Biuret reagent is a combination of copper sulfate, potassium iodide in sodium hydroxide, and potassium sodium tartrate. The copper sulfate is the key to the reaction because it is the cupric ion that complexes with the peptide bonds of protein. To keep the copper in solution until its use, potassium sodium tartrate is employed as a complexing agent, whereas the autoreduction of copper is prevented by potassium iodide.

91.

D. The majority of the plasma proteins are manufactured by the liver. Albumin, fibrinogen, and most of the alpha- and beta-globulins are produced by the liver. The immunoglobulins, including IgG, IgA, IgM, IgD, and IgE, are produced by the lymphoid cells.

92.

D. The immunoglobulins, IgG, IgA, IgM, IgD, and IgE, migrate electrophoretically with the gamma-globulin fraction. The normal serum levels of the IgD and IgE classes are so low that these two immunoglobulins do not normally contribute to the intensity of the stained gamma-globulin electrophoretic fraction. The primary component of the gamma fraction consists of IgG, with IgA and IgM contributing to the intensity of the stained fraction to a lesser degree. In disease states the concentration relationship between the immunoglobulins may be significantly altered from the normal.

93.

D. All the immunoglobulins consist of heavy- and light-chain polypeptides. The heavy chains are designated as gamma (γ), alpha (α), mu (μ), delta (Δ), and epsilon (ε) and are specific for the immunoglobulins IgG, IgA, IgM, IgD, and IgE, respectively. The light chains are designated as kappa (κ) and lambda (λ), with both types being found in each of the immunoglobulin classes, although the two light chains attached to a particular set of heavy chains must be of the same type. Therefore, IgG consists of two heavy chains of the gamma type and two light chains of either the kappa or lambda type. The immunoglobulins IgA, IgD, and IgE have a structure similar to that of IgG in that they consist of two light chains and two heavy chains of the respective type. IgM is a macromolecule with a pentamer type of structure. IgM consists of five sets of two heavy-chain and two light-chain units, with the basic units being linked to each other by peptide fragments.

94.

A. The immunoglobulin class IgA is found in both plasma and body secretions, with the two types being differentiated by their sedimentation coefficients. Plasma IgA has an average sedimentation coefficient of 7S, and secretory IgA has a sedimentation coefficient of 11S. Secretory IgA is present in saliva, tears, and secretions of nasal, gastrointestinal, and tracheolbronchial origin. Secretory IgA is dimeric in structure and possesses a glycoprotein secretory component attached to its heavy chains and a J polypeptide. The principal immunoglobulin found in secretions is IgA, with only trace amounts of IgG being present. The presence of IgM, IgD, or IgE in secretions has not been detected.

95.

D. The only immunoglobulin class that is able to cross the placenta from the mother's circulation to the fetus is IgG. Therefore, at birth, there is very little immunoglobulin present in the infant except for the maternal IgG. After birth, as the infant comes in contact with antigens, the levels of IgG, IgA, and IgM slowly increase.

96.

D. α_1-Antitrypsin is an acute-phase reactant protein whose concentration increases in response to inflammation. α_1-Antitrypsin inhibits the self-destruction of one's own tissue by forming inactive complexes with proteolytic enzymes. In this way the enzymes are inhibited, and tissue destruction through self-digestion is avoided. α_1-Antitrypsin has been found to have the highest concentration in serum of any of the plasma proteolytic inhibitors. It is an effective inhibitor of the enzymes chymotrypsin, plasmin, thrombin, collagenase, and elastase. The primary effect of α_1-antitrypsin may be seen in the respiratory tract and the closed spaces of the body where physiological pH values are maintained. α_1-Antitrypsin is least effective in the stomach and intestines.

97.

A. Ceruloplasmin, a metalloprotein, is the principal transport protein of copper in the plasma. In the plasma, copper is primarily bound to ceruloplasmin, with only very small amounts of copper bound to albumin or in a dialyzable free state. When subjected to an electric field, ceruloplasmin migrates as an alpha$_2$-globulin.

98.

C. The liver of a fetus and the yolk sac produce a protein known as α_1-fetoprotein (AFP). The concentration of AFP in the blood of a fetus reaches a maximum concentration at approximately 16–18 weeks gestation. Blood levels decline from this point and finally disappear approximately 5 weeks after birth. In cases of open spina bifida or anencephaly, the fetus leaks large amounts of AFP into the amniotic fluid. By means of an amniocentesis, the amount of AFP present in the amniotic fluid may be quantified by enzyme-labeled immunoassay and other immunoassay techniques.

99.

C. Fibronectin is an adhesive glycoprotein that functions with collagen to support cell adhesion. It is a normal constituent in the placenta and amniotic fluid. As labor begins, a change occurs in cell adhesion that affects the placenta and uterine wall. The level of fetal fibronectin increases in the secretions of the cervix and vagina. When this occurs prematurely, the increase in fetal fibronectin is used to predict risk of premature birth. Inhibin A, α_1-fetoprotein, human chorionic gonadotropin, and unconjugated estriol are used together in the quadruple test to assess risk for such disorders as Down syndrome.

100.

D. The immunoglobulins are composed of both heavy and light chains. In Bence Jones proteinuria, there is an overproduction of one type of light chain by a single clone of plasma cells. Therefore, the plasma cells produce either an excessive amount of kappa light chains or an excessive amount of lambda light chains. The light-chain type produced is in such abundance that the renal threshold is exceeded, resulting in the excretion of free light chains of the kappa or lambda type in the urine. The type of light chain excreted in the urine may be identified by performing immunoelectrophoresis on a concentrated urine specimen. In addition, immunoturbidimetric and immunonephelometric methods may also be used.

101.

C. In multiple myeloma, there is an abnormal proliferation of plasma cells. These plasma cells produce a homogeneous immunoglobulin protein that stains as a well-defined peak in the gamma region. Because of the presence of this monoclonal protein, the serum total protein will be elevated. Bone destruction is commonly seen in this disorder, with the plasma cells forming densely packed groups in the lytic areas. Hypercalcemia is primarily the result of bone destruction.

102.

A. Immunonephelometric and immunoturbidimetric techniques are used to quantify specific immunoglobulin classes. Nephelometric techniques used to quantify the immunoglobulins are based on the measurement of light scatter by the antigen-antibody complexes formed. This method also calls for the comparison of unknowns with standards. Although radial immunodiffusion can be used to quantify the immunoglobulins, it is not a method of choice. Serum protein electrophoresis, immunoelectrophoresis, and isoelectric focusing cannot be used to quantify the immunoglobulins.

103.

C. Portal cirrhosis is a chronic disease of the liver in which fibrosis occurs as a result of tissue necrosis and diffuse small nodules form as liver cells regenerate, with a concomitant distortion of liver structure. The cause of this disorder may include alcoholism, malnutrition, or submassive hepatic necrosis. When a serum protein electrophoresis is performed, the characteristic pattern seen in portal cirrhosis is an elevation of both the gamma- and beta-globulin regions, with these two regions showing a bridging or fusing appearance. This beta-gamma bridging effect is due to an increased level of IgA, which migrates with beta mobility. It should also be noted that the albumin level is depressed.

104.

D. Although microbiological analysis and chemical analysis may be employed to detect and quantify a specific amino acid, chromatographic analysis is preferred as a screening technique for amino acid abnormalities or when differentiation among several amino acids is necessary. Thin-layer chromatography, either one- or two-dimensional, is being used in conjunction with a mixture of ninhydrin-collidine for color development. To quantify amino acids high- performance liquid chromatography, ion-exchange chromatography, and tandem mass spectrometry are used.

105.

C. Protein electrophoresis is performed on a serum specimen. If plasma is substituted for serum, the electrophoresis will show an extra fraction in the beta-gamma region, because fibrinogen is a $beta_2$-globulin. This extra fraction represents the protein fibrinogen that is present in a plasma specimen. Fibrinogen contributes approximately 0.2–0.4 g/dL to the total protein concentration.

106.

A. When serum proteins are exposed to a buffer solution of pH 8.6, the proteins take on a net negative charge. The negatively charged proteins will migrate toward the anode (+) when exposed to an electrical field. Albumin migrates the fastest toward the anode whereas the gamma-globulins remain close to the point of application and actually move slightly in a cathodic (−) direction because of the effects of endosmosis. The order of migration of the serum proteins, starting at the anode with the fastest-moving fraction, is albumin, $alpha_1$-globulin, $alpha_2$-globulin, beta-globulin, and gamma-globulin.

107.

D. α_1-Fetoprotein, synthesized by the fetus, peaks at 13 weeks and declines at 34 weeks of gestation. When concern exists for the well-being of the fetus, maternal serum AFP is measured between 15 and 20 weeks of gestation. An increased AFP level in maternal serum is associated with such disorders as neural tube defects, spina bifida, and fetal distress. A decreased AFP level in maternal serum is characteristic of Down syndrome.

108.

C. The normal range for total PSA is referenced as less than 4.0 ng/mL. However, early-detection guidelines may endorse a lower cutoff for total PSA up to 2.5 ng/mL and recommend that values that fall in the indeterminate range (2.5–4.0 ng/mL) be taken on a patient-by-patient basis. Men with prostate cancer tend to have lower % free PSA (free PSA/total PSA) than men with benign disease; thus lower % free PSA is associated with a higher risk of prostate cancer. In the case presented, the patient's total PSA was 3.1 ng/mL with a free PSA of 0.3 ng/mL, which is 10% free PSA. This low percentage is suggestive of a higher probability of cancer, whereas a percentage >25% is associated with lower risk of cancer.

109.

B. Carcinoembryonic antigen (CEA), a glycoprotein, is found in increased amounts in serum when malignant tumors of the colon, lung, pancreas, stomach, and breast are present. Care must be exercised in treating CEA as a diagnostic test, because elevated values are also seen in people who smoke, people with hepatitis, and people with several other nonmalignant disorders. Clinically, CEA is more valuable in prognosis and treatment monitoring. Enzyme immunoassay and other types of immunoassays are available for the quantification of CEA.

110.

B. AFP is normally produced only by the fetus, with blood levels disappearing shortly after birth. However, in the adult, such conditions as hepatoma or teratoma stimulate the production of this primitive protein by the tumor cells. The quantification of AFP may be used both diagnostically and as a monitor of chemotherapy.

111.

D. PSA is a single-chain glycoprotein whose function aids in the liquefaction of seminal coagulum. PSA is found specifically in the prostate gland, and elevated levels are associated with prostate cancer and benign prostatic hyperplasia (BPH). Thus, combining the quantification of PSA with the performance of the digital rectal examination is more beneficial for prostate cancer detection. Immunoassays using enzyme, fluorescent, and chemiluminescent labels are available to quantify PSA. According to the American Cancer Society, the traditional PSA level of 4.0 ng/mL is recommended as a reasonable threshold for further evaluation. Values that fall in the indeterminate range (2.5–4.0 ng/mL) be taken on a patient-by-patient basis.

112.

B. CA 125 is an oncofetal antigen, glycoprotein in nature, that is produced by ovarian epithelial cells. The majority of individuals with nonmucinous epithelial ovarian cancer exhibit elevated levels of CA 125. CA 125 is also increased in other malignancies, including endometrial, breast, colon, pancreas, and lung cancers. Several benign disorders also exhibit CA 125 elevated levels. It appears that the primary usefulness of CA 125 is in monitoring the success of therapy in treating ovarian carcinoma.

113.

A. CA 19-9 is an oncofetal protein that is a sialylated Lewis blood group antigen. It is found in increased levels in colorectal carcinoma as well as in gastric, hepatobiliary, and pancreatic cancers. CA 19-9 is also elevated in several benign disorders, including pancreatitis, extra-hepatic cholestasis, and cirrhosis. The combination use of CA 19-9 and CEA (carcinoembryonic antigen) is helpful in monitoring the recurrence of colorectal cancer.

114.

B. Elevations of serum levels of AFP are found in a number of malignant as well as benign disorders. Although AFP is considered the most specific laboratory test for hepatocellular carcinoma, increased levels are also found in benign liver disease, including viral hepatitis, chronic active hepatitis, and cirrhosis. Other malignant disorders associated with increased levels of AFP include testicular and ovarian germ cell tumors, pancreatic carcinoma, gastric carcinoma, and colonic carcinoma. Thus, AFP is not a tissue-specific tumor marker. AFP is not elevated in prostatic cancer, which is characterized by an elevation in PSA. The use of AFP in conjunction with human chorionic gonadotropin (hCG) is effective in monitoring treatment and identifying recurrence of testicular cancer.

115.

D. hCG is a dimer consisting of alpha and beta polypeptide chains, with the β subunit conferring immunogenic specificity. Although hCG is more commonly associated with testing to confirm pregnancy, it is also associated with certain forms of cancer. β-hCG is used as a tumor marker for hydatidiform mole, gestational choriocarcinoma, and placental-site trophoblastic tumor. hCG's utility also extends to monitoring the success of therapy in testicular and ovarian germ cell tumors. In addition, increased levels of hCG have been identified in hematopoietic malignancy, melanoma, gastrointestinal tract neoplasms, sarcoma, and lung, breast, and renal cancers.

116.

D. CA 15-3 and CA 549 are oncofetal antigens that are glycoprotein in nature. CA 15-3 is found on mammary epithelium. Increased serum levels of CA 15-3 are found in breast, pancreatic, lung, colorectal, and liver cancers. CA 549 is found in the cell membrane and luminal surface of breast tissue. Increased serum levels of CA 549 are found in breast, lung, prostate, and colon cancers. Although both CA 15-3 and CA 549 are elevated in more advanced stages of breast cancer, neither is helpful in detecting early stages of breast cancer.

Nonprotein Nitrogenous Compounds

117.

D. Constituents in the plasma that contain the element nitrogen are categorized as being protein- or nonprotein-nitrogen compounds. The principal substances included among the nonprotein-nitrogen compounds are urea, amino acids, uric acid, creatinine, creatine, and ammonia. Of these compounds, urea is present in the plasma in the greatest concentration, comprising approximately 45% of the nonprotein-nitrogen fraction.

118.

D. Because the substances classified as non protein-nitrogen (NPN) compounds were quantified by assaying for their nitrogen content, it became customary to express urea as urea nitrogen. When urea was expressed as urea nitrogen, a comparison could be made between the concentration of urea and the concentration of other NPN compounds. When it is necessary to convert urea nitrogen values to urea, the concentration may be calculated easily by multiplying the urea nitrogen value by 2.14. This factor is derived from the molecular mass of urea (60 daltons) and the molecular weight of its two nitrogen atoms (28):

$$\frac{60}{28} = 2.14$$

119.

B. In addition to the fact that sodium fluoride is a weak anticoagulant, it also functions as an antiglycolytic agent and is used as a preservative for glucose in blood specimens. With the urease reagent systems for the quantification of urea, the use of sodium fluoride must be avoided because of its inhibitory effect on this system. Additionally, contamination from the use of ammonium oxalate and ammonium heparin must be avoided, because urease catalyzes the production of ammonium carbonate from urea. In several methods, the ammonium ion formed reacts proportionally to the amount of urea originally present in the sample. Anticoagulants containing ammonium would contribute falsely to the urea result.

120.

B. In the diacetyl method, acidic diacetyl reacts directly with urea to form a yellow-diazine derivative. Thiosemicarbazide and ferric ions are reagents used to intensify the color of the reaction. Because urea is quantified directly, the method does not suffer from interferences from ammonia contamination, as do some of the urea methods.

121.

A. Adequate specificity is generally obtained when using the urease/glutamate dehydrogenase method. Because urease hydrolyzes urea to ammonia and water, a positive interference from endogenous ammonia will occur with elevated blood levels of ammonia. Such interference may occur from use of aged blood specimens and in certain metabolic diseases.

122.

B. An enzymatic method for quantifying urea employs urease and glutamate dehydrogenase (GLDH) in a coupled enzymatic reaction. Urease catalyzes the production of ammonium carbonate from urea. The ammonium ion produced reacts with 2-oxoglutarate and NADH in the presence of GLDH with the formation of NAD^+ and glutamate. The decrease in absorbance, as NADH is oxidized to NAD^+, is followed kinetically at 340 nm using a spectrophotometer. In the conductimetric method, the formation of ammonium ions and carbonate ions, from the ammonium carbonate, causes a change in conductivity that is related to the amount of urea present in the sample.

123.

C. The Berthelot reaction is based on the production of a blue-indophenol compound when ammonia reacts in an alkaline medium with phenol and sodium hypochlorite. This basic colorimetric reaction can be used to quantify both urea and blood ammonia levels. Therefore, any ammonia contamination (i.e., in the distilled water used to make reagents for the urea procedure and on glassware) must be avoided so that falsely elevated urea values will not be obtained.

124.

A. The catabolism of some amino acids involves a transamination reaction in which the α-amino group of the amino acid is enzymatically removed. After its removal, the α-amino group is transferred to an α-keto acid (α-ketoglutarate) with the formation of l-glutamate. Glutamate, which is the common product formed by most transaminase reactions, then may undergo oxidative deamination in the liver mitochondria with the formation of ammonia. The ammonia thus formed leaves the mitochondria as the amino group of citrulline. Citrulline, in turn, condenses with aspartate, which contains the second amino group needed for urea synthesis, forming argininosuccinate, which ultimately leads to the formation of urea. Therefore, the formation of urea and its excretion in the urine provide the principal means by which the body is able to free itself of excess ammonia.

125.

D. It is necessary that certain precautions in specimen handling be exercised because the enzymatic process of deamination of amides continues at room temperature after a blood sample is drawn. When blood is drawn for ammonia analysis, it is critical that any *in vitro* ammonia formation be prevented. It is recommended that the tube containing the blood specimen be placed in an ice bath immediately after the blood is drawn, because the cold environment will help retard metabolic processes. It is also important that the chemical analysis of the specimen be started within 20 minutes of drawing the specimen.

126.

C. There is no reference method for the measurement of ammonia in biological fluids, however the preferred method to measure plasma ammonia on current automated analyzers uses GLDH with either NADH or NADPH. The ammonia concentration is proportional to the decrease in absorbance at 340 nm.

$$NH_4^+ + \text{2-oxoglutarate} + NADH + H^+ \xrightarrow{\text{glutamate dehydrogenase}} \text{glutamate} + NAD^+ + H_2O$$

127.

D. Ion-exchange, ion-selective electrode, and enzymatic methods have been employed for the analysis of ammonia in plasma specimens. Because the enzymatic method is a direct assay, prior separation of ammonium ions is not required. The enzymatic reaction catalyzed by glutamate dehydrogenase follows:

$$\text{2-Oxoglutarate} + NH_4^+ + NADPH \rightleftharpoons \text{Glutamate} + NADP^+ + H_2O$$

The rate of oxidation of NADPH to $NADP^+$ is followed as a decreasing change in absorbance at 340 nm.

128.

D. The gastrointestinal tract is the primary source of blood ammonia. With normal liver function, ammonia is metabolized to urea for urinary excretion. When blood ammonia levels become elevated, toxicity of the central nervous system occurs. Diseases associated with elevated blood ammonia levels include Reye syndrome, renal failure, chronic liver failure, cirrhosis, and hepatic encephalopathy.

129.

A. Creatinine is a waste product of muscle metabolism and as such its production is rather constant on a daily basis. Creatinine is freely filtered by the glomerulus, with only a very small amount secreted by the proximal tubule. Thus, measurement of creatinine is a reflection of glomerular filtration. An increase in the serum creatinine level would be indicative of decreased glomerular filtration. Although uric acid, urea, and ammonia levels may be increased with decreased glomerular filtration, increased levels of these analytes are associated with a number of specific metabolic diseases and, therefore, they are not used as indicators of the glomerular filtration rate.

130.

D. In a renal pathologic state, both BUN and creatinine would be elevated. The elevation in creatinine should be approximately equal to the elevation in BUN because BUN and creatinine elevate in equal amounts in a renal pathologic state. With a creatinine of 6.0 (a result 5 times higher than normal) one would expect a BUN result to be five times higher as well.

131.

C. Creatine is synthesized from the amino acids arginine, glycine, and methionine. In tissues that include the kidneys, small intestinal mucosa, pancreas, and liver, arginine and glycine form guanidoacetate through a transaminidase reaction. The guanidoacetate is transported in the blood to the liver, where it reacts with *S*-adenosylmethionine through a transmethylase reaction to form creatine. Creatine is transported in the blood to muscle tissue. Creatine in the form of phosphocreatine is a high-energy storage compound that provides the phosphate needed to produce adenosine triphosphate (ATP) for muscle metabolism. When ATP is formed from phosphocreatine, free creatine is also released. Creatine, through a spontaneous and irreversible reaction, forms creatinine. Creatinine serves no functional metabolic role. It is excreted in the urine as a waste product of creatine.

132.

A. The Jaffe reaction, which was described in 1886, is still used for creatinine analysis. The Jaffe reaction employs the use of an alkaline picrate solution that reacts with creatinine to form a bright orange-red complex. A drawback to this procedure is its lack of specificity for creatinine, because noncreatinine chromogens, glucose, and proteins are also able to react with alkaline picrate.

133.

A. Because protein will interfere with the Jaffe reaction, serum for a manual creatinine analysis is treated with sodium tungstate and sulfuric acid to precipitate the proteins. The use of tungstic acid to make a protein-free filtrate is known as the Folin-Wu method. The protein-free filtrate, which still contains creatinine and other reducing substances, is then mixed with alkaline picrate reagent to yield the characteristic Jaffe reaction. Automated methods have replaced manual methods. These kinetic methods using the alkaline picrate reagent system have been adapted to use small volumes of serum and have readings taken within a short interval of 25–60 sec following initiation of the reaction. Because of the speed at which the analysis is performed and the small serum sample requirement, serum may be used directly, alleviating the need for a protein-free filtrate.

134.

D. The creatinine clearance test is used to assess the glomerular filtration rate. An accurately timed 24-hour urine specimen and a blood sample, drawn in the middle of the 24-hour urine collection, are required. The creatinine concentrations of the urine specimen and the plasma are determined, and these values, along with the urine volume, are used to determine the creatinine clearance. The body surface area will not be used in the calculation because the clearance is being done on an average-size adult. The following general mathematical formula is used to calculate creatinine clearance:

$$\frac{U}{P} \times V = \text{Creatinine clearance (mL/min)}$$

where U = urine creatinine concentration in milligrams per deciliter, P = plasma creatinine concentration in milligrams per deciliter, and V = volume of urine per minute, with volume expressed in milliliters and 24 hours expressed as 1440 minutes. Applying this formula to the problem presented in the question:

$$\frac{120 \text{ mg/dL}}{1.2 \text{ mg/dL}} \times \frac{1520 \text{ mL/24 h}}{1440 \text{ min/24 h}} = 106 \text{ mL/min}$$

It should be noted that both the size of the kidney and the body surface area of an individual influence the creatinine clearance rate. Because normal values for creatinine clearance are based on the average adult body surface area, it is necessary that the clearance rate be adjusted when the body surface area of the individual being tested differs significantly from the average adult area. This type of adjustment is especially critical if the individual is an infant, a young child, or an adolescent. The body surface area may be calculated from an individual's height and weight, or it may be determined from a nomogram. The average body surface area is accepted as being 1.73 m^2. The mathematical formula used to calculate a creatinine clearance when the body surface area of the individual is required follows:

$$\frac{U}{P} \times V \times \frac{1.73}{A} = \text{Creatinine clearance}$$
$$\text{(mL/min/standard surface area)}$$

where 1.73 = standard adult surface area in square meters and A = body surface area of the individual in square meters.

135.

C. Creatinine assays are preferably performed on fresh urine specimens. If an acid urine specimen is kept for a time, any creatine in the urine will be converted to creatinine. In alkaline urine, an equilibrium situation will occur between the creatine and creatinine present in the specimen. To avoid either of these situations, it is recommended that the urine be adjusted to pH 7.0 and that the specimen be frozen. It is thought that at a neutral pH, the integrity of the urine specimen will be maintained because it will require days or even weeks for equilibrium to occur between the two compounds.

136.

D. Creatine is predominantly found in muscle cells, where the quantity of creatine is proportional to muscle mass. As muscle metabolism proceeds, creatine is freed from its high-energy phosphate form, and the creatine, thus liberated, forms the anhydride creatinine. The quantity of creatinine formed daily is a relatively constant amount because it is related to muscle mass. Therefore, it has been customary to quantify the creatinine present in a 24-hour urine specimen as an index of the completeness of the collection.

137.

A. In addition to the endpoint and kinetic methods, which use the Jaffe reaction (picric acid), several methods have been developed that use coupled enzymatic reactions for the quantification of creatinine. In one such method, creatinine amidohydrolase (creatininase) catalyzes the conversion of creatinine to creatine and subsequently to sarcosine and urea. Sarcosine oxidase catalyzes the oxidation of sarcosine to glycine, formaldehyde, and hydrogen peroxide. The hydrogen peroxide reacts with the reduced form of a chromogenic dye in the presence of peroxidase to form an oxidized colored dye product that is read spectrophotometrically.

138.

C. Creatinine is an endogenous substance that is filtered by the glomeruli and normally is neither reabsorbed nor secreted by the tubules. When plasma levels of creatinine rise, some secretion of creatinine by the tubules will occur. The filtration properties of creatinine and the fact that it is a substance normally present in blood make the creatinine clearance test the method of choice for assessing the glomerular filtration rate.

139.

B. Through a sequence of enzymatic reactions, the purine nucleosides, adenosine and guanosine, are catabolized to the waste product uric acid. The catabolism of purines occurs primarily in the liver, with the majority of uric acid being excreted as a urinary waste product. The remaining amount of uric acid is excreted in the biliary, pancreatic, and gastrointestinal secretions through the gastrointestinal tract. In the large intestine, uric acid is further degraded by bacteria and excreted in the stool.

140.

D. Uric acid may be quantified by reacting it with phosphotungstic acid reagent in alkaline solution. In this reaction, uric acid is oxidized to allantoin and the phosphotungstic acid is reduced, forming a tungsten blue complex. The intensity of the tungsten blue complex is proportional to the concentration of uric acid in the specimen.

141.

B. Uric acid absorbs light in the ultraviolet region of 290–293 nm. When uricase is added to a uric acid mixture, uricase destroys uric acid by catalyzing its degradation to allantoin and carbon dioxide. On the basis of these two characteristics, differential spectrophotometry has been applied to the quantification of uric acid. This type of method is used on analyzers that are capable of monitoring the decrease in absorbance as uric acid is destroyed by uricase. The decrease in absorbance is proportional to the concentration of uric acid in the specimen.

142.

A. As renal function continues to be lost over time, chronic renal failure develops. Chronic renal failure is manifested by loss of excretory function, inability to regulate water and electrolyte balance, and increased production of parathyroid hormone, all of which contribute to the abnormal laboratory findings. The decreased production of erythropoietin causes anemia to develop.

143.

D. Gout is a pathological condition that may be caused by a malfunction of purine metabolism or a depression in the renal excretion of uric acid. Two of the major characteristics of gout are hyperuricemia and a deposition of uric acid as monosodium urate crystals in joints, periarticular cartilage, bone, bursae, and subcutaneous tissue. Such a deposition of urate crystals causes inflammation of the affected area and precipitates an arthritic attack.

144.

A. An increase in serum uric acid levels may be seen during chemotherapy for leukemia. The cause of this is the accelerated breakdown of cell nuclei in response to the chemotherapy. Other proliferative disorders that may respond similarly are lymphoma, multiple myeloma, and polycythemia. It is important that serum uric acid be monitored during chemotherapy to avoid nephrotoxicity.

Carbohydrates

145.

D. When two monosaccharides condense with loss of a molecule of water, a disaccharide is formed. Disaccharides, therefore, can be hydrolyzed into two monosaccharides. The most important disaccharides are maltose, lactose, and sucrose. On hydrolysis, sucrose will yield one molecule of glucose and one molecule of fructose. Maltose can be hydrolyzed into two molecules of glucose. Lactose can be hydrolyzed into glucose and galactose.

146.

A. Glycogen is a polysaccharide composed of many glucose molecules. In contrast to the amylopectin molecule, a glycogen molecule is more highly branched and more compact. Glycogen is found in a variety of animal tissues, particularly in the liver, and provides the storage form for carbohydrates in the body. When energy requirements warrant it, glycogen may be broken down to glucose by a series of phosphorylating and related enzymes.

147.

A. There are three major classifications of carbohydrates: monosaccharides, disaccharides, and polysaccharides. Starch is classified as a polysaccharide because its structure is composed of many molecules of glucose (a monosaccharide) condensed together. Monosaccharides (e.g., glucose) are carbohydrates with the general molecular formula $C_n(H_2O)_n$ that cannot be broken down to simpler substances by acid hydrolysis. Disaccharides (e.g., sucrose, lactose) are condensation products of two molecules of monosaccharides with loss of one molecule of water.

148.

A. The level of glucose in the blood is a result of a variety of metabolic processes. Processes that increase the blood glucose include ingestion of sugar, synthesis of glucose from noncarbohydrate sources, and breakdown of glycogen. Processes that decrease blood glucose include metabolizing glucose to produce energy and converting glucose to glycogen or fat. Glycogen is a polysaccharide, which is the storage form of carbohydrates in animals. *Glycogenesis* refers to the formation of glycogen in the liver from blood glucose. This occurs in response to increased blood glucose levels. In response to decreasing blood glucose levels, glycogen in the liver is broken down to glucose. This process is called *glycogenolysis*. When glucose is metabolized, for example, to produce energy, it is converted to lactate or pyruvate. This process is called *glycolysis*. When the body synthesizes glucose from noncarbohydrate sources—that is, amino acids, glycerol, or lactate—the process is called *gluconeogenesis*. When the body uses glucose to synthesize fat, this process is called *lipogenesis*.

149.

A. When highly specific analytical methods are used, the glucose concentration in fasting whole blood is approximately 12–15% lower than in plasma or serum. Although glucose diffuses freely between the water phase of plasma and red blood cells, there is a higher concentration of water in plasma (approximately 12%) than in whole blood, accounting for the increased glucose concentration in plasma. The water content of whole blood depends on the hematocrit.

150.

D. Renal threshold is defined as the plasma level that must be exceeded in order for the substance to appear in the urine. The renal threshold for glucose is 180 mg/dL. This means that the blood glucose level must exceed 180 mg/dL in order for glucose to be excreted in the urine.

151.

D. *Glycated hemoglobin* is a collective term encompassing the three glycated hemoglobin fractions—hemoglobin A_{1a}, hemoglobin A_{1b}, and hemoglobin A_{1c}. Hb A_{1c} is the fraction of Hb A_1 that is present in the greatest concentration. Some commercially available column chromatography methods measure the three fractions collectively. *Glycated hemoglobin* refers to the specific red cell hemoglobin A types to which a glucose molecule becomes irreversibly attached. The greater the glucose concentration in the plasma, the greater the number of hemoglobin molecules that will become glycated. Because red blood cells have an average life span of 120 days and the glycation is irreversible, measurement of glycated hemoglobin reflects the average plasma glucose level of an individual during the previous 2- to 3-month period. This test is used as a monitor of diabetic control.

152.

B. The patient presents as having diabetes mellitus. The American Diabetes Association (ADA) published updated standards in 2007 for the classification and diagnosis of diabetes mellitus. Three criteria have been defined, with only one needing to be present to establish the diagnosis of diabetes mellitus. The three criteria include classic diabetic symptoms and a casual plasma glucose of ≥200 mg/dL, a fasting plasma glucose of ≥126 mg/dL, and a 2-hour postload plasma glucose (part of OGTT) of ≥200 mg/dL. It is recommended that any positive test be repeated on a subsequent day, if possible, to confirm the diagnosis. It should be noted that the OGTT is not recommended for routine clinical use and would be used only in special circumstances.

153.

C. Increased insulin resistance is commonly seen in the late second and third trimesters of pregnancy. Most women are able to compensate by secreting additional insulin and, thus, are able to maintain normal blood glucose levels. In cases of gestational diabetes mellitus, women are unable to make sufficient insulin to meet their needs. In the screening test, serum glucose is assessed at 1 hour following the ingestion of a 50-g glucose load (glucose challenge test). If the serum glucose is ≥140 mg/dL, the next step is to perform an oral glucose tolerance test.

154.

D. Sodium fluoride is a weak anticoagulant that acts as a preservative for glucose. It functions as a glucose preservative by inhibiting glycolysis. However, it is not suitable for use with many enzyme procedures. In the determination of BUN, where urease activity is utilized, the high concentration of fluoride in the plasma acts as an enzyme inhibitor, preventing the necessary chemical reaction.

155.

D. Based on the biochemistry of the disease, diabetes mellitus has been classified as type 1 and type 2. Type 1 occurs more commonly in individuals under 20 years of age. Studies suggest that type 1 is associated with autoimmune destruction of β-cells, and it is characterized by insulin deficiency and thus a dependency on injection of insulin. Unlike people afflicted with type 2, type 1 individuals are prone to ketoacidosis and to such complications as angiopathy, cataracts, nephropathy, and neuropathy.

156.

C. The protein hormone insulin is synthesized in the pancreas by the β-cells of the islets of Langerhans. Insulin, a two-chain polypeptide, consists of 51 amino acids. A single-chain preproinsulin is cleaved to proinsulin, which is the immediate precursor of insulin. Proinsulin is hydrolyzed to form insulin, a two-chain polypeptide, and inactive C-peptide. Insulin promotes the entry of glucose into tissue cells.

157.

D. Insulin may be described as an anabolic, polypeptide hormone. Insulin stimulates glucose uptake by muscle cells (which increases protein synthesis), by fat cells (which increases triglyceride synthesis), and by liver cells (which increases lipid synthesis and glycogenesis). If cellular uptake of glucose is stimulated, the glucose concentration in the circulation decreases.

158.

D. In uncontrolled diabetes mellitus, the blood glucose level exceeds the renal threshold of approximately 180 mg/dL for glucose, leading to glycosuria and polyuria. The excess secretion of glucagon stimulates lipolysis, with increased formation of acetoacetic acid. In the blood, the ketoacids dissociate, with the hydrogen ions being buffered by bicarbonate. This causes the bicarbonate to become depleted and leads to metabolic acidosis.

159.

D. Glucose determinations are generally performed on serum or plasma rather than whole blood. Serum or plasma is more convenient to use than whole blood in most automated systems because serum does not require mixing before sampling. Glucose stability is greater in separated plasma than in whole blood because glycolysis is minimized. Specificity for glucose is higher when plasma or serum is used because variations attributable to interfering substances in the red cells are avoided.

160.

D. Research has demonstrated that there is a correlation between blood glucose levels in diabetes mellitus and the development of long-term complications. These complications may include such disorders as retinopathy, neuropathy, atherosclerosis, and renal failure. Thus, quantifying such blood analytes as urea, creatinine, and lipids as well as urinary albumin can aid in monitoring people with diabetes.

161.

D. There are greater than 100 causes of hypoglycemia. Among the causes is the ingestion of certain drugs. Use of ethanol, propranolol, and salicylate has been linked to the occurrence of hypoglycemia.

162.

B. The diagnostic test for hypoglycemia is the 72-hour fast, which requires the analysis of glucose, insulin, C-peptide, and proinsulin at 6-hour intervals. The test should be concluded when plasma glucose levels drop to ≤45 mg/dL, when hypoglycemic symptoms appear, or after 72 hours have elapsed. In general, hypoglycemic symptoms occur when the plasma glucose level falls below 55 mg/dL. Such symptoms may include headache, confusion, blurred vision, dizziness, and seizures. The term "neuroglycopenia" has been applied to these central nervous system disorders. Although decreased hepatic glucose production and increased glucose utilization may cause hypoglycemia, there are over 100 causes of this disorder.

163.

B. Glucose in the presence of oxygen is oxidized to gluconic acid and hydrogen peroxide. This reaction is catalyzed by glucose oxidase. By using a polarographic oxygen electrode, the rate of oxygen consumption is measured and related to the concentration of glucose in the sample.

164.

C. The hexokinase method for quantifying glucose uses two coupled enzymatic reactions. In the first reaction, which is catalyzed by hexokinase, glucose is phosphorylated by adenosine triphosphate, forming glucose-6-phosphate and adenosine diphosphate. In the second reaction, glucose-6-phosphate dehydrogenase (derived from yeast) catalyzes the oxidation of glucose-6-phosphate and the reduction of nicotinamide adenine dinucleotide phosphate. The amount of reduced NADPH formed is proportional to the glucose concentration in the sample. Thus, the greater the absorbance reading of NADPH at 340 nm, the greater is the glucose concentration. If bacterial G-6-PD is used, the cofactor is NAD^+ with the production of NADH.

165.

A. The glucose oxidase method for quantifying glucose employs two coupled enzymatic reactions. In the first reaction, which is catalyzed by glucose oxidase, glucose in the presence of oxygen is oxidized to gluconic acid and hydrogen peroxide. In the second reaction, peroxidase catalyzes a reaction between hydrogen peroxide and the reduced form of a chromogenic oxygen acceptor, such as *o*-dianisidine, forming an oxidized colored product that is read spectrophotometrically.

166.

C. The glucose dehydrogenase method uses only one enzymatic reaction for the measurement of glucose in a sample. Glucose dehydrogenase catalyzes the oxidation of glucose and the reduction of nicotinamide adenine dinucleotide. The amount of reduced NADH formed is proportional to the glucose concentration in the sample. When measuring blood glucose levels during the administration of an oral xylose tolerance test, the glucose dehydrogenase method should not be used, because the relative rate of reaction of d-xylose as compared to glucose is 15% with this method. In contrast, d-xylose will not react in the hexokinase and glucose oxidase methods, thus allowing glucose to be measured accurately.

The d-xylose absorption test is useful in distinguishing two types of malabsorption: intestinal malabsorption and malabsorption resulting from pancreatic insufficiency. When d-xylose is administered orally, it is absorbed by passive diffusion into the portal vein from the proximal portion of the small intestine. Because d-xylose is not metabolized by the liver, it is excreted unchanged by the kidneys. In intestinal malabsorption, the amount of d-xylose excreted, as measured in a 5-hour urine specimen, is less than normal because of decreased absorption of d-xylose. In malabsorption caused by pancreatic insufficiency, the absorption of d-xylose is normal.

167.

C. Although there are several reliable enzymatic glucose methods available, the hexokinase method is the reference method for quantifying glucose. The reference method requires that a protein-free filtrate be made using barium hydroxide and zinc sulfate. The clear supernatant is then used as the sample in the hexokinase/glucose-6-phosphate dehydrogenase coupled enzyme reactions. For routine clinical use, serum is used directly in the hexokinase method because deproteinization is too time-consuming.

168.

C. The reference interval for glucose in CSF is 60% of the normal plasma value. For a plasma glucose of 110 mg/dL, the expected CSF glucose level would be 66 mg/dL. The equilibration of CSF with plasma glucose takes several hours. The reference interval for the CSF glucose level is 40–70 mg/dL as compared with a normal fasting plasma glucose level. Low levels of CSF glucose are associated with a number of diseases including bacterial meningitis and tuberculous meningitis, whereas viral disease generally presents with a normal level of CSF glucose.

169.

C. The reference interval for fasting serum glucose in an adult expressed in conventional units is 74–99 mg/dL. To convert conventional units to SI units (Système International d'Unités), multiply the conventional units in mg/dL by the 0.0555 conversion factor to obtain SI units in mmol/L. Thus, 74 mg/dL × 0.0555 = 4.1 mmol/L and 99 mg/dL × 0.0555 = 5.5 mmol/L. Although conventional units are used commonly in the United States, many scientific journals require the use of SI units in their publications and many foreign countries use SI units routinely in clinical practice. To identify additional conversion factors for other analytes, consult the appendix of a clinical chemistry textbook.

170.

B. It is currently recommended by the ADA that hemoglobin A_{1c} should be lowered to an average of approximately 7% in individuals with diabetes mellitus. When hemoglobin A_{1c} is reduced to this level or less, there is a reduction in microvascular and neuropathic complications of diabetes and to some degree macrovascular disease. Therefore, the ADA recommends that nonpregnant adults be maintained at a hemoglobin A_{1c} level of <7%. There is some discussion that 6% would be better. Hemoglobin A_{1c} is the major component of the glycated hemoglobins. Quantification of hemoglobin A_{1c} may be performed using high-performance liquid chromatography, ion-exchange chromatography (manual), isoelectric focusing, and immunoassay techniques.

171.

D. Regulation of the blood glucose concentration depends on a number of hormones. These include insulin, glucagon, cortisol, epinephrine, growth hormone, adrenocorticotropic hormone, and thyroxine. Of these hormones, *insulin* is the only one that decreases the blood glucose level. *Glucagon* is produced in the pancreas by the alpha cells. Glucagon promotes an increase in the blood glucose concentration by its stimulatory effect on glycogenolysis in the liver. *Cortisol* is produced by the adrenal cortex. It stimulates gluconeogenesis, thus increasing the blood level of glucose. *Epinephrine* is produced by the adrenal medulla. It promotes glycogenolysis, thus increasing blood glucose. *Growth hormone* and *adrenocorticotropic hormone* are produced by the anterior pituitary gland. Both hormones are antagonistic to insulin and hence increase blood glucose. *Thyroxine* is produced by the thyroid gland. It not only stimulates glycogenolysis but also increases the intestinal absorption rate of glucose.

172.

B. Epinephrine is produced by the adrenal medulla. It promotes glycogenolysis, thus increasing the blood glucose level. Epinephrine also inhibits the secretion of insulin and stimulates the secretion of glucagon.

173.

A. In Cushing syndrome, the adrenal cortex secretes an excessive amount of the hormone cortisol. Because cortisol has a stimulatory effect on gluconeogenesis, hyperglycemia commonly occurs as a secondary disorder. Hypoglycemia frequently characterizes Addison disease in which there is decreased production of cortisol.

174.

B. When a fasting plasma glucose test is performed and the glucose value is between 100–125 mg/dL, the individual is considered to have impaired fasting glucose (IFG). This is less than the value associated with diagnosis of diabetes mellitus, which is a fasting plasma glucose ≥126 mg/dL. IFG is considered a risk factor and a stage between normal glucose metabolism and development of diabetes mellitus.

175.

B. Because of the critical reasons for aspirating a CSF specimen, the testing is performed as soon as possible upon receipt of the specimen in the laboratory. In this case, the cloudy appearance would be most likely due to the presence of bacteria. Both bacteria and red blood cells can use glucose *in vitro*. Thus any delay in glucose testing could result in a falsely low result. The CSF specimen should be centrifuged to remove cellular material and assayed immediately.

176.

A. In the glucose oxidase/peroxidase method, the second coupled enzyme reaction involves peroxidase catalyzing the reaction between hydrogen peroxide and a chromogenic oxygen acceptor, which is oxidized to its colored form. Several blood constituents, including uric acid, ascorbic acid, bilirubin, tetracycline, hemoglobin, and glutathione, when present in increased concentrations can interfere with the assay by competing for the hydrogen peroxide produced in the first coupled enzyme reaction. This loss of hydrogen peroxide would result in falsely low plasma glucose results. Because of the high levels of uric acid normally found in urine, the glucose oxidase/peroxidase method would not be suitable for measuring urine glucose.

177.

D. A casual plasma glucose should be less than 200 mg/dL. The reference range for glycated hemoglobin (Hb A_{1c}) is 4–6%. Because the individual is a postmenopausal, 57-year-old female, with abnormal test results being found as part of an annual physical examination, the most likely diagnosis is type 2 diabetes mellitus. The ADA recommends that in the absence of unequivocal hyperglycemia, the glucose result should be confirmed by repeating the casual glucose or performing a fasting plasma glucose on a subsequent day. The ADA does not recommend HbA_{1c} as a screening test for diabetes mellitus.

178.

A. Carbohydrate is stored in the body in the form of glycogen. There are many enzymes involved in the metabolism of glycogen. A deficiency of any one of the enzymes involved will result in what are called glycogen storage diseases, or glycogenoses. There are at least 10 distinct types of glycogen storage diseases, and all of them are rare. All are hereditary. Diagnosis of each type can be made by the assay of the deficient enzyme from the appropriate tissue and by microscopic study of the affected tissues.

- Type I—von Gierke disease is clinically characterized by severe fasting hypoglycemia and lactic acidosis. This is due to a deficiency of the enzyme glucose-6-phosphatase. Glucose cannot be transported from the liver as glucose-6-phosphate during the breakdown of glycogen. It is metabolized to lactic acid and thus results in lactic acidosis.
- Type II—Pompe disease is caused by a deficiency of lysosomal α-1,4-glucosidase. This results in an increase of glycogen in all organs and abnormally large lysosomes. The glycogen cannot be degraded because of the deficiency of α-1,4-glucosidase.
- Type III—Cori disease is caused by the absence of a debrancher enzyme. This disease is characterized by hypo glycemia, hepatomegaly, seizures, and growth retardation.
- Type IV—Andersen disease is caused by a deficiency of brancher enzyme. It is a rare disease characterized by progressive liver enlargement or cirrhosis and muscular weakness by the age of 2 months. Storage glycogen is not usually found, but unbranched amylopectin accumulates in this disease.

Lipids and Lipoproteins

179.

C. Bile acids are synthesized in the hepatocytes of the liver. They are C_{24} steroids that are derived from cholesterol. With fat ingestion, the bile salts are released into the intestines, where they aid in the emulsification of dietary fats. Thus bile acids also serve as a vehicle for cholesterol excretion. A majority of the bile acids, however, are reabsorbed from the intestines into the enterohepatic circulation for reexcretion into the bile. The two principal bile acids are cholic acid and chenodeoxycholic acid. These acids are conjugated with one of two amino acids, glycine or taurine. Measurement of bile acids is possible via immunotechniques and may aid in the diagnosis of some liver disorders such as obstructive jaundice, primary biliary cirrhosis, and viral hepatitis.

180.

C. After fat ingestion, lipids are first degraded, then reformed, and finally incorporated by the intestinal mucosal cells into absorbable complexes known as chylomicrons. These chylomicrons enter the blood through the lymphatic system, where they impart a turbid appearance to serum. Such lipemic plasma specimens frequently interfere with absorbance or cause a change in absorbance measurements, leading to invalid results.

181.

C. Total cholesterol consists of two fractions, free cholesterol and cholesteryl ester. In the plasma, cholesterol exists mostly in the cholesteryl ester form. Approximately 70% of total plasma cholesterol is esterified with fatty acids. The formation of cholesteryl esters is such that a transferase enzyme catalyzes the transfer of fatty acids from phosphatidylcholine to the carbon-3 alcohol function position of the free cholesterol molecule. Laboratories routinely measure total cholesterol by first using the reagent cholesterol esterase to break the ester bonds with the fatty acids.

182.

D. A "routine" lipid profile would most likely consist of the measurement of total cholesterol, triglyceride, HDL cholesterol, and LDL cholesterol. These measurements are most easily adapted to today's multichannel chemistry analyzers. Both total cholesterol and triglyceride use enzymatic techniques to drive the reaction to completion. HDL cholesterol and LDL cholesterol are commonly requested tests to help determine patient risk for coronary heart disease. The HDL is separated from other lipoproteins using a precipitation technique, immunotechniques, and/or polymers and detergents. The nonprecipitation techniques are preferred because they can give better precision, be adapted to an automated chemistry analyzer, and be run without personnel intervention. LDL cholesterol may be calculated using the Friedewald equation, or it may be assayed directly using selective precipitation methods or direct homogeneous techniques.

183.

D. Blood specimens for lipid studies should be drawn in the fasting state at least 9–12 hours after eating. Although fat ingestion only slightly affects cholesterol levels, the triglyceride results are greatly affected. Triglycerides peak at about 4–6 hours after a meal, and these exogenous lipids should be cleared from the plasma before analysis. The presence of chylomicrons, as a result of an inadequate fasting period, must be avoided because of their interference in spectrophotometric analyses.

184.

A. Total cholesterol screenings are commonly performed on nonfasting individuals. Total cholesterol is only slightly affected by the fasting status of the individual, whereas triglycerides, fatty acids, and lipoproteins are greatly affected. Following a meal, chylomicrons would be present, which are rich in triglycerides and fatty acids and contain very little cholesterol. The majority of cholesterol is produced by the liver and other tissues. High levels of exogenous triglycerides and/or fatty acids will interfere with the measurement of lipoproteins. Chylomicrons are normally cleared from the body 6 hours after eating.

185.

B. The long-chain fatty acids of triglycerides can be broken down to form energy through the process of beta/oxidation, also known as the fatty acid cycle. In this process, two carbons at a time are cleaved from long-chain fatty acids to form acetyl-coenzyme A. Acetyl-coenzyme A, in turn, can enter the Krebs cycle to be converted to energy or be converted to acetoacetyl-Co-A and converted to energy by an alternate pathway, leaving behind the acidic by-product ketones composed of beta-hydroxybutyrate, acetoacetate, and acetone. Under proper conditions, pyruvate can be converted to acetyl-coenzyme A at the end of glycolysis of glucose. Bile is a breakdown product of cholesterol used in the digestion of dietary cholesterol.

186.

D. The kinetic methods used for quantifying serum triglycerides use a reaction system of coupling enzymes. It is first necessary to hydrolyze the triglycerides to free fatty acids and glycerol. This hydrolysis step is catalyzed by the enzyme lipase. The glycerol is then free to react in the enzyme-coupled reaction system that includes glycerokinase, pyruvate kinase, and lactate dehydrogenase or in the enzyme-coupled system that includes glycerokinase, glycerophosphate oxidase, and peroxidase.

187.

C. In the enzymatic method for quantifying total cholesterol in serum, the serum specimen must initially be treated with cholesteryl ester hydrolase. This enzyme hydrolyzes the cholesteryl esters into free cholesterol and fatty acids. Both the free cholesterol, derived from the cholesteryl ester fraction, and any free cholesterol normally present in serum may react in the cholesterol oxidase/peroxidase reactions for total cholesterol. The hydrolysis of the cholesteryl ester fraction is necessary because cholesterol oxidase reacts only with free cholesterol.

188.

C. Chylomicrons are protein-lipid complexes composed primarily of triglycerides and containing only small amounts of cholesterol, phospholipids, and protein. After food ingestion, the chylomicron complexes are formed in the epithelial cells of the intestines. From the epithelial cells, the chylomicrons are released into the lymphatic system, which transports chylomicrons to the blood. The chylomicrons may then carry the triglycerides to adipose tissue for storage, to organs for catabolism, or to the liver for incorporation of the triglycerides into very-low-density lipoproteins (VLDLs). Chylomicrons are normally cleared from plasma within 6 hours after a meal.

189.

B. Beta-hydroxybutyric acid, acetoacetic acid, and acetone are collectively referred to as ketone bodies. They are formed as a result of the process of beta-oxidation in which liver cells degrade fatty acids with a resultant excess accumulation of acetyl-coenzyme A (CoA). The acetyl-CoA is the parent compound from which ketone bodies are synthesized through a series of reactions.

190.

D. Sphingolipids, most notably sphingomyelin, are the major lipids of the cell membranes of the central nervous system (i.e., the myelin sheath). Like phospholipids, sphingolipids are amphipathic and contain a polar, hydrophilic head and a nonpolar, hydrophobic tail, making them excellent membrane formers. Although sometimes considered a subgroup of phospholipids, sphingomyelin is derived from the amino alcohol sphingosine instead of glycerol.

191.

B. All the lipoproteins contain some amount of triglyceride, cholesterol, phospholipid, and protein. Each of the lipoprotein fractions is distinguished by its unique concentration of these substances. The beta-lipoprotein fraction is composed of approximately 50% cholesterol, 6% triglycerides, 22% phospholipids, and 22% protein. The beta-lipoproteins, which are also known as the low-density lipoproteins (LDLs), are the principal transport vehicle for cholesterol in the plasma. Both the chylomicrons and the prebeta-lipoproteins are composed primarily of triglycerides. The chylomicrons are considered transport vehicles for exogenous triglycerides. In other words, dietary fat is absorbed through the intestine in the form of chylomicrons. After a meal, the liver will clear the chylomicrons from the blood and use the triglyceride component to form the prebeta-lipoproteins. Therefore, in the fasting state triglycerides are transported in the blood primarily by the prebeta-lipoproteins. The prebeta-lipoproteins are composed of approximately 55% triglycerides.

192.

B. The 27-carbon, ringed structure of cholesterol is the backbone of steroid hormones. The nucleus is called the cyclopentanoperhydrophenanthrene ring. The steroid hormones having this ring include estrogens (18 carbons), androgens (19 carbons), glucocorticoids (21 carbons), and mineralocorticoids (21 carbons).

193.

C. The majority of the lipid (lysosomal) storage diseases are inherited as autosomal recessive mutations. This group of diseases is characterized by an accumulation of sphingolipids in the central nervous system or some other organ. Such lipid accumulation frequently leads to intellectual disability or progressive loss of central nervous system functions. The cause of such lipid accumulation has been attributed either to specific enzyme deficiencies or to nonfunctional enzyme forms that inhibit the normal catabolism of the sphingolipids.

194.

B. Pancreatic insufficiency, Whipple disease, cystic fibrosis, and tropical sprue are diseases characterized by the malabsorption of lipids from the intestines. This malabsorption results in an excess lipid accumulation in the feces that is known as steatorrhea. When steatorrhea is suspected, the amount of lipid material present in the feces may be quantified. A 24- or 72-hour fecal specimen should be collected, the latter being the specimen of choice. The lipids are extracted from the fecal specimen and analyzed by gravimetric or titrimetric methods.

195.

B. A double nomenclature exists for the five principal lipoprotein fractions. The nomenclature is such that the various fractions have been named on the basis of both the electrophoretic mobilities and the ultracentrifugal sedimentation rates. The chylomicrons are known as chylomicrons by both methods. The chylomicrons are the least dense fraction, exhibiting a solvent density for isolation of less than 0.95 g/mL, and have the slowest electrophoretic mobility. The HDLs, also known as the alpha-lipoproteins, have the greatest density of 1.063–1.210 g/mL and move the fastest electrophoretically toward the anode. The VLDLs, also known as the prebeta-lipoproteins, move slightly slower electrophoretically than the alpha fraction. The VLDLs have a density of 0.95–1.006 g/mL. The IDLs, intermediate-density lipoproteins, have a density of 1.006–1.019 g/mL and migrate as a broad band between beta- and prebeta-lipoproteins. The LDLs, also known as the beta-lipoproteins, have an electrophoretic mobility that is slightly slower than that of the IDL fraction. The LDLs have an intermediate density of 1.019–1.063 g/mL, which is between the IDLs and the HDLs. To summarize the electrophoretic mobilities, the alpha-lipoprotein fraction migrates the farthest toward the anode from the origin, followed in order of decreasing mobility by the prebeta-lipoprotein, broad band between beta- and prebeta-lipoprotein, beta-lipoprotein, and chylomicron fractions. The chylomicrons remain more cathodal near the point of serum application.

196.

C. The quantification of the HDL cholesterol level is thought to contribute in assessing the risk that an individual may develop coronary artery disease (CAD). There appears to be an inverse relationship between HDL cholesterol and CAD. With low levels of HDL cholesterol, the risk of CAD increases. It is thought that the HDL facilitates the removal of cholesterol from the arterial wall, therefore decreasing the risk of atherosclerosis. In addition, LDL cholesterol may be assessed, because increased LDL cholesterol and decreased HDL cholesterol are associated with increased risk of CAD.

197.

D. Respiratory distress syndrome (RDS), also referred to as hyaline membrane disease, is commonly seen in preterm infants. A deficiency of pulmonary surfactant causes the infant's alveoli to collapse during expiration, resulting in improper oxygenation of capillary blood in the alveoli. Currently, the surfactant/albumin ratio by fluorescence polarization is performed using amniotic fluid to assess fetal lung maturity. The amniotic fluid is mixed with a fluorescent dye. When the dye binds to albumin there is a high polarization, and when the dye binds to surfactant there is a low polarization. Thus the surfactant/albumin ratio is determined. The units are expressed as milligrams of surfactant per gram of albumin, with fetal lung maturity being sufficient with values greater than 50 mg/g. Older methodologies have employed the determinations of phosphatidylglycerol, foam stability, and lecithin/sphingomyelin (L/S) ratio. The L/S ratio is based on the physiological levels of lecithin and sphingomyelin. Lecithin is a surfactant that prepares lungs to expand and take in air. Sphingomyelin is incorporated into the myelin sheath of the central nervous system of the fetus. The amounts of lecithin and sphingomyelin produced during the first 34 weeks of gestation are approximately equal; however, after the 34th week, the amount of lecithin synthesized greatly exceeds that of sphingomyelin. At birth, an L/S ratio of 2:1 or greater would indicate sufficient lung maturity.

198.

C. The VLDL fraction is primarily composed of triglycerides and lesser amounts of cholesterol and phospholipids. Protein components of VLDL are mostly apolipoprotein B-100 and apolipoprotein C. VLDL migrates electrophoretically in the prebeta region.

199.

A. The patient has a history as diabetes and has been experiencing chest pain and shortness of breath with activity. The ECG was normal. The most likely diagnosis is angina pectoris. The LDL cholesterol result does not correlate with the other lipid results, and it appears to be less than what would be expected. Using the formula LDL cholesterol = total cholesterol − [HDL cholesterol + triglycerides/5], the calculated LDL cholesterol would be 192 mg/dL. The total cholesterol, HDL cholesterol, and triglyceride results correlate and indicate hyperlipidemia. The elevated fasting glucose indicates poor carbohydrate metabolism, and the elevated hemoglobin A_{1c} indicates a lack of glucose control during the previous 2–3 months. The elevated glucose and lipid results support an increased risk of coronary artery disease, as does the hs-CRP value, which falls in the high risk range (>3.0 mg/L).

200.

C. Either a dextran sulfate-magnesium chloride mixture or a heparin sulfate-manganese chloride mixture may be used to precipitate the LDL and VLDL cholesterol fractions. This allows the HDL cholesterol fraction to remain in the supernatant. An aliquot of the supernatant may then be used in a total cholesterol procedure for the quantification of the HDL cholesterol level.

201.

B. Both the direct and the heparin sulfate- manganese chloride precipitation methods measure HDL cholesterol. The direct or homogeneous method for HDL cholesterol uses a mixture of polyanions and polymers that bind to LDL and VLDL and chylomicrons, causing them to become stabilized. The polyanions neutralize ionic charges on the surface of the lipoproteins, and this enhances their binding to the polymer. When a detergent is added, HDL goes into solution, where as the other lipoproteins remain attached to the polymer/polyanion complexes. The HDL cholesterol then reacts with added cholesterol enzyme reagents while the other lipoproteins remain inactive. The reagents, polymer/polyanions, and detergent can be added to the specimen in an automated way without the need for any manual pretreatment step. Furthermore, the direct HDL cholesterol procedure has the capacity for better precision than the manual precipitation methods. Both the adaptability to automated instruments and the better precision make the direct method a preferred choice for quantifying HDL cholesterol.

202.

A. A number of risk factors are associated with developing coronary heart disease. Notable among these factors are increased total cholesterol and decreased HDL cholesterol levels. Although the reference ranges for total cholesterol and HDL cholesterol vary with age and sex, reasonable generalizations can be made: An HDL cholesterol less than 40 mg/dL and a total cholesterol value ≥240 mg/dL are undesirable and the individual is at greater risk for coronary heart disease. Total cholesterol values between 200 and 239 mg/dL are borderline high.

203.

B. Once the total cholesterol, triglyceride, and HDL cholesterol are known, LDL cholesterol can be quantified by using the Friedewald equation

$$\text{LDL cholesterol} = \text{Total cholesterol} - (\text{HDL cholesterol} + \text{Triglyceride}/5)$$

In this example, all results are in mg/dL:

$$\begin{aligned}\text{LDL cholesterol} &= 300 - (50 + 200/5)\\ &= 300 - (90)\\ &= 210 \text{ mg/dL}\end{aligned}$$

This estimation of LDL cholesterol has been widely accepted in routine clinical laboratories and can be easily programmed into laboratory computers. In addition, LDL methods are available for direct measurement of serum levels. *Note:* The equation should not be used with triglyceride values exceeding 400 mg/dL because the VLDL composition is abnormal, making the [triglyceride/5] factor inapplicable.

204.

D. Both total cholesterol and HDL cholesterol are independent measurable indicators of risk of coronary heart disease (CHD). By relating total and HDL cholesterol in a mathematical way, physicians can obtain valuable additional information in predicting risk for CHD. Risk of CHD can be quantified by the ratio of total cholesterol to HDL cholesterol along the following lines:

Ratio	Risk CHD
3.43	half average
4.97	average
9.55	two times average
24.39	three times average

Thus this patient shows approximately twice the average risk for CHD. Risk ratios for CHD can easily be calculated by instrument and/or laboratory computers given the total and HDL cholesterol values. Reports indicating level of risk based on these results can be programmed by the laboratory and/or manufacturer.

205.

C. A number of immunochemical assays can be used to quantify the apolipoproteins. Some of the techniques that can be used include immunonephelometric assay, enzyme-linked immunosorbent assay (ELISA), and immunoturbidimetric assay. Commercial kits are available for the quantification of Apo A-I and Apo B-100. Measuring the apolipoproteins can be of use in assessing increased risk for coronary heart disease.

206.

A. Lipoprotein (a) is an apolipoprotein that is more commonly referred to as Lp(a). Although it is related structurally to LDL, Lp(a) is considered to be a distinct lipoprotein class with an electrophoretic mobility in the prebeta region. Lp(a) is believed to interfere with the lysis of clots by competing with plasminogen in the coagulation cascade, thus increasing the likelihood of atherosclerotic cardiovascular disease.

207.

B. Historically, total cholesterol levels of Americans have been below 300 mg/dL. Other countries, however, have relatively lower population cholesterol levels. The prevalent diet of these countries, however, may be vegetarian or fish, as opposed to meat, oriented. Higher total cholesterol resulting from a meat diet has been established. Clinical studies have also shown an increased risk of CAD in individuals with total cholesterol greater than 200 mg/dL. Thus, the upper reference interval of acceptable total cholesterol was artificially lowered to 200 mg/dL to reflect the lower risk of CAD associated with it.

208.

D. The Abell-Kendall assay is commonly used to separate HDL cholesterol from other lipoproteins. In this precipitation technique a heparin sulfate-manganese chloride mixture is used to precipitate the LDL and VLDL cholesterol fractions. This technique works well as long as there is no significant amount of chylomicrons or lipemia in the specimen and/or the triglyceride is under 400 mg/dL. Incomplete sedimentation is seen as cloudiness or turbidity in the supernatant after centrifugation. It indicates the presence of other lipoproteins and leads to overestimation of HDL cholesterol. The lipemic specimens maybe cleared and the HDL cholesterol separated more effectively by using ultrafiltration, extraction, latex immobilized antibodies, and/or ultracentrifugation. These techniques are usually not available in a routine laboratory.

209.

A. Hyperlipoproteinemia can be genetically inherited or secondary to certain diseases such as diabetes mellitus, hypothyroidism, or alcoholism. If the alcoholism has advanced to the state where there is liver damage, the liver can become inefficient in its metabolism of fats, leading to an increase of total cholesterol, triglyceride, LDL, and/or VLDL in the bloodstream. The elevation of these lipids along with the previous liver damage (e.g., cirrhosis) leads to a poor prognosis for the patient.

210.

D. In evaluating lipid profile results, it is important to start with the integrity of the sample. From the case history, it is doubtful that a 10-year-old healthy, active boy would be suffering from a lipid or glucose disorder manifesting these kinds of results. Furthermore, the boy came in for testing after school. It is improbable that a 10-year-old boy would be able to maintain a 9- to 12-hour fast during the school day. In this case, the boy should have been thoroughly interviewed by the laboratory staff before the blood test to determine if he was truly fasting. Specimen integrity is the first thing that must be ensured before running any glucose or lipid tests.

211.

C. In this case, the child fits the description of a suspected patient with dyslipidemia. He is known to have diabetes mellitus, and the mother has assured the laboratory that the boy has followed the proper fasting protocol before the test. Hyperlipoproteinemia can be secondary to diabetes mellitus. The boy has a relatively high risk to develop CAD, and, with a history of diabetes, should never undergo an oral 3-hour glucose tolerance test.

Enzymes and Cardiac Assessment

212.

D. Enzymes are often measured using a coupled reaction that converts NAD (oxidized) to NADH (reduced) or NADH to NAD. Both NAD and NADH have maximum absorptions associated with them and during enzyme assays the absorbance readings will increase over time when measuring NADH at 340 nm and will decrease over time when measuring NAD at 340 nm. This is because NAD has an absorbance maximum at 265 nm and NADH has a absorbance peak at 265 and 340 nm.

213.

B. Enzymes are proteins that act as catalysts. It is not practical to measure enzyme concentrations in a body fluid specimen, but rather to assay enzymes according to their activity in catalyzing an appropriate reaction; that is, the conversion of substrate to product. An enzyme acts by combining with a specific substrate to form an enzyme-substrate complex, which then breaks down into product plus free enzyme, which is reused. A general form of the reaction is

$$[E] + [S] \rightleftarrows [ES] \longrightarrow [P] + [E]$$

where [E] = concentration of enzyme, [S] = concentration of substrate, [ES] = concentration of enzyme-substrate complex, and [P] = concentration of product of the reaction. Because the rate of such a reaction is used as a measure of enzyme activity, it is important to consider the effect of substrate concentration on the rate of the reaction. The kinetics of the reaction are initially of the first order (i.e., the rate varies with the concentration of substrate as well as the concentration of enzyme) until there is sufficient substrate present to combine with all enzyme. The reaction rate then becomes zero order (i.e., the rate is independent of concentration of substrate and directly proportional to concentration of enzyme as measured by reaction rate) when substrate is present in excess. Hence it is desirable to use conditions that provide zero-order kinetics when assaying enzyme activity.

214.

B. Michaelis and Menten proposed a basis for the theory of enzyme-substrate complexes and rate reactions. By measuring the velocity of the reaction at varying substrate concentrations, it is possible to determine the Michaelis constant (K_m) for any specific enzymatic reaction. K_m represents the specific concentration of substrate that is required for a particular reaction to proceed at a velocity that is equal to half of its maximum velocity. The K_m value tells something about the affinity of an enzyme for its substrate. When $[S] = K_m$, the velocity of the reaction is expressed as $V = 1/2\ V_{max}$. In the graph shown with this question, the K_m of the reaction is represented by *b*. Because substrate must be present in excess to obtain zero-order kinetics, the substrate concentration necessary would have to be at least 10 times the K_m, which is represented by *d*. Usually substrate concentrations 20–100 times the K_m are used to be sure that substrate is present in excess. Thus it is critical that the K_m value be determined experimentally.

215.

A. Factors that affect enzyme assays include temperature, pH, substrate concentration, and time of incubation. For each clinically important enzyme, the optimum temperature and pH for its specific reaction are known. When lower than optimum temperature or pH is employed, the measured enzyme activity will be lower than the expected activity value. As temperature increases, the rate of the reaction increases. Generally, a twofold increase in reaction rates will be observed with a 10°C rise in temperature. However, once the optimum temperature is exceeded, the reaction rate falls off as enzyme denaturation occurs at temperatures ranging from 40 to 70°C.

216.

D. An international unit (IU) is defined as the enzyme activity that catalyzes the conversion of 1 μmol of substrate in 1 minute under standard conditions. For determination of enzyme activity when a rate method is employed, the following equation is used:

$$\frac{\Delta A/\text{min} \times \text{total assay volume (mL)} \times 10^6 \mu\text{mol/mol}}{\text{Absorptivity coefficient} \times \text{light path (cm)} \times \text{specimen volume (mL)}} = \text{IU/L}$$

$$\frac{0.077 \times 3.02\ \text{mL} \times 10^6\ \mu\text{mol/mol}}{6.22 \times 10^3 \text{L/mol} \cdot \text{cm} \times 1\ \text{cm} \times 0.02\ \text{mL}} = 1869 \text{IU/L}$$

It is important to remember that the total assay volume includes the volume of reagent, diluent, and sample used in the particular assay and that the total assay volume and specimen volume should be expressed in the same units.

217.

B. Enzymes are protein in nature. Like all proteins, they may be denatured with a loss of activity as a result of several factors (e.g., heat, extreme pH, mechanical agitation, strong acids, and organic solvents). Enzymes act as catalysts for the many chemical reactions of the body. Enzymes increase the rate of a specific chemical reaction by lowering the activation energy needed for the reaction to proceed. They do not change the equilibrium constant of the reaction; but rather, enzymes affect the rate at which equilibrium occurs between reactants and products.

218.

C. Serum alkaline phosphatase is elevated in several disorders, including hepatobiliary and bone diseases. For an accurate assay of most serum enzymes, the presence of hemolyzed red blood cells must be avoided because many enzymes are present in red cells. Serum aspartate transaminase (formerly known as glutamate-oxaloacetate transaminase, GOT) and lactate dehydrogenase are both enzymes that are elevated in acute myocardial infarction and liver disease.

219.

D. There are six major classes of enzymes. The International Commission of Enzymes of the International Union of Biochemistry has categorized all enzymes into one of these classes: oxidoreductases, transferases, hydrolases, lyases, isomerases, and ligases. Transferases are enzymes that catalyze the transfer of groups, such as amino and phosphate groups, between compounds. Transferases frequently need coenzymes, such as pyridoxal-5′-phosphate (P-5′-P), for the amino transfer reactions. Aspartate and alanine aminotransferases, creatine kinase, and gamma- glutamyltransferase are typical examples.

220.

D. Lactate dehydrogenase (LD) is a hydrogen transfer enzyme that catalyzes the oxidation of L-lactate (L) to pyruvate (P) with the mediation of NAD^+ as a hydrogen acceptor. The reaction is reversible, and the reaction equilibrium is pH dependent, with alkaline pH favoring the conversion P→L and neutral pH favoring the reverse reaction.

221.

C. The oxidoreductases are enzymes that catalyze the addition or removal of hydrogen from compounds. These enzymes need a coenzyme, such as nicotinamide adenine dinucleotide (NAD^+) or its phosphorylated derivative $NADP^+$, as a hydrogen acceptor or donor in order to function. Lactate dehydrogenase and glucose-6-phosphate dehydrogenase are examples of oxi doreductases. Isomerases are those enzymes that catalyze intramolecular conversions such as the oxidation of a functional group by an adjacent group within the same molecule. Glucose phosphate isomerase is an example of this class of enzymes. Ligases are those enzymes that catalyze the union of two molecules accompanied by the breakdown of a phosphate bond in adenosine triphosphate (ATP) or a similar triphosphate. An example is glutamine synthetase.

222.

B. Aspartate and alanine aminotransferases catalyze the transfer of amino groups between amino acids and α-oxoacids. A prosthetic group, pyridoxal-5′-phosphate (P-5′-P), is required for the transfer of the amino group. In the aspartate aminotransferase (AST) reaction, AST catalyzes the transfer of an amino group from l-aspartate to α-oxoglutarate, with the amino group transfer mediated by P-5′-P, which is bound to the apoenzyme. The products formed are oxaloacetate and l-glutamate. By coupling this reaction with a malate dehydrogenase reaction, the decrease in absorbance of NADH as it is oxidized to NAD^+ can be followed at 340 nm. The change in absorbance will be proportional to the AST activity present in the serum specimen.

223.

D. Alanine aminotransferase (ALT), formerly known as glutamate pyruvate transaminase (GPT), and aspartate aminotransferase (AST), formerly known as glutamate oxaloacetate transaminase (GOT), are categorized as transferase enzymes. These older designations are still seen in conjunction with the current terminology on reagent packaging, on physician test request forms, and on laboratory test result forms. Through the transfer of amino groups, ALT and AST catalyze the interconversion of amino acids and keto acids. ALT catalyzes the interconversion of alanine and oxoglutarate to pyruvate and glutamate. The reaction is reversible. In viral hepatitis, both ALT and AST are elevated. In acute myocardial infarction, AST is elevated and ALT is normal or slightly increased.

$$\text{L-Alanine} + \alpha\text{-oxoglutarate} \xrightleftharpoons{\text{ALT P-5}'\text{-P}} \text{pyruvate} + \text{L-glutamate}$$

224.

D. When measuring CK-MB, the mass immunoassay is more sensitive because it is quantifying the amount of enzyme present. This is in contrast to a kinetic method, which measures enzyme activity by means of the enzyme catalyzing a reaction and the product of that reaction being measured. Electrophoretic methods also measure enzyme activity based on colored product or fluorescent product formation.

225.

A. Lactate dehydrogenase (LD, also abbreviated LDH) is found in all body tissues and is especially abundant in red and white blood cells. Hence hemolyzed serum will give falsely elevated results for LD. The enzyme catalyzes the conversion of lactate to pyruvate at pH 8.8–9.8 and pyruvate to lactate at pH 7.4–7.8, mediated by nicotinamide adenine dinucleotide (NAD^+). Each of these reactions is associated with its own unique reference range. LD exists in five isomeric forms called isoenzymes. The isoenzymes can be separated by electrophoresis. Serum specimens for LD isoenzyme determinations can be stored at room temperature for 2–3 days without appreciable loss of activity. Room temperature storage is necessary because LD-4 and LD-5 are labile in the cold. This is in contrast to most enzymes, which are more stable when refrigerated or frozen.

226.

C. C-reactive protein is an acute-phase reactant that is increased in the presence of inflammation. High-sensitivity C-reactive protein (hs-CRP) refers to a sensitive method that is able to measure low levels of CRP in serum. One theory is that elevated levels of CRP contribute to the damage of arterial walls that precedes plaque formation. hs-CRP is considered a good predictor test for assessing cardiovascular risk. However, it is also elevated in other conditions, including infection, stress, and trauma. CK-MB, troponin, and myoglobin are tests used to assess if a myocardial infarction has occurred.

227.

C. Enzymes catalyze specific reactions or closely related groups of reactions. Lactate dehydrogenase (LD), with nicotinamide adenine dinucleotide (NAD^+) as a hydrogen acceptor, catalyzes the oxidation of l-lactate to pyruvate and the reduction of NAD^+ to NADH. Because NAD^+ does not absorb light at 340 nm but NADH does, the production of NADH can be monitored as an increase in absorbance at 340 nm and related to the LD activity present in the specimen. Because this reaction is reversible, either the forward or reverse reaction can be used in the laboratory to quantify LD activity. Although the reaction equilibrium favors the formation of lactate from pyruvate, this reaction is less commonly used. It should be noted that the reference ranges for the two reactions are considerably different. Elevation of serum LD is associated with acute myocardial infarction, liver disease, pernicious anemia, malignant disease, and pulmonary embolism. It is also seen in some cases of renal disease, especially where tubular necrosis or pyelonephritis exists.

228.

B. In acute myocardial infarction (AMI), the initial increase in serum myoglobin levels occurs in 1–3 hours following onset of symptoms. Serial measurements need to be made because a single value is not diagnostic. When doubling of the initial value occurs within 1–2 hours, this is suggestive of AMI. In AMI, the myoglobin level will peak within 5–12 hours, with serum levels returning to normal within 18–30 hours. Because myoglobin is found in other tissues and is not cardiac specific, it is usually used in conjunction with cardiac troponin and CK-MB to assess the occurrence of AMI.

229.

C. Increased serum creatine kinase (CK), formerly called creatine phosphokinase (CPK), values are caused primarily by lesions of cardiac muscle, skeletal muscle, or brain tissue. CK increases in the early stages of Duchenne-type progressive muscular dystrophy. Assays of total CK and CK isoenzymes are commonly used in the diagnosis of myocardial infarction. Hypothyroidism causes a moderate increase in CK values. Elevation of this enzyme also occurs after vigorous muscular activity, in cases of cerebrovascular accidents (stroke), and after repeated intramuscular injections. In addition to quantifying total CK activity, isoenzymes may be determined by using electrophoretic, immunologic, or ion-exchange chromatography methods. Three isoenzymes have been identified: CK-1 or BB, primarily found in brain and nerve tissues with some in thyroid, kidney, and intestine; CK-2 or MB, primarily found in heart muscle; and CK-3 or MM, primarily found in skeletal muscle but present in all body tissues. CK is not elevated in bone disease.

230.

C. Creatine kinase (CK) is found mainly in skeletal muscle, cardiac muscle, and brain tissue. CK catalyzes the following reversible reaction:

$$\text{creatine} + \text{adenosine triphosphate (ATP)} \underset{\text{pH 6.7}}{\overset{\text{pH 9.0}}{\rightleftarrows}} \text{phosphocreatine} + \text{adenosine diphosphate (ADP)}$$

Mg^{2+} is required as an activator. The direction in which the reaction takes place, and hence the equilibrium point, depends on the pH. Measurement of CK activity is valuable in the early diagnosis of acute myocardial infarction. Its level rises 4–6 hours after infarction, reaches its peak at 12–24 hours, and returns to normal by the third day. In addition to quantifying total CK activity, electrophoresis may be performed to ascertain the presence of an MB band, which represents the heart tissue isoenzyme. Electrophoretically, the MB band moves to an intermediary position between the BB and the MM bands. The BB band travels fastest toward the anode and the MM band travels slowest, remaining in the gamma-globulin region. Electrophoretic separation of CK-MB has been widely replaced by immunologic methods that can be performed on automated instruments.

231.

B. The function of amylase to catalyze the hydrolysis of starch to dextrins, maltose, and glucose has been used as the basis for several methods over the years. The more commonly used methods today employ small oligosaccharides and 4-nitrophenylglycoside as substrates. In general, these methods can be automated, using an oxygen electrode system and UV or visible wavelength spectrophotometry to determine amylase activity.

232.

D. Gamma-glutamyltransferase (GGT) catalyzes the transfer of gamma-glutamyl groups from peptides to an appropriate acceptor. GGT is found in almost all cells. The highest amount of GGT is found in the kidney, and slightly less is found in the liver and pancreas. Diagnostically, the assay of GGT is widely used to investigate hepatic disease. Increased values are seen in a variety of liver disorders and in conditions that are characterized by secondary liver involvement, including acute pancreatitis, pancreatic carcinoma, infectious mononucleosis, alcoholism, and cardiac insufficiency. Normal GGT levels are seen in bone disorders, in growing children, and during pregnancy.

233.

C. The main sources of alkaline phosphatase are liver, bone, intestine, and placenta. Elevated serum alkaline phosphatase is associated with liver disease and with both obstructive jaundice and intrahepatic jaundice. In most cases, the serum alkaline phosphatase value in obstructive jaundice is higher than in intrahepatic jaundice. Increased serum values are also found in bone diseases such as Paget disease; in pregnant women (placental origin), especially in the third trimester of a normal pregnancy; and in normal growing children. In the presence of the latter conditions, when liver disease is also suspected, a GGT assay may be performed to aid in a differential diagnosis. Serum GGT levels are normal in these conditions but are elevated in liver disease.

234.

B. Alanine aminotransferase, aspartate aminotransferase, alkaline phosphatase, gamma- glutamyltransferase, and lactate dehydrogenase are enzymes for which the serum activities may be assayed to assess liver function. At the cellular level, alkaline phosphatase functions in the membrane border, gamma-glutamyltransferase functions in the cell membrane, and alanine aminotransferase functions both in the cytoplasm and mitochondria. With tissue damage and necrosis, the cells disintegrate and leak their contents into the blood. Because these enzymes are cellular enzymes, any increase in their activity levels in serum is indicative of tissue destruction. It is important to remember that these enzyme levels must be used in conjunction with other clinical data because enzymes generally are not organ specific; they are found in several tissues.

235.

B. Amylase and lipase are the two most important enzymes in evaluating pancreatic function. The values of amylase and lipase activity are significantly elevated in acute pancreatitis and obstruction of the pancreatic duct. In most cases of acute pancreatitis, the lipase activity stays elevated longer than amylase activity.

236.

B. The quantification of serum prostate-specific antigen has replaced measurement of serum acid phosphatase for assessing carcinoma of the prostate. PSA measurement in conjunction with the digital rectal examination is recommended for prostate cancer screening. In addition, PSA can be used to stage and monitor therapy of prostatic cancer.

237.

B. Cholinesterase is a serum enzyme synthesized by the liver. It is also known as pseudocholinesterase to distinguish it from "true" cholinesterase (acetylcholinesterase) of erythrocytes. Although a number of disease states are associated with abnormal levels of this enzyme, cholinesterase levels are especially important in detecting organic insecticide poisoning of workers in the chemical industry and agriculture. Decreased cholinesterase levels and atypical enzyme forms are associated with prolonged apnea after succinylcholine administration during surgery. Propionylthiocholine is a commonly used substrate for measuring serum cholinesterase activity.

238.

D. The heme protein myoglobin can bind oxygen reversibly and is found in cardiac and striated muscles. In cases of acute myocardial infarction, myoglobin increases within 1–3 hours of the infarct. Myoglobin is not cardiac specific, and increased serum levels also occur in vigorous exercise, intramuscular injections, rhabdomyolysis, and muscular dystrophy. Because myoglobin is a relatively small protein and able to be excreted by the kidneys, elevated serum levels occur in renal failure.

239.

D. Troponin is a group of three proteins that function in muscle contraction by binding to the thin filaments of cardiac and skeletal striated muscle. The three proteins are known as troponin T (TnT), troponin I (TnI), and troponin C (TnC). With AMI, the cardiac-specific isoforms of troponin are released into the blood; the two of clinical interest are cTnI and cTnT. Cardiac troponin I (cTnI) will show an increase that exceeds the reference interval in approximately 3–6 hours following an AMI. Quantification should be done serially starting with an initial measurement at presentation followed by testing at 3–6, 6–9, and 12–24 hours. cTnI will remain elevated for 5–10 days. Unlike cTnT, which is expressed in small quantities in regenerating and diseased skeletal muscle, cTnI is not, which makes it specific for cardiac muscle.

240.

C. For many years, the diagnosis of an AMI was facilitated by assaying serum levels of aspartate aminotransferase (AST), lactate dehydrogenase (LD), creatine kinase (CK), and LD and CK isoenzymes. Today the clinical usefulness of AST and LD has been replaced primarily by cardiac troponin and to a lesser degree by myoglobin, whereas CK isoenzymes continue to play a role. Although myoglobin will increase above the upper reference interval in 1–3 hours following AMI, it is not tissue specific for cardiac muscle and its application has found limited usefulness. Myoglobin will also be increased following skeletal muscle trauma. Troponin I and troponin T have proven to be useful markers, because each has a cardiac-specific isoform, cTnI and cTnT. cTnI appears to be more specific for cardiac muscle, because it has not been identified in regenerating or diseased skeletal muscle, whereas cTnT is made in small amounts by skeletal muscle. Total CK is elevated in AMI and takes 4–6 hours to rise above the upper reference interval. It is the increased level of CK-2 (CK-MB) that is more helpful in diagnosing AMI, but caution needs to be exercised here, because skeletal muscle injury can cause a similar increase.

241.

D. Osteitis deformans, also known as Paget disease, is a chronic disorder of bone. This disorder is characterized by a significant increase in the serum alkaline phosphatase level. Gamma- glutamyltransferase will be normal in bone disease, because this enzyme is not found in bone tissue. However, in hepatobiliary disease both enzymes would characteristically be elevated.

242.

C. Obstruction of the biliary tree is also referred to as intrahepatic cholestasis. This disorder is characterized by significant elevations in the serum levels of alkaline phosphatase and gamma-glutamyltransferase. The serum levels of alanine and aspartate aminotransferases and lactate dehydrogenase are only slightly elevated. Early in the disease, the serum bilirubin level may be normal or only slightly elevated. In alcoholic cirrhosis, viral hepatitis, and infectious mononucleosis, only a slight to moderate elevation of alkaline phosphatase would be seen.

243.

A. Acute hepatitis is characterized by markedly elevated levels of serum alanine aminotransferase and aspartate aminotransferase, which may range from 10- to 100-fold greater than the reference values. Although alkaline phosphatase and gamma-glutamyltransferase are increased, their elevations are less notable than the aminotransferases. Alkaline phosphatase may range up to two times the reference range whereas gamma-glutamyltransferase may go as high as five times the reference range in acute hepatitis. Due to leakage of conjugated bilirubin from the hepatocytes, the urine bilirubin will be positive. With less conjugated bilirubin reaching the intestines, fecal urobilinogen will be less than normal.

244.

A. To aid in the diagnosis of skeletal muscle disease, measurement of creatine kinase would be most useful. CK yields the most reliable information when skeletal muscle disease is suspected. Other enzymes that are also useful to measure are aspartate aminotransferase and lactate dehydrogenase. Both of these enzymes will be moderately elevated, whereas CK is significantly increased.

245.

C. When an AMI occurs, CK is the first enzyme to become elevated in the blood, rising within 4–6 hours following chest pain. AST exhibits a rise in the serum level within 6–8 hours. LD shows an increase in 8–12 hours following infarction. Measurement of these three enzymes to assess acute myocardial infarction has been replaced by cardiac troponin, myoglobin, and CK-MB. However, awareness of the CK, AST, and LD patterns as well as other biochemical tests is useful in assessing organ complications that may arise during the period of AMI.

246.

C. Quantification of serum total creatine kinase, CK-MB (or CK-2) isoenzyme, and cardiac troponin I (cTnI) or cardiac troponin T (cTnT) is very useful in determining an AMI. Determining the presence and activity level of CK-MB is valuable, because CK-MB levels can increase following an infarct, ranging from 6 to 30% of the total CK. Serial assessment of serum specimens is recommended, with the initial specimen obtained at presentation, followed by blood collection at 3–6, 6–9, and 12–24 hours from the initial time. Because alkaline phosphatase isoenzymes are associated with liver, bone, intestinal, and placental tissues, their analysis would not contribute any significant information to determining the occurrence of an AMI.

247.

D. Symptoms are sometimes nonspecific, making it difficult to diagnose congestive heart failure. B-type (brain) natriuretic peptide (BNP) is used to determine if physical symptoms are related to congestive heart failure. BNP is synthesized in and secreted by myocardial ventricles in response to ventricular volume expansion and pressure overload. An increase in BNP causes dilation of blood vessels and promotes sodium and water loss by the kidneys. This reduces fluid load on the heart in an attempt to improve cardiac function. Albumin cobalt binding is a test that measures ischemia-modified albumin, which is a marker for ischemic heart disease.

248.

B. The child's symptoms are consistent with Duchenne dystrophy, which is an X-linked recessive disorder. It is characterized by muscle weakness, which is caused by destruction of muscle fibers. Symptoms are seen in male children starting at three to 7 years of age. The most notable enzyme increase is in creatine kinase, which may increase 50–100 times the reference range. Aspartate transaminase and lactate dehydrogenase would also be increased, because both enzymes are present in skeletal muscle tissue. Alkaline phosphatase is not present in skeletal muscle tissue and is measured to assess hepatobiliary and bone disorders.

249.

B. The controls were within acceptable limits, so it is assumed that all test results are accurate. The elevated myoglobin, total CK, and CK-MB with a troponin I that showed no change and remained in the reference range suggest that the elevated results were due to the skeletal muscle injuries sustained in the car crash. Myoglobin is not tissue specific and may be increased in skeletal muscle injuries, muscular dystrophy, and AMI. The same is true for creatine kinase, which is not tissue specific and may be increased in skeletal muscle disorders as well as cardiac muscle disorders. CK-MB, although it is associated with cardiac muscle and the occurrence of AMI, is not tissue specific and will increase with skeletal muscle injury (but to a lesser degree than CK-MM). Cardiac troponin I is tissue specific and not expressed by skeletal muscle; thus it would remain within the reference range in the absence of an AMI. Total CK and CK-MB do not provide information to assess if a stroke has occurred.

250.

A. Elevated homocysteine levels are associated with increased risk for coronary heart disease. Increased homocysteine contributes to the damage of arterial walls preceding formation of plaques. Individuals at risk need to be evaluated for vitamin B levels, because low levels of folic acid, vitamin B_6, and vitamin B_{12} are associated with increased levels of homocysteine.

251.

C. N-terminal proBNP is released when BNP (B-type or brain natriuretic peptide) is cleaved from precursor proBNP. NT-proBNP is released in a 1:1 ratio to BNP; however, NT-proBNP has a half-life of hours as compared to BNP's short half-life of approximately 22 minutes. The longer half-life of NT-proBNP contributes to its clinical utility. In addition, when measuring NT-proBNP, there is no interference when an individual is being treated with nesiritide, which is human recombinant BNP used in treating congestive heart failure.

252.

D. Reye syndrome is associated with viral infections, exogenous toxins, and salicylate use. The disorder generally manifests itself in children from 2 to 13 years of age. The laboratory findings that support a diagnosis of Reye syndrome include increased levels of serum aspartate and alanine transaminases (greater than three times the reference range), increased plasma ammonia level (can exceed 100 μg/dL), and prolonged prothrombin time (3 sec or more than the control). In Reye syndrome the serum bilirubin level is generally within the reference range.

253.

B. A primary reference procedure for amylase measurement at 37°C was established by IFCC Scientific Division, Committee on Reference Systems for Enzymes (C-RSE) using a chromolytic technique. The chromalytic technique uses the substrate 4,6-ethylidene(G1)-*p*-nitrophenyl(G7)-α-D-maltoheptaoside at 30°C.

254.

D. Cystic fibrosis is inherited as an autosomal recessive trait. It is a systemic disease that affects the exocrine glands, causing gastrointestinal malabsorption, pancreatic insufficiency, and pulmonary disease. Cystic fibrosis is characterized by increased concentrations of chloride and sodium in sweat. With pancreatic insufficiency, the amount of lipase, amylase, trypsin, and bicarbonate secreted into the duodenum is decreased. Because the three enzymes contribute to digestion of fats, starches, and proteins, respectively, children with this disorder suffer from malabsorption.

Liver Function and Porphyrin Formation

255.

D. The biochemical synthesis of the porphyrins consists of a series of reactions. Succinyl coenzyme A and glycine are the two compounds that originally condense to form aminolevulinic acid (ALA). Through a second condensation reaction, two molecules of ALA condense and cyclize to form porphobilinogen. Porphobilinogen is a monopyrrole structure and the precursor of porphyrin synthesis.

256.

D. Heme is derived from a series of biochemical reactions that begin with the formation of porphobilinogen from succinyl coenzyme A and glycine. Because porphobilinogen is a monopyrrole, four molecules of porphobilinogen condense and cyclize to form the porphyrinogen precursors of protoporphyrin IX. Protoporphyrin IX chelates iron to form heme and is, therefore, the immediate precursor of heme formation.

257.

D. Porphobilinogen is a precursor compound in the biosynthesis of heme. In acute intermittent porphyria, excess amounts of porphobilinogen are excreted in the urine. The Watson-Schwartz test employs *p*-dimethylaminobenzaldehyde reagent (also known as Ehrlich's aldehyde reagent) to form a red condensation product with porphobilinogen.

258.

D. The porphyrins that are of clinical significance include uroporphyrin, coproporphyrin, and protoporphyrin. These three porphyrin compounds may be detected in acid solution by irradiating the solution with long-wave ultraviolet light, which causes the porphyrins to fluoresce. The intense orange-red fluorescence of the porphyrins is due to the conjugated unsaturation of the tetrapyrrole ring structure.

259.

B. When measurement of aminolevulinic acid, porphobilinogen, uroporphyrin, or coproporphyrin is requested, a 24-hour urine specimen should be collected. The urine should be refrigerated during collection and stored in a brown bottle to protect light-sensitive compounds. Because porphobilinogen is more stable under alkaline conditions and aminolevulinic acid is more stable under acid conditions, sodium bicarbonate should be added as a compromise to maintain the pH near 7.

260.

D. In the catabolic process of hemoglobin degradation, the alpha-carbon methene bridge of the tetrapyrrole ring structure of heme opens oxidatively to form verdohemoglobin. Verdohemoglobin is a complex composed of biliverdin, iron, and the protein globin. This complex then undergoes degradation in which iron is removed and returned to the body iron stores, the globin portion is returned to the amino acid pool, and the biliverdin undergoes reduction to form bilirubin. It is biliverdin, therefore, that is the immediate precursor of bilirubin formation. Mesobilirubinogen and urobilinogen represent intestinal breakdown products of bilirubin catabolism.

261.

B. Diazo reagent is a mixture of sulfanilic acid, sodium nitrite, and hydrochloric acid. The mixing of sodium nitrite with hydrochloric acid forms nitrous acid, which in turn reacts with sulfanilic acid to form a diazonium salt. This diazotized sulfanilic acid mixture, when mixed with solubilized bilirubin, forms a red azobilirubin complex. The azobilirubin complexes are isomeric structures formed from the splitting of the bilirubin compound in half. Each half then reacts with the diazo reagent to form two isomeric azobilirubin complexes.

262.

C. In order for the bilirubin-albumin complex to reach the parenchymal cells of the liver, the complex must be transported from the sinusoids to the sinusoidal microvilli and into the parenchymal cell. The microsomal fraction of the parenchymal cell is responsible for the conjugation of bilirubin. It is here that bilirubin reacts with uridine diphosphate glucuronate in the presence of the enzyme uridine diphosphate glucuronyltransferase to form bilirubin diglucuronide.

263.

B. Bilirubin that has been secreted through the bile into the small intestine is reduced by anaerobic microorganisms to urobilinogen. One of the possible fates of urobilinogen is its conversion to urobilin. In the colon, a portion of the urobilinogen is oxidized by the action of microorganisms to urobilin, which is excreted in the feces as an orange-brown pigment.

264.

A. The cells of the reticuloendothelial system are able to phagocytize aged red blood cells and convert the hemoglobin to the excretory product bilirubin. It is then necessary for the bilirubin to be transported to the liver, where it is conjugated for excretion in the bile. Albumin acts as the transport vehicle for unconjugated bilirubin in the blood, with each mole of albumin capable of binding 2 moles of bilirubin.

265.

A. When total bilirubin levels exceed 2.5 mg/dL, the clinical manifestation of jaundice develops. Characteristically, such body areas as the skin and sclera develop a yellow-pigmented appearance. Jaundice may be caused by an increase in either the unconjugated or conjugated form of bilirubin. Such increases in bilirubin levels may be caused by prehepatic, hepatic, or posthepatic disorders.

266.

A. An abnormal accumulation of bilirubin in the body may be due to increased production or decreased excretion of bilirubin. Terms frequently associated with a buildup of bilirubin include "jaundice," "kernicterus," and "icterus." Both jaundice and icterus are characterized by the yellow coloration of the skin, sclera, and mucous membranes that results from increased plasma concentrations of either conjugated or unconjugated bilirubin or both. This yellow coloration is also visible in serum and plasma specimens *in vitro*. *Kernicterus* refers to the accumulation of bilirubin in brain tissue that occurs with elevated levels of unconjugated bilirubin. This condition is most commonly seen in newborns with hemolytic disease resulting from maternal-fetal Rh incompatibility. Newborns afflicted with kernicterus will exhibit severe neural symptoms.

267.

B. In the small intestine, urobilinogen is formed through the enzymatic reduction process of anaerobic bacteria on bilirubin. The fate of urobilinogen is such that some of the urobilinogen will be excreted unchanged in the stool, a portion will be oxidized to urobilin for excretion in the stool, and up to 20% will be absorbed from the intestine into the portal circulation. This circulating urobilinogen is almost completely picked up by the liver, with only a small amount excreted in the urine. The liver oxidizes a small part of the recycled urobilinogen to bilirubin. This newly formed bilirubin and any unchanged urobilinogen are transported through the bile canaliculi into the bile for reexcretion by the intestines. This recycling of urobilinogen is part of the enterohepatic circulation.

268.

A. As chronic hepatitis progresses to cirrhosis, the platelet count will decrease, prothrombin time will increase, albumin will decrease, and ALP will increase.

269.

C. Four bilirubin fractions represented by Greek letters have been identified: unconjugated (alpha), monoconjugated (beta), diconjugated (gamma), and unconjugated bilirubin covalently bound to albumin (delta). Delta-bilirubin is normally present in low concentration in the blood, and it is known to react directly with diazotized sulfanilic acid. Increased serum levels of delta-bilirubin are associated with liver-biliary disease.

270.

A. The cells of the reticuloendothelial system are responsible for the removal of old red blood cells from the peripheral circulation. As the red blood cells reach the end of their 120-day life span, the specialized cells mainly of the spleen phagocytize the aged cells and convert the released hemoglobin into the excretory pigment bilirubin. The bone marrow is also responsible for the destruction of a small number of red blood cells that have not completed the maturation process. The bilirubin produced by the reticuloendothelial cells is indirect bilirubin, which, as a protein-bound compound, is transported to the liver for conjugation into direct bilirubin.

271.

C. Bilirubinometer, bilirubin oxidase, and Jendrassik-Grof are methods that have been used to quantify serum bilirubin concentrations. The bilirubinometer is used for direct spectrophotometric assay in which the bilirubin concentration is read directly at 454 nm. In the bilirubin oxidase method, bilirubin is oxidized to biliverdin and the reaction is followed at 405–460 nm. The Jendrassik-Grof method utilizes a caffeine-sodium benzoate mixture to accelerate the coupling reaction of unconjugated bilirubin with diazo reagent to form an azobilirubin complex. Because of a high recovery rate, the Jendrassik-Grof method is considered to be the method of choice for bilirubin analysis.

272.

A. Direct bilirubin was so named because of its ability in the van den Bergh method to react directly with diazotized sulfanilic acid without the addition of alcohol. Such a direct reaction is possible because direct bilirubin is conjugated in the liver with glucuronic acid, thereby making it a polar, water-soluble compound. Because conjugated bilirubin is both water soluble and not protein bound, it may be filtered through the glomerulus and excreted in the urine of jaundiced patients. Indirect bilirubin is a protein-bound unconjugated compound that is soluble in alcohol but not in water, and because of these properties, it is unable to be excreted in the urine.

273.

C. Ehrlich's diazo reagent consists of sulfanilic acid, hydrochloric acid, and sodium nitrite. Sulfanilic acid is dissolved in hydrochloric acid and diluted to volume with deionized water. Sodium nitrite is dissolved in deionized water and diluted to volume. Aliquots of these two reagent mixtures are combined to prepare Ehrlich's diazo reagent, which must be prepared fresh before use because of its unstable nature.

274.

C. Unlike direct bilirubin, indirect-reacting bilirubin is insoluble in deionized water and dilute hydrochloric acid. Indirect-reacting bilirubin must first be mixed with methanol or caffeine-sodium benzoate to solubilize it before proceeding with the diazo reaction. Because of these properties, total bilirubin and direct bilirubin are usually chemically analyzed, and the indirect, or unconjugated, fraction is calculated from the difference between the total and direct values. The total value represents the reaction of both conjugated and unconjugated bilirubin, whereas the direct value represents only the reaction of conjugated bilirubin.

275.

B. In the bilirubin oxidase method, the enzyme bilirubin oxidase catalyzes the oxidation of bilirubin to the product biliverdin, which is colorless. This is seen as a decrease in absorbance and is monitored between 405 and 460 nm. This method has an advantage over diazo methods in that hemoglobin does not interfere in the assay and cause falsely low results.

276.

A. Conjugated bilirubin and a small amount of unconjugated bilirubin will pass from the bile into the small intestine. In the small intestine, enzyme systems of anaerobic bacteria are able to reduce bilirubin to the reduction products mesobilirubinogen, stercobilinogen, and urobilinogen. These three reduction products of bilirubin catabolism are collectively referred to as urobilinogen.

277.

D. "Obstructive jaundice" is a term applied to conditions in which the common bile duct is obstructed because of gallstone formation, spasm, or neoplasm. Such an obstruction blocks the flow of bile from the gallbladder into the small intestine. This impedance of bile flow will result in a backflow of bile from the gallbladder into the sinusoids of the liver and ultimately into the peripheral circulation. Because the liver is not initially involved and the disorder is of posthepatic origin, the increased levels of bilirubin in the blood are caused by the backflow of conjugated bilirubin. If the disorder is allowed to progress, the continued backflow of bile will cause parenchymal cell destruction. Such cellular necrosis will result in a depression of the conjugating ability of the liver, and an elevation of unconjugated bilirubin levels in the blood will ensue.

278.

A. Hemolytic jaundice is also referred to as prehepatic jaundice. It is caused by excessive destruction of erythrocytes at a rate that exceeds the conjugating ability of the liver. As a result, increased levels of unconjugated bilirubin appear in the blood. The amount of conjugated bilirubin being formed in the liver is proportionately greater than normal; this is reflected in the increased levels of urobilinogen and urobilin found in the stool. Because of the enterohepatic circulation, the increased urobilinogen levels in the small intestines are reflected by an increase in the circulating blood levels of urobilinogen. Because the liver is unable to pick up all the circulating urobilinogen, the urinary levels of urobilinogen are increased. Urinary bilirubin levels are negative because the blood level of conjugated bilirubin is usually normal.

279.

D. The enzyme uridine diphosphate glucuronyltransferase catalyzes the conjugation of bilirubin with glucuronic acid. In newborns, especially premature infants, this liver enzyme system is not fully developed or functional. Because of this deficiency in the enzyme system, the concentration of unconjugated bilirubin rises in the blood, because only the conjugated form may be excreted through the bile and urine. The increased levels of unconjugated bilirubin will cause the infant to appear jaundiced. Generally, this condition persists for only a short period because the enzyme system usually becomes functional within several days after birth. Neonatal physiological jaundice resulting from an enzyme deficiency is hepatic in origin. Hemolytic jaundice resulting from either Rh or ABO incompatibility is a prehepatic type of jaundice, whereas a stricture of the common bile duct is classified as posthepatic jaundice.

280.

C. With complete obstruction of the common bile duct, bilirubin diglucuronide would be unable to pass from the bile into the intestines. Such obstruction to the flow of bile will cause the conjugated bilirubin to be regurgitated into the sinusoids and the general circulation. Because conjugated bilirubin is water soluble, it will be excreted in the urine. However, because of the lack of bile flow into the intestines, neither urobilinogen nor urobilin will be present in the feces. The lack of urobilin in the feces will be apparent from the light brown to chalky-white coloration of the stools. Because there is no urobilinogen in the intestines to be picked up by the enterohepatic circulation, the urinary excretion of urobilinogen will be negative. Because the obstruction may sometimes be only partial, this description would be somewhat altered. Provided that some bile was able to flow into the intestines, the fecal urobilinogen and urobilin concentrations would be present but depressed, the urinary urobilinogen excretion would be below normal, and the urinary bilirubin level would be increased.

281.

B. In disorders such as viral hepatitis, toxic hepatitis, and cirrhosis, hepatocellular damage occurs. The damaged parenchymal cells lose their ability either to conjugate bilirubin or to transport the bilirubin that is conjugated into the bile. Because of loss of conjugating ability by some parenchymal cells, the early stage of viral hepatitis is characterized by an increase in the unconjugated bilirubin fraction in the blood. An increase of lesser magnitude in the conjugated fraction is also demonstrated. The increase in conjugated bilirubin is due to the fact that some cells are able to conjugate but are damaged in such a way that there is leakage of conjugated bilirubin into the sinusoids and the general circulation. Because of this increase in the conjugated fraction, urinary bilirubin excretion is positive. Because the amount of conjugated bilirubin reaching the intestines is less than normal, it follows that the fecal urobilinogen and urobilin levels will also be less than normal. However, the urinary urobilinogen levels will be greater than normal because the urobilinogen that does reach the enterohepatic circulation is not efficiently removed by the liver but, rather, is excreted by the urinary system.

282.

B. Both Crigler-Najjar syndrome and neonatal jaundice, a physiological disorder, are due to a deficiency in the enzyme-conjugating system. With a deficiency in uridine diphosphate glucuronyltransferase, the liver is unable to conjugate bilirubin, and both of these conditions are characterized by increased levels of unconjugated bilirubin. Unlike Crigler-Najjar syndrome, which is a hereditary disorder, neonatal physiological jaundice is a temporary situation that usually corrects itself within a few days after birth.

283.

D. Gilbert syndrome is a preconjugation transport disturbance. In this disorder the hepatic uptake of bilirubin is defective because the transportation of bilirubin from the sinusoidal membrane to the microsomal region is impaired. Gilbert syndrome is inherited as an autosomal dominant trait characterized by increased levels of unconjugated bilirubin.

284.

C. In Dubin-Johnson syndrome, the transport of conjugated (direct) bilirubin from the microsomal region to the bile canaliculi is impaired. In this rare familial disorder, plasma conjugated bilirubin levels are increased because of defective excretion of bilirubin in the bile. Because conjugated bilirubin is water soluble, increased amounts of bilirubin are found in the urine.

285.

D. Abnormal conditions characterized by jaundice may be classified according to their type of liver involvement. The three types of jaundice are prehepatic, hepatic, and posthepatic. Hepatic jaundice may be subdivided into two groups on the basis of the type of excessive bilirubin: conjugated bilirubin or unconjugated bilirubin. Gilbert syndrome and Dubin-Johnson syndrome are disorders in which the process of bilirubin transport is malfunctioning. Both Crigler-Najjar syndrome and neonatal jaundice, a physiological disorder, are due to a deficiency in the enzyme-conjugating system. Disorders such as viral hepatitis, toxic hepatitis, and cirrhosis cause damage and destruction of liver cells so that the ability of the liver to remove unconjugated bilirubin from the blood and to conjugate it with glucuronic acid becomes impaired. As these disorders progress, the level of unconjugated bilirubin in the blood rises. There is also an increase, although not as great as that of unconjugated bilirubin, in blood levels of conjugated bilirubin. The cause is a leakage of conjugated bilirubin from damaged parenchymal cells into the sinusoids. Neoplasm of the common bile duct is a form of posthepatic jaundice.

286.

A. Prehepatic jaundice is also known as hemolytic jaundice, a term that is descriptive of the cause of the disorder. Any disorder that causes the destruction of erythrocytes at a faster rate than the liver is able to conjugate the bilirubin being formed by the reticuloendothelial system will exhibit hyperbilirubinemia. The increased concentration of bilirubin and the ensuing jaundice is not due to any hepatic malfunction but only to the inability of the liver to handle the conjugation of such a bilirubin overload. Therefore, the jaundice is caused by an increased concentration of unconjugated bilirubin. Disorders that follow this type of course are acute hemolytic anemia, chronic hemolytic anemia, and neonatal jaundice. Causes of hemolytic anemia may be genetic or acquired and include hereditary spherocytosis, sickle-cell anemia, and blood trans fusion reactions. Neonatal jaundice may be due to an ABO or Rh incompatibility, as seen in erythroblastosis fetalis.

287.

B. Posthepatic jaundice is caused by an obstruction in the common bile duct, extrahepatic ducts, or the ampulla of Vater. Such an obstruction may be caused by gallstones, neoplasms, or strictures. In this type of jaundice, the liver is functioning properly in its conjugation of bilirubin, but the obstruction causes a blockage so that the conjugated bilirubin is unable to be excreted through the intestines. Therefore, there is a backup of bile into the sinusoids and an overflow into the blood. The circulating blood will characteristically contain excessive amounts of conjugated bilirubin, which will cause increased amounts of bilirubin to be excreted in the urine. Because the blockage prevents proper excretion of bilirubin into the intestines, the formation of urobilinogen and urobilin is impeded. This pattern will continue until the regurgitation of bile causes hepatocellular damage. With destruction of the parenchymal cells, conjugation of bilirubin will be depressed and the blood levels of unconjugated bilirubin will also rise.

288.

D. The laboratory test results suggest that the woman has posthepatic biliary obstruction. The diagnosis is supported by the greater increase in alkaline phosphatase in contrast to the lesser increases in ALT and AST, the greater increase in the direct (conjugated) bilirubin level, and the decrease in urine urobilinogen. In biliary obstruction, increased synthesis of alkaline phosphatase is induced, with more produced in hepatocytes adjacent to biliary canaliculi. When an obstruction occurs in the biliary system, which may be caused by such disorders as gallstones in the common bile duct or a tumor in the region of the ampulla of Vater, the conjugated bilirubin made in the liver is unable to pass into the intestines. This will increase the bilirubin level in the blood, as well as result in less production of urobilinogen in the intestines. Thus, less urobilinogen will be transported in the enterohepatic circulation and less urobilinogen will be excreted in the urine. The other choices, viral hepatitis, exposure to toxic chemicals, and cirrhosis, are hepatic disorders that affect the hepatocytes directly and thus liver function. In such cases, there would be hepatocyte injury or tissue necrosis resulting in greater elevation of ALT and AST as compared to alkaline phosphatase, and the unconjugated bilirubin would be the fraction with the more significant increase because hepatocyte function is compromised. Urobilinogen would also be increased in the urine because of the inability of the liver to process it.

289.

A. In viral hepatitis, hepatocyte injury and necrosis cause the release of cellular contents. ALT is more specific for hepatocyte injury because it is significantly present in liver tissue, whereas AST is less specific because of its significant presence not only in liver but also in many other tissues. In viral hepatitis, both ALT and AST are significantly elevated in serum. Because liver function is compromised in viral hepatitis, the liver will be unable to pick up urobilinogen from the enterohepatic circulation to process, resulting in increased urobilinogen excretion in the urine. Although serum total bilirubin will be elevated, the indirect bilirubin (unconjugated) will comprise the larger fraction and the direct bilirubin (conjugated) will be the lesser fraction. Liver function is compromised, as is the ability of the liver to pick up bilirubin and conjugate it.

Electrolytes and Osmolality

290.

C. Sodium is the principal cation found in the plasma. The normal serum sodium level is 136–145 mmol/L, whereas in urine the sodium con centration ranges between 40 and 220 mmol/day, being dependent on dietary intake. Because sodium is a threshold substance, it is normally excreted in the urine when the serum sodium concentration exceeds 110–130 mmol/L. When serum levels fall below 110 mmol/L, all the sodium in the glomerular filtrate is virtually reabsorbed in the proximal and distal tubules. This reabsorption process is influenced by the hormone aldosterone.

291.

D. Osmolality is a measure of the total number of solute particles per unit weight of solution and is expressed as milliosmoles per kilogram of water. The normal osmolality of serum is in the range of 275–295 mOsm/kg water. For monovalent cations or anions the contribution to osmolality is approximately 92%. Other serum electrolytes, serum proteins, glucose, and urea contribute to the remaining 8%.

292.

B. Hemolysis of blood specimens because of physiological factors is often difficult to differentiate from hemolysis produced by the blood collection itself. In either case, the concentration of potassium will be increased in the serum because of the release of the very high level of intracellular potassium from the erythrocytes into the plasma. When hemolysis is present, the serum concentrations of sodium, bicarbonate, chloride, and calcium will be decreased because their concentrations are lower in erythrocytes than in plasma.

293.

D. The largest fractions of the anion content of serum are normally provided by chloride and bicarbonate. The third largest anion fraction is contributed by the proteins that are negatively charged at physiological pH and that provide about 16 mmol ion charge per liter. Of the remaining organic anions, the largest contribution is generally from lactate, which ranges normally from 1 up to 25 mmol/L in lactic acidosis. The ketone bodies, including acetoacetate, normally constitute only a small fraction of the total anions, but their total contribution may increase to 20 mmol/L in diabetic acidosis. Iron is present in the serum as a cation and does not contribute.

294.

D. In contrast to sodium, which is the principal plasma cation, potassium is the principal cellular cation. After absorption in the intestinal tract, potassium is partially filtered from the plasma by the kidneys. It is then almost completely reabsorbed from the glomerular filtrate by the proximal tubules and subsequently reexcreted by the distal tubules. Unlike sodium, potassium exhibits no renal threshold, being excreted into the urine even in K^+-depleted states. In acidotic states, as in renal tubular acidosis in which the exchange of Na^+ for H^+ is impaired, the resulting retention of potassium causes an elevation in serum K^+ levels. Hemolysis must be avoided in blood specimens that are to be used for K^+ analysis because erythrocytes contain a potassium concentration 23 times greater than serum K^+ levels. If the red blood cells are hemolyzed, a significant increase in serum K^+ will result.

295.

A. Chloride can be quantified by the spectrophotometric ferric perchlorate method. The reagent reacts with chloride to form a colored complex. Other methods employed are the spectrophotometric mercuric thiocyanate method, the coulometric-amperometric titration method, and the ion-selective electrode method, which is employed by many automated analyzers.

296.

C. Chloride is the principal plasma anion. The average concentration of chloride in plasma is 103 mmol/L. In the kidneys, chloride ions are removed from the blood through the glomerulus and then passively reabsorbed by the proximal tubules. The chloride pump actively reabsorbs chloride in the thick ascending limb of the loop of Henle. In the lungs, chloride ions participate in buffering the blood by shifting from the plasma to the red blood cells to compensate for ionic changes that occur in the alveoli when the HCO_3^- from the red blood cells enters the plasma. This is termed the chloride shift. Chloride can be measured in a variety of body fluids, including serum, plasma, urine, and sweat.

297.

A. The calculation of the anion gap may be used both to assess instrument performance and as a quality assurance tool for electrolyte analyses. The following is one of the several equations that may be used to calculate the anion gap: anion gap $(mmol/L) = (Na^+ + K^+) - (Cl^- + HCO_3^-)$. The acceptable reference range for this method of calculation is 10–20 mmol/L. If the values of a particular patient fall within this acceptable level, it is presumed that there are no gross problems with the electrolyte measurements. In this case, the anion gap is 18 mmol/L and within the reference range. When using the anion gap it is important to remember that values are affected not only by measurement errors but also by such disease processes as renal failure, ketoacidosis, and salicylate poisoning. Therefore, it is important to differentiate between laboratory errors and true disease states.

298.

C. Addison disease is characterized by the hyposecretion of the adrenocortical hormones by the adrenal cortex. Both aldosterone, a mineralocorticoid, and cortisol, a glucocorticoid, are inadequately secreted in this disorder. The decreased secretion of aldosterone will affect body electrolyte balance and extracellular fluid volume. The decrease in sodium reabsorption by the renal tubules will be accompanied by decreased chloride and water retention. This loss of sodium, chloride, and water into the urine will cause the extracellular fluid volume to be decreased. Additionally, the decreased reabsorption of sodium will interfere with the secretion of potassium and hydrogen ions in the renal tubules, causing an increase in the serum potassium ion and hydrogen ion (acidosis) concentrations.

299.

D. Primary aldosteronism is characterized by the hypersecretion of aldosterone, a mineralocorticoid, by the zona glomerulosa cells of the adrenal cortex. Excessive secretion of aldosterone will increase renal tubular reabsorption of sodium, resulting in a decrease in the loss of sodium in the urine. The net result of this mechanism is increased sodium in the extracellular fluid. Additionally, there will be increased renal excretion of potassium, causing a decrease of potassium in the extracellular fluid.

300.

D. A decreased serum sodium concentration, or hyponatremia, is associated with a variety of disorders, including (1) *Addison disease,* which involves the inadequate secretion of aldosterone, resulting in decreased reabsorption of sodium by the renal tubules; (2) *diarrhea,* which involves the impaired absorption from the gastrointestinal tract of dietary sodium and of sodium from the pancreatic juice, causing an excessive quantity of sodium to be excreted in the feces; (3) *diuretic therapy,* which causes a loss of water with concurrent loss of electrolytes, including sodium; and (4) *renal tubular disease,* which involves either the insufficient reabsorption of sodium in the tubules or a defect in the Na^+–H^+ tubular exchange mechanism. A diagnosis of Cushing syndrome is incorrect because the disorder is associated with hypernatremia.

301.

C. Free ionized calcium normally accounts for about 50% of total serum calcium, with the remainder being made up of complexed calcium (about 10%) and calcium bound to proteins (about 40%). The main factors that affect the free ionized calcium fraction are the protein concentration and the pH of the blood. Calcium ions are bound mainly to albumin, but they also bind to globulins. Because the binding is reversible, factors that decrease the protein concentration will increase the free ionized fraction of calcium in the blood. A decrease in blood pH will also increase the fraction of free ionized calcium.

302.

D. The renal tubular reabsorption of phosphate is controlled by the action of parathyroid hormone (PTH) on the kidney. Increased PTH secretion from any cause will lead to a decreased tubular reabsorption of phosphate (increased urine phosphate and decreased serum phosphate). The test is useful in distinguishing serum hypercalcemia that is a result of excess PTH production by the parathyroid glands from hypercalcemia due to other causes (e.g., bone disease).

303.

D. PTH, calcitonin, vitamin D, plasma proteins, and plasma phosphates are factors that influence plasma calcium levels. *PTH* is a hormone important in maintaining plasma calcium levels. It mobilizes calcium from bones. It increases the synthesis of one of the vitamin D derivatives, thereby causing an increase in bone resorption and intestinal absorption of calcium. When normal calcium levels are restored, PTH secretion is cut off (negative-feedback mechanism). *Calcitonin* (thyrocalcitonin) is a hormone secreted by the thyroid gland in response to elevated levels of plasma calcium. It acts by inhibiting bone resorption of calcium, thereby preventing significant variations in plasma calcium concentrations. Hydroxylation of *vitamin D* gives a derivative that will increase the intestinal absorption of calcium and phosphates.

304.

D. PTH has physiological actions on bone, kidney, and intestine. Its overall effect is to raise serum ionized calcium levels and lower serum phosphorus levels. Its actions on various organs are the result of a combination of both direct and indirect effects. In bones, PTH directly acts to increase bone resorption, thereby increasing both calcium and phosphorus in the blood. In the kidneys, PTH directly acts on the renal tubules to decrease phosphate reabsorption. In combination with the effect on bone, the overall result is a decrease in blood phosphorus levels. In the intestines, PTH acts to increase absorption of calcium by its action in increasing 1,25-dihydroxyvitamin D_3 synthesis in the kidneys, which in turn stimulates intestinal absorption of calcium.

305.

A. Primary hyperparathyroidism is a disorder characterized by increased secretion of PTH into the blood, without the stimulus on the parathyroid gland of a decreased level of ionized calcium. The increase in PTH produces increased blood calcium and vitamin D_3 levels, along with a decreased blood phosphorus level. The hypersecretion is most often caused by a single parathyroid adenoma. PTH secretion can usually, but not in all cases, be suppressed by calcium infusion. The decreased blood phosphate level is a result of the action of PTH on the kidneys, which decreases tubular reabsorption of phosphate ions. The increased blood level of 1,25-dihydroxyvitamin D_3 is also caused by PTH action on the kidneys in that PTH stimulates increased renal synthesis of this compound.

306.

C. Secondary hyperparathyroidism is a disorder that represents the response of a normally functioning parathyroid gland to chronic hypocalcemia. Inmost patients, the hypocalcemia is the result of renal disease or vitamin D deficiency. Vitamin D deficiency decreases intestinal calcium absorption, resulting in hypocalcemia. The hypocalcemia resulting from renal disease is more complex. It can result either from the increased serum phosphate level caused by decreased glomerular filtration or from the decreased synthesis of 1,25-dihydroxyvitamin D_3 in kidney disease.

307.

B. Serum inorganic phosphate concentrations are determined most commonly by reacting with ammonium molybdate reagent. The molybdenum-phosphate complexes can be quantified at 340 nm. Alternately, treatment of the phosphomolybdate compound formed with a reducing agent leads to the formation of molybdenum blue, which can be measured spectrophotometrically. Use of the anticoagulants EDTA, oxalate, and citrate should be avoided, because they interfere with the formation of phosphomolybdate.

308.

A. Total serum calcium concentration is often determined by the spectrophotometric quantification of the color complex formed with cresolphthalein complexone. Magnesium will also form a color complex and, therefore, is removed by reacting the serum with 8-hydroxyquinoline. Calcium concentration is determined with the use of a variety of other reagents and most reliably by means of atomic absorption spectrophotometry.

309.

B. Plasma phosphates influence plasma calcium levels. Case studies show that there is a reciprocal relationship between calcium and phosphorus. A decrease in plasma calcium will be accompanied by an increase in plasma inorganic phosphate.

310.

B. Similarly to potassium, which is a major intracellular cation, phosphate is a major intracellular anion. Therefore, when blood is drawn for serum inorganic phosphate measurement, hemolysis of the specimen must be avoided. Also, serum should be removed from the clot as soon after collection as possible to avoid leakage of phosphate into the serum. Both of these situations would contribute to falsely increased serum phosphate levels. Conversely, serum phosphate levels will be depressed following meals, during the menstrual period, and during intravenous glucose and fructose therapy.

311.

B. Copper is found in the plasma mainly in two forms: a minor fraction loosely bound to albumin and the majority, representing about 80–95%, firmly bound to the enzyme ceruloplasmin, an α_2-globulin, which is important in the oxidation of iron from the ferrous to the ferric state. Copper is also an essential constituent of a variety of other enzymes found in erythrocytes and in other sites throughout the body. The major clinical usefulness of determining serum copper or ceruloplasmin levels is that the decreased level of both is associated with Wilson disease. Decreased levels of copper are also found in protein malnutrition and malabsorption and in nephrosis.

312.

A. Transferrin is a glycoprotein that reversibly binds serum iron that is not combined with other proteins such as hemoglobin and ferritin. Transferrin concentration in serum is rarely determined directly but, rather, in terms of the serum iron content after saturation with iron. This is the total iron-binding capacity (TIBC). The percent saturation of transferrin is determined by dividing the serum iron level by the serum TIBC and expressing this value as a percentage. Normally in adults the percent saturation of transferrin is in the range of 20–50%, whereas in iron-deficiency anemia, the saturation is expected to be less than 15%. In iron-deficiency anemia complicated by other disorders that either increase serum iron concentration or decrease the TIBC, the percent saturation may remain within the reference range.

313.

C. In adults the total body iron content averages 3–4 g. The majority of this iron is found in the active pool as an essential constituent of hemoglobin, with a much lesser amount being an integral component of myoglobin and a number of enzymes. Approximately 25% of the body iron is found in inactive storage forms. The major storage form of iron is ferritin, with a lesser amount being stored as hemosiderin. Ferritin may be found in most body cells but especially in reticuloendothelial cells of the liver, spleen, and bone marrow.

314.

D. In cases of iron-deficiency anemia uncomplicated by other diseases, serum ferritin levels correlate well with the evidence of iron deficiency obtained by marrow examination for stainable iron. This indicates that ferritin is released into the serum in direct proportion to the amount stored in tissues. In iron deficiency, serum ferritin levels fall early in the disease process. However, in certain disorders there is a disproportionate increase in serum ferritin in relation to iron stores. Examples include chronic infections, chronic inflammation, malignancies, and liver disease. For individuals who have these chronic disorders or iron deficiency, it is common for their serum ferritin levels to appear normal.

315.

B. Serum iron concentrations are most often determined by the colorimetric reaction with ferrozine, bathophenanthroline, or tripyridyltriazine. The same reagent is usually used in the determination of serum TIBC by saturating the transferrin in the serum with an excess of iron, removing any unbound iron, and measuring the iron bound to transferrin. This measurement of TIBC provides a measure of transferrin concentration. Several magnesium methods require the precipitation of magnesium as part of the analysis, and 8-hydroxyquinoline effectively precipitates magnesium.

316.

A. Transferrin is the iron transport protein in serum and is normally saturated with iron to the extent of approximately 20–50%. An increased percent saturation of transferrin is expected in patients with hemochromatosis, an iron overload disease, and iron poisoning. The increased saturation is due to the increased iron concentration in the serum. In patients with chronic infections and malignancies, there is impairment of iron release from body storage sites, leading to a decreased percent saturation of transferrin. In myocardial infarction the serum iron levels are depressed, but the TIBC levels are normal. Iron-deficiency anemia because of poor absorption, poor diet, or chronic loss results in decreased serum iron, increased transferrin, and decreased percent saturation of transferrin in most cases.

317.

C. In order to differentiate among diseases, it is necessary to perform several laboratory determinations to properly assess iron metabolism. In iron-deficiency anemia, the serum iron is decreased whereas the TIBC is increased. Thus it follows that the transferrin saturation is decreased. The serum ferritin level, which represents stored body iron, is depressed, and the free erythrocyte protoporphyrin (FEP) level is increased. FEP is not a specific test for iron-deficiency anemia, but it can function as a screening test.

318.

A. A low ionized serum magnesium level is characteristic of a magnesium deficiency tetany. The serum magnesium level usually ranges between 0.15 and 0.5 mmol/L when tetany occurs. In addition, the serum calcium level and blood pH are normal, whereas the serum potassium level is decreased. This type of tetany is treated with $MgSO_4$ to increase the level of serum magnesium, thus alleviating the tetany and convulsions that accompany this disorder.

319.

A. Magnesium measurements are commonly done spectrophotometrically using reagent systems such as calmagite, methylthymol blue, and chlorophosphonazo III. Calcium will interfere and is eliminated by complexing with a chelator that binds calcium and not magnesium. Atomic absorption is a specific and sensitive method for analysis of magnesium, with the only significant interference being phosphate ions, which are removed by complexing with a lanthanum salt.

320.

D. Plasma lactate concentrations are increased in cases of lactic acidosis. The accumulation of lactate in the blood results from any mechanism that produces oxygen deprivation of tissues and, thereby, anaerobic metabolism. Lactate concentrations in whole blood are extremely unstable because of the rapid production and release of lactate by erythrocytes as a result of glycolysis. One method of stabilizing blood lactate levels in specimen collection is to add an enzyme inhibitor such as fluoride or iodoacetate to the collection tubes. Heparin, ethylenediaminetetra-acetic acid (EDTA), and oxalate will act as anticoagulants but will not prevent glycolysis in the blood sample.

321.

C. Measuring the concentration of chloride in sweat is a commonly used diagnostic procedure for determining the disorder of cystic fibrosis (CF). The majority of patients with CF will present with increased concentrations of sodium and chloride in their sweat. Generally, children with CF will manifest sweat chloride levels that are two to five times the reference interval. In sweat testing, sweat production is stimulated by iontophoresis with pilocarpine. Then the sweat is either collected and analyzed for chloride or an ion-selective electrode is applied to the skin surface to quantify chloride. It has been established that the gene abnormality causing CF is located on chromosome 7.

322.

A. Colligative properties of a solution are those properties that depend only on the number of particles in solution, not on the nature of the particles. The colligative properties are boiling point, freezing point, osmotic pressure, and vapor pressure. Terms used to describe the concentration of particles in solution are "osmole" (the number of particles, 6.0224×10^{23}, that lowers the freezing point 1.86°C) and "osmolal" (a concentration of 1 Osm of solute per kilogram of water). One mole of an unionized solute dissolved in 1 kg of water lowers the freezing point 1.86°C. Thus it is an osmolal solution. For nonionized substances such as glucose, 1 mol equals 1 Osm. For substances that ionize, such as sodium chloride, wherein each molecule in solution becomes two ions and thus two particles, 1 mol of sodium chloride theoretically equals 2 Osm. In reality, however, this is not always the case; an osmotic activity coefficient factor is used to correct for the deviation. In practice, three types of osmometers are available. They are the freezing point, vapor pressure, and colloid osmotic pressure osmometers.

323.

D. The freezing point of an aqueous solution is lowered 1.86°C for every osmole of dissolved particles per kilogram of water. These particles may be ions (e.g., Na^+ and Cl^-), or undissociated molecules such as glucose. The freezing point osmometer is an instrument designed to measure the freezing point of solutions. It uses a thermistor that is capable of measuring very small changes in temperature.

324.

D. When the osmolality has been both measured in the laboratory and calculated, the osmolal gap may then be determined by subtracting the calculated osmolality from the measured. Plasma osmolality may be calculated when the plasma sodium, glucose, and urea nitrogen values are known. The equation for calculating osmolality expresses Na^+, glucose, and urea nitrogen in mmol/L (SI units). To convert glucose and urea nitrogen from mg/dL to mmol/L, the conversion factors 0.056 and 0.36 are used, respectively. For sodium, the factor 2 is used to count the cation (sodium) once and its corresponding anion once. Because glucose and urea nitrogen are undissociated molecules, they are each counted once. Use the following equation:

$$\text{Calculated osmolality (mOsm/kg)} = 2.0\,Na^+(\text{mmol/L}) + \text{Glucose (mmol/L)} + \text{Urea nitrogen (mmol/L)}$$

$$= 2.0\,(142\ \text{mmol/L}) + (0.056 \times 130\ \text{mg/dL}) + (0.36 \times 18\ \text{mg/dL})$$

$$284 + 7.3 + 6.5 = 298\ \text{mOsm/kg}$$

325.

C. The colloid osmotic pressure (COP) osmometer is composed of a semipermeable membrane that separates two chambers, a mercury manometer, a pressure transducer, and a meter. When a serum sample is introduced into the sample chamber, saline solution from the reference chamber moves across the membrane by osmosis. This causes the development of a negative pressure on the saline side that is equivalent to the COP, which represents the amount of protein in the serum sample. COP osmometers measure the serum protein contribution to the total osmolality in terms of millimeters of mercury. COP levels are helpful in monitoring intravenous fluid therapy.

Acid-Base Metabolism

326.

A. Because of its high concentration in blood, the bicarbonate/carbonic acid pair is the most important buffer system in the blood. This buffer system is also effective in the lungs and in the kidneys in helping to regulate body pH. The other buffers that also function to help maintain body pH are the phosphate, protein, and hemoglobin buffer systems. The acetate buffer system is not used by the body to regulate pH.

327.

C. PCO_2 is an indicator of carbonic acid (H_2CO_3). The PCO_2 millimeters of mercury value (mm Hg) multiplied by the constant 0.03 equals the millimoles per liter (mmol/L) concentration of H_2CO_3 ($PCO_2 \times 0.03 = H_2CO_3$). PCO_2 can be measured using a pH/blood gas analyzer.

328.

A. The concentration of total CO_2 ($ctCO_2$) or carbon dioxide content is a measure of the concentration of bicarbonate, carbonate, carbamino compounds, carbonic acid, and dissolved carbon dioxide gas (PCO_2) in the plasma. Bicarbonate makes up approximately 95% of the total CO_2 content, but most laboratories are not equipped to directly measure bicarbonate. Therefore, total CO_2 is generally quantified. The bicarbonate concentration may be estimated by subtracting the H_2CO_3 concentration (measured in terms of PCO_2 and converted to H_2CO_3) from the total CO_2 concentration.

329.

B. The most important buffer pair in the plasma is bicarbonate with carbonic acid. Use of the Henderson-Hasselbalch equation

$$pH = pK' + \log\frac{[salt]}{[acid]}$$

shows that the pH changes with the ratio of salt to acid—that is, bicarbonate to carbonic acid—because pK′ is a constant. For this buffer pair, apparent pK′ = 6.1. When the ratio of the concentrations of bicarbonate to carbonic acid is 20:1 (log of 20 = 1.3), the pH is 7.4; that is,

$$pH = 6.1 + \log 20$$
$$7.4 = 6.1 + 1.3$$

The carbonic acid designation represents both the undissociated carbonic acid and the physically dissolved carbon dioxide found in the blood. Because the concentration of the undissociated carbonic acid is negligible compared to the concentration of physically dissolved carbon dioxide, the expression for carbonic acid concentration is usually written ($PCO_2 \times 0.03$).

330.

D. The acid-base equilibrium of the blood is expressed by the Henderson-Hasselbalch equation:

$$pH = pK' + \log\frac{cHCO_3^-}{(PCO_2 \times 0.03)}$$

In this buffer pair, pK′ = 6.1. Normally, the ratio of the concentration of bicarbonate ions $cHCO_3^-$ to the concentration of carbonic acid expressed as ($PCO_2 \times 0.03$) in the plasma is 20:1. The bicarbonate component of the equation is considered to be the "metabolic" component, controlled by the kidneys. The carbonic acid component is considered the "respiratory" component, controlled by the lungs. An excess of bicarbonate without a change in PCO_2 will increase the ratio of bicarbonate to carbonic acid. Therefore, the pH will increase; that is, the plasma becomes more alkaline.

331.

C. The normal ratio of bicarbonate ions to dissolved carbon dioxide is 20:1 and pH = 6.1 + log 20/1. An excess of dissolved CO_2 (e.g., increase in PCO_2) will increase the denominator in the equation or decrease the ratio of bicarbonate ions to dissolved CO_2. The pH will decrease; that is, the plasma becomes more acidic. The amount of dissolved CO_2 (PCO_2) in the blood is related to respiration. Hence, this condition is termed "respiratory acidosis."

332.

B. It is possible to use arterial, venous, or capillary blood for blood gas analysis. The specimen of choice for determining pulmonary dysfunction in adults is arterial blood. Analysis of arterial blood is the best indicator of pulmonary function, the capacity of the lungs to exchange carbon dioxide for oxygen. PO_2 and PCO_2 measurements from capillary blood are usually confined to infant sampling, and they are dependent on the patient preparation and sampling site. Venous blood should not be used for blood gas studies involving pulmonary problems because venous blood gas values also reflect metabolic processes. Furthermore, the reference range for PO_2 in venous blood varies drastically from arterial blood. Urine cannot be used to determine the acid/base status of a patient.

333.

B. Heparin is the best anticoagulant to use in drawing blood for blood gas analyses because it does not affect the value of the blood pH. This is also critical to PO_2 measurements because alterations in blood pH will cause concomitant changes in PO_2 values. Several heparin salts are available for use as anticoagulants. Sodium heparinate, 1000 U/mL, is commonly used. Ammonium heparinate may be substituted for the sodium salt when it is necessary to perform additional testing, such as electrolyte analysis, on the blood gas sample.

334.

A. When a blood specimen is drawn for gas analysis, it is important to avoid exposure of the specimen to air because of the differences in the partial pressures of carbon dioxide and oxygen in air and in blood. The PCO_2 in blood is much greater than the PCO_2 in air. Hence on exposure of blood to air, the total CO_2 and the PCO_2 both decrease, causing an increase in pH. Similarly, the PO_2 of air is much greater than that of blood, thus, the blood PO_2 increases on exposure to air.

335.

C. Glycolysis and other oxidative metabolic processes will continue *in vitro* by red blood cells when a whole blood specimen is left standing at room temperature. Oxygen is consumed during these processes, resulting in a decrease in PO_2 levels. A decrease of 3–12 mm Hg/hour at 37°C has been observed for blood specimens exhibiting normal PO_2 ranges. This rate of decrease is accelerated with elevated PO_2 levels. Additionally, carbon dioxide is produced as a result of continued metabolism. An increase in PCO_2 levels of approximately 5 mm Hg/hour at 37°C has been demonstrated. The increased production of carbonic acid and lactic acid during glycolysis contributes to the decrease in blood pH.

336.

D. The solubility coefficient of CO_2 gas (dissolved CO_2) in normal blood plasma at 37°C is 0.03 mmol/L/mm Hg. The concentration of dissolved CO_2 found in plasma is calculated by multiplying the PCO_2 blood level by the solubility coefficient (0.03). The predominant components of total CO_2 are bicarbonate (95%) and carbonic acid (5%). The bicarbonate ion concentration in millimoles per liter can be calculated by subtracting the product of (0.03 mmol/L/mm Hg $\times$ PCO_2 mm Hg), which represents carbonic acid, from the total CO_2 concentration (millimoles per liter).

337.

C. The red blood cell membrane is permeable to both bicarbonate and chloride ions. Chloride ions participate in buffering the blood by diffusing out of or into the red blood cells to compensate for the ionic change that occurs when bicarbonate enters or leaves the red blood cell. This is called the chloride shift.

338.

B. In a person with diabetes, diabetic ketoacidosis is one of the complications that may require emergency therapy. Blood glucose levels are usually in the range of 500–700 mg/dL but may be higher. The result is severe glycosuria that produces an osmotic diuresis, leading to loss of water and depletion of body electrolytes. Lipolysis is accelerated as a result of insulin deficiency. The free fatty acids produced are metabolized to acetyl-coenzyme A units, which are converted in the liver to ketone bodies. Hydrogen ions are produced with ketone bodies (other than acetone), contributing to a decrease in blood pH. Ketoacids are also excreted in the urine, causing a decrease in urinary pH.

339.

D. One of the primary reasons for metabolic alkalosis, especially in infants, is vomiting. Hydrogen ions are lost in the vomit, and the body reacts to replace them in the stomach. Consequently, hydrogen is lost from the plasma. This loss of hydrogen is due to a metabolic as opposed to a respiratory reason. Salicylate poisoning, uncontrolled diabetes mellitus, and renal failure all lead to metabolic acidosis either through an overproduction of ketone bodies, such as acetoacetic acid and beta-hydroxybutyric acid, or because of a reduced excretion of acid by the kidneys.

340.

D. Laboratory results from arterial blood gas studies in partially compensated respiratory alkalosis are as follows: pH slightly increased, PCO_2 decreased, HCO_3^- decreased, and total CO_2 decreased. Respiratory alkalosis is a disturbance in acid-base balance that is caused by hyperventilation associated with such conditions as fever, hysteria, and hypoxia. Respiratory alkalosis is characterized by a primary deficiency in physically dissolved CO_2 (decreased PCO_2). This decrease in the level of PCO_2 is due to hyperventilation, causing the accelerated loss of CO_2 by the lungs. This loss of CO_2 alters the normal 20:1 ratio of $cHCO_3^-/PCO_2$, causing an increase in the blood pH level. In respiratory alkalosis, because the initial defect is in the lungs, the kidneys respond as the major compensatory system. Ammonia production in the kidneys is decreased, $Na^+–H^+$ exchange is decreased with the retention of H^+, and bicarbonate reabsorption is decreased. By decreasing the bicarbonate reabsorption into the bloodstream, the kidneys attempt to reestablish the 20:1 ratio and normal blood pH. In a partially compensated state, as the blood bicarbonate level decreases, the blood pH begins to return toward normal but continues to be slightly alkaline. In a fully compensated state the blood pH is normal.

341.

C. Respiratory acidosis is a disturbance in acid-base balance that is caused by the retention of CO_2 by the lungs. This imbalance is associated with such conditions as bronchopneumonia, pulmonary emphysema, pulmonary fibrosis, and cardiac insufficiency. Respiratory acidosis is characterized by a primary excess in physically dissolved CO_2, which is quantified by measuring the blood PCO_2 level. The primary problem leading to an increase in the PCO_2 level is hypoventilation. This retention of CO_2 alters the normal 20:1 ratio of $cHCO_3^-/PCO_2$, causing a decrease in blood pH level. In respiratory acidosis, because the initial defect is associated with the lungs, the kidneys respond as the major compensatory system. The production of ammonia, the exchange of Na^+ for H^+ with the excretion of H^+, and the reabsorption of bicarbonate are all increased in the kidneys to compensate for the malfunction of the lungs. In cases where the defect is not within the respiratory center, the excess of PCO_2 in the blood can actually have a stimulatory effect on the center, causing an increase in the respiration rate. Thus compensation can also occur through CO_2 elimination by the lungs.

342.

A. There is a wide variety of conditions that will cause a shift of the dissociation curve of oxyhemoglobin to the left or to the right. A shift to the left will mean an increase in the affinity of hemoglobin for oxygen. Because of this increased affinity, there is also less oxygen delivered to the tissue for a given percent saturation of hemoglobin. When the curve is shifted to the right, there is a decrease in the affinity of hemoglobin for oxygen. Hence there is increased oxygen delivered to tissues for a given hemoglobin oxygen saturation. Oxyhemoglobin is a stronger acid than deoxyhemoglobin. Both exist in equilibrium in the blood. Increased hydrogen ion concentration shifts the equilibrium toward the deoxygenated form. This shift results in increased oxygen delivery to the tissue. The higher the concentration of 2,3-bisphosphoglycerate in the cell, the greater is the displacement of oxygen, thus facilitating the release of oxygen at the tissue level. Increased PCO_2 and increased temperature will also have this same effect.

343.

A. Carbonic anhydrase (CA) is an enzyme found in red blood cells that catalyzes the reversible hydration of CO_2 to bicarbonate and a proton:

$$H_2O + CO_2 \xrightleftharpoons{CA} HHCO_3$$

The proton, in turn, is buffered by the histidine portion of the hemoglobin molecule that activates the release of oxygen. It is at this point that oxyhemoglobin is converted to deoxyhemoglobin. In the alveoli of the lungs, CA catalyzes the conversion of H_2CO_3 to CO_2 and H_2O. The CO_2 is then exhaled. Carbonic anhydrase is an intracellular enzyme of erythrocytes and renal tubular cells, and it is not found normally in any significant concentration in the plasma. It is not associated with the oxygen dissociation curve.

344.

B. Base excess is a measure of the nonrespiratory buffers of the blood. They are hemoglobin, serum protein, phosphate, and bicarbonate. Therefore, base excess reflects an abnormality in the buffer base concentration. Bicarbonate has the greatest influence on base excess, which is an indicator of metabolic function. The normal range for base excess is ± 2.5 mmol/L. A quick estimation of base excess is to subtract the average "normal" reference bicarbonate level set by the laboratory from the measured bicarbonate level (e.g., if laboratory reference bicarbonate = 25 and patient's bicarbonate = 30, then base excess = (30 − 25) = +5; if patient's bicarbonate = 20, then base excess = (20 − 25) = −5). As demonstrated, a positive base excess is associated with metabolic alkalosis, and a negative base excess is associated with metabolic acidosis.

345.

C. The acid-base equilibrium of the blood is expressed by the Henderson-Hasselbalch equation:

$$pH = pK' + \log \frac{cHCO_3^-}{(PCO_2 \times 0.03)}$$

For the stated problem, convert PCO_2 in mm Hg to dissolved CO_2, multiplying by the solubility coefficient of CO_2 gas: 44 mm Hg × 0.03 mmol/L/mm Hg = 1.32 mmol/L. Next, determine the bicarbonate concentration by finding the difference between the total CO_2 and dissolved CO_2 concentrations: 29 mmol/L − 1.32 mmol/L = 27.68 mmol/L. pK′ for the bicarbonate buffer system is 6.1. Therefore,

$$pH = 6.1 + \log\frac{27.68}{1.32}$$

$$pH = 6.1 + \log 20.97$$

$$pH = 6.1 + \log 21$$

$$pH = 6.1 + 1.32$$

$$pH = 7.42$$

346–349.

In evaluating acid-base balance, the pH, PCO_2, and total CO_2 of an arterial blood specimen are measured. The reference values of arterial whole blood at 37°C for adults are as follows:

$$pH = 7.35\text{–}7.45$$

$$PCO_2 = 35\text{–}45 \text{ mm Hg}$$

$$cHCO_3^- = 22\text{–}26 \text{ mmol/L}$$

$$ctCO_2 = 23\text{–}27 \text{ mmol/L}$$

$$PO_2 = 80\text{–}110 \text{ mm Hg}$$

Acid-base disturbances can be characterized into four basic disorders: metabolic alkalosis, metabolic acidosis, respiratory alkalosis, and respiratory acidosis.

$$pH = pK' + \log \frac{cHCO_3^-}{H_2CO_3}$$

or

$$pH = pK' + \log \frac{cHCO_3^-}{(PCO_2 \times 0.03)}$$

Normally, the average ratio of bicarbonate to the concentration of carbonic acid is 20:1, resulting in a blood pH of 7.4. The $cHCO_3^-$ is represented in the measurement of total CO_2 value because 95% of the total CO_2 is HCO_3^-. The concentration of carbonic acid is calculated by multiplying the PCO_2 value by 0.03 (the solubility coefficient of CO_2 gas). The bicarbonate (base) represents the renal component of the acid-base balance. It is related to metabolic function. The dissolved carbon dioxide, measured as PCO_2, represents the respiration component and is related to respiratory function. Thus respiratory acidosis is characterized by an increase in blood PCO_2, whereas respiratory alkalosis is characterized by a decrease of blood PCO_2. Metabolic acidosis is characterized by a decrease in the blood bicarbonate levels, whereas metabolic alkalosis is related to an increase in blood bicarbonate levels. In acid-base disorders, the compensatory changes occur in the component that is not the original cause of the imbalance if compensation can occur. Thus in an acid-base imbalance of respiratory origin, the kidneys exert the major corrective action. In an acid-base imbalance of metabolic origin, the lungs exert the major corrective action. Sometimes a "mixed" or "double" problem of acidosis and alkalosis may exist due to more than one pathological process (e.g., a diabetic with asthma where both the respiratory and metabolic components indicate acidosis). If neither the respiratory nor the metabolic components indicate the condition of the patient (e.g., acidosis or alkalosis), then, most likely, there is something wrong with one or more of the blood gas results. In approaching acid-base problems, one should first key on the pH to determine the general condition (acidosis or alkalosis), then ask what is causing it—for example, a change in bicarbonate or PCO_2—to determine if the problem is metabolic or respiratory, and finally look at the remaining component to see if there is compensation bringing the pH closer to 7.4. If there is no movement in the remaining component from the reference value, then there is no compensation or uncompensation.

346.

A. In this case the pH is increased indicating alkalosis. HCO_3^- is increased, which means it is a metabolic problem. The PCO_2 is also increased, which indicates that the lungs are trying to compensate by retaining PCO_2 thus bringing the pH closer to 7.4.

347.

B. Here the pH is decreased indicating acidosis. The PCO_2 is increased, which indicates that the problem is respiratory in nature. The HCO_3^- is unchanged from the reference range, which indicates that there is no compensation; thus the patient has uncompensated respiratory acidosis.

348.

C. The pH clearly indicates acidosis. Both the metabolic (decreased HCO_3^-) and respiratory (increased PCO_2) components, however, indicate acidosis. There is no compensation seen in the results. Thus the patient has a double or mixed problem of acidosis.

349.

D. Here the pH and case information indicate alkalosis, but both the metabolic (decreased HCO_3^-) and respiratory (increased PCO_2) components indicate acidosis. Most likely there is a problem/error in one or more of the measurements.

Endocrinology

350.

C. The hypothalamus produces releasing factors or hormones that affect the release and synthesis of anterior pituitary hormones. The releasing hormones could have a stimulatory effect, as in the case of luteinizing hormone-releasing hormone (LH-RH), or an inhibitory effect, as in the case of prolactin-inhibiting factor (PIF). The posterior lobe of the pituitary acts only as a storage area for vasopressin and oxytocin, which are manufactured in the hypothalamus. The posterior lobe of the pituitary gland does not affect any feedback control on the anterior lobe. The intermediate lobe secretes beta-melaninophore-stimulating hormone, which acts on the skin. It also does not affect any control over the anterior lobe. The adrenal medulla secretes catecholamines, which are not involved in any feedback mechanism to the pituitary gland.

351.

B. Adrenocorticotropic hormone (ACTH) stimulates the adrenal cortex to secrete cortisol and, to a certain extent, aldosterone. However, aldosterone is also regulated by sodium and potassium levels and, more importantly, by the renin-angiotensin system. Cortisol alone has an inhibitory effect or a negative feedback relationship to ACTH secretion by the pituitary. A low level of cortisol stimulates the hypothalamus to secrete corticotropin- releasing hormone (CRH), which in turn stimulates release of ACTH from the pituitary gland and causes the adrenal cortex to secrete more cortisol. Elevated levels of cortisol reverse this process. ACTH secretion is not inhibited by estrogen or progesterone levels.

352.

A. The corticosteroids, produced by the adrenal cortex, may be classified as glucocorticoids or mineralocorticoids. Cortisol is the primary glucocorticoid, and aldosterone is the primary mineralocorticoid. Aldosterone functions as a regulator of salt and water metabolism. Aldosterone promotes water retention and sodium resorption with potassium loss in the distal convoluted tubules of the kidney.

353.

B. Renin is a proteolytic enzyme secreted by the juxtaglomerular cells of the kidneys. In the blood, renin acts on renin substrate (angiotensinogen) to produce angiotensin I. An angiotensin-converting enzyme secreted by endothelial cells then converts angiotensin I to angiotensin II. It is the latter that is responsible for the vasoconstrictive action of renin release. Angiotensin III is a product of aminopeptidase on angiotensin II, and the action of angiotensin II and III is directed at modulating aldosterone secretion. Plasma renin activity, determined by immunoassay, is assessed by quantifying the amount of angiotensin I produced by the action of renin on angiotensinogen using an initial kinetic assay. In addition, renin can be measured directly by an immunometric-mass assay that utilizes a monoclonal antibody.

354.

A. A low-salt diet, upright position, and diuretics cause a decrease in effective plasma volume. This decrease stimulates the renin-angiotensin system, which increases aldosterone secretion. Aldosterone promotes sodium retention and potassium loss.

355.

B. The hypothalamus, which secretes CRH, is sensitive not only to cortisol levels and stress but also to sleep-wake patterns. Thus plasma ACTH and cortisol levels exhibit diurnal variation or circadian rhythm. Cortisol secretion peaks at the time of awakening between 6 A.M. and 8 A.M. and then declines to the lowest level between early evening and midnight. After midnight the level again begins to increase. Specimens should be taken at 8 A.M. and 8 P.M. The evening cortisol level should be at least 50% lower than the morning result. In 90% of patients with Cushing syndrome there is no diurnal variation. However, absence of the normal drop in the evening cortisol level is not specific for Cushing syndrome. Other conditions, such as ectopic ACTH syndrome, blindness, hypothalamic tumors, obesity, acute alcoholism, and various drugs, alter normal circadian rhythm in cortisol secretion. To confirm Cushing syndrome, a dexamethasone suppression test may be performed.

356.

D. For differentiation of primary and secondary adrenal dysfunction, stimulation or suppression tests that depend on the feedback mechanism between cortisol and ACTH are performed. In the ACTH stimulation test, a patient with a low baseline serum cortisol level is given ACTH. The level of cortisol will increase slightly if the problem lies with the anterior pituitary gland, thus secondary adrenal insufficiency. This increase will be less than normal and may be somewhat delayed due to atrophy of the adrenal cortex as a result of the primary pituitary dysfunction. If the serum cortisol level does not change from baseline, the dysfunction is with the adrenal cortex, thus primary adrenal insufficiency.

357.

C. Only very small quantities, normally less than 2%, of the total adrenal secretion of cortisol appear in the urine as free cortisol. The majority of cortisol is either metabolized in various tissues or conjugated in the liver and excreted. It is only the serum unconjugated cortisol not bound to corticotropin binding globulin (CBG) or the conjugated cortisol that can be cleared by glomerular filtration in the kidney. Therefore, the measurement of free cortisol in the urine is a sensitive reflection of the amount of unbound cortisol in the serum. It is not a reflection of the amount of conjugated cortisol or the serum total cortisol but, rather, only the increased cortisol production that is not accompanied by an increase in serum levels of CBG.

358.

C. The probable diagnosis is Cushing syndrome caused by adrenocortical carcinoma. In adrenocortical carcinoma, the urinary free cortisol and the serum cortisol levels would be elevated and the plasma ACTH level would be decreased. The carcinoma produces excess cortisol that, because of the feedback loop, turns off pituitary production of ACTH. Neither the low-dose dexamethasone suppression test nor the high-dose test is able to suppress cortisol production. Because dexamethasone is a cortisol analogue, it would normally suppress ACTH and cortisol levels in a healthy individual. All these data support primary adrenal dysfunction caused by an adrenal carcinoma. If the elevated cortisol level was due to a pituitary adenoma or ectopic ACTH lung cancer, the ACTH level would also be increased. Addison disease is caused by hypofunction of the adrenal cortex.

359.

B. The adrenogenital syndrome, congenital adrenal hyperplasia, is due to a deficiency in specific enzymes needed for the synthesis of cortisol and aldosterone. Because cortisol production is blocked, the pituitary increases its secretion of adrenocorticotropic hormone (ACTH), causing adrenal hyperplasia and hypersecretion of cortisol precursors. There are eight recognized types of inherited enzyme defects in cortisol biosynthesis. The most common type of defect is the lack of 21-hydroxylase, occurring in 95% of the cases. Conversion of 17α-hydroxyprogesterone to 11-deoxycortisol is impaired, causing accumulation of 17α-hydroxyprogesterone, which is metabolized to pregnanetriol. An increased plasma 17α-hydroxyprogesterone level is diagnostic and can be determined by radioimmunoassay. Determinations of serum testosterone and urinary pregnanetriol elevations are also diagnostic of this disorder. Virilization takes place in this syndrome because cortisol precursors are shunted to produce weak androgens [e.g., dehydroepiandrosterone (DHEA) and androstenedione]. These androgens are converted peripherally to testosterone in large-enough amounts to create this condition. The second most common defect is 11β-hydroxylase deficiency with an accumulation of 11-deoxycortisol. 3β-Hydroxysteroid dehydrogenase-isomerase deficiency and C-17,20-lyase/17α-hydroxylase deficiency are examples of other enzyme defects seen in this disorder. A testicular or adrenal tumor may cause symptoms similar to this syndrome; however, these tumors would be acquired in contrast to congenital disorders.

360.

D. Testosterone is the most potent of the body's androgens. One of the major functions of the testes is to produce testosterone. It is metabolized to the 17-ketosteroids, etiocholanolone, and androsterone, but testosterone is not itself a 17-ketosteroid. The 17-ketosteroids, dehydroepiandrosterone (DHEA), androsterone, and androstenedione, all have androgenic properties but are much weaker than testosterone.

361.

B. The pituitary gland produces protein hormones such as adrenocorticotropic hormone, thyroid-stimulating hormone, follicle-stimulating hormone, growth hormone, and prolactin. Steroid hormones include C_{21} corticosteroids and progesterone, C_{19} androgens, and C_{18} estrogens. The mineralo- and gluco-corticosteroids are secreted only by the adrenal glands, but the other steroids listed are secreted by the ovaries, testes, adrenal glands, and placenta to a varying extent, depending on the individual's sex.

362.

C. 17β-Estradiol (E_2) is the most potent estrogen. 17β-Estradiol is considered to be the true ovarian hormone because it is secreted almost entirely by the ovaries. In contrast, estrone (E_1) is produced from circulating C_{19} neutral steroids (e.g., androstenedione) and is also synthesized from 17β-estradiol. Estriol (E_3) is derived almost exclusively from 17β-estradiol and has little clinical significance except in pregnancy. The measurement of 17β-estradiol is used to evaluate ovarian function.

363.

C. In pregnant women the level of human chorionic gonadotropin (hCG) is highest during the first trimester, then it stabilizes to a lower level during the rest of the pregnancy. In the first trimester, the level of pregnanediol is slightly higher than that found in nonpregnant women during the luteal phase of the menstrual cycle. As pregnancy progresses, the placenta secretes more progesterone, which peaks midway into the third trimester and then levels off. It should be noted that pregnanediol is a biologically inactive metabolite of progesterone that is sometimes measured in urine. After the second month of pregnancy, estriol levels steadily increase as the placenta takes over estrogen production.

364.

C. The triple test for Down syndrome includes quantification of α_1-fetoprotein (AFP), unconjugated estriol (uE_3), and human chorionic gonadotropin (hCG) in the maternal serum. These measurements should be done between 16 and 18 weeks gestation, and they are useful in detecting neural tube defects and Down syndrome. In Down syndrome, the AFP and uE_3 levels are low, whereas the hCG level is elevated. These test results are related to gestational age and are expressed as a multiple of the median (MoM), meaning the maternal serum result is divided by the median result of the corresponding gestational population.

365.

A. Progesterone production can be monitored by measuring plasma progesterone or urinary pregnanediol, the major metabolite of progesterone. In the follicular stage of the menstrual cycle, only a small amount of progesterone is secreted. In the luteal stage, or the time from ovulation to menstruation, progesterone levels rapidly increase. Hence, serial assays of plasma progesterone or urinary pregnanediol can be used to identify the time of ovulation. If pregnancy does not occur, progesterone quickly decreases approximately 24 hours before menstruation. If there is no ovulation, then there is no corpus luteum formation and no cyclic rise in progesterone levels.

366.

D. Luteinizing hormone (LH) is secreted only by the anterior pituitary. A protein hormone, human chorionic gonadotropin (hCG), appears soon after conception and is thus used for early detection of pregnancy. Human placental lactogen (HPL), also a protein hormone, is produced only by the placenta and is measurable between the seventh and ninth weeks. HPL steadily increases throughout pregnancy and peaks near term. Analysis of HPL for placental dysfunction has been successful; however, it is not widely used for this purpose. During pregnancy the placenta is the main source of estrogen and progesterone. Both hormones are needed for the maintenance of pregnancy.

367.

D. The formation of estriol during pregnancy involves mainly the fetoplacental unit. Dehydroepiandrosterone sulfate (DHEA-S) and its 16α-hydroxy-DHEA-S derivative are formed mainly by the fetal adrenal glands and to a lesser degree by the liver. The fetus possesses 16α-hydroxylase activity, which is needed to convert dehydroepiandrosterone sulfate (DHEA-S) to 16α-hydroxy-DHEA-S. The 16α-hydroxy-DHEA-S compound is metabolized by the placenta to estriol. The placenta lacks certain enzymes needed for the conversion of simple precursors such as acetate, cholesterol, and progesterone to estrogens. Thus, the placenta must rely on immediate precursors produced in the fetus. In the case of estriol, the placenta utilizes the 16α-hydroxy-DHEA-S precursor made in the adrenal glands of the fetus. The latter compound crosses into the placenta, which takes over with the necessary enzymes to complete the synthesis of estriol. This estriol produced in the placenta is rapidly reflected in the maternal plasma and far exceeds maternal synthesis of estriol. Thus measurement of estriol in the maternal blood or urine is a sensitive indicator of the integrity of the fetoplacental unit. A defect in either the fetus or the placenta will be reflected by a decrease in estriol production.

368.

D. The concentration of estriol in maternal plasma or in a 24-hour sample of maternal urine is often used as an indicator of fetal distress or placental failure. A single value of either serum or urine estriol has relatively little value unless it can be related accurately to the gestational week. When sequential estriol determinations are made during pregnancy, a pattern of stable or steadily falling values may indicate a problem pregnancy. For serum or urine estriols, any individual value that is 30–50% less than the previous value or the average of the previous 3 days' values is significant.

369.

D. The testes are comprised of two anatomical units: seminiferous tubules and interstitium. The seminiferous tubules contain sertoli cells and these cells are responsible for sperm production.

370.

C. During the menstrual cycle, follicle- stimulating hormone (FSH) levels decrease in the later part of the follicular stage. Luteinizing hormone (LH) gradually increases during the follicular stage. At midcycle, both FSH and LH levels spike. Following this spike, in the luteal stage or second-half of the menstrual cycle, FSH and LH levels gradually decrease. In postmenopausal women the ovaries stop secreting estrogens. In response the gonadotropins, FSH and LH, rise to their highest levels. The reason is the feedback system between estrogen secretion by the gonads and the secretion of releasing factors by the hypothalamus; a decreased estrogen level causes increased secretion of FSH-releasing factor and LH-releasing factor.

371.

C. Ectopic hormones are hormonal substances produced by benign and malignant tumors derived from tissues that do not normally secrete those hormones. Examples of ectopic hormone production would be ACTH production by oat cell carcinoma of the lung and growth hormone production by bronchogenic carcinomas of the lung. Cortisol and growth hormone are normally secreted by the adrenal gland and anterior pituitary gland, respectively. Ectopic hormones are not in all cases chemically identical to the native hormone but may be similar enough to cross-react in immunoassay methods for the native hormone.

372.

D. At the cellular level, the site of action of the peptide and catecholamine hormones is different from that of the steroid and thyroid hormones. The peptide and catecholamine hormones bring about their effects by combining with receptors on or in the cell membranes of the target cells. In some cases, this binding to the membrane results in activation of adenylate cyclase, which sets in motion the so-called second-messenger mechanism of hormone action. On the other hand, steroid and thyroid hormones act predominantly by diffusing through the target cell membranes and combining with cytoplasmic or nucleic receptors to form a complex that then brings about the hormone's action.

373.

C. The adrenal medulla produces 80% epinephrine and 20% norepinephrine (noradrenalin). Metanephrine is a metabolite of epinephrine. Dopamine, a catecholamine, is a precursor of norepinephrine. Norepinephrine is converted to epinephrine by an enzyme, *N*-methyltransferase, which is present almost exclusively in the adrenal medulla. A tumor of the chromaffin tissue, called a pheochromocytoma, secretes excessive amounts of epinephrine. Ninety percent of pheochromocytomas are in the adrenal medulla. The increased levels of epinephrine from the pheochromocytoma cause hypertension. Although hypertension caused by a pheochromocytoma is rare, a correct diagnosis is very important because pheochromocytoma is one of the few causes of hypertension that is curable by surgery.

374.

A. The majority of pheochromocytomas (rare tumors) occur in the adrenal medulla, causing increased secretion of the catecholamines. As a screening test for this disorder, quantification of urinary metanephrine, the methylated product of epinephrine, is suggested because false negatives seldom occur. Follow-up testing should include measurement of urinary vanillylmandelic acid (VMA), because VMA is the primary metabolite of epinephrine and norepinephrine.

375.

B. Antidiuretic hormone (ADH), also known as vasopressin, is a peptide hormone secreted by the posterior pituitary gland under the influence of three major stimuli: decreased serum osmolality, increased blood volume, or psychogenic factors. ADH increases the renal reabsorption of water by increasing the permeability of the collecting ducts, with the result that body water is retained and urine osmolality increases. Diabetes insipidus is the syndrome that results from decreased secretion of ADH from any cause. Serum levels of ADH can be measured, but usually the measurement of serum and urine osmolality is sufficient to indicate the severity of the disease.

376.

D. Neuroblastoma is a solid malignant tumor found in the medulla of the adrenal gland, or it may arise from the extra-adrenal sympathetic chain. More commonly the disease occurs in children under the age of 5 years. Metastasis may occur to the liver, bone, bone marrow, or brain. Neuroblastoma is characterized by tumor production of epinephrine, norepinephrine, and dopamine, so all three hormones will be increased in the blood. The end-product of dopamine metabolism is homovanillic acid (HVA). The end-product of the catecholamines, epinephrine and norepinephrine, is vanillylmandelic acid (VMA). Both HVA and VMA will be excreted in excess in the urine.

377.

C. Serotonin (5-hydroxytryptamine or 5-HT) is synthesized from tryptophan in a variety of tissues, with the majority found in the argentaffin (enterochromaffin) cells of the intestine. Abdominal carcinoid is a metastasizing tumor of those cells and is associated with excessive production of serotonin. Serotonin in the blood is found almost exclusively in the platelets and is rapidly oxidized in the lungs to 5-hydroxyindoleacetic acid (5-HIAA), its major urinary metabolite. Urinary levels of 5-HIAA may also be increased by eating foods such as bananas and avocados, which are rich in serotonin; by the use of certain drugs such as the phenothiazines; and by carcinoid tumors.

378.

D. Somatostatin is also known as growth hormone-inhibiting hormone (GHIH). Somatostatin is a 14-amino-acid peptide that is secreted by the hypothalamus and is an inhibitor of growth hormone (somatotropin) secretion by the pituitary. It is also secreted by a variety of other organs and is a powerful inhibitor of insulin and glucagon secretion by the pancreas. Somatostatin can be measured by immunoassay methods, but its concentration in the peripheral circulation is extremely low, making it likely that its action is mostly at or near the site of secretion.

379.

B. Growth hormone (somatotropin) is a polypeptide secreted by the anterior pituitary. It is essential to the growth process of cartilage, bone, and a variety of soft tissues. It also plays an important role in lipid, carbohydrate, and protein metabolism of adults. During the growth phase of humans, hyposecretion of somatotropin results in dwarfism, whereas hypersecretion, conversely, causes pituitary gigantism. After the growth phase, hypersecretion of somatotropin causes acromegaly. Diagnosis of hypersecretion or hyposecretion of growth hormone usually requires the use of suppression or provocative tests of growth hormone release. Growth hormone levels may be quantified using immunoassay methods, including chemiluminescence immunoassay.

380.

C. Somatomedins, insulin-like growth factors I and II, is the designation given to a family of small peptides whose formation in the liver is under the control of growth hormone. The somatomedins exhibit similar activity as insulin and are active in stimulating many aspects of cell growth, particularly that of cartilage. Blood levels of somatomedin have been determined by radioimmunoassay methods, and acromegalic adults have been shown to have significantly elevated levels in comparison with normal adults.

381.

A. Calcitonin is a calcium-lowering hormone secreted by the parafollicular or C cells of the thyroid. Calcitonin acts as an antagonist to parathyroid hormone (PTH) action on the bone and kidneys. Medullary carcinoma of the thyroid is a neoplasm of the parafollicular cells that usually results in elevated serum levels of calcitonin. If the fasting calcitonin level is within the normal reference interval in a patient with suspected medullary carcinoma, a provocative calcium infusion test is often useful in improving the sensitivity of the test.

382.

A. Thyroglobulin is a glycoprotein in which the thyroid hormones are stored in the thyroid gland. When tyrosine residues of the thyroglobulin are iodinated, monoiodotyrosine (MIT) and diiodotyrosine (DIT) are formed. These iodotyrosine residues are not hormones. Triiodothyronine (T_3) and thyroxine (T_4) are the hormones produced by the thyroid, being formed by the coupling of either MIT or DIT residues. T_4 is the predominant form of the thyroid hormones secreted into the circulation, having a concentration in the plasma significantly greater than T_3. However, in terms of physiological activity, T_3 must be considered because it is four to five times more potent than T_4. Thus the overall contribution of T_3 to the total physiological effect of the thyroid hormones on the body is very significant.

383.

B. The thyroid gland is composed of two lobes connected by a structure called the isthmus. The lobes consist of many follicles. The follicle, in the shape of a sphere, is lined with a single layer of epithelial cells. The epithelial cells produce T_3 and T_4, which are stored as a component of the thyroglobulin. Within the lumen of the follicle is colloid. Thyroglobulin, secreted by the epithelial cells, makes up 90% of the colloid. As the epithelial cells synthesize the thyroid hormones, the hormones are stored in the thyroglobulin molecule. Thyroglobulin is then secreted into the colloid of the follicular lumen. When the thyroid hormones are needed, they are absorbed by the epithelial cells from their storage site, and through proteolysis, the hormones are released from fragments of the thyroglobulin molecule. T_3 and T_4 are then secreted by the cells into the blood.

384.

A. A small amount of reverse T_3 (rT_3) is made in the thyroid gland, but the majority is made from peripheral deiodination of T_4. rT_3 varies from T_3 in that rT_3 contains one iodine atom in the tyrosyl ring and two iodines in the phenolic ring, whereas T_3 has two iodines in the tyrosyl ring and one iodine in the phenolic ring. rT_3 does not have any physiological action as it is metabolically inactive. However, increased levels of rT_3 are associated with nonthyroidal illness (NTI), which also manifests with decreased levels of total T_3.

385.

C. Currently, the suggested term for autoantibodies that bind to TSH receptor sites is thyrotropin-receptor antibodies (TRAb). The thyrotropin-receptor antibodies (TRAb) are thyroid-stimulating immunoglobulins (TSI) that are IgG autoantibodies and are able to bind to the thyroid-stimulating hormone (TSH) receptor sites on thyroid cell membranes, thus preventing TSH from binding. These autoantibodies interact with the receptors similarly to TSH, thus stimulating the thyroid to secrete thyroid hormones. Because these autoantibodies do not respond to the negative feedback system as does TSH, hyperthyroidism is the end result. The majority of patients with Graves hyperthyroid disease exhibit high titers of TRAb.

386.

C. Graves disease is a name given to a diffusely hyperactive thyroid that produces thyrotoxicosis. Thyrotoxicosis results from elevated levels of thyroid hormone; therefore, laboratory results for free thyroxine (FT_4) and free triiodothyronine (FT_3) would be increased, thyroid hormone binding ratio (THBR) increased, and thyroid-stimulating hormone (TSH) decreased. In hyperthyroidism, the THBR is increased because thyroxine-binding globulin (TBG) is saturated with endogenous T_4. TSH levels are decreased because of the negative-feedback control of the thyroid hormones on the anterior pituitary.

387.

C. Hypothyroidism is a systemic disorder in which the thyroid gland does not secrete sufficient thyroid hormone. Myxedema is commonly used synonymously for hypothyroidism. Hypothyroidism can result from various diseases. If the disease affects the thyroid itself, it is referred to as primary hypothyroidism. If there is TSH deficiency of the pituitary gland, it is termed secondary hypothyroidism. Tertiary hypothyroidism is caused by hypothalamic failure that results in a decreased secretion of thyrotropin-releasing hormone. Thyroid failure in the newborn is termed cretinism. The free T_4 level and the thyroid hormone binding ratio (THBR) are decreased because of inadequate secretion of hormones. Since the thyroid hormones are low in concentration, the feedback mechanism to the anterior pituitary gland is triggered to increase production of TSH.

388.

B. To distinguish between a hypothalamic disorder and a disorder of the pituitary gland, thyroid-releasing hormone (TRH) is administered. In the case of a hypothalamic disorder (tertiary hypothyroidism), the TRH administered will cause an increased excretion of pituitary hormone, TSH. However, if the disorder originates in the pituitary gland (secondary hypothyroidism), the administration of TRH will have no effect on the pituitary gland and thus no increased excretion of TSH. Because the values of TSH were low before and remained low after administration of TRH, the disorder is secondary hypothyroidism. Primary hypothyroidism is caused by failure of the thyroid gland itself and is not evaluated by use of the TRH stimulation test. Iodine deficiency would cause high levels of TSH, and administration of TRH is not used to evaluate this disorder.

389.

B. Antibodies to thyroglobulin (TgAb) and thyroid cell peroxidase (TPOAb) are produced in several thyroid diseases. Very high antibody titers for antithyroglobulin antibodies and the detection of antithyroid peroxidase antibodies are highly suggestive of Hashimoto thyroiditis (a type of hypothyroidism). These antibodies are also frequently detected in primary myxedema and Graves' disease by means of hemagglutination methods. It should be noted that antithyroid antibodies do occur in other thyroid diseases, but their prevalence is less. These antibodies have also been detected in 5–10% of the normal population.

390.

B. Almost all the triiodothyronine (T_3) and thyroxine (T_4) hormones are reversibly bound to the serum proteins, thyroxine-binding globulin (TBG), thyroxine binding prealbumin (TBPA), and albumin. Most T_3 is bound to TBG, whereas 70% of T_4 is bound to TBG, 20% to TBPA, and 10% to albumin. T_3 has a lower affinity for TBG and TBPA than T_4. Thyroglobulin is manufactured and stored in the thyroid follicle and is not released into the circulation.

391.

C. Due to increased protein synthesis, the binding capacity of thyroxine-binding globulin (TBG) is increased in situations such as pregnancy and administration of oral contraceptives. The increased total thyroxine (total T_4) levels in these situations do not reflect the functional state of the thyroid gland. It is important when interpreting total T_4 levels to take into consideration situations such as these. Free T_4 is not affected by variations in thyroxine-binding proteins and better reflects the metabolic state that is euthyroid. However, use of the thyroid hormone binding ratio (THBR), which measures the unoccupied binding sites of TBG, in conjunction with the free and total T_4 levels permits a better interpretation of thyroid function. By this process it can be seen where the primary change occurs, whether in the level of T_4 or in TBG-binding capacity.

392.

B. In cases of peptic ulcer, treatment may include surgery that severs the vagus nerve. This severing is known as vagotomy, which, if complete, prevents the secretion of gastrin and HCl by the stomach. The Hollander insulin test is performed to assess the completeness of the vagotomy. If the vagotomy is complete, the hypoglycemia caused by the administration of insulin will not exert its normal stimulatory effect on gastric HCl and pepsinogen secretion.

393.

C. Gastrin is the designation given to a family of protein hormones produced by the mucosal cells of the gastric antrum. Once secreted, gastrin is carried in the blood to the fundic cells, causing release of hydrochloric acid. Serum gastrin levels are markedly elevated in the Zollinger-Ellison syndrome, a neoplastic proliferation of the nonbeta cells of the pancreatic islets. Gastrin levels may also be elevated in pernicious anemia, duodenal ulcer disease, and gastric ulcer disease.

394.

B. Measurement of PTH during surgery for adenoma resection of the parathyroid glands assists the surgeon in determining completeness of the resection based on the rapid fall of PTH. At least three samples are needed: first, a preincision baseline sample as surgery starts; a second baseline sample following exposure of the gland because PTH will increase with any manipulation of the tissue; and a postexcision sample drawn 10 minutes following gland removal (some surgical protocols may require multiple sampling at 5, 10, and 20 minutes postexcision). In general, at 10 minutes postexcision, the PTH level should fall to 50% or less of the preincision value or the value at the time of gland resection. If the PTH value remains increased and such a decrease does not occur or if the PTH rises again after what initially appeared to be a decrease, multigland disease or ectopic production need to be investigated.

Therapeutic Drug Monitoring and Toxicology

395.

D. The term "carboxyhemoglobin saturation" refers to the fraction of circulating hemoglobin combined with carbon monoxide. People who do not smoke generally have carboxyhemoglobin saturations ranging from 0.5 to 1.5%. Fatal carbon monoxide poisoning is usually associated with carboxyhemoglobin saturations of more than 60%, and acute symptoms begin to appear at saturations of 20%. People who smoke cigarettes exhibit levels of 8–9% carboxyhemoglobin, but occasionally saturations of greater than 16% have been reported in people who smoke heavily.

396.

D. Gas-liquid chromatography (GLC) is one of the few methods that can quantify ethanol reliably in the presence of isopropanol (2-propanol) or other alcohols. Examples of the analytical problems associated with quantifying alcohols are as follows: Isopropanol significantly cross-reacts (6%) in the widely used alcohol dehydrogenase (ADH) method for ethanol; other alcohols will cross-react with dichromate methods for ethanol; and other alcohols will cross-react with the permanganate-chromotropic acid method, which is sometimes used for the identification of methanol. Because GLC is not generally available in stat laboratories, for patients with suspected exposure to alcohols other than ethanol, a variety of other laboratory and clinical findings are often used.

397.

A. A significant fraction of absorbed isopropanol is metabolized to acetone and rapidly excreted in the urine. Because of isopropanol's relatively low molecular weight, exposure to this compound will in most cases significantly increase the patient's serum osmolality. Of course, other alcohols will have a similar effect. Urine osmolality exhibits a wide variability throughout the day and, therefore, would be of little use in determining isopropanol exposure. Serum sodium would be only secondarily affected by isopropanol exposure.

398.

D. The Reinsch test is applied to urine and is based on the ability of copper to reduce most metal ions to their metallic states in the presence of acid. Cyanide is not a metal and, therefore, will not be reduced. Increased urinary levels of arsenic, bismuth, antimony, and mercury will coat the copper with dull black, shiny black, blue-black, and silver-gray deposits, respectively. The test is intended as a rapid screening method only, and results should be confirmed by more sensitive and specific methods.

399.

B. Heroin (diacetylmorphine), an abused drug, is a derivative of morphine. The morphine used in its synthesis is generally obtained from opium. Although heroin itself is not pharmacologically active, it does have a rapid onset of action. It is converted quickly to 6-acetylmorphine and then hydrolyzed to morphine, both of which are pharmacologically active. So heroin abuse can be detected by measuring its metabolite morphine in the blood or urine.

400.

B. Morphine, codeine, and heroin are collectively referred to as opiates. Codeine is found in many prescription medicines and is rapidly metabolized after absorption into morphine and norcodeine. Because blood concentrations of most opiates are low even in overdose, screening is usually done on the urine. Immunoassay or colorimetric methods can be used for screening purposes, but chromatography is generally required for quantification of specific compounds. Gas chromatography/mass spectroscopy (GC/MS) is useful for the quantification of morphine and codeine.

401.

B. THC (Δ^9-tetrahydrocannabinol) is the principal active component of marijuana. Homogeneous enzyme immunoassay methods test for the presence of THC metabolites, especially 11-nor-Δ^9-THC-9-carboxylic acid, which is the primary urinary metabolite. Metabolites appear in urine within hours of smoking and continue to be detectable for 3–5 days following exposure.

402.

B. Cocaine is an abused drug and not available for therapeutic use. After absorption, cocaine in the blood is rapidly converted into ecgonine and benzoylecgonine. Because of the kidney's concentrating effect, examination of the urine for the metabolites is a sensitive method of determining exposure to cocaine.

403.

C. After absorption, lead is distributed into an active pool in the blood and soft tissue and a storage pool in bone, teeth, and hair. In blood, the majority is found in erythrocytes, with only minor quantities in plasma or serum. Lead is mainly excreted by the kidney; hence urine or whole blood would be appropriate specimens for determining lead exposure. Provision for lead-free sample containers is a major requirement. Lead analysis can be done accurately by flameless atomic absorption or anodic stripping voltammetry.

404.

B. Lead interferes in heme biosynthesis at several stages, the last of these being the incorporation of iron into the tetrapyrrole ring. This alteration in biosynthesis results in the formation and accumulation of zinc protoporphyrin (ZPP), with zinc replacing the iron in the tetrapyrrole ring. Free erythrocyte protoporphyrin is the extraction product of the zinc metabolite and is a sensitive screening method for determining lead exposure above 25 μg/dL. The test is not as specific as accurate determination of lead content, however, because iron-deficiency anemia and erythropoietic protoporphyria give false-positive results. Caution must be exercised in monitoring children under 6 years of age, because the Centers for Disease Control and Prevention has defined the acceptable blood level for lead to be less than 10 μg/dL in young children. At this level, ZPP and erythrocyte protoporphyrin assays are not sufficiently sensitive.

405.

D. After absorption, mercury rapidly accumulates in many organs and in the central nervous system, with only minor quantities found in the blood. The excretion of mercury by the kidney generally forms the basis for measurement of exposure. The preferred specimen in screening for exposure to methanol or acetaminophen is serum. Whole blood is required for determining carbon monoxide exposure, because practically all the inhaled carbon monoxide is found in erythrocytes bound to hemoglobin. Following release of carbon monoxide from hemoglobin, the CO gas can be measured using gas chromatography. The percent carboxyhemoglobin saturation of whole blood can be determined by differential spectrophotometry or by using an automated, wavelength system such as a CO-oximeter.

406.

C. The term "half-life" refers to the time required for a 50% decrease in serum drug concentration after absorption and distribution are complete. The more complete descriptive term is "drug elimination half-life." It requires five to seven half-life periods for drug concentration to reach steady state. At steady state, the drug concentration is in equilibrium with the dose administered rate and the elimination rate. Knowledge of a drug's half-life is important both for planning therapy and for monitoring drug concentration. In disease states, particularly involving the kidney and liver, half-life may be significantly altered and lead to accumulations of the drug or its metabolites in the blood.

407.

C. The Trinder reaction or modification is used almost routinely in the determination of salicylate and is based on the colorimetric reaction with ferric ions. The availability of rapid quantification in cases of salicylate overdose has been particularly useful because of the necessity of determining the drug's elimination half-life. Most clinically used thin-layer chromatographic methods are insensitive to the presence of salicylate. Because the colorimetric reaction used for determining the presence of phenothiazines with ferric perchloricnitric (FPN) reagent is dependent on ferric ions also, false-positive reactions in the ferric ion methods for salicylate may be expected.

408.

D. Hepatotoxicity is common in acetaminophen overdose. It is particularly important to be able to determine the acetaminophen serum level rapidly so that the elimination half-life of the drug can be estimated. Hepatic necrosis is more common when the half-life exceeds 4 hours and is very likely when it exceeds 12 hours. The concentration of acetaminophen can be measured by HPLC, colorimetric, EMIT, and fluorescence polarization methods.

409.

A. The barbiturates are classified pharmacologically according to their duration of action. Phenobarbital is long acting, amobarbital and butabarbital are intermediate acting, and pentobarbital and secobarbital are short acting. In general, the long-acting barbiturates have higher therapeutic and toxic levels than the shorter-acting barbiturates. In cases of overdose, it is important to be able to identify the type of barbiturate in the blood for correct therapy. Measurement of specific barbiturates usually requires chromatography or immunoassay.

410.

B. Tobramycin and gentamicin are examples of aminoglycoside antibiotics. Their use has been associated with both nephrotoxicity and ototoxicity. Drug concentration monitoring of patients taking the aminoglycosides requires an analytic system with good precision and accuracy over a wide range because both peak and trough levels are usually monitored. The trough level is used mainly as a measure of nephrotoxicity, whereas the peak level is useful in determining whether adequate therapy is being given to eliminate the causative organism.

411.

C. Although digoxin, nortriptyline, and quinidine have various effects on cardiac arrhythmias, they do not have metabolites with similar activity. Procainamide is an antiarrhythmic drug and has at least one metabolite with the same activity, namely, *N*-acetylprocainamide (NAPA). Because of differences in half-life, NAPA may accumulate in the blood and produce toxic effects even with therapeutic levels of procainamide. Therefore, both procainamide and NAPA need to be quantified for therapeutic drug monitoring.

412.

A. Drugs in the free state are able to elicit a pharmacologic response. It is the free drug that is able to cross cell membranes and to bind at receptor sites. In the protein-bound state, drugs are unable to enter tissues and interact at receptor sites.

413.

B. Acute glomerulonephritis is characterized by hematuria and albuminuria. The hypoalbuminemia results in less protein-bound drug and an increase in free drug. Thus, more free drug is available in the circulation to enter the tissues. Such a situation may result in severe side effects and even toxic effects. Therefore, to properly regulate drug dosages, it is advisable to measure free drug levels in blood, rather than total drug levels, whenever possible.

414.

B. The term "free drug" refers to the fraction of drug in the plasma not bound to protein. For the determination of free drug concentrations, urine would not be the proper specimen because the rate of drug excretion depends mainly on conjugation or metabolism and not on protein binding. In preparation of a protein-free filtrate of plasma, the drugs bound to protein would also enter the filtrate because they are dissociated when the protein is denatured. Saliva is a form of plasma ultrafiltrate and with some restrictions as to sampling and type of drug analyzed can be used for free-drug monitoring. Methods for equilibrium dialysis and for preparation of ultrafiltrates of plasma are now available and can provide excellent samples for free-drug analyses of some compounds.

415.

C. Tacrolimus (Prograf) is an antibiotic that functions as an immunosuppressant in organ transplantation, especially in liver transplants. By inhibiting interleukin production, it blocks lymphocyte proliferation. Adverse reactions to the drug include nephrotoxicity, nausea, vomiting, and headaches. Other immunosuppressant drugs include cyclosporine, mycophenolic acid, and sirolimus. Methotrexate is an antineoplastic drug, amiodarone is an antiarrhythmic drug, and paroxetine is an antidepressant drug.

416.

B. Theophylline, a xanthine with bronchodilator activity, is widely used in the treatment of asthma. Because of its availability and potential toxicity, it can also be subject to accidental overdose. Chromatographic methods are effective in separating theophylline from caffeine and theobromine, which are two commonly occurring and potentially interfering xanthines. However, most clinical thin-layer chromatographic methods are relatively insensitive to the xanthines, and suspected theophylline overdose should be confirmed by HPLC or immunoassay methods.

417.

D. Following absorption, primidone is metabolized primarily to phenobarbital and secondarily to phenylethylmalonamide (PEMA). Both metabolites have anticonvulsant activity, and both have a longer half-life than primidone. Generally, only serum phenobarbital and primidone concentrations are monitored. Determination of phenobarbital is particularly important when another anticonvulsant phenytoin is also administered because the metabolic rate of primidone conversion to phenobarbital may be increased, with a resulting accumulation of phenobarbital in the blood.

418.

A. Amitriptyline, doxepin, and imipramine and their active metabolites nortriptyline, nordoxepin, and desipramine, respectively, are tricyclic compounds particularly useful in the treatment of endogenous depression. These compounds are lipid soluble and, therefore, highly protein bound in the plasma. Although toxic concentrations of these drugs often lead to cardiac arrhythmias, low concentrations have been found to have antiarrhythmic activity. Because of these varying biological effects at differing serum concentrations, there is a need both for monitoring in cases of therapy and screening for toxic effects in cases of overdose.

419.

B. Lithium is used in the treatment of manic depression. Because of the small difference between therapeutic and toxic levels in the serum, accurate measurements of lithium concentrations are essential. It is also important to standardize the sample drawing time in relation to the previous dose. Measurement is made by ion-selective electrode electrochemical analysis or by atomic absorption spectrophotometric analysis.

420.

C. The collection of blood samples for therapeutic drug monitoring requires both the selection of the proper time for sampling and the recording of that time on the report. It is essential that the drug level be related in time to the time of the previous and/or the next drug administration. Collection of blood samples is generally avoided during the drug's absorption and distribution phases. When peak levels of the drug are required, the blood sample must be drawn at a specified time after drug administration. Trough levels are most reliably determined by collecting the blood sample before the next drug administration.

421.

C. Persons involved in therapeutic drug monitoring should consider not only the properties of the various drugs but also the populations to which they are administered. The neonate is particularly susceptible to drug toxicity because of renal and hepatic immaturity, which leads to an increased drug half-life in comparison with that seen in adults. The neonatal pattern of drug elimination is reversed rapidly several weeks after birth, and children generally metabolize drugs more rapidly than adults. With the onset of puberty, the rate of drug metabolism generally slows and approaches the adult rate of drug use.

422.

C. Within the systemic circulation a drug will either remain free or will bind to protein. Generally, acidic drugs bind to albumin, and basic drugs bind to such globulins as alpha$_1$-acid glycoprotein (AAG). Occasionally, a particular drug may bind to both types of protein.

423.

D. Chlorpromazine (Thorazine®) and thioridazine are examples of phenothiazines and are used in the treatment of psychoses. Although the drugs themselves have a relatively short half-life, metabolites may be found in the urine for many weeks after cessation of therapy. Screening for phenothiazines is often done by specific chromatographic techniques or by the less specific ferric perchloricnitric (FPN) colorimetric reagent. Quantification is done by HPLC and fluorescent polarization immunoassay (FPIA).

424.

A. Phenytoin is the recommended name for the anticonvulsant diphenylhydantoin. Because of its wide use and toxicity at high concentrations, phenytoin is often the subject of overdose. Thin-layer chromatography or spectrophotometry is used for screening. Quantification usually requires gas- or high-performance liquid chromatography or immunoassay (e.g., EMIT, FPIA).

425.

D. Diazepam (Valium®) is an example of a benzodiazepine. This group of drugs is used for the treatment of anxiety. Oxazepam is an active metabolite of diazepam and is also available as a prescribed drug (Serax®). Detection of oxazepam glucuronide in the urine is used as a screening method for diazepam. Quantification of the benzodiazepines may be achieved using HPLC.

426.

D. The major active metabolite of procainamide is *N*-acetylprocainamide (NAPA). Procainamide is an antiarrhythmic drug that is used to treat such disorders as premature ventricular contractions, ventricular tachycardia, and atrial fibrillation. Because procainamide and its metabolite NAPA exhibit similar and cumulative effects, it is necessary that both be quantified to assess therapy. Methods for their analysis include GC, HPLC, FPIA, and EMIT.

427.

A. Theophylline is a bronchodilator that is used to treat asthma. The therapeutic range is 10–20 μg/mL, and use must be monitored to avoid toxicity. Use of theophylline has been replaced where possible with β-adrenergic agonists, which are available in the inhaled form.

Vitamins

428.

A. HPLC is a commonly used technique for the measurement of vitamins. Measurement by HPLC tends to be rapid, sensitive, and specific. Other techniques employed include spectrophotometric, fluorometric, and microbiological assays.

429.

B. Ascorbic acid is commonly known as vitamin C. Because humans are unable to synthesize ascorbic acid, it is necessary that it be taken in through the diet. If ascorbic acid is not ingested in a sufficient amount, a deficiency develops that leads to the disease known as scurvy. Scurvy is characterized by bleeding gums, loose teeth, and poor wound healing.

430.

B. The term "lipid" encompasses a large group of compounds, including the sterols, fatty acids, triglycerides, phosphatides, bile pigments, waxes, and fat-soluble vitamins. Vitamins A, D, E, and K are classified as fat-soluble vitamins. Thiamine (B_1), riboflavin (B_2), pyridoxine (B_6), cyanocobalamin (B_{12}), niacin, pantothenic acid, lipoic acid, folic acid, inositol, and ascorbic acid (C) are classified as water-soluble vitamins and as such are not lipid compounds.

431.

C. The definitive test for the diagnosis of steatorrhea (fat malabsorption) is the fecal fat determination that usually is done with a 72-hour collection. Carotenoids are a group of fat-soluble compounds that are precursors of vitamin A (retinol). The carotenoids are not synthesized in humans, and their absorption depends on intestinal fat absorption. Therefore, the serum carotene level is sometimes used as a simple screening test for steatorrhea. In addition to steatorrhea, other conditions, such as poor diet, liver disease, and high fever, can result in below-normal carotene levels. Folic acid and vitamins C and B_{12} are water soluble and would not be useful for determining fat absorption.

432.

C. Vitamin B_{12} (cyanocobalamin) is a cobalt-containing vitamin that is necessary for normal erythropoiesis. Intrinsic factor is a gastric protein that specifically binds vitamin B_{12} and carries it to the ileum for absorption. The transcobalamins are a group of plasma proteins, some of which bind vitamin B_{12} and some of which bind both vitamin B_{12} and cobalamin analogs. The cobalophilins (R proteins) are those transcobalamins that can also bind the cobalamin analogs.

433.

A. Vitamin B_{12} is a water-soluble vitamin. It is absorbed in the gastrointestinal tract by way of a substance called intrinsic factor. Deficiency of vitamin B_{12} produces a megaloblastic anemia. Anemia caused by a deficiency of vitamin B_{12} because of a lack of intrinsic factor (IF) is called pernicious anemia. The Schilling test (with and without IF) is used to diagnose pernicious anemia. It is helpful in distinguishing pernicious anemia from other malabsorption syndromes. A positive Schilling test indicates low absorption of B_{12} without IF and normal absorption with IF. However, in diseases of the small bowel, low absorption occurs with and without IF.

434.

A. The designation "vitamin D" applies to a family of essential fat-soluble sterols that includes vitamin D_3 or cholecalciferol. This compound can either be absorbed directly or synthesized in the skin from 7-dehydrocholesterol with the help of ultraviolet irradiation. For physiological functioning, vitamin D_3 must be metabolized first by the liver to 25-hydroxyvitamin D_3 and then by the kidney to the final hormonal product, 1,25-dihydroxyvitamin D_3 (calcitriol). The kidney also synthesizes 24,25-dihydroxyvitamin D_3 by an alternate pathway. This compound does not have the hormonal activity of calcitriol, but because of its similar structure and relatively high concentration in the serum, it has complicated the determination of serum calcitriol.

435.

D. Adequate amounts of vitamin K are required for the synthesis of prothrombin by the liver. Because prothrombin is an essential component of the clotting system, a deficiency of vitamin K leads to a deficiency of prothrombin, which results in a delayed clot formation. Several closely related compounds having vitamin K properties include phylloquinones, which are synthesized in plants, and menaquinones, which are synthesized by bacteria. Because the intestinal flora may not be developed sufficiently in the newborn, vitamin K (menaquinone) deficiency can occur. This leads to increased clotting time, which may result in hemorrhagic disease in infancy.

436.

B. Riboflavin (vitamin B_2) is a constituent of two redox coenzymes, flavin mononucleotide (FMN) and flavin-adenine dinucleotide (FAD). These coenzymes, in combination with appropriate proteins, form the flavoprotein enzymes, which participate in tissue respiration as components of the electron-transport system. The property that enables them to participate in electron-transport is their ability to exist in the half-reduced form (FADH) and in the fully reduced form ($FADH_2$).

437.

A. A deficiency in thiamin (vitamin B_1) is associated with beriberi and Wernicke-Korsakoff syndrome. In general, thiamin deficiency affects the nervous and cardiovascular systems. Thiamin deficiency is sometimes seen in chronic alcoholics and in the elderly.

REFERENCES

Bishop, M. L., Fody, E. P., and Schoeff, L. (Eds.) (2005). *Clinical Chemistry Principles, Procedures, Correlations*, 5th ed. Philadelphia: Lippincott Williams & Wilkins.

Burtis, C. A., Ashwood, E. R., and Bruns, D. E. (Eds.) (2008). *Tietz Fundamentals of Clinical Chemistry*, 6th ed. Philadelphia: Saunders.

Haven, M. C., Tetrault, G. A., and Schenken, J. R. (Eds.) (1995). *Laboratory Instrumentation*, 4th ed. New York: Van Nostrand Reinhold.

Kaplan, L. A., Pesce, A. J., and Kazmierczak, S. C. (Eds.) (2003). *Clinical Chemistry Theory, Analysis, Correlation*, 4th ed. St. Louis: Mosby.

Westgard, J. O., Quam, E., and Barry, T. (Eds.) (1998). *Basic QC Practices*. Madison, WI: WesTgard® Quality Corporation.

CHAPTER

2 Hematology

contents

I. FUNDAMENTAL HEMATOLOGY PRINCIPLES

A. Blood Composition

1. **Whole blood** includes erythrocytes, leukocytes, platelets, and plasma. When a specimen is centrifuged, leukocytes and platelets make up the **buffy coat** (small white layer of cells lying between the packed red blood cells and the plasma).
2. **Plasma** is the liquid portion of unclotted blood or it is the component produced when blood is combined with a chemical known as an anticoagulant (e.g., EDTA). **Serum** is the fluid that remains after coagulation has occurred and a clot has formed.
   a. Plasma is composed of 90% water and contains proteins, enzymes, hormones, lipids, and salts.
   b. Plasma (contains all coagulation proteins) normally appears hazy and pale yellow, and serum (lacks fibrinogen group coagulation proteins) normally appears clear and straw colored.

B. Basic Hematology Terminology

a-	without
-blast	youngest/nucleated
-chromic	colored
-cyte	cell
dys-	abnormal
-emia	in the blood
ferro-	iron
hyper-	increased
hypo-	decreased
iso-	equal
macro-	large
mega-	very large/huge
micro-	small
myelo-	marrow
normo-	normal
-oid	like
-osis	increased
pan-	all
-penia	decreased
-plasia	formation
-poiesis	cell production
poly-	many
pro-	before
thrombo-	clot

C. Formed Elements and Sizes

Formed Element	Size
1. Thrombocytes (platelets)	2–4 μm
2. Erythrocytes (RBCs)	6–8 μm
3. Normal lymphocytes	6–9 μm
4. Reactive lymphocytes	10–22 μm
5. Basophils	10–15 μm
6. Segmented neutrophils	10–15 μm
7. Band neutrophils	10–15 μm
8. Eosinophils	12–16 μm
9. Monocytes	12–20 μm

D. Basic Homeostasis

1. **Homeostasis** is the body's tendency to move toward physiological stability. *In vitro* testing of blood and other body fluids must replicate exact environmental body conditions. These conditions should include the following:
   a. **Osmotic concentration** is the body/cellular water concentration, composed of 0.85% sodium chloride. This normal osmotic concentration is termed **isotonic.** In a **hypotonic** solution (greater amount of H_2O in relationship to lesser amount of solutes), water enters the cell; the cell **swells** and may lyse. In a **hypertonic** solution (lesser amount of H_2O in relationship to greater amount of solutes), water leaves the cell; the cell may **crenate.**
   b. **pH reference range:** Venous blood range 7.36–7.41; arterial blood range 7.38–7.44.
   c. **Temperature:** Normal body temperature is 37.0°C. Blood specimens should be analyzed as soon as possible to prevent cellular breakdown (refer to individual tests for specimen collection requirements, stability times, and storage temperature).

E. RBC Indices

1. **MCV (mean corpuscular volume):** Reference range (SI/conventional units) is 80–100 femtoliters (fL), and it is an indicator of the average/mean volume of erythrocytes (RBCs). Calculate using the hematocrit (Hct) and RBC count:

$$\text{MCV (fL)} = \frac{\text{Hct (\%)} \times 10}{\text{RBC count} \ (\times 10^{12}/\text{L})}$$

   a. **Increased** in megaloblastic anemia, hemolytic anemia with reticulocytosis, liver disease, and normal newborn. May be falsely increased in cold agglutinin disorder
   b. **Decreased** in iron deficiency anemia, thalassemia, sideroblastic anemia, and lead poisoning

2. **MCH (mean corpuscular hemoglobin):** Reference range (SI/conventional units) is 26–34 picograms (pg), and it is an indicator of the average weight of hemoglobin in individual RBCs. Calculate using the hemoglobin (Hgb) and RBC count:

$$\text{MCH (pg)} = \frac{\text{Hemoglobin (g/dL)} \times 10}{\text{RBC count} (\times 10^{12}/\text{L})}$$

   a. **Increased** in macrocytic anemia
   b. **Decreased** in microcytic, hypochromic anemia

3. **MCHC (mean corpuscular hemoglobin concentration):** Reference range (conventional units) is 32–37 g/dL (SI units 320–370 g/L), and it is a measure of the average concentration of hemoglobin in grams per deciliter. Calculate using the hemoglobin and hematocrit values:

$$\text{MCHC (g/dL)} = \frac{\text{Hemoglobin (g/dL)}}{\text{Hct}} \times 100$$

   a. 32–37 g/dL MCHC indicates **normochromic** RBCs.
   b. Lesser than (<) 32 g/dL MCHC indicates **hypochromic** RBCs, which is seen in iron deficiency and thalassemia.
   c. Greater than (>) 37 g/dL MCHC indicates a possible error in RBC or hemoglobin measurement, or the presence of **spherocytes.**

F. Other RBC Parameters

1. **RDW (RBC distribution width):** Reference range (conventional units) is 11.5–14.5%.
   a. Determined from the RBC histogram
   b. Increased proportional to the degree of anisocytosis (variation in size); coefficient of variation of the mean corpuscular volume
   c. High RDW: Seen post-transfusion, post-treatment (e.g., iron, B_{12}, and folic acid therapy), idiopathic sideroblastic anemia, in the presence of two concurrent deficiencies (iron and folic acid deficiencies)

2. **Hct (Hematocrit):** Reference range for males (conventional units) is 41–53% (SI units 0.41–0.53 L/L). Reference range for females (conventional units) is 36–46% (SI units 0.36–0.46 L/L). Reference range for hematocrit is age and sex dependent. Hematocrit is the percentage of RBCs in a given volume of whole blood.
   a. Spun **microhematocrit** is the reference manual method.
   b. The buffy coat layer of leukocytes and platelets, not included in the measurement, can be seen between plasma (upper) and RBC (lower) layers.
   c. Hematocrit is calculated by many automated cell counters using the MCV and RBC count:

$$\text{Hct \%} = \frac{\text{MCV (fL)} \times \text{RBC count} (\times 10^{12}/\text{L})}{10}$$

3. **Hgb (Hemoglobin):** Reference range for males (conventional units) is 13.5–17.5 g/dL (SI units 135–175 g/L). Reference range for females (conventional units) is 12.0–16.0 g/dL (SI units 120–160 g/L). Reference range for hemoglobin is age and sex dependent.

G. Platelets

1. **PLT (Platelets):** Reference range (SI units) is 150−450 × 10^9/L (conventional units 150,000−450,000/μL).
2. **MPV (mean platelet volume):** Reference range (SI/conventional units) is 6.8–10.2 fL. MPV is analogous to the MCV for erythrocytes.

H. Relative and Absolute Blood Cell Counts

1. **Relative count** is the amount of a cell type in relation to other blood components. **Relative lymphocytosis** is an increase in the **percentage** of lymphocytes; this is frequently associated with neutropenia. In **relative polycythemia**, RBCs appear increased due to a decreased plasma volume.
2. **Absolute count** is the actual number of each cell type without respect to other blood components. **Absolute lymphocytosis** is a true increase in the **number** of lymphocytes. **Absolute polycythemia** is a true increase in **red cell mass.**

I. Hematology Stains

1. **Nonvital (dead cell) polychrome stain (Romanowsky)**
   a. Most commonly used routine peripheral blood smear stain is **Wright stain.**
   b. **Wright stain** contains **methylene blue**, a basic dye, which stains acidic cellular components (DNA and RNA) blue, and **eosin**, an acidic dye, which stains basic components (hemoglobin and eosinophilic cytoplasmic granules) red-orange.
   c. **Methanol fixative** is used in the staining process to fix the cells to the slide.
   d. Staining does not begin until a **phosphate buffer** (pH between 6.4 and 6.8) is added.
   e. Causes of **RBCs too red** and **WBC nuclei poorly stained:** Buffer or stain below pH 6.4, excess buffer, decreased staining time, increased washing time, thin smear, expired stains
   f. Causes of **RBCs and WBC nuclei too blue:** Buffer or stain above pH 6.8, too little buffer, increased staining time, poor washing, thick smear, increased protein, heparinized blood sample
   g. Examples of polychrome stains include: Wright, Giemsa, Leishman, Jenner, May-Grünwald, and various combinations of them
2. **Nonvital monochrome stain**
   a. Stains specific cellular components
   b. **Prussian blue** stain is an example.
      1) Contains potassium ferrocyanide, HCl, and a safranin counterstain
      2) Used to visualize **iron granules** in RBCs (siderotic iron granules), histiocytes, and urine epithelial cells

3. **Supravital** (living cell) **monochrome stain**
   a. Used to stain specific cellular components
   b. No fixatives are used in the staining process.
   c. Includes:
      1) **New methylene blue** used to precipitate RNA in **reticulocytes**; measure of bone marrow **erythropoiesis**
      2) **Neutral red** with **brilliant cresyl green** as a counterstain is used to visualize **Heinz bodies**; clinical disorders associated with Heinz bodies include **G6PD deficiency** and other **unstable hemoglobin** disorders.

II. HEMATOPOIESIS

A. Hematopoiesis

1. Production and differentiation of blood cells
2. Blood cell production, maturation, and death occur in organs of the **reticuloendothelial system** (RES).
   a. RES includes bone marrow, spleen, liver, thymus, lymph nodes.
   b. RES functions in **hematopoiesis, phagocytosis**, and **immune defense.**
3. **Intrauterine hematopoiesis** includes three phases:
   a. **Mesoblastic (yolk sac) phase** begins at ~19 days gestation. The **yolk sac** is located outside the developing embryo. The first cell to be produced is a **primitive nucleated erythroblast.** This cell produces embryonic hemoglobins: **Portland, Gower I and Gower II.** Alpha-globin chain production begins at this phase and continues throughout life.
   b. **Hepatic** (liver) **phase** begins at 6 weeks gestation with production of mainly **red blood cells**, but also granulocytes, monocytes, and megakaryocytes. Alpha- and gamma-globin chain production predominates forming **Hgb F**; detectable Hgb A and A_2 are also present.
   c. **Myeloid/medullary phase** begins around the fifth month of gestation, with the **bone marrow** producing mainly **granulocytes.** The M:E (myeloid:erythroid) ratio approaches the adult level of 3:1. Alpha- and gamma-globin chain production predominates at birth, forming **Hgb F**; Hgb A and A_2 are also present. Hgb A will not predominate until 6 months of age when the gamma-beta globin chain switch is complete.
4. At birth, the bone marrow is very cellular with mainly **red marrow**, indicating very active blood cell production. Red marrow is gradually replaced by inactive **yellow marrow** composed of fat. Under physiological stress, yellow marrow may revert to active red marrow.

B. Pediatric and Adult Hematopoiesis

1. **Bone marrow**
   a. Newborn: 80–90% of bone marrow is active red marrow.
   b. Young adult (age 20): 60% of bone marrow is active. Hematopoiesis is confined to the proximal ends of large flat bones, pelvis, and sternum.

c. Older adult (age 55): 40% of bone marrow is active; 60% is fat.

d. **Cellularity** is the ratio of marrow cells to fat (red marrow/yellow marrow) and is described in adults as:

1) **Normocellular**—Marrow has 30–70% hematopoietic cells.
2) **Hypercellular/hyperplastic**—Marrow has >70% hematopoietic cells.
3) **Hypocellular/hypoplastic**—Marrow has <30% hematopoietic cells.
4) **Aplastic**—Marrow has few or no hematopoietic cells.

e. **M:E (myeloid:erythroid) ratio** is the ratio of granulocytes and their precursors to nucleated erythroid precursors. A normal ratio is between **3:1** and **4:1.** Granulocytes are more numerous because of their short survival (1–2 days) as compared to erythrocytes with a 120-day life span. Lymphocytes and monocytes are excluded from the M:E ratio.

f. Stem cell theory

1) Hematopoiesis involves the production of **pluripotential stem cells** that develop into **committed progenitor cells (lymphoid or myeloid)** and finally mature blood cells.

a) **Progenitor cells**

i) **Lymphoid:** Differentiate into either **B or T lymphocytes** in response to cytokines/lymphokines/interleukins/CSFs/growth factors

ii) **Myeloid:** Gives rise to the multipotential progenitor **CFU-GEMM (colony-forming-unit-granulocyte-erythrocyte-macrophage-megakaryocyte)**, which will differentiate into **committed progenitor cells** and finally **mature blood cells** in response to cytokines/interleukins/colony stimulating factors/growth factors:

Committed Progenitor Cell		Growth Factors/Interleukins	Mature Cell
CFU-MEG		Thrombopoietin, GM-CSF	Thrombocytes
CFU-GM	CFU-M	GM-CSF, M-CSF, IL-3	Monocytes
CFU-GM	CFU-G	GM-CSF, G-CSF, IL-3	Neutrophils
BFU-E	CFU-E	Erythropoietin, GM-CSF, IL-3	Erythrocytes
CFU-Eo		GM-CSF, IL-3, IL-5	Eosinophils
CFU-Ba		IL-3, IL-4	Basophils

2. **Lymphoid tissue**

a. **Primary lymphoid tissue**

1) Bone marrow: Site of pre–B cell differentiation
2) Thymus: Site of pre–T cell differentiation
3) This is antigen-**independent** lymphopoiesis.

b. **Secondary lymphoid tissue**

1) B and T lymphocytes enter the blood and populate secondary lymphoid tissue, where antigen contact occurs.

2) Includes lymph nodes, spleen, gut-associated tissue (Peyer's patches)
3) Antigen-**dependent** lymphopoiesis depends on antigenic stimulation of T and B lymphocytes.

C. Introduction to Leukocytes

1. Classified as **phagocytes** (granulocytes, monocytes) or **immunocytes** (lymphocytes, plasma cells, and monocytes). WBCs can also be classified based on morphology.
2. **WBC reference range** (SI units) is $4.0–11.0 \times 10^9/L$ (conventional units $4.0–11.0 \times 10^3/\mu L$).
3. **Granulocytes** include neutrophils, polymorphonuclear (PMN) or segmented, eosinophils, and basophils.
4. **Neutrophils** are the first to reach the tissues and **phagocytize** (destroy) bacteria. In the process, they die.
5. **Monocytes** differentiate into **macrophages**, and as such they work in the tissues to **phagocytize** foreign bodies. They arrive at the site of inflammation after neutrophils and do not die in the process.
6. **T lymphocytes** provide **cellular immunity.** They represent 80% of lymphocytes in the blood. When activated, they proliferate and produce **cytokines/interleukins.**
7. **B lymphocytes** develop into **plasma cells** in the tissue and produce **antibodies** needed for **humoral immunity.** B lymphocytes represent 20% of the lymphocytes in the blood.
8. **NK** (natural killer) **lymphocytes** destroy tumor cells and cells infected with viruses. They are also known as **large granular lymphocytes** (LGLs).
9. **Eosinophils** modulate the allergic response caused by basophil degranulation.
10. **Basophils** mediate immediate hypersensitivity reactions (type I, anaphylactic).
11. **CD markers** are surface proteins expressed by **specific cell lines** at different maturation stages. As a cell matures, some markers vanish and new ones appear. More than 200 CD markers have been identified. Commonly used markers include the following:

CD2, CD3	Lymphoid, pan T cells
CD4	Helper/inducer T cells
CD8	Suppressor/cytotoxic T cells
CD13	Pan myeloid
CD11c, CD14	Monocytes
CD19, CD20	Lymphoid, pan B cells
CD33	Pan myeloid cells
CD34	Stem cell marker (lymphoid and myeloid precursor)
CD16, CD56	NK cells

D. Medullary versus Extramedullary Hematopoiesis

1. **Medullary hematopoiesis:** Blood cell production **within** the bone marrow
   a. Begins in the fifth month of gestation and continues throughout life
2. **Extramedullary hematopoiesis:** Blood cell production **outside** the bone marrow
   a. Occurs when the bone marrow cannot meet body requirements
   b. Occurs mainly in the liver and spleen; hepatomegaly and/or splenomegaly often accompany this

E. Basic Cell Morphology

1. **Nucleus**
   a. Contains **chromatin** composed of **DNA** and proteins
   b. Contains **nucleoli** rich in **RNA**
2. **Cytoplasm**
   a. **Golgi complex** forms lysosomes.
   b. **Lysosomes** contain hydrolytic enzymes that participate in phagocytosis.
   c. **Ribosomes** assemble amino acids into protein.
   d. **Mitochondria** furnish the cell with energy (ATP).
   e. **Endoplasmic reticulum** is a system of interconnected tubes for protein and lipid transport.

F. General Cell Maturation Characteristics for Leukocytes

Immature Cells	Mature Cells
Cell is large	Cell becomes smaller
Nucleoli present	Nucleoli absent
Chromatin fine and delicate	Chromatin coarse and clumped
Nucleus round	Nucleus round, lobulated, or segmented
Cytoplasm dark blue (rich in RNA)	Cytoplasm light blue (less RNA)
High N:C ratio	Low N:C ratio

III. GRANULOCYTES

A. Basic Review

1. The myeloid progenitor cell gives rise to a committed progenitor cell that is acted on by growth factors to form granulocytes.

B. Maturation and Morphology of Immature Granulocytes

1. **Myeloblast:** Earliest recognizable granulocyte precursor
   a. 14–20 μm
   b. N:C ratio 7:1–4:1
   c. Round/oval nucleus with fine reddish-purple staining chromatin
   d. Two to five nucleoli
   e. Dark blue cytoplasm

f. **No cytoplasmic granules**
g. 1% of the nucleated cells in the bone marrow

2. **Promyelocyte**
   a. 15–21 μm
   b. N:C ratio 3:1
   c. Round/oval nucleus with slightly coarsening chromatin
   d. One to three nucleoli
   e. Dark blue cytoplasm
   f. Cytoplasm has large, **nonspecific/primary granules** containing **myeloperoxidase.**
   g. 2–5% of the nucleated cells in the bone marrow
3. **Myelocyte:** First stage where granulocyte types can be differentiated into eosinophils, basophils, and neutrophils
   a. 12–18 μm
   b. N:C ratio 2:1
   c. Round nucleus with coarse chromatin
   d. Early myelocytes may have visible nucleoli.
   e. Light blue to light pink cytoplasm
   f. Prominent **golgi apparatus—clear area** located in the cytoplasm next to the nucleus
   g. Cytoplasm has **specific/secondary granules** that contain **hydrolytic enzymes**, including **alkaline phosphatase** and **lysozyme.**
   h. **Nonspecific/primary granules** are present and may still stain.
   i. Last stage capable of cell division
   j. **Neutrophilic myelocyte** makes up 13% of the nucleated cells in the bone marrow.
4. **Metamyelocyte**
   a. 10–18 μm
   b. N:C ratio 1.5:1
   c. Nucleus is indented in a **kidney bean** shape and has coarse, clumped chromatin.
   d. Nuclear indent is **less than** half the width of a hypothetical round nucleus.
   e. Cytoplasm is pink and filled with pale blue to pink **specific/secondary granules.**
   f. **Nonspecific/primary granules** are present but usually do not stain.
   g. **Neutrophilic metamyelocyte** makes up 16% of the nucleated cells in the bone marrow.
5. **Band neutrophil**
   a. 10–15 μm
   b. N:C ratio 1:2
   c. Nucleus is "C" or "S" shaped with coarse, clumped chromatin **lacking segmentation.**

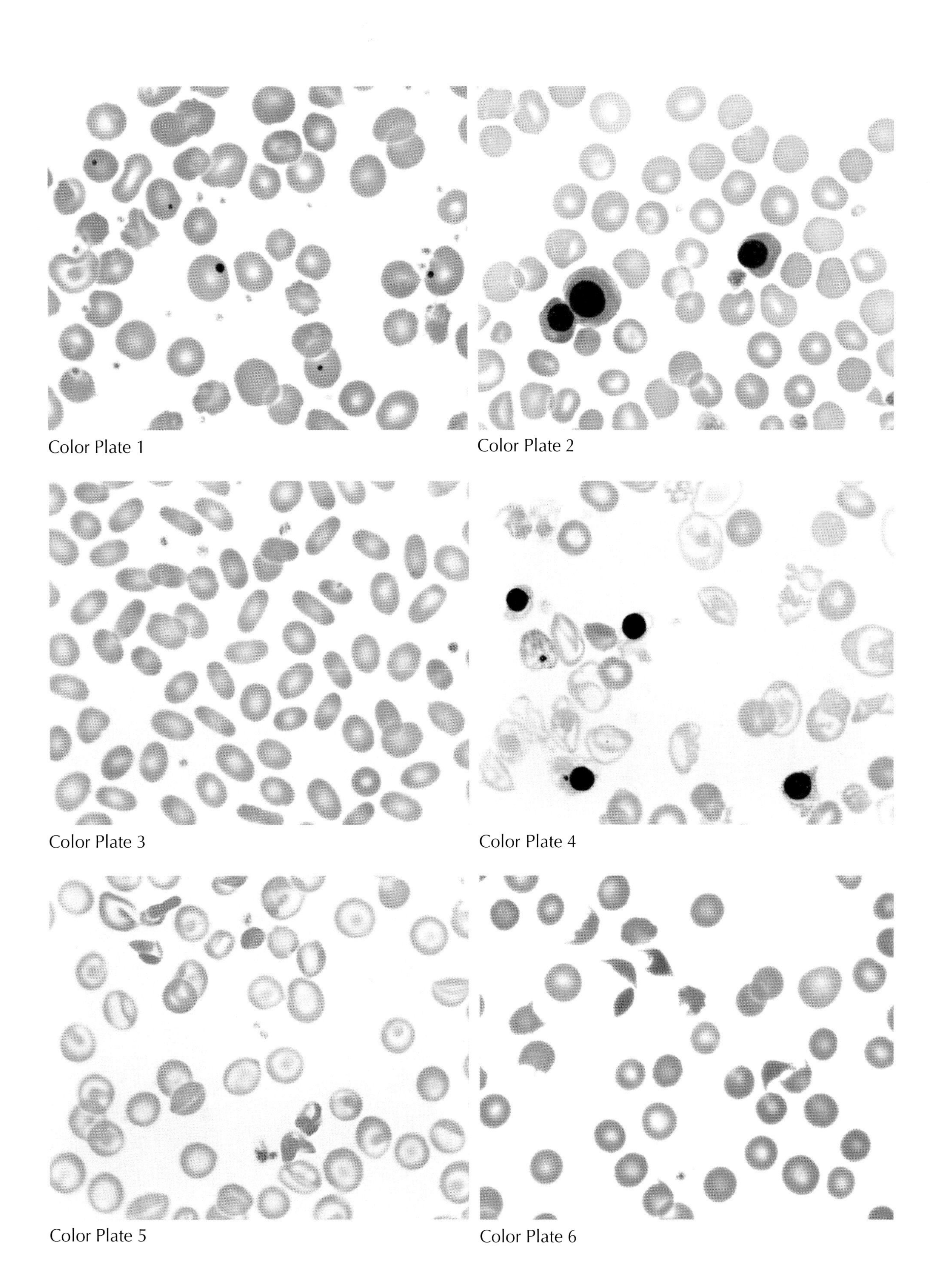

Color Plate 1

Color Plate 2

Color Plate 3

Color Plate 4

Color Plate 5

Color Plate 6

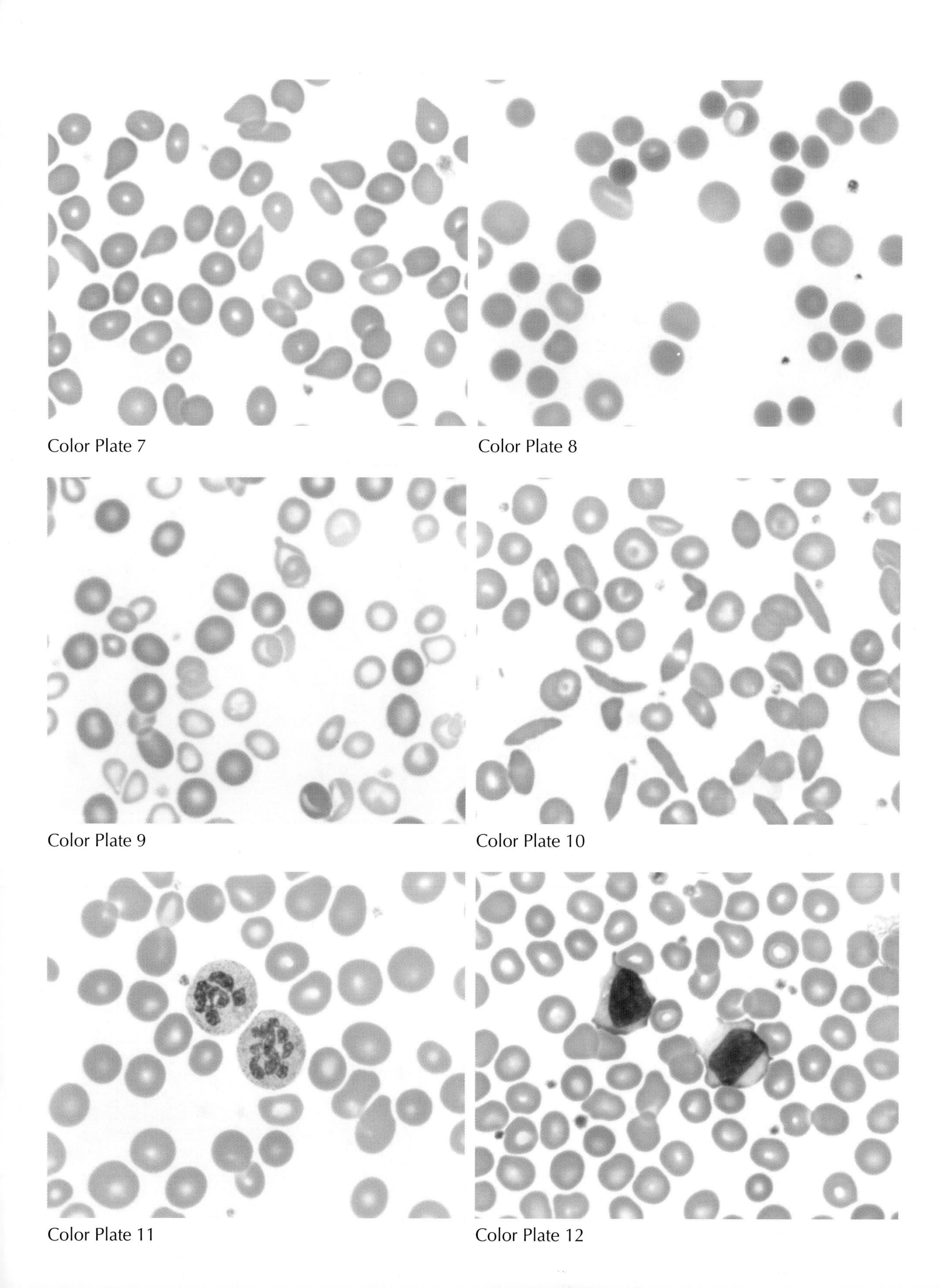

Color Plate 7

Color Plate 8

Color Plate 9

Color Plate 10

Color Plate 11

Color Plate 12

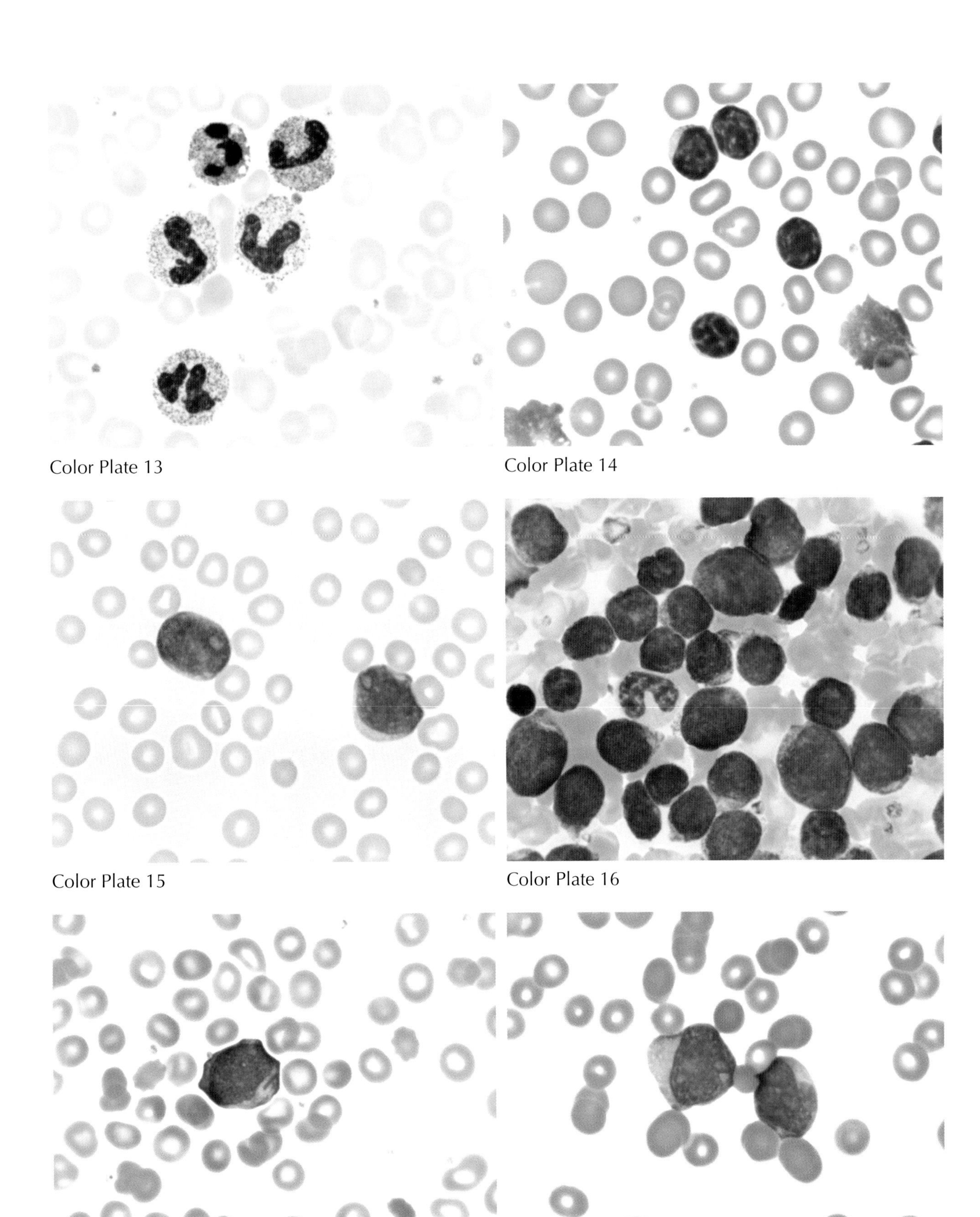

Color Plate 13

Color Plate 14

Color Plate 15

Color Plate 16

Color Plate 17

Color Plate 18

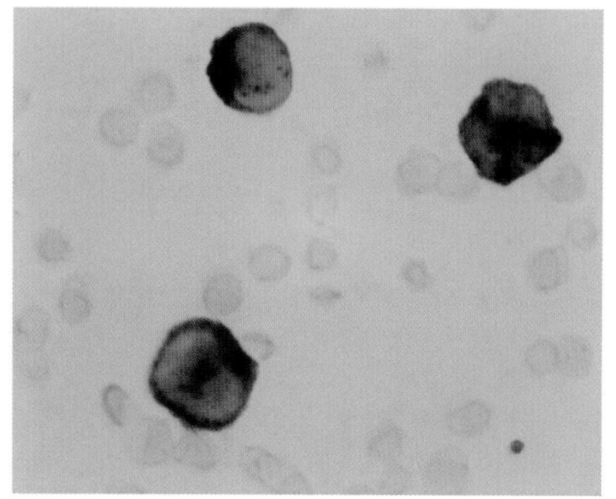

Color Plate 19

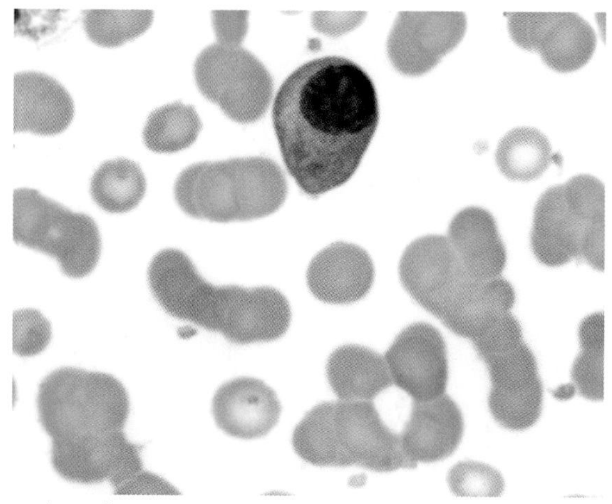

Color Plate 20

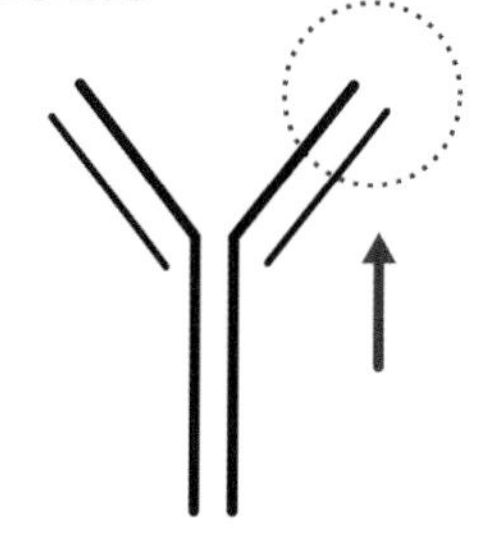

Color Plate 21

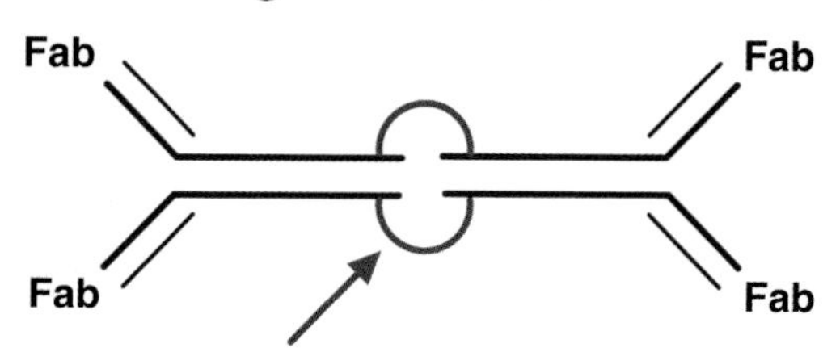

Color Plate 22

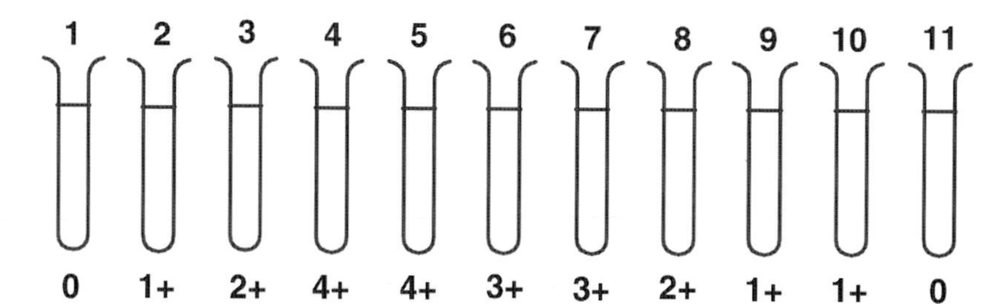

Color Plate 23

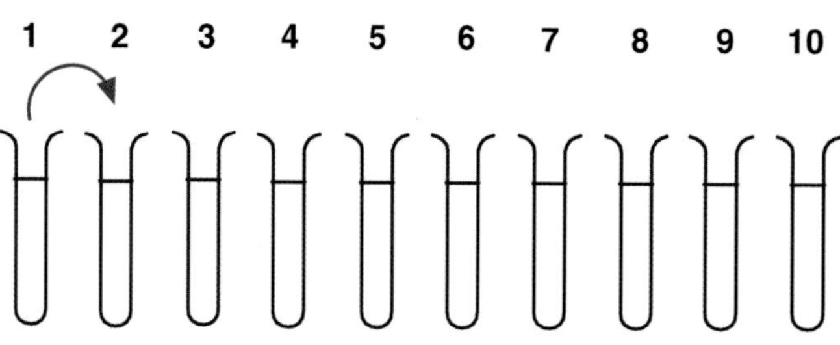

Color Plate 24

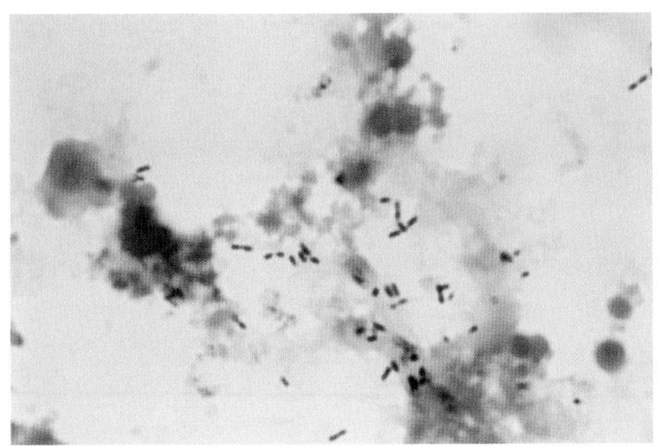
Color Plate 25

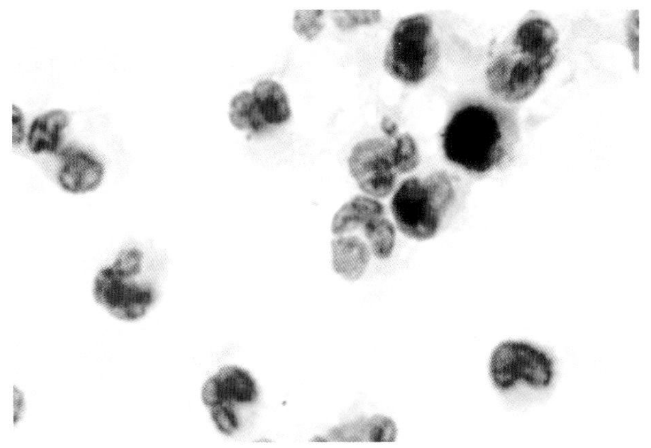
Color Plate 26

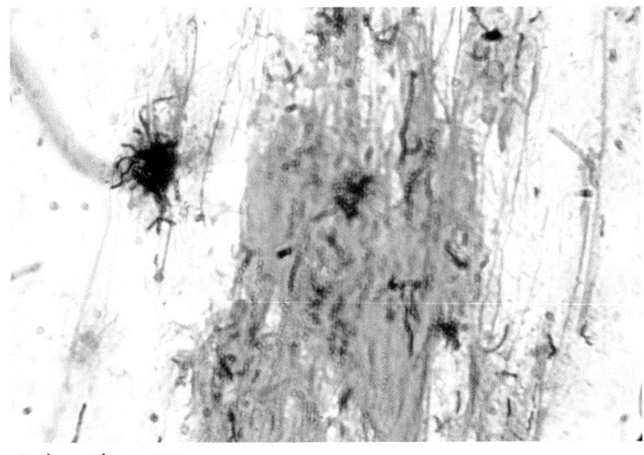
Color Plate 27

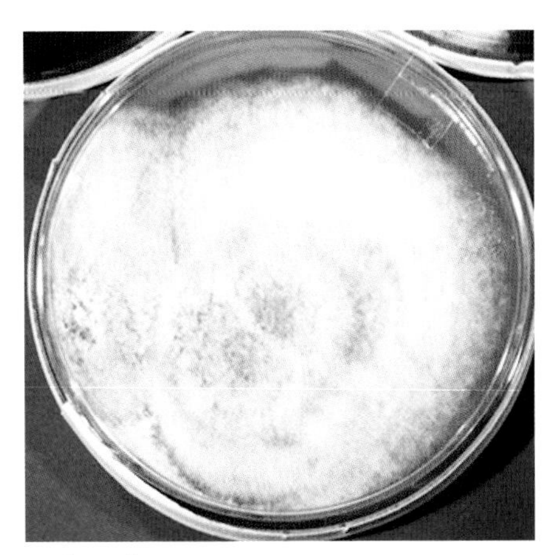
Color Plate 28

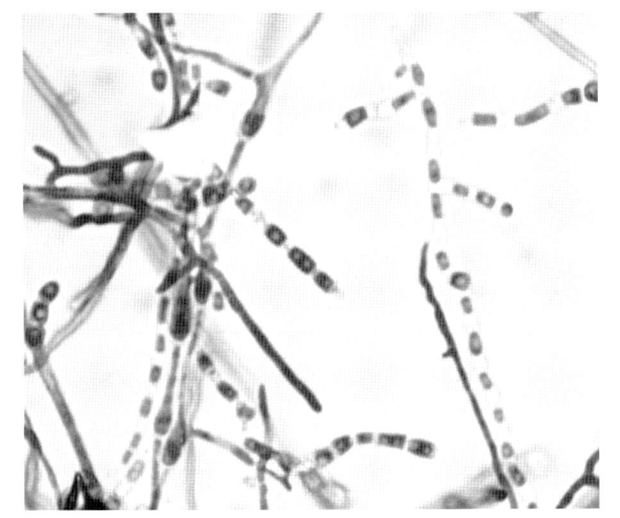
Color Plate 29

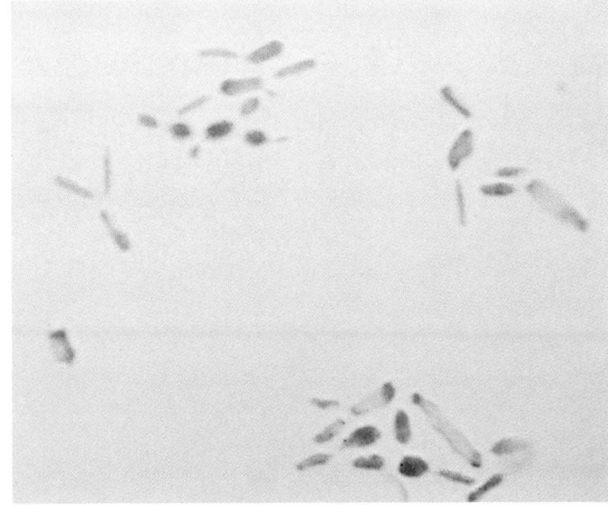
Color Plate 30

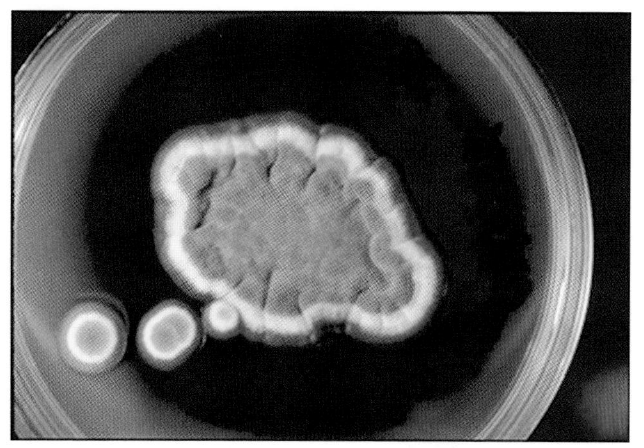

Color Plate 31

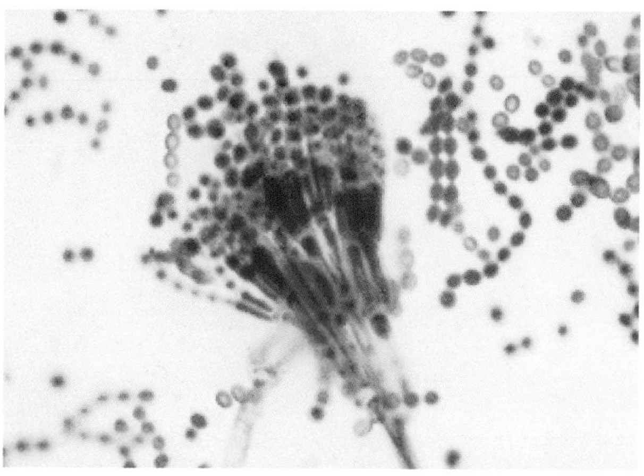

Color Plate 32

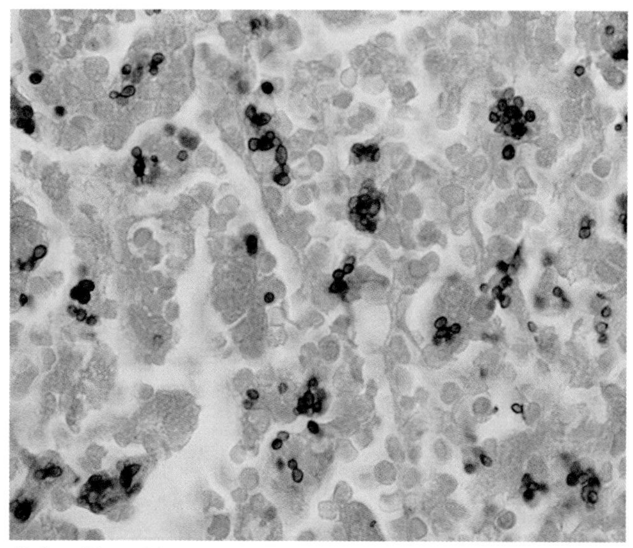

Color Plate 33

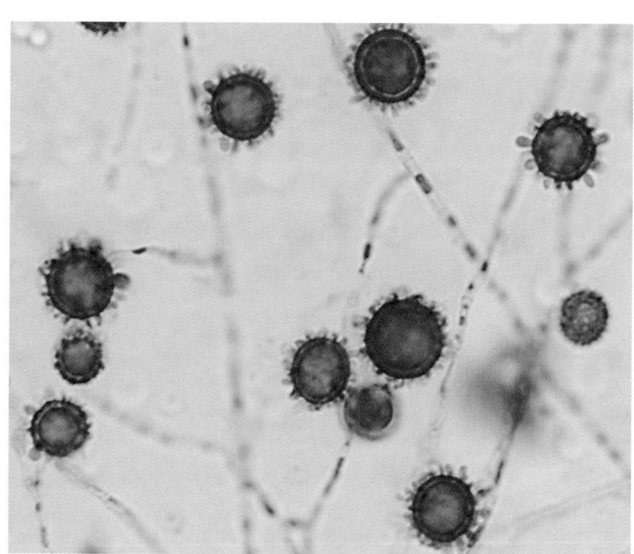

Color Plate 34

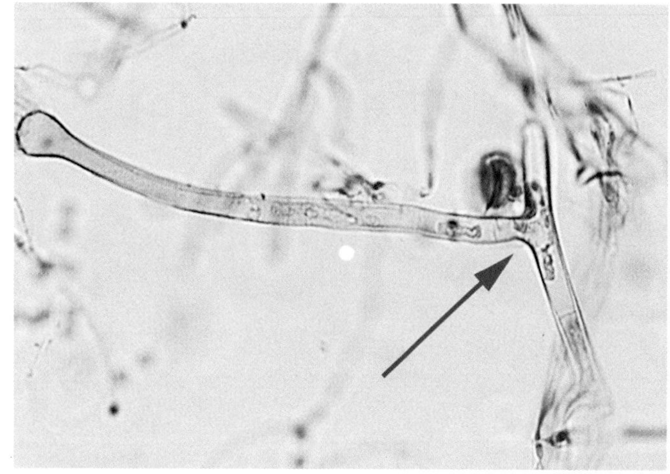

Color Plate 35

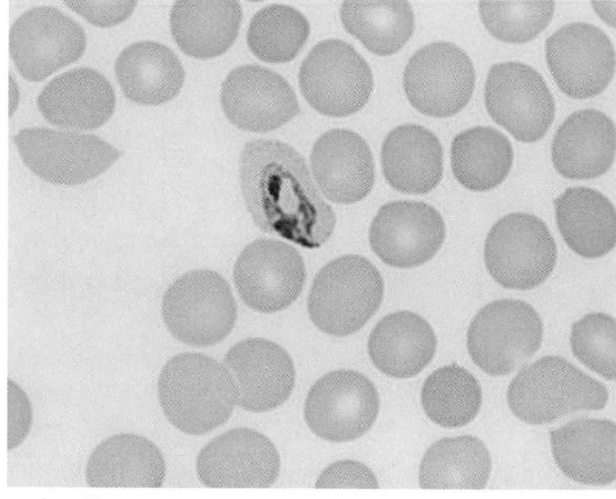

Color Plate 36

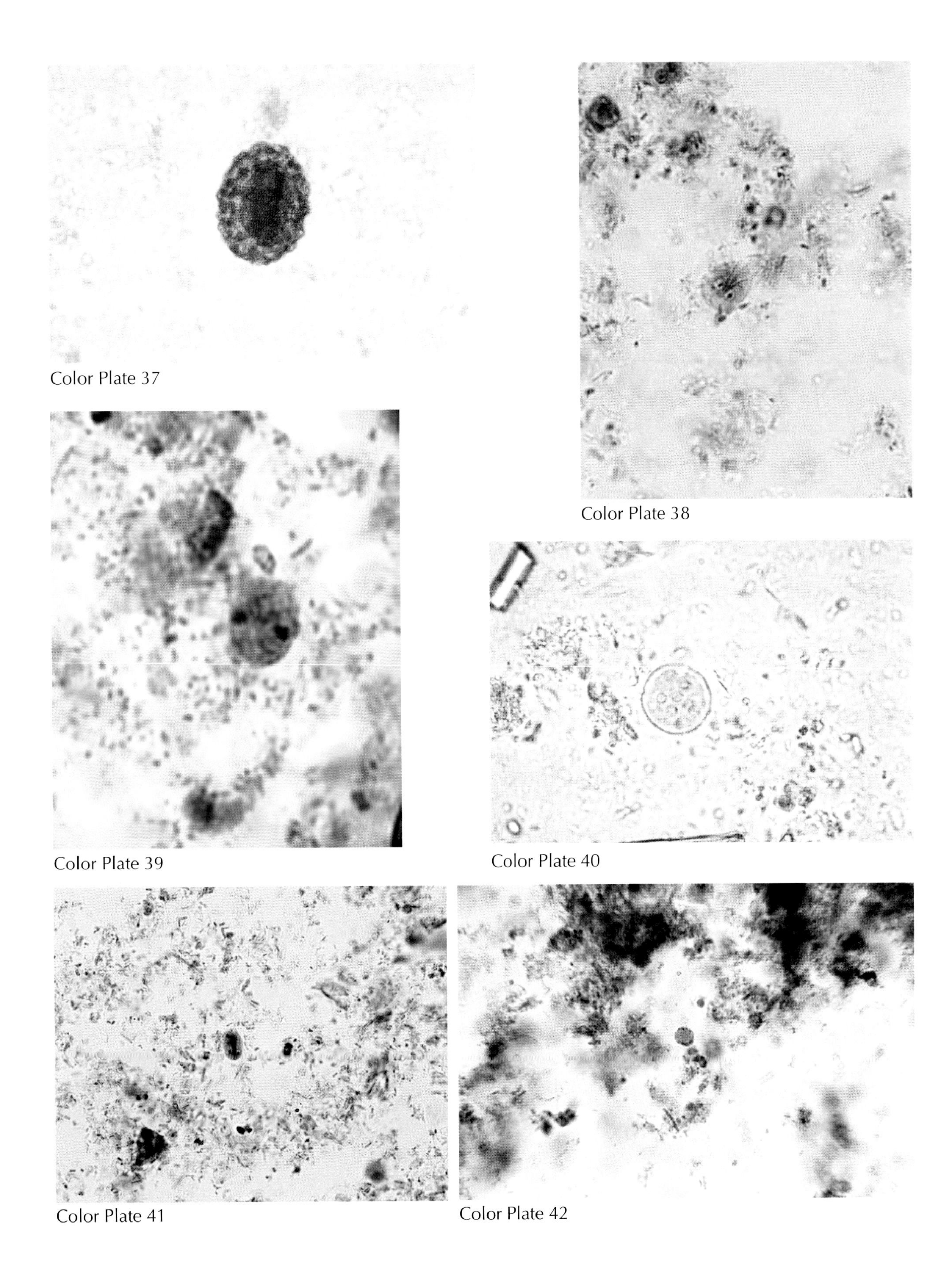

Color Plate 37

Color Plate 38

Color Plate 39

Color Plate 40

Color Plate 41

Color Plate 42

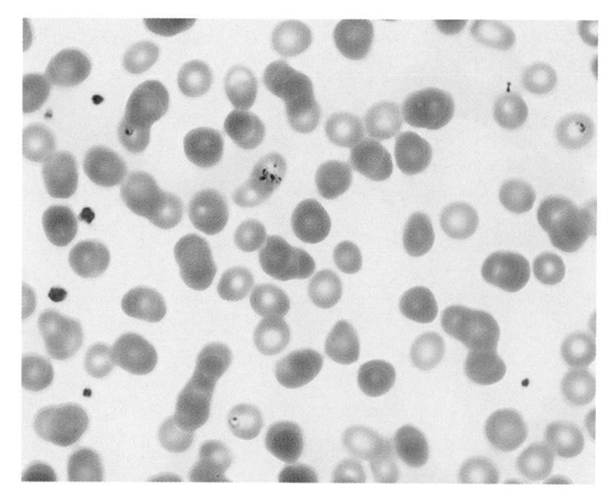

Color Plate 43

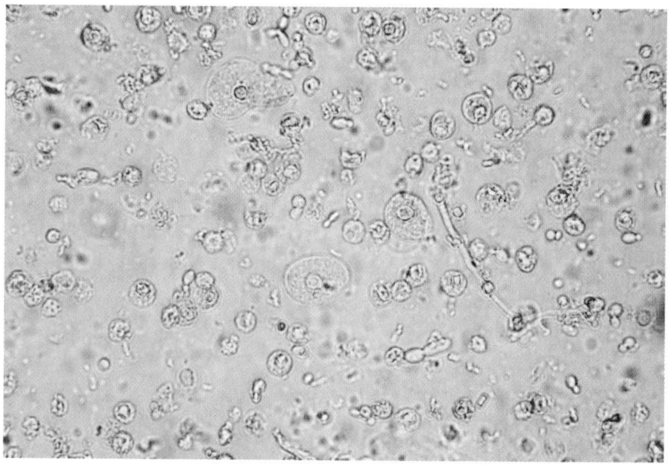

Color Plate 44

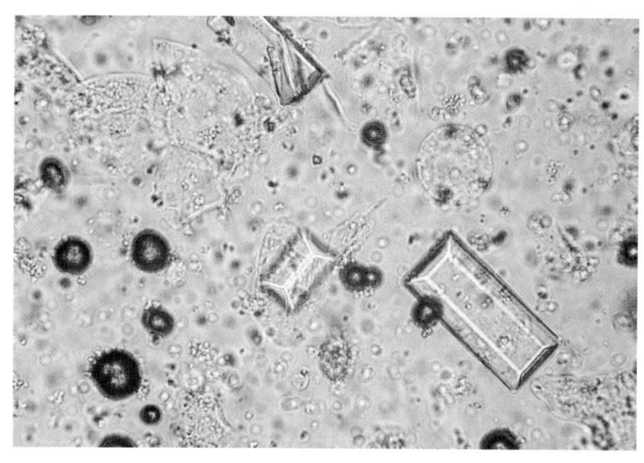

Color Plate 45

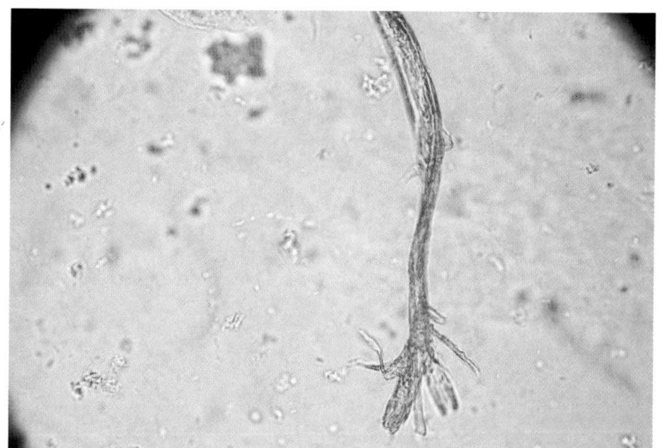

Color Plate 46

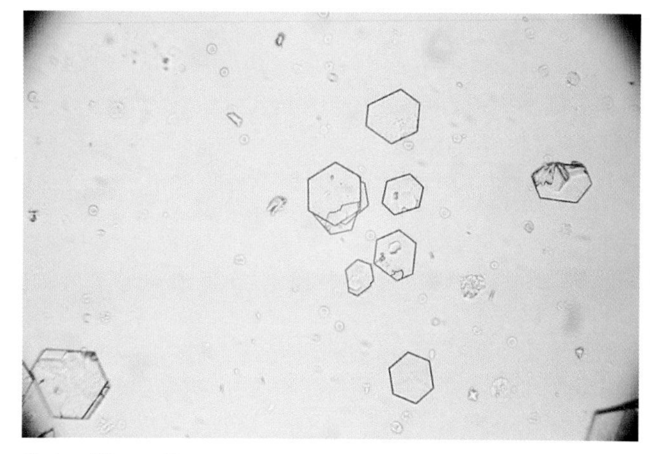

Color Plate 47

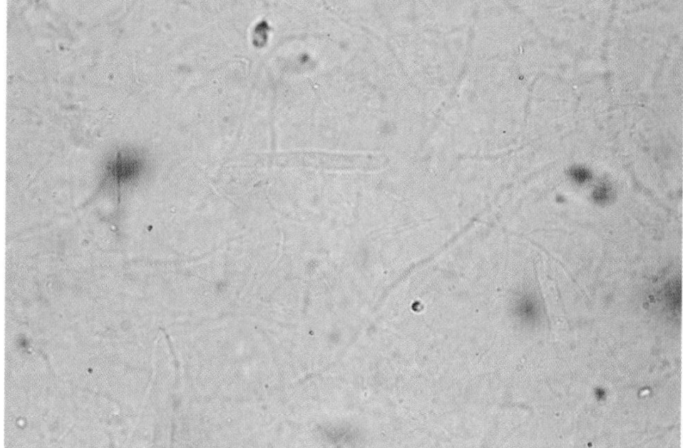

Color Plate 48

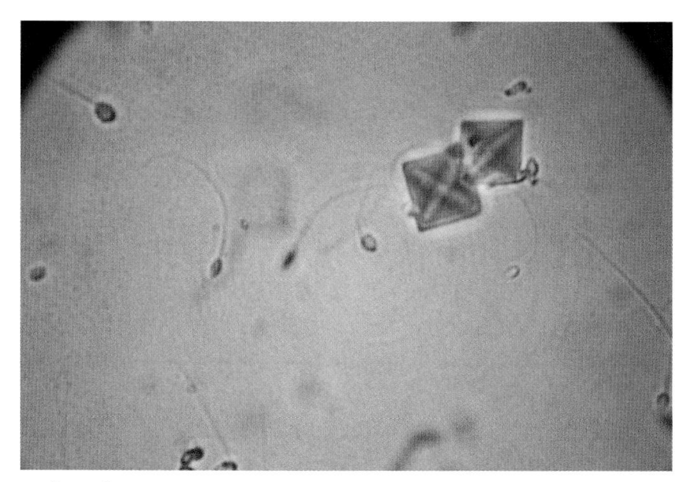
Color Plate 49

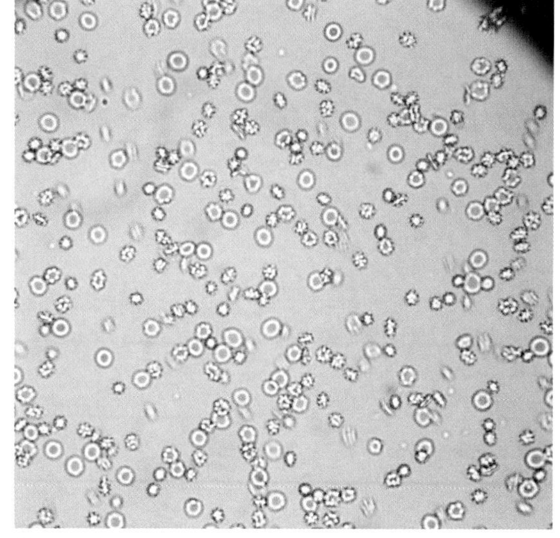
Color Plate 50

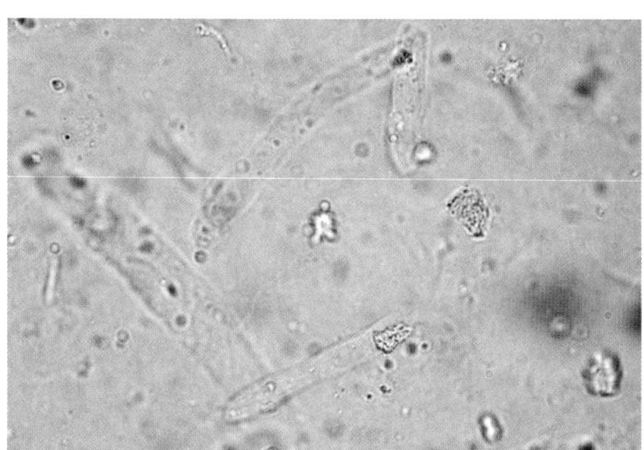
Color Plate 51

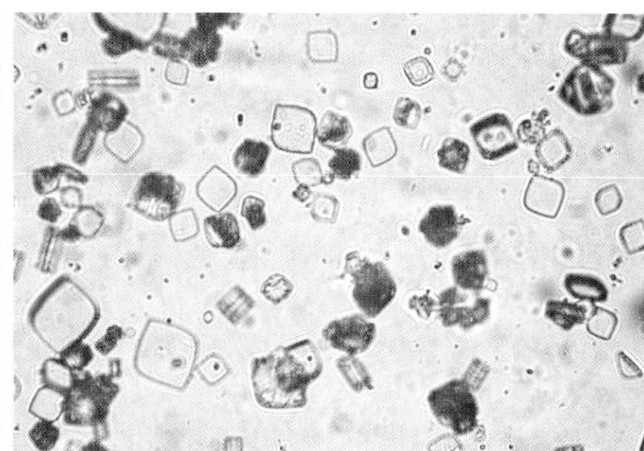
Color Plate 52

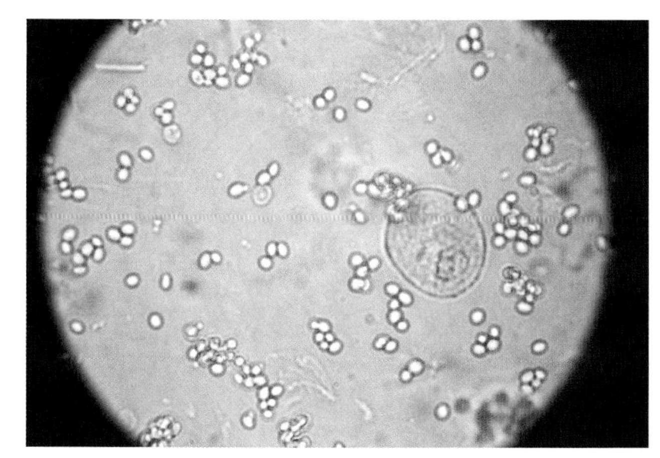
Color Plate 53

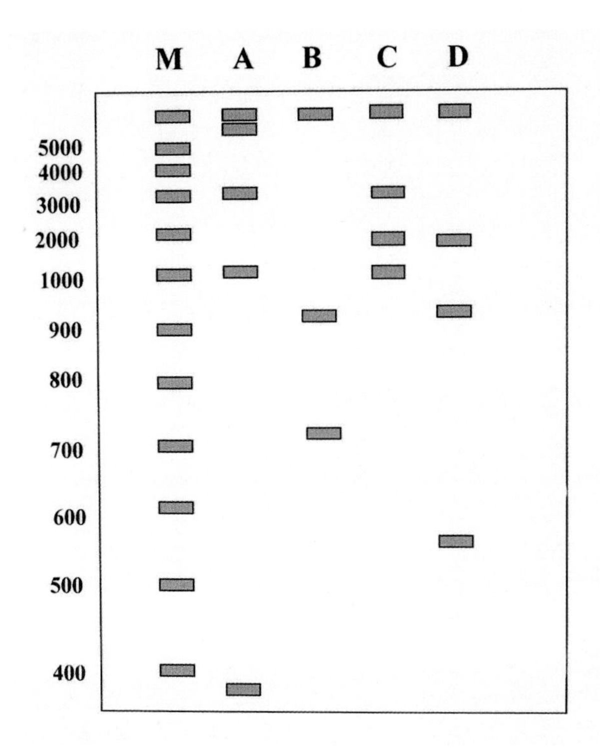

Color Plate 54

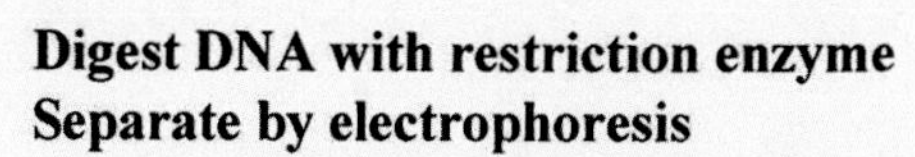

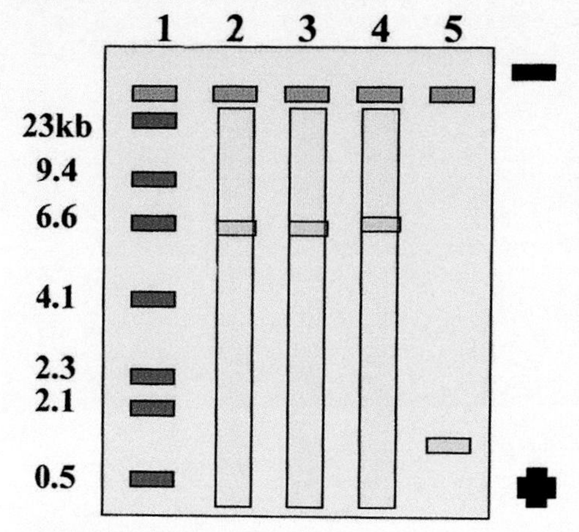

Chemical depurination
Denaturation
Neutralization

Transfer to membrane

Bind DNA to membrane

Hybridize membrane with ^{32}P labeled probe
Wash off excess probe
Expose to X-ray film
Develop autoradiogram

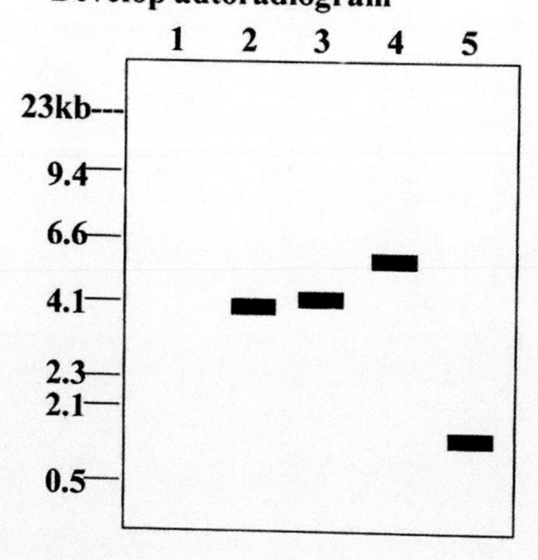

Color Plate 55

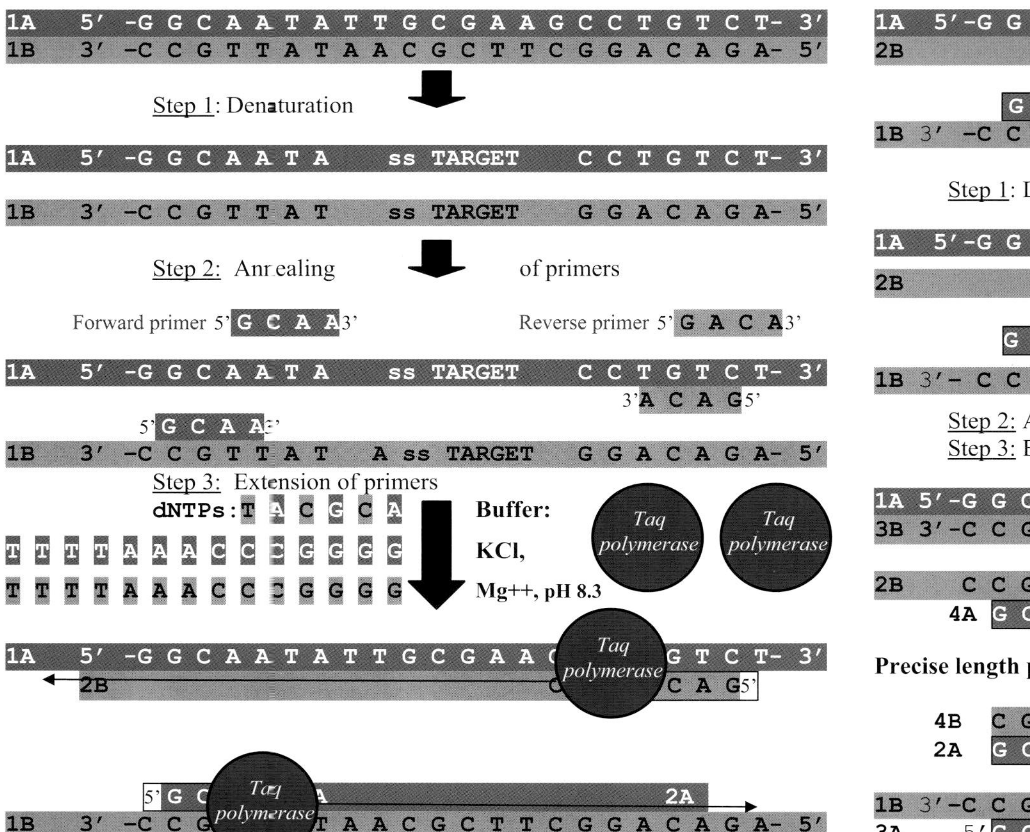

Color Plate 56a

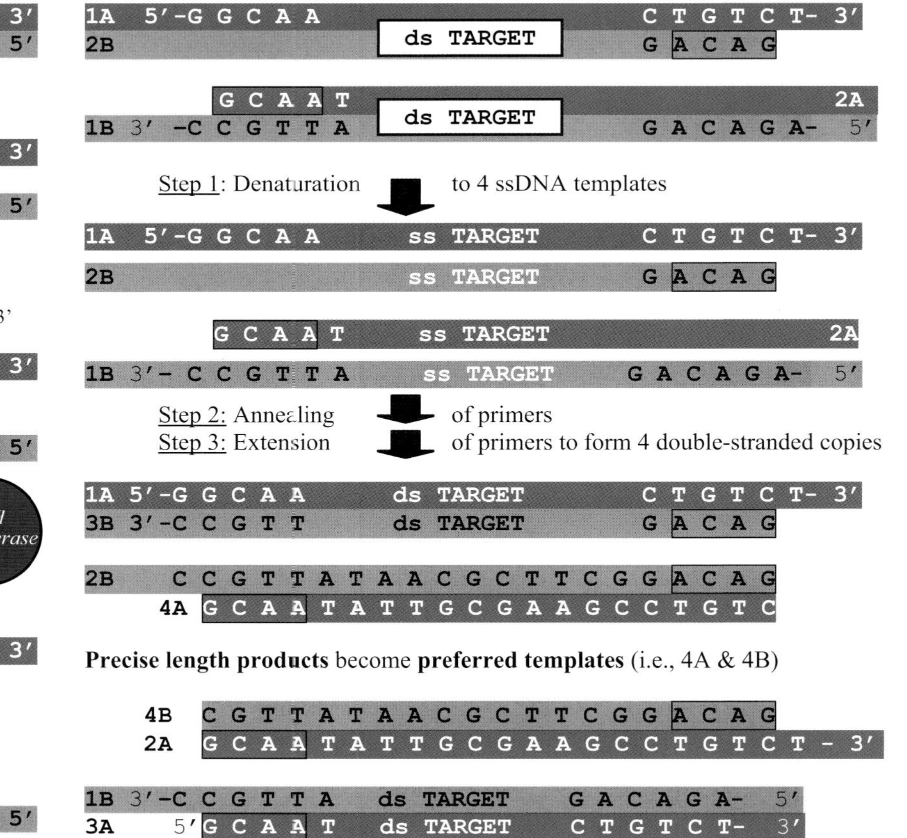

Color Plate 56b

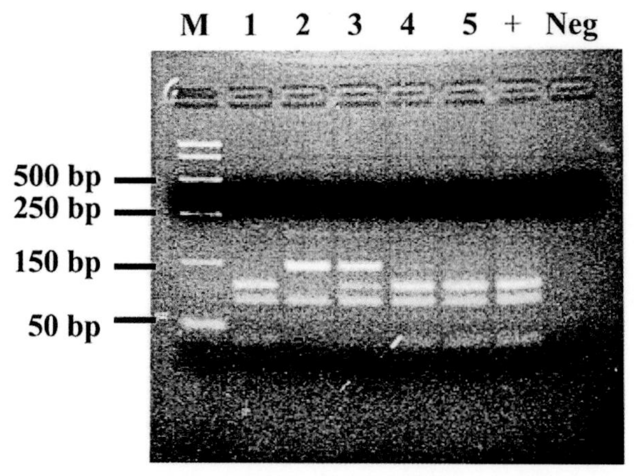

Color Plate 57

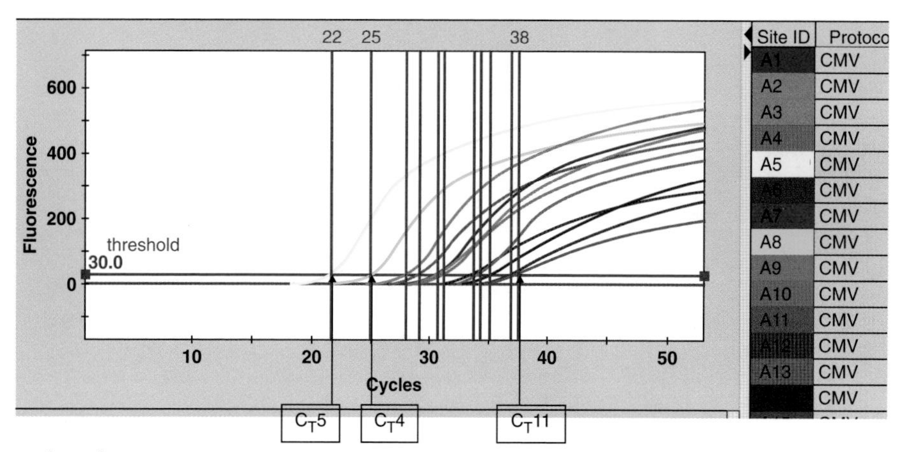

Color Plate 58

d. Nuclear indent is **greater than** half the width of a hypothetical round nucleus.
e. Cytoplasm is pink and filled with pale blue to pink **specific/secondary granules.**
f. **Nonspecific/primary granules** are present but usually don't stain.
g. **Band neutrophil** makes up 12% of the nucleated cells in the bone marrow, and 0–5% of peripheral white blood cells (WBCs).
h. Stored in the bone marrow and released when there is an increased demand for neutrophils

C. Morphology of Mature Granulocytes

1. **Segmented neutrophil** (Referred to as: seg, polymorphonuclear cell (PMN), and poly)
   a. 10–15 μm
   b. N:C ratio 1:3
   c. Nucleus has coarse, clumped chromatin with **three to five lobes** connected by thin filaments.
   d. Cytoplasm is pink and filled with small pale blue to pink **specific/secondary granules.**
   e. **Nonspecific/primary granules** are present but usually do not stain unless in response to infection or growth factor.
   f. **Segmented neutrophils** make up 12% of the nucleated cells in the bone marrow, and 50–80% of peripheral WBCs.
2. **Eosinophil**
   a. Recognizable maturation stages include the eosinophilic myelocyte, eosinophilic metamyelocyte, eosinophilic band, and eosinophil (segmented form).
   b. Eosinophils are 12–16 μm.
   c. Nucleus is usually bilobed.
   d. Cytoplasm contains large **bright red-orange** secondary granules that contain **enzymes** and **proteins.**
   e. Eosinophils make up less than 1% of the nucleated cells in the bone marrow and 5% of peripheral WBCs
3. **Basophil**
   a. Recognizable maturation stages include the basophilic myelocyte, basophilic metamyelocyte, basophilic band, and basophil (segmented form).
   b. Basophils are 10–15 μm.
   c. Cytoplasm contains large **purple-black** secondary granules that contain **heparin** and **histamine.**
   d. Granules may be numerous and obscure the nucleus, or they may "**wash out**" in staining (because the granules are water soluble) and leave empty areas in the cytoplasm.

e. Basophils make up less than 0.1% of the nucleated cells in both the bone marrow and peripheral blood.

4. Relative and Absolute WBC counts:

WBCs: 4.5–11.5 (Adult)

Cells	Relative	Absolute
PMNs	50–80	2.3–9.2
BANDs	0–5	0–0.6
LYMPHs	18–42	0.8–4.8
Eos	1–5	0–0.6
BASOs	0–1	0–0.2

D. Granulocyte Function

1. **Neutrophils**
   a. Blasts, promyelocytes, and myelocytes are in the bone marrow **mitotic pool** 3–6 days, and that is where they **divide.**
   b. Metamyelocytes, bands, and segmented neutrophils are in the bone marrow **post-mitotic pool** about 6 days, and that is where they **mature.**
   c. Released into circulation when mature or when needed
   d. Total blood granulocyte pool
      1) Contains 50% **circulating granulocyte pool** (mainly neutrophils) that is measured when a WBC count is performed
      2) Contains 50% **marginating granulocyte pool** (mainly neutrophils) that adheres to vessel walls
      3) There is a rapid and free exchange of neutrophils between the circulating granulocyte pool and marginating granulocyte pool.
      4) Neutrophils **diapedese** into the **tissues** from the marginating pool in response to **antigenic stimulation.**
      5) **Chemotactic factors** attract the neutrophil to the site of inflammation; include **complement, bacterial products, injured tissue,** and **hemostatic components.**
      6) **Opsonins** such as **IgG** and complement component **C3b** help neutrophils recognize a substance as foreign.
      7) **Phagocytosis** involves neutrophil attachment to the foreign object, formation of a vacuole around it, and neutrophilic degranulation to release lytic enzymes (**respiratory burst**) in an effort to kill the organism.
      8) Neutrophils are sensitive to the oxidants they secrete and are destroyed in the process.
   e. Blood and tissue cells in the body undergo **cell death** through **necrosis** or **apoptosis.**
      1) **Necrosis** is induced by **extracellular** forces such as lethal chemical, biological, or physical events. The blood cell is "killed."

2) **Apoptosis** is "**programmed cell death**" due to extracellular or **intracellular** processes that depend on a signal.

2. **Visible response to infection by neutrophils (toxic changes)**
   a. Toxic changes are associated with **bacterial infection** or **growth factor therapy.** Any combination of these changes may be seen in some but not necessarily all of the neutrophils.
   b. **Toxic granulation** is prominent granulation due to persistent staining of **primary granules.** Neutrophilic cytoplasm normally contains only visible, small, **secondary granules.**
   c. **Toxic vacuolation:** Colorless areas in the cytoplasm that indicate phagocytosis and degranulation have occurred
   d. **Döhle bodies:** Small oval inclusions **(RNA)** located in the cytoplasm that stain light blue
   e. **Shift to the left** refers to an increased number of myelocytes, metamyelocytes, and/or bands in the peripheral blood. It is associated with either increased or decreased WBC counts.
      1) **Regenerative shift to the left** is an appropriate bone marrow response to increased demand for neutrophils. It is seen in infection or in other physiological or pathological conditions requiring neutrophils.
         a) WBC count above the reference range
         b) Most common type of left shift
      2) **Degenerative shift to the left** is seen after an overwhelming infection in which bone marrow production cannot keep up with increased need for neutrophils.
         a) Associated with a poor prognosis
         b) WBC count below the reference range
3. **Eosinophils**
   a. They are in the blood only a few hours before seeking a tissue site such as nasal passages, skin, or urinary tract.
   b. They can degranulate like neutrophils. They express Fc receptors for **IgE,** which is a response to **parasitic infections.**
   c. They release substances that can neutralize products released by basophils and mast cells; eosinophils modulate the **allergic** response.
4. **Basophils**
   a. In the blood only a few hours before migrating to the site of inflammation in the tissues
   b. They express membrane receptors for **IgE.** Once activated, degranulation releases histamine. This initiates the classic signs **of immediate hypersensitivity reactions (Type I).**
   c. Basophils release a chemotactic factor that attracts eosinophils to the site.

E. Nonmalignant Granulocytic Disorders

1. **Shift/physiologic/pseudoneutrophilia**
   a. Redistribution of blood pools causes a short-term **increase** in the total WBC count and in the absolute number of neutrophils in the **circulating granulocyte pool.**
   b. Caused by exercise, stress, pain, pregnancy
   c. It is not a response to tissue damage. The **total blood granulocyte pool** in the body has not changed. The bone marrow has not released immature neutrophils. There are no toxic changes and there is **no shift to the left.**
2. **Pathologic neutrophilia**
   a. Neutrophils leave the circulating pool, enter the marginating pool, and then move to the tissues in response to tissue damage.
   b. Bone marrow reserves are released into the blood to replenish the circulating pool. The **WBC count can increase up to 50.0 $\times$ 10^9/L**, and there is a **shift to the left** with toxic changes to the neutrophils.
   c. Bone marrow **increases production** of neutrophils to replenish reserves.
   d. Occurs in response to **bacterial** and other infections, **tissue destruction**, drugs or toxins, **growth factor**, etc.
3. **Neutrophilic leukemoid reaction (NLR)**
   a. Blood picture mimics that seen in **chronic myelogenous leukemia.**
   b. **Benign**, extreme response to a specific agent or stimulus
   c. The **WBC count can increase to between 50.0 and 100.0 $\times$ 10^9/L**, and there is a **shift to the left** with toxic changes to the neutrophils.
4. **Leukoerythroblastic reaction**
   a. Presence of **immature leukocytes** and **immature (nucleated) erythrocytes** in the blood
   b. Occurs in marrow replacement disorders, such as **myelofibrosis**
5. **Neutropenia**
   a. **Decrease** in absolute number of **neutrophils; risk of infection** increases as neutropenia worsens
   b. Due to **bone marrow production defects:**
      1) Chronic or severe infection depletes available neutrophil reserves. **Use exceeds bone marrow production.**
      2) **Hypersplenism** causes neutrophils to be removed from circulation.
      3) Bone marrow **injury** (aplastic anemia), bone marrow **infiltration** (leukemia, myelodysplastic syndromes, or metastatic cancer), bone marrow **suppression** by chemicals or drugs (chemotherapy)
      4) **DNA synthesis** defects due to vitamin B_{12} or folate deficiency
      5) Many **viral infections** are associated with neutropenia.

6. **Eosinophilia**
   a. **Increase** in the absolute number of **eosinophils**
   b. Associated with:
      1) **Parasitic infections, allergic reactions, chronic inflammation**
      2) Chronic myelogenous leukemia, including early maturation stages, Hodgkin disease, tumors
7. **Eosinopenia**
   a. **Decrease** in the absolute number of **eosinophils**
   b. Seen in **acute inflammation** and inflammatory reactions that cause release of glucocorticosteroids and epinephrine
8. **Basophilia**
   a. **Increase** in the absolute number of **basophils**
   b. Associated with:
      1) **Type I hypersensitivity reactions**
      2) **Chronic myelogenous leukemia**, including **early maturation stages**, polycythemia vera
      3) **Relative transient basophilia** can be seen in patients on hematopoietic growth factors.
9. **Basopenia**
   a. **Decrease** in the absolute number of **basophils** associated with inflammatory states and following immunologic reactions
   b. Difficult to diagnose because of their normally low reference range
10. **Functional disorders of neutrophils**
   a. **Chronic granulomatous disease (CGD)**
      1) Both **sex-linked** and autosomal recessive inheritance with the ratio of affected males to females being 6:1
      2) Morphologically normal, but functionally abnormal because of enzyme deficiency that results in an inability to degranulate, which causes inhibited bactericidal function
      3) Fatal early in life
   b. **Chédiak-Higashi syndrome**
      1) Autosomal recessive disorder causes large, gray-green, peroxidase positive granules in the cytoplasm of leukocytes; abnormal fusion of primary and secondary neutrophilic granules
      2) Both **morphologically** and **functionally abnormal** leukocytes; WBCs unable to degranulate and kill invading bacteria
      3) Patients will present with photophobia and skin hypopigmentation.
      4) Fatal early in life
11. **Nuclear abnormalities of neutrophils**
   a. **Hypersegmentation** characterized by **five or more lobes** in the **neutrophil;** associated with **megaloblastic anemia** due to vitamin B_{12} or folic acid deficiencies

b. **Hyposegmentation** refers to a tendency in **neutrophils** to have **one or two lobes**; may indicate an anomaly or a shift to the left.
   1) **Pelger-Huët anomaly**
      a) **Autosomal dominant** inheritance
      b) Nucleus is hyperclumped and it does not mature past the two-lobed stage.
      c) Nucleus dumbbell- or peanut shaped; referred to as "pince-nez"
      d) Morphologically abnormal but **functionally normal**
      e) Must **differentiate from a shift to the left** associated with an infection (toxic changes); infection requires treatment but Pelger-Huët anomaly (no toxic changes) does not.
   2) **Pseudo Pelger-Huët**
      a) **Acquired** abnormality associated with **myeloproliferative disorders** and **myelodysplastic syndromes**; can also be drug induced
      b) **Nucleus** is usually **round** instead of the dumbbell shape that is seen in the anomaly.
      c) Frequently accompanied by **hypogranulation**

12. **Inherited cytoplasmic anomalies**
   a. **May-Hegglin anomaly**
      1) **Autosomal dominant** inheritance
      2) Large, crystalline, **Döhle-like inclusions** in the cytoplasm of neutrophils on Wright stain; gray-blue and spindle (cigar) shaped
      3) Morphologically abnormal but **functionally normal**
      4) **Giant platelets, thrombocytopenia**, and clinical bleeding are also associated with this anomaly.
   b. **Alder-Reilly anomaly**
      1) **Autosomal recessive** inheritance
      2) **Large azurophilic** granules appear in cytoplasm of **all or only one cell line.** Granules contain degraded mucopolysaccharides due to an enzyme defect.
      3) Morphologically abnormal but **functionally normal**
      4) Must differentiate from **toxic granulation** present in **neutrophils only** in infectious conditions

IV. MONOCYTES AND MACROPHAGES

A. Basic Review

1. The **myeloid progenitor cell** gives rise to a committed progenitor cell, **CFU-GM** (colony-forming-unit-granulocyte-macrophage), that is acted on by growth factors (GM-CSF) and interleukins (ILs) to form **monocytes.** Monocytes form in the bone marrow, pass through the peripheral blood, and then migrate into the tissues **(macrophages)**, where they fight infection. Macrophages are named according to their location in the body.

a. **Monocytes**—peripheral blood
b. **Kupffer cells**—liver
c. **Microglial cells**—central nervous system
d. **Osteoclasts**—bone
e. **Langerhans cells**—skin
f. **Alveolar cells**—lung

B. Maturation and Morphology of Monocytes

1. **Monoblast:** Earliest recognizable monocyte precursor
   a. 12–18 μm; N:C ratio 4:1
   b. Round/oval eccentric nucleus with fine chromatin; 1–2 nucleoli
   c. Dark blue cytoplasm; may have a gray tint; **no cytoplasmic granules**
2. **Promonocyte**
   a. 12–20 μm; N:C ratio 3:1
   b. Irregularly shaped, indented nucleus with fine chromatin; 0–1 nucleoli
   c. Blue to gray cytoplasm; fine azurophilic granules
3. **Monocyte**
   a. 12–20 μm
   b. Horseshoe- or kidney-bean-shaped nucleus, often with "brainlike" convolutions
   c. Fine, lacy chromatin
   d. Blue-gray cytoplasm; may have pseudopods and vacuoles
   e. Many fine azurophilic granules give the appearance of "ground glass."
   f. Transitional cell because it migrates into the tissue and becomes a fixed or free macrophage
4. **Macrophage:** "Tissue monocyte"
   a. 15–80 μm
   b. Indented, elongated, or egg-shaped nucleus with fine chromatin
   c. Blue-gray cytoplasm with many vacuoles and coarse azurophilic granules; may contain ingested material

C. Monocyte Characteristics

1. Granules are lysosomes that contain hydrolytic enzymes, including peroxidase and acid phosphatase.
2. Highly motile cell that marginates against vessel walls and into the tissues
3. Reference range is 2–10% in peripheral blood.

D. Monocyte/Macrophage Function

1. Play a major role in **initiating** and **regulating** the **immune response**
2. They process ingested material and also **process antigenic information**, which is relayed to the **T helper (CD4)** lymphocyte. The T helper lymphocyte coordinates the immune response to foreign antigens.

3. They arrive at the site of inflammation after neutrophils. Unlike neutrophils, the phagocytic process does not kill the monocyte.
4. Very efficient **phagocytic** cells with receptors for IgG or complement-coated organisms
5. Known as "**scavenger cells**" because of their ability to ingest foreign material
   a. Blood monocytes ingest **antigen-antibody complexes** and **activated clotting factors,** limiting the coagulation response.
   b. Splenic macrophages remove **old/damaged RBCs** and conserve iron for recycling.
   c. Liver macrophages remove **fibrin degradation products.**
   d. Bone marrow macrophages remove abnormal RBCs, ingest bare **megakaryocyte nuclei** or **extruded RBC nuclei**, and store and supply **iron** for hemoglobin synthesis.
6. Monocytes secrete **cytokines/interleukins** and **tumor necrosis factor.**

E. Nonmalignant Monocytic Disorders

1. **Monocytosis**
   a. **Increase** in the absolute number of **monocytes** associated with:
      1) Recovery stage from acute bacterial infections and recovery following marrow suppression by drugs
      2) Tuberculosis, syphilis, subacute bacterial endocarditis
      3) Autoimmune disorders (systemic lupus erythematosus, rheumatoid arthritis)
2. **Lipid storage disorders**
   a. **Gaucher disease** is the most common lipid storage disorder and has an autosomal recessive inheritance pattern. A deficiency in glucocerebrosidase causes glucocerebroside to accumulate in macrophages of the bone marrow, spleen, and liver, with **Gaucher cells** more commonly seen in the bone marrow.
   b. **Niemann-Pick disease** has an autosomal recessive inheritance pattern. A deficiency in sphingomyelinase causes sphingomyelin to accumulate in macrophages in multiple organs and bone marrow, where **Niemann-Pick cells** can be seen.
   c. **Sea-blue histiocytosis** is caused by an unknown deficiency. Sea-blue macrophages are found in the spleen and bone marrow.
   d. Others include Tay-Sachs and Fabry diseases
3. **Monocytopenia**
   a. **Decrease** in the absolute number of **monocytes**
   b. Associated with stem cell disorders such as **aplastic anemia**

V. LYMPHOCYTES AND PLASMA CELLS

A. Basic Review

1. The pluripotential stem cell gives rise to the **lymphoid progenitor cell** that is acted on by colony stimulating factors/interleukins/cytokines to form **B** and **T lymphocytes. Pre–B lymphocytes** differentiate in the **bone marrow**, and

pre–T lymphocytes differentiate in the **thymus** through **antigen-independent lymphopoiesis.**

2. Bone marrow and thymus are **primary lymphoid tissues.**
3. B and T cells enter the blood and populate the **secondary lymphoid tissues** (lymph nodes, spleen, and Peyer's patches in the intestine), where antigen contact occurs.

B. Maturation and Morphology of Lymphocytes

1. **Lymphoblast:** Earliest recognizable lymphocyte precursor
   a. 10–18 μm; N:C ratio 4:1
   b. Round/oval eccentric nucleus with fine chromatin; 1 or more nucleoli
   c. Dark blue cytoplasm; **no cytoplasmic granules**
2. **Prolymphocyte**
   a. 9–18 μm; N:C ratio 3:1
   b. Round or indented nucleus with coarsening chromatin; 0–1 nucleoli
   c. Basophilic cytoplasm; **no cytoplasmic granules**
3. **Lymphocyte**
   a. 7–18 μm
   b. Round, oval, or slightly indented nucleus; condensed chromatin
   c. Scant to moderate amount of blue cytoplasm; **few azurophilic granules**
4. **Reactive lymphocytes** have become activated as part of the immune response. Associated with **lymphocytosis** and can show the following characteristics:
   a. Generally larger cell with increased amount of dark blue cytoplasm (RNA)
   b. Fine chromatin pattern with nucleoli
   c. Irregular shape to the nucleus
   d. Irregular shape to the cytoplasm (tags, sharp ridges); indented by red cells

C. T Lymphocytes (T cells)

1. Become immunocompetent in the secondary lymphoid tissue; **dependent on antigenic stimulation**
   a. Acquire specific receptors for antigens
   b. Make up **80%** of the peripheral blood lymphocytes
2. They are identified by membrane markers **CD2, CD3**, and others. The markers appear, disappear, and then reappear throughout cell development.
3. **T lymphocyte function**
   a. T cells provide **cellular immunity.** They are responsible for graft rejections and lysis of neoplastic cells, and they attack/destroy viral and fungal organisms.
   b. Obtain antigenic information from monocytes; this information is passed to other T cells and B cells
   c. Regulate humoral response by helping antigens activate B cells
   d. End products of activation are **cytokines/lymphokines/interleukins**
4. Three **T cell subsets** are involved in the immune response and are differentiated by cluster designation **(CD)** markers.

a. **T helper/inducer cell (T-h, T_4)**
   1) Identified by **CD4** membrane marker
   2) Promotes activation of B cells by antigens
b. **T suppressor cell (T-s, T_8)**
   1) Identified by **CD8** membrane marker
   2) Suppresses activation of B cells by antigens
c. **Cytotoxic T cell (T-c, T_8)**
   1) Identified by **CD8** membrane marker
   2) Functions in viral infections and organ rejections
d. The normal **T_4:T_8 ratio** in circulating blood is **2:1.** This ratio must be maintained for proper immune response. It is used to monitor people living with HIV. T helper (CD4) cells are destroyed by the HIV virus, which decreases the ratio as the infection spreads.

D. B Lymphocytes (B cells)

1. Become immunocompetent in the secondary lymphoid tissue; **dependent on antigenic stimulation.**
   a. Acquire specific receptors for antigens
   b. Make up **20%** of the peripheral blood lymphocytes
2. Identified by membrane markers **CD19, CD20**, and others
3. **B lymphocyte function**
   a. Contact with foreign antigens stimulates B lymphocytes to become **reactive lymphocytes**, with the characteristic morphology associated with reactivity.
   b. Reactive lymphocytes transform into **immunoblasts**, and then **plasma cells** that produce **antibodies** to provide **humoral immunity.**
   c. **Plasma cells**
      1) End stage of B lymphocyte; dominant in lymph nodes; not normally seen in circulation
      2) 10–20 μm
      3) Abundant blue cytoplasm with prominent **perinuclear (golgi) zone**
      4) **Eccentric nucleus** with a very coarse, clumped chromatin pattern
      5) Make up less than 4% of nucleated cells in the bone marrow

E. Natural Killer (NK)/Large Granular Lymphocytes (LGLs)

1. Large cells with low N:C ratio, large cytoplasmic granules, and pale blue cytoplasm
2. Lack B cell or T cell membrane markers; are **CD16 and CD56 positive**
3. Responsible for surveillance of cells for surface alterations such as tumor cells or cells infected with viruses
4. Activated by IL-2 to express nonspecific cytotoxic functions
5. Attack antigens with attached IgG; called **antibody-dependent cytotoxic cells**

F. Nonmalignant Lymphocytosis Associated with Viral Infections

1. **Infectious mononucleosis**
   a. **Epstein-Barr** virus (EBV) infects **B lymphocytes.**

b. Common in the 14–24 age group with symptoms ranging from malaise and fever to pharyngitis, lymphadenopathy, and splenomegaly
c. Transmitted through nasopharyngeal secretions
d. Lymphocytes usually >50% of the WBCs, with 20% being **reactive T lymphocytes** attacking affected B lymphocytes
e. **Positive heterophile antibody** test

2. **Cytomegalovirus (CMV)**
   a. Symptoms similar to infectious mononucleosis
   b. Transmission is by blood transfusions and saliva exchange.
   c. 90% of lymphocytes can be reactive.
   d. Negative heterophile antibody test
   e. Transfused blood products are often tested for CMV.
3. **Infectious lymphocytosis**
   a. Associated with **adenovirus** and **coxsackie A** virus
   b. Contagious disease mostly affecting young children
   c. After a 12- to 21-day incubation period, symptoms appear and include vomiting, fever, rash, diarrhea, and possible CNS involvement.
   d. Lymphocytosis with **no reactive lymphocytes**

G. Other Conditions Associated with Lymphocytosis

1. **Viral**—hepatitis, influenza, mumps, measles, rubella, and varicella
2. **Nonviral**—*Bordetella pertussis* (whooping cough), brucellosis, toxoplasmosis

VI. MALIGNANT LEUKOCYTE DISORDERS

A. Basic Review

1. Malignant clones of cells proliferate that do not respond to normal regulatory mechanisms.
   a. **Leukemia** originates in the bone marrow and is initially **systemic.**
   b. **Lymphoma** originates in lymphoid tissue and is initially **localized.**
2. **Etiology remains unclear.** Multiple theories exist about **oncogene activation**, which most likely includes multiple factors:
   a. **Viral**—Viruses can suppress immune function or activate oncogenes (HTLV-I, II, V) and HIV-1.
   b. **Bone marrow damage**—Radiation, chemicals, and malignancies secondary to cancer treatments
   c. **Chromosome defects**—Some chromosomal abnormalities are diagnostic for leukemic subtypes; **t(15;17)** is diagnostic for **acute promyelocytic leukemia.**
   d. **Genetic factors**—Increased incidence in Down syndrome, Fanconi, and others
   e. **Immune dysfunction**—Hereditary and acquired defects in the immune system
3. Can be classified by **stem cell involved** and **length of clinical course**
   a. **Lymphoproliferative disorders**—acute or chronic
   b. **Myeloproliferative disorders**—acute or chronic

4. **Bone marrow examination** used to aid in diagnosis
    a. Indications include:
        1) Investigation of **peripheral blood abnormalities**, such as unexplained cytopenias
        2) **Staging** and **management** of patients with certain lymphomas or solid tumors
        3) **Ongoing monitoring** of response to therapy in patients with malignancy
    b. Optimal sample for examination includes both the **aspirate** and **core biopsy specimen.**
    c. **Posterior superior iliac crest** most commonly used; less commonly used is the **anterior iliac crest** or **sternum**
    d. Routinely assessed for **cellularity, M:E ratio, megakaryocyte evaluation, iron stores, differential**
    e. Assessment may also include flow cytometry, cytogenetics, molecular, and microbiology testing.

B. Comparison of Acute and Chronic Leukemias

1. **Duration**
    a. **Acute**—Survival is **weeks to months** without treatment; death is due to infection and bleeding.
    b. **Chronic**—Survival is **years** without treatment.
2. **Predominant cell type**
    a. **Acute**—Immature/blast cells predominate.
        1) **AML** has **myeloblasts.**
        2) **ALL** has **lymphoblasts.**
    b. **Chronic**—Maturing or mature cells predominate
        1) **CML** has **granulocytes.**
        2) **CLL** has **lymphocytes.**
3. **Clinical manifestations and laboratory findings**
    a. **Acute—sudden onset**; affects all ages
        1) Weakness and fatigue due to **anemia**
        2) Petechiae and bruising due to **thrombocytopenia**
        3) Fever and infection due to **neutropenia**
        4) Variable **leukocyte** count
        5) **Marrow blasts ≥20% based on World Health Organization classification or >30% based on French-American-British classification with cellularity >70%**
    b. **Chronic**—frequently **asymptomatic** initially; affects adults
        1) **Anemia** mild or absent
        2) Normal to slightly increased **platelet count**
        3) **WBC count** usually **high**
        4) Marrow cellularity is >70%.

c. **Both acute and chronic**
    1) Unexplained weight loss or night sweats
    2) Splenomegaly, hepatomegaly, lymphadenopathy

4. **Treatment**
    a. **Chemotherapy** used is dependent on the type of leukemia. Proper diagnosis is crucial.
    b. Radiation
    c. Bone marrow/stem cell transplant
    d. Supportive with transfusions of red blood cells and platelets, antibiotics, growth factors

C. French-American-British (FAB) and World Health Organization (WHO)

1. Hematopoietic malignancy classifications
2. **FAB classification** is based on **cellular morphology** and **cytochemical stain** results. FAB defines **acute leukemia as >30% bone marrow blasts.**
3. **WHO classification** is based on cellular morphology and cytochemical stains, but also utilizes information obtained from immunologic probes of **cell markers, cytogenetics, molecular genetic abnormalities**, flow cytometry, and **clinical syndrome.** WHO defines **acute leukemia as ≥20% bone marrow blasts.**
4. **WHO classification** is now the **standard for diagnosis.**
5. **FAB classification** is easier to use and is still widely taught.

D. Cytochemical Stains—Used in Diagnosis of Hematologic Disorders

1. **Myeloperoxidase (MPO)**
    a. Cells of the **granulocytic series** and, to a lesser degree, the **monocytic series** contain the enzyme **peroxidase** in their granules that is detected by this stain. Auer rods also stain positive; **lymphocytic cells** are **negative** for this stain.
    b. Used to **differentiate blasts** of acute myelogenous leukemias **(AMLs)** from acute lymphoblastic leukemias **(ALLs)**
2. **Sudan black B**
    a. Stains **phospholipids** and **lipoproteins**
    b. **Granulocytic cells** and **Auer rods** stain **positive** (blue-black granulation); **lymphocytic cells** are **negative** for Sudan black B (reaction parallels MPO).
    c. Used to **differentiate blasts** of **AML from ALL**
3. **Esterases**
    a. **Specific esterase stain** (naphthol AS-D chloroacetate esterase stain)
        1) **Detects esterase** enzyme present in primary **granules** of **granulocytic cells; monocytic cells negative** for this stain
    b. **Nonspecific esterase stains** (alpha-naphthyl acetate and alpha-naphthyl butyrate)
        1) **Detects esterase** enzyme present in **monocytic cells; granulocytic cells negative** for these stains

c. The **esterase stains** may be useful in **distinguishing acute leukemias** that are of **myeloid origin** (FAB M1, M2, M3, M4) **from** those **leukemias** that are primarily cells of **monocytic origin** (FAB M5).

4. **Periodic acid–Schiff (PAS)**
   a. PAS stains intracellular **glycogen** bright pink.
   b. Immature lymphoid cells, malignant erythroblasts, and megakaryocytic cells **stain positive** with this stain; myeloblasts and normal erythrocytic cells are **negative** with this stain.
   c. Useful in diagnosis of **erythroleukemia** (FAB M6) and **acute lymphoblastic leukemia**
5. **Leukocyte alkaline phosphatase (LAP)**
   a. Detects **alkaline phosphatase** enzyme activity in primary **granules** of **neutrophils**
   b. A positive stain will show dark precipitate when alkaline phosphatase activity is present; color is dependent on dye used.
   c. Used to differentiate **chronic myelogenous leukemia** (**CML**) from a **neutrophilic leukemoid reaction** (NLR). CMLs show low LAP score and NLR will show a high LAP score
   d. **LAP score**
      1) 100 neutrophils are graded on a scale from 0 to 4+ based on stain intensity and size of granules. Number of cells counted in each grade are multiplied by their grades and the products summed to obtain total LAP score.
      2) Reference range is 13–130.
   e. **Clinical significance**
      1) **Decreased LAP score:** CML, paryoxysmal nocturnal hemoglobinuria
      2) **Normal LAP score:** CML in remission or with infection, Hodgkin lymphoma in remission, secondary polycythemia
      3) **Increased LAP score:** Neutrophilic leukemoid reaction, polycythemia vera, CML in blast crisis, late trimester pregnancy
6. **Tartrate-resistant acid phosphatase (TRAP) stain**
   a. Almost all blood cells contain the acid phosphatase enzyme and show positivity with acid phosphatase stain. Once tartrate is added, staining is inhibited in most cells.
   b. Only hairy cells from **hairy cell leukemia** are resistant to inhibition with tartrate and continue to stain positive; all other cells stain negative.
7. **Perl's Prussian blue stain**
   a. Free iron precipitates into small blue/green granules in mature erythrocytes; cells are called **siderocytes.** Iron inclusions are called siderotic granules or **Pappenheimer bodies** when visible with Wright's stain.
   b. **Sideroblasts** are nucleated RBCs in bone marrow that contain iron granules. These are normal. Ringed sideroblasts contain iron that encircles the nucleus. These are abnormal.

c. **Increased percentage of siderocytes** is seen in severe hemolytic anemias (e.g., beta-thalassemia major), iron overload, sideroblastic anemia, and post-splenectomy; **ringed sideroblasts** are seen in bone marrow of myelodysplastic syndrome (refractory anemia with ringed sideroblasts [RARS]) and sideroblastic anemias.

E. Acute Lymphoproliferative Disorders

1. Unregulated proliferation of the **lymphoid stem cell**; classified morphologically using **FAB** criteria, or immunologically using **CD markers** to determine cell lineage (T or B cell)
2. **Clinical symptoms:** Fever, bone/joint pain, bleeding, hepatosplenomegaly
3. **Laboratory:** Neutropenia, anemia, and thrombocytopenia; variable WBC count, hypercellular marrow with bone marrow blasts ≥ 20% (WHO) or >30% (FAB)
4. **Lymphoblasts** stain **PAS positive**; Sudan black B and myeloperoxidase negative
5. **FAB classification of acute lymphoblastic leukemia (ALL)**
   a. **FAB L1**
      1) Most common **childhood** leukemia (2- to 10-year peak); also found in young adults
      2) **Small lymphoblasts, homogeneous** appearance
      3) Best prognosis
      4) Most T cell ALLs are FAB L1.

   b. **FAB L2**
      1) Most common in **adults**
      2) **Large lymphoblasts, heterogeneous** appearance

   c. **FAB L3**
      1) Leukemic phase of Burkitt lymphoma
      2) Seen in both **adults and children**
      3) **Lymphoblasts** are **large and uniform** with prominent nucleoli; cytoplasm stains deeply basophilic and may show vacuoles.
      4) Poor prognosis
      5) ALL FAB L3s are of **B cell lineage.**

   d. **Burkitt lymphoma**
      1) High-grade non-Hodgkin lymphoma phase of **FAB L3 leukemia**
      2) Endemic in East Africa with high association with **Epstein-Barr virus**; children present with jaw/facial bone tumors
      3) U.S. variant seen in children and young adults; present with abdominal mass
6. **Immunophenotyping of ALL**
   a. **CD marker characteristics of B cell lineage**
      1) Expressed by specific cell lines at different maturation stages; as cell matures, loses some antigens and expresses new ones
      2) **Progenitor B cells** are **CD19, CD34,** and **TdT** (terminal deoxynucleotidyl transferase) **positive; CD10** (CALLA) **negative.** This is the least mature B cell.

3) **Early-pre–B cells ALL** are **CD10** (CALLA), **CD19, CD34,** and **TdT positive.** This is the most common subtype.
4) **Pre–B cells ALL** are **CD10** (CALLA), **CD19, CD20,** and **TdT positive.** This is the second most common subtype.
5) **B cells ALL** (early B) are **CD19, CD20 positive; TdT negative.** This is the most mature B cell and least common subtype.
6) **CD19** is the only marker **expressed** through **all stages of B cells.**

b. **CD marker characteristics of T cell lineage**
1) Differentiated from B cells using **markers present on all T cells, including CD2, CD3, CD5,** and **CD7** (pan T cell markers). **Immature T cells** are **TdT positive.**
2) **Immature T cells** can have **both or neither CD4 and CD8. Mature T cells** have **one or the other, but not both.**
3) **T cell ALL** occurs most often in **males; mediastinal mass** is a common finding.

7. **Genetic translocations** are helpful in diagnosis. Common ones include:
a. **FAB L3/Burkitt lymphoma—t(8;14)** with a rearrangement of the **MYC oncogene**
b. **Pre–B cell ALL** associated with **t(9;22); B cell ALL** associated with **t(4;11)**
c. **T cell ALL** associated with **t(7;11)**

F. Chronic Lymphoproliferative Disorders

1. **Chronic lymphocytic leukemia (CLL)**
a. Found in adults over 60 years of age; more common in males (2:1); survival rate of 5–10 years
b. **B cell** malignancy **(CD19, CD20 positive)**
c. Often asymptomatic and diagnosed secondary to other conditions
d. **Laboratory:** Bone marrow is **hypercellular**; blood shows absolute **lymphocytosis** of $>5.0 \times 10^9$/L; **homogeneous, small, hyperclumped lymphocytes** and **smudge cells**
e. **Anemia** is **not usually present** unless **secondary to warm autoimmune hemolytic anemia** (frequent complication).
f. **Small lymphocyte lymphoma** (SLL) is the lymphoma phase of CLL.

2. **Hairy cell leukemia (HCL)**
a. Found in adults over 50 years of age; more common in males (7:1)
b. **B cell** malignancy **(CD19, CD20 positive)**
c. Massive splenomegaly; extensive bone marrow involvement results in **dry tap** on bone marrow aspiration
d. **Laboratory:** Pancytopenia; cytoplasm of lymphocytes shows hair-like projections; hairy cells are tartrate-resistant, acid phosphatase (TRAP) stain positive

3. **Prolymphocytic leukemia (PLL)**
a. Found in adults; more common in males
b. Can be **either B cell** (most common) or **T cell** malignancy

c. Marked splenomegaly
d. **Laboratory:** Characterized by **lymphocytosis** ($>100 \times 10^9/L$) with many **prolymphocytes;** anemia and thrombocytopenia
e. Both B and T cell types are aggressive and respond poorly to treatment.

G. Other Lymphoid Malignancies

1. **Plasma cell neoplasms**
   a. **Multiple myeloma**
      1) **Monoclonal gammopathy** causes **B cell** production of **excessive IgG** (most common) **or IgA**, with decreased production of the other immunoglobulins.
      2) Found in adults over 60 years of age; incidence higher in males
      3) Multiple **skeletal system tumors** of **plasma cells** (myeloma cells) cause **lytic bone lesions** and hypercalcemia.
      4) Identified on serum protein electrophoresis by an "M"-spike in the gamma-globulin region; immunoglobulin class determined using immunoelectrophoresis and quantified using an immunoassay method
      5) Excessive IgG or IgA production by myeloma cells causes **increased blood viscosity.**
      6) Abnormal immunoglobulin binds to platelets, blocking receptor sites for coagulation factor binding; this results in **prolonged bleeding**.
      7) **Laboratory:** Bone marrow **plasma cells** >30%, marked rouleaux, increased erythrocyte sedimentation rate (ESR), blue background to blood smear, plasma cells and lymphocytes on blood smear
      8) **Bence Jones** proteins **(free light chains—kappa or lambda)** found in the urine; toxic to tubular epithelial cells; cause **kidney damage**
   b. **Waldenström macroglobulinemia**
      1) **Monoclonal gammopathy** causes **B cell** production of **excessive IgM** (macroglobulin) and decreased production of the other immunoglobulins.
      2) Found in adults over 60 years of age
      3) **Lymphadenopathy** and **hepatosplenomegaly**; no bone tumors
      4) Identified on serum protein electrophoresis by an "M"-spike in the gamma-globulin region; immunoglobulin class determined using immunoelectrophoresis and quantified using an immunoassay method
      5) Excessive IgM production causes **increased blood viscosity.**
      6) Abnormal immunoglobulin may interfere with platelet function, fibrin polymerization, and the function of other coagulation proteins.
      7) **Laboratory:** Marked rouleaux, increased ESR, blue background to blood smear; plasmacytoid lymphocytes, plasma cells, and lymphocytes on blood smear
2. **Lymphoma**
   a. Proliferation of malignant cells in **solid lymphatic tissue**
   b. Initially **localized; may spread** to bone marrow and blood

c. **Clinical symptom:** Lymphadenopathy
d. **Diagnosis:** Tissue biopsy, CD surface markers, cytogenetics, DNA analysis/PCR
e. World Health Organization **(WHO)** groups the lymphomas into **Hodgkin, B cell**, and **T/NK cell** (non-Hodgkin) neoplasms.
f. **Hodgkin lymphoma** (classical)
   1) **40% of lymphomas**; seen in patients between 15 and 35 years of age and over 55 years of age; seen more frequently in males; certain subtypes have an **Epstein-Barr virus (EBV)** association
   2) **Reed-Sternberg (RS)** cells found in lymph node biopsy are large, multinucleated cells each with prominent, large nucleoli; **B cell lineage**
   3) Hodgkin lymphoma subtypes using **WHO** classification:
      a) Nodular sclerosis—**70% are this subtype**; lowest EBV association
      b) Mixed cellularity—20% are this subtype; **highest EBV association**
      c) Lymphocyte rich
      d) Lymphocyte depleted—uncommon
      e) All subtypes are associated with RS cells
   4) **Laboratory: Mild anemia, eosinophilia**, and **monocytosis; increased LAP score** and **ESR** during active disease
g. **Non-Hodgkin lymphoma**
   1) **WHO** separates B cell and T/NK cell neoplasms into conditions with precursor cells or mature cells.
   2) **Sixty percent of lymphomas**; seen in patients over 50 years of age; seen more frequently in males
   3) Enlarged lymph nodes or gastrointestinal (GI) tumors
   4) **B cell neoplasms** are more common; include Burkitt (lymphoma phase of Burkitt leukemia), mantle cell, follicular, and other lymphomas
   5) Cells can be small and mature (e.g., small lymphocytic lymphoma) or large and primitive (e.g., Precursor B cell lymphoblastic lymphoma).
   6) Can be slow growing or very aggressive
h. **Mycosis fungoides (cutaneous T cell lymphoma)**
   1) Classified by WHO as a **T/NK cell neoplasm** (non-Hodgkin lymphoma)
   2) Seen in patients over 50 years of age
   3) **Cutaneous lymphoma** causes skin itching, leading to ulcerative tumors.
   4) **Sézary syndrome**, a variant of mycosis fungoides, presents as a disseminated disease with widespread skin involvement and circulating lymphoma cells.
   5) CD2, CD3, and CD4 positive

H. Acute Myeloproliferative Disorders

1. Unregulated proliferation of the **myeloid stem cell**; classified using morphology, cytochemical stains, CD markers, cytogenetics; **WHO classification standard for diagnosis; FAB** classification still widely taught

2. Platelets, erythrocytes, granulocytes, and/or monocytes can be affected.
3. Found mainly in **middle-aged adults**; also children <1 year old
4. **Clinical symptoms:** Fever, malaise, weight loss, petechiae, bruises, mild hepatosplenomegaly
5. **Laboratory: Neutropenia, anemia**, and **thrombocytopenia**; variable WBC count; **hypercellular marrow** with **bone marrow blasts ≥20% (WHO) or >30% (FAB)**
6. **Acute myelogenous leukemia (AML)**
   a. **FAB M0—Blasts** exhibit myeloid markers **CD13, CD33**, and **CD34** but **stain negatively** with the usual cytochemical stains, myeloperoxidase (MPO), and Sudan black B (SBB). Constitutes <5% of AMLs.
   b. **FAB M1 (AML without maturation)** shows **90%** or more **marrow myeloblasts**; may have **Auer rods** (fused primary granules)
   c. **FAB M2 (AML with maturation)** shows **<90% marrow myeloblasts**; may have **Auer rods**; chromosome abnormality **t(8;21) (q22;q22)**
      1) Both **FAB M1** and **FAB M2** are **SBB, MPO**, and **specific esterase positive.**
      2) FAB M1 and FAB M2 account for **50%** of the AMLs.
      3) **CD13** and **CD33 positive** (pan myeloid markers)
   d. **Acute promyelocytic leukemia (APL; FAB M3)**
      1) Characterized by **>30% marrow promyelocytes** with bundles of **Auer rods (faggot cells)**; heavy azurophilic granulation. WHO: Acute promyelocytic leukemia (APL) with t(15;17) (q22;q12) is an AML in which abnormal promyelocytes predominate.
      2) **Clinical symptoms:** Severe bleeding, hepatomegaly, and disseminated intravascular coagulation (promyelocytes have procoagulant activity)
      3) Accounts for 5–8% of the AMLs
      4) **SBB, MPO**, and **specific esterase positive**
      5) **CD13** and **CD33 positive; diagnostic** chromosome abnormality **t(15;17);** PML/RARA oncogene involved
   e. **Acute myelomonocytic leukemia (AMML; FAB M4)**
      1) Characterized by **≥20% (WHO) or >30% (FAB) marrow myeloblasts** with **>20% cells of monocytic origin;** may have **Auer rods**
      2) Proliferation of unipotential stem cell **CFU-GM** that gives rise to both granulocytes and monocytes
      3) Accounts for 5–10% of the AMLs
      4) Increased urine/serum lysozyme because of the monocytic proliferation.
      5) **SBB, MPO, and specific** and **nonspecific esterase positive**
      6) **CD13** and **CD33 positive** (myeloid) and **CD14 positive** (monocytes)
      7) **M4Eo** is a **subclass of AMML** that presents with **eosinophilia.**
   f. **Acute monocytic leukemia (AMoL; FAB M5)**
      1) Characterized by **≥20% (WHO) or >30% (FAB) marrow monoblasts**
      2) Accounts for 10% of the AMLs

3) **Nonspecific esterase positive; CD14 positive**
4) Contains two variants:
   a) **M5a** is seen in children with **>80% monoblasts** in the bone marrow.
   b) **M5b** is seen in middle-aged adults with **<80% monoblasts** in the bone marrow.

g. **Acute erythroleukemia (AEL, Di Guglielmo syndrome; FAB M6)**
1) Characterized by **≥20% (WHO) or >30% (FAB) marrow myeloblasts** and **>50% dysplastic marrow normoblasts**
2) Accounts for 5% of the AMLs
3) **Malignant normoblasts** are **PAS positive.** The **myeloblasts** are **SBB and MPO positive.**
4) Malignant **normoblasts** are **CD45** and **CD71** (glycophorin A) **positive.** The **myeloblasts** are **CD13, CD15**, and **CD33 positive.**
5) **Peripheral blood poikilocytosis, anisocytosis, and anemia with a large number of nucleated erythrocytes that are dysplastic with megaloblastoid nuclei**
6) **The BM erythroblasts are distinctly abnormal with bizarre morphological features.**

h. **Acute megakaryocytic leukemia (AMkL; FAB M7)**
1) Characterized by a proliferation of **megakaryoblasts** and **atypical megakaryocytes** in the bone marrow; **blasts** may have **cytoplasmic blebs**
2) Accounts for<5% of the AMLs
3) Marrow aspiration results in dry tap; blood shows pancytopenia
4) Difficult to diagnose with cytochemical stains
5) **CD41, CD42**, and **CD61** (platelet markers) **positive**

i. **Bilineage leukemias** contain two cell populations. One population expresses **myeloid antigens**; the other population expresses **lymphoid antigens.**

j. **Biphenotypic leukemias** occur when **myeloid and lymphoid antigens** are expressed on the **same cell**; poor prognosis

k. The **WHO classification** of **acute myeloid leukemias** has more than **20 subtypes**; all have **≥20% marrow blasts.**

I. Chronic Myeloproliferative Disorders

1. Characterized by **hypercellular marrow, erythrocytosis, granulocytosis, and thrombocytosis**
   a. Defect of the **myeloid stem cell**
   b. Named for the cell line most greatly affected
   c. All may **terminate** in **acute leukemia.**
2. Molecular diagnostic studies are helpful in identifying oncogenes.
   a. **JAK2 oncogene** is implicated in polycythemia vera (80%), chronic idiopathic myelofibrosis (50%), and essential thrombocythemia (40%).
   b. The **BCR/ABL** oncogene is associated with chronic myelogenous leukemia.

3. **Chronic myelogenous leukemia (CML)** presents with **proliferation of granulocytes.**
   a. Found mainly in adults 45 years of age and older; often diagnosed secondary to other conditions
   b. **Clinical symptoms:** Weight loss, splenomegaly, fever, night sweats, and malaise
   c. Bone marrow has an **increased M:E ratio.**
   d. **Laboratory:** Blood findings include mild anemia and WBC between 50 and $500 \times 10^9/L$, with all stages of granulocyte production (shift to the left), including early forms of eosinophils and basophils. Myelocytes predominate; may have a few circulating blasts.
   e. CML can mimic a neutrophilic leukemoid reaction (NLR). LAP score is used to differentiate; **LAP** is **low in CML** and high in NLR.
   f. **Philadelphia chromosome, t(9;22)**, is present in virtually all patients. All cell lines are affected except lymphocytes. The few who lack the chromosome have a worse prognosis.
   g. **Chronic phase** can last up to 5 years; **accelerated phase** (blast crisis) ultimately leads to acute leukemia in most patients. Recent therapies are improving the prognosis.
4. **Essential thrombocythemia (ET)**
   a. Characterized by **proliferation of megakaryocytes**
   b. Found mainly in adults 60 years of age and older
   c. **Laboratory:** Platelets commonly greater than $1000 \times 10^9/L$, giant forms, platelet function abnormalities, leukocytosis
   d. Must differentiate from reactive thrombocytosis and polycythemia vera
5. **Polycythemia vera (PV)**
   a. **Malignant hyperplasia** of the **multipotential myeloid stem cell** causes **increase in all cell lines** (polycythemia); **erythrocytes** most greatly **increased** despite **decreased erythropoietin** (EPO); inappropriate erythropoiesis
   b. **High blood viscosity** can cause high blood pressure, stroke, and heart attack.
   c. Found in adults 50 years of age and older
   d. **Laboratory:** Increased RBC ($7–10 \times 10^{12}/L$), hemoglobin (>20 g/dL), and hematocrit (>60%) along with increased leukocytes and platelets indicate polycythemia. RBC mass is increased with a normal plasma volume.
   e. **Treatment** is therapeutic phlebotomy, splenectomy, and chemotherapy. PV is a chronic disease with a life expectancy after diagnosis of up to 20 years.
   f. Must differentiate from other forms of polycythemia
      1) **Secondary polycythemia**
         a) **Increase in RBC mass** is an appropriate response to **increased EPO** or **tissue hypoxia.** Plasma volume, leukocyte count, and platelet count are normal.
         b) Can be caused by smoking, emphysema, or high altitude

2) **Relative (pseudo-) polycythemia**
   a) **Decreased plasma volume** with a **normal RBC mass** caused by **dehydration** (diarrhea, diuretics, or burns)
   b) Increased **hemoglobin**, normal leukocyte and platelet count, **normal EPO**

6. **Chronic idiopathic myelofibrosis**
   a. **Myeloid stem cell disorder** characterized by **proliferation of erythroid, granulocytic**, and **megakaryocytic precursors** in marrow with dyspoiesis
   b. Progressive **marrow fibrosis**
   c. Found in adults 50 years of age and older
   d. **Clinical symptoms:** Bleeding due to abnormal platelet function; extramedullary hematopoiesis causes splenomegaly and hepatomegaly
   e. **Laboratory:** Anisocytosis, poikilocytosis with teardrop cells, leukoerythroblastic anemia (immature neutrophils and nucleated RBCs in circulation); abnormal morphology associated with all cell lines

J. Myelodysplastic Syndromes (MDSs)

1. **Basic Review**
   a. Group of **acquired clonal disorders** affecting the **pluripotential stem cell**; characterized by progressive **blood cytopenias** despite **bone marrow hyperplasia. Can also be considered preleukemia.**
   b. **Dyspoiesis** affects erythroid, myeloid, and megakaryocytic cell lines. High incidence of terminating in acute myelogenous leukemia occurs.
   c. MDS development can be triggered by chemotherapy, radiation, and chemicals.
   d. Found in older adults; rarely found in children and young adults
   e. Hematologic evidence of dyspoiesis:
      1) **Erythroid:** Variable anemia; erythrocytes can be macrocytic (with oval macrocytes) or microcytic and hypochromic; dimorphic erythrocytes, poikilocytosis, Howell-Jolly bodies, basophilic stippling, Cabot rings, nucleated RBCs
      2) **Myeloid:** Neutropenia, hypogranulation, hyposegmentation of neutrophils, shift to the left
      3) **Thrombocytes:** Variable platelet count, giant platelets, hypogranulation, micromegakaryocytes
   f. Five subgroups of MDS using the FAB classification scheme; **up to 30% blasts in the bone marrow**
2. **Refractory anemia (RA)**
   a. Anemia that is **refractory** (not responsive) **to therapy**
   b. **Laboratory:** Oval macrocytes, reticulocytopenia, dyserythropoiesis; bone marrow blasts <5% and peripheral blood blasts <1%
3. **Refractory anemia with ringed sideroblasts (RARS)**
   a. Ringed sideroblasts comprise more than 15% of bone marrow nucleated cells. Signs of dyserythropoiesis, neutropenia

b. **Laboratory:** Similar to RA; dimorphic erythrocytes
c. This is the primary/idiopathic sideroblastic anemia discussed with the anemias.

4. **Chronic myelomonocytic leukemia (CMML)**
   a. The one MDS that usually presents with **leukocytosis**
   b. **Laboratory:** Bone marrow blasts 5–20% and peripheral blood blasts <5%; absolute monocytosis greater than 1.0 $\times 10^9$/L
5. **Refractory anemia with excess blasts (RAEB)**
   a. Trilineage cytopenias common
   b. **Laboratory:** Bone marrow and peripheral blood blasts are the **same as** with **CMML**, but there is **no** absolute monocytosis.
   c. The higher the blast percent, the worse is the prognosis.
6. **Refractory anemia with excess blasts in transformation (RAEB-t)**
   a. **Laboratory:** bone marrow blasts >20% but less than 30%; peripheral blood blasts >5%
   b. **WHO** classification **reassigns RAEB-t** as an **acute leukemia** instead of a myelodysplastic syndrome because of the bone marrow blast percent.
7. WHO classification of MDS has additional groups (e.g., refractory cytopenia with multilineage dysplasia, 5q deletion syndrome).
8. WHO created the new category of **myelodysplastic/myeloproliferative disease**, which includes the FAB's **CMML.**

VII. ERYTHROCYTES

A. General Characteristics

1. **Oxygen transport, removal of metabolic waste**
2. **Loss of nucleus** is required for function.
3. Normal life span is **120 days.**

B. Erythropoietin

1. Produced mainly by the **kidneys**
2. **Growth factor** that **stimulates erythrocyte production from myeloid progenitor cell**; influences colony-forming unit-erythrocytes (CFU-Es) to differentiate into erythroblasts

C. Erythrocyte Maturation

1. **Pronormoblast (rubriblast)**
   a. Earliest RBC, size up to 20 μm, with an N:C ratio of 8:1
   b. One to three nucleoli, nucleus has dark areas of DNA
   c. Chromatin is fine and uniform and stains intensely
   d. Deep blue cytoplasm with no granules
2. **Basophilic normoblast (prorubricyte)**
   a. Size up to 16 μm with an N:C ratio of 6:1
   b. Centrally located nucleus with 0–1 nucleoli
   c. Chromatin is coarsening.
   d. Cytoplasm is less blue but intensely basophilic (RNA).

3. **Polychromatophilic normoblast (rubricyte)**
   a. Size up to 12 μm with an N:C ratio of 4:1
   b. Eccentric nucleus with no nucleoli
   c. Chromatin shows significant clumping.
   d. Begins to produce hemoglobin, resulting in gray-blue cytoplasm
4. **Orthochromic normoblast (metarubricyte)**
   a. Size up to 10 μm with an N:C ratio of 0.5:1
   b. Eccentric nucleus with small, fully condensed (pyknotic) nucleus; no nucleoli
   c. Pale blue to salmon cytoplasm
   d. Hemoglobin synthesis decreases
5. **Reticulocyte**
   a. Size up to 10 μm
   b. A reticulocyte contains **no nucleus** but has mitochondria and ribosomes.
   c. Last stage to synthesize hemoglobin
   d. Last stage in bone marrow before release to the blood
   e. Reference ranges are 0.5–1.5% for adults and 2.5–6.5% for newborns, with slightly increased ranges at higher altitudes
   f. A **supravital stain** is used to enumerate reticulocytes.
   g. **Reticulocyte count** is one of the best indicators of bone marrow function.
   h. **Stress reticulocytes** are young cells released from bone marrow after older reticulocytes have been released. This is a response to increased need.
   i. Hemoglobin continues to be produced by reticulocytes for approximately 24 hours after exiting the bone marrow.
6. **Mature erythrocyte**
   a. Size range is 6–8 μm.
   b. Round, biconcave discocyte
   c. Salmon with central pallor (clearing in the center) when a blood smear is Wright stained
      1) **Normal cells** have a **central pallor** that is one-third the diameter of the cell.
      2) **Decreased central pallor** is seen with **spherocytic** disorders, including thermal injury and liver disease.
      3) **Central pallor greater** than one-third the diameter of the cell is seen in **microcytic anemias.**
   d. **RBC reference ranges** in SI units:
      1) Females 4.0–5.4 $\times 10^{12}$/L (conventional units 4.0–5.4 $\times 10^{6}$/μL)
      2) Males 4.6–6.0 $\times 10^{12}$/L (conventional units 4.6–6.0 $\times 10^{6}$/μL)
   e. Erythropoiesis is regulated by **erythropoietin** produced in the kidney. Additional regulation includes:
      1) Hypoxia due to high altitudes, heart or lung dysfunction, anemia
      2) Androgens (male hormones that appear to enhance the activity of erythropoietin) and hemolytic anemias (increased erythrocyte destruction)

D. Erythrocyte Physiology

1. Early RBCs get energy from oxidative phosphorylation. During maturation, the mitochondria are lost, and energy is derived from glycolysis.
2. Erythrocytes need proper volume ratio for exchange of blood gases and flexibility to travel through capillaries. This is accomplished by the cation pump, a mechanism that keeps sodium outside and potassium inside the cell.
3. Erythrocyte membrane is 50–60% lipid (phospholipids, cholesterol, and glycolipids) and 40–50% protein.

E. Substances Needed for Erythropoiesis

1. **Iron:** Must be in the ferrous state (Fe^{2+}) to transport oxygen
2. **Amino acids:** Globin-chain synthesis
3. **Folic acid/vitamin B_{12}:** DNA replication/cell division
4. **Others:** Erythropoietin, vitamin B_6 (pyridoxine), trace minerals

F. Erythrocytic Morphology and Associated Disease (Size and Shape)

1. **Normocytes (discocytes)** are normal erythrocytes that are approximately the same size as the nucleus of a small lymphocyte.
2. **Macrocytes**
   a. RBCs greater than 8 µm in diameter; **MCV greater than 100 fL**
   b. Seen in **megaloblastic anemias**, such as B_{12}/folate deficiency
   c. Seen in non-megaloblastic anemia of liver disease or accelerated erythropoiesis; also seen in normal newborns
3. **Microcytes**
   a. RBCs less than 6 µm in diameter; **MCV less than 80 fL**
   b. Seen in iron-deficiency anemia, thalassemias, sideroblastic anemia, and anemia of chronic disease
4. **Anisocytosis**
   a. **Variation in RBC size**, indicating a heterogeneous RBC population (dimorphism)
   b. Correlates with RDW (red blood cell distribution width), especially when the RDW exceeds 15.0%
   c. Seen post-transfusion, post-treatment for a deficiency (e.g., iron), presence of two concurrent deficiencies (e.g., iron and vitamin B_{12}), and idiopathic sideroblastic anemia
5. **Poikilocytosis**
   a. General term to describe **variation in shape**
   b. Associated with a variety of pathologic conditions
6. **Echinocytes** include **crenated** and **burr cells**
   a. Have evenly spaced **round** projections; central pallor area present
   b. Seen in liver disease, uremia, heparin therapy, pyruvate kinase deficiency, or as an artifact
   c. Caused by changes in osmotic pressure

7. **Acanthocytes (spur cells)**
   a. Have unevenly spaced **pointed** projections; **lack** a central pallor area
   b. Associated with alcoholic liver disease, post-splenectomy, and abetalipoproteinemia
   c. Caused by excessive cholesterol in the membrane
8. **Target cells (codocytes or Mexican hat cells)**
   a. Show a central area of hemoglobin surrounded by a colorless ring and a peripheral ring of hemoglobin; cells have an **increased surface-to-volume ratio**
   b. Seen in liver disease, hemoglobinopathies, thalassemia, iron-deficiency anemia
   c. Caused by excessive cholesterol in the membrane or a hemoglobin distribution imbalance
9. **Spherocytes**
   a. Disc-shaped cell with a smaller volume than a normal erythrocyte; cells have a **decreased surface-to-volume ratio**
   b. **Lack** a central pallor area
   c. Associated with defects of the red cell membrane proteins
   d. **MCHC may be >37%**; increased osmotic fragility
   e. **Damaged RBC**; seen in hereditary spherocytosis, G6PD deficiency, and immune hemolytic anemias
   f. **Microspherocytes** (<4 μm) are frequently seen in severe thermal injury (burns).
10. **Teardrops (dacryocytes)**
    a. **Pear-shaped** cell with **one blunt projection**
    b. Seen in megaloblastic anemias, thalassemia, and extramedullary hematopoiesis (myelofibrosis, myelophthisic anemia)
11. **Sickle cells (drepanocytes)**
    a. Shapes vary but show **thin, elongated, pointed ends** and will appear **crescent shaped;** usually lack a central pallor area
    b. Contain polymers of abnormal **hemoglobin S**
    c. Seen in hemoglobinopathies SS, SC, SD, and S/β-thalassemia
    d. Cell shape is caused by **cell membrane alterations** due to an amino acid substitution
12. **Helmet cells (horn cells or keratocytes)**
    a. Interior portion of cell is hollow, resembling a horn or helmet
    b. Seen in microangiopathic hemolytic anemias
13. **Schistocytes (RBC fragments)**
    a. **Damaged RBC**; fragments of various sizes and shapes are present, often with **pointed projections**
    b. Seen in microangiopathic hemolytic anemias (e.g., DIC, HUS, TTP), thermal injury, renal transplant rejection, and G6PD deficiency
14. **Stomatocytes (mouth cells or coin slot)**
    a. Characterized by an elongated or slit-like area of central pallor

b. Seen in liver disease, hereditary stomatocytosis, or as an artifact
c. Caused by osmotic changes due to cation imbalance (Na^+/K^+)

15. **Elliptocytes (ovalocytes)**
    a. Cigar- to egg-shaped erythrocytes
    b. Associated with defects of the red cell membrane proteins
    c. Seen in hereditary elliptocytosis, iron-deficiency anemia (pencil forms), megaloblastic anemia (macro-ovalocytes), thalassemia major

G. Erythrocyte Inclusions and Associated Diseases

1. **Nucleated RBCs (nRBCs, nucRBCs)**
    a. Usually **orthochromic normoblasts** (metarubricyte) but can appear in any erythrocytic stage of maturation
    b. Indicate **bone marrow stimulation** or **increased erythropoiesis**
    c. Associated with thalassemia major, sickle cell anemia, and other hemolytic anemias, erythroleukemia, and myeloproliferative disorders
    d. Normal newborns can have a few.
    e. Healthy individuals should have **none** on a peripheral blood smear.
2. **Howell-Jolly bodies**
    a. Small, round **DNA fragments** (0.5–1.0 μm in diameter) usually **one** per cell, but can be **multiple**
    b. Stain **dark purple to black** with **Wright stain**
    c. Not seen in normal erythrocytes; normally **pitted** by splenic macrophages
    d. Seen in sickle cell anemia, beta-thalassemia major, and other severe hemolytic anemias, megaloblastic anemia, alcoholism, post-splenectomy
3. **Basophilic stippling**
    a. Multiple, tiny, fine, or coarse **inclusions** (ribosomal RNA remnants) **evenly dispersed throughout the cell**; "blueberry bagel" appearance
    b. Stain **dark blue** with **Wright stain**
    c. Seen in thalassemias, megaloblastic anemias, sideroblastic anemia, lead poisoning, and alcoholism
4. **Pappenheimer bodies**
    a. Small, irregular, **dark-staining iron granules** usually **clumped together at periphery of the cell**
    b. Stain with **Perl's Prussian blue stain**; appear **dark violet with Wright stain**
    c. Caused by an accumulation of ribosomes, mitochondria, and iron fragments
    d. Seen in sideroblastic anemia, hemoglobinopathies, thalassemia, megaloblastic anemia, myelodysplastic syndrome (RARS)
5. **Cabot rings**
    a. Thin, **red-violet**, single to multiple **ringlike structures** that may appear in **loop or figure-eight shapes**
    b. Seen in megaloblastic anemia, myelodysplastic syndromes, lead poisoning
    c. Composed of **fragments of nuclear material**

6. **Hemoglobin C crystals**
   a. Condensed, intracellular, rod-shaped crystal
   b. Seen in hemoglobin C or SC disease, but not in trait
7. **Hemoglobin SC crystals (Washington monument)**
   a. One to two blunt, fingerlike projections extending from the cell membrane
   b. Seen in hemoglobin SC disease
8. **Heinz bodies**
   a. Multiple inclusions ranging in size from 0.3 to 2.0 μm
   b. Invisible with Wright stain; must use a **supravital stain to visualize**
   c. Seen in G6PD deficiency, beta-thalassemia major, Hgb H disease, unstable hemoglobinopathies, drug-induced anemias
   d. Represent **denatured hemoglobin**
9. **Malarial parasites**—include *P. vivax, P. falciparum, P. malariae*, and *P. ovale*

H. Erythrocyte Hemoglobin Content and Associated Diseases

1. **Normochromasia:** Cells have the normal one-third clear, central pallor area
2. **Hypochromasia**
   a. Central pallor area is greater than one-third the diameter of the cell
   b. **MCH** and **MCHC** usually **decreased**
   c. Often associated with **microcytosis**
   d. Seen in iron-deficiency anemia, thalassemias, anemia of chronic disease, sideroblastic anemia, myelodysplastic syndromes
3. **Polychromasia**
   a. Variation in hemoglobin content showing a **slight blue tinge** when stained with **Wright stain; residual RNA**
   b. Indicates **reticulocytosis;** supravital reticulocyte stain to enumerate
   c. Usually slightly macrocytic
4. **Hyperchromasia** (term no longer used)
   a. Current terminology is **spherocyte**; lacks a central pallor area

I. Abnormal Erythrocyte Distributions and Associated Diseases

1. **Rouleaux**
   a. **Stacking** or "coining" pattern of erythrocytes due to **abnormal or increased plasma proteins**
   b. May see excessively blue color to smear macroscopically and microscopically
   c. Seen in hyperproteinemia, multiple myeloma, Waldenström macroglobulinemia, and conditions that produce increased fibrinogen (chronic inflammation)
   d. May be artifact; considered normal in thicker area of the peripheral smear
   e. True rouleaux formation is determined in the thin area of the peripheral smear.
2. **Agglutination**
   a. Characterized by clumping of erythrocytes with **no pattern**
   b. Occurs when **erythrocytes** are **coated with IgM antibodies and complement**

c. Seen in cold autoimmune hemolytic anemia (cold agglutinin disease)
d. Warm blood to 37°C to correct a false low RBC and hematocrit, and false high MCHC (>37 g/dL) when using an automated cell counting instrument

VIII. HEMOGLOBIN

A. Introduction

1. Hemoglobin is an **oxygen-transporting protein** contained within erythrocytes.
2. The heme portion of hemoglobin gives erythrocytes their characteristic red color.

B. Hemoglobin Structure

1. **Four identical heme** groups, each consisting of a **protoporphyrin ring** and **ferrous (Fe^{2+}) iron**
2. **Four globin** (polypeptide) **chains**
   a. Alpha chains have 141 amino acids.
   b. Beta, gamma, and delta chains have 146 amino acids.
3. The **amino acid sequence** of the globin chain determines the type of hemoglobin; normal adult hemoglobin consists of two alpha and two non-alpha chains in pairs.

C. Hemoglobin Synthesis

1. 65% hemoglobin synthesis occurs in immature nRBCs.
2. 35% hemoglobin synthesis occurs in reticulocytes.
3. **Heme synthesis** occurs in the **mitochondria of normoblasts** and is dependent on glycine, succinyl coenzyme A, aminolevulinic acid synthetase, and vitamin B_6 (pyridoxine).
4. **Globin synthesis** occurs in the **ribosomes,** and it is controlled on **chromosome 16** for alpha chains and **chromosome 11** for all other chains.
5. Each **globin** chain **binds to a heme** molecule in the cytoplasm of the immature RBC.

D. Hemoglobin/Erythrocyte Breakdown

1. **Intravascular hemolysis** (10%)
   a. Occurs when **hemoglobin breaks down in the blood** and **free hemoglobin** is released into **plasma**
   b. **Free hemoglobin** binds to **haptoglobin** (major free hemoglobin transport protein), **hemopexin,** and **albumin**, and it is phagocytized by liver macrophages.
   c. **Laboratory:** Increased plasma hemoglobin, serum bilirubin, serum LD, and urine urobilinogen; hemoglobinuria and hemosiderinuria present; decreased serum haptoglobin
2. **Extravascular hemolysis** (90%)
   a. Occurs when **senescent/old RBCs** are **phagocytized** by macrophages in the liver or spleen

b. **Protoporphyrin ring** metabolized to **bilirubin** and **urobilinogen**; excreted in urine and feces
c. **Globin chains** are recycled into the **amino acid pool** for protein synthesis.
d. **Iron** binds to **transferrin** and is transported to bone marrow for new RBC production, or it is stored for future use in the form of **ferritin** or **hemosiderin.**

E. Hemoglobin and Iron

1. Most iron in the body is in hemoglobin and must be in the ferrous state (Fe^{2+}) to be used. **Fe^{2+} binds to oxygen** for transport to lungs and body tissues. Ferric iron (Fe^{3+}) is not able to bind to hemoglobin, but does bind to transferrin. Iron is an **essential** mineral and is not produced by the body.
   a. **Serum iron** measures the amount of Fe^{3+} bound to transferrin.
   b. **Total iron-binding capacity (TIBC)** measures the total amount of iron that transferrin can bind when fully saturated.
   c. Serum ferritin is an indirect measurement of storage iron in tissues and bone marrow.

F. Types of Hemoglobin

1. **Hgb F** contains two alpha- and two gamma-globin chains. Hgb F functions in a reduced oxygen environment. **Hgb F predominates at birth** (80%). Gamma chain production switches over to beta chain production and is complete by 6 months of age.
   a. **Laboratory:** Alkali denaturation test and Kleihauer-Betke acid elution stain (Hgb F is resistant to denaturation/elution), column chromatography, radial immunodiffusion
   b. Hgb F is a compensatory hemoglobin and can be increased in homozygous hemoglobinopathies and beta-thalassemia major.
2. **Adult**
   a. **Hgb A** contains two alpha- and two beta-globin chains.
      1) Hgb A is subdivided into glycosylated fractions. The **A_{1c}** fraction (the predominant fraction) reflects glucose levels in the blood and is used to monitor individuals with diabetes mellitus.
   b. **Hgb A_2** contains two alpha- and two delta-globin chains.
   c. Reference range for a normal adult is **97% Hb A, 2% Hb A_2, and 1% Hb F.**

G. Different Forms of Normal Hemoglobin

1. **Oxyhemoglobin:** Hemoglobin with Fe^{2+} + O_2; seen in arterial circulation
2. **Deoxyhemoglobin:** Hemoglobin with Fe^{2+} but no O_2; seen in venous circulation
3. **Carboxyhemoglobin:** Hemoglobin with Fe^{2+} and carbon monoxide (CO); hemoglobin has 200 × more affinity for CO than O_2, so CO is carried instead of O_2; can result in death, but is reversible if given pure O_2

4. **Sulfhemoglobin:** Hemoglobin with S; cannot transport O_2; seldom reaches fatal levels; caused by drugs and chemicals; irreversible, not measured by the cyanmethemoglobin method
5. **Methemoglobin:** Hemoglobin with Fe^{3+}; cannot transport O_2; increased levels cause cyanosis and anemia

H. Oxygen Dissociation Curve

1. **Oxygen affinity** is the ability of hemoglobin to bind or release oxygen. Expressed in terms of the oxygen tension at which hemoglobin is 50% saturated with oxygen.
2. The relationship between oxygen tension and hemoglobin saturation with oxygen is described by the **oxygen dissociation curve.**
   a. **Right shift** decreases oxygen affinity, **more** O_2 release to the tissues—high 2,3-bisphosphoglycerate (formerly 2,3-diphosphoglycerate/2,3-DPG) level or increased body temperature; decreased body pH
   b. **Left shift** increases oxygen affinity, **less** O_2 release to the tissues—low 2,3-bisphosphoglycerate (2,3-BPG) level or decreased body temperature; increased body pH

IX. ANEMIAS

A. Introduction: Anemia is defined as a decrease in erythrocytes and hemoglobin, resulting in decreased oxygen delivery to the tissues. The anemias can be classified **morphologically** using RBC indices (MCV, MCH, and MCHC). They can also be classified based on **etiology/cause.** Anemia is suspected when the hemoglobin is **<12 g/dL in men** or **<11 g/dL in women.**

1. **Relative (pseudo) anemia**
   a. RBC mass is normal, but **plasma volume** is **increased.**
   b. Secondary to an unrelated condition and can be transient in nature
   c. Causes include conditions that result in hemodilution, such as pregnancy and volume overload.
   d. **Reticulocyte** count **normal; normocytic/normochromic** anemia
2. **Absolute anemia**
   a. **RBC mass** is **decreased**, but plasma volume is normal. This is indicative of a true decrease in erythrocytes and hemoglobin.
   b. **Mechanisms** involved include:
      1) **Decreased delivery** of red cells into circulation
         a) Caused by impaired or defective production
         b) Bone marrow fails to respond; **reticulocytopenia**
      2) **Increased loss** of red cells from the circulation
         a) Caused by acute bleeding or accelerated destruction (hemolytic)
         b) Bone marrow can respond; **reticulocytosis**

B. Impaired or Defective Production Anemias

1. **Iron-deficiency anemia**
   a. Most common form of anemia in the United States
   b. Prevalent in infants and children, pregnancy, excessive menstrual flow, elderly with poor diets, malabsorption syndromes, chronic blood loss (GI blood loss, hookworm infection)
   c. **Laboratory: Microcytic/hypochromic anemia**; serum iron, ferritin, hemoglobin/hematocrit, RBC indices, and reticulocyte count low; RDW and total iron-binding capacity (TIBC) high; smear shows ovalocytes/pencil forms
   d. **Clinical symptoms:** Fatigue, dizziness, pica, stomatitis (cracks in the corners of the mouth), glossitis (sore tongue), and koilonychia (spooning of the nails)
2. **Anemia of chronic disease (ACD)**
   a. Due to an **inability to use available iron** for hemoglobin production
   b. Impaired release of storage iron associated with increased **hepcidin** levels
      1) Hepcidin is a liver hormone and a positive acute-phase reactant. It plays a major role in body iron regulation by influencing intestinal iron absorption and release of storage iron from macrophages.
      2) Inflammation and infection cause hepcidin levels to increase; this decreases release of iron from stores.
   c. **Laboratory: Normocytic/normochromic anemia**, or **slightly microcytic/hypochromic anemia**; increased ESR; normal to increased ferritin; low serum iron and TIBC
   d. Associated with persistent infections, chronic inflammatory disorders (SLE, rheumatoid arthritis, Hodgkin lymphoma, cancer)
   e. Anemia of chronic disease is second only to iron deficiency as a common cause of anemia.
3. **Sideroblastic anemia**
   a. Caused by **blocks** in the **protoporphyrin pathway** resulting in defective hemoglobin synthesis and iron overload
   b. Excess iron accumulates in the mitochondrial region of the immature erythrocyte in the bone marrow and encircles the nucleus; cells are called **ringed sideroblasts.**
   c. Excess iron accumulates in the mitochondrial region of the mature erythrocyte in circulation; cells are called **siderocytes**; inclusions are siderotic granules (**Pappenheimer bodies** on Wright stained smears).
   d. **Siderocytes** are best demonstrated using **Perl's Prussian blue stain.**
   e. Two types of sideroblastic anemia:
      1) **Primary**—irreversible; cause of the blocks unknown
         a) Two RBC populations **(dimorphic)** are seen.
         b) This is one of the myelodysplastic syndromes—refractory anemia with ringed sideroblasts (RARS).
      2) **Secondary**—reversible; causes include alcohol, anti-tuberculosis drugs, chloramphenicol

   f. **Laboratory: Microcytic/hypochromic anemia** with increased ferritin and serum iron; TIBC is decreased
4. **Lead poisoning**
   a. **Multiple blocks** in the **protoporphyrin pathway** affect heme synthesis.
   b. Seen mostly in children exposed to lead-based paint
   c. **Clinical symptoms:** Abdominal pain, muscle weakness, and a **gum lead line** that forms from blue/black deposits of lead sulfate
   d. **Laboratory: Normocytic/normochromic anemia** with characteristic coarse **basophilic stippling**
5. **Porphyrias**
   a. These are a group of **inherited disorders** characterized by a **block** in the **protoporphyrin pathway** of heme synthesis. Heme precursors before the block accumulate in the tissues, and large amounts are excreted in urine and/or feces.
   b. **Clinical symptoms:** Photosensitivity, abdominal pain, CNS disorders
   c. Hematologic findings are insignificant.
6. **Megaloblastic anemias**
   a. **Defective DNA synthesis** causes abnormal nuclear maturation; RNA synthesis is normal, so the cytoplasm is not affected. The nucleus matures slower than the cytoplasm (asynchronism). **Megaloblastic** maturation is seen.
   b. Caused by either a vitamin **B_{12}** or **folic acid deficiency**
   c. **Laboratory:** Pancytopenia, **macrocytic/normochromic anemia** with oval macrocytes and teardrops, hypersegmented neutrophils; inclusions include Howell-Jolly bodies, nucleated RBCs, basophilic stippling, Pappenheimer bodies, and Cabot rings; elevated LD, bilirubin, and iron levels due to destruction of fragile, megaloblastic cells in the blood and bone marrow
   d. **Vitamin B_{12} deficiency (cobalamin)**
      1) Intrinsic factor is secreted by parietal cells and is needed to bind vitamin B_{12} for absorption into the intestine.
         a) **Pernicious anemia:** Caused by deficiency of **intrinsic factor**, antibodies to intrinsic factor, or antibodies to parietal cells
         b) Prevalent in older adults of English, Irish, and Scandinavian descent
         c) Characterized by **achlorhydria** and atrophy of gastric parietal cells
      2) Other causes of vitamin B_{12} deficiency include malabsorption syndromes, *Diphyllobothrium latum* tapeworm, total gastrectomy, intestinal blind loops, and a total vegetarian diet.
      3) **Clinical symptoms:** Jaundice, weakness, sore tongue (glossitis), and gastrointestinal (GI) disorder, numbness and other **CNS problems**
      4) Vitamin B_{12} deficiency takes 3–6 years to develop because of high body stores.
   e. **Folic acid deficiency** causes a **megaloblastic anemia** with a blood picture and clinical symptoms similar to vitamin B_{12} deficiency, except there is **no CNS involvement.** It is associated with poor diet, pregnancy, or chemotherapeutic anti-folic acid drugs such as **methotrexate.** Folic acid has low body stores.

7. **Non-megaloblastic macrocytic anemias** include alcoholism, liver disease, and conditions that cause accelerated erythropoiesis. The **erythrocytes** are **round**, not oval as is seen in the megaloblastic anemias.
8. **Aplastic anemia**
   a. Bone marrow failure causes **pancytopenia.**
   b. **Laboratory:** Decrease in hemoglobin/hematocrit and reticulocytes; **normocytic/normochromic anemia**; no response to erythropoietin
   c. Most commonly affects people around the age of 50 and above. It can occur in children.
   d. Patients have a poor prognosis with complications that include bleeding, infection, and iron overload due to frequent transfusion needs.
   e. **Treatment** includes bone marrow or stem cell transplant and immunosuppression.
   f. Can be genetic, acquired, or idiopathic
      1) **Genetic aplastic anemia (Fanconi anemia)**
         a) **Autosomal recessive** trait
         b) Dwarfism, renal disease, intellectual disability
         c) Strong association with malignancy development, especially acute lymphoblastic leukemia
      2) **Acquired aplastic anemia** (secondary) caused by:
         a) Antibiotics: Chloramphenicol and sulfonamides
         b) Chemicals: Benzene and herbicides
         c) About 30% of acquired aplastic anemias are due to **drug exposure.**
         d) Viruses: B19 parvovirus secondary to hepatitis, measles, CMV, and Epstein-Barr virus
         e) Radiation or chemotherapy
         f) Myelodysplastic syndromes, leukemia, solid tumors, paroxysmal nocturnal hemoglobinuria
      3) **Idiopathic** (primary): 50–70% of aplastic anemias have **no known cause.**
   g. Diamond-Blackfan anemia
      1) **True red cell aplasia** (leukocytes and platelets normal in number)
      2) Autosomal inheritance
9. **Myelophthisic** (marrow replacement) **anemia**
   a. **Hypoproliferative anemia** caused by replacement of bone marrow hematopoietic cells by malignant cells or fibrotic tissue
   b. Associated with cancers (breast, prostate, lung, melanoma) with bone metastasis
   c. **Laboratory: Normocytic/normochromic anemia**; leukoerythroblastic blood picture
10. Hemochromatosis
   a. Describes the clinical disorder that results in parenchymal tissue damage from progressive iron overload
   b. Classified as hereditary or secondary

c. Some causes of hereditary iron overload
   1) Classical hemochromatosis: HFE- associated mutation (type 1)
   2) Juvenile hemochromatosis (type 2)
   3) Hepcidin (HAMP) mutations (type 2B)
   4) Transferrin-receptor 2 deficiency (type 3)
   5) Ferroportin deficiency (type 4)
d. Some causes of secondary iron overload
   1) Anemia with ineffective erythropoiesis (e.g., sickle cell anemia)
   2) Chronic transfusions
   3) Chronic liver disease
   4) Viral hepatitis
   5) Dietary overload

C. Blood Loss Anemia

1. **Acute blood loss anemia**
   a. Characterized by a **sudden loss of blood** resulting from trauma or other severe forms of injury
   b. **Clinical symptoms:** Hypovolemia, rapid pulse, low blood pressure, pallor
   c. **Laboratory: Normocytic/normochromic anemia**; initially normal reticulocyte count, hemoglobin/hematocrit; in a few hours, increase in platelet count and leukocytosis with a left shift, drop in hemoglobin/hematocrit and RBC; reticulocytosis in 3–5 days
2. **Chronic blood loss anemia**
   a. Characterized by a **gradual, long-term loss of blood**; often caused by gastrointestinal bleeding
   b. **Laboratory: Initially normocytic/normochromic anemia** that over time causes a decrease in hemoglobin/hematocrit; **gradual loss** of **iron** causes **microcytic/hypochromic anemia**

D. Hemolytic Anemias Due to Intrinsic Defects

1. All cause a **normocytic/normochromic anemia**; usually hereditary with reticulocytosis due to accelerated destruction
2. **Hereditary spherocytosis**
   a. **Most common membrane defect**; autosomal dominant; characterized by splenomegaly, variable degree of anemia, **spherocytes** on the peripheral blood smear
   b. Increased permeability of the membrane to sodium
   c. Results in loss of membrane fragments; erythrocytes have **decreased surface area-to-volume ratio**; rigid spherocytes culled/removed by splenic macrophages
   d. **Laboratory:** Spherocytes, **MCHC may be >37 g/dL**, increased osmotic fragility, and increased serum bilirubin

3. **Hereditary elliptocytosis (ovalocytosis)**
   a. Autosomal dominant; most persons **asymptomatic** due to normal erythrocyte life span; **>25% ovalocytes** on the peripheral blood smear
   b. Membrane defect is caused by polarization of cholesterol at the ends of the cell rather than around pallor area.
4. **Hereditary stomatocytosis**
   a. Autosomal dominant; variable degree of anemia; **up to 50% stomatocytes** on the blood smear
   b. Membrane defect due to abnormal permeability to both sodium and potassium; causes erythrocyte swelling
5. **Hereditary acanthocytosis (abetalipoproteinemia)**
   a. Autosomal recessive; mild anemia associated with steatorrhea, neurological and retinal abnormalities; 50–100% of erythrocytes are **acanthocytes**
   b. Increased cholesterol:lecithin ratio in the membrane due to abnormal plasma lipid concentrations; absence of serum β-lipoprotein needed for lipid transport
6. **G6PD (glucose-6-phosphate dehydrogenase) deficiency**
   a. **Sex-linked enzyme defect**; most common enzyme deficiency in the **hexose monophosphate shunt**
   b. Reduced glutathione levels are not maintained because of decreased NADPH generation.
   c. Results in oxidation of hemoglobin to **methemoglobin** (Fe^{3+}); denatures to form **Heinz bodies**
   d. Usually not anemic until oxidatively challenged (primaquine, sulfa drugs); then severe hemolytic anemia with reticulocytosis
7. **Pyruvate kinase (PK) deficiency**
   a. Autosomal recessive; most common enzyme deficiency in **Embden-Meyerhof pathway**
   b. Lack of ATP causes impairment of the cation pump that controls intracellular sodium and potassium levels.
   c. Decreased erythrocyte deformability reduces their life span.
   d. Severe hemolytic anemia with reticulocytosis and echinocytes
8. **Paroxysmal nocturnal hemoglobinuria (PNH)**
   a. An **acquired** membrane defect in which the red cell membrane has an increased sensitivity for **complement binding** as compared to normal erythrocytes
   b. Etiology unknown
   c. All cells are abnormally sensitive to lysis by complement.
   d. **Characterized by:** Pancytopenia; chronic intravascular hemolysis causes hemoglobinuria and hemosiderinuria at an acid pH at night; PNH noted for low leukocyte alkaline phosphatase (LAP) score; Ham's and sugar water tests used in diagnosis; increased incidence of acute leukemia
   e. Although Ham's and sugar water tests have been traditionally used in diagnosis of PNH, the standard now used is flow cytometry to detect deficiencies for surface expression of glycosyl phosphatidylinositol (GPI)-linked proteins such as CD55 and CD59.

E. Hemolytic Anemias Due to Extrinsic/Immune Defects

1. All cause a **normocytic/normochromic anemia** due to defects extrinsic to the RBC. All are acquired disorders that cause **accelerated destruction** with **reticulocytosis.**
2. **Warm autoimmune hemolytic anemia (WAIHA)**
   a. RBCs are coated with **IgG and/or complement.** Macrophages may phagocytize these RBCs, or they may remove the antibody or complement from the RBC's surface, causing membrane loss and spherocytes.
   b. 60% of cases are idiopathic; other cases are secondary to diseases that alter the immune response (e.g., chronic lymphocytic leukemia, lymphoma); can also be drug induced.
   c. **Laboratory:** Spherocytes, MCHC may be >37 g/dL, increased osmotic fragility, bilirubin, reticulocyte count; occasional nRBCs present; positive direct antiglobulin test (DAT) helpful in differentiating from hereditary spherocytosis.
3. **Cold autoimmune hemolytic anemia (CAIHA or cold hemagglutinin disease)**
   a. RBCs are coated with **IgM and complement** at temperatures below 37°C. RBCs are lysed by complement or phagocytized by macrophages. Antibody is usually anti-I but can be anti-i.
   b. Can be **idiopathic**, or secondary to ***Mycoplasma pneumoniae***, lymphoma, or infectious mononucleosis
   c. **Laboratory:** Seasonal symptoms; RBC clumping can be seen both macroscopically and microscopically; MCHC >37 g/dL; increased bilirubin, reticulocyte count; positive DAT detects complement-coated RBCs
   d. If antibody titer is high enough, sample must be warmed to 37°C to obtain accurate RBC and indices results.
4. **Paroxysmal cold hemoglobinuria (PCH)**
   a. An **IgG biphasic Donath-Landsteiner antibody** with **P specificity** fixes complement to RBCs in the cold (less than 20°C); the complement-coated RBCs lyse when warmed to 37°C.
   b. Can be **idiopathic**, or secondary to viral infections (e.g., measles and mumps) and non-Hodgkin lymphoma
   c. **Laboratory:** Variable anemia following hemolytic process; increased bilirubin and plasma hemoglobin, decreased haptoglobin; DAT may be positive; Donath-Landsteiner test positive
5. **Hemolytic transfusion reaction**
   a. Recipient has antibodies to antigens on donor RBCs; donor cells are destroyed.
   b. **ABO incompatibility** causes an immediate reaction with massive intravascular hemolysis that is complement induced.
      1) Usually **IgM** antibodies
      2) Can trigger **DIC** due to release of tissue factor from the lysed RBCs
   c. **Laboratory:** Positive DAT, increased plasma hemoglobin

6. **Hemolytic disease of the newborn (HDN)**
   a. **May be** due to **Rh incompatibility** (erythroblastosis fetalis)
      1) Rh-negative woman is exposed to Rh antigen from fetus and forms IgG antibody; this antibody will cross the placenta and destroy RBCs of the **next fetus** that is Rh positive.
      2) **Laboratory:** Severe anemia, nRBCs, positive DAT; very high bilirubin levels cause **kernicterus** leading to brain damage
      3) Exchange transfusions *in utero* or shortly after birth
      4) No longer a common problem with the use of Rh immunoglobulin (RhoGam)
   b. May be due to **ABO incompatibility**
      1) Group O woman develops IgG antibody that crosses the placenta and **coats** fetal RBCs when fetus is group A or B. The coated RBCs are phagocytized.
      2) **Laboratory:** Mild or no anemia, few spherocytes, weakly positive DAT, slightly increased bilirubin

F. Hemolytic Anemias Due to Extrinsic/Nonimmune Defects

1. All cause a **normocytic/normochromic anemia** caused by trauma to the RBC. All are **acquired** disorders that cause intravascular hemolysis with **schistocytes** and **thrombocytopenia.**
2. **Microangiopathic hemolytic anemias (MAHAs)**
   a. **Disseminated intravascular coagulation (DIC)**
      1) Systemic clotting is initiated by activation of the coagulation cascade due to toxins or conditions that trigger release of procoagulants (tissue factor). Multiple organ failure can occur due to clotting.
      2) Fibrin is deposited in small vessels, causing RBC fragmentation.
   b. **Hemolytic uremic syndrome (HUS)**
      1) Occurs most often in children following a gastrointestinal infection (e.g., *E. coli*)
      2) Clots form, causing **renal damage.**
   c. **Thrombotic thrombocytopenic purpura (TTP)**
      1) **TTP** occurs most often in adults.
      2) It is likely due to a deficiency of the enzyme **ADAMTS 13** that is responsible for breaking down large von Willebrand factor multimers. When multimers are not broken down, clots form, causing RBC fragmentation and central nervous system impairment.
3. **March hemoglobinuria:** Transient hemolytic anemia that occurs after forceful contact of the body with hard surfaces (e.g., marathon runners and tennis players)
4. **Other causes**
   a. Infectious agents (e.g., *P. falciparum* and *Clostridium perfringens*) damage the RBC membrane. **Schistocytes** and **spherocytes** are seen on the blood smear.
   b. Mechanical trauma, caused by prosthetic heart valves (Waring blender syndrome), chemicals, drugs, and snake venom, damage the RBCs through various mechanisms.

c. Thermal burns (third degree) cause direct damage to the RBC membrane, producing acute hemolysis, which is characterized by severe anemia with many schistocytes and micro-spherocytes.

X. HEMOGLOBINOPATHIES

A. Introduction: These are a group of inherited disorders causing **structurally abnormal** globin chain synthesis due to **amino acid substitutions** (qualitative defect); changes in RBC deformability and electrophoretic mobility can occur. Homozygous (disease) conditions (both globin chains affected) are more serious than heterozygous(trait) conditions (only one globin chain affected). **Target cells** are associated with the hemoglobinopathies. Hemoglobin electrophoresis, isoelectric focusing, and/or DNA (PCR) analysis may be used to confirm the diagnosis. The amino acid substitution causing formation of **Hgb S** is the **most common, Hgb C** is the **second** most common, and **Hgb E** is the third most common.

B. Sickle Cell Disease (Hgb SS)

1. **Sickle cell disease** is caused when **valine** replaces **glutamic acid** at position 6 on **both beta chains.** It results in a decrease in hemoglobin solubility and function. Defect is inherited from **both parents.**
2. Occurs most commonly in African-American, African, Mediterranean, and Middle East populations
3. **No Hgb A** is produced, and approximately 80% **Hgb S** and 20% **Hgb F** (the compensatory hemoglobin) are seen. Hgb A_2 is variable.
4. Hemoglobin insolubility results when deoxyhemoglobin is formed. Hemoglobin crystallizes in erythrocytes. It is characterized by the classic **sickled shape** of erythrocytes.
5. **Clinical findings**
   a. Erythrocytes become rigid and trapped in capillaries; blood flow restriction causes lack of oxygen to the tissues, resulting in **tissue necrosis.**
   b. All organs are affected, with **kidney failure** being a common outcome; hyposplenism and joint swelling also occur.
   c. **Vaso-occlusive crisis** occurs with increased bone marrow response to the **hemolytic anemia.** Crisis can be initiated by many physiological factors, including surgery, trauma, pregnancy, high altitudes, etc.
   d. Apparent immunity to *Plasmodium falciparum*
6. Diagnosis is made after 6 months of age (time of beta-gamma globin chain switch), with life expectancy of 50 years with proper treatment. Death usually results from infection or congestive heart failure.
7. **Laboratory**
   a. Severe **normochromic/normocytic hemolytic anemia** with polychromasia resulting from premature release of reticulocytes; bone marrow erythroid hyperplasia (M:E ratio decreases)
   b. Sickle cells, target cells, nucleated RBCs, Pappenheimer bodies, and Howell-Jolly bodies are seen. Increased bilirubin and decreased haptoglobin are characteristic due to hemolysis.

c. Positive hemoglobin solubility screening test
d. **Hgb S** migrates with hemoglobins **D and G** on alkaline hemoglobin electrophoresis; can differentiate using acid electrophoresis.

C. Sickle Cell Trait (Hgb AS)

1. **Sickle cell trait** is caused when **valine** replaces **glutamic acid** at position 6 on **one beta chain.** Defect is inherited from **one parent.** One normal beta chain can produce some Hgb A.
2. Approximately 60% Hgb A and 40% Hgb S are produced, with normal amounts of Hgbs A_2 and F.
3. This **heterozygous trait** is the most common hemoglobinopathy in the United States.
4. Sickle cell trait generally produces no clinical symptoms. Anemia is rare but, if present, will be normochromic/normocytic, and sickling can occur during rare crisis states (same as in Hgb SS).
5. Positive hemoglobin solubility screening test
6. Apparent immunity to *Plasmodium falciparum*

D. Hgb C Disease/Hgb CC

1. **Hgb C disease** is caused when **lysine** replaces **glutamic acid** at position 6 on **both beta chains.** Defect is inherited from **both parents.**
2. Occurs in the African-American and African populations
3. **No Hgb A** is produced; approximately **90% Hgb C, 2% Hgb A_2,** and **7% Hgb F** are produced. Mild anemia may be present.
4. **Laboratory: Normochromic/normocytic anemia** with target cells; characterized by intracellular rod-like **C crystals**
5. **Hgb C** migrates with hemoglobins **A_2, E,** and **O** on alkaline hemoglobin electrophresis; can differentiate hemoglobins using acid electrophoresis.
6. A person living with heterozygous Hgb C trait is asymptomatic, with no anemia; the one normal beta chain is able to produce approximately 60% Hgb A and 40% Hgb C, with normal amounts of Hgb A_2 and Hgb F.

E. Hgb SC Disease

1. **Hgb SC disease** is a double **heterozygous** condition where an abnormal sickle gene from one parent and an abnormal C gene from the other parent are inherited.
2. Seen in African, Mediterranean, and Middle Eastern populations; symptoms less severe than sickle cell anemia but more severe than Hgb C disease
3. **No Hgb A** is produced; approximately **50% Hgb S** and **50% Hgb C** are produced. Compensatory Hgb F may be elevated up to 7%.
4. **Laboratory:** Moderate to severe **normocytic/normochromic anemia** with target cells; characterized by SC crystals; may see rare sickle cells or C crystals; positive hemoglobin solubility screening test

F. Other Hemoglobinopathies

1. **Hemoglobin E**
   a. Caused when **lysine** replaces **glutamic acid** at position 26 on the **beta chain**
   b. Found more commonly in Southeast Asian, African, and African-American populations
   c. Homozygous condition results in mild anemia with microcytes and target cells; heterozygotes are asymptomatic.
   d. **Hgb E** migrates with hemoglobins **A_2, C,** and **O** on alkaline hemoglobin electrophoresis.
2. **Hemoglobin D**
   a. Caused when **glycine** replaces **glutamic acid** at position 121 on the **beta chain**
   b. Found more commonly in Middle Eastern and Indian populations
   c. Both homozygous and heterozygous conditions are asymptomatic.
   d. **Hgb D migrates** with **Hgb S** and **Hgb G** on alkaline hemoglobin electrophoresis.

XI. THALASSEMIAS

A. Introduction: Group of inherited disorders causing **decreased rate of synthesis** of a structurally normal globin chain (quantitative defect); characterized by **microcytic/hypochromic** RBCs and **target cells**

1. Classified according to the globin chain affected
2. Found in Mediterranean (beta), Asian (alpha), and African (alpha and beta) populations
3. **Severity varies** from no clinical abnormalities to transfusion-dependent to fatal
4. **Thalassemia major: Severe anemia**; either no alpha or no beta chains produced
5. **Thalassemia minor/trait: Mild anemia**; sufficient alpha and beta chains produced to make normal hemoglobins **A, A_2,** and **F**, but may be in **abnormal amounts**

B. Beta-Thalassemia

1. **Major/homozygous (Cooley anemia)**
   a. Markedly decreased rate of synthesis or absence of both beta chains results in an excess of alpha chains; no **Hgb A** can be produced; compensate with up to 90% **Hgb F.**
   b. Excess alpha chains precipitate on the RBC membrane, form Heinz bodies, and cause rigidity; destroyed in the bone marrow or removed by the spleen
   c. Symptomatic by 6 months of age; hepatosplenomegaly, stunted growth, jaundice; prominent facial bones, especially the cheek and jaw; iron overload from RBC destruction and multiple transfusions cause organ failure

d. **Laboratory:** Severe **microcytic/hypochromic anemia**, target cells, teardrops, many nRBCs, basophilic stippling, Howell-Jolly bodies, Pappenheimer bodies, Heinz bodies; increased serum iron and increased bilirubin reflect the hemolysis

2. **Minor/heterozygous**
   a. Decreased rate of synthesis of one of the beta chains; other beta chain normal
   b. **Laboratory:** Mild **microcytic/hypochromic anemia**, with a normal or slightly elevated RBC count; target cells, basophilic stippling
   c. Hgb A is slightly decreased, but **Hgb A_2** is slightly **increased** to compensate

C. Alpha-Thalassemia

1. **Major (hydrops fetalis)**
   a. All **four alpha genes** are **deleted; no normal hemoglobins** are produced.
   b. 80% **hemoglobin Bart's (γ_4)** produced; cannot carry oxygen; incompatible with life; die *in utero* or shortly after birth
2. **Hgb H disease**
   a. **Three alpha genes** are **deleted.** Decrease in alpha chains leads to beta chain excess.
   b. **Hemoglobin H (β_4)**, an unstable hemoglobin, is produced. **Heinz bodies** form and rigid RBCs are destroyed in the spleen. Distinguishing characteristics include: moderate **microcytic/hypochromic anemia**; up to 30% Hgb H; the rest is Hgb A.
3. **Minor/trait**
   a. **Two alpha genes** are **deleted.** Patients are usually asymptomatic and discovered accidentally. Up to 6% **Hgb Bart's** in newborns may be helpful in diagnosis; absent by 3 months of age
   b. Mild **microcytic/hypochromic anemia** often with a high RBC count and target cells
4. **Silent carrier**
   a. **One alpha gene** is **deleted.** Patients are asymptomatic and are often not diagnosed unless gene analysis is done.
   b. Borderline low MCV may be the only sign.

D. Thalassemia/Hemoglobinopathy Interactions

1. Caused by the inheritance of a thalassemia gene from one parent and a hemoglobin variant gene from the other parent
2. Severity and symptoms depend on the specific interactions.
3. Common interactions include Hgb S/beta-thalassemia, Hgb C/beta-thalassemia, and Hgb E/beta-thalassemia.

XII. HEMATOLOGY TESTS

A. Blood Cell Enumeration—Manual Methods

1. Manual **WBC count** using a hemacytometer
   a. Dilute a well-mixed, EDTA, whole blood sample 1:20 with 3% glacial acetic acid; allow 10 minutes for complete RBC lysis; fill both sides of hemacytometer; allow 1–2 minutes for settling.
   b. Use bright field or phase microscopy, count WBCs seen in the four 1-mm^2 corner squares on both sides of the hemacytometer, use the 10 × objective. Total area counted is **8 mm^2.**
   c. **Formula**

$$\text{WBC/mm}^3 = \frac{\text{Total WBCs counted} \times \text{dilution (20)}}{\text{Total area counted (mm}^2) \times \text{depth (0.1)}}$$

   d. Alternate dilution factor and area counted can be used; appropriate adjustments must be made to the formula. Other diluents (1% ammonium oxalate) can also be used.
   e. **Correction for presence of nucleated RBCs**

$$\text{Corrected WBC/mm}^3 = \frac{100 \times \text{uncorrected WBCs}}{100 + \#\text{nRBCs per 100 WBCs}}$$

2. **Platelet count**
   a. Dilute a well-mixed, EDTA, whole blood sample 1:100 with 1% ammonium oxalate; allow 10 minutes for complete RBC lysis; fill both sides of hemacytometer; allow 10 minutes for complete settling in a humidified chamber to prevent evaporation.
   b. Use phase (preferred) or bright field microscopy; count platelets seen in the **center** 1-mm^2 square on both sides of the hemacytometer; use the 40× objective. Total area counted is **2 mm^2.**
   c. **Formula**

$$\text{PLT count/mm}^3 = \frac{\text{Total PLTs counted} \times \text{dilution (100)}}{\text{Total area counted (mm}^2) \times \text{depth (0.1)}}$$

3. **Sources of error** involving manual cell counts
   a. Specimen clotted
   b. Sample inadequately mixed before diluting
   c. Equipment not thoroughly cleaned or dried
   d. Technical errors due to evaporation on the hemacytometer, diluting/plating, following procedure, counting of cells, calculating results

B. Blood Cell Enumeration—Automated Methods

1. **Electrical impedance**
   a. Cells pass through an aperture with an electrical current flowing through simultaneously. Cells do not conduct current but rather they change electrical resistance, which is then counted as voltage pulses.
   b. The number of pulses generated is proportional to the number of cells present; amplitude of the pulse generated is proportional to the size of the cell.
   c. Sample is diluted in isotonic conductive solution that preserves cell shape and characteristics.
      1) Dilutions used are dependent on instrument/methodology used.
      2) Platelets are counted simultaneously with RBCs.
      3) Sample for counting WBCs is mixed with reagent to lyse RBCs. A commercially available reagent, which both lyses RBCs and converts hemoglobin to cyanmethemoglobin, can be used to determine hemoglobin and WBCs in one dilution.
   d. Thresholds are used to separate cell populations and subpopulations.
   e. Hydrodynamic focusing is utilized to reduce **cell coincidence** (chance of one cell being counted more than once).
2. **Light scattering optical method**
   a. Uses a flow cytometer with laser to measure light-scattering properties of cells
      1) Forward angle light scatter measures **cell size.**
      2) Side angle light scatter provides information on cell **granularity** and **lobularity.**
      3) Number of pulses generated is proportional to the number of cells present.
   b. Dilutions used are dependent on instrument/methodology used.
3. Interpretative reports give relative percentages and absolute counts for the five leukocyte subpopulations (most instruments).
4. Suspect "**flags**" indicate problems: Exceeding linearity, lack of agreement among apertures, unacceptable distribution caused by unusual cell populations.
5. Automated cell count errors
   a. WBC counts exceeding instrument linearity limits result in increased cell turbidity and may falsely increase the hemoglobin, MCH, and MCHC.
   b. Glucose over 600 mg/dL (hyperosmolarity) may increase the MCV and hematocrit and decrease the MCHC.
   c. Cold agglutinins increase the MCV, MCH, and MCHC and decrease the RBC count and hematocrit.
   d. Lipemia increases the hemoglobin, MCH, and MCHC.
   e. Repeat the analysis if:
      1) **Rule of three** (shown below) failure on a normocytic sample (especially MCHC >37 g/dL)
         a) RBC $\times$ 3 = Hgb
         b) RBC $\times$ 9 = Hct
         c) Hgb $\times$ 3 = Hct

2) Any result outside linearity limits established by manufacturer (dilute into linearity range)
3) Unexplained **delta check failures** (e.g., results do not correlate with recent previous results, especially MCV)

C. Histograms and Scatterplots

1. A **histogram** utilizes **impedance technology**, and it is a representation of cell number versus one measured property, usually cell size. It is used for WBCs, RBCs, and platelets.
   a. **WBC histogram**
      1) 35–450 fL is the reference size range for **WBCs.**
      2) First peak: 35–90 fL is the range for **lymphocytes.**
      3) Second peak: 90–160 fL is the range for **mononuclear cells (monocytes, reactive lymphocytes,** and **immature WBCs).**
      4) Third peak: 160–450 fL is the range for **granulocytes.**
   b. **Abnormal WBC histogram**
      1) Population before 35 fL may indicate nucleated RBCs **(nRBCs), giant** or **clumped platelets.**
      2) Peak overlap at 90 fL may indicate **reactive lymphocytes** or **blast cells.**
      3) Peak overlap at 160 fL may indicate an increase in **bands, immature neutrophils, eosinophils**, or **basophils.**
      4) Population after 450 fL may indicate a **high granulocyte** count.
   c. **RBC histogram**
      1) 36 fL and above is the reference size range for **RBCs.**
      2) A normal RBC histogram will show a single peak between 70 and 110 fL that will correlate with the MCV.
   d. **Abnormal RBC histogram**
      1) Two peaks indicate a **dimorphic** erythrocyte population.
      2) Increased curve width will correlate with an increased RDW **(anisocytosis).**
      3) Shift to the right indicates an increased MCV **(macrocytic).**
      4) Shift to the left indicates a decreased MCV **(microcytic).**
   e. **Platelet histogram**
      1) 2–20 fL is the reference size range for **platelets.**
      2) **Lower region interference** (<2 fL) indicates electrical interference; **upper region interference** (>20 fL) indicates microcytic RBCs or schistocytes, giant or clumped platelets.
2. A **scatterplot/scattergram** is a two-dimensional representation of two or more cell properties or characteristics plotted against each other (e.g., size vs. granularity or lobularity). Scatterplots of WBCs are displayed on a monitor and are color coded for different subpopulations.
   a. Methodologies include radio frequency, fluorescence, and cytochemistry.
   b. Correlation between abnormal cell populations and suspect flags is generally very good.

D. Hemoglobin Measurement

1. Blood oxygen capacity: Measures functional hemoglobin

$$\frac{\text{Oxygen capacity in mL/dL blood}}{\text{1.34 (Hgb oxygen capacity)}} = \text{grams of Hgb/dL blood}$$

2. Cyanmethemoglobin method is the **reference method**; it will measure all hemoglobins except sulfhemoglobin.
   a. Uses **Drabkin** reagent (potassium ferricyanide and KCN) to lyse RBCs and convert heme iron to the ferric state (Fe^{3+}), forming methemoglobin. KCN in the reagent converts methemoglobin to cyanmethemoglobin; read spectrophotometrically at **540 nm.**
   b. Automated cell counters use some modification of the cyanmethemoglobin method to determine hemoglobin concentration.

E. Reticulocyte Counts

1. **Supravital new methylene blue stain** is used to demonstrate reticulum in reticulocytes.
2. Reticulocyte (retic) formulas:
   a. Relative count

$$\text{Retics (\%)} = \frac{\text{\# of retics}}{\text{1000 RBCs observed}} \times 100$$

   b. Absolute count

$$\text{Absolute retic } (\times 10^9/\text{L}) = \text{Retic \%} \times \text{RBC count } (¥\ 10^{12}/\text{L})/100$$

3. Corrected reticulocyte counts are calculated to account for the degree of anemia by using a standard normal hematocrit of 45% expressed in SI units.

$$\text{Corrected retic count} = \text{Retic \%} \times \frac{\text{Hct (L/L)}}{\text{0.45 L/L}}$$

4. Immature reticulocyte fraction (IRF) is an instrument calculated parameter that indicates the ratio of immature reticulocytes to total reticulocytes.

F. Erythrocyte Sedimentation Rate: ESR measures degree of settling of RBCs in plasma in an anticoagulated specimen during a specific time, usually 1 hour. High fibrinogen or protein levels increase the ESR.

1. **Reference range:** Approximately 0–20 mm/hr; age and sex dependent
2. ESR is **increased** in chronic inflammatory conditions, including rheumatoid arthritis and pregnancy (increased fibrinogen), bacterial infection, malignancy, tissue damage, multiple myeloma, Waldenström macroglobulinemia, and severe anemia.

a. **Sources of error** causing **falsely increased** results: Tilted column, hemolysis, increased room temperature

3. ESR is **normal to decreased** in polycythemia, sickle cell anemia, spherocytosis, and other conditions with poikilocytosis (prevents rouleaux formation).
   a. **Sources of error** causing **falsely decreased** results: Clotted sample, excess anticoagulant, "old" blood (spherocytes form)

G. Hemoglobin F (Kleihauer-Betke method): Count dense-staining Hgb F cells and the number of ghost cells containing Hgb A to obtain percentage.

1. It is used to detect the presence of fetal cells in the maternal circulation during problem pregnancies because Hgb F in fetal cells resists acid elution.
2. It differentiates hereditary persistence of fetal hemoglobin from other conditions associated with high Hgb F levels.
3. Normal newborns have 70–90% Hgb F levels.

H. Solubility Test for Hemoglobin S (Sickle Cell Prep)

1. Hemoglobin S is insoluble when combined with a reducing agent (sodium dithionite).
2. Hgb S will crystallize and give a turbid appearance to the solution.
3. The test will **not** differentiate homozygous from heterozygous conditions containing Hgb S.
4. Follow up a positive solubility test with hemoglobin electrophoresis.

I. Hemoglobin Electrophoresis

1. Procedure for the identification of normal and abnormal hemoglobins
2. Methodology is based on net negative charges, which cause hemoglobins to migrate from the negative **(cathode)** region toward the positive **(anode)** region. The distance a particular hemoglobin molecule migrates is due to its net electrical charge.
3. Two types of electrophoresis: **Cellulose acetate** at **pH 8.6** and **citrate agar** at **pH 6.2**
4. Migration of hemoglobin is dependent on net negative charge and buffer pH.
5. **Cellulose Acetate (pH 8.6) Hemoglobin Electrophoresis**

Cathode (–)				Anode (+)
(x) origin	A_2	S	F	A
	C	D		
	E	G		
	O			

   a. At pH 8.6, Hgb A migrates the fastest, and Hgb A_2, C, E, and O migrate the slowest.

6. **Citrate Agar (pH 6.2) Hemoglobin Electrophoresis**

Anode (+)				Cathode (–)
C S	(x) origin	A	F	
		A_2		
		D		
		G		
		E		
		O		

a. At pH 6.2, Hgb S is differentiated from Hgb D and G.
b. At pH 6.2, Hgb C is differentiated from Hgb A_2, E, and O.

J. Flow Cytometry

1. **Principle: Cells** in a suspension of buffered solution are **labeled with** one to several **fluorescent compounds.** This cell suspension is run under high pressure and in a single, narrow stream through a laser, causing excitation of the fluorescent compound(s) and resulting in the emission of light energy. This energy is amplified by a photomultiplier tube and is subsequently converted into computerized data, which upon analysis provides information regarding number, size, and cellular composition of the population assayed.
2. Major components of a **flow cytometer**
   a. **Fluidics**—Flow chamber for single cell separation, sheath fluid, and hydrodynamic focusing
   b. **Optics**—Excitation light sources include lasers (argon, krypton, helium-neon, helium-cadmium, diode) or lamps (mercury, xenon-mercury). Light is separated by dichroic mirrors and filters.
   c. **Electronics**—Photomultiplier tube amplifies light energy, then coverts this to voltage pulses; computers translate pulses into data files.
3. Hydrodynamic focusing uses laminar flow to line the cells up single file.
4. **Light** is **scattered** at 90 degrees or forward.
5. **Fluorescent dyes** used in flow cytometry include, but are not limited to, allophycocyanin (APC), acridine orange (AO), chromomycin A3, cyanine dye (Cy), fluorescein isothiocyanate (FITC), peridinin chlorophyll protein (PerCP), phycoerythrin (PE), propidium iodine (PI), pyronin Y, rhodamine isothiocyanate, and sulforhodamine 101 acid chloride.
6. **Specimens analyzed** by flow cytometry: Leukocytes, erythrocytes, lymph nodes, peripheral whole blood, bone marrow, tumors, and other tissues
7. **Clinical applications:** Differentiation of T and B cells; cell cycle analysis; diagnosing and following patients with leukemia, lymphoma, and autoimmune or deficiency diseases; karyotyping; and monitoring a patient's response to drug therapy

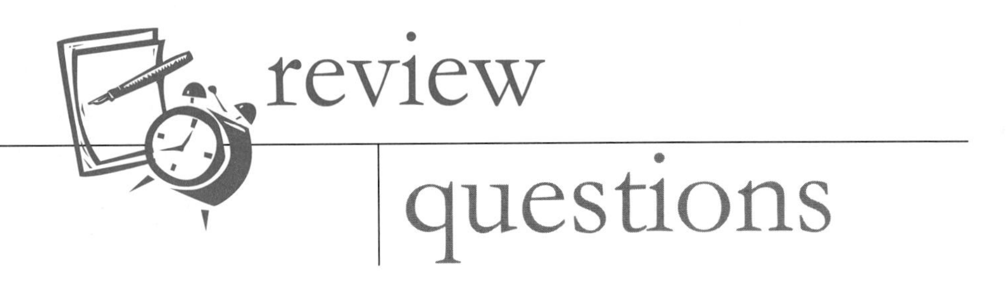

INSTRUCTIONS Each of the questions or incomplete statements that follow is comprised of four suggested responses. Select the *best* answer or completion statement in each case.

Hematopoiesis

1. What is the first type of cell produced by the developing embryo?
   A. Erythrocyte
   B. Granulocyte
   C. Lymphocyte
   D. Thrombocyte
2. What percentage of tissue located in the bone marrow cavities of adults is fat?
   A. 10%
   B. 25%
   C. 50%
   D. 75%
3. Which of the following is a characteristic of pluripotent hematopoietic stem cells?
   A. Does possess self-renewal ability
   B. Produce progenitor cells that are not restricted to any specific cell lineage
   C. Express the stem cell marker CD23
   D. Are morphologically recognizable
4. In an adult, what are the two best areas for obtaining active bone marrow by aspiration?
   A. Vertebra, tibia
   B. Sternum, vertebra
   C. Anterior iliac crest, tibia
   D. Posterior iliac crest, sternum
5. What is the normal ratio of myeloid to erythroid precursors in bone marrow (M:E ratio)?
   A. 1:1
   B. 1:3
   C. 4:1
   D. 8:1
6. Which of the following accurately describe hematopoietic growth factors?
   A. Bind to target cell receptors to express activity
   B. Action of majority is lineage restricted
   C. Does not promote or suppress cell death
   D. Does not stimulate or inhibit cell proliferation

7. In the third month of gestation, what is the primary site of hematopoiesis?
   A. Liver
   B. Marrow of long bones
   C. Spleen
   D. Yolk sac

8. The mechanism that relays information about tissue oxygen levels to erythropoietin-producing sites is located in the
   A. Brain
   B. Kidney
   C. Liver
   D. Spleen

9. Antigen-independent lymphopoiesis occurs in primary lymphoid tissue located in the
   A. Liver and kidney
   B. Spleen and lymph nodes
   C. Peyer's patches and spleen
   D. Thymus and bone marrow

10. Programmed cell death is called
    A. Necrosis
    B. Apoptosis
    C. Cellular senescence
    D. Terminal differentiation

11. In what area of the bone marrow does hematopoiesis take place?
    A. Cords
    B. Endosteum
    C. Endothelium
    D. Sinuses

12. Bone marrow cellularity refers to the ratio of
    A. Red cell precursors to white cell precursors
    B. Hematopoietic tissue to adipose tissue
    C. Granulocytic cells to erythrocytic cells
    D. Extravascular tissue to intravascular tissue

13. New research has shown that interleukins and colony stimulating factors can be produced by many different cells including:
    A. B lymphocytes and erythrocytes
    B. Erythrocytes and thrombocytes
    C. Monocytes and T lymphocytes
    D. Neutrophils and monocytes

14. What is the approximate total blood volume in an adult?
    A. 1 L
    B. 2 L
    C. 6 L
    D. 12 L

15. The myeloid progenitor cell can produce cells committed to
    A. Granulocytic, erythrocytic, monocytic, or megakaryocytic lineages
    B. Granulocytic, monocytic, lymphocytic, or megakaryocytic lineages
    C. Erythrocytic, granulocytic, monocytic, or lymphocytic lineages
    D. Erythrocytic, granulocytic, lymphocytic, or megakaryocytic lineages

16. The largest hematopoietic cells in normal bone marrow are
    A. Osteoblasts
    B. Osteoclasts
    C. Megakaryocytes
    D. Plasma cells

17. When evaluating a bone marrow aspirate smear, which finding is considered abnormal?
    A. A predominance of granulocyte precursors as compared to nucleated red cells
    B. Detection of stainable iron in macrophages and erythroid precursors with Prussian blue
    C. An average of three megakaryocytes seen per low power (10×) field
    D. The presence of 10% myeloblasts on the cell differential count

18. As most blood cell lines mature, which of the following is characteristic?
    A. Cell diameter increases
    B. Nucleus to cytoplasm ratio (N:C) decreases
    C. Nuclear chromatin becomes less condensed
    D. Basophilia of the cytoplasm increases
19. Which of the following describes thrombopoietin (TPO)?
    A. Renal hormone that regulates marrow red cell production
    B. Marrow hormone secreted by developing megakaryoblasts
    C. Hormone produced by the liver that stimulates megakaryopoiesis
    D. Pituitary hormone that controls platelet sequestration by the spleen
20. When the hepatic phase of fetal life is reactivated in an adult, hematopoiesis can be termed
    A. Myeloid or medullary
    B. Myeloid metaplasia or extramedullary
    C. Myelophthisis or myelodysplasia
    D. Mesoblastic or mesenchymal

Erythrocytes

21. What is the average life span of a normal red blood cell?
    A. 1 day
    B. 10 days
    C. 60 days
    D. 120 days
22. The Na^+–K^+ cation pump is an important mechanism in keeping the red blood cell intact. Its function is to maintain a high level of
    A. Intracellular Na^+
    B. Intracellular K^+
    C. Plasma Na^+
    D. Plasma K^+
23. Which of the following depicts the structure of the hemoglobin molecule?
    A. Two heme groups, two globin chains
    B. Four heme groups, two globin chains
    C. Two heme groups, four globin chains
    D. Four heme groups, four globin chains
24. Which of the following describes the process known as *culling?*
    A. Release of red cells from the bone marrow
    B. Binding of free hemoglobin by transport proteins
    C. Incorporation of iron into protoporphyrin IX
    D. Removal of abnormal red cells by the spleen
25. Hemoglobin forms that are incapable of oxygen transport include
    A. Deoxyhemoglobin and oxyhemoglobin
    B. Oxyhemoglobin and carboxyhemoglobin
    C. Carboxyhemoglobin and methemoglobin
    D. Methemoglobin and deoxyhemoglobin
26. The majority of iron found in an adult is a constituent of
    A. Ferritin
    B. Myoglobin
    C. Hemoglobin
    D. Peroxidase
27. A common source of interference in the cyanmethemoglobin method is
    A. Hemolysis
    B. Very high WBC count
    C. Cold agglutinin
    D. Clumped platelets
28. What red cell morphologic abnormality is described by the term "poikilocytosis"?
    A. Variations in size
    B. Deviations from normal shape
    C. Presence of inclusions
    D. Alterations in hemoglobin concentration

29. Howell-Jolly bodies are composed of
   A. DNA
   B. Iron
   C. Reticulum
   D. RNA

30. When spherocytes are reported, what is observed on the peripheral blood smear?
   A. Red cells without a central pallor
   B. Red cells with blunt projections
   C. Red cells with sharp projections
   D. Red cells with intracellular rod-shaped crystals

31. The red cells found in lead poisoning characteristically exhibit coarse granules composed of _______ that are reported as _______.
   A. precipitated hemoglobin; Pappenheimer bodies
   B. aggregated ribosomes; basophilic stippling
   C. nuclear fragments; Pappenheimer bodies
   D. excess iron deposits; basophilic stippling

32. The most characteristic peripheral blood smear finding in multiple myeloma is:
   A. Plasmacytic satellitosis in the bone marrow
   B. Many plasma cells in the peripheral blood
   C. Many mott cells in the peripheral blood
   D. Rouleaux formation of the red cells

33. Which of the following is most frequently associated with the inclusion bodies seen in Color Plate 1■?
   A. Iron-overload state
   B. Post-transfusion
   C. Post-splenectomy
   D. Iron-deficient state

34. Which of the following statements about iron absorption is *true?*
   A. Absorption occurs in the ileum.
   B. The mucosal cell always absorbs the correct amount of iron to meet needs.
   C. Absorption increases when erythropoietic activity increases.
   D. Alkaline pH favors absorption.

35. What term describes a mature red blood cell that contains iron granules or deposits?
   A. Siderosome
   B. Sideroblast
   C. Ringed sideroblast
   D. Siderocyte

36. Which of the following is associated with a "shift to the left" in the oxygen dissociation curve of hemoglobin?
   A. Decreased pH and elevated temperature
   B. Decreased oxygen affinity
   C. Decreased oxygen release
   D. Presence of 2,3-bisphosphoglycerate (2,3-BPG)

37. Which of the following statements does *not* characterize erythropoietin (EPO)?
   A. Transforms the CFU-E into the earliest recognizable RBC precursor
   B. Increases the rate of red blood cell production by the bone marrow
   C. Shortens the maturation time of developing erythroid precursors
   D. Decreases stimulation of erythropoiesis when cellular hypoxia increases

38. Which of the following factors will result in an immediate increase in oxygen delivery to the tissues?
   A. Increased pH
   B. High altitudes
   C. Increased hemoglobin binding of 2,3-BPG
   D. Increased renal release of erythropoietin

39. Periods of intense erythropoietin activity cause premature release of marrow reticulocytes into the blood. Which of the following is *not* true of these early reticulocytes?
    A. Loss of residual RNA occurs immediately upon marrow release
    B. Circulate longer than usual before reaching maturity
    C. May be termed "shift or stress reticulocytes"
    D. Show diffuse basophilia with Wright's stain
40. Which of the following inclusions is *only* visible with supravital staining?
    A. Basophilic stippling
    B. Cabot rings
    C. Heinz bodies
    D. Pappenheimer bodies
41. The presence of schistocytes on the peripheral blood smear is commonly associated with
    A. Increased iron mobilization
    B. Increased red cell destruction
    C. Decreased erythropoietin activity
    D. Decreased red cell proliferation
42. Which of the following may be a sign of accelerated bone marrow erythropoiesis?
    A. Hypercellular marrow with a decreased number of RBC precursors
    B. Bone marrow M:E ratio of 6:1
    C. Nucleated red cells in the peripheral circulation
    D. Low erythrocyte, hemoglobin, and hematocrit levels
43. Microcytic, hypochromic red cells are most often associated with impaired
    A. DNA synthesis
    B. RNA metabolism
    C. Hemoglobin synthesis
    D. Enzyme metabolism
44. When in bone marrow, the nucleated red cells present in Color Plate 2■ would be staged as
    A. Basophilic normoblasts
    B. Polychromatophilic normoblasts
    C. Orthochromic normoblasts
    D. Pronormoblasts
45. When acanthocytes are found on the blood smear, it is usually the result of
    A. Abnormal membrane permeability
    B. Altered membrane lipids
    C. Mechanical trauma
    D. Polymerization of hemoglobin molecules
46. Which erythrocyte metabolic pathway generates adenosine triphosphate (ATP) via glycolysis?
    A. Embden-Meyerhof
    B. Hexose monophosphate
    C. Rapoport-Luebering
    D. Methemoglobin reductase
47. Which of the following red blood cell precursors is the last stage to undergo mitosis?
    A. Pronormoblast
    B. Basophilic normoblast
    C. Polychromatophilic normoblast
    D. Orthochromic normoblast
48. The major adult hemoglobin requires the synthesis of alpha-globin chains and
    A. Beta-globin chains
    B. Delta-globin chains
    C. Epsilon-globin chains
    D. Gamma-globin chains
49. Defective nuclear maturation commonly results in the production of red cells that are
    A. Normocytic
    B. Hypochromic
    C. Macrocytic
    D. Microcytic

50. The major storage form of iron is
    A. Ferritin
    B. Transferrin
    C. Hemosiderin
    D. Hemachromatin

51. The red cells observed on a peripheral blood smear show extreme anisocytosis with an equal number of macrocytes and microcytes. Which of the following values correlate with this finding?
    A. MCV 108.0 fL, RDW 14.0%
    B. MCV 90.0 fL, RDW 25.0%
    C. MCV 75.0 fL, RDW 16.0%
    D. MCV 88.0 fL, RDW 12.0%

52. Excessive extravascular red cell destruction is associated with
    A. Hemoglobinemia
    B. Bilirubinemia
    C. Hemoglobinuria
    D. Hemosiderinuria

53. Which protein is primarily responsible for transport of hemoglobin dimers resulting from intravascular hemolysis?
    A. Hemopexin
    B. Albumin
    C. Hemosiderin
    D. Haptoglobin

54. The morphologic abnormality characteristically found in hemoglobinopathies is
    A. Elliptocytes
    B. Dacryocytes
    C. Codocytes
    D. Discocytes

55. Where do the early and late stages of heme synthesis occur?
    A. On ribosomes
    B. In mitochondria
    C. In cytoplasm
    D. In nucleoli

56. Spectrin is a protein that occupies a major role in
    A. Red cell membrane structure
    B. Reducing ferric iron
    C. Red cell transport and removal of CO_2
    D. Iron recovery during hemoglobin degradation

57. What is the function of reduced glutathione (GSH) in the red blood cell?
    A. Promotes Kreb's cycle activity
    B. Maintains anion balance during the "chloride shift"
    C. Neutralizes intracellular oxidants that accumulate
    D. Prevents oxygen uptake by hemoglobin

58. What does measuring the total iron-binding capacity (TIBC) represent?
    A. Amount of free iron in serum
    B. Circulating protein-bound iron
    C. Amount of iron that transferrin can bind
    D. Indirect measurement of iron stores

59. Serum ferritin is a good indicator of the amount of
    A. Cytochrome iron
    B. Storage iron
    C. Hemoglobin iron
    D. Transferrin saturation

60. Fetal hemoglobin differs from adult hemoglobin in that hemoglobin F
    A. Has a lower oxygen affinity
    B. Resists elution from red cells with acid solutions
    C. Is no longer synthesized after birth in a normal individual
    D. Has four gamma-globin chains

Erythrocyte Disorders

61. Impaired DNA metabolism is characteristic of
    A. Hemoglobin C disease
    B. Iron-deficiency anemia
    C. Sideroblastic anemia
    D. Megaloblastic anemia

62. Which of the following is associated with glucose-6-phosphate dehydrogenase (G6PD) deficiency?
    A. G6PD gene is located on the X chromosome.
    B. Ongoing intravascular hemolysis occurs.
    C. All circulating red cells, including reticulocytes, lack enzyme activity.
    D. Splenectomy can relieve the rate of red cell destruction.

63. In regard to variant hemoglobin E, $\alpha_2\beta_2^{26\,Glu \rightarrow Lys}$, which of the following statements is *false?*
    A. There are two normal alpha chains.
    B. Glutamic acid replaces lysine on position 26 of the beta chains.
    C. Hemoglobin E is the second most common hemoglobin variant known.
    D. Glutamic acid is normally found at position 26 of the beta chain.

64. Color Plate 3■ shows the peripheral blood of a 16-year-old female with a sporadic history of dizzy spells, fainting, and jaundice. This patient also had a history of periodic abdominal pain related to gallstones. Upon physical examination, she exhibited mild splenomegaly. Her hemoglobin was 107 g/L (10.7 g/dL), hematocrit was 0.32 L/L (32%), red cell indices were normal, and the direct antiglobulin test was negative. Based on history and peripheral blood morphology, which of the following statements is most likely *true?*
    A. Hemoglobin S will be revealed by electrophoresis.
    B. Tests to confirm iron deficiency should be ordered.
    C. An intrinsic hereditary defect of red cells should be suspected.
    D. The anemia is secondary to spleen and gallbladder disorders.

65. A 9-month-old male was seen in the Emergency Department with a femur fracture that had occurred from a fall down the stairs. Upon physical examination, the physician noted hepatosplenomegaly, extreme pallor, and a slight arrhythmia. A complete blood count revealed the following:

WBC	$12.2 \times 10^9/L$ ($12.2 \times 10^3/\mu L$)
RBC	$3.05 \times 10^{12}/L$ ($3.05 \times 10^6/\mu L$)
Hemoglobin	61 g/L (6.1 g/dL)
Hematocrit	0.20 L/L (20%)
MCV	65.5 fL
MCH	20 pg
MCHC	305 g/L (30.5 g/dL)
RDW	25%

The Wright stained blood smear showed the findings seen in Color Plate 4■. Hemoglobin electrophoresis was ordered with results as follows:

Hgb A	0%
Hgb A_2	3%
Hgb F	97%

Which condition is most likely causing the hematologic abnormalities?
A. Alpha-thalassemia major
B. Cooley beta-thalassemia major
C. Hemoglobin H disease
D. Hereditary persistence of hemoglobin F

66. A 14-year-old African-American male was seen in the clinic for abdominal pain. A complete blood count revealed the following:

WBC	$7.0 \times 10^9/L$ ($7.0 \times 10^3/\mu L$)
RBC	$2.90 \times 10^{12}/L$ ($2.90 \times 10^6/\mu L$)
Hemoglobin	85 g/L (8.5 g/dL)
Hematocrit	0.25 L/L (25%)
MCV	86.2 fL
MCH	29.3 pg
MCHC	340 g/L (34.0 g/dL)
RDW	21%

The perapheral smear showed the red blood cell morphology seen in Color Plate 5■. What condition is suggested by these findings?
A. Hemoglobin E disease
B. Hemoglobin S disease
C. Hemoglobin SC disease
D. Hemoglobin C disease

67. Pica is most commonly associated with which of the following conditions?
A. Pyridoxine deficiency
B. Lack of erythrocyte folate
C. Iron deficiency
D. Porphyrias

68. Of the following, the leading cause of folate deficiency is
A. Increased requirements
B. Dietary insufficiency
C. Drug inhibition
D. Malabsorption

69. Which of the following statements about sickle cell syndrome is *false?*
    A. Asplenism may result from repeated sickling crises in the homozygous state.
    B. Heterozygous persons may be partly protected from infection by falciparum malaria.
    C. Hemoglobin S is more soluble in dithionite than is normal hemoglobin.
    D. Trait conditions arc gcncrally asymptomatic with no sickle cell formation.

70. The findings seen in Color Plate 6■ can be found in patients with microangiopathic hemolytic anemia (MAHA). Which of the following conditions could *not* be responsible for this type of red cell destruction?
    A. Disseminated intravascular coagulation (DIC)
    B. Hemolytic uremic syndrome (HUS)
    C. Thrombotic thrombocytopenic purpura (TTP)
    D. Idiopathic thrombocytopenic purpura (ITP)

71. Which one of the following blood findings correlates with the presence of ringed sideroblasts in the bone marrow?
    A. Pappenheimer bodies
    B. Basophilic stippling
    C. Increased MCHC
    D. Increased spherocytes

72. Which one of the following conditions is usually associated with marked reticulocytosis?
    A. hereditary elliptocytosis
    B. Drug-induced autoimmune hemolytic anemia
    C. Vitamin B_{12} deficiency
    D. Pernicious anemia

73. Hereditary stomatocytosis manifests physiologically by changes in
    A. Hemoglobin oxygen affinity
    B. Membrane cation permeability
    C. Efficiency of hemoglobin reduction
    D. Glycolytic ATP production

74. In addition to an increase in red blood cells, which of the following is characteristic of polycythemia vera?
    A. Decreased platelets, decreased granulocytes, decreased erythropoietin level
    B. Decreased platelets, decreased granulocytes, increased erythropoietin level
    C. Increased platelets, increased granulocytes, increased erythropoietin level
    D. Increased platelets, increased granulocytes, decreased erythropoietin level

75. Which of the following is *not* characteristic of aplastic anemia?
    A. Extramedullary hematopoiesis
    B. Bone marrow hypoplasia
    C. Absolute reticulocytopenia
    D. Blood findings of pancytopenia

76. What values would you expect to obtain on hemoglobin and hematocrit determinations done immediately after a major hemorrhage, if hemoglobin and hematocrit values were normal prior to the hemorrhage?
    A. Both normal
    B. Both decreased
    C. Hemoglobin decreased, hematocrit normal
    D. Hemoglobin normal, hematocrit decreased

77. Results from a 1-day-old infant include a hemoglobin of 201 g/L (20.1 g/dL), hematocrit of 0.60 L/L (60.0%), MCV of 110.2 fL, and four nucleated red cells/100 WBCs. How should these results be interpreted?
    A. The elevated hemoglobin and hematocrit values indicate possible dehydration.
    B. The nucleated red cells suggest accelerated erythropoiesis due to a hemolytic process.
    C. Testing should be done to identify the cause of the macrocytosis.
    D. No further testing is indicated.

78. When viewing Color Plate 7■, the red blood cells with a single elongated projection are known as _______ and may be seen in _______
    A. acanthocytes; liver disease
    B. echinocytes; liver disease
    C. drepanocytes; myelofibrosis
    D. dacryocytes; myelofibrosis

79. A patient with normocytic, normochromic anemia secondary to small cell carcinoma may be exhibiting an anemia designated as
    A. Hemolytic
    B. Megaloblastic
    C. Myelophthisic
    D. Sideroblastic

80. Idiopathic aplastic anemia is best defined as a form of anemia that
    A. Has no identifiable cause
    B. Is caused by a physician's treatment
    C. Follows exposure to ionizing radiation
    D. Develops after a viral infection

81. Which of the following is a true red blood cell aplasia?
    A. Marrow replacement anemia
    B. Fanconi anemia
    C. Diamond-Blackfan anemia
    D. Donath-Landsteiner anemia

82. Which one of the following is a cause of absolute secondary erythrocytosis?
    A. Defective cardiac or pulmonary function
    B. Extreme heat
    C. Dehydration secondary to diuretic use
    D. Hemoglobins with decreased oxygen affinity

83. A cellulose acetate hemoglobin electrophoresis (alkaline pH), performed on the blood of a stillborn infant, revealed a single band that migrated farther toward the anode than did the Hb A control. What is the most likely composition of the stillborn infant's hemoglobin?
    A. Four beta chains
    B. Four gamma chains
    C. Two alpha and two beta chains
    D. Two alpha and two gamma chains

84. The most likely cause of the stillborn infant's condition in question 83 is
    A. Erythroblastosis fetalis
    B. Rh hemolytic disease of the fetus
    C. Hydrops fetalis
    D. ABO hemolytic disease of the newborn

85. Which of the following conditions show similar CBC and blood smear findings?
    A. Beta-thalassemia major and minor
    B. Folic acid and vitamin B_{12} deficiencies
    C. Acute and chronic blood loss
    D. Sickle cell disease and trait

86. Which of the following would be useful in identifying the cause of the blood profile seen in Color Plate 8■?
    A. Osmotic fragility test
    B. Reticulocyte count
    C. Direct antiglobulin test
    D. Urine urobilinogen level

87. Which of the following conditions is *not* associated with the presence of schistocytes and spherocytes?
    A. Clostridial septicemia
    B. Prosthetic heart valves
    C. Severe thermal burns
    D. Aplastic anemia

88. A 30-year-old woman who has been vomiting for 3 days has a hemoglobin value of 180 g/L (18.0 g/dL) and a hematocrit of 0.54 L/L (54.0%). Her results suggest the presence of
    A. Absolute erythrocytosis
    B. Primary polycythemia
    C. Secondary polycythemia
    D. Relative polycythemia

89. An excessive accumulation of iron in body tissues is called
    A. Hemochromatosis
    B. Erythroblastosis
    C. Megaloblastosis
    D. Acrocyanosis

90. Abetalipoproteinemia is characterized by mild anemia and numerous ________ on the peripheral blood smear.
    A. acanthocytes
    B. elliptocytes
    C. echinocytes
    D. stomatocytes

91. What is the most common cause of iron deficiency?
    A. Bleeding
    B. Gastrectomy
    C. Inadequate diet
    D. Intestinal malabsorption

92. Which one of the following is acharacteristic of beta-thalassemia major?
    A. Transfusion-dependent anemia
    B. Decreased alpha chains result in excess beta chains.
    C. Iron chelation therapy is not necessary.
    D. Common in persons of Scandinavian ancestry

93. In the anemia of chronic disease, what are the usual serum iron and transferrin levels?
    A. Serum iron decreased, transferrin decreased
    B. Serum iron decreased, transferrin increased
    C. Serum iron normal, transferrin normal
    D. Serum iron increased, transferrin increased

94. In children, the most important effect of lead poisoning is on the
    A. Liver
    B. Kidney
    C. Neurologic system
    D. Development of erythrocytes

95. Which of the following would *not* result in the dual population of red cells represented in Color Plate 9■?
    A. Blood transfusion
    B. Oral iron therapy
    C. Spleen removal
    D. Coexisting deficiencies

96. What is the most likely genetic defect in the hemoglobin of cells seen in Color Plate 10■?
    A. Substitution of valine for glutamic acid in position 6 of the alpha-globin chain
    B. Substitution of valine for glutamic acid in position 6 of the beta-globin chain
    C. Substitution of lysine for glutamic acid in position 6 of the alpha-globin chain
    D. Substitution of lysine for glutamic acid in position 6 of the beta-globin chain

97. On what criteria below is the classification of sickle cell trait versus sickle cell disease based?
    A. Severity of the clinical symptoms
    B. Number of irreversibly sickled cells (ISCs)
    C. Level of compensatory hemoglobin F
    D. Percentage of hemoglobin S on electrophoresis

98. Which of the following is the most appropriate treatment for sickle cell anemia?
    A. Hydroxyurea
    B. Supportive therapy
    C. Hyperbaric oxygen
    D. Iron

99. Which of the following values can be used to indicate the presence of a hemolytic anemia?
    A. Hemoglobin level
    B. Hematocrit level
    C. Erythrocyte count
    D. Reticulocyte count

100. A pre-operative, 20-year-old female has a mild microcytic anemia, with target cells and stippled red cells observed on the blood smear. Her hemoglobin A_2 level is quantified at 5%. What do these findings suggest?
    A. Iron-deficiency anemia
    B. Heterozygous alpha-thalassemia
    C. Heterozygous beta-thalassemia
    D. Hemoglobin S/beta-thalassemia

101. What causes the hemolytic process in glucose-6-phosphate dehydrogenase deficiency following oxidant exposure?
    A. Coating of red cells by antibody
    B. Osmotic pressure changes
    C. Complement attachment
    D. Precipitation of denatured hemoglobin

102. In clinically severe hereditary spherocytosis, which of the following findings would *not* be found post-splenectomy?
    A. Rise in the red cell count and hemoglobin level
    B. Higher number of circulating reticulocytes
    C. Increased number of Howell-Jolly bodies
    D. Transient elevation in the platelet count

103. Which of the following laboratory results is consistent with accelerated red cell destruction?
    A. Increased serum sodium
    B. Increased plasma hemoglobin
    C. Increased serum chloride
    D. Increased serum haptoglobin

104. Acquired hemolytic anemias are usually due to
    A. Extracorpuscular factors
    B. Defects within the bone marrow
    C. Intracellular factors
    D. Changes in hemoglobin stability

105. The antibody associated with paroxysmal cold hemoglobinuria shows specificity for
    A. ABO antigens
    B. I antigens
    C. P antigens
    D. Rh antigens

106. A 69-year-old male is admitted with pallor, mild tachycardia, and difficulty walking because of numbness in the extremities. His CBC reveals a hemoglobin of 78 g/L (7.8 g/dL), a hematocrit of 0.25 L/L (25.0%), and MCV of 118.5 fL. This patient's symptoms and the blood findings seen in Color Plate 11■ are most suggestive of anemia due to a lack of
    A. Folic acid
    B. Vitamin B_{12}
    C. Vitamin B_6
    D. Ascorbic acid

107. A clinical laboratory scientist examined a Wright stained peripheral smear and saw what appeared to be small, dark-staining granules in the mature erythrocytes. A second smear was stained with Prussian blue and a positive result was obtained. Based on this information, which of the following would you expect to be abnormal?
    A. Plasma hemoglobin level
    B. Serum ferritin level
    C. Hemoglobin electrophoresis
    D. Test for parietal cell antibodies

108. Hemoglobinopathies are characterized by
    A. Absent or reduced rate of globin-chain synthesis
    B. Inability to transport and release oxygen to the tissues
    C. Inhibition of iron chelation needed for heme biosynthesis
    D. Production of structurally abnormal hemoglobin variants

109. Which of the following statements about hereditary spherocytosis is *true?*
    A. Abnormally shaped cells are produced in the bone marrow.
    B. Cells have a decreased mean cell hemoglobin concentration (MCHC).
    C. Membrane loss and red cell trapping occur in the splenic microcirculation.
    D. Red cell osmotic fragility is decreased.

110. Which of the following statements about hereditary elliptocytosis (HE) is *true?*
    A. Characteristic oval shape occurs in mature erythrocytes.
    B. Heterogeneous group of disorders linked to Rh-null individuals.
    C. Cellular defect involves the lipid composition of the membrane.
    D. HE cells are abnormally permeable to calcium.

111. Which of the following disorders is commonly linked to the development of anemia of chronic disease?
    A. Cardiovascular disease
    B. Leukemoid reaction
    C. Chronic gastrointestinal blood loss
    D. Malignancy

112. The most appropriate screening test for detecting hemoglobin F is:
    A. Osmotic fragility
    B. Dithionite solubility
    C. Kleihauer-Betke
    D. Heat instability test

113. Which of the following is associated with sickle cells?
    A. Increased oxygen tension promotes sickling.
    B. There is decreased mechanical fragility.
    C. There is increased deformability.
    D. Increased sickling occludes vessels.

114. A bone marrow M:E ratio of 4:1 would be an expected finding for
    A. Sickle cell anemia
    B. Aplastic anemia
    C. Beta-thalassemia major
    D. Megaloblastic anemia

115. An elderly man with a 10-year history of chronic lymphocytic leukemia presented with jaundice and fatigue that was attributed to a recent 3-gram drop in his hemoglobin. Many spherocytes and polychromatophilic red cells were found on his Wright stained blood smear. Which type of immune hemolytic anemia is most likely?
    A. Idiopathic warm autoimmune hemolytic anemia
    B. Secondary warm autoimmune hemolytic anemia
    C. Primary cold hemagglutinin disease
    D. Paroxysmal cold hemoglobinuria

116. A person experiencing moderate anemia with suspected pernicious anemia (PA) shows intrinsic factor antibodies and a low cobalamin level. Which of the following would *not* support the diagnosis of PA?
    A. Gastric atrophy and achlorhydria
    B. Oval macrocytes and Howell-Jolly bodies
    C. Bone marrow erythroid precursors exhibit normoblastic maturation.
    D. Elevated serum lactate dehydrogenase (LD) and bilirubin levels

117. A cellulose acetate electrophoresis revealed a large band of hemoglobin in the hemoglobin S position. This band quantified at 95%. The peripheral smear revealed 70% target cells, and the solubility test was negative. Based on this information, what is the hemoglobin?
   A. Hemoglobin C
   B. Hemoglobin D
   C. Hemoglobin E
   D. Hemoglobin S

118. A previously healthy man experiences weakness and hemoglobinuria after taking the antimalarial agent primaquine. This hemolytic attack most likely occurred because of a deficiency of
   A. Pyruvate kinase
   B. Glucose-6-phosphate dehydrogenase
   C. 2,3-Bisphosphoglycerate
   D. Methemoglobin reductase

119. Which of the following is an acquired red cell membrane defect that results in increased sensitivity to complement binding?
   A. March hemoglobinuria
   B. Paroxysmal nocturnal hemoglobinuria
   C. Paroxysmal cold hemoglobinuria
   D. Methemoglobinemia

120. A screening test for paroxysmal nocturnal hemoglobinuria is:
   A. Osmotic fragility test
   B. Heat instability test
   C. Sucrose hemolysis
   D. Dithionite solubility

121. Which of the following statements about the relative anemia of pregnancy is *true?*
   A. It is due to a reduction in the number of erythrocytes.
   B. It is normocytic and normochromic.
   C. It produces an oxygen deficit for the fetus.
   D. It is associated with a decreased in plasma volume.

122. The anemia found in chronic renal failure is most likely caused by
   A. Loss of erythropoietin synthesis
   B. Lack of cellular oxygen demand
   C. Defective iron absorption
   D. Destruction of red cells by uremic metabolites

123. Which of the following phrases about aplastic anemia is *false?*
   A. Stem cell disorder
   B. Risk of life-threatening infection
   C. Frequent bleeding complications
   D. Reduced red cell survival

124. The fish tapeworm *Diphyllobothrium latum* is associated with the development of
   A. Microcytic anemia
   B. Macrocytic anemia
   C. Hemolytic anemia
   D. Hypoproliferative anemia

125. An increase in erythropoietin is *not* a normal compensating mechanism in which of the following conditions?
   A. Renal tumors
   B. Heavy smoking
   C. Cardiovascular disease
   D. Pulmonary disease

126. Thalassemias are the result of a
   A. Structural defect in the heme portion of hemoglobin
   B. Quantitative defect in globin-chain synthesis
   C. Qualitative defect in globin-chain structure
   D. Change in hemoglobin solubility properties

127. Which of the following characterizes iron-deficiency anemia?
   A. Decreased serum iron, decreased transferrin saturation, normal ferritin
   B. Decreased serum transferrin, decreased transferrin saturation, decreased ferritin
   C. Increased serum transferrin, decreased transferrin saturation, decreased ferritin
   D. Increased serum transferrin, increased transferrin saturation, decreased serum iron

128. Clinical manifestations of a homozygous mutation involving the beta-globin gene will most likely appear
    A. During embryonic development
    B. In the neonate at birth
    C. No later than 3 weeks after birth
    D. By 6 months of age

129. The hemolysis associated with infection by malaria organisms is due to the
    A. Release of merozoites from erythrocytes
    B. Invasion of erythrocytes by merozoites
    C. Host's immunologic response to infected erythrocytes
    D. Toxins produced by the malarial organism

130. A clinical laboratory scientist received a 5 mL EDTA tube that contained 0.5 mL of anticoagulated blood. A smear was prepared and stained with Wright stain. When examined microscopically, the majority of cells appeared to have many evenly distributed, blunt spicules on the surface. How should this cellular appearance be interpreted?
    A. An anemic condition requiring further testing
    B. Spur cells caused by using incorrect technique during slide preparation
    C. Artifact caused by a dirty spreader slide
    D. Crenated cells caused by incorrect blood to anticoagulant ratio

131. A failure to generate sufficient ATP is characteristic of red blood cells with
    A. Pyruvate kinase deficiency
    B. Glucose-6-phosphate dehydrogenase deficiency
    C. Lipoprotein deficiency
    D. Hexokinase deficiency

132. When iron use exceeds absorption, which of the following occurs *first?*
    A. Hemoglobin level decreases.
    B. Iron stores are depleted.
    C. Transferrin synthesis increases.
    D. Excretion of iron decreases.

133. The major mechanism responsible for the anemia of chronic disease is
    A. A key iron regulator called hepcidin
    B. Damaged bone marrow stem cells
    C. Immune destruction caused by red cell autoantibodies
    D. Increased erythropoietin response by committed red cell progenitor cells

134. Which of the following is a characteristic of the idiopathic type of sideroblastic anemia?
    A. Refractory to treatment
    B. Blocks in heme synthesis are readily known
    C. Reversible with intramuscular vitamin B_{12} injections
    D. Subtype of myelogenous leukemia

135. Thinning of bones and deformation of facial bone structure seen in homozygous beta-thalassemia is a
    A. Consequence of disturbances in calcium metabolism
    B. Result of hyperplastic marrow activity
    C. Secondary disorder due to immunologic response
    D. Result of increased fibroclast activity

136. Which of the following does *not* accurately describe cold autoimmune hemolytic anemia?
    A. Red cell agglutination in extremities induces Raynaud's phenomenon.
    B. It may occur secondary to *Mycoplasma* pneumonia.
    C. Hemolysis is complement-mediated or via removal of coated cells.
    D. The autoantibody is usually an IgG type directed against Rh antigens.

137. Which of the following represents an anemia that would have a high red cell distribution width (RDW)?
A. Sickle cell disease during crisis
B. Thalassemia minor
C. Aplastic anemia
D. Anemia of chronic disorders

138. In which of the following disorders would splenomegaly *not* be a common finding?
A. Homozygous beta-thalassemia
B. Hereditary spherocytosis
C. Hemoglobin SC disease
D. Folic acid deficiency

Leukocytes

139. Functionally, white blood cells are divided into
A. Granulocytes, nongranulocytes
B. Polymorphonuclears, mononuclears
C. Phagocytes, immunocytes
D. Granulocytes, lymphocytes

140. The term "left shift" refers to:
A. A microscopic adjustment
B. Immature cell forms in the peripheral blood
C. A trend on the Levy-Jennings chart
D. A calibration adjustment on the instrument

141. What is the approximate amount of time a granulocyte spends in the circulation before migrating into the tissues?
A. Less than 1 day
B. About 3 days
C. Up to 5 days
D. More than 10 days

142. What percentage of neutrophils in the peripheral blood constitutes the circulating pool?
A. 100%
B. 80%
C. 50%
D. 30%

143. What is the major phagocytic cell involved in the initial defense against bacterial pathogens?
A. Neutrophil
B. Lymphocyte
C. Basophil
D. Monocyte

144. What is the growth factor that is primarily responsible for regulating granulocyte and monocyte production?
A. Erythropoietin
B. Colony stimulating factor
C. Interleukin
D. Thrombopoietin

145. What does the granulocyte mitotic pool in the bone marrow contain?
A. Myeloblasts and promyelocytes
B. Band and segmented forms
C. The majority of marrow granulocytes
D. Myelocytes and metamyelocytes

146. Cells that produce antibodies and lymphokines are:
A. Erythrocytes
B. Granulocytes
C. Lymphocytes
D. Thrombocytes

147. Which of the following is characteristic of agranulocytosis in the peripheral blood and bone marrow?
A. Neutrophils without granules
B. Decreased numbers of granulocytes, red cells, and platelets
C. Immature granulocytes in the peripheral blood
D. Decreased numbers of granulocytes

148. Which of the following is a characteristic of T lymphocytes?
A. Produce B Cells
B. Stimulate leukopoiesis
C. Comprise majority of cells in the blood lymphocyte pool
D. Regulate the immune response

149. An adult has a total white blood cell count of $4.0 \times 10^9/L$ $(4.0 \times 10^3/\mu L)$. The differential count is as follows: polymorphonuclear neutrophils (PMNs) 25%, bands 5%, lymphocytes 65%, and monocytes 5%. The absolute value reference range for lymphocytes is $1.0-4.0 \times 10^9/L$. Which of the following is *true?*
   A. The percentage of lymphocytes is normal.
   B. There is an absolute lymphocytosis.
   C. There is a relative lymphocytosis.
   D. There is both an absolute and a relative lymphocytosis.

150. Which of the following statements is *correct?*
   A. Hypersegmented neutrophils have four nuclear lobes.
   B. Auer rods are composed of fused primary (nonspecific) granules.
   C. Toxic granules are prominent secondary granules.
   D. Döhle bodies are agranular patches of DNA.

151. Which of the following factors is *not* associated with variations in the total white blood cell count?
   A. Age
   B. Exercise
   C. Emotional stress
   D. Sex

152. Of the following, an absolute neutrophil count of $1.0 \times 10^9/L$ would be associated with
   A. Shortness of breath
   B. Bleeding tendencies
   C. Risk of infection
   D. No clinical symptoms

153. Which of the following statements about basophils is *true?*
   A. Morphologically, basophils resemble mott cells.
   B. Membrane receptors bind IgG, initiating anaphylactic reactions.
   C. Basophilic granules contain heparin and histamine.
   D. Granules are non–water soluble.

154. The most mature granulocyte precursor that can undergo mitosis is the
   A. Myeloblast
   B. Promyelocyte
   C. Myelocyte
   D. Band

155. Production of primary granules ceases and production of secondary granules commences with what cell stage?
   A. Myeloblast
   B. Promyelocyte
   C. Myelocyte
   D. Metamyelocyte

156. Which of the following statements about eosinophils is *true?*
   A. They contain a type of peroxidase that is distinct from that of neutrophils.
   B. Eosinophilic granules contain lysozyme.
   C. Eosinophils are an important line of defense against bed sores
   D. Major basic protein is a component of sederotic granules.

157. Which of the following is characteristic of secondary granules?
   A. Coated with a phospholipid membrane
   B. Called specific granules appearing in the myelocyte stage
   C. Contain myeloperoxidase, lysozyme, and acid phosphatase
   D. Present in the promyelocyte stage only

158. The peripheral blood monocyte is an intermediate stage in the formation of the:
A. Plasmacyte
B. Osteoclast
C. Fibroblast
D. Hairy cell

159. What is the term for cell movement through blood vessels to a tissue site?
A. Diapedesis
B. Opsonization
C. Margination
D. Chemotaxis

160. Vasodilation and bronchoconstriction are the result of degranulation by which of the following blood cells?
A. Eosinophils
B. Monocytes
C. Neutrophils
D. Basophils

161. Multipotent stem cells are capable of producing
A. Daughter cells of only one cell line
B. Only T Lymphocytes and B Lymphocytes
C. Erythropoietin, thrombopoietin, and leukopoietin
D. Lymphoid and myeloid stem cells

162. Cells that provide cellular (cell mediated) immunity are:
A. Natural killer cells
B. T lymphocytes
C. Virocytes
D. Thymocytes

163. Which of the following statements about neutrophils is *true?*
A. Suppress allergic reactions caused by basophils
B. Have surface receptors for IgM and complement components
C. Contain alkaline phosphatase and muramidase
D. Act in specific phagocytosis and are destined to live for a long time

164. Which of the following characteristics would be *least* likely to distinguish reactive lymphocytes from monocytes?
A. Sharp indentation of the cytoplasmic margin by adjacent red blood cells
B. Presence of large azurophilic granules
C. Irregular, indented nuclear shape
D. Abundant, deeply basophilic cytoplasm

165. Which of the following can differentiate a metamyelocyte from a band?
A. Presence of specific granules
B. Indentation of nucleus less than 50%
C. Absence of nucleoli
D. Color of cytoplasm

166. Lymphocyte concentrations in the peripheral blood are greatest during what age interval?
A. 1 to 4 years
B. 4 to 15 years
C. 16 to 40 years
D. 40 to 70 years

167. Which of the following is the *least* likely to be expressed by early B cell precursors?
A. SIgM, a surface membrane immunoglobulin
B. CD34, a hematopoietic stem cell marker
C. TdT (terminal deoxynucleotidyl transferase), a nuclear enzyme
D. CD10 (CALLA), a surface antigen

168. Which of the following statements about macrophages is *correct?*
A. They are mature tissue forms of blood lymphocytes.
B. They serve as antigen-presenting cells to the immune system.
C. Their quantity of lysosomes and acid hydrolases decreases during maturation.
D. They are not active in removing cellular debris.

169. Antigen-dependent lymphopoiesis occurs in secondary lymphoid tissue located in the
   A. Liver and kidney
   B. Spleen and lymph nodes
   C. Lungs and Peyer's patches
   D. Thymus and bone marrow

170. Which of the following is associated with pseudo-Pelger-Huet anomaly?
   A. Aplastic anemia
   B. IDA
   C. Myelogenous leukemia
   D. Chediak-Higashi syndrone

Leukocyte Disorders

171. In patients with infectious mononucleosis, which blood cells are infected by which causative agent?
   A. Monocytes
   B. T lymphocytes
   C. B lymphocytes
   D. Histiocytes

172. Which of the following statements about hairy cell leukemia is *true?*
   A. It is an acute disease, primarily affecting young adults.
   B. Splenomegaly is an unusual finding.
   C. Hairy cells contain tartrate-resistant acid phosphatase.
   D. Hairy cells are abnormal T lymphocytes.

173. Based on the WHO classification system, B cell ALL (FAB type L3) and _______ represent different clinical presentations of the same disease entity.
   A. Burkitt lymphoma
   B. Hodgkin lymphoma
   C. mycosis fungoides
   D. small lymphocytic lymphoma

174. Biochemical abnormalities characteristic of polycythemia vera include:
   A. Increased serum B12 binding capacity
   B. Hypouricemia
   C. Hypohistaminemia
   D. Decreased LAP activity

175. In which anomaly is a failure of granulocytes to divide beyond the band or two-lobed stage observed?
   A. Pelger-Huët
   B. May-Hegglin
   C. Alder-Reilly
   D. Chédiak-Higashi

176. In which of the following are eosinophils decreased?
   A. Cushing syndrome
   B. Allergic disorders
   C. Skin disorders
   D. Parasitic infection

177. Which of the following represents the principal defect in chronic granulomatous disease (CGD)?
   A. Chemotactic migration
   B. Phagocytosis
   C. Lysosomal formation and function
   D. Oxidative respiratory burst

178. The blood shown in Color Plate 11■ is from a patient with leukemia following treatment. These findings are most suggestive of therapy with
   A. Corticosteroids (e.g., prednisone)
   B. A folate antagonist (e.g., methotrexate)
   C. Recombinant erythropoietin
   D. Chloramphenicol

179. A patient with normal hemoglobin and WBC count values, a persistently elevated platelet count (over 1000×10^9/L), increased marrow megakaryocytes, and a history of frequent bleeding and clotting episodes most likely has
   A. Polycythemia vera
   B. Chronic myelofibrosis
   C. Essential thrombocythemia
   D. Chronic myelogenous leukemia

180. An adult patient with massive splenomegaly has mild anemia, a slightly elevated WBC count, and an LAP score of 10. These findings are most consistent with
   A. Chronic myelogenous leukemia
   B. Idiopathic myelofibrosis
   C. Primary polycythemia
   D. Primary thrombocythemia

181. Which of the following infections does *not* reveal a blood picture as seen in Color Plate 12■?
   A. Epstein-Barr virus (EBV)
   B. *Bordetella pertussis* (whooping cough)
   C. Cytomegalovirus (CMV)
   D. *Toxoplasma gondii* (toxoplasmosis)

182. A rare and more aggressive type of chronic lymphocytic leukemia (CLL) in the United States involves the
   A. B cell
   B. NK cell
   C. T cell
   D. Plasma cell

183. Which of the following are characteristic findings in Waldenström disease?
   A. Increased IgA and hepatosplenomegaly
   B. Increased IgE and renal failure
   C. Increased IgG and bone fracture
   D. Increased IgM and blood hyperviscosity

184. Which of the following would *not* cause a total WBC count of 62.2×10^9/L ($62.2 \times 10^3/\mu L$) and the blood findings seen in Color Plate 13■?
   A. Treatment with myeloid growth factors
   B. Gram-negative septicemia
   C. Human immunodeficiency virus (HIV)
   D. Systemic fungal infection

185. The peripheral blood shown in Color Plate 14■ is from a 69-year-old female. Her WBC count was 83.0×10^9cells/L ($83.0 \times 10^3/\mu L$) and her platelet count was normal. Based on the cell morphology and this information, what is the most likely diagnosis?
   A. Acute lymphoblastic leukemia
   B. Chronic lymphocytic leukemia
   C. Waldenström macroglobulinemia
   D. Viral infection

186. In which of the following is progression to acute leukemia *least* likely?
   A. Chronic myelogenous leukemia (CML)
   B. Refractory anemia with excess blasts (RAEB)
   C. Refractory anemia with ringed sideroblasts (RARS)
   D. Chronic lymphocytic leukemia (CLL)

187. A Gaucher cell is best described as a macrophage with
   A. "Wrinkled" cytoplasm due to an accumulation of glucocerebroside
   B. "Foamy" cytoplasm filled with unmetabolized sphingomyelin
   C. Pronounced vacuolization and deposits of cholesterol
   D. Abundant cytoplasm containing storage iron and cellular remnants

188. Which of the following suggests a diagnosis of Hodgkin disease rather than other lymphoproliferative disorders?
   A. Presence of a monoclonal population of large lymphoid cells
   B. Predominance of immature B cells with irregular nuclear clefts
   C. Circulating T cells with a convoluted, cerebriform nucleus
   D. Presence of giant binucleated Reed-Sternberg cells with prominent nucleoli

189. The M:E ratio in acute myelocytic leukemia is usually
   A. Normal
   B. High
   C. Low
   D. Variable

190. The presence of the chromosomal abnormality t(15;17) and a high incidence of disseminated intravascular coagulation (DIC) is diagnostic of
   A. Acute myeloblastic leukemia without maturation (FAB type M1)
   B. Acute myeloblastic leukemia with maturation (FAB type M2)
   C. Acute promyelocytic leukemia (FAB type M3)
   D. Acute myelomonocytic leukemia (FAB type M4)

191. Which of the following is *not* commonly found in acute myelogenous leukemias?
   A. Neutropenia
   B. Thrombocytopenia
   C. Hepatosplenomegaly
   D. Lymphadenopathy

192. The child whose blast cells are shown in Color Plate 15■ has acute lymphoblastic leukemia that is precursor B cell type and CALLA positive. Analysis by flow cytometry would likely show cells that immunophenotype for
   A. CD2, CD7
   B. CD10, CD19
   C. CD13, CD33
   D. CD14, CD34

193. The patient whose bone marrow is shown in Color Plate 16■ most likely has a(n)
   A. Acute leukemia
   B. Chronic leukemia
   C. Myelodysplastic syndrome
   D. Aplastic anemia

194. Multiple myeloma is characterized by the presence in urine and serum of
   A. Cryoglobulins
   B. IgG heavy chains
   C. M spike on protein electrophoresis
   D. Beta microglobulins

195. Which of the following is *not* classified as a myeloproliferative disorder?
   A. Polycythemia vera
   B. Essential thrombocythemia
   C. Multiple myeloma
   D. Chronic myelogenous leukemia

196. Which of the following gene mutations correlates with the t(9;22) that is present in Philadelphia chromosomepositive chronic myelogenous leukemia?
   A. MYC/IGH
   B. BCR/ABL
   C. PML/RARA
   D. JAK2

197. Which of the following statements correctly describes the WHO (World Health Organization) classification of hematopoietic neoplasms?
   A. Acute leukemia is defined as the presence of at least 5% bone marrow blasts.
   B. Diagnosis is based on cellular morphology and cytochemistry.
   C. It groups lymphoid disorders into B cell, T/NK cell, and Hodgkin lymphoma.
   D. Diagnostic criteria include PCR testing features

198. Which of the following would be helpful in distinguishing chronic myelogenous leukemia (CML) from a neutrophilic leukemoid reaction?
   A. An extreme leukopenia with increased neutrophilic bands, metamyelocytes, and myelocytes
   B. Leukocyte alkaline phosphatase score
   C. Presence of a normal spleen
   D. Monocytes with Döhle bodies and toxic granulation

199. The cytoplasmic inclusion present in the cell shown in Color Plate 17■
   A. Excludes a diagnosis of acute myelogenous leukemia
   B. Stains positive with leukocyte alkaline phosphatase (LAP)
   C. Stains positive with myeloperoxidase (MPO)
   D. Identifies the cell as a malignant lymphoblast

200. 50–90% myeloblasts in a peripheral blood is typical of which of the following?
   A. CML
   B. MMM
   C. Erythroleukemia
   D. AML

201. In what condition would a LAP score be elevated?
   A. Viral infection
   B. Late pregnancy
   C. Decreased red cell count
   D. Chronic myelogenous leukemia

202. Which of the following is associated with neutrophilia?
   A. Cirrhosis
   B. Infectious mononucleosis
   C. Infectious hepatitis
   D. Neoplasms (tumors)

203. In which of the following would an absolute monocytosis be seen?
   A. Tuberculosis
   B. Recovery stage of non-acute bacterial infection
   C. Hemolytic disorders
   D. Infectious mononucleosis

204. Coarse PAS positivity may be found in the leukemic cells of
   A. Acute myeloblastic leukemia (FAB type M1)
   B. Acute lymphoblastic leukemia (FAB type L1)
   C. Acute myelomonocytic leukemia (FAB type M4)
   D. Acute monocytic leukemia (FAB type M5)

205. Which of the following are among the diagnostic criteria used for classifying the myelodysplastic syndromes?
   A. Unexplained anemia of chronic disease
   B. Hypergranular and hypersegmented neutrophils
   C. Abnormal platelet size and granulation
   D. Hypocellular bone marrow with 25% blasts

206. Naphthol AS-D chloroacetate esterase (specific) is usually positive in _______ cells, and alpha-naphthyl acetate esterase (nonspecific) is useful for identifying blast cells of _______ lineage.
    A. granulocytic; monocytic
    B. monocytic; granulocytic
    C. granulocytic; lymphocytic
    D. monocytic; lymphocytic

207. The familial disorder featuring pseudo-Döhle bodies, thrombocytopenia, and large platelets is called
    A. May-Hegglin anomaly
    B. Chédiak-Higashi syndrome
    C. Pelger-Huët anomaly
    D. Alder-Reilly anomaly

208. Alder-Reilly anomaly is an abnormality of
    A. Lysosomal fusion
    B. Nuclear maturation
    C. Oxidative metabolism
    D. Mucopolysaccharide metabolism

209. What is the initial laboratory technique for the diagnosis of monoclonal gammopathies?
    A. Immunologic markers of marrow biopsy cells
    B. Cytochemical staining of marrow and peripheral blood cells
    C. Serum and urine protein electrophoresis
    D. Cytogenetic analysis of marrow cells

210. Which of the following statements about Hodgkin disease is *false?*
    A. Peak incidence occurs in young adults.
    B. Staging determines extent of disease and treatment course.
    C. Stage IV has the best prognosis.
    D. Almost a 2:1 male predominance over females is characteristic.

211. The blast cells shown in Color Plate 18■ are CD14 and CD33 positive, Sudan black B positive, specific esterase positive, and nonspecific esterase positive. Which type of acute leukemia is most consistent with the immunophenotyping and cytochemical staining results?
    A. Acute lymphoblastic leukemia, T cell type
    B. Acute erythroleukemia
    C. Acute myelomonocytic leukemia
    D. Acute monocytic leukemia

212. Which type of leukemia is associated with the best prognosis for a cure?
    A. Chronic lymphocytic leukemia in the elderly
    B. Acute lymphoblastic leukemia in children
    C. Acute myelogenous leukemia in children
    D. Chronic myelogenous leukemia in young adults

213. What is the key diagnostic test for Hodgkin lymphoma?
    A. Bone marrow biopsy
    B. Lymph node biopsy
    C. Spinal tap
    D. Skin biopsy

214. A bone marrow with 90% cellularity and myeloid:erythroid (M:E) ratio of 10:1 is most characteristic of
    A. Chronic myelogenous leukemia
    B. Primary polycythemia
    C. Beta-thalassemia major
    D. Aplastic anemia

215. A 60-year-old patient presents with extreme fatigue. Her blood and bone marrow findings are as follows: severe anemia with a dual RBC population, 3% marrow blasts, and numerous ringed sideroblasts. This information is most consistent with
   A. Refractory anemia (RA)
   B. Refractory anemia with ringed sideroblasts (RARS)
   C. Refractory anemia with excess blasts (RAEB)
   D. Chronic myelomonocytic leukemia (CMML)

216. Which of the following is *not* a mechanism by which neutropenia may be produced?
   A. Hypersplenism
   B. Marrow injury or replacement
   C. Recent strenuous exercise
   D. Drug-induced antibodies

217. Which of the following is a characteristic findings in polycythemia vera?
   A. Blood cytopenia
   B. Increased red cell mass
   C. Increased erythropoietin level
   D. decreased blood viscosity

218. In what disorder is significant basophilia most commonly seen?
   A. Hairy cell leukemia
   B. Plasma cell leukemia
   C. Acute lymphoblastic leukemia
   D. Chronic myelogenous leukemia

219. Acute erythroleukemia (FAB type M6) is characterized by increased
   A. Promyelocytes and lysozyme activity
   B. Marrow megakaryocytes and thrombocytosis
   C. Marrow erythroblasts and multinucleated red cells
   D. Marrow monoblasts and immature monocytes

220. The blood findings present in Color Plate 20■ are from a patient with complaints of fatigue and severe lower back pain. Which of the following would *not* be typical of this disease?
   A. Bone tumors of plasma cells
   B. Hypercalcemia
   C. Progressive renal impairment
   D. Normal sedimentation rate

221. Myeloid metaplasia refers to
   A. Displacement of normal marrow cells by fibrous tissue
   B. Hematopoietic failure
   C. Extramedullary hematopoiesis
   D. Tumors (neoplasms) of the bone marrow

222. Which of the following statements about non-Hodgkin types of lymphoma is *true?*
   A. Lymphadenopathy is the most common presenting symptom.
   B. Initially, they present as a systemic disease rather than a localized tumor.
   C. They are often associated with multiple bone lesions.
   D. They are characterized by proliferation of malignant cells primarily involving the bone marrow.

Methodology

223. What combination of reagents is used to measure hemoglobin?
   A. Hydrochloric acid and *p*-dimethylaminobenzaldehyde
   B. Potassium ferricyanide and potassium cyanide
   C. Sodium bisulfite and sodium metabisulfite
   D. Sodium citrate and hydrogen peroxide

224. The slowest-moving hemoglobin(s) on an alkaline electrophoresis at pH 8.6 is(are)
   A. A
   B. A_2, C, E, and O
   C. F
   D. S, D, and G

225. A patient with suspected sickle cell trait has negative solubility test results, but hemoglobin electrophoresis at pH 8.6 shows an apparent A-S pattern. What is the most likely explanation?
   A. Patient has hemoglobin AS, and the solubility test is incorrect.
   B. Patient has hemoglobin AA, and the electrophoresis is incorrect.
   C. Patient has hemoglobin AD or AG, and both procedures are correct.
   D. Tests need to be repeated; impossible to determine which procedure is correct.

226. Which of the following is an *incorrect* statement about the solubility test for Hemoglobin S?
   A. Hemoglobin S polymerizes when deoxygenated.
   B. Testing performed on a 2-day-old infant can result in a false-negative result.
   C. Sickle cell trait can be differentiated from sickle cell anemia with this test.
   D. The test is positive in hemoglobin C_{Harlem}.

227. Which of the following is *not* associated with causing a falsely low ESR?
   A. Column used is slanted.
   B. EDTA tube is clotted.
   C. EDTA tube is one-third full.
   D. EDTA specimen is 24 hours old.

228. A platelet count is performed on an automated instrument from an EDTA blood sample. Smear evaluation reveals the presence of platelet clumps. The specimen is redrawn using sodium citrate as the anticoagulant, and a count of $300 \times 10^9/L$ is obtained. What is the correct platelet count to report?
   A. $270 \times 10^9/L$
   B. $300 \times 10^9/L$
   C. $330 \times 10^9/L$
   D. $360 \times 10^9/L$

229. To best preserve cellular morphology, differential smears from an EDTA specimen should be made no more than ____ hour(s) after collection.
   A. 1
   B. 5
   C. 12
   D. 24

230. The blood smear made on a patient with polycythemia vera is too short. What should be done to correct this problem?
   A. Decrease the angle of the spreader slide.
   B. Increase the angle of the spreader slide.
   C. Adjust the angle of the spreader slide to 45 degrees.
   D. Use a smaller drop of blood.

231. The components of Wright stain include
   A. Crystal violet and safranin
   B. Brilliant green and neutral red
   C. New methylene blue and carbolfuchsin
   D. Methylene blue and eosin

232. What is the reason for red blood cells to be bright red and the WBC nuclei to be poorly stained when using Wright's stain?
   A. The staining time is too long.
   B. The stain or buffer is too alkaline.
   C. The stain or buffer is too acidic.
   D. The smear was not washed long enough.

233. If 60 reticulocytes are counted in 1000 red blood cells, what is the reticulocyte count?
   A. 0.06%
   B. 0.6%
   C. 6.0%
   D. 60.0%

234. Using the percent reticulocyte from question 233 and an RBC count of $3.00 \times 10^{12}/L$ ($3.00 \times 10^6/\mu L$), the calculated absolute reticulocyte count reported in SI units is
A. $1.8 \times 10^9/L$
B. $18 \times 10^9/L$
C. $180 \times 10^9/L$
D. $180 \times 10^3/\mu L$

235. The Sudan black B stain shown in Color Plate 19■ is a stain for
A. Glycogen
B. Lipids
C. Myeloperoxidase
D. Acid phosphatase

236. The following numbers were obtained in evaluating leukocyte alkaline phosphatase (LAP) activity in neutrophils. What is the score?

0	1	2	3	4
15	20	30	20	15

A. 100
B. 115
C. 200
D. 215

237. Perl's Prussian blue is a stain used to detect
A. DNA
B. RNA
C. Iron
D. Glycogen

238. Which of the following red cell inclusions stain with *both* Perl's Prussian blue and Wright's stain?
A. Howell-Jolly bodies
B. Basophilic stippling
C. Pappenheimer bodies
D. Heinz bodies

239. What is the depth between the counting platform and the coverslip on a hemacytometer?
A. 0.01 mm
B. 0.10 mm
C. 1.00 mm
D. 0.1 cm

240. A WBC count is performed on a hemacytometer using a 1:20 dilution. 308 cells are seen in a total area of 8 mm^2. What is the WBC count?
A. $3.8 \times 10^9/L$
B. $7.7 \times 10^9/L$
C. $15.4 \times 10^9/L$
D. $38.5 \times 10^9/L$

241. Which set of results indicates that an error in measurement has occurred?

	RBC $\times 10^{12}/L$	Hgb (g/dL)	Hct (%)
A.	2.50	7.6	22.9
B.	2.75	9.5	24.8
C.	3.40	10.0	31.0
D.	3.75	11.1	34.0

242. Which of the following would *not* be the cause of a *falsely* high MCHC of 38.3 g/dL on an automated instrument?
A. Hereditary spherocytosis
B. Lipemia
C. Presence of a cold agglutinin
D. Instrument sampling or mixing error

243. What is the principle of automated impedance cell counters?
A. Angle of laser beam scatter by cells
B. Amplification of an electrical current by cells
C. Interruption of an electrical current by cells
D. Change in optical density of the solution containing cells

244. A clinically significant difference between two electronic cell counts is indicated when the standard deviation is greater than
  A. ± 1.0
  B. ± 1.5
  C. ± 2.0
  D. ± 3.0

245. Foward angle scatter in a laser-based cell counting system is used to measure
  A. Relative cell size
  B. Cytoplasmic granularity
  C. Cell number
  D. Immunologic (antigenic) identification

246. A white blood cell count is done on an automated impedance cell counter from a patient with the blood picture seen in Color Plate 4■. The WBC count is most likely
  A. Falsely increased because of nRBCs
  B. Falsely increased because of red cell fragments
  C. Falsely decreased because of nRBCs
  D. Accurate; no error with this methodology

247. The hemoglobin A_2 quantification using anion exchange chromatography will be valid in
  A. Hemoglobin C disease
  B. Hemoglobin E trait
  C. Hemoglobin O trait
  D. Beta-thalassemia minor

248. Which of the following is associated with a decreased osmotic fragility and an increased surface area-to-volume ratio?
  A. Beta-thalassemia major
  B. Hereditary spherocytosis
  C. Target cells associated with thalassemias
  D. Burn victims

249. A clotted EDTA tube can falsely affect which tests except?
  A. Erythrocyte sedimentation rate
  B. Solubility test for hemoglobin S
  C. Hematocrit
  D. Platelet count

250. The test value range that includes 95% of the normal population is the
  A. Reference interval
  B. Linearity limit
  C. Reportable range
  D. Critical range

251. To establish a standard curve for reading hemoglobin concentration,
  A. A commercial control material is used.
  B. A wavelength of 640 nm is employed.
  C. Certified standards are used.
  D. A patient blood sample of known hemoglobin concentration is used.

252. Which of the following is a source of error when measuring hemoglobin by the cyanmethemoglobin method?
  A. Excessive anticoagulant
  B. White blood cell count that exceeds linearity limits
  C. Sodium citrate plasma
  D. Clear glass hemoglobin measuring cell

253. Which of the following statements about microhematocrits is *false?*
  A. Improper sealing of the capillary tube causes an increase in Hct readings as a result of loss of blood during centrifugation.
  B. A tube less than half full causes falsely low results.
  C. Hemolysis causes falsely low results.
  D. Trapped plasma causes falsely high results.

254. The erythrocyte sedimentation rate (ESR) is influenced by the red cell phenomenon seen in Color Plate 20■. Which of the following factors will neither contribute to this phenomenon nor affect the ESR?
  A. Size of the red blood cells
  B. Shape of the red blood cells
  C. Hemoglobin content of the red blood cells
  D. Composition of the plasma

255. An EDTA blood sample run on an automated impedance cell counter has generated a warning flag at the upper region of the platelet histogram illustrated below. Which of the following would *not* be a cause of this warning flag?
A. Nucleated RBCs
B. Microcytic RBCs
C. EDTA-dependent platelet agglutinins
D. Giant platelets

256. To evaluate normal platelet numbers in an appropriate area of a blood smear, approximately how many platelets should be observed per oil immersion field?
A. 1–4
B. 4–10
C. 8–20
D. 20–50

257. Which of the following statements about manual reticulocyte counts is *true?*
A. The blood/stain mixture is incubated for 5–10 minutes.
B. New Prussian blue, a supravital stain, is used.
C. RBC inclusions can result in falsely decreased counts.
D. An erythrocyte must have at least four blue particles to be counted as a reticulocyte.

258. When are automated cell counters required to have a calibration check performed?
A. At least every 3 months
B. After replacement of any major part
C. After performing monthly maintenance
D. When the control values are greater than two standard deviations from the mean

259. A blood sample was run through an automated cell counter and the following results were obtained: WBC 6.9×10^9/L ($6.9 \times 10^3/\mu L$), RBC 3.52×10^{12}/L ($3.52 \times 10^6/\mu L$), Hgb 120 g/L (12.0 g/dL), Hct 0.32 L/L (32.0%), MCH 34.1 pg, MCHC 37.5 g/dL. Which of the troubleshooting steps that follows should be performed to obtain reportable results?
A. Perform a saline replacement procedure.
B. Warm the specimen to 37°C and rerun.
C. Perform a microhematocrit.
D. None; the results are reportable.

260. Which of the following tests could be performed on a hemolyzed blood sample?
A. Hemoglobin only
B. Hemoglobin and platelet count
C. RBC count and hematocrit
D. No results would be reportable.

261. For which of the following procedures would heparin be a recommended anticoagulant?
A. Platelet count
B. Coagulation tests
C. Smear-based red cell morphology
D. Osmotic fragility

262. In the platelet count procedure using phase microscopy,
A. Platelets appear dark against a light background.
B. The entire ruled counting surface of the hemacytometer is used.
C. Ammonium oxalate will lyse the WBCs.
D. Platelets should be counted immediately after plating on the hemacytometer.

263. What is the quality control term used to describe the reproducibility of a test?
A. Accuracy
B. Precision
C. Standard deviation
D. Specificity

Case Histories

Use the following information to answer questions 264–268.

The peripheral blood shown in Color Plate 4■ is from a 10-month-old Greek boy with the following results on an automated impedance counter: WBC $35.0 \times 10^9/L$ ($35.0 \times 10^3/\mu L$); RBC $2.50 \times 10^{12}/L$ ($2.50 \times 10^6/\mu L$); hemoglobin 45 g/L (4.5 g/dL); hematocrit 0.16 L/L (16%); platelet count250 $\times 10^9/L$ ($250,000/\mu L$); reticulocyte count 8.0%; 110 nucleated red blood cells/100 WBCs and many targets are seen. Other laboratory results are as follows: serum iron elevated; total iron-binding capacity (TIBC) decreased; serum ferritin elevated.

264. What is the corrected white blood cell count expressed in SI units of $\times 10^9/L$?
A. 4.6
B. 12.5
C. 16.7
D. 18.4

265. What would be the appearance of the child's red blood cells on a peripheral smear?
A. Microcytic, hypochromic
B. Normocytic, hypochromic
C. Normocytic, normochromic
D. Microcytic, normochromic

266. The CBC, serum iron, total iron-binding capacity, and serum ferritin levels are most characteristic of
A. Beta-thalassemia minor
B. Iron-deficiency anemia
C. Alpha-thalassemia minor
D. Beta-thalassemia major

267. What type(s) of hemoglobin will be detected on this child using hemoglobin electrophoresis?
A. A only
B. A and F
C. A, increased A_2, F
D. F only

268. Why is it difficult to diagnose this disorder in a newborn?
A. The liver is immature.
B. The beta chains are not fully developed at birth.
C. It is similar to hemolytic disease of the newborn (HDN) because of ABO incompatibility.
D. There are normally many erythrocyte precursors in the peripheral blood.

Use the following information to answer questions 269–271.

A 75-year-old man with rheumatoid arthritis complains to his physician of pain and fatigue. His CBC results are as follows: WBC 6.8×10^9/L ($6.8 \times 10^3/\mu L$); RBC 3.49×10^{12}/L ($3.49 \times 10^6/\mu L$); hemoglobin 97 g/L (9.7 g/dL); hematocrit 0.29 L/L (29%); MCV 83 fL; MCHC 33.9 g/dL. Other laboratory results are as follows: serum iron and total iron-binding capacity (TIBC) both decreased, serum ferritin slightly elevated.

269. If the serum iron is 22 μg/dL and the TIBC is 150 μg/dL, what is the percent transferrin?
A. 7%
B. 10%
C. 12%
D. 15%

270. The results of the CBC and iron studies in this case are most characteristic of
A. Beta-thalassemia minor
B. Iron deficiency
C. Sideroblastic anemia
D. Anemia of chronic disease

271. Which of the following is *not* associated with the anemia described in question 270?
A. Chronic gastrointestinal blood loss
B. Hodgkin lymphoma
C. Tuberculosis
D. Systemic lupus erythematosus

Use the following information to answer questions 272–274.

The peripheral blood shown in Color Plate 11■ is from a 19-year-old female college student who has been living primarily on tea, beer, and cereal for the past 9 months because she finds dining hall food distasteful. She visits student health complaining of fatigue. Her CBC results are as follows: WBC 2.5×10^9/L ($2.5 \times 10^3/\mu L$); RBC 2.10×10^{12}/L ($2.10 \times 10^6/\mu L$); hemoglobin 85 g/L (8.5 g/dL); hematocrit 0.24 L/L (24%); platelet count 110×10^9/L (110,000/μL); MCV 114 fL; MCHC 35.0 g/dL; reticulocyte count 0.8%.

272. What test(s) should be done *first* to determine a diagnosis in this patient?
A. Vitamin B_{12} and folate levels
B. Iron studies
C. Bone marrow examination
D. Osmotic fragility

273. In the absence of neurological symptoms, the anemia in this patient is most likely caused by a lack of
A. An enzyme
B. Iron
C. Folic acid
D. Intrinsic factor

274. Which of the following is *not* a laboratory finding in this general classification of anemia?
A. Target cells and schistocytes
B. Teardrop cells and macro-ovalocytes
C. Howell-Jolly bodies and Cabot rings
D. Elevated serum LD and iron levels

Use the following information to answer questions 275–277.

A 45-year-old Scandinavian woman with white hair appears older than her age. She complains to her physician of weakness, a tingling sensation in her lower extremities, and shortness of breath. Her CBC results are as follows: WBC $3.4 \times 10^9/L$ ($3.4 \times 10^3/\mu L$); RBC $1.90 \times 10^{12}/L$ ($1.90 \times 10^6/\mu L$); hemoglobin level 86 g/L (8.6 g/dL); hematocrit 0.25 L/L (25%); MCV 132 fL; MCHC 34.4 g/dL; platelet count $100 \times 10^9/L$ ($100{,}000/\mu L$). Cabot rings are noted on the peripheral smear.

275. The clinical and laboratory findings are most consistent with
   A. Liver disease
   B. Pernicious anemia
   C. Folic acid deficiency
   D. Aplastic anemia

276. Which of the following is *not* associated with this disorder?
   A. Alcoholism
   B. Antibodies to intrinsic factor or parietal cells
   C. *Diphyllobothrium latum* infection
   D. Achlorhydria

277. Which of the following statements about megaloblastic anemia is *true?*
   A. Oral folate therapy reverses the neurologic symptoms of PA.
   B. Intramuscular injections of vitamin B_{12} will reverse the neurologic symptoms of PA.
   C. Methotrexate (chemotherapeutic agent) is a vitamin B_{12} antagonist.
   D. Folate deficiency takes years to develop.

Use the following information to answer questions 278–280.

A 32-year-old African-American traveling to Africa on business had been healthy until he began taking primaquine for prevention of malaria. He went to his physician because he felt faint and his urine was black. His CBC results are as follows: WBC $6.5 \times 10^9/L$ ($6.5 \times 10^3/\mu L$); RBC $1.67 \times 10^{12}/L$ ($1.67 \times 10^6/\mu L$); hemoglobin level 50 g/L (5.0 g/dL); hematocrit 0.15 L/L (15%); MCV 89.8 fL; MCHC 33.3 g/dL; platelet count $175 \times 10^9/L$ ($175{,}000/\mu L$); reticulocyte 25.0%.

278. The most likely cause of this hemolytic episode is
   A. G6PD deficiency
   B. Hereditary spherocytosis
   C. Sickle cell disease
   D. Pyruvate kinase deficiency

279. The defect in this disorder is caused by an
   A. Amino acid substitution
   B. Intrinsic red blood cell membrane defect
   C. Enzyme deficiency in the hexose monophosphate shunt
   D. Enzyme deficiency in the Embden-Meyerhof pathway

280. Inclusions that form when the patient is oxidatively challenged are composed of
   A. RNA
   B. Denatured hemoglobin
   C. DNA
   D. Iron

Use the following information to answer questions 281–283.

A 15-month-old malnourished child is brought to the clinic for a routine examination. Her CBC results are as follows: WBC 9.5×10^9/L (9.5×10^3/µL); RBC 2.70×10^{12}/L (2.70×10^6/µL); hemoglobin 67 g/L (6.7 g/dL); hematocrit 0.25 L/L (25%); MCV 73.5 fL; MCHC 26.8 g/dL; reticulocyte 0.2%; RDW 19%. Abnormal RBC morphology present included pencil forms and target cells.

281. What is this toddler's most probable diagnosis?
   A. Folic acid deficiency
   B. Hereditary spherocytosis
   C. Iron deficiency
   D. Erythroblastosis fetalis

282. The earliest indicator of this disease state is
   A. Decreased folic acid
   B. Decreased serum iron
   C. Decreased serum ferritin
   D. Increased bilirubin

283. What is the toddler's absolute reticulocyte count?
   A. 0.05×10^9/L
   B. 0.5×10^9/L
   C. 5×10^9/L
   D. 50×10^9/L

Use the following information to answer questions 284–288.

An 8-year-old girl is seen by the family physician. On physical examination, the physician notes fever, sore throat, bruising, petechiae, and pallor. A CBC is drawn and the results are as follows: WBC 110×10^9/L (110×10^3/µL); RBC 1.70×10^{12}/L (1.70×10^6/µL); hemoglobin 55 g/L (5.5 g/dL); hematocrit 0.16 L/L (16%); differential count shows 93% blasts and 7% lymphocytes. A bone marrow examination is performed and reveals 85% blasts. All of the blasts are small with no variation in their appearance.

284. Which of the following would you expect to most accurately reflect the child's platelet count?
   A. 10×10^9/L
   B. 100×10^9/L
   C. 200×10^9/L
   D. 400×10^9/L

285. What is this child's most probable diagnosis?
   A. Acute lymphoblastic leukemia
   B. Acute myelogenous leukemia
   C. Hairy cell leukemia
   D. Myelodysplastic syndrome

286. Which of the following cytochemical stains would most likely be positive in the blast cells of this patient?
   A. Myeloperoxidase
   B. Leukocyte alkaline phosphatase
   C. Periodic acid–Schiff
   D. Nonspecific esterase

287. Terminal deoxyribonucleotidyl transferase (TdT) is present in
   A. Precursor B and precursor T lymphoid cells
   B. Mature B and T lymphocytes
   C. Precursor B cells and precursor T myeloid cells
   D. Precursor T cells and mature T lymphocytes

288. The presence of CD2, CD5, CD7 and the *absence* of CD10 (CALLA) are associated with
   A. B lymphocytes
   B. T lymphocytes
   C. Myeloid cells
   D. Monocytic cells

Use the following information to answer questions 289–292.

The peripheral blood smear in Color Plate 17■ and the Sudan black B stain in Color Plate 19■ are from a 90-year-old man complaining of fatigue and nosebleeds. The physician noted the patient was febrile and had petechiae. CBC results were as follows: WBC $20.0 \times 10^9/L$ ($20.0 \times 10^3/\mu L$); RBC $2.58 \times 10^{12}/L$ ($2.58 \times 10^6/\mu L$); hemoglobin 77 g/L (7.7 g/dL); hematocrit 0.24 L/L (24%); platelet count $32 \times 10^9/L$ ($32{,}000/\mu L$); differential count shows 75% blasts, 20% lymphocytes, and 5% segmented neutrophils. A bone marrow examination revealed 80% cellularity with 80% blasts. The blasts were myeloperoxidase and specific esterase positive; nonspecific esterase and PAS negative.

289. What is this patient's most likely diagnosis?
   A. Acute myelogenous leukemia without maturation (FAB type M1)
   B. Acute myelogenous leukemia with maturation (FAB type M2)
   C. Acute monocytic leukemia (FAB type M5)
   D. Myelodysplastic syndrome

290. Cytogenetic studies would most likely show which of the following chromosome abnormalities?
   A. t(8;21)
   B. t(8;14)
   C. t(9;22)
   D. t(15;17)

291. Using FAB classification (FAB) criteria for the diagnosis of acute leukemia, the percentage of bone marrow blasts must be at least
   A. 5
   B. 20
   C. 30
   D. 50

292. Which of the following is *not* considered an underlying condition that predisposes a patient to acute leukemia?
   A. Viral infections
   B. Bacterial infections
   C. Chronic bone marrow dysfunction
   D. Congenital chromosome abnormalities

Use the following information to answer questions 293–296.

An 83-year-old woman is seen in the emergency department complaining of fatigue and recent weight loss. Her CBC results are as follows: WBC $2.6 \times 10^9/L$ ($2.6 \times 10^3/\mu L$); RBC $2.79 \times 10^{12}/L$ ($2.79 \times 10^6/\mu L$); hemoglobin 92 g/L (9.2 g/dL); hematocrit 0.28 L/L (28%); MCV 100.0 fL; RDW 23.5%; platelet count $42 \times 10^9/L$ ($42{,}000/\mu L$); differential count shows 42% segmented neutrophils, 45% band neutrophils, 3% lymphocytes, 3% metamyelocytes, 4% myelocytes, 3% blasts, and 4 nRBC/100 WBC. Morphologic changes noted on the differential smear include poor granulation and hyposegmentation of the neutrophils, giant platelets that display poor granulation, oval macrocytes, basophilic stippling, Cabot rings, Pappenheimer bodies, and Howell-Jolly bodies. Three micromegakaryocytes are seen per 100 WBCs. Serum B_{12} and folate levels are normal.

293. The peripheral blood findings are most consistent with
   A. Myelodysplastic syndrome
   B. Degenerative left shift
   C. Megaloblastic anemia
   D. Chronic myelogenous leukemia

294. The expected bone marrow findings in this disorder using WHO criteria are
   A. Hypocellular; blasts $\geq 20\%$
   B. Hypocellular; blasts $<20\%$
   C. Hypercellular; blasts $\geq 20\%$
   D. Hypercellular; blasts $<20\%$

295. If the bone marrow in this patient had 18% blasts, the most likely disorder would be
   A. Chronic myelomonocytic leukemia (CMML)
   B. Chronic myelogenous leukemia (CML)
   C. Refractory anemia with ringed sideroblasts (RARS)
   D. Refractory anemia with excess blasts (RAEB)

296. Which of the following is a *false* statement about myelodysplastic syndromes?
   A. MDS is "preleukemic" and frequently terminates in acute leukemia.
   B. Treatment for MDS is only supportive and not a cure.
   C. Median survival for all types of MDS is 5 years.
   D. The lower the blast percent, the longer is the survival rate.

Use the following information to answer questions 297–300.

A 53-year-old man reported to the laboratory for routine blood work as part of a yearly physical. He had been feeling tired for the last few months. Physical examination revealed splenomegaly. His CBC results are as follows: WBC $80.0 \times 10^9/L$ ($80.0 \times 10^3/\mu L$); RBC $4.10 \times 10^{12}/L$ ($4.10 \times 10^6/\mu L$); hemoglobin 123 g/L (12.3 g/dL); hematocrit 0.37 L/L (37.0%); platelet count $650 \times 10^9/L$ ($650{,}000/\mu L$); differential count shows 40% polymorphonuclear neutrophils, 18% bands, 5% metamyelocytes, 7% myelocyte, 28% lymphocytes, and 2% monocytes. No RBC or WBC morphologic abnormalities are seen.

297. The peripheral blood findings are most consistent with a diagnosis of
    A. Neutrophilic leukemoid reaction
    B. Chronic myelogenous leukemia
    C. Acute myelogenous leukemia
    D. Regenerative left shift

298. Which of the following would yield the most diagnostic information for this patient?
    A. Sudan black B (SBB)
    B. Periodic acid–Schiff (PAS)
    C. Tartrate-resistant acid phosphatase (TRAP)
    D. Leukocyte alkaline phosphatase (LAP)

299. Which of the following myeloproliferative disorders is characterized by the presence of a t(9;22) chromosome abnormality and the BCR/ABL oncogene?
    A. Polycythemia vera
    B. Acute myelogenous leukemia
    C. Chronic myelogenous leukemia
    D. Chronic idiopathic myelofibrosis

300. How does the presence of this chromosome abnormality affect the prognosis?
    A. It is not a prognostic indicator.
    B. The prognosis is worse when the abnormality is present.
    C. The prognosis is better when the abnormality is present.
    D. Progression to acute lymphoblastic leukemia occurs more often when the abnormality is present.

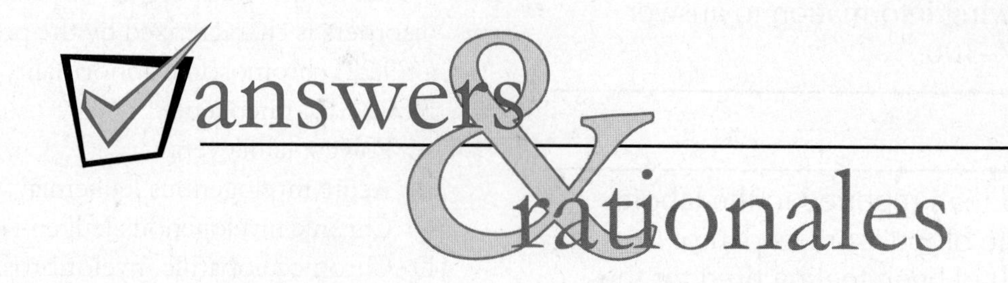

Hematopoiesis

1.

A. The need for oxygen delivery to developing tissues results in the production of erythrocytes before other blood cells. Erythropoiesis commences in the yolk sac as early as the fourteenth day of embryonic development. These primitive red cells produce embryonic hemoglobins that temporarily serve oxygen needs of the fetus. Myelopoietic and lymphopoietic activities begin when the liver and spleen become sites of production at 6–9 weeks of gestation; however, erythropoiesis still predominates. At this time, the red cells produce hemoglobin F, which is the chief oxygen carrier during fetal life.

2.

C. In the infant, there is an increased demand for blood formation because of the rate of growth. At birth, all bone marrow cavities are filled with hematopoietic tissue (active red marrow). As the growth rate slows, there is less need for active marrow. Fatty infiltration of the marrow becomes noticeable at about 4 years of age as cell production diminishes within the shafts of the long bones and is filled with yellow inactive tissue. Fat comprises 50% of the total marrow space in the adult. Except for lymphopoiesis, hematopoiesis is confined to the flat bones and pelvic area by the age of 25 years.

3.

A. Hematopoietic stem cells can make copies of themselves to maintain the stem cell pool and possess the ability to generate cells of all lineages (pluripotential). These stem cells give rise to multipotential myeloid and lymphoid progenitor cells, which ultimately produce progenitor cells that are restricted to a specific cell lineage. With appropriate cytokine stimulus, the committed progenitor cells undergo proliferation to recognizable precursors that produce an amplified number of mature end-stage cells. Stem cells and progenitor cells cannot be morphologically distinguished (look similar to small lymphocytes) but can be identified phenotypically by markers such as the stem cell marker CD34. CD34 expression is lost as antigens for a specific cell lineage are expressed. CD13 is a marker expressed by myeloid precursors.

4.

D. Unlike the infant, in which all bone marrow is capable of forming blood cells, the active marrow in an adult is confined to the flat bones of the skeleton such as the sternum and posterior iliac crest. Although the spinous processes of the vertebrae contain active marrow, these sites are rarely used for aspiration in adults because of the danger of damage to the spinal cord. Sternal puncture also presents a possibility of serious damage to underlying structures, but this site may be used because of easy accessibility or if the aspirate is a "dry tap" in the iliac crest. To obtain both a bone marrow aspirate and core biopsy, most marrow specimens are taken from the posterior iliac crest. The anterior iliac crest may occasionally be used in adults and sometimes the tibia in children less than 2 years of age.

5.

C. The ratio between all granulocytes and their precursors and all nucleated red cell precursors represents the myeloid:erythroid ratio. Myeloid precursors outnumber erythroid precursors by about three or four to one in the normal bone marrow. Although there are many more red blood cells in the peripheral blood than granulocytes, red blood cells have a much longer life span in circulation (120 days) as compared to granulocytes (about 8 hours). Granulocytes, therefore, require a more continual production than erythrocytes and are the most numerous marrow precursors. Alterations in the M:E ratio, such as 1:1 or 8:1, may indicate erythroid hyperplasia or granulocytic hyperplasia, respectively.

6.

A. A diverse group of growth factors (cytokines) regulate and maintain hematopoiesis in a steady state. Most hematopoietic growth factors are not lineage restricted but can act on more than one cell type and have multiple functions. For example, interleukins (IL-3) and colony stimulating factors (GM-CSF) affect multiple cell lines, whereas erythropoietin action is limited to erythroid cells. Cytokines are glycoproteins that usually express activity by binding to specific receptors on target cells. The action of growth factors on hematopoietic progenitor and precursor cells can stimulate or inhibit cell proliferation and differentiation as well as promote or suppress cell death. Growth factors may act alone or together to exert a positive or negative influence on hematopoiesis as well as on the function of mature cells. A determining factor for controlling the rate of cell production is cytokine stimulation in response to physiologic need.

7.

A. The liver of the fetus assumes responsibility for hematopoiesis about the second month of gestation. From 3 to 6 months of fetal development, the spleen, thymus, and lymph nodes are also involved, but the principal site of hematopoiesis remains the liver. By the seventh gestational month, the bone marrow becomes the primary hematopoietic site. Around birth, the liver and spleen have ceased hematopoiesis (except for splenic lymphopoiesis) but maintain the potential for reactivation of hematopoiesis.

8.

B. Erythropoietin (EPO) is a hormone that stimulates red cell production in the bone marrow by its action on the committed RBC progenitor cells. To maintain optimal erythrocyte mass for tissue oxygenation, the body's mechanism for sensing tissue oxygen levels is located in the kidney. Erythropoietin production increases when hypoxia is detected by renal oxygen sensors, with 90% being synthesized in the kidney and 10% in the liver. EPO levels in the blood vary according to the oxygen carrying capacity of the blood (e.g., EPO levels rise in anemia and fall when tissue oxygen levels return to normal).

9.

D. The marrow-derived common lymphoid progenitor cell ultimately gives rise to lymphocytes of T, B, or NK (presumably) cell lineages. Antigen-independent lymphopoiesis occurs in primary lymphoid tissue located in the thymus and bone marrow. The formation of immunocompetent T and B cells from precursor cells is influenced by environment (thymus, bone marrow) and several interleukins. Antigen-dependent lymphopoiesis occurs in secondary lymphoid tissue (spleen, lymph nodes, Peyer's patches of the gastrointestinal tract) and begins with antigenic stimulation of immunocompetent cells.

10.

B. Apoptosis is physiologically programmed cell death that can be induced by deprivation of growth factors or prevented by growth-promoting cytokines. Apoptosis plays an important role in the regulation of cell number and is deregulated in certain malignancies. Necrosis is accidental cell death by phagocytic cells and is associated with lethal physical damage. Cellular senescence describes cells that have lived their life span and will die of old age. Terminal differentiation refers to mature end-stage cells that are no longer capable of replication.

11.

A. Bone marrow consists of vessels, nerves, hematopoietic cells at various levels of maturation, and stromal cells encased in a membrane lining called the endosteum. The vascular system empties into a system of sinuses (venous sinusoids). A layer of endothelium lines these sinusoids. Blood cell formation occurs in hematopoietic cords located outside of the sinusoids and between the trabeculae of spongy bone. The bone marrow stroma (macrophages, adipocytes, fibroblasts, endothelial cells) forms an optimal microenvironment for developing cells by providing support and secreting cytokines. Mature differentiated cells can deform to penetrate the vessel wall and enter the sinuses and blood circulation.

12.

B. Bone marrow cellularity in the normal adult is approximately 50% hematopoietic tissue and 50% adipose tissue (fat), with a range of 30–70% cellularity being normocellular. Marrow cellularity is usually estimated from the core biopsy. An intact bone marrow can respond to demand by increasing its activity several times the normal rate if sufficient supplies and growth factors are available. The marrow becomes hypercellular when inactive fatty tissue is replaced by active hematopoietic marrow. In contrast, bone marrow failure may result in hypocellularity or aplasia with increased fat and a reduced number of hematopoietic cells.

13.

C. Interleukins and colony stimulating factors are cytokines produced by a variety of cells, including monocytes/macrophages, T lymphocytes, fibroblasts, and endothelial cells. It is essential that cytokines are continuously supplied by cells present in the bone marrow microenvironment during hematopoietic cell development, or cells will die. Erythropoietin functions as a true hormone because it is produced by the kidney, released into the blood, and carried to the bone marrow, where it stimulates red cell production.

14.

C. In a normal adult, the total blood volume is approximately 12 pints or 6 liters. Cells account for about 45% (44% is red cell mass) and plasma accounts for 55%. Alterations in red cell mass or plasma volume are reflected in the RBC count and in measurements of hemoglobin and hematocrit. True anemia or polycythemia is due to a decrease or increase in total RBC mass, respectively. A reduction in plasma volume with a normal RBC mass may cause relative (pseudo) polycythemia. Conversely, an increase in plasma volume with normal RBC mass may cause relative (pseudo) anemia.

15.

A. The pluripotent hematopoietic stem cell gives rise to lymphoid and myeloid progenitor cells. The lymphoid progenitor produces cells destined to become lymphocytic cells, whereas the myeloid progenitor cell produces progenitors committed to differentiation into granulocytic, erythrocytic, monocytic, or megakaryocytic lineages with appropriate stimulus. The cells produced by progenitor cells can be demonstrated using *in vitro* culture techniques; thus, the myeloid progenitor cell is termed "CFU (colony forming unit)-GEMM" based on the cell colonies formed.

16.

C. The mature megakaryocyte, the largest hematopoietic cell in normal bone marrow, has a multilobed nucleus and abundant, granular cytoplasm. Plasma cells are characterized by a round, eccentric nucleus and intensely blue cytoplasm. Osteoblasts and osteoclasts are nonhematopoietic cells that may be present in normal bone marrow. Osteoblasts are cells involved in bone formation that resemble plasma cells but are larger and often found in groups. Osteoclasts reabsorb bone and are similar to megakaryocytes in size but are multinucleated.

17.

D. In normal adult marrow, about 50% is fat, 40% is myeloid (granulocytic) cells, and 10% is erythroid cells. The M:E ratio is determined by performing a differential count of marrow precursor cells. The presence of 10% myeloblasts is an abnormal finding (reference range 0–2%), and a hematologic disease is likely. Megakaryocytes should be seen when scanning and are usually reported as normal, increased, or decreased in number. Marrow iron is assessed with Perl's Prussian blue stain, and it is normal to see stainable iron in macrophages, as well as iron granules in the cytoplasm of developing red cell precursors.

18.

B. The nucleus:cytoplasm ratio decreases as blood cell lines mature. With maturation, cells generally become smaller, the nuclear chromatin becomes clumpy and condensed, nucleoli disappear, and the cytoplasm loses its deep blue basophilia when stained with Wright's stain. Exceptions include megakaryocytes (because of endomitosis they grow larger as cytoplasm accumulates) and plasma cells (increased RNA and protein synthesis produces a deep basophilia).

19.

C. Thrombopoietin (TPO) is the major regulator of platelet production in the bone marrow by its action on committed progenitor and precursor cells of the megakaryocytic line. It is primarily produced by hepatocytes and possibly by the kidney. After marrow release, about 70% of platelets are in the blood circulation and 30% are sequestered in the spleen. Unlike erythropoietin, which is manufactured for routine therapeutic use, recombinant TPO is still being evaluated.

20.

B. Hematopoiesis within the medulla or inner part of the bone marrow is termed "medullary or myeloid." Hematopoiesis that occurs in the liver and spleen (reactivation of fetal life) is called extramedullary or myeloid metaplasia (organs may enlarge). Cell production outside of the marrow space takes place when the bone marrow is unable to meet its production demands. This may occur in severe hemolytic anemias when the maximal capacity of the bone marrow to increase activity is exceeded. Myeloid metaplasia may also be an extension of a disease process such as myelofibrosis. Myelophthisis refers to the replacement of normal marrow hematopoietic tissue by fibrotic tissue or cancer cells, whereas myelodysplasia describes abnormal maturation of erythrocytic, granulocytic, and/or megakaryocytic cell lines. The period of intrauterine life when cell production occurs in the yolk sac may be termed "mesoblastic."

Erythrocytes

21.

D. Normal red blood cells survive about 4 months, or 120 days. The entire life span of the red cell is spent inside the vascular tree, making it easier to determine the rate of production and destruction. Red cell survival depends upon an intact RBC membrane, sufficient cellular energy, and normal hemoglobin function. As red cells circulate for 120 days, enzymes are depleted and the ability to deform decreases. Under normal conditions, red cell loss due to aging (~1%) is equal to daily replacement. Most destruction of aged red cells occurs extravascularly by macrophages of the reticuloendothelial system (spleen, liver).

22.

B. The erythrocyte has a semipermeable membrane that allows water and some anions, such as chloride (Cl^-) and bicarbonate HCO_3^-, to enter the cell rapidly. Sodium ions (Na^+) enter the cell and potassium ions (K^+) leave the cell slowly but continuously. In order to maintain a high intracellular K^+ concentration and remove excess Na^+, ATP-dependent cationic pumps expel Na^+ and take in K^+. This regulation of intracellular cations allows the red cell to control its volume and water content.

23.

D. A molecule of hemoglobin is composed of four globular, protein subunits, and each subunit contains a heme group bound within a convoluted globin chain. Heme groups are identical and consist of protoporphyrin IX with a central iron atom, made largely in the mitochondria. Amino acids are sequenced on ribosomes to produce four types of globin chains (alpha, beta, delta, and gamma) that combine in identical pairs. A normal hemoglobin molecule consists of two alpha-globin chains and two non-alpha-globin chains, each of which binds a heme group. The different globin chains determine the hemoglobin type (A, A_2, or F).

24.

D. Culling is the process of removing aged or abnormal red blood cells from the circulation by the spleen. Red cells (7 μm) enter the spleen through the splenic artery and must squeeze back into active circulation through 2- to 4-μm clefts in the venous sinusoids. Aged or abnormally shaped red cells with impaired membrane flexibility are trapped in the splenic microcirculation and ingested by macrophages. The spleen is the largest filter of blood in the body and has an essential role in the "quality control" of red cells.

25.

C. Each hemoglobin molecule has four heme groups located at its surface, and oxygen binds to the central ferrous iron (Fe^{2+}) in heme. Deoxyhemoglobin (not carrying O_2) and oxyhemoglobin (carrying up to four O_2) are normal physiologic forms of hemoglobin with iron in the ferrous state. Hemoglobin in which the ferrous iron (Fe^{2+}) has been oxidized to the ferric state (Fe^{3+}) is known as methemoglobin and is unable to carry O_2. Carboxyhemoglobin is hemoglobin with carbon monoxide (CO) attached to ferrous iron rather than O_2. Both methemoglobin and carboxyhemoglobin are reversible.

26.

C. Of the total body iron present in a normal adult, approximately 70% is contained in hemoglobin (in red cells of the blood and marrow). Most of the remainder, ~25%, is found in storage sites as ferritin or hemosiderin. A much smaller amount of iron is contained in muscle myoglobin (4%) and respiratory enzymes such as peroxidase (1%). The structures of hemoglobin and myoglobin are similar (both consist of globin and heme), but myoglobin functions as an oxygen trap in the tissues.

27.

B. A very high WBC causes turbidity in cyanmethemoglobin reagent-patient specimen that will result in falsely elevated hemoglobin values.

28.

B. "Poikilocytosis" is a general term that refers to deviations from the normal red cell shape (biconcave, discoid). "Anisocytosis" is the term used when differences in the sizes of red cells are described. Color in red cells is designated as normochromic (normal) or hypochromic (indicating a decreased hemoglobin concentration). Abnormally shaped red cells and red cell inclusions are associated with rigid red cells that have reduced deformability and shortened survival.

29.

A. Howell-Jolly bodies are nuclear (DNA) remnants that remain in the red cell after the nucleus has been extruded and may represent nuclear instability. These inclusions are associated with the defective nuclear maturation found in megaloblastic anemias and the rapid cell division that occurs in severe hemolytic anemias. Under normal circumstances, the spleen effectively pits these bodies from the cell. Pitting is a process that removes inclusions while leaving the rest of the red cell intact. It may be that the pitting mechanism is overwhelmed and cannot keep pace with inclusion formation in hemolytic anemias. Howell-Jolly bodies can also be seen in individuals after splenectomy who lack the normal pitting function.

30.

A. Spherocytes appear smaller and more densely staining than normal red cells and lack a central pallor area. Because they are the result of membrane loss, their surface area-to-volume ratio is decreased. Spherocytes should be distinguished from acanthocytes, which also lack a pallor area but have sharp, irregular projections. Echinocytes have a central pallor area and blunt, short projections. Red cells with intracellular rod- or bar-shaped crystals contain hemoglobin C crystals.

31.

B. The presence of lead causes an inhibition of several of the enzymes important in heme synthesis. Among these is pyrimidine 5´-nucleotidase, which is normally responsible for degradation of ribosomal ribonucleic acid (RNA). The lack of this enzyme apparently allows aggregates of incompletely degraded RNA to remain in the cell cytoplasm. It is this ribosomal material that appears on Wright's stain as punctate basophilic stippling. Precipitated hemoglobin forms Heinz bodies (not visible with Wright's stain), nuclear fragments are called Howell-Jolly bodies, and iron deposits are Pappenheimer bodies.

32.

D. Rouleaux is the stacking of red cells like coins and is caused by increased amounts of immunoglobulins in the blood causing the RBCs to adhere to each other.

33.

C. In viewing Color Plate 1■, the inclusions in the red blood cells are Howell-Jolly bodies. During passage through the microvessels of the spleen, the red cell is examined for intracellular inclusions or membrane-bound antibodies, which, if present, are removed. Abnormal red cells circulate longer, and inclusions such as Howell-Jolly bodies or Pappenheimer bodies will be seen post-splenectomy (or in conditions with splenic atrophy). The phagocytic removal of abnormal red cells is assumed by the liver, but the liver is not as efficient as the spleen. Howell-Jolly bodies are not associated with iron-deficient or iron-overload states.

34.

C. One of the reasons for increased intestinal absorption of iron is an accelerated rate of erythropoiesis (another is depletion of iron stores). Although the mucosal cell does act as a barrier in normal circumstances, this function is not absolute and controls break down in the presence of large amounts of iron, causing an excess to be absorbed. An acid pH is required for iron absorption, and sites of maximal absorption are the duodenum and upper jejunum. The body has no effective means for iron excretion.

35.

D. The presence of iron granules or deposits can be detected with Perl's Prussian blue iron stain. Siderocytes are mature red blood cells that contain stainable iron granules (abnormal). Sideroblasts are bone marrow nucleated red cells (normoblasts) that contain small amounts of iron in the cytoplasm (normal). Ringed sideroblasts are marrow normoblasts that contain iron in the mitochondria that forms a ring around the nucleus (abnormal). Siderocytes and ringed sideroblasts are associated with iron overload problems, particularly sideroblastic anemia. Reticulocytes may contain small amounts of unused iron that is normally removed by the spleen.

36.

C. A "shift to the left" in the oxygen dissociation curve of hemoglobin means that a higher percentage of hemoglobin will retain more of its oxygen at a given pressure. Thus, affinity will be greater and oxygen delivery will be reduced. A higher or more alkaline pH and a lower temperature are associated with decreased oxygen dissociation. With conditions in the lungs (increased pH, decreased 2,3-BPG, decreased temperature), hemoglobin affinity for oxygen is increased, which favors oxygen uptake. With conditions in the tissues (decreased pH, increased 2,3-BPG, increased temperature), hemoglobin affinity for oxygen is decreased, which favors release of oxygen to the tissues.

37.

D. Erythropoietin (EPO) is a hormone produced by the kidney that increases erythropoiesis in the bone marrow in response to tissue hypoxia. The CFU-E (colony-forming unit–erythroid) is a committed erythroid progenitor cell with many receptors for erythropoietin. EPO stimulation of the CFU-E produces the recognizable pronormoblast and promotes differentiation of RBC precursors. The maturation time of erythrocyte precursors (5–7 days) can be reduced in times of increased need for red cells by the action of erythropoietin.

38.

C. Increased binding of 2,3-BPG (2,3-bisphosphoglycerate) decreases the affinity of hemoglobin for oxygen, which promotes oxygen release to the tissues, a compensatory mechanism in people presenting with anemia. Increased pH (alkalinity) enhances oxygen affinity and thus inhibits delivery to the tissues. Less oxygen is available at higher altitudes, and this affects blood saturation and delivery to tissues. An increase in erythropoietin release will affect red cell production but does not have an immediate or direct impact on oxygen delivery.

39.

A. After the nucleus is extruded, reticulocytes spend about 2 days in the bone marrow before release into the blood, where maturation continues for another day. Intense erythropoietin stimulus can cause early release of bone marrow reticulocytes. These reticulocytes are larger and contain more filamentous reticulum than a more mature reticulocyte. These "shift" or "stress" reticulocytes exhibit diffuse basophilia on the wright stained smear and will need more than the usual 1 day in circulation to mature (to lose RNA). A very high number of reticulocytes in the blood circulation can increase the MCV. The level of reticulocyte maturity is best assessed by the immature reticulocyte fraction (IRF), an index reported by automated cell counters that is based on RNA content.

40.

C. Heinz bodies do not stain with wright stain and appear as "normal" hemoglobin even though their presence causes cell rigidity and membrane damage. They can be visualized on wet preps with phase microscopy or by using supravital stains, such as crystal violet or brilliant green. Heinz bodies consist of intracellular globin or hemoglobin precipitate that results from hemoglobin denaturation (G6PD deficiency, unstable hemoglobin variants) or excess globin chains (certain thalassemic syndromes). Basophilic stippling, Cabot rings, and Pappenheimer bodies are visible with both Wright's and supravital stains.

41.

B. The presence of schistocytes (schizocytes) on the smear indicates that red cells have been subjected to some form of physical trauma that causes damage. Red cell fragmentation can be the result of impact with fibrin strands, mechanical trauma by artificial surfaces, injury by heat, partial phagocytosis, or damage by toxins and drugs. Schistocytes are characteristic of the increased red blood cell destruction that occurs in severe hemolytic anemias but are not associated with anemias that result from defective bone marrow delivery of red cells to the blood.

42.

C. Tissue hypoxia associated with low erythrocyte and hemoglobin levels causes increased renal release of erythropoietin to stimulate bone marrow erythropoiesis. Depending on severity, the bone marrow responds by increasing its activity six to eight times normal and becomes hypercellular because of an increase in RBC precursors (erythroid hyperplasia); and the M:E ratio falls. Nucleated red cells may be released into the blood along with the outpouring of reticulocytes. The number of nucleated red cells tends to correlate with anemia severity.

43.

C. Millions of hemoglobin molecules are produced in the red cell cytoplasm during maturation. When developing erythroid cells are deprived of essential hemoglobin components, the result is the production of microcytic, hypochromic red cells. It is thought that during maturation, extra cell divisions occur until a certain hemoglobin concentration is reached. Impaired hemoglobin synthesis may be the result of heme defects (involving iron or protoporphyrin) or may be caused by globin defects. Impaired DNA synthesis is associated with macrocytic red cells, and normocytic red cells are characteristic of enzyme defects.

44.

C. The nucleated red cells seen in Color Plate 2■ would be staged as orthochromic normoblasts (metarubricytes) when in the bone marrow. This is the last stage of red cell maturation that contains a nucleus. The pyknotic, degenerated nucleus is normally extruded out of the red cell in the marrow to yield the anucleate reticulocyte. The release of nucleated red cells into the blood before reaching maturity usually indicates a high demand for red cells.

45.

B. The red cell membrane consists of a protein shell heavily coated with lipids. The membrane lipid bilayer is maintained by constant interchange with plasma lipids. Acanthocytes are the result of abnormal plasma lipids that have altered the lipid composition of the membrane, often involving increased cholesterol content. Acanthocytes (spur cells) are associated with a congenital form of acanthocytosis and with liver disease, or are seen following splenectomy.

46.

A. The mature red cell, which lacks mitochondria and Kreb's cycle activity, depends on glucose metabolism for cellular energy. The end product of the anaerobic Embden-Meyerhof pathway (EMP) is ATP, which is necessary for membrane maintenance and volume control (cation pumps). The hexose monophosphate (HMP) pathway is aerobic and reduces oxidants by providing NADPH and glutathione. The Rapoport-Luebering shunt controls the amount of 2,3-bisphosphoglycerate that regulates hemoglobin affinity for oxygen. Oxidized hemoglobin (methemoglobin) is reduced to functional hemoglobin by the methemoglobin reductase pathway.

47.

C. The polychromatophilic normoblast (rubricyte) is the last red cell stage capable of mitosis. With cellular divisions, each pronormoblast produces up to 16 erythrocytes. The polychromatophilic normoblast is also the stage in which hemoglobin is first visible. The gray-blue color of the cytoplasm when Wright's stained is due to a mixture of hemoglobin and RNA, hence the name "polychromatophilic." The reticulocyte is the last stage able to synthesize hemoglobin.

48.

A. The major adult hemoglobin, Hb A, consists of two alpha- and two beta-globin chains. The switch from gamma chains (Hb F) to beta chains occurs 3–6 months after birth, and Hb A reaches adult levels (about 97%) around 6 months of age. Most globin chains produced in a normal adult are alpha and beta types (1:1 ratio) for hemoglobin A production. Hemoglobin A_2 contains delta chains and comprises about 2% of hemoglobin in normal adults. Epsilon chains are found in early embryonic hemoglobins only.

49.

C. Impaired DNA synthesis results in nuclear maturation that lags behind cytoplasmic development (asynchrony), decreased cellular divisions, and the production of macrocytic red cells. Defective nuclear maturation (megaloblastic) is almost always caused by a deficiency of vitamin B_{12} or folic acid, which are DNA coenzymes. Macrocytic red cells that are not due to vitamin B_{12} or folic acid deficiency (nonmegaloblastic) may be seen in liver disease or when reticulocytosis is pronounced. Microcytic, hypochromic red cells are the result of impaired hemoglobin synthesis.

50.

A. When iron is removed from the heme of destroyed red blood cells, it is bound to transferrin and recycled for hemoglobin production or goes to storage. The major storage form of iron is ferritin, which is a water-soluble iron complex bound in a protein shell called apoferritin. Hemosiderin is a water-insoluble complex of iron aggregates and is a protein that is derived from ferritin. The main site of iron stores is the liver, but storage iron is also found in the bone marrow and spleen.

51.

B. RBC indices are average values, so they have less meaning in heterogeneous RBC populations with wide size variations. Because the MCV is a mean red cell volume measurement, the presence of both microcytes and macrocytes would yield a falsely normal MCV value. One would expect the RDW (red blood cell distribution width) to be high because it is an index of variation in red cell size or anisocytosis. The RDW is low when red cells are of uniform size (a homogeneous population). The RDW is high when a heterogeneous population of red cells is present.

52.

B. Bilirubin is formed when hemoglobin degradation occurs in the reticuloendothelial system, primarily in the spleen. Unconjugated bilirubin is transported by albumin in the plasma to the liver, where it is conjugated. When excessive extravascular red cell destruction occurs, the plasma bilirubin levels rise, exceed the capacity for albumin, and remain as unconjugated bilirubin. When acute intravascular red cell destruction occurs, hemoglobin is released into the plasma and findings may include hemoglobinemia, hemoglobinuria, and hemosiderinuria.

53.

D. Haptoglobin forms a 1:1 complex with alpha-beta dimers of hemoglobin. The large size of this complex prevents filtration of the hemoglobin through the kidneys, where it can cause renal damage. Haptoglobin can be depleted in the plasma during major hemolytic events, such as malarial attacks, transfusion reactions, and other causes of severe intravascular red cell destruction.

54.

C. Codocytes (target cells) have an increased surface area-to-volume ratio and are associated with abnormal hemoglobin synthesis. They are found in hemoglobinopathies, especially hemoglobin S or C disorders, as well as thalassemias and iron deficiency. Target cells can also result from an increase in membrane lipids and may be seen in liver disease. Discocytes are normal biconcave red cells, and elliptocytes (ovalocytes) can be found in varying sizes. The teardrop shape of dacryocytes may occur when a red cell is stretched in the spleen and cannot regain its original shape.

55.

B. Heme synthesis begins in the mitochondria with the formation of aminolevulinic acid. Formation of the pyrrole ring structure occurs in the cytoplasm, resulting in the synthesis of coproporphyrinogen III. The final stages of porphyrin synthesis occur again in the mitochondria, culminating in the formation of heme when ferrous iron is incorporated into protoporphyrin IX in the presence of ferrochelatase.

56.

A. The red cell membrane consists of an outer bilayer of lipids with embedded, integral proteins and an underlying skeleton. Spectrin is the predominant skeletal protein that forms a cytoskeleton with other proteins, such as actin, protein 4.1, and ankyrin. The skeletal proteins are responsible for cell shape, deformability, and stability. Any defect in structure or extensive damage to the membrane cannot be repaired and may lead to premature red cell death.

57.

C. Reduced glutathione (GSH) counteracts oxidants that accumulate in the red cell. These occur as a result of normal metabolic activities and increase during infections or as a result of treatment by certain drugs. In the absence of GSH or as a result of enzyme deficiencies in the hexose monophosphate pathway (HMP), oxidant accumulation can lead to oxidation and precipitation of hemoglobin.

58.

C. Total iron-binding capacity (TIBC) represents the amount of iron that circulating transferrin could bind when fully saturated. In this test, the amount of transferrin protein in the serum is indirectly measured by adding ferric (Fe^{3+}) iron to the serum and allowing it to bind to the unsaturated sites on transferrin. Unbound iron is then removed and the sample analyzed for the remaining iron that is bound to transferrin. The serum iron level measures iron bound to transferrin. Under normal conditions, about one-third of the binding sites on transferrin are occupied with iron.

59.

B. The amount of circulating ferritin indirectly reflects the amount of storage iron in the tissues. A bone marrow exam is not essential to assess iron stores, except in complicated cases, because the serum ferritin test is considered a good indicator of iron storage status in most individuals. Because ferritin is an acute-phase reactant, it may be increased in chronic inflammatory disorders regardless of iron stores. Therefore, the serum ferritin should be interpreted with other iron tests. The percent transferrin saturation is the serum iron divided by the serum TIBC.

60.

B. Fetal hemoglobin can be distinguished from adult hemoglobin in red blood cells by the acid elution technique of Kleihauer and Betke. Only hemoglobin F remains in red blood cells after exposure to a citric acid–phosphate buffer solution at pH 3.3. Hb F has a higher oxygen affinity than Hb A (less binding of 2,3-BPG), so it carries oxygen well *in utero*. Hemoglobin F production decreases after birth, composing less than 1% of total hemoglobin in normal adults. In certain conditions (thalassemias, hemoglobinopathies), defective beta-chain production can be compensated for by increased production of gamma chains and formation of hemoglobin F (two alpha and two gamma chains).

Erythrocyte Disorders

61.

D. Deficiencies of folic acid (folate) and vitamin B_{12} result in abnormal DNA synthesis and a resultant delay in nuclear maturation in comparison to cytoplasmic development. These anemias are categorized as megaloblastic because of the giant red cell precursors observed in the bone marrow. The other anemias are characterized by defects of heme (sideroblastic anemia and iron-deficiency anemia) or globin synthesis (hemoglobin C disease).

62.

A. G6PD deficiency has a sex-linked inheritance pattern and is the most common enzyme deficiency in the hexose monophosphate (HMP) shunt. Individuals are asymptomatic unless exposed to oxidants, which compromise the ability of the glutathione reduction pathway to prevent the oxidation of hemoglobin. The oxidized hemoglobin precipitates in the form of Heinz bodies, which cause acute intravascular hemolysis. In the most common G6PD variant, the hemolytic episode is self-limiting, with old red cells that lack enzyme being destroyed and young red cells with some enzyme activity unaffected.

63.

B. Hemoglobin nomenclature indicates a number of things. The symbol α_2 or α_2^{A} indicates the presence of normal adult, or A, alpha chains. The designation $\beta_2^{26\ Glu \rightarrow Lys}$ indicates that lysine residues have replaced glutamic acid on position 26 of the beta chains. All types of E hemoglobin show a similar electrophoretic mobility and migrate closely to hemoglobins C and A_2 on cellulose acetate (alkaline pH). Hemoglobin E occurs with the greatest frequency in Southeast Asia.

64.

C. The peripheral blood as seen in Color Plate 3■ shows numerous elliptocytes (ovalocytes). If they were artifact due to smear preparation, they would be oriented in the same direction. Hereditary elliptocytosis (HE) is associated with symptomatic hemolytic anemia in only about 10–15% of the cases, but the presence of an enlarged spleen is evidence of ongoing extravascular destruction. In patients with chronic hemolysis, gallstones are a common complication because of excess bilirubin catabolism. In most persons with HE, anemia does not develop because bone marrow production of red cells compensates for the mild shortening of red cell life span.

65.

B. Cooley anemia, or beta-thalassemia major, would be the appropriate diagnosis in this case. In this condition, two beta-thalassemia genes are inherited that result in virtually no hemoglobin A production because no beta-globin chains are produced. The primary hemoglobin made is hemoglobin F. The severe microcytic anemia results from the destruction of red cell precursors in the bone marrow (ineffective erythropoiesis) and rigid red cells in the blood that contain unused alpha-globin chains. Nucleated red blood cells and target cells, as seen in Color Plate 4■, are common, as well as basophilic stippling. Infants with alpha-thalassemia major die *in utero* or shortly after birth. Hemoglobin H disease (three-gene deletion alpha-thalassemia) results from deficient, alpha-chain synthesis that leads to production of Hb H (four beta chains), an unstable hemoglobin that forms Heinz bodies and causes chronic hemolysis. No clinical manifestations are seen in patients with hereditary persistence of fetal hemoglobin (HPFH).

66.

C. As seen in Color Plate 5■, the presence of numerous target cells and SC crystals on the peripheral blood smear suggests the presence of hemoglobin SC disease. These bizarre crystals are distinguished by one or more blunt, fingerlike projections that protrude from the cell membrane. Clinically, hemoglobin SC disease is not usually as severe as sickle cell disease, and electrophoresis shows equal amounts of Hb S and Hb C. Codocytes, in varying numbers, are typical of hemoglobin S, C, and E disorders.

67.

C. Pica is a clinical finding seen in some patients with iron deficiency. Pica is unusual cravings for nonfood items that may include dirt, clay, laundry starch, or, most commonly, ice. Among some cultures, pica is a custom (eating dirt) that may contribute to iron deficiency. In children, lead poisoning often results from the ingestion of dirt or lead-based paint from toys and may be related to iron deficiency. Porphyrias are a group of inherited disorders characterized by enzyme deficiencies and abnormal porphyrin metabolism. The presence of pyridoxine (pyridoxal-5'-phosphate or vitamin B_6) is important to early porphyrin synthesis.

68.

B. Folate deficiency is most commonly a result of poor dietary intake of folate alone or in combination with increased requirements as during pregnancy. Daily requirements for folate are high, and depletion of folate stores can occur within 4 months as compared to vitamin B_{12}, in which deficiency takes at least 2 years to develop (there are high stores). Thus, dietary deficiency of vitamin B_{12} is rare, but folate supplements are commonly required during pregnancy or in hemolytic anemias with excess cell turnover.

69.

C. The hemoglobin solubility test can detect the presence of hemoglobin S, which is insoluble in the dithionite reagent, whereas normal hemoglobin A is soluble. A positive screening test, however, does not distinguish between patients with hemoglobin AS trait, hemoglobin SC disease, and hemoglobin SS disease, so results must be confirmed by electrophoresis. Sickle cell trait is clinically asymptomatic with target cells only. Disorders prevalent in the malarial belt (sickle cell trait, G6PD deficiency, hereditary ovalocytosis, thalassemia minor) are thought to impart resistance to falciparum malaria. Repeated splenic infarctions by sickle cell masses in hemoglobin SS disease cause autosplenectomy by adulthood.

70.

D. The schistocytes in Color Plate 6■ are found in microangiopathic hemolytic anemia and caused by red cells shearing on fibrin strands deposited in small vessels. Widespread or localized (e.g., kidney) fibrin deposition in DIC, HUS, and TTP results in red cell fragmentation. In addition, thrombocytopenia is a usual feature of MAHA. ITP is characterized by severe thrombocytopenia that results from destruction of platelets by autoantibodies, but it is not associated with red cell damage or anemia.

71.

A. Ringed sideroblasts result from the accumulation of iron deposits in the mitochondria surrounding the nucleus of erythroid precursors. The deposits are secondary to a defect in heme synthesis and a pathological finding in sideroblastic anemia. Blocks in the protoporphyrin pathway required for heme synthesis may be hereditary (rare) or acquired and result in iron overload with increased marrow iron. Pappenheimer bodies and basophilic stippling are frequent findings on the blood smear, and increased serum iron, decreased TIBC, increased percent transferrin saturation, and increased serum ferritin are usual.

72.

B. Reticulocytosis is indicative of increased erythropoietic activity by the bone marrow. This is a normal response in conditions involving premature red cell destruction in the circulation or following blood loss due to acute hemorrhage. The reticulocyte count is consistently increased in active hemolytic disease because the marrow speeds up red cell production to supply replacement cells. Anemia develops when the rate of red cell destruction exceeds the marrow's ability to replace red cells (uncompensated hemolytic disease). The reticulocyte count is not usually elevated in pernicious anemia even though increased marrow erythropoiesis occurs. The defective cellular maturation that occurs in megaloblastic anemias results in the death of many red cells in the bone marrow (ineffective erythropoiesis).

73.

B. The major defect in hereditary stomatocytosis is altered permeability of the red cell membrane to Na^+ and K^+ ions. A net gain of sodium within the cell leads to increased water entry and the appearance of a swollen cell with a slit-like area of pallor. This is a heterogeneous group of disorders, in that a number of specific membrane defects have been postulated, and anemia varies from mild to severe. One autosomal dominant disorder is associated with Rh-null individuals.

74.

D. Polycythemia vera (PV) belongs to the group of disorders that are hematopoietic stem cell defects and commonly characterized as myeloproliferative disorders. Although the major increase in PV is in red blood cells, there is also an overproduction of granulocytes and platelets, particularly in the early stages of the disease. The increased production of red cells in PV is not due to the activity of erythropoietin. The production of erythropoietin is almost completely suppressed in this malignant condition.

75.

A. Aplastic anemia can be defined as blood pancytopenia resulting from bone marrow failure. This stem cell disorder results in a hypocellular marrow with few developing precursors and decreased production of all cell lines. The anemia is generally normocytic or slightly macrocytic with reticulocytopenia. The "defect" also affects resting hematopoietic cells in the liver and spleen, so extramedullary hematopoiesis does not occur to compensate for marrow failure.

76.

A. Because red blood cells and plasma are lost together, the hemoglobin and hematocrit will not reflect the severity of an acute hemorrhage until the lost blood volume begins to be replaced by the formation of plasma. The restoration of a normal blood volume is usually complete by 24 hours. It is then that the hemoglobin and hematocrit will reach their lowest point and will begin to rise only with the release of newly formed red cells, usually within 3–4 days.

77.

D. Elevated RBC, hemoglobin, and hematocrit values in a newborn are a carryover from intrauterine life, when a high number of red cells were needed to carry oxygen. Erythropoiesis is suppressed in response to the marked increase in oxygenation of tissues after birth, and the reticulocyte count, which is initially high, will fall along with a slow decline in the hemoglobin level. A hemoglobin value below 140 g/L (14.0 g/dL) is abnormal for a neonate. Newborn red cells are macrocytic and up to 10 nucleated red cells per differential may be seen.

78.

D. The red blood cells with single elongated projections, seen in Color Plate 7■, are dacryocytes or teardrops. Dacryocytes are often seen in disorders of marrow replacement that affect bone marrow architecture, especially myelofibrosis. Teardrops can also result from the splenic removal of inclusions and may be present in a variety of anemias. Drepanocytes or sickle cells are observed during a sickling crisis of sickle cell anemia. Acanthocytes, echinocytes, and/or codocytes can be found in liver disease (presence varies with disease severity).

79.

C. Myelophthisic anemia is an anemia of bone marrow failure. It is seen in patients who are experiencing bone marrow replacement of normal hematopoietic tissue by metastatic cancer cells, fibrosis, or leukemia. The anemia is considered a hypoproliferative anemia because there is no hemolysis involved and the cells are normocytic, normochromic. Disruption of the bone marrow by abnormal cells can result in the release of immature cells (nucleated red cells and immature neutrophils) into the blood and may involve blood cell production in extramedullary sites.

80.

A. Any idiopathic disorder is one for which there is no apparent cause. Ionizing radiation is a well-known cause of aplasia, as is chemical exposure (pesticides, benzene). Iatrogenic disorders are those that result from treatments for a different disorder; for example, aplasia can result from chloramphenicol treatment for bacterial disease. Aplastic anemia may develop as a complication from infections such as Epstein-Barr or hepatitis viruses.

81.

C. Diamond-Blackfan anemia is a congenital disorder that depresses only red blood cell production. Fanconi anemia is a congenital form of aplastic anemia that results in aplasia of all cell lines and has a high risk of developing acute myeloid leukemia or other cancers. The bone marrow distinguishes Diamond-Blackfan from the hypocellular marrow seen in aplastic anemia because there is a lack of erythroid precursors but a normal number of myeloid and megakaryocytic precursor cells.

82.

A. Dehydration is a cause of relative (pseudo) erythrocytosis due to plasma loss. High altitude adjustment, cardiac or pulmonary disease, and defective oxygen transport are all causes of absolute secondary erythrocytosis. Secondary erythrocytosis (polycythemia) is a compensatory increase in red cells, produced in an attempt to increase the amount of oxygen available to the tissues.

83.

B. In infants with homozygous alpha-thalassemia, no alpha-globin chains are produced (because of the deletion of all four alpha genes). Consequently, the infants have nearly 100% hemoglobin Bart's, which consists of four gamma-globin chains. This hemoglobin migrates farther toward the anode than Hb A. Because Hb Bart's has a very high oxygen affinity, it is useless for delivery of oxygen to the tissues, making its presence incompatible with life. Hemoglobin H, composed of four beta chains, also migrates farther than Hb A, but Hb H disease is not fatal.

84.

C. Bart's hydrops fetalis (homozygous alpha-thalassemia major) is a lethal condition in which all normal hemoglobins are absent and the presence of Bart's hemoglobin results in death due to hypoxia. Severe cases of Rh hemolytic disease of the newborn/fetus (erythroblastosis fetalis) are characterized by hemolytic anemia, high numbers of nucleated red blood cells, and hyperbilirubinemia that can cause brain damage (kernicterus). The bilirubin level is elevated but anemia is mild, if present, in ABO hemolytic disease of the newborn.

85.

B. The blood profile alone cannot distinguish folic acid and vitamin B_{12} deficiencies, because both are characterized by macrocytic ovalocytes, Howell-Jolly bodies, and hypersegmented neutrophils. Clinical severity generally differentiates the heterozygous (mild) and homozygous (severe) conditions of thalassemic and sickle cell syndromes. The anemia of acute blood loss is usually normocytic, whereas the anemia of chronic blood loss becomes microcytic due to the development of iron deficiency.

86.

C. The cause of the many spherocytes and polychromatophilic red cells seen in Color Plate 8■ would be best determined with the direct antiglobulin test (DAT). The differential diagnosis is hereditary spherocytosis (negative DAT) and warm autoimmune hemolytic anemia (positive DAT). Both of these hemolytic disorders are the result of membrane injury and would show an increased osmotic fragility result due to the spherocytes, elevated reticulocyte counts, and elevated urine urobilinogen, as well as elevated serum bilirubin levels.

87.

D. Schistocytes and spherocytes are associated with red cell destruction and would be found in clostridial septicemia (toxins), prosthetic heart valves (mechanical trauma), and thermal burns (heat). Microspherocytes can also result from the direct membrane damage caused by clostridial toxins and heat. Aplastic anemia is not a hemolytic anemia but is caused by decreased bone marrow production. Aplastic anemia is usually normocytic, with no evidence of red cell damage on the blood smear, and red cell destruction tests such as serum bilirubin would be normal.

88.

D. Erythrocytosis (polycythemia) is either absolute or relative. Absolute erythrocytosis occurs when the RBC mass increases, taking up a larger than usual proportion of the blood volume. Relative polycythemia occurs when the RBC mass stays normal but the amount of fluid volume decreases, thus increasing the proportion of the blood occupied by red cells as compared to the total blood volume which has decreased. Primary polycythemia is a condition of erythrocytosis without an underlying or contributing condition. The body produces an increased number of red cells without an increase in erythropoietin (an inappropriate response). Secondary polycythemia occurs when some underlying condition causes an increase in erythropoietin, so erythrocytosis occurs secondary to the condition (an appropriate response).

89.

A. Hemochromatosis is an excessive deposition of iron in body tissues that results in iron-laden macrophages, expansion of storage sites, and serious damage to organs (heart, liver). Iron overload can be hereditary or acquired as a complication of severe hemolytic anemias, frequent blood transfusions, or sideroblastic anemia. Hereditary hemochromatosis is caused by a mutation of the HFE gene that results in increased absorption of iron from the gastrointestinal tract and leads to iron overload. It is associated with low levels of hepcidin, an iron regulator, which causes increased iron absorption and release of iron from macrophages. The treatment for hereditary hemochromatosis is phlebotomy, and molecular testing is done for diagnosis.

90.

A. Abetalipoproteinemia, or hereditary acanthocytosis, is a rare autosomal recessive disorder of lipid metabolism. An absence of serum beta lipoprotein, a transport protein, causes abnormal plasma lipids. The numerous acanthocytes (spur cells) are the result of an alteration in the lipid content of the red cell membrane. The anemia is mild, but this disorder is associated with progressive neurologic disease.

91.

A. The majority of body iron is found in the hemoglobin of circulating erythrocytes. This means that any form of bleeding will lead to excessive iron loss. Iron balance is normally very tightly controlled through absorption rather than excretion. Iron deficiency in males is rare but, if present, it is usually the result of chronic gastrointestinal bleeding (ulcers, cancer).

92.

A. The severe transfusion-dependent anemia, which is typical of homozygous beta-thalassemia, is the result of imbalanced globin-chain synthesis and massive red cell destruction that far exceeds the rate of production. Decreased or absent beta chains lead to excess alpha chains that precipitate in red cells and subsequently are destroyed. The response is intense marrow erythroid hyperplasia, bone expansion, and erythropoiesis in extramedullary sites. A complication of continuous red cell hemolysis and repeated blood transfusions is iron overload. Patients require iron chelation therapy to prevent liver and heart failure. Splenectomy may be needed to reduce blood requirements, but it is not done before 4 years of age because of the increased risk of infection.

93\.

A. Serum iron is low in both iron-deficiency anemia and the anemia of chronic disorders. The total iron-binding capacity (TIBC), which is an indirect measure of the amount of transferrin protein, is low in the anemia of chronic disease, whereas it is high in iron deficiency. Synthesis of transferrin is regulated by iron availability. Usually, when storage iron decreases, serum iron levels decrease and transferrin levels (TIBC) increase. In the anemia of chronic disorders, storage iron is normal or increased (but unavailable), and transferrin levels (TIBC) are decreased.

94\.

C. Although the punctate basophilic stippling found in lead poisoning in erythrocytes is considered a classic finding, the anemia present is usually not severe unless accompanied by iron deficiency. The presence of lead inhibits several enzymes involved in the formation of heme, with a consequent increase in erythrocyte protoporphyrin and urinary aminolevulinic acid. The most significant effect of lead toxicity is the resulting neurological deficit and impairment of mental development.

95\.

C. In Color Plate 9■, the dual population of red blood cells represented may also be termed dimorphic. This blood picture could be seen in a patient with microcytic, hypochromic anemia after the transfusion of normal red cells or when new normocytic, normochromic red cells are produced after successful treatment for iron deficiency. Concurrent deficiencies, such as coexisting iron and folate deficiency during pregnancy, would result in the production of both microcytic and macrocytic red cells.

96\.

B. The cells visualized in Color Plate 10■ are sickle cells in the presence of target cells. The substitution of a valine for the glutamic acid normally found in the sixth position of the beta-globin chain causes red cells containing hemoglobin S to undergo the characteristic shape change that gives the sickle cell its name. A defect of both beta genes results in sickle cell disease, whereas a single gene mutation causes the sickle cell trait. Hemoglobin C results from the substitution of lysine for glutamic acid in the sixth position of the beta-globin chain.

97\.

D. The number of irreversibly sickled cells (ISCs) and the proportion of S hemoglobin within the cells contribute collectively to the severity of sickle cell disorders. The classification of "trait" versus "disease" is not based on the severity of symptoms. The absence of Hb A and the presence of over 80% Hb S on electrophoresis would be classified as homozygous sickle cell disease (SS), whereas the heterozygous condition (AS) would show approximately 60% Hb A and 40% Hb S. Sickling is rare in the trait condition because of the lower concentration of Hb S. Sickle cell disease typically shows increased levels of compensatory Hb F, as does hemoglobin SC disease.

98\.

B. Hyperbaric oxygen will reverse the sickling process, but it will also suppress erythropoietin, which stimulates the bone marrow to produce adequate replacement erythrocytes. Hydroxyurea reduces sickling by increasing Hb F levels and has been shown to improve the clinical course of patients plagued by painful crises. Treatment is primarily supportive and symptomatic, with efforts made to avoid those factors known to precipitate a crisis.

99.

D. In response to premature red cell destruction, the normal bone marrow can speed up red cell production. Hemolytic anemias typically have high reticulocyte counts, because the marrow can respond to the need for red cells. Generally, anemias caused by defective maturation or decreased production have inappropriately low reticulocyte counts, because the marrow fails to respond due to injury or lack of essential hematopoietic components. Low hemoglobin and hematocrit values reveal the presence of anemia but do not indicate etiology. The reticulocyte count is particularly useful in distinguishing hemolytic anemias from other normocytic anemias that are not hemolytic.

100.

C. Both iron deficiency and heterozygous thalassemia can present with a mild microcytic, hypochromic anemia. Target cells may be seen in both, but basophilic stippling is only found in thalassemia. The hemoglobin A_2 is normal in heterozygous alpha-thalassemia but is frequently twice the normal level in heterozygous beta-thalassemia, because these individuals compensate with increased delta-chain production due to deficient beta-globin chain synthesis. In this case, iron deficiency would likely be ruled out first with iron tests. Beta-thalassemia with hemoglobin S trait (Hb S/beta-thalassemia) produces a severe clinical picture similar to sickle cell anemia, with sickling of red cells.

101.

D. Oxidative denaturation is the primary mechanism of the hemolytic process. When glucose-6-phosphate dehydrogenase (G6PD) is deficient, the red blood cells cannot generate sufficient reduced glutathione (GSH) to detoxify hydrogen peroxide. Hemoglobin is oxidized to methemoglobin, denatures, and precipitates, forming Heinz bodies. The Heinz bodies cause the rigidity of the red cells, and hemolysis occurs as the cells try to pass through the microcirculation.

102.

B. In hereditary spherocytosis, the rigid spherocytes are being destroyed in the splenic microcirculation. Following splenectomy, the hemoglobin level should rise as the spherocytes circulate longer. Consequently, there is less need for increased red cell production by the bone marrow, and the number of reticulocytes released into the blood will fall. Approximately, 30% of platelets are normally sequestered by the spleen, so a transient increase in the platelet count occurs and red cell inclusions (Howell-Jolly and Pappenheimer bodies), normally pitted out of red cells by the spleen, will be observed.

103.

B. Unconjugated bilirubin levels will rise when either excessive intravascular or extravascular hemolysis is occurring. When hemolysis is intravascular, the free hemoglobin released into the circulation is bound by haptoglobin, and the complex is transported to the liver, where it is metabolized to bilirubin. Depletion of the haptoglobin protein will occur if use exceeds production, and then hemopexin binds hemoglobin for removal. When both haptoglobin and hemopexin are depleted, plasma hemoglobin levels will increase. The serum lactate dehydrogenase rises when red cells are broken down and intracellular LD enzymes are released.

104.

A. Hemolytic anemias can be classified by the mode of transmission (hereditary or acquired) and by the type of defect (intrinsic or extrinsic). With the exception of paroxysmal nocturnal hemoglobinuria (PNH), intrinsic defects are hereditary, and the defect that shortens survival is within the abnormal red cell. Hemolytic anemias due to extrinsic defects are acquired and caused by external agents or extracorpuscular factors that destroy the intrinsically normal red cell.

105.

C. Paroxysmal cold hemoglobinuria (PCH) is caused by an IgG biphasic antibody with P specificity known as the Donath-Landsteiner antibody. This autoantibody fixes complement to the red cells in the cold, and the complement-coated red cells lyse when warmed. PCH can be idiopathic or follow a viral infection and is characterized by acute intravascular hemolysis and hemoglobinuria after cold exposure. Cold autoantibodies usually show I specificity, whereas warm autoantibodies are often directed against Rh antigens on the red cells.

106.

B. The hypersegmented neutrophils and macrocytic ovalocytes seen in Color Plate 11■ suggest the presence of megaloblastic anemia. The two most common causes are lack of folic acid or vitamin B_{12}, which are coenzymes required for normal DNA synthesis. This patient's neurological symptoms are indicative of a vitamin B_{12} deficiency, because that vitamin is also needed for myelin synthesis (CNS).

107.

B. Pappenheimer bodies observed with Wright stain can be confirmed with the Prussian blue stain and are composed of iron. The presence of siderotic granules in the red cells is associated with iron overload, and the serum ferritin test, which reflects the amount of storage iron, would be elevated. The test for parietal cell antibodies can be done to determine the cause of vitamin B_{12} deficiency.

108.

D. Hemoglobinopathies are a hereditary group of qualitative disorders in which genetic mutations cause the production of structurally abnormal globin chains. The three most common variant hemoglobins are Hb S, Hb C, and Hb E, all of which are due to an amino acid substitution in the beta-globin chain. Hemoglobin C is the second most common hemoglobin variant, after hemoglobin S, seen in the United States. Thalassemias are characterized by an absent or reduced rate of globin-chain synthesis.

109.

C. The structurally abnormal red cells in hereditary spherocytosis (HS) are deficient in spectrin and are abnormally permeable to sodium. The bone marrow produces red cells of normal biconcave shape, but HS cells lose membrane fragments and become more spherical as they go through the spleen and encounter stress in the blood circulation. The membrane defect is accentuated by the passage of red cells through the spleen, where they are deprived of glucose and are unable to generate sufficient ATP to pump sodium out of the cell. Ultimately, the red cells are trapped and destroyed in the spleen. The osmotic fragility is increased because of the membrane loss (reduced surface area-to-volume ratio), and the MCHC value may be increased.

110.

A. In hereditary elliptocytosis (HE), the red blood cells show increased permeability to sodium and may have one of several membrane defects linked to this heterogeneous disorder. These include deficiencies in skeletal proteins such as protein 4.1 or spectrin. The characteristic oval or elliptical shape is seen only in mature red blood cells, and it occurs in the circulation when HE red cells cannot return to a normal biconcave shape.

111.

D. The anemia of chronic disease (ACD) is very common and develops in patients with chronic infections (tuberculosis), chronic inflammatory disorders (rheumatoid arthritis, systemic lupus), and malignant disease (cancer, lymphoma). ACD has a complex etiology that includes impaired release of storage iron for erythropoiesis and a reduced response to erythropoietin. The anemia may be normocytic or microcytic, and severity depends on the underlying disorder.

112.

C. The Kleihauer-Betke procedure is commonly used as a screening test to determine the amount of fetal blood that has mixed with maternal blood.

113.

D. Red cells that contain a high concentration of hemoglobin S will assume the sickle shape when deprived of oxygen (which can be reversed if reoxygenated). After repeated sickling, reversion capabilities are lost and irreversibly sickled cells (ISCs) are seen. Sickle cells are mechanically brittle, nondeformable cells that become impeded in circulation, causing blocks that restrict blood flow in vessels and leading to organs (vascular occlusive disease). They are easily trapped in the small vessels of the spleen, leading to obstructive ischemia and eventual destruction of splenic tissue.

114.

B. Aplastic anemia is bone marrow failure characterized by hypocellularity and decreased production of all cell lines. The normal M:E ratio (4:1) does not change in aplasia, because the number of both myeloid and erythroid precursors is decreased. In anemias such as sickle cell anemia, beta-thalassemia major, or megaloblastic anemia, the marrow becomes hypercellular because of an increase in erythroid precursors, and the M:E ratio falls.

115.

B. The immune hemolytic anemia indicated by the smear findings is warm autoimmune hemolytic anemia (WAIHA). Antibody-coated red cells are being partially phagocytized by macrophages (with receptors for IgG and complement), causing loss of membrane fragments. The spherocytes are ultimately destroyed, primarily in the spleen. The cause of the autoantibody production may be unknown (idiopathic), develop secondary to a disease that alters the immune response (chronic lymphocytic leukemia or lymphoma), or can be drug induced. Cold hemagglutinin disease is characterized by red cell agglutination due to a cold autoantibody.

116.

C. Intrinsic factor is a glycoprotein secreted by the parietal cells, along with HCl, that is needed to bind vitamin B_{12} for absorption. Pernicious anemia (PA), which is a megaloblastic anemia caused by the lack of intrinsic factor, is most common cause of vitamin B_{12} deficiency (cobalamin). PA is characterized by atrophy of the gastric parietal cells and achlorhydria (absence of HCl). Autoimmune factors are involved because a high percentage of patients produce autoantibodies to intrinsic factor (50%) and/or parietal cells (90%). The bone marrow erythroid precursors exhibit megaloblastic maturation, with nuclear maturation lagging behind cytoplasmic maturation (asynchrony is also seen in developing granulocytes and platelets). Many fragile red cells die in the bone marrow, and those released into the circulation have a very short survival, which causes a marked increase in lactate dehydrogenase levels.

117.

B. Hemoglobin D migrates in the same location as hemoglobin S on cellulose acetate at alkaline pH but does not cause sickling. The negative solubility test rules out the presence of hemoglobin S. Target cells are seen in large numbers in homozygous hemoglobin D disease. The quantification of 95% differentiates homozygous from heterozygous states where less than 50% hemoglobin D would be seen.

118.

B. G6PD deficiency compromises the ability of the glutathione reduction pathway to prevent the oxidation of hemoglobin. Oxidative stress may occur from infections, ingestion of mothballs, ingestion of fava beans, and certain drugs, including primaquine or sulfonamides. The oxidized hemoglobin precipitates in the form of Heinz bodies, which leads to a hemolytic crisis characterized by intravascular red cell destruction, removal of Heinz bodies by splenic macrophages, and the presence of spherocytes and fragmented red cells on the smear.

119.

B. Paroxysmal nocturnal hemoglobinuria (PNH) is an acquired defect of membrane structure in which red cells have a high affinity for complement binding. PNH is characterized by pancytopenia and chronic intravascular hemolysis with hemoglobinuria and hemosiderinuria. A stem cell mutation causes production of red cells, white cells, and platelets that are sensitive to complement lysis because of the loss of a membrane glycolipid (GPI). The sucrose hemolysis test can be used to screen for PNH red cells, but the Ham's acid serum test has been replaced by immunophenotyping for confirmation of PNH. Paroxysmal cold hemoglobinuria (PCH) is characterized by intravascular hemolysis and hemoglobinuria after cold exposure that is due to a complement-binding autoantibody. A transient finding of hemoglobinuria following forceful contact of the body with hard surfaces (as may be seen in joggers and soldiers) describes March hemoglobinuria.

120.

C. The sucrose hemolysis test is still sometimes used for screening; however, the most accurate measurement is immunophenotyping.

121.

B. Although iron deficiency may be the most common cause of anemia in pregnancy, there is a mild form of anemia that develops during the third trimester in pregnant women with adequate iron levels. Although both erythrocytes and plasma increase during pregnancy, the plasma increases in a higher proportion, causing a relative (pseudo) anemia. This increased blood volume actually increases oxygen delivery to both the mother and the fetus.

122.

A. The anemia of chronic renal failure results from decreased production and release of erythropoietin from the diseased kidney. The drop in erythropoietin results in decreased red blood cell production by the marrow. Recombinant erythropoietin is of great value in treating anemia resulting from end-stage renal disease. Iron or folate supplements may be needed to maximize the response, especially in patients on dialysis. Uremic metabolites may cause reduced red cell survival and impairment of platelet function.

123.

D. Aplastic anemia is a stem cell defect that leads to decreased production of erythrocytes, leukocytes, and platelets (pancytopenia). The survival of red cells released into the circulation is normal. Infection is a serious problem because of the lack of neutrophils. The reduced number of platelets is responsible for the bleeding often seen. Treatment includes blood and platelet transfusions, antibiotics, growth factors, and steroids. Bone marrow transplantation may be necessary.

124.

B. The fish tapeworm competes for vitamin B_{12}, and a macrocytic (megaloblastic) anemia may develop. Hookworm infestation causes chronic blood loss and a microcytic anemia due to iron deficiency. A variety of organisms are associated with hemolysis, including malaria and clostridial infections. Viral hepatitis can cause marrow suppression and a normocytic, hypoproliferative anemia.

125.

A. A need for the increased oxygen carrying capacity provided by additional red blood cells is found in conditions such as pulmonary disease, where normal oxygenation is inhibited. A decrease in the ability of the cardiovascular system to appropriately circulate cells is another reason for increased erythrocytes. Individuals with a high level of methemoglobin, such as heavy smokers or persons with genetic disorders, cannot effectively unload oxygen. This results in a need for increasing the number of red blood cells to compensate. Renal tumors are associated with excess production of erythropoietin, leading to an inappropriate polycythemia.

126.

B. Thalassemias are a group of congenital disorders characterized by quantitative defects in globin-chain synthesis. Alpha-thalassemias result from gene deletions that cause a reduced rate of alpha-globin chain production. Beta-thalassemias result from point mutations that cause a reduced rate of beta-globin chain synthesis. Normally, equal amounts of alpha- and beta-globin chains are produced for Hb A synthesis. In alpha- or beta-thalassemias, synthesis of globin chains is imbalanced, because a decreased production rate of one type of globin chain causes an excess of the other (consequences will depend on the thalassemia type).

127.

C. Low serum iron and iron stores (represented by serum ferritin) characterize iron deficiency that is severe enough to result in anemia. The production of transferrin, the iron transport protein, increases as iron stores decrease. Transferrin saturation decreases dramatically so that transferrin is less than 15% saturated with iron.

128.

D. The switch from gamma-globin chain production for Hb F to beta-globin chain synthesis for Hb A occurs 3–6 months after birth. Clinical symptoms of a homozygous beta-globin chain defect, such as sickle cell disease or homozygous beta-thalassemia, will not be evident until about 6 months of age or shortly after. Alpha-globin chain production is normally high throughout fetal and adult life. A homozygous defect involving the alpha-globin chain will affect the infant *in utero*.

129.

A. The hemolytic crisis of malaria results from the rupture of erythrocytes containing merozoites. This event becomes synchronized to produce the fever and chill cycles that are characteristic of this infection. In severe infections, particularly those caused by *Plasmodium falciparum*, the massive intravascular hemolysis results in significant hemoglobinuria.

130.

D. The incorrect ratio of blood to anticoagulant caused the cells to shrink. This produced the crenated appearance of the red cells. This is an artifact as opposed to a significant clinical finding and can also be the result of prolonged blood anticoagulation. Spur cells (or acanthocytes) lack a central pallor area and have sharp projections, as opposed to crenated cells (or echinocytes), which have a pallor area and blunt projections.

131.

A. Pyruvate kinase (PK) is an enzyme of the Embden-Meyerhof pathway (anaerobic glycolysis). A deficiency of PK results in decreased ATP generation, which causes impairment of the cation pump and a loss of normal membrane deformability. PK-deficient cells have a shortened survival time, but clinical manifestations vary widely.

132.

B. When iron use exceeds absorption, iron stores (serum ferritin) are depleted first. At this early stage, there is no anemia (normal hemoglobin) and the transferrin level is normal. This is followed by increased transferrin synthesis (TIBC) and decreased serum iron. Finally, a microcytic, hypochromic anemia develops.

133.

A. In the anemia of chronic disease (ACD), a chronic illness causes impaired release of iron from storage. These patients have iron but are unable to use it for bone marrow erythropoiesis. Hepcidin, a hormone produced by the liver, plays a major role in the regulation of body iron by influencing intestinal absorption and release of storage iron from macrophages. Hepcidin levels increase during inflammation (positive acute-phase reactant), which causes decreased release of iron from stores. There is also impaired response of marrow red cell precursors to erythropoietin stimulation in ACD. The impaired response is thought to be related to the effects of inflammatory cytokines. Recombinant erythropoietin improves the anemia in some cases.

134.

A. In the idiopathic or primary type of sideroblastic anemia, the blocks in the protoporphyrin pathway (heme synthesis) that lead to iron overload are unknown and, therefore, are irreversible. The anemia is refractory (unresponsive) to treatment other than transfusion. Ringed sideroblasts and increased stainable iron will be found in the bone marrow when stained with Prussian blue. This primary, acquired form of sideroblastic anemia is also known as refractory anemia with ringed sideroblasts (RARS) and is classified as a myelodysplastic syndrome.

135.

B. The demand for red blood cell replacement in beta-thalassemia major during early childhood development results in a hyperproliferative marrow. Expansion of the marrow causes the bones to be thin and narrow. This may result in pathologic fractures. Facial bones show prominence of the forehead, cheek bones, and upper jaw appearance.

136.

D. Cold autoimmune hemolytic anemia (CAIHA), or cold hemagglutinin disease, is characterized by the production of IgM cold autoantibodies that often show I specificity. The cause of the autoantibody production may be unknown (primary) or occur secondary to *Mycoplasma* pneumonia or lymphoma. Significantly high titers can result in agglutination of red cells in the extremities called Raynaud's phenomenon (acrocyanosis).

137.

A. The red blood cell distribution width (RDW) is an index of red cell size variation or anisocytosis. The RDW will be high when a heterogeneous cell population consisting of red cells with varying sizes is present (sickle cell anemia with compensation). The RDW is low when a homogeneous or single population of red cells is present that are of uniform size (thalassemia minor, anemia of chronic disease).

138.

D. Splenomegaly is a common finding in hemolytic anemias, because the spleen is the major site of extravascular red cell destruction. Patients with hereditary spherocytosis and hemoglobin SC disease often have enlarged spleens for this reason. Patients with beta-thalassemia major exhibit splenomegaly because of active splenic removal of red cells, but the spleen may also be a site of extramedullary erythropoiesis. Splenomegaly can also be due to extramedullary hematopoiesis in malignant disorders such as polycythemia vera or myelofibrosis. Splenomegaly would not be a characteristic finding in megaloblastic anemia.

Leukocytes

139.

C. The major function of leukocytes is defense, either by phagocytosis or by immune mechanisms. The phagocytic cells are the granulocytes and monocytes. The immune response is mediated by lymphocytes; however, monocytes play a role in immunity as antigen-presenting cells. Leukocytes may be classified according to granularity as granulocytes and nongranulocytes or divided based on nuclear segmentation as polymorphonuclears (PMNs) and mononuclears.

140.

B. Definition of left shift.

141.

A. After granulocytes are released from the bone marrow, they remain in the circulation 1 day or less. Their major function takes place in the tissues. They migrate through the vessel walls to reach areas of inflammation very soon after release. The life span of the granulocyte is short; however, eosinophils and basophils appear to survive longer in the tissues than neutrophils.

142.

C. Approximately 50% of the neutrophils in the peripheral blood are found in the circulating pool. This is the pool measured when a total WBC count is done. Another 50% are found adhering to vessel walls (marginal pool). These pools are in constant exchange. Emotional or physical stimuli can cause a shift of cells from the marginating pool to the circulating pool, causing a transient rise in the total WBC count. The total WBC count can double but returns to normal within several hours.

143.

A. Although some phagocytic activity has been attributed to the eosinophil, it is the segmented neutrophil and monocyte that have the greatest phagocytic activity. The neutrophil is the most important because of numbers and its ability to respond quickly, especially against bacterial pathogens. Monocytes arrive at the site of injury after the neutrophil to "clean up."

144.

B. The growth factor mainly responsible for regulating the production of granulocytes and monocytes is granulocyte/monocyte colony-stimulating factor (GM-CSF), which acts on the committed bipotential progenitor cell CFU-GM (colony-forming unit–GM). GM-CSF stimulation of granulocyte or monocyte production increases in response to need and can also affect the production of erythrocytic and megakaryocytic lineages. G-CSF induces granulocyte differentiation, and M-CSF supports monocyte differentiation. Erythropoietin (EPO) is a lineage-specific growth factor responsible for stimulating erythrocyte production, and thrombopoietin (TPO) is mainly responsible for regulating platelet production. Interleukins, particularly IL-3, influence multiple cell lines, including granulocytes and monocytes.

145.

A. The granulocyte mitotic pool contains the cells capable of division, which are the myeloblasts, promyelocytes, and myelocytes. The post-mitotic pool, or reserve, is the largest bone marrow pool and contains metamyelocytes, band and segmented forms. This pool is available for prompt release into the blood if needed (e.g., infection), and its early release is the cause of a "left shift." If released, the bone marrow mitotic pool can dramatically increase its activity to replenish this reserve (cytokine stimulation increases).

146.

C. The function of lymphocytes is to produce antibodies and lymphokines.

147.

D. "Agranulocytosis" refers to an absence of granulocytes in both the peripheral blood and bone marrow. A deficiency of granulocytes is found in cases of aplastic anemia, in which deficiencies in red cells and platelets also occur. The early release of cells from the bone marrow will result in immature cells in the blood but is not referred to as agranulocytosis. Neutrophils that exhibit little or no granulation may be called hypogranular or agranular and are a sign of abnormal growth (dyspoiesis).

148.

C. Antibodies are synthesized by plasma cells, which are end-stage B lymphocytes that have transformed to plasma cells following stimulation by an antigen. An end product of T cell activation is the production of cytokines (lymphokines) such as interleukins and colony-stimulating factors. T cells are surveillance cells that normally comprise the majority (about 80%) of lymphocytes in the blood. T cells regulate the immune response by helping (T helper or inducer cells) or suppressing (T suppressor cells) the synthesis of antibody by plasma cells.

149.

C. Absolute values for cell types are obtained by multiplying the percentage of the cell type by the total number of cells. In this case, $4000/mm^3 \times 0.65 = 2600/\mu L$ or $2.6 \times 10^9/L$. Although reference ranges vary, the normal absolute count for lymphocytes is from 1.0 to $4.0 \times 10^9/L$ and the normal percentage of lymphocytes is 20–44%. In this case, there is a relative lymphocytosis (increase in percentage), but the absolute lymphocyte value is normal. Percentages can be misleading, so the absolute number of a particular cell type should always be evaluated.

150.

B. Auer rods are seen in the cytoplasm of malignant cells, most often myeloblasts, and are composed of fused primary (nonspecific, azurophilic) granules. Hypersegmented neutrophils have five lobes or more and are associated with vitamin B_{12} or folate deficiency. Toxic granules are primary granules with altered staining characteristics that stain in late-stage neutrophils due to toxicity. Döhle bodies are agranular patches of RNA present in neutrophil cytoplasm and associated with toxic states.

151.

D. The total white blood cell count reference ranges for males and females are equivalent. WBC counts do change with age, being higher in newborns and children than in adults. Any change from basal conditions, such as exercise or emotional stress, will cause a transient leukocytosis due to a redistribution of blood pools. WBC values are lower in the morning and higher in the afternoon (diurnal variation).

152.

C. Neutropenia is associated with a risk of infection. The degree of neutropenia correlates with the infection risk from high susceptibility ($<1.0 \times 10^9/L$) to great risk ($<0.5 \times 10^9/L$). Infection increases with the degree and duration of the neutropenia. Shortness of breath and bleeding tendencies are clinical symptoms associated with severe anemia and thrombocytopenia, respectively.

153.

C. Basophils and tissue mast cells have receptors for IgE and complement components, which trigger degranulation when appropriate antigens are present and are responsible for severe hypersensitivity reactions (anaphylaxis). Basophils and tissue mast cells have morphologic similarities but represent distinct cell types. Basophils possess water-soluble granules that contain, among other substances, heparin and histamine (a vasodilator and smooth muscle contractor). Basophils have a segmented nucleus, and the granules, although often scanty, overlie the nucleus. The mast cell has a single round nucleus, contains many more granules than the basophil, and can be found in the bone marrow.

154.

C. The last stage in the granulocytic series that divides is the myelocyte. Cells before and including this stage constitute the bone marrow mitotic pool and undergo multiple cellular divisions. Nuclear chromatin progressively clumps and nucleoli are no longer present in the nondividing metamyelocyte stage that follows the myelocyte.

155.

C. The precursor cell that can first be recognized as granulocytic is the myeloblast and has no granules. Primary or nonspecific granule production begins and ends during the promyelocyte stage. The granules are distributed between daughter cells as mitotic divisions occur. Secondary or specific granule production begins with the myelocyte stage and continues during succeeding cell stages with the synthesis of products specific to the function of the particular granulocyte (neutrophil, eosinophil, or basophil).

156.

A. Eosinophils lack lysozyme, which is present in neutrophils and monocytes, and contain a distinctive peroxidase that differs biochemically from the myeloperoxidase of neutrophils and monocytes. Major basic protein is a component of the granules and is very important to the ability of eosinophils to control parasites. In addition, eosinophils play a role in modifying the allergic reactions caused by degranulation of basophils. Basophils release eosinophil chemotactic factor of anaphylaxis (ECF-A), which calls eosinophils to the site.

157.

B. Primary granules, which appear in the promyelocyte stage, may be called azurophilic or nonspecific granules. Specific or secondary granules (neutrophilic, eosinophilic, basophilic) appear in the myelocyte stage. Primary granules contain hydrolytic enzymes (e.g., myeloperoxidase, lysozyme, acid phosphatase) and are coated with a phospholipid membrane. Lactoferrin is a component of neutrophil granules. Primary granules are visible in the myelocyte stage, but in later stage cells the primary granules, although present, are less visible by light microscopy under normal conditions.

158.

C. The intermediate stage in the formation of the fibroblast is the peripheral blood monocyte.

159.

A. Diapedesis is the movement of cells (usually referring to neutrophils) from the blood stream into the tissues by squeezing through endothelial cells of the vessel wall. Chemotaxis is the movement of cells directed by chemotactic stimuli such as bacterial products, complement components, or injured tissue. Opsonization is the coating of an organism or foreign particle by IgG or complement for recognition and phagocytosis by neutrophils or monocytes. The ingestion of red cells, often coated with IgG or complement, is called erythrophagocytosis. Margination is the attachment of neutrophils to the endothelial lining of the blood vessels.

160.

D. Basophil granules contain histamine, a potent vasodilator and smooth muscle contractor, that is responsible for the systemic effects seen in immediate hypersensitivity reactions (type I), which are also termed "anaphylaxis." Degranulation occurs when basophils are coated with an IgE type of antibody that recognizes a specific allergen, such as bee venom, certain plant pollens, or latex. The resulting anaphylactic shock can be life threatening.

161.

D. Definition of multipotent stem cell.

162.

B. Plasma cells are the mature end stage of the B lymphocyte, producing immunoglobulins (antibodies) in response to activation by a specific antigen (humoral immunity). The antibody produced by a single plasma cell is of one immunoglobulin type. Natural killer (NK) cells recognize and kill tumor cells or cells infected with virus through direct contact. Virocytes are reactive lymphocytes, and thymocytes are immature T cells. T lymphocytes provide cellular (cell mediated) immunity.

163.

C. A function of the eosinophil is to modify the severe allergic reactions caused by degranulation of the basophil. Neutrophils have receptors for the opsonins IgG and complement and are the most important cell in the initial defense against acute bacterial infection. Neutrophils are nonspecific phagocytes, ingesting bacteria, fungi, dead cells, etc., and they contain hydrolytic enzymes, including muramidase (lysozyme) and alkaline phosphatase. Neutrophils die in the performance of their function and are removed by macrophages.

164.

C. The nucleus in both monocytes and reactive lymphocytes can be irregular in shape, with indentations, although a monocyte nucleus often has folds and lobulations. Reactive lymphocytes characteristically have an increased amount of dark blue cytoplasm, whereas monocyte cytoplasm is usually a blue-gray color. Lymphocytes lack the many fine granules that give monocytes a typical "ground glass" appearance of the cytoplasm, but monocytes can occasionally have larger granules. Sharp indentation of the cytoplasm by adjacent red cells and an increased number of large granules are features of reactive lymphocytes. Vacuoles, although more commonly present in monocytes, can also be seen in reactive lymphocytes.

165.

B. Indentation of the nucleus (kidney shape) is the feature that characterizes the metamyelocyte stage. Specific granules begin forming in the myelocyte and persist through later stages. Cytoplasmic color is not a reliable feature, because it is variable and may not differ significantly from the myelocyte or band stage. Nucleoli are absent in metamyelocytes and may not be visible in myelocytes (they may be indistinct).

166.

A. Young children have the highest peripheral lymphocyte concentrations, ranging from 4.0 to 10.5×10^9 cells/L at 1 year of age and declining to $2.0–8.0 \times 10^9$ cells/L by 4 years of age. Lymphocyte counts decrease with age because of a decrease in lymphocyte stimulation and processing of antigens, ranging from 1.0 to 4.0×10^9 cells/L in adults. In addition to the difference in lymphocyte number in children, the normal morphology of children's lymphocytes differs from that of adults. Patient age should be considered when deciding between normal and abnormal lymphocytes.

167.

A. Early B cell precursors would be expected to express TdT, CD10, and CD34. TdT, the enzyme marker for terminal deoxynucleotidyl transferase, and the stem cell marker CD34 are present on the earliest B or T lymphoid cells. Surface immunoglobulin (SIgM) can only be detected on B cells at later stages of development. TdT can be used to differentiate the leukemic cells of acute lymphoid leukemia from acute myeloid leukemia. CALLA (CD10 or common ALL antigen) is a marker found in precursor types of B cell ALL.

168.

B. Acid hydrolases and the number of lysosomes increase as the blood monocyte matures into a tissue macrophage. Macrophages are widely dispersed in body tissues and organs of the reticuloendothelial (RE) system (also known as the mononuclear phagocyte system). Macrophages have receptors for IgG and complement, and they serve as phagocytes by ingesting debris and dead cells (usually neutrophils) at sites of inflammation. Macrophages act in the immune response as antigen-presenting cells by ingesting and exposing antigens for recognition by lymphocytes. Monocytes/macrophages secrete complement components and cytokines, including colony stimulating factors and interleukins.

169.

B. Antigen-*independent* lymphopoiesis occurs in primary lymphoid tissue located in the thymus and bone marrow. The formation of immunocompetent T and B cells from the lymphoid progenitor cell is influenced by environment (thymus, marrow) and several interleukins. Antigen-*dependent* lymphopoiesis occurs in secondary lymphoid tissue (spleen, lymph nodes, Peyer's patches) and begins with antigenic stimulation of immunocompetent T and B cells. Lymphocytes are the only white cells that recirculate (i.e., return to the blood from the tissues).

170.

C. Differentiates leukemia with classic granulocyte anomaly.

Leukocyte Disorders

171.

C. The Epstein-Barr virus (EBV) attaches to receptors on B lymphocytes, and is incorporated into the cell. The infection generates an intense immune response of T cells directed against infected B cells. It is the activated T lymphocytes that comprise the majority of reactive lymphocytes seen in the blood of patients with infectious mononucleosis. Other B cells produce nonspecific polyclonal (heterophile) antibody in response to the EBV infection.

172.

C. The malignant cells of hairy cell leukemia (HCL) stain positive with acid phosphatase in the presence of tartaric acid; that is, hairy cells contain tartrate-resistant acid phosphatase (TRAP). Normal cells stain acid phosphatase positive, but staining is inhibited by the addition of tartrate. HCL is a chronic disorder, mainly confined to the elderly. The spleen usually shows marked enlargement, but enlarged lymph nodes are very uncommon. Hairy cells are malignant B cells, and pancytopenia is usual at presentation.

173.

A. The lymphoid cells of B cell acute lymphoblastic leukemia (FAB type L3) are morphologically identical to the malignant B cells of Burkitt lymphoma (large cells with basophilic cytoplasm and cytoplasmic lipid vacuoles). Although the site of origin is the bone marrow in B cell ALL and the tissues in Burkitt lymphoma, the World Health Organization (WHO) classifies them as the same disease entity with different clinical presentations (Burkitt leukemia/lymphoma). Both chronic lymphocytic leukemia (CLL) and small lymphocytic lymphoma (SLL) are malignant proliferations of small, mature lymphocytes, and diagnosis is based on the predominant site of involvement. Mycosis fungoides and Sézary syndrome are different stages of a cutaneous T cell lymphoma in which the skin is the early site of involvement, with subsequent progression to the bone marrow and blood.

174.

A. Lab findings are reflective of erythroid rather than myeloid metaplasia.

175.

A. "True" Pelger-Huët anomaly is a benign autosomal dominant trait characterized by hyposegmentation of the granulocytes, coarse nuclear chromatin, and normal cytoplasmic granulation. The cells have no functional defect. It is of practical importance to recognize this anomaly so that it is not confused with a shift to the left due to infection. Acquired or "pseudo" Pelger-Huët is commonly associated with myeloproliferative disorders, myelodysplastic syndromes, or drug therapy. Pelgeroid cells are hyposegmented and the cytoplasm is frequently hypogranular.

176.

A. Eosinophils are decreased in Cushing syndrome, in which the adrenal glands secrete large amounts of adrenocorticosteroids. Eosinophils are increased in allergic disorders, various skin diseases, and certain types of parasitic infections (especially those due to intestinal and tissue-dwelling worms). Eosinophilia is also seen in chronic myelogenous leukemia and Hodgkin lymphoma.

177.

D. Chronic granulomatous disease (CGD) is a hereditary disorder in which neutrophils are incapable of killing most ingested microbes. The disease is usually fatal because of defective generation of oxidative metabolism products, such as superoxide anions and hydrogen peroxide, which are essential for killing. Chemotaxis, lysosomes, phagocytosis, and neutrophil morphology are normal. Several variants of CGD have been described, with specific enzyme defects and different modes of inheritance. The more common type of CGD has a sex-linked inheritance pattern.

178.

B. A drug-induced megaloblastic blood profile with macrocytic ovalocytes and hypersegmented neutrophils is shown in Color Plate 11■. This is a common finding in patients receiving antifolate chemotherapeutic drugs such as methotrexate. Recombinant erythropoietin is associated with a reticulocyte response and used to treat a variety of conditions, such as renal disease, anemia of chronic disease, or anemia caused by chemotherapy. Chloramphenicol is an antibiotic with a known association for aplasia due to marrow suppression.

179.

C. Primary or essential thrombocythemia (ET) is a chronic myeloproliferative disorder in which the main cell type affected is the platelet. An extremely high number of platelets are produced, but abnormal platelet function leads to both bleeding and clotting problems. The bone marrow shows megakaryocytic hyperplasia. The hemoglobin value and platelet count are increased in polycythemia vera, and CML is characterized by a high WBC count. Malignant thrombocythemia must be differentiated from a reactive thrombocytosis seen in patients with infection or following surgery. In reactive causes, the platelet count is rarely over 1 million $\times 10^9$/L, platelet function is normal, and thrombocytosis is transient.

180.

A. The bone marrow is progressively replaced by fibrotic tissue in myelofibrosis, a chronic myeloproliferative disorder. Attempts to aspirate bone marrow usually result in a "dry tap." A biopsy stain demonstrates increased fibrosis (fibroblasts are thought to be stimulated by megakaryocytes). The presence of teardrop-shaped red blood cells is an important feature of myelofibrosis. In addition, abnormal platelets, a leukoerythroblastic blood profile and myeloid metaplasia in the spleen and liver are often associated with this disease. A high LAP score (reference range 13–160) and increased RBC mass are found in polycythemia vera, but the LAP score is low in chronic myelogenous leukemia.

181.

B. A striking lymphocytosis may be seen in children with pertussis, but normal lymphocytes, rather than reactive lymphocytes, are present. A relative and/or absolute lymphocytosis with reactive lymphocytes in various stages of activation, as seen in Color Plate 12■, is characteristic of infection caused by Epstein-Barr virus (EBV), cytomegalovirus (CMV), and toxoplasmosis. A positive heterophile antibody test can help distinguish infectious mononucleosis caused by EBV from conditions with a similar blood picture. Epstein-Barr virus is also linked to Burkitt and Hodgkin lymphomas.

182.

C. B cell chronic lymphocytic leukemia (CLL) is by far the most common type found in the United States. Immune dysfunction because of hypogammaglobulinemia occurs in later stages of the disease, as does thrombocytopenia. Development of warm autoimmune hemolytic anemia is a frequent occurrence in patients with CLL. Treatment for B cell CLL is conservative and aimed at controlling symptoms. T cell CLL is a rare and is a more aggressive disease.

183.

D. Waldenström macroglobulinemia is caused by a proliferation of transitional B lymphocytes (lymphoplasmacytic or plasmacytoid lymphs) that secrete high amounts of monoclonal IgM. Because IgM is a macroglobulin, blood hyperviscosity is the cause of many of the symptoms found in this disease (bleeding and visual impairment). Plasmapheresis can reduce the IgM protein concentration. Hepatosplenomegaly is common in Waldenström disease (rather than bone lesions).

184.

C. The elevated WBC count and toxic neutrophils seen in Color Plate 13■ indicate an extreme response to severe infection (bacterial septicemia, fungal) or treatment with recombinant myeloid growth factors. GM-CSF and G-CSF are used to increase cells for peripheral stem cell transplant and reduce infection in patients after high-dose chemotherapy or during transplant. A leukemoid reaction is one that mimics the type of blood picture seen in leukemia. It is associated with extremely high leukocyte counts (often greater than 50×10^9 cells/L) and is usually found in severe infection. The most common type of leukemoid reaction is neutrophilic, but lymphocytic leukemoid reactions also occur. HIV infection is associated with leukopenia and lymphocytopenia.

185.

B. The blood shown in Color Plate 14■ is from an elderly patient with chronic lymphocytic leukemia (CLL), which is characterized by an absolute lymphocytosis and a predominance of small, mature lymphocytes with hyperclumped nuclear chromatin. Elevated leukocyte counts are usual, as are fragile, smudged lymphocytes. Acute lymphoblastic leukemia (ALL) typically occurs in children and is characterized by immature lymphoid cells. Plasmacytoid lymphocytes and red cell rouleaux may be found in the blood of individuals with Waldenström disease. Viral infections are associated with a lymphocytosis and the presence of reactive lymphocytes that are heterogeneous in morphology. Reactive lymphocytes exhibit a variety of forms with regard to size and cytoplasmic staining intensity as compared to the homogeneous cell populations present in malignant disorders such as CLL and ALL.

186.

D. Progression to acute leukemia is a very unlikely event for patients with chronic lymphocytic leukemia, even though there is no cure. Patients with chronic myelogenous leukemia typically progress to "blast crisis," most often of myeloid type, unless treated with imatinib mesylate (Gleevec®) in the chronic phase. Refractory anemia with excess blasts (RAEB) is the most likely type of myelodysplastic syndrome to develop acute myelogenous leukemia. Refractory anemia with ringed sideroblasts (RARS) is "preleukemic" but fairly stable.

187.

A. Gaucher disease is a lipid storage disorder in which there is an accumulation of glucocerebroside in the macrophages because of a genetic lack of glucocerebrosidase, an enzyme required for normal lipid metabolism. Gaucher cells are found in the liver, spleen, and bone marrow. Niemann-Pick disease is caused by a deficiency of sphingomyelinase in which "foamy" macrophages, called Niemann-Pick cells, are filled with sphingomyelin. Normal macrophages may contain iron and other cellular debris.

188.

D. The presence of Reed-Sternberg cells is the diagnostic feature of Hodgkin disease (lymphoma). The Reed-Sternberg giant cell is usually binucleated, and each lobe has a prominent nucleolus. Studies suggest that this neoplastic cell is of B cell lineage. It is not found in the blood but only in the tissues. Circulating T cells with a convoluted nucleus describe the Sézary cells seen in Sézary syndrome, the leukemic phase of mycosis fungoides. A monoclonal population of large lymphoid cells or immature B cells with nuclear clefts is most descriptive of lymphoma cells, present in certain types of peripheralized non-Hodgkin lymphoma, that have spread from the tissues to the bone marrow and blood.

189.

B. The myeloid predominance in acute myelocytic leukemia would increase from the normal (2:1 to 4:1) myeloid:erythroid ratio.

190.

C. The abnormal cells found in acute promyelocytic leukemia (FAB type M3) contain large numbers of azurophilic granules. These granules contain procoagulants that on release hyperactivate coagulation, resulting in disseminated intravascular coagulation. Although other acute leukemias may trigger DIC, M3 is the one most frequently associated with this life-threatening bleeding complication. If DIC is resolved, many patients with acute promyelocytic leukemia respond favorably to therapy with retinoic acid, which causes maturation of the malignant promyelocytes. The presence of t(15;17) has diagnostic and prognostic significance, and acute promyelocytic leukemia is classified with "acute myeloid leukemias with recurrent cytogenetic translocations" by the World Health Organization (WHO). Acute myeloblastic leukemia with t(8;21) is also included in this WHO category (correlates with FAB type M2).

191.

D. Although a hallmark of acute lymphoblastic leukemias (ALLs), lymphadenopathy is not associated with acute myelogenous leukemias. ALL is also more likely to have central nervous system involvement, and the CNS is a potential site of relapse. Hepatomegaly and splenomegaly are associated with both types of acute leukemia, as well as with the presence of anemia, neutropenia, and thrombocytopenia. Common presenting symptoms are fatigue, infection, or bleeding. If untreated, both acute myelogenous and lymphoblastic leukemias have a rapidly fatal course.

192.

B. The blast cells shown in Color Plate 15■ are from a child with CALLA positive, precursor B acute lymphoblastic leukemia. The malignant cells would be expected to express CD10, the common ALL antigen marker; the B cell lineage marker CD19; and TdT (terminal deoxynucleotidyl transferase), a marker on early lymphoid cells. Precursor T acute lymphoblastic leukemia would express TdT and the T cell markers CD2 and CD7. CD13 and CD33 are myeloid markers, and CD14 is a marker for monocytic cells.

193.

A. The "packed" bone marrow with predominantly immature blast cells and few normal precursor cells, as seen in Color Plate 16■, is most indicative of a patient with acute leukemia. Although chronic leukemias usually have a hypercellular marrow, the malignant cells are more mature or differentiated (i.e., able to mature beyond the blast stage). Myelodysplastic syndromes are associated with a hypercellular bone marrow, but the marrow blast percent is less than 20% (using WHO criteria). Aplastic anemia is characterized by a hypocellular bone marrow with few cells.

194.

C. The secretion of large amounts of monoclonal IgG or other immunoglobulin light chains by a malignant clone of plasma cells produces a characteristic M spike on serum and urine protein electrophoresis. In some cases, only the light chains are produced in excess. Because the light chains are easily cleared by the kidneys, they may appear only in the urine (Bence-Jones proteinuria). Renal impairment in multiple myeloma is associated with the toxic effects of filtered light chains. High levels of serum beta microglobulin correlate with the myeloma tumor burden. Cryoglobulins are proteins that precipitate in the cold and may be seen in multiple myeloma and Waldenström macroglobulinemia.

195.

C. Multiple myeloma is a malignant lymphoproliferative disorder characterized by a clonal proliferation of plasma cells and multiple bone tumors. Myeloproliferative disorders are characterized by a proliferation of bone marrow cells (granulocytic, monocytic, erythrocytic, megakaryocytic), with usually one cell type primarily affected. For example, the main cell type affected in polycythemia vera is the erythrocyte, and the platelet is mainly affected in essential thrombocythemia. Transformation among the myeloproliferative disorders is frequent.

196.

B. The Philadelphia chromosome, t(9;22), is detected in almost all cases of CML (depends on detection method) and results in a mutated BCR/ABL fusion gene. The resulting fusion protein causes increased tyrosine kinase activity, which promotes cell proliferation. Imatinib mesylate (Gleevec®) is a therapeutic agent that targets the molecular defect by blocking tyrosine kinase activity and is now a first-line drug used in the chronic phase of CML. The t(15;17) that is diagnostic of promyelocytic leukemia results in a PML/RARA (retinoic acid receptor alpha) fusion gene that blocks maturation. Many people with PML respond to retinoic acid therapy, which induces promyelocyte differentiation. Nearly all cases of Burkitt lymphoma have t(8;14), which is a translocation of the MYC gene from chromosome 8 to the Ig heavy chain (IgH) region on chromosome 14. JAK2 (Janus kinase) is a point mutation in a gene regulating cell proliferation, and it is present in over 90% of polycythemia vera cases and approximately 50% of those with essential thrombocythemia and myelofibrosis. Detection of cytogenetic and molecular mutations has diagnostic and prognostic significance and is an important tool in monitoring response to treatment.

197.

C. The French-American-British (FAB) classification of acute leukemias, myeloproliferative disorders, and myelodysplastic diseases was originally based on cellular morphology and cytochemistry (immunophenotyping was later added). Using FAB criteria, acute leukemia was defined as greater than 30% bone marrow blasts. The diagnostic criteria used by the World Health Organization (WHO) includes morphologic, cytochemical, immunologic, cytogenetic, and molecular features, as well as clinical findings, to better characterize all hematologic malignancies (myeloid and lymphoid) and predict disease course. The WHO classification defines acute leukemia as the presence of 20% or more bone marrow blasts and includes diagnostic categories with recurrent cytogenetic abnormalities. According to the WHO classification, lymphoid disorders are grouped into B cell, T/NK cell, and Hodgkin lymphoma. Further division of the B and T cell neoplasms considers site of involvement and precursor cell versus mature cell conditions.

198.

B. The blood profile of both chronic myelogenous leukemia (CML) and a neutrophilic leukemoid reaction is characterized by extremely high leukocyte counts with immature neutrophils. Splenomegaly is a manifestation of the malignant disease process and associated with CML rather than a leukemoid reaction. The presence of toxic granules and Döhle bodies would be typical of a leukemoid reaction caused by a severe bacterial infection. The LAP score is low in CML and high in a neutrophilic leukemoid reaction.

199.

C. In Color Plate 17■, the malignant blast cell contains an Auer rod, composed of fused primary granules, which stains positive with both myeloperoxidase and Sudan black B. Auer rods are not seen in lymphoblasts, and their presence can be diagnostic of acute myelogenous leukemia, such as acute myeloblastic leukemia (FAB types M1 and M2) or acute myelomonocytic leukemia (FAB type M4). Multiple Auer rods may be seen in acute promyelocytic leukemia (FAB type M3). Auer rods stain negatively with LAP, which detects the enzyme alkaline phosphatase in neutrophil granules.

200.

D. Acute myelocytic leukemia will show >20% myeloblasts without other immature stages. It will also differentiate AML from CML and myeloid metaplasia. Erythroleukemia requires at least 50% erythroid precursors in the marrow.

201.

B. Leukocyte alkaline phosphatase (LAP) scores are usually low in patients with chronic myelogenous leukemia (CML). The LAP reflects alkaline phosphatase activity in neutrophils, and the score is usually elevated in conditions where neutrophils are activated and/or increased in number, such as late pregnancy, bacterial infection, and polycythemia vera. The primary use of the LAP is to distinguish between the malignant cells of CML and a severe bacterial infection (leukemoid reaction). It may also be used to distinguish between CML and other chronic myeloproliferative disorders such as polycythemia vera. The LAP may be called NAP (neutrophil alkaline phosphatase) stain.

202.

D. Acute viral hepatitis and other liver infections are associated with lymphocytosis. The major causes of neutrophilia are bacterial infection, neoplastic tumors, and inflammatory responses to tissue injury. "Toxic" neutrophils may be present (toxic granulation, Döhle bodies, vacuolization). Infection with organisms other than bacteria (fungi, some parasites, certain viruses) may also cause neutrophilia.

203.

A. Monocytes must be distinguished from reactive lymphocytes, which are the characteristic feature of infectious mononucleosis. Monocytosis occurring in the recovery stage of acute infections is considered a favorable sign. An increase in monocytes is associated with collagen disorders (e.g., rheumatoid arthritis), tuberculosis, and malignant conditions such as myelodysplastic syndromes and monocytic leukemias.

204.

B. The periodic acid–Schiff (PAS) stain can be used to detect intracellular glycogen deposits in the lymphoblasts of acute lymphoblastic leukemia (ALL), in which coarse clumps of PAS positive material may be observed. Myeloblasts and monoblasts usually show a faint staining reaction. The immunophenotype has a much greater diagnostic value for ALL than the cytochemical stain results. The PAS may also be used to distinguish the malignant erythroid precursors of acute erythroleukemia, which show strong PAS positivity, from normal erythrocytic cells that stain negative.

205.

C. Myelodysplastic syndromes (MDSs) are characterized by a hypercellular bone marrow and up to 20% marrow blasts that distinguish MDS from acute leukemia (using WHO criteria). The blood and bone marrow blast percentages differ, and the risk of transformation to acute leukemia varies with the types of MDSs. These disorders are characterized by one or more peripheral blood cytopenias along with features of abnormal growth (dyspoiesis) in the bone marrow. A consistent feature in all types of myelodysplasia is unexplained and refractory anemia. Abnormalities may be morphologic and/or functional. Criteria that help define the types of myelodysplastic syndromes include megaloblastoid maturation of erythroid precursors, presence of multinucleated red cells, ringed sideroblasts, hypogranular and/or hyposegmented neutrophils, monocytosis, abnormal platelet morphology, circulating micromegakaryocytes, and degree of dyspoiesis.

206.

A. Naphthol AS-D chloroacetate esterase (specific) reacts strongly in granulocytic cells, and alpha-naphthyl acetate esterase (nonspecific) stains positively in monocytic cells. The esterase stains are used to distinguish between subtypes of acute myelogenous leukemia. The cells of acute myeloblastic leukemia (FAB types M1 and M2) will stain positive with specific esterase and negative with nonspecific esterase. The cells of acute monocytic leukemia (FAB type M5) will stain positive with nonspecific esterase and negative with specific esterase. The cells of acute myelomonocytic leukemia (FAB type M4) will show positivity with both specific and nonspecific esterase. Stain results are correlated with cell morphology, immunophenotype, and karyotype for diagnosis.

207.

A. May-Hegglin anomaly is an autosomal dominant disorder in which large blue cytoplasmic structures that resemble Döhle bodies are found in the granulocytes and possibly the monocytes. Leukocytes are normal in function. Platelets are decreased in number and abnormally large. About one-third of patients have mild to severe bleeding problems because of abnormal platelet function.

208.

D. Alder-Reilly anomaly is a hereditary autosomal recessive disorder caused by a deficiency of enzymes involved in the metabolism of mucopolysaccharides. Partially degraded mucopolysaccharides accumulate in various tissues, organs, and the leukocytes that are characterized by the presence of large azurophilic granules resembling toxic granulation. The inclusions do not affect leukocyte function and are referred to as Alder-Reilly bodies. The anomaly is often associated with facial and skeletal abnormalities, such as those seen in Hunter syndrome and Hurler syndrome. Lysosomal fusion with impaired degranulation is the defect in Chédiak-Higashi syndrome and is associated with early death due to abnormal leukocyte function.

209.

C. Serum and urine protein electrophoresis detects the presence of an M spike, the first essential step in establishing the disorder as a monoclonal gammopathy such as multiple myeloma or Waldenström disease. This can be followed by immunoelectrophoresis to determine the class of immunoglobulin or chain type. Immunologic markers, cytochemical stains, and/or cytogenetics are used in conjunction with cell morphology to diagnose malignant conditions.

210.

C. The prognosis is poor for patients with stage IV Hodgkin disease, in which there is widespread disease including bone marrow involvement. Stage I and II Hodgkin disease both have a very good prognosis for cure. The clinical course and treatment varies with the extent of disease and morphologic subtype (Rye classification). The peak incidence for Hodgkin lymphoma occurs in young adults (late twenties). Men have a 50% higher incidence of the disease than women. The CRP level and ESR are increased during active disease and can be used to monitor remission status.

211.

C. The acute leukemia indicated by these results is acute myelomonocytic leukemia (AMML), which has both granulocytic and monocytic features. Note the monocytic characteristics of the blast cells in Color Plate 18■. CD14 is a monocytic marker and CD33 is a marker for primitive myeloid cells. The SBB shows positive staining in both granulocytic and monocytic cells, the specific esterase stains positive in granulocytic cells, and the nonspecific esterase is positive in monocytic cells.

212.

B. Acute lymphoblastic leukemia (ALL) of children has the best prognosis. Other favorable factors include children between ages 3 and 7, mild to moderate increases in the peripheral white blood count prior to treatment, and precursor B ALL, CALLA-positive type (rather than T cell ALL). Certain cytogenetic and molecular abnormalities are also associated with a better prognosis. Acute leukemia in adults is less favorable because remissions are shorter and more difficult to induce, especially in those over 70 years of age. Prognosis is poor in adults with ALL.

213.

B. The test that would be the most beneficial for the diagnosis of Hodgkin lymphoma is a lymph node biopsy. Lymphadenopathy is the major clinical presentation of Hodgkin disease, and early stages do not have bone marrow involvement. A skin biopsy would be indicated for diagnosis of mycosis fungoides, a T cell lymphoma of the skin. A bone marrow exam and spinal tap are important to the diagnosis of acute leukemias.

214.

A. A hypercellular bone marrow and high M:E ratio are most characteristic of the excessive granulocyte production that occurs in chronic myelogenous leukemia. Polycythemia vera typically has a hypercellular marrow with panhyperplasia and a normal or low M:E ratio. Beta-thalassemia major is a severe hemolytic anemia in which RBC hyperplasia of the marrow is pronounced and a low M:E ratio is usual. Aplastic anemia is associated with a hypocellular marrow with a reduction of all cell lines and normal M:E ratio.

215.

B. Refractory anemia with ringed sideroblasts (RARS) is a myelodysplastic syndrome (MDS) that may also be referred to as primary or idiopathic sideroblastic anemia. The main findings that characterize this type of MDS include refractory anemia with a heterogeneous population of red cells, a hypercellular bone marrow with <5% blasts, and the presence of >15% ringed sideroblasts in the marrow (demonstrated with Prussian blue stain). RA and RARS are the least likely MDS types to progress to acute myelogenous leukemia.

216.

C. Recent strenuous exercise or other physical and emotional stimuli cause a transient increase in the leukocyte count. This is due to a redistribution of the blood pools. Marrow injury to stem cells or marrow replacement by malignant cells causes neutropenia of varying degrees. Neutropenia may be caused by immune mechanisms (antibodies) or an overactive spleen that sequesters neutrophils. Chemotherapeutic drugs also suppress bone marrow production of neutrophils.

217.

B. Primary polycythemia (vera) is a malignant myeloproliferative disorder characterized by autonomous marrow production of erythrocytes in the presence of low erythropoietin levels. Usual findings include increased RBC mass with elevated hemoglobin values and variable degrees of leukocytosis and thrombocytosis (pancytosis). Splenomegaly, a high LAP score, thrombotic tendencies, and problems caused by blood viscosity are typical. Phlebotomy is done to reduce red cell mass.

218.

D. Basophilia (and eosinophilia) is a typical finding in patients with chronic myelogenous leukemia (CML). A progressive increase in basophil number suggests transformation of the disease to a more accelerated phase. Myeloproliferative disorders such as CML, polycythemia vera, or AML are often associated with peripheral basophilia, which is not a feature of lymphoproliferative disorders such as acute lymphoblastic leukemia, hairy cell leukemia, or plasma cell leukemia.

219.

C. More than 50% of the marrow cells are erythroid in acute erythroleukemia (FAB type M6). Giant erythroid precursors, bizarre and multinucleated red cells, and increased myeloblasts are found in the marrow and may appear in the blood. Acute erythroid leukemia is rare, and the disease typically evolves into acute myeloblastic leukemia (FAB types M1 or M2).

220.

D. Plasma cell myeloma is a clonal disease involving malignant end-stage B cells, in which overproduction of immunoglobulin is a hallmark and the presence of red cell rouleaux is a characteristic finding on the blood smear, as shown in Color Plate 20■. Excessive amounts of a monoclonal immunoglobulin result in the deposition of proteins on circulating red cells that causes red cell "coining." The erythrocyte sedimentation rate is extremely elevated because of spontaneous rouleaux formation. Multiple myeloma is characterized by bone pain and spontaneous bone fractures caused by tumors of plasma cells. Bone destruction leads to elevated calcium levels, and renal impairment can result from damage by excess light chains. Plasma cells progressively crowd out normal bone marrow precursors and may be found in the blood circulation in advanced disease. Treatment with thalidomide has improved survival.

221.

C. The production of hematopoietic cells in sites outside of the bone marrow can be referred to as myeloid metaplasia or extramedullary hematopoiesis. Hematopoiesis, with the exception of lymphopoiesis, is normally confined to the bone marrow during postnatal life. Production of erythroid, myeloid, and megakaryocytic elements can be established in the liver and spleen, similar to that which occurs during embryonic development. Myeloid metaplasia is frequently associated with myelofibrosis, a condition in which the marrow is gradually replaced by fibrotic tissue.

222.

A. Prominent lymphadenopathy is the most consistent finding in non-Hodgkin types of lymphoma at presentation, but lymphoma may also arise in the spleen, liver, or GI tract (abdominal tumor). Lymphomas begin as localized tumors involving lymphoid tissue that spread to the bone marrow and blood (depends on type). The malignant lymphoid cells are immunologically classified as B cell (most common) or T/NK cell. Clonality can also be established by demonstrating gene rearrangements via molecular analysis. Some common subtypes of non-Hodgkin lymphoma are small lymphocytic, Burkitt, follicular, and mantle cell lymphomas. Leukemias are initially systemic disorders primarily involving the bone marrow and blood at onset. Bone lesions are associated with multiple myeloma.

Methodology

223.

B. The standard assay for hemoglobin utilizes potassium ferricyanide. This solution, formerly called Drabkin's reagent, is now called cyanmethemoglobin (HiCN) reagent. The ferricyanide oxidizes hemoglobin iron from ferrous (Fe^{2+}) to ferric (Fe^{3+}), and the potassium cyanide stabilizes the pigment as cyanmethemoglobin for spectrophotometric measurement.

224.

B. The band containing hemoglobin A_2 is the slowest-migrating, staying closest to the cathode. The band containing hemoglobin A has a net negative charge at an alkaline pH, and it moves the farthest toward the anode. An adult patient without a hemoglobinopathy will have only these two bands appearing on a cellulose acetate electrophoresis.

225.

C. Hemoglobins S, D, and G all migrate to the same location on the hemoglobin electrophoresis gel at an alkaline pH. However, because hemoglobins D and G are nonsickling hemoglobins, tests based on sickle formation under decreased oxygen tension will have negative results. These hemoglobins can be further differentiated by their movement on agar gel at an acid pH, whereas hemoglobins D and G will migrate with hemoglobin A, not with hemoglobin S.

226.

C. When the sample is deoxygenated, reduced hemoglobin S polymerizes, resulting in a cloudy solution. A false negative can be obtained if the quantity of hemoglobin S is below the sensitivity of the method, which can be seen in newborns and anemic patients. Although this procedure is a screening test for hemoglobin S detection, it is positive in the presence of any sickling hemoglobin, such as hemoglobin C_{Harlem}.

227.

A. A slanted column increases the ESR. A clotted sample, which lacks fibrinogen, causes a falsely decreased ESR. Fibrinogen is the plasma protein that most greatly affects the ESR. The EDTA tube for ESR must be at least half-full, and the test must be set up within 4 hours of draw; failure to follow these guidelines results in poikilocytosis that will inhibit rouleaux formation.

228.

C. Some patients develop EDTA-dependent platelet agglutinins caused by an IgM or IgG platelet-specific antibody. To correct for this, the sample can be redrawn in sodium citrate and rerun. The dilution factor of blood to anticoagulant in sodium citrate is 9:1. To compensate for the 10% dilutional loss of platelets, the platelet count obtained must be multiplied by 1.1 ($300 \times 10^9/L \times 1.1 = 330 \times 10^9/L$).

229.

B. Blood smears should be made within 5 hours of collection from blood anticoagulated with EDTA. Although some of the blood cells may still be normal in blood kept longer, others (especially granulocytes) may deteriorate. Vacuolation of neutrophils can appear as an artifact in blood kept past this time. The age of the blood may also affect the visual quality when the slide is stained.

230.

A. Decreasing the angle will produce a longer, thinner smear. Increasing the angle or using a smaller drop of blood will produce a shorter, thicker smear. The angle normally used for the spreader slide when making a smear is 30–45 degrees.

231.

D. One type of Romanowsky stain is the Wright's stain. It is a polychrome stain consisting of methylene blue and eosin. This combination causes multiple colors to appear on staining. Another commonly used Romanowsky stain is the Wright-Giemsa stain. Brilliant green and neutral red are used in a supravital stain for Heinz bodies. Crystal violet and safranin are used in Gram's stain for bacteria.

232.

C. When red blood cells are stained correctly with Wright stain, their color is pink to orange-red. They will appear bright red in the presence of an acid buffer and stain. Staining elements such as white cells, which stain with a more basic pH, will not take up the stain adequately in this instance. Inadequate washing and an alkaline stain or buffer mixture results in a smear that is excessively blue.

233.

C. The formula for calculating a reticulocyte count in percent is

$$\frac{\text{Number of reticulocytes counted}}{\text{Total number of RBCs counted}} \times 100$$

In the case described in question 233,

$$\%\text{Reticulocytes} = \frac{60}{1000} \times 100 = 6.0\%$$

Because the error in reticulocyte counts is high, it is desirable to count a larger number of cells or use a standardized counting method such as the Miller disk.

234.

C. The formula used to calculate the absolute reticulocyte count is

$$\frac{\text{Reticulocyte percent}}{100} \times \text{RBC}\,(10^{12}/\text{L}) \times 1000$$

Multiplication by 1000 is done to report the results in SI units of $10^9/\text{L}$.

In this case, $$\frac{6.0 \times 3.00}{100} \times 1000 = 180 \times 10^9/\text{L}$$

$180 \times 10^3/\mu\text{L}$ is not expressed in SI units.

235.

B. As visualized in Color Plate 19■, Sudan black B is a cytochemical stain for lipids, including steroids, phospholipids, and neutral fats. It is widely used as a tool to differentiate the blasts of acute lymphoblastic leukemia (ALL) from those of acute myelogenous leukemia (AML). Blasts in ALL are SBB negative, whereas those in AML will show some degree of positivity.

236.

C. An LAP score is determined by first multiplying the number of cells found by the degree of positivity (i.e., $20 \times 1 = 20$). These numbers are then added together to obtain a final score. In this instance, $0 + 20 + 60 + 60 + 60 = 200$.

237.

C. When stained with a mixture of potassium ferricyanide and hydrochloric acid, nonheme iron stains bright blue. This is the most common stain used for storage iron. It can be used on bone marrow to identify sideroblasts, peripheral blood to identify the presence of siderocytes, or urine to perform hemosiderin testing.

238.

C. Pappenheimer bodies are iron deposits associated with mitochondria, and they stain with both Perl's Prussian blue and Wright stain. A cell that contains Pappenheimer bodies is called a siderocyte. Howell-Jolly bodies and basophilic stippling can be visualized with Wright's stain, whereas Heinz bodies require a supravital stain to be seen.

239.

B. Depth on a standard counting chamber is 0.10 mm. The formula to calculate volume is $V = A \times D$, where V is volume, A is area, and D is depth. When the counting chamber is used, the area may change, depending on the number of ruled squares counted, but the depth remains constant.

240.

B. The standard formula for hemacytometer counts expressed in mm^3 is

$$\frac{\text{Total number cells counted} \times \text{dilution factor}}{\text{Area counted} \times \text{depth}}$$

In this instance,

$$\frac{308 \times 20}{8\ mm^2 \times 0.10\ mm} = \frac{6160}{0.8\ mm^3} = 7700/mm^3$$
$$= 7.7 \times 10^9/L$$

241.

B. The Rule of Three states that RBC $\times$ 3 = Hgb and Hgb $\times$ 3 = Hct ± 3 in error-free results. These rules apply only for normocytic, normochromic erythrocytes. One check to determine if an error has occurred is to determine the MCHC. An MCHC should be less than 37 g/dL in error-free results. The MCHC is calculated by dividing hemoglobin by hematocrit and multiplying by 100. In instance (B), the MCHC is 38.3 g/dL and the Rule of Three is broken. All other answers follow the Rule of Three.

242.

A. The only *true* cause of a high MCHC is the presence of spherocytes, as may be seen in hereditary spherocytosis. Because the MCHC is a calculation using the hemoglobin and hematocrit, anything causing those parameters to be wrong will affect the MCHC. The occurrence of a falsely high MCHC is much more common than the presence of spherocytes, and specimen troubleshooting procedures must be undertaken to obtain reportable results.

243.

C. Blood cells are nonconductors of electrical current; they create a resistance/impedance of current in a diluent solution that is conductive. When the suspension is forced through a small aperture, the current flow is interrupted by the presence of the cells. A pulse is generated. The number of pulses generated is proportional to the number of particles present, and the size of the pulse generated is proportional to the size of the cell.

244.

C. Using ±2 *s*, 95% confidence limits are achieved; 95% confidence limits predict a range that values should fall within 95% of the time. For example, if a WBC count is $12.0 \times 10^9/L$ with 2 *s* of ±0.5, then a succeeding count must be less than $11.5 \times 10^9/L$ or greater than $12.5 \times 10^9/L$ to be considered significantly different.

245.

A. Side angle scatter of a laser beam increases with granularity of the cytoplasm. Forward angle scatter is used to determine relative size. The number of signals is proportional to the number of cells. The presence of specific antigens in the cytoplasm or on the cell surface is determined by immunofluorescence after reactions with appropriate antibodies.

246.

A. An impedance counter cannot differentiate between the nucleus of a white blood cell and the nucleus of an nRBC. Both will be counted as WBCs. The presence of five or more nRBCs/100 WBCs can result in a falsely elevated white blood cell count, and a correction must be made as follows:

Corrected WBC count =

$$\text{Observed count} \times \frac{100}{100 + \#\text{nRBCs}/100\,\text{WBCs}}$$

247.

D. Hemoglobin A_2 values up to 3.5% are considered normal. Values between 3.5 and 8.0% are indicative of beta-thalassemia minor. Hemoglobins C, E, and O have net electrical charges similar to hemoglobin A_2. They elute off with hemoglobin A_2 using anion exchange (column) chromatography, causing an invalid hemoglobin A_2 result. If the hemoglobin A_2 quantification using column chromatography yields a result greater than 8.0%, one of these interfering hemoglobins should be considered.

248.

C. Any condition with spherocytes can cause an increased osmotic fragility, dependent on the number of spherocytes present. Spherocytes are seen in hereditary spherocytosis, immune hemolytic anemias, and severe burns. Target cells, associated with thalassemias and hemoglobinopathies, have an increased surface area-to-volume ratio and a decreased osmotic fragility.

249.

B. The solubility test for hemoglobin S is not quantitative; it is reported as positive or negative. A clotted specimen will not affect the result. A clotted specimen will falsely decrease the other tests listed: ESR due to low fibrinogen, hematocrit due to a false low RBC count, and platelets are trapped in the clot.

250.

A. Hematology reference intervals are available in many textbooks. They are influenced by patient population, instrumentation, and reagents used. Therefore, it is ideal for each laboratory to establish its own reference intervals. The reference interval excludes the upper and lower 2.5% of the values. The remaining 95% represent the reference interval.

251.

C. Standards are commercially available to generate a hemoglobin concentration curve. The absorbance of each solution is read against a reagent blank at 540 nm on a spectrophotometer. Patient blood samples and commercial control materials can be used to assess precision and other quality control parameters.

252.

B. Anything that causes an increase in absorbance will cause a hemoglobin that is detected spectrophotometrically to be falsely high. It is necessary to correct for this type of error, such as making a plasma blank in the case of lipemia or icterus. WBCs are present in the hemoglobin dilution and usually do not interfere. When the WBC count is extremely high, their presence will cause cloudiness, increasing the absorbance in the hemoglobin measuring cell and resulting in a falsely high hemoglobin concentration. Excessive anticoagulant does not affect hemoglobin readings.

253.

A. When a microhematocrit is spun at 10,000–15,000 × *g* for 5 minutes, maximum packing is achieved. Spinning a longer time has no affect on the result. A tube that is not full causes RBC shrinkage and a falsely decreased hematocrit. Improper sealing of the capillary tube causes a decreased Hct reading as a result of loss of blood during centrifugation. Trapped plasma is present when optimal packing is not achieved due to inadequate speed or time of centrifugation, causing a falsely high hematocrit.

254.

C. The erythrocyte sedimentation rate (ESR) measures the rate of fall of red cells through plasma. ESR increases when cells become stacked (rouleaux, as seen in Color Plate 20■). ESR decreases when cells are not normal discocytes. Larger cells (macrocytes) and fewer cells (anemia) fall faster. Plasma containing increased proteins, such as fibrinogen and globulins, promote rouleaux formation and an elevated ESR. Hemoglobin content does not affect the ESR.

255.

A. Impedance counters measure RBCs and platelets using the same dilution. To differentiate the two, sizing thresholds are used. Particles between 2 and 20 fL are counted as platelets, and particles larger than 35 fL are counted as RBCs. Small RBCs, clumped platelets, and giant platelets fall in the overlap area between platelets and RBCs, generating a warning flag. Nucleated RBCs are larger than normal RBCs and are not mistaken for platelets.

256.

C. A platelet estimate is obtained by multiplying the average number of platelets per oil immersion field (in an erythrocyte monolayer) by 20,000. The reference range for a platelet count is 150–450 × 10^9/L. Approximately 8–20 platelets per oil immersion field will represent a normal platelet concentration of approximately 160–400 × 10^9/L. This method assumes that the red blood cell count is normal. If it is not, alternate platelet estimate procedures may need to be performed.

257.

A. A living cell stain using new methylene blue is performed for reticulocyte counts. Reticulocytes should not be stained for less than 5 minutes. Howell-Jolly bodies, Pappenheimer bodies, crenated cells, and refractile artifact can be mistaken for reticulocyte inclusions. Two or more particles of reticulum constitute a reticulocyte.

258.

B. All accredited laboratories are required to perform calibration with commercially available calibrators at least once every 6 months. Calibration must be checked if any major part is replaced or if optical alignment is adjusted. A calibration procedure can be verified using commercially available controls.

259.

A. An MCHC >37 g/dL is most likely caused by an error in measurement. In this instance, the Rule of Three shows that the RBC × 9 matches the hematocrit, but the RBC × 3 does not match the hemoglobin. The hemoglobin does not match either the RBC or hematocrit. This indicates a hemoglobin problem, and it can be corrected with a saline replacement procedure. This specimen may be lipemic or icteric. Warming the specimen is useful in troubleshooting a high MCHC due to a cold agglutinin. A microhematocrit would be indicated if the hematocrit result was invalid.

260.

A. Hemoglobin is valid on a hemolyzed specimen, because RBC lysis is the first step in the cyanmethemoglobin method. The red blood cell count depends on the presence of intact red blood cells. Red blood cell fragments caused by hemolysis may be as small as platelets and affect instruments that use sizing criteria to differentiate the two. Therefore, samples for these procedures should be recollected.

261.

D. Heparin is recommended for osmotic fragility and red cell enzyme studies, because it results in less lysis and less membrane stress than other anticoagulants. Heparin induces platelet clumping and is unacceptable for the platelet count. Heparin is unacceptable for coagulation test procedures because it binds with antithrombin to neutralize many enzymes, especially thrombin. This would cause very long coagulation test results. EDTA is recommended for most routine hematology procedures, especially for Wright stained smears. Sodium citrate or EDTA can be used for sedimentation rates.

262.

A. When counting platelets, the center square (1 mm^2) is counted on each side of the hemacytometer. Platelets appear round or oval and may have dendrites. These characteristics can help distinguish them from debris, which is irregularly shaped and often refractile. White cells are not lysed; they may be counted, using a different ruled area of the hemacytometer. Platelets will be easier to count if allowed to settle for 10 minutes, because they will have settled into one plane of focus.

263.

B. "Precision" is the term used to describe the reproducibility of a method that gives closely similar results when one sample is run multiple times. An accurate method is one that gives results that are very close to the true value. Laboratories must have procedures that are both accurate and precise.

Case Histories

264.

C. WBC counts done by an impedance cell counter must be corrected when nucleated red blood cells (nRBCs) are present (see Color Plate 4■), because such instruments do not distinguish between white and red nucleated cells. This correction is done according to the following formula:

$$\text{Corrected WBC count} = \text{Observed count} \times \frac{100}{100 + \#\text{nRBCs per 100 WBCs}}$$

In this instance,

$$35.0 \times \frac{100}{100 + 110} = 16.7 ¥ 10^9/L$$

265.

A. The appearance of red cells on a differential smear may be predicted by calculating the red cell indices.

$$\text{MCV} = \frac{\text{Hct} \times 10}{\text{RBC}} = \frac{16\% \text{ ¥ } 10}{2.50 \text{ ¥ } 10^{12}/\text{L}} = 64.0 \text{ fL}$$

$$\text{MCH} = \frac{\text{Hgb} \times 10}{\text{RBC}} = \frac{4.5 \text{ g/dL ¥ } 10}{2.50 \text{ ¥ } 10^{12}/\text{L}} = 18.0 \text{ pg}$$

$$\text{MCHC} = \frac{\text{Hgb} \times 100}{\text{Hct}} = \frac{4.5 \text{ g/dL ¥ } 100}{16\%}$$

$$= 28.1 \text{ g/dL} \, (281 \text{ g/L})$$

The mean corpuscular volume (MCV), mean corpuscular hemoglobin (MCH), and mean corpuscular hemoglobin concentration (MCHC) are all below the reference range. This indicates a cell that is small (microcytic) with a reduced hemoglobin concentration (hypochromic). These indices refer to averages and do not necessarily reflect the actual appearance of cells in which there is great diversity in size and shape.

266.

D. Children with beta-thalassemia major, also known as Cooley anemia, do not use iron effectively to make heme. This occurs because of a genetic defect that causes a decreased rate of production of structurally normal globin chains. In addition, these children receive frequent transfusions due to the severe hemolytic anemia. The result is hemochromatosis with a high serum iron and storage iron. None of the other anemias listed would elicit the bone marrow response seen by the high number of nucleated RBCs, because they are not hemolytic.

267.

D. Beta-thalassemia major is characterized by an inability to produce beta-globin chains, resulting in a decrease or complete absence of hemoglobin A. Hemoglobin F, a compensatory hemoglobin that contains two alpha- and two gamma-globin chains, is frequently the only hemoglobin present. Hemoglobin A_2 is classically increased in heterozygous beta-thalassemia, but it is variable in homozygous beta-thalassemia.

268.

B. The predominant hemoglobin present at birth is hemoglobin F, which consists of two alpha- and two gamma-globin chains. It is not until about 6 months of age that beta-chain production is at its peak. At this point, hemoglobin A (two alpha and two beta chains) replaces hemoglobin F as the predominant hemoglobin. A deficiency in the production of these chains will not be apparent until this beta-gamma switch has occurred.

269.

D. The formula for calculation of transferrin saturation is as follows:

$$\text{Transferrin saturation \%} = \frac{\text{Serum iron } (\mu\text{g/dL}) \times 100}{\text{TIBC } (\mu\text{g/dL})}$$

In this case,

$$\text{Transferrin saturation \%} = \frac{22 \times 100}{150} = 15\%$$

Because the reference range for saturation is 20–45%, this is a low saturation.

270.

D. In the anemia of chronic disease, patients have iron but are unable to utilize it. Hepcidin, a hormone produced by the liver, plays a role in body iron regulation. Intestinal iron absorption and release of iron from macrophages both decrease in response to increased hepcidin levels. Hepcidin is a positive acute-phase reactant, so increased levels are seen in anemia of chronic disease due to inflammation. This adversely affects iron availability.

271.

A. The most common anemia among hospitalized patients is anemia of chronic disease. Patients with chronic infections, inflammatory disorders, and neoplastic disorders develop this type of anemia. The typical presentation is a normocytic, normochromic anemia, but microcytic and hypochromic anemia can develop in long-standing cases. Chronic blood loss can cause iron deficiency and microcytic/hypochromic anemia.

272.

A. Both megaloblastic anemias and some nonmegaloblastic anemias are characterized by the presence of macrocytic, normochromic red cells. Vitamin B_{12} and folic acid are coenzymes necessary for DNA synthesis. Lack of either one causes megaloblastic anemia. Maturation asynchrony is evident in both the peripheral blood and bone marrow. The bone marrow examination is done after vitamin B_{12} and folate levels because of the test's invasive nature. Vitamin B_{12} and folic acid levels are normal or increased in nonmegaloblastic anemias. Iron studies are useful in the diagnosis of microcytic/hypochromic anemias.

273.

C. The common causes of megaloblastic anemia are pernicious anemia and folic acid deficiency. Neurological symptoms are not associated with folic acid deficiency. Folic acid is a water-soluble vitamin for which there are low body stores. A diet low in green vegetables and meat products or high in alcohol can result in folate deficiency in 2–4 months. Alcohol is a folate antagonist.

274.

A. The general classification of anemia described here is megaloblastic anemia. A deficiency of vitamin B_{12} or folic acid affects DNA production. All dividing cells will show nuclear abnormalities, resulting in megaloblastic changes. In the neutrophil, as seen in Color Plate 11■, this takes the form of hypersegmentation (five lobes or more). Enlarged, fragile cells are formed, many of which die in the bone marrow. This destruction leads to increased LD, bilirubin, and iron levels. Oval macrocytes and teardrop cells are seen. Pancytopenia and inclusions are common findings. One cause of a nonmegaloblastic macrocytic anemia, which has round cells such as target cells instead of oval cells, is liver disease.

275.

B. The pancytopenia and red blood cell morphologic findings are all consistent with megaloblastic anemia. Further investigation of serum folate and vitamin B_{12} levels is warranted. Pernicious anemia (PA) is noted for neurological complications and is seen more commonly among people of British and Scandinavian ancestry. PA is caused by a lack of intrinsic factor production in the stomach, which is necessary for the absorption of vitamin B_{12}. Because there are large body stores of vitamin B_{12}, it takes from 1 to 4 years for the deficiency to manifest itself. Aplastic anemia is also associated with pancytopenia, but not the red cell morphologic changes seen in this patient.

276.

A. Alcohol is a folic acid, not a vitamin B_{12}, antagonist. Patients with pernicious anemia (PA) are incapable of absorbing vitamin B_{12} due to a lack of intrinsic factor or antibodies to intrinsic factor or parietal cells. PA is characterized by achlorhydria and atrophy of gastric parietal cells that secrete intrinsic factor. Achlorhydria is not diagnostic for PA, because it may occur in other disorders (such as severe iron deficiency), but it is confirmatory evidence of the problem. *D. latum* competes for B_{12} in the intestines.

277.

B. Because intrinsic factor is necessary for absorption of vitamin B_{12} from the ileum, intramuscular injections of vitamin B_{12} are used to treat PA. Although oral doses of folic acid will correct the megaloblastic blood profile seen in PA, the neurological symptoms will not improve. For this reason, correct diagnosis is crucial. Methotrexate is a folic acid antagonist. Because body folic acid stores are low, a deficiency can develop quickly.

278.

A. The adult red blood cell in glucose-6-phosphate dehydrogenase (G6PD) deficiency is susceptible to destruction by oxidizing drugs. This occurs because the mechanism for providing reduced glutathione, which keeps hemoglobin in the reduced state, is defective. The anti-malarial drug primaquine is one of the best-known drugs that may precipitate a hemolytic episode. Ingestion of fava beans can also elicit a hemolytic episode in some patients.

279.

C. G6PD deficiency, a sex-linked disorder, is the most common enzyme deficiency in the hexose monophosphate shunt. Most patients are asymptomatic and go through life being unaware of the deficiency unless oxidatively challenged. Pyruvate kinase, an enzyme in the Embden-Meyerhof pathway, is necessary to generate ATP. ATP is needed for red blood cell membrane maintenance. Patients with a pyruvate kinase deficiency have a chronic mild to moderate anemia.

280.

B. Reduced glutathione levels are not maintained due to a decrease in NADPH production. Methemoglobin (Fe^{3+}) accumulates and denatures in the form of Heinz bodies. Heinz bodies cause rigidity of the RBC membrane, resulting in red cell lysis. Döhle bodies are composed of RNA; Howell-Jolly bodies are composed of DNA; Pappenheimer bodies are iron deposits.

281.

C. Iron-deficiency anemia (IDA) causes a microcytic, hypochromic anemia. It is the most common anemia found in children. IDA develops quickly in children because of rapid growth with increased dietary iron requirements. Hereditary spherocytosis results in RBCs that are normal to low-normal in size, with an MCHC possibly greater than 37.0 g/dL. Folic acid deficiency causes a macrocytic/normochromic anemia. Erythroblastosis fetalis is a hemolytic disease of the newborn caused by red blood cell destruction by antibodies from the mother; such antibodies are no longer in the circulation of a 15-month-old child.

282.

C. The development of iron deficiency occurs in stages: the iron depletion stage, the iron-deficient erythropoiesis stage, and the iron-deficiency anemia stage. Iron stores are the first to disappear, so the serum ferritin level is the earliest indicator of iron-deficiency anemia. This is followed by decreased serum iron and increased TIBC. The last abnormality seen is microcytic, hypochromic red blood cells.

283.

C. In iron-deficiency anemia, red blood cell production is restricted because of lack of iron, and the reticulocyte absolute value reflects this ineffective erythropoiesis. The formula used to calculate the absolute reticulocyte count is

Absolute reticulocytes =

$$\frac{\text{Reticulocytes \%}}{100} \times \text{RBC}\,(10^{12}/\text{L}) \times 1000$$

The 1000 in the calculation is to convert to SI units (10^9/L).

In this case,

$$\frac{0.2}{100} \times 2.70\,(10^{12}/\text{L}) \times 1000 = 5\,\text{¥}\,10^{9}/\text{L}$$

The reference interval for the absolute reticulocyte count is approximately 18–158 $\times 10^9$/L.

284.

A. Petechiae and ecchymoses (bruises) are primary hemostasis bleeding symptoms seen in quantitative and qualitative platelet disorders. Although estimates vary, spontaneous bleeding does not usually occur until platelet numbers are less than 50 $\times 10^9$/L. The malignant disorder represented in this case is noted for thrombocytopenia.

285.

A. The bone marrow blast percent indicates the presence of an acute leukemia. The triad of symptoms seen in acute leukemia is neutropenia, anemia, and thrombocytopenia. Acute lymphoblastic leukemia is the leukemia most likely to be found in this age group. Hairy cell leukemia does not present with blasts. Myelodysplastic syndrome presents with less than 20/30 (WHO/FAB, respectively) percent marrow blasts.

286.

C. Periodic acid–Schiff stains glycogen in lymphoblasts. The myeloperoxidase stain is positive in myeloid cells. Monocytes show a positive reaction to the nonspecific esterase stain. Leukocyte alkaline phosphatase is useful in the diagnosis of chronic myelogenous leukemia.

287.

A. Terminal deoxyribonucleotidyl transferase (TdT) is a nuclear enzyme (DNA polymerase) found in stem cells and precursor B and T lymphoid cells. High levels of TdT are found in 90% of ALLs. TdT has been found in up to 10% of cases of AML (FAB M0 and M1), but in lower levels than are present in ALL. This enzyme is not found in mature lymphocytes.

288.

B. There are now more than 200 recognized human leukocyte antigens, each of which has been given a CD (cluster designation) number. CDs 2, 5, and 7 are seen on T cells. CALLA, the common acute lymphoblastic leukemia antigen, is seen in early pre–B cells. Distinct CD markers have been identified for cells of both lymphoid and myeloid stem cell lineage.

289.

B. The bone marrow blast percent is high enough to indicate an acute leukemia. Sudan black B, myeloperoxidase, and specific esterase stains are positive, indicating the presence of the myeloid cell line. The nonspecific esterase stain is negative, indicating the absence of a monocytic cell line. The bone marrow blast percent is too low for FAB M1, but it is in the range for FAB M2.

290.

A. Chromosome analysis is an important diagnostic tool in clinical medicine. Nonrandom chromosome abnormalities are recognized in many forms of cancer. t(8;21) is associated with acute myelogenous leukemia FAB M2; t(15;17) is only seen in FAB M3. The Philadelphia chromosome, t(9;22), is seen in at least 90% of patients with chronic myelogenous leukemia; t(8;14) is associated with Burkitt lymphoma.

291.

C. When a diagnosis of AML or myelodysplastic syndrome is suspected, a bone marrow examination is performed. The WHO approach to the diagnosis of acute leukemia requires the presence of >20% blasts in the bone marrow; the FAB classification requires >30%. The reference interval for bone marrow blast percent is 0–2%. Myelodysplastic syndromes have increased bone marrow blast percentages, but <20% using WHO criteria and <30% using FAB criteria.

292.

B. HTLV-I is implicated in T cell leukemia and lymphoma in Japan. The Epstein-Barr virus is associated with Burkitt lymphoma in Africa. Chronic bone marrow dysfunction can be caused by exposure to radiation, drugs, and chemicals such as benzene. Myelodysplastic syndromes and myeloproliferative disorders are "preleukemic" because they have a high incidence of terminating in acute leukemia. Paroxysmal nocturnal hemoglobinuria, aplastic anemia, multiple myeloma, and lymphoma are stem cell disorders that are particularly noted for transformation into acute leukemia. Genetic susceptibility is associated with Klinefelter and Down syndromes, both of which have chromosomal abnormalities. It is likely that more than one factor is responsible for the evolution of an acute leukemia.

293.

A. The myelodysplastic syndromes (MDSs) are pluripotential stem cell disorders characterized by one or more peripheral blood cytopenias. Bone marrow examination is necessary for diagnosis. There are prominent maturation abnormalities in all three cell lines in the bone marrow. Megaloblastoid erythrocyte maturation is present that is not responsive to B_{12} or folic acid therapies. Although many of the red blood cell inclusions noted in this case can be seen in a megaloblastic anemia such as pernicious anemia, this patient has a normal vitamin B_{12} and folate level. This patient has hyposegmentation of neutrophils, whereas megaloblastic anemias present with hypersegmentation of neutrophils. Of the disorders listed, the only one associated with dyshematopoiesis of all cell lines is myelodysplastic syndrome.

294.

D. In most cases of MDS, the bone marrow is hypercellular with erythroid hyperplasia. MDS is considered a disease of the elderly. Because normal cellularity decreases with age, interpretation of cellularity must take the age of the patient into account. WHO criteria for a diagnosis of MDS are related to bone marrow blast percent, which must be <20%.

295.

D. In RAEB at least two cell lines exhibit cytopenia, and all cell lines show evidence of dyshematopoiesis. Poor granulation and pseudo-Pelger-Huët anomaly is seen. There are less than 5% blasts in the peripheral blood, and between 5 and 19% blasts in the bone marrow. Platelets exhibit poor granulation, giant forms, and the abnormal maturation stage of micromegakaryocytes. The five FAB classifications of myelodysplastic syndrome are RA, RARS, RAEB, CMML, and RAEB-t. CML is a myeloproliferative disorder, not a myelodysplastic syndrome.

296.

C. The myelodysplastic syndromes are refractory to treatment, and patients are supported using blood products dependent on their cytopenias. The median survival rate for all types of MDSs is less than 2 years. RAEB and RAEB-t have the highest percentage of blasts and the lowest survival rates. At this time, bone marrow transplant offers the only chance for a cure, and it is the treatment of choice in patients below 50 years of age. Studies have shown that the incidence of MDS is greater than the incidence of AML in the 50–70-year-old age group. Up to 40% of the myelodysplastic syndromes transform into acute leukemia.

297.

B. Chronic myelogenous leukemia (CML) is a myeloproliferative disorder, a malignant proliferation of leukocytes not in response to infection; the leukocyte count is often greater than $100.0 \times 10^9/L$. No toxic changes are present in CML. Thrombocytosis is seen in more than half of the patients with CML. A neutrophilic leukemoid reaction represents a normal body response to a severe infection. It is a benign proliferation of WBCs with a high leukocyte count but usually less than $50.0 \times 10^9/L$. Toxic changes to the neutrophils such as toxic granulation, vacuoles, and Döhle bodies are present. These two disorders both display a "left" shift, and they can be confused with each other.

298.

D. Leukocyte alkaline phosphatase activity is increased in severe infections such as the neutrophilic leukemoid reaction and polycythemia vera, and during the last trimester of pregnancy. It is greatly reduced in chronic myelogenous leukemia, although it may increase during blast crisis of this disease. Periodic acid–Schiff and Sudan black B are used to differentiate ALL from AML. The TRAP stain is useful in the diagnosis of hairy cell leukemia.

299.

C. The Philadelphia chromosome, t(9;22), is found in the precursor cells for erythrocytes, granulocytes, and platelets in at least 90% of the cases of CML. It is an acquired chromosome abnormality that results from a reciprocal translocation between chromosomes 9 and 22, and it can be detected even when the patient is in remission. The BCR/ABL oncogene is also associated with CML.

300.

C. Patients who have the Philadelphia chromosome have a less aggressive disease and better prognosis than the rare cases that do not have the abnormality. Some cases of CML terminate in an acute lymphoblastic leukemia. However, this outcome cannot be predicted by the presence or absence of the Philadelphia chromosome.

REFERENCES

Anderson, S. C., and Poulsen, K. B. (2014). *Atlas of Hematology*, Philadelphia: Lippincott Williams & Wilkins.

Carr, J. H., and Rodak, B. F. (2016). *Clinical Hematology Atlas*, 5th ed. St. Louis: Elsevier.

Harmening, D. M. (Ed.) (2009). *Clinical Hematology and Fundamentals of Hemostasis*, 5th ed. Philadelphia: F. A. Davis.

Hoffbrand, V., Moss, P., and Pettit, J. (2016). *Essential Haematology*, 7th ed. Malden, MA: Wiley-Blackwell.

McKenzie, S. B. (2004). *Clinical Laboratory Hematology*, Upper Saddle River, NJ: Pearson Prentice Hall.

McKenzie, S. B., and Williams, L. J. (2015). *Clinical Laboratory Hematology*, 3rd ed. Upper Saddle River, NJ: Pearson Prentice Hall.

Rodak, B. F., Fritsma, G. A., and Doig, K. (2007). *Hematology Clinical Principles and Applications*, 3rd ed. St. Louis: Elsevier.

CHAPTER

3 Hemostasis

contents

I. INTRODUCTION TO THE VASCULAR SYSTEM

A. Vascular Structure and Function

1. **Endothelium**
   a. Vascular permeability and blood flow rate are controlled by a single layer of endothelial cells that line the vessel wall.
   b. Vascular lining is nonreactive to platelets and plasma proteins until damaged.
   c. Upon injury, increased vascular permeability occurs, allowing leakage of plasma proteins and blood cell migration to site of injury.
   d. Damage causes vasoconstriction to minimize blood loss and allows interaction among vessels, platelets, and plasma proteins.
2. **Subendothelium**
   a. Composed of smooth muscle cells and connective tissue with collagen fibers
   b. Exposure of collagen causes platelet activation and activates the intrinsic pathway of secondary hemostasis.
3. **Vascular endothelium** produces or releases substances important in hemostasis.
   a. **Produces von Willebrand factor (vWF),** necessary for platelet **adhesion** to collagen; carrier protein for coagulation factor VIII:C
   b. **Tissue factor** in vessels is **exposed** during vessel damage and activates the **extrinsic pathway** of secondary hemostasis.
   c. **Tissue plasminogen activator** is released during vessel damage and activates the **fibrinolytic system.**
   d. Produces **prostacyclin**, a platelet aggregation inhibitor and vasodilator
   e. The endothelial surface receptor **thrombomodulin** forms a complex with **thrombin** to inhibit factors V and VIII in secondary hemostasis through the protein C system.

II. DISEASES AND CONDITIONS ASSOCIATED WITH THE VASCULAR SYSTEM

A. Hereditary Vascular Defects

1. **Hemorrhagic telangiectasia:** Thin vessel walls cause mucous membrane bleeding.
2. **Ehlers-Danlos syndrome:** Abnormal collagen production causes hyperelastic skin and joint abnormalities.
3. **Pseudoxanthachroma elastica:** Accumulation of deposits of calcium and other minerals in elastic fibers.
4. **Marfan syndrome:** Genetic disorder of the connective tissue which may lead to cardiovascular issues such as mitral valve prolapse and aortic aneurysm.

B. Acquired Vascular Defects

1. **Vitamin C deficiency:** Vitamin C is needed for proper collagen synthesis and vessel integrity. Deficiency causes **scurvy.**
2. Drug induced (steroids)
3. Age induced (senile purpura)
4. Inadequate platelet support because of quantitative or qualitative platelet defects

C. Vascular Defect Bleeding Symptoms

1. Superficial, resulting in easy bruising and petechiae

III. INTRODUCTION TO THROMBOCYTES

A. Thrombocyte Maturation

1. **Megakaryoblast**
   a. Committed **myeloid progenitor cell**, in response to growth factor **thrombopoietin**, gives rise to megakaryocytes.
   b. Earliest thrombocyte stage where the nucleus divides without cytoplasmic division; process known as **endomitosis**
   c. Results in the formation of **giant cells**, with a size range of 20–50 μm
   d. Round nucleus contains 2–6 nucleoli and fine chromatin.
   e. The scant basophilic cytoplasm contains **no granules**; irregularly shaped with **cytoplasmic tags** (blunt extensions of cytoplasm)
2. **Promegakaryocyte**
   a. **Increases** size with a range of 20–80 μm
   b. Indented or lobulated nucleus contains variable number of nucleoli with coarsening chromatin.
   c. Basophilic cytoplasm with **granules** beginning to appear; cytoplasmic tags present
   d. **Demarcating membrane system (DMS)** begins to form.
      1) DMS is an invagination of the plasma membrane that becomes the future site of platelet fragmentation.
3. **Megakaryocyte**
   a. **Increases** in size up to 100 μm; **largest cell in the body**
   b. It contains a **multilobulated nucleus** with very **coarse chromatin** and variable number of **nucleoli.**
   c. Cytoplasm has many **small granules** that stain purple with Wright's stain.
   d. Represents 1% of nucleated bone marrow cells with a reference range of 5–10 megakaryocytes on low (10X) power
   e. Increased number indicates increased demand for platelets; acute bleeding episodes
   f. Approximately 2000–4000 platelets per megakaryocyte are shed into the marrow sinuses and enter circulation as cytoplasmic fragments. The nucleus remains in marrow and is phagocytized by marrow macrophages.
4. **Mature platelets (thrombocytes)**
   a. **2–4 μm** in size, appearing as **pale blue** cells with **azurophilic granules**
   b. Mature **platelets** have **no nucleus.**
   c. **Platelet zones**
      1) **Peripheral zone**
         a) Glycocalyx is the exterior coat and contains glycoprotein receptor sites.

b) Submembrane area contains the phospholipid membrane (PF3), which serves as a surface for interaction of coagulation factors in **secondary hemostasis.**

2) **Sol-gel (structural) zone** contains microtubules, cytoskeleton, actin, and myosin.

3) **Organelle zone** contains the granules, lysosomes, mitochondria, peroxisomes, and glycogen. It controls platelet function in response to coagulation.

a) **Alpha granules** predominate and contain a number of different proteins, with some of the most prominent being fibrinogen, von Willebrand factor, beta thromboglobulin, platelet-derived growth factor (PDGF), and PF4 (platelet factor 4).

b) **Dense bodies** (delta granules) contain ADP, ATP, serotonin, and calcium.

c) **Lysosomes** (third type of granule) contain hydrolase enzymes.

d. Membrane systems

1) **Dense tubular system** (DTS): Regulator of intracellular calcium concentration

2) **Open canalicular system** (OCS): Releases granular contents through channels leading to the surface of the platelet

B. Platelet Characteristics

1. The reference range for healthy individuals is **150–450 10^9/L** or approximately 7–21 per high-power field. Two-thirds of available platelets are in **circulation**; one-third is stored in the **spleen.**
2. **Life span** of 8–12 days; shorter in certain disease states
3. With Wright's stain, platelets stain gray-blue with purple granules.
4. Platelets are found in the bone marrow, spleen, and blood vessels; in the blood vessels platelets function in hemostasis.
5. Originate from the same progenitor cell as the erythroid and myeloid series
6. **Giant platelets** indicate premature release from the bone marrow and result from increased demand or certain disease states.
7. **Immature platelets** are found in the peripheral blood in certain diseases (e.g., acute megakaryocytic leukemia and myelodysplastic syndrome).

C. Thrombocyte Function

1. Platelet function is dependent on **platelet secreted proteins, ATP, ADP, calcium, and platelet factors.**
2. **Platelet-secreted proteins**

a. **Serotonin** stimulates vasoconstriction when vessel injury occurs.

b. **Thromboxane A_2** stimulates platelet aggregation and vasoconstriction.

c. **Actomyosin** contracts the thrombus at the end of the coagulation process.

3. **Platelet factors**
   a. **PF4:** Neutralizes heparin
   b. **PF3:** Platelet phospholipid needed for proper platelet function and coagulation
      1) Needed in the production of **thromboxane A_2**
      2) Provides a surface for fibrin formation, limiting the hemostatic response to the site of injury
4. Proper platelet function involves **adhesion, release of granule contents, aggregation, and clot retraction.**
   a. **Adhesion**
      1) Platelets undergo a shape change and adhere to vascular surfaces.
      2) Response to collagen exposure in subendothelium caused by vascular injury
      3) Dependent on binding of **von Willebrand factor** at the GPIb receptor site
      4) Can be activated by thrombin
   b. The **contents** of the platelet **storage granules** are **released** into the open canalicular system in response to internal, cellular contraction.
   c. **Aggregation**
      1) **Fibrinogen** attaches at the **IIb/IIIa receptor** of adjoining platelets, forming the initial platelet plug.
      2) Platelets release nonmetabolic **ADP** (platelet agonist), **serotonin,** and **PF4.**
      3) During aggregation, **PF3** is released to provide the phospholipid surface needed for binding of clotting factors in secondary hemostasis.
   d. **Clot retraction**
      1) Follows clot formation
      2) Dependent on **thrombasthenin** and **glycoprotein receptors IIb/IIIa**
      3) Restores normal blood flow to the vessel

D. Laboratory Analysis of Platelets

1. Quantitative
   a. Platelet numbers: Automated instrumentation, hemacytometer counts with phase contrast microscopy, blood smear estimates
2. Qualitative
   a. **Bleeding time (BT)** will detect defects in adhesion, release, and aggregation. The general **reference interval (RI)** for the BT is 1–9 minutes. Patients with platelet counts less than usually have a prolonged BT. The BT has been discredited in recent years as being an unreliable screening test. It lacks reproducibility and is affected by location of the incision, pressure applied when performing the incision, operator experience, and patient factors such as age, gender, diet, hematocrit, skin elasticity (tissue turgor), medications, and platelet count.

b. **Platelet aggregation studies** detect platelet function abnormalities. Aggregating agents used include ADP, epinephrine, collagen, thrombin, and ristocetin. Some aggregometers can measure adenosine triphosphate (ATP) secreted from dense granules, either by whole blood or by PRP-optical methodologies. Luminescence assays improve the diagnosis of storage pool or storage release defects because an actual amount of ATP, directly proportional to the dense granule content, is measured. Measuring the amount of ATP is more accurate than evaluating whether the platelet aggregation curve is biphasic.

c. **vWF:Ag (antigenic), vWF:RCo (activity) assays, Collagen binding assay (vWF:CB), vWF activity assay: (VWF:Act)** may be used to measure von Willebrand factor activity.

d. **PFA-100, PFA-200**
   - Is a method developed to replace the bleeding time
   - Uses shear force to measure closure time with three types of cartridges using whole blood: EPI/COLL, ADP/COLL, and P2Y12
   - The EPI/COLL screens for aspirin-like products and von Willebrand disease.
   - The ADP/COLL screens for platelet disorders and the P2Y12 detects a Plavix-like defect response.
   - The normal ranges are established locally in seconds.

IV. DISEASES AND CONDITIONS ASSOCIATED WITH THROMBOCYTES

A. Hereditary Adhesion Defects

1. **von Willebrand disease**
   a. Lacks von Willebrand factor, which is needed for platelets to adhere to collagen in damaged vessels and is a carrier protein for coagulation factor VIII:C.
   b. Decreased platelet adhesion causes mucous membrane bleeding that is variable in severity.
   c. **Laboratory:** Normal **platelet count**, prolonged **bleeding time (if available)**, decreased **aggregation response to ristocetin**, variable **aPTT**, normal **PT**, decreased **vWF:RCo, vWF:Ag, VIII:C, VWF:CB, VWF:Act**
   d. **Most common hereditary hemorrhagic disorder**; autosomal-dominant inheritance.
2. **Bernard-Soulier syndrome**
   a. Giant platelets (increased MPV) that **lack glycoprotein Ib receptor**; adhesion defect due to faulty binding of the platelet to von Willebrand factor.
   b. **Laboratory:** Variable **platelet count, platelet anisocytosis** (increased PDW). prolonged **bleeding time**, decreased **aggregation response to ristocetin**, normal **aPTT and PT**, normal **vWF:RCo, vWF:Ag, and VIII:C**

B. Hereditary Aggregation and Clot Retraction Defect

1. **Glanzmann thrombasthenia**
   a. **Hemorrhagic disorder** seen in populations where consanguinity is prevalent
   b. Lack of **glycoprotein IIb/IIIa**, the fibrinogen-binding receptor

c. Inability of fibrinogen to bind with platelets causes aggregation defect; lack of thrombasthenin/actomyosin causes clot retraction defect.
d. **Laboratory:** Decreased **aggregation response** with ADP, epinephrine, and collagen, normal response with ristocetin

C. Storage Pool Defects: Deficiency of One or More Types of Storage Granules

1. **Gray-platelet syndrome** is characterized by large platelets, thrombocytopenia, and an absence of **alpha granules.** Patients are prone to lifelong mild bleeding tendencies.
2. **Wiskott-Aldrich syndrome** is characterized by small platelets (low MPV), thrombocytopenia, and a decreased amount of **alpha granules and dense bodies.** Patients are prone to hemorrhage and recurrent infections.
3. **Hermansky-Pudlak syndrome** is characterized by a lack of **dense body granules.** Patients exhibit oculocutaneous albinism and are prone to hemorrhage.

D. Acquired Defects

1. **Drugs**
   a. Aspirin and nonsteroidal anti-inflammatory drugs interfere with the cyclooxygenase enzymes, preventing **thromboxane A_2** synthesis and subsequent aggregation.
   b. P2Y12 inhibitors such as Clopidogrel bisulfate (Plavix®), ticlopidine, prasugrel, and ticagrelor are adenosine diphosphate (ADP) receptor inhibitors. The blockage of this receptor inhibits platelet aggregation.
   c. Eptifibatide and similar antiplatelet medications block IIb/IIIa glycoprotein receptors, preventing aggregation.
2. **Myeloproliferative disorders and uremia** are examples of diseases that can cause platelet dysfunction.

E. Quantitative Platelet Disorders

1. **Primary thrombocytosis**
   a. Uncontrolled, **malignant proliferation** of platelets, **not** in response to thrombopoietin; can be caused by **essential thrombocythemia, polycythemia vera**, and **chronic myelocytic leukemia**
   b. Platelet counts can be **$>$1000 10^9/L.**
   c. Associated with either hemorrhagic or thrombotic complications
2. **Secondary (reactive) thrombocytosis**
   a. It is characterized by increased platelet production, usually in response to **thrombopoietin.** Platelet count is elevated, but usually **$<$1000 10^9/L.** Can result from:
      1) Chronic and acute **inflammatory disease** (e.g., tuberculosis and cirrhosis)
      2) **Iron deficiency:** Iron regulates thrombopoiesis by inhibiting thrombopoietin; deficiency causes increased thrombopoietin and stimulates thrombopoiesis.
      3) **Rapid blood regeneration** due to hemolytic anemia and acute blood loss

4) Exercise, prematurity, and response to drugs
5) **Other conditions:** Cytotoxic drug withdrawal, postoperative state from tissue damage, and splenectomy

3. **Thrombocytopenia**
   a. **Decrease** in the **number of platelets**, which can result from the following:
      1) **Megakaryocyte hypoproliferation:** Caused by chemotherapy, marrow replacement by malignant cells, aplastic anemia, drug and alcohol abuse
      2) **Ineffective thrombopoiesis:** Caused by megaloblastic anemias
      3) **Increased loss/destruction**
         a) **Nonimmune** loss is due to severe hemorrhage, extensive transfusion (dilution loss), and increased consumption seen in the microangiopathic hemolytic anemias (e.g., DIC, hemolytic uremic syndrome, and thrombotic thrombocytopenic purpura [ADAMTS 13 deficiency]).
         b) **Immune** loss can be due to neonatal purpura, posttransfusion purpura, immune/idiopathic thrombocytopenic purpura, and heparin-induced thrombocytopenia.
      4) **Splenic sequestration**
         a) **Hypersplenism** may result in up to 90% of platelets being sequestered.
         b) Increased destruction of damaged and normal platelets
         c) **Splenomegaly** occurs in leukemia, lymphoma, Gaucher and other storage diseases, cirrhosis of the liver, and sarcoidosis.
      5) **Hereditary conditions:** May-Hegglin anomaly, Bernard-Soulier, Wiskott-Aldrich, and Glanzmans syndromes
      6) **Falsely low platelet counts**
         a) **Platelet satellitosis:** Platelets can adhere to neutrophils when exposed to EDTA. Redraw in sodium citrate to correct; multiply obtained platelet count by 1.1 to correct for dilution factor in sodium citrate tube.
         b) **EDTA-dependent platelet agglutinins:** Platelets can adhere to each other when exposed to EDTA. Correction of the problem is the same as for platelet satellitosis.

F. Vessel and Platelet Defect Bleeding Symptoms

1. Superficial, resulting in easy bruising, petechiae, ecchymoses, purpura, epistaxis, mucous membrane, or gingival bleeding

V. INTRODUCTION TO HEMOSTASIS

A. Primary Hemostasis

1. **Vascular system and platelets** are involved; primary hemostasis starts when platelets come in contact with exposed collagen, microfilaments, and the basement membrane of endothelial tissue.
2. **Small blood vessels constrict,** allowing platelets to adhere to exposed tissue, which causes **ADP/ATP** release (promotes platelet aggregation and acts as an

energy source) and synthesis of **thromboxane A_2** from arachidonic acid (promotes activation, release, and aggregation).

3. **Platelets** begin to **aggregate**, which causes the release of additional ADP, ATP, and **serotonin** (substance that promotes vasoconstriction).
4. **Platelet receptor sites** are **exposed**, which allows binding of coagulation proteins from **secondary hemostasis** (e.g., fibrinogen binds at the glycoprotein IIb/IIIa receptor).

B. Secondary Hemostasis (see Figure 3-1■)

1. The goal is **generation** of sufficient **thrombin** to **convert fibrinogen to fibrin clot.** Secondary hemostasis involves **activation** of **intrinsic, extrinsic**, and **common coagulation pathway factors.**
2. **Fibrin clot** includes the **platelet plug** formed in **primary hemostasis** and **fibrin** formed in **secondary hemostasis.**

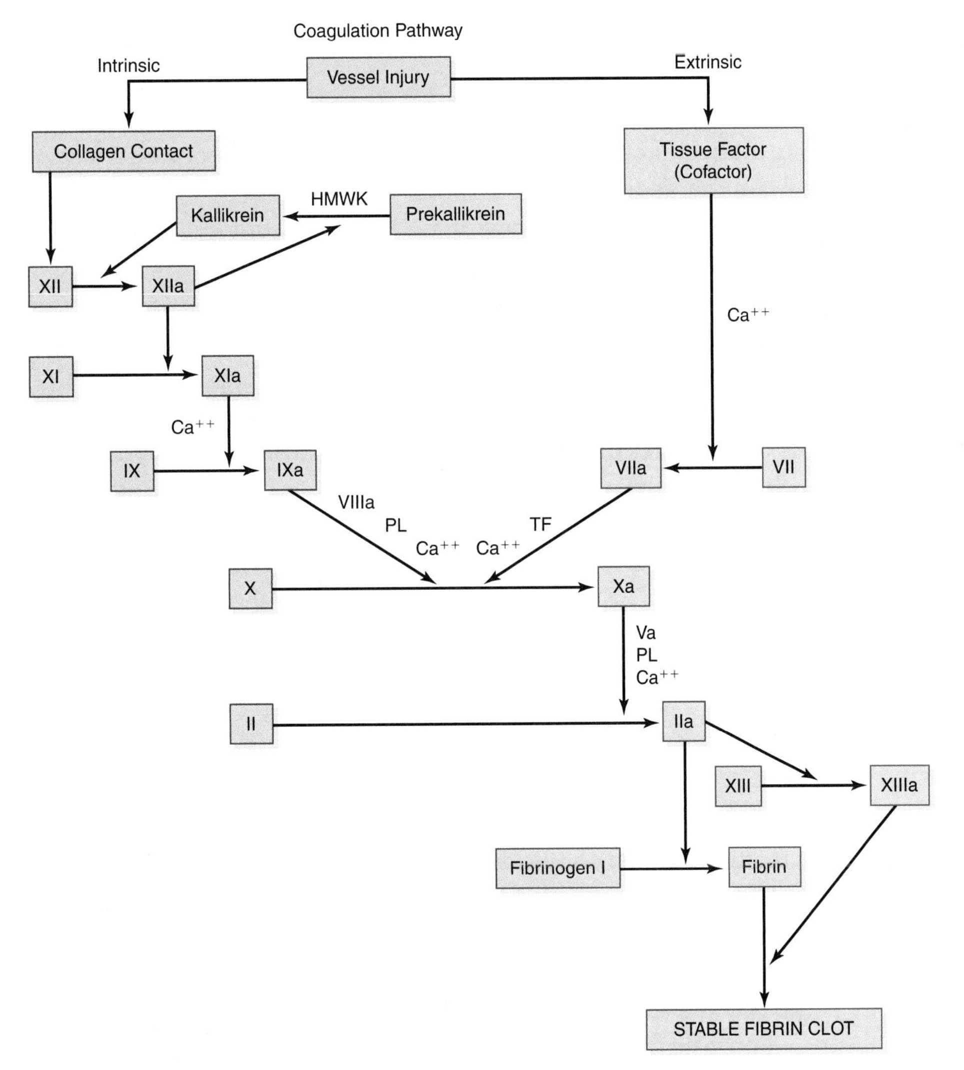

FIGURE 3–1 ■ Coagulation pathway.

3. **Intrinsic pathway** is activated when coagulation proteins are exposed to subendothelial collagen. The intrinsic pathway includes factors **XII** (Hageman), **XI** (plasma thromboplastin antecedent), **prekallikrein** (Fletcher), **HMWK** (Fitzgerald), **IX** (plasma thromboplastin component/Christmas factor), and **VIII** (antihemophiliac).
4. **Extrinsic pathway (dominant *in vivo* pathway)** starts with the **release of tissue factor** from injured blood vessel endothelial cells and subendothelium. Tissue factor is found in most tissues, organs, and large blood vessels. **Factor VII** (stable factor) is in this pathway.
5. **Common pathway** begins with **factor X activation** by either the extrinsic (main *in vivo*) or intrinsic pathway. It includes factors **X** (Stuart-Prower), **V** (proaccelerin/labile factor), **II** (prothrombin), and **I** (fibrinogen).
6. Alternative pathways link the extrinsic, intrinsic, and common pathways.
7. Additional synonyms include **tissue factor** (III), **calcium** (IV)**, fibrin stabilizing factor** (XIII), and **ristocetin cofactor** (von Willebrand factor).

C. Coagulation Factors (Coagulation Proteins)

1. **Coagulation factors** are also known as **enzyme precursors** or **zymogens.** They are found in the plasma, along with nonenzymatic cofactors and calcium.
2. **Zymogens** are substrates having **no biologic activity** until converted by enzymes to **active forms** called **serine proteases.**
   a. The **zymogens** include **II, VII, IX, X, XI, XII**, and **prekallikrein.**
   b. The **serine proteases** are **IIa, VIIa, IXa, Xa, XIa, XIIa**, and **kallikrein.**
3. **Cofactors** assist in the **activation of zymogens** and include **V, VIII, tissue factor**, and **high-molecular-weight kininogen (HMWK).**
4. In its active form, **factor XIII** is a **transglutaminase (FXIIIa).**
5. **Fibrinogen** is the only substrate in the cascade that does **not** become **an activated enzyme. It is the only one of the coagulation proteins that as a substrate does not further participate in the coagulation cascade.**

D. The Coagulation Groups

1. **Contact group**
   a. Includes **prekallikrein, HMWK,** and **factors XI** and **XII**
   b. Produced in the **liver**
   c. Requires contact with a foreign surface for activation (e.g., collagen *in vivo* and kaolin *in vitro*)
   d. Functions of the contact group:
      1) **XII** and **prekallikrein** reciprocally **activate each other; HMWK** is a **cofactor** for this process.
      2) All play a **role in intrinsic coagulation activation.**
      3) **XIIa, kallikrein**, and **HMWK** play a role in the inflammatory response, intrinsic fibrinolytic activation, kinin formation, and activation of the complement system.

2. **Prothrombin group**
   a. Includes factors **II, VII, IX,** and **X**
   b. Produced in the **liver**
   c. **Vitamin K** is required for synthesis of functional factors, with **calcium-binding sites** necessary for binding to phospholipid (PF3) surfaces.
   d. Causes for synthesis of **nonfunctional factors:**
      1) **Vitamin K deficiency** or **antibiotics** that kill the intestinal bacterial flora responsible for vitamin K synthesis
      2) **Oral anticoagulants** (warfarin) that interfere with the metabolism of vitamin K (vitamin K antagonists)
3. **Fibrinogen group**
   a. Includes factors **I, V, VIII,** and **XIII**
   b. Produced in the **liver**
   c. Consumed in the clotting process
   d. **Thrombin feedback** on fibrinogen group factors depends on its concentration.
      1) **Low thrombin levels activate** factors **V, VIII** (positive feedback on the cascade), and **XIII** and induce platelet aggregation.
      2) When **thrombin levels** are **high,** thrombin **binds to thrombomodulin** on the endothelial cell surface and **activates** the **protein C pathway.**
      3) **Activated protein C** and its cofactor, **protein S,** inhibit factors V and VIII (negative feedback on the cascade).
   e. Factors I, V, and VIII serve as substrates for the fibrinolytic enzyme plasmin.
   f. Factors I and V are found in platelets.
   g. Conversion of **fibrinogen to fibrin** is a three-step process.
      1) **Fibrinogen alpha and beta fibrinopeptides** are cleaved by thrombin, forming soluble fibrin monomers.
      2) **Fibrin monomers** spontaneously polymerize, forming **soluble fibrin polymers.** This is the endpoint for clot-based tests.
      3) **Clot stabilization** occurs, requiring thrombin activation of **XIII** and **calcium.**
   h. **VIII/vWF complex**
      1) Factor **VIII** is synthesized in the **liver** and is composed of two fractions.
         a) **VIII:C** (antihemophilic factor) is the coagulation portion that acts as a cofactor in the intrinsic coagulation pathway.
         b) **VIII:Ag** is the antigenic property of factor VIII.
         c) **VIII:C** is deficient in hemophilia A. **VIII:Ag** is usually normal.
      2) **von Willebrand factor** (vWF) is synthesized by **endothelial cells** and **megakaryocytes** and is composed of two fractions.
         a) **vWF:RCo** (ristocetin cofactor) is needed for **platelet adhesion** to collagen *in vivo*; it is needed for a normal response to ristocetin on aggregation studies *in vitro.*

b) **vWF:Ag** is the **antigenic property** of vWF.
c) Both **vWF:RCo** and **vWF:Ag** are **deficient** in classical **von Willebrand disease.**

3) **vWF subunits** polymerize to form **multimers** of varying sizes that complex with and act as the **carrier protein for factor VIII:C.**

E. Complement System and Coagulation System Interaction

1. The **complement system** is activated during coagulation and fibrinolysis.
2. Contains more than 30 circulating blood proteins, primarily to mediate inflammatory response and immune and allergic reactions
3. Complement functions in **lysing antibody–coated cells**
4. **Plasmin** (in association with antibody-antigen complexes) **activates C1** and causes **cleavage of C3** to C3a and C3b. **C3a** increases vascular permeability, and **C3b** causes immune adherence of erythrocytes to neutrophils, which enhances phagocytosis.
5. Complement activation is regulated by **C1 inactivator**, which also inhibits several coagulation factors.

F. Kinin System and Coagulation System Interaction

1. The **kinin system** contains four plasma proteins: factors **XII** and **XI, prekallikrein** (Fletcher factor), and **HMWK** (Fitzgerald factor).
2. Generates **bradykinin**, an active peptide, and **kallikrein**, a proteolytic enzyme
3. Involved in chemotaxis and pain sensation
4. **Function:** Mediate inflammatory responses, promote vasodilation, and activator of intrinsic coagulation and complement pathways

VI. THE FIBRINOLYTIC SYSTEM

A. Fibrinolytic System: Keeps blood vessels clear and is important in **clot dissolution.** During this process, **plasminogen** is activated to **plasmin.**

B. Plasminogen

1. Glycoprotein produced in the **liver**
2. **Zymogen** (inert) found in the plasma
3. **Converted to plasmin** by plasminogen activators:
   a. **Intrinsic activators** are **XIIa, kallikrein**, and **HMWK.**
   b. **Extrinsic activators** are **tissue-type plasminogen activator** (t-PA) and **urokinase-type plasminogen activator** (u-PA).
   c. **Exogenous activators** (therapeutic agents) include **t-PA, streptokinase**, and **urokinase.** They are administered to **lyse**-existing clots.

C. Plasmin

1. **Not normally found in circulation**; the precursor plasminogen is found in circulation
2. **Degrades** fibrin clots (fibrinolysis), fibrinogen (fibrinogenolysis), factors V and VIII
3. **Activates** the complement system

VII. REGULATORY PROTEINS OF COAGULATION AND FIBRINOLYSIS

A. Antithrombin (AT)

1. Produced in the **liver**
2. Principal **inhibitor of coagulation**
3. **Inhibits** the **serine proteases**
4. Therapeutic **heparin enhances** the action of antithrombin.

B. Proteins C and S

1. **Vitamin K–dependent** regulatory proteins
2. Activated when thrombin binds to thrombomodulin on the endothelial cell surface
3. Inhibit factors V and VIII to provide **negative feedback** on the cascade

C. Tissue Factor Pathway Inhibitor: Inhibits factor VIIa–tissue factor complex

D. α_2-Macroglobulin: Inhibits thrombin, Xa, kallikrein, and plasmin

E. α_1-Antitrypsin: Inhibits XIa and inactivates plasmin

F. C1 Inhibitor: Inhibits C1 from the complement cascade, and XIIa, XIa, kallikrein, and plasmin

G. α_2-Antiplasmin: Principal inhibitor of fibrinolysis; neutralizes plasmin

H. PAI-1 (plasminogen activator inhibitor-1)

1. Important **inhibitor** of fibrinolysis
2. Prevents activation of plasminogen by t-PA; released from endothelial cells upon damage

VIII. THROMBOTIC DISORDERS

A. Primary Thrombotic Disorders

1. **Deficiency in regulatory proteins**
   a. **Antithrombin (AT) deficiency**
      1) **Genetic deficiency** occurs about 1:2000 in the general population; associated with **deep vein thrombosis** and **pulmonary embolism**
      2) Serine proteases not inhibited; negative feedback to cascade impaired
      3) **Laboratory:** Antithrombin activity assay, both clottable and chromogenic (antigenic testing less common)

   b. **Protein C or Protein S deficiencies**
      1) Vitamin K–dependent **regulatory proteins** that **inactivate** factors V and VIII
      2) Can **cause** superficial and deep vein **thrombosis** and/or pulmonary **embolism**
      3) **Laboratory:** Immunologic and functional testing to diagnose

2. **Decreased activation of the fibrinolytic system**
   a. **XII, prekallikrein,** and **HMWK** are contact factors in secondary hemostasis, but their most important role is the **intrinsic activation** of the **fibrinolytic system. Deficiencies** are associated with thrombosis, **not** hemorrhage.
   b. All have an autosomal recessive inheritance pattern.
   c. **Factor XII (Hageman factor) deficiency** causes a **prolonged aPTT**; factor XII assay confirms.
   d. **Prekallikrein (Fletcher factor) deficiency** causes a **prolonged aPTT** that shortens in patient plasma incubated with **kaolin.**
   e. **HMWK (Fitzgerald factor) deficiency** causes a **slightly prolonged aPTT.**
   f. **Plasminogen deficiency** is characterized by thrombosis due to an inability to generate plasmin.
3. **Genetic mutations**
   a. **Factor V Leiden** (Activated Protein C Resistance—APCR)
      1) **Most common hereditary cause of thrombosis**; caused by an amino acid substitution
      2) **Protein C is incapable of inactivating factor V Leiden**, causing thrombin generation and subsequent fibrin clot formation.
      3) **Laboratory:** PCR-based molecular assay to single-point mutation in the gene for factor V
   b. **Prothrombin gene mutation 20210**
      1) **Second most common hereditary cause of thrombosis**; caused by an amino acid substitution
      2) May have slightly elevated prothrombin level
      3) **Laboratory:** PCR-based molecular assay
   c. **Dysfibrinogenemia**
      1) Autosomal-dominant trait; abnormal structure of fibrinogen; caused by gene mutations
      2) Associated with either bleeding or thrombosis; dependent on the specific gene mutation
   d. ABO Blood groups: Non-O groups such as B and A1 have been associated with venous thrombosis. Connected with ABO locus glycotransferases connected with vWF and FVIII elevated proteins.

B. Secondary Thrombotic Disorders

1. **Lupus anticoagulant, anticardiolipin antibodies, anti-β2 GP1 antibodies, anti-prothrombin antibodies:** The body develops autoantibodies against platelet phospholipids; etiology is unknown.
2. **Postoperative status:** Thrombotic event starts after tissue factor release during surgery, activating the extrinsic coagulation (dominant *in vivo*) pathway.
3. **Malignancy:** Risk of malignancy increases because of the release of thromboplastic substances by neoplastic cells.

4. **Pregnancy**
   a. The placenta is rich in tissue factor, which may enhance thrombosis during pregnancy, especially high-risk patients having cesarian section delivery.
   b. Factor V and VIII and VWF levels increase, contributing to clot formation.
5. **Estrogen/oral contraceptives:** Increase risk of venous thrombosis and renal artery thrombosis (decreases AT levels).
6. **Morbid obesity:** Results in decreased AT levels and increased PAI-1, causing thrombosis
7. **Hyperhomocysteinemia:** This disorder is linked to atherosclerosis, resulting in arterial and venous thromboembolism. Mechanisms are not fully understood but may be associated with a reduction in the localized activation of the protein C pathway.

IX. HEMORRHAGIC DISORDERS

A. Inherited Disorders: Generally affect only **one** hemostatic component (e.g., factor VIII). There are, however, case reports of FV- and FVIII-combined deficiencies.

B. Acquired Disorders: Involve **multiple** hemostatic components or pathways (e.g., warfarin therapy and liver disease)

C. Hemorrhagic Symptoms: Associated with defects in secondary hemostasis; include bleeding into deep tissues, joints, and abdominal and other body cavities

D. Inherited Intrinsic Pathway Hemorrhagic Disorders

1. **von Willebrand disease**
   a. Autosomal-dominant trait
   b. **Most common hereditary bleeding disorder**; abnormalities in **both** primary and secondary hemostasis
   c. Caused by a defect in von Willebrand factor that is needed for **platelet adhesion** to collagen in primary hemostasis. vWF is also the **carrier protein for factor VIII:C** in secondary hemostasis.
   d. **Clinical:** Mild to moderate bleeding dependent of vWF and VIII:C levels; menorrhagia common symptom in women
   e. **Laboratory:** Decreased **vWF:RCo, vWF:Ag, vWF:CB, abnormal vWF multimers** and **VIII:C**; abnormal **platelet aggregation with ristocetin**, variable **aPTT** (often prolonged because of decreased VIII:C), and prolonged **bleeding time if available.**
   f. **Treatment:** Factor **VIII** concentrate such as Alphanate, Humate P, Wilate, and non-Vendi (recombinate); **DDAVP** (deamino-D-arginine-vasopressin) used to raise plasma levels of vWF and VIII:C
2. **Factor VIII:C (hemophilia A, classic hemophilia) deficiency**
   a. Sex-linked disorder transmitted on the **X chromosome** by carrier women to their sons

b. Accounts for 80% of the hemophilias; **second most common hereditary bleeding disorder**
c. Many new cases of hemophilia A result from spontaneous mutations.
d. **Clinical:** Bleeding symptoms are proportional to the degree of the factor deficiency. Spontaneous bleeding occurs often and is especially bad in joint regions (hemarthrosis).
e. **Laboratory:** Prolonged **aPTT** only, factor VIII:C assay to confirm
f. **Treatment: Cryoprecipitate** and factor **VIII** concentrates are used; in mild cases, DDAVP can be used to stimulate the release of VIII:C and vWF from stored reserves.
g. **Plasma factor concentrates. Theoretical risk of HBV, HCV, HIV transmission**
   – Hemofil-M, Monoclate-P, Alphanate, Humate-P
   – Human plasma matrix
   – Purification: immunoaffinity column,
   – solvent-detergent, Pasteurization,
   – viral inactivation
      • No lipid-envelope virus transmission, but may transmit hepatitis A, parvovirus B19
      • <25% of FVIII concentrates used in industrialized countries
h. **Recombinant factor concentrates. Serum or albumin in culture medium**
   – Helixate FS, Kogenate FS, Recombinate, Nuwiq
   – Abundant, may be used for prophylaxis
   – No HBV, HCV, HIV seroconversions
      • No protein in culture or preparation
   – No viral risk: Advate, abundant supplies
      • B-domain-deleted FVIII concentrate,
   – Human albumin in culture: ReFacto
   – No protein: Xyntha
   – Extended half-life: Eloctate Adynovate, Afstyla

   Gene Therapy is showing great promise but is not yet FDA cleared.
i. About 15–20% of patients will develop a factor VIII inhibitor; it is associated with a bleeding tendency and a worse prognosis.
   – Treatment for inhibitors: NovoSeven RT is a recombinant product that can be given on demand for treatment of subjects with FVIII and FIX inhibitors. It has been associated with clotting issues if given improperly in off-label situations.

3. **Factor IX (hemophilia B, Christmas disease) deficiency**
   a. Sex-linked recessive trait
   b. Accounts for 20% of the hemophilias; **third most common hereditary bleeding disorder**
   c. **Clinical:** Bleeding symptoms are similar to those seen in hemophilia A.

d. **Laboratory:** Prolonged **aPTT** only; factor IX assay to confirm
e. **Treatment:** Factor **IX** concentrates such as recombinant FIX (Benefix), prothrombin complex concentrates (Konyne, Proplex), FIX concentrates such as Mononine and gene therapy shows great promise.
f. Between 1 and 3% of patients will develop a factor IX inhibitor; it is associated with a bleeding tendency and worse prognosis.

4. **Factor XI (hemophilia C) deficiency**
   a. Mainly seen in the Ashkenazi Jewish population
   b. Characterized by clinical bleeding that is asymptomatic until surgery or trauma
   c. **Laboratory:** Prolonged **aPTT** only; factor XI assay to confirm
5. Deficiencies of factors XII, prekallikrein, and HMWK in the intrinsic pathway have already been discussed with the thrombotic disorders.

E. Inherited Extrinsic and Common Pathway Hemorrhagic Disorders

1. **Factor VII (stable factor) deficiency**
   a. Autosomal-recessive trait
   b. **Clinical:** Soft tissue bleeding
   c. **Laboratory:** Prolonged **PT** only with decreased levels of FVII
2. **Factor X (Stuart-Prower) deficiency**
   a. Autosomal-recessive trait
   b. **Clinical:** Soft tissue bleeding and chronic bruising
   c. **Laboratory:** Prolonged **PT** and **aPTT with decreased levels of FX**
3. **Factor V (Owren disease, labile factor) deficiency**
   a. Autosomal-recessive trait
   b. **Clinical:** Mild to moderate bleeding symptoms
   c. **Laboratory:** Prolonged **PT** and **aPTT with decreased levels of FV**
   d. May develop severe inhibitors in response to certain medications (cephlasporins and bovine thrombin).
4. **Factor II (prothrombin) deficiency**
   a. Autosomal-recessive trait
   b. **Clinical:** Mild bleeding symptoms
   c. **Laboratory:** Prolonged **PT** and **aPTT with decreased levels of FII**
5. **Factor I (fibrinogen) deficiency**
   a. Autosomal-recessive trait; results from the following inherited disorders:
      1) **Afibrinogenemia:** Inherited **lack** of fibrinogen; severe bleeding symptoms
      2) **Hypofibrinogenemia:** Inherited **deficiency** of fibrinogen; bleeding symptoms correlate with fibrinogen concentration
   b. **Clinical:** Spontaneous bleeding of mucosa, intestines, and intracranial sites
   c. **Laboratory:** Prolonged **bleeding time** (fibrinogen bridges do not form; platelet aggregation defect), decreased **fibrinogen** concentration, and prolonged **PT, aPTT**, and **thrombin time**
6. **Factor XIII (fibrin-stabilizing factor) deficiency**

a. Autosomal-recessive trait
b. **Clinical:** Spontaneous bleeding, delayed wound healing, and unusual scar formation; increased incidence of spontaneous abortion
c. **Laboratory: 5.0 M urea test** abnormal, **PT** and **aPTT** normal, and enzymatic and immunologic studies can be done
d. **Quantitative factor XIII** activity assays are based on either ammonia release or covalent linkage of amines in a protein substrate. Quantitative factor XIII antigen can be measured using latex particles coated with monoclonal antibodies directed against A subunits. Performed in special coagulation laboratories. Elisa testing is also available.

F. Acquired Disorders of Coagulation and Fibrinolysis

1. **Hepatic disease**
   a. The **liver** is the major site of **hemostatic protein synthesis.**
   b. Hepatic disease can result in **decreased synthesis** of coagulation or regulatory proteins; it also causes **impaired clearance** of activated hemostatic components.
   c. **Laboratory:** Prolonged **PT, aPTT, bleeding time**, and possibly decreased **platelet counts** because of hypersplenism, alcohol toxicity, and disseminated intravascular coagulation (DIC)
2. **Vitamin K deficiency**
   a. **Vitamin K** is needed for **liver synthesis** of functional factors **II, VII, IX,** and **X.**
   b. Vitamin K is produced by normal intestinal flora.
   c. **Deficiencies** in vitamin K can result from oral antibiotics, vitamin K antagonists (warfarin), or decreased absorption resulting from obstructive jaundice.
   d. Breast-fed babies are more prone to vitamin K deficiency because breast milk is sterile, which allows no bacterial intestinal colonization to occur.
   e. **Laboratory:** Prolonged **PT** (VII, X, II) and prolonged **aPTT** (IX, X, II)
3. **Disseminated intravascular coagulation with secondary fibrinolysis**
   a. Predisposing condition triggers **systemic clotting**; leads to systemic **fibrinolysis** and **bleeding**
   b. Triggering events include gram-negative septicemia, acute promyelocytic leukemia (FAB M3), obstetrical complications, massive tissue damage.
   c. Fibrinogen group factors (I, V, VIII, XIII) and platelets are consumed in clotting.
   d. **Laboratory**
      1) **PT, aPTT,** and **thrombin time** are prolonged.
      2) **Platelet count, antithrombin,** and **fibrinogen** concentrations are decreased.

3) **Fibrin degradation products** and **fibrinogen degradation products** are present (abnormal **D-dimer** and **FDP** tests[if available]).
4) **Schistocytes** form when RBCs are fragmented by intravascular clots.

e. **Clinical:** A systemic thrombotic event causes multiple organ failure; systemic lysis ultimately leads to severe hemorrhage.

f. **Treatment:** Treat the underlying condition with **FFP, platelet transfusions, antithrombin concentrates, antithrombolytics**, and **heparin** to stop systemic clotting.

4. **Primary fibrinogenolysis**
   a. Plasminogen is inappropriately activated to plasmin in the **absence** of clot formation. **Plasmin circulates** free in plasma and destroys factors I, V, and VIII.
   b. Caused by certain malignancies (e.g., prostate cancer) or massive tissue damage that causes release of plasminogen activators
   c. **Laboratory**
      1) **PT, aPTT**, and **thrombin time** are prolonged, and **fibrinogen** concentration is low (plasmin degrades fibrinogen, V, and VIII).
      2) **Platelet** count, **RBC morphology**, and **antithrombin** concentration are normal because there is no clot formation.
      3) **Fibrinogen degradation products** are present (abnormal FDP test), but **fibrin degradation products** are **absent** (normal D-dimer because there is **no clot formation**). Rare condition that the FDP assay may be appropriate.
   d. **Clinical: Hemorrhagic** symptoms occur that may resemble DIC.
   e. **Treatment:** Epsilon aminocaproic acid (**EACA**) is used to turn off inappropriate systemic lysis.
5. **Inhibitors** to factors VIII and IX in the intrinsic pathway have already been discussed with factor VIII and IX deficiencies. These inhibitors are associated with bleeding.

X. SAMPLE COLLECTION, HANDLING, AND PROCESSING FOR COAGULATION TESTING

A. Nontraumatic Venipuncture: It is ***essential*** that **trauma be avoided** because it may cause hemolysis that Interferes with photo-optical testing. The old laboratory legend of **tissue thromboplastin interference** produced in a traumatic draw is an "urban lab legend" that has never been proven. There are no references of data demonstrating this issue, only opinion.

B. Order of Draw: It is ***important*** that proper order of draw be followed. Collect tube for coagulation testing **before** any tubes containing heparin, EDTA, sodium fluoride, or clot-promoting additives.

C. Use Plastic- or Silicone-Coated Glass Tubes: **Plain glass** tubes will **activate** the **intrinsic pathway**, including the activation of the **contact factors** prekallikrein, XI, and XII. Do not use foreign objects such as applicator sticks to check for clots because these objects can activate platelets and contact factors. Check visually for clots. If a clot is suspected because of suspicious results check for clot after centrifuging and initial testing.

D. Ratio of Blood to Anticoagulant: The ratio in blood collection tubes is **critical**, and it must be maintained at a **9:1** ratio of **blood** to 3.2% sodium citrate **anticoagulant** or excess citrate will bind calcium chloride in the reagents for PT and aPTT, causing falsely long coagulation times.

E. **Specimen Processing**: Specimens must be processed as soon as possible following blood collection. Recommendations include processing within **4 hours** for **aPTT** and **24 hours** for **PT.** Centrifuge at 2500g for at least 10 minutes to obtain platelet-poor plasma (PPP), and remove plasma from cells. Freeze plasma at preferably –70°C. Platelet-poor plasma platelet counts must be less than 10×10^9L to prevent residual platelet interference. Centrifuges must be checked every 6 months by checking the platelet counts in PPP.

F. Temperature: **Testing** must be performed at **37°C.** Enzyme reactions work best at 37°C. Labile factors V and VIII will break down at temperatures above 37°C.

XI. EVALUATION TESTS FOR SECONDARY HEMOSTASIS

A. Activated Partial Thromboplastin Time (aPTT)

1. Screening test for factors **XII, XI, prekallikrein, HMWK, IX, VIII, X, V, II, and I (intrinsic/common pathways)**
2. Monitors unfractionated **heparin therapy**
3. Two reagents needed:
   a. **Platelet phospholipid substitute** with an **activator** (kaolin, celite, silica, or ellagic acid)
   b. Calcium chloride
4. **Principle:** Add phospholipid/activator reagent to citrated platelet-poor plasma and incubate to allow for contact factor activation. Add calcium chloride; measure the time required for clot formation.
5. Run normal and abnormal controls (essential for quality control).
6. **Reference range:** 23.0–35.0 sec; established by each institution according to reagent/instrument combination being used
7. **Prolonged aPTT** can indicate:
   a. **Factor deficiencies** in the **intrinsic/common pathways**; factor activity less than 25–30% will prolong aPTT
   b. **Acquired** circulating inhibitor: Heparin, direct oral anticoagulants (DOACs), Vitamin K antagonists, lupus anticoagulant, or antibody to a specific factor
8. **Sources of error**
   a. Improper sample collection, preparation, and inherent patient problems
      1) **Falsely long aPTT:** Blood collection tube not full or wrong selection of specimen collection tube, large clot in tube, heparin contamination from line draw, hematocrit >55.0%, and lipemia/icterus only if optical method used
      2) **Falsely short aPTT:** Hemolysis, small clot in tube, and plasma containing platelets (not platelet poor)

b. Incorrect **reagent** preparation: Incorrect dilution, water impurities, or improper storage
c. **Instrumentation:** Problems with temperature, light source, bubbles in sample

B. Prothrombin Time (PT)

1. Screening test for factors **VII, X, V, II, and I (extrinsic/common pathways)**
2. **Monitors** anticoagulation **therapy** by vitamin K antagonists (**warfarin/coumarin**)
3. **Reagents: Thromboplastin** source (tissue factor/TF) with **calcium chloride**
4. **Principle:** Add thromboplastin reagent containing calcium chloride to citrated platelet-poor plasma; measure the time required for clot formation.
5. Run normal and abnormal controls (essential for quality control).
6. **Reference range:** 10.0–14.0 sec; established by each institution
7. **INR:** International normalized ratio
   a. Means of **standardizing PT reporting** worldwide; not dependent on thromboplastin reagent or instrument used
   b. **INR** values are used to **monitor warfarin/coumarin therapy.** There is no reference range. The therapeutic range is dependent on the condition being treated, but it is generally considered to be between **2.0** and **3.0.**
   c. Formula

$$\text{INR} = \left[\frac{\text{Patient PT in sec}}{\text{Reference interval in sec}}\right]^{\text{ISI}}$$

   d. **ISI** is the **international sensitivity index** for the thromboplastin reagent; this number is provided by the manufacturer and is lot number and instrument specific.
   e. The most sensitive thromboplastin reagents have an ISI value of 1.00, based on World Health Organization (WHO) standards.
8. **Prolonged PT** can indicate **factor deficiencies** in the **extrinsic/common pathways**; DOACs, factor activity less than 25–30% or warfarin therapy will prolong the PT.
9. **Sources of error**
   a. Improper sample collection, improper preparation, and inherent patient problems
      1) **Falsely long PT:** Same as for aPTT
      2) **Falsely short PT:** Small clot in tube
   b. **Reagent** preparation and **instrumentation** problems are the same as for aPTT.

C. Other Laboratory Tests

1. **Mixing study** is performed when the PT or aPTT is prolonged to **differentiate a factor deficiency from a circulating inhibitor.** Patient plasma is mixed with normal pooled plasma and test(s) is(are) repeated.
   a. **Shortening of the time** into the reference range (correction) indicates a **factor deficiency** (hereditary, or acquired causes such as warfarin therapy or liver disease).

   b. **Partial or no correction** indicates a **circulating inhibitor** (heparin, lupus anticoagulant, V, VIII, or IX inhibitor).
2. **Fibrinogen level** is a quantitative test for fibrinogen. **Thrombin reagent** is added to **diluted** citrated patient plasma. Thrombin clotting time obtained is read using a standard curve and is inversely proportional to fibrinogen concentration.
3. **Thrombin time** is a qualitative/quantitative **test for fibrinogen. Thrombin reagent** is added to **undiluted** patient plasma and result is reported in seconds. Presence of **heparin, degradation products,** or **low fibrinogen** level will **prolong** the result.
4. Reptilase time (RT) is qualitative assay test for the presence of heparin usually used in conjunction with the thrombin time. In the presence of heparin, the RT is normal and the thrombin time is abnormal.
5. **Factor assays** are used to **confirm** a suspected **factor deficiency**, as suggested by a mixing study that shows correction. Test measures the ability of patient plasma to correct the PT or aPTT result obtained with plasma known to be factor deficient (compared to known standards). The **factor activity percent** is reported.
6. **5.0 M urea clot solubility test:** The unstable clot that forms in factor XIII deficiency dissolves in 5.0 M urea; a factor XIIIa-stabilized clot remains intact in 5.0 M urea for at least 24 hours. Quantitative XIII assays are performed in special coagulation laboratories. Elisa testing is also available.
7. **Dilute Russell viper venom test (DRVVT)** is a sensitive test that uses snake venom as the reagent to activate factor X in the cascade. If the **lupus inhibitor** is present, the venom is neutralized, and the test is prolonged. **Dilute Russell Viper venom confirm (DRVVC)** assay uses a higher phospholipid to correct the prolonged **DRVVT** and a ratio is determined to detect the presence of a lupus inhibitor. Usually the ratio >greater than 1.3 is indicative a lupus inhibitor is present.
8. **Hexagonal phospholipids.** The hexagonal-phase phospholipids (HPPs) test uses egg phosphatidylethanolamine in a hexagonal-phase configuration. This configuration will neutralize most lupus inhibitors and not react to factor deficiencies or inhibitors. The system is aPTT based with a degree of correction.
9. **Activated clotting time (ACT)**
   a. Whole blood is placed in a glass tube containing activator. Determine time it takes the clot to form; blood is kept at 37°C during testing.
   b. Point-of-care test performed at a clinic, cardiac catheterization laboratory, or surgical suite. Most often used to **monitor high-dose heparin therapy** during coronary artery bypass surgery.
10. **Thromboelastography (TEG) and rotational thromboelastometry (ROTEM)** are the continuous assessment of torque created from clotting blood onto an oscillating pin or cup. The interpretation of the torque created clotting curves from these methods will depend on (a) patient history (e.g., surgical, trauma, and hemophilia), (b) type of sample used (e.g., native whole blood and citrated whole blood), and (c) type of activator used (e.g., kaolin and tissue factor). These are classified as global hemostasis systems.

XII. EVALUATION TESTS FOR THE FIBRINOLYTIC SYSTEM

A. Fibrin Degradation Products (FDPs): Latex particles are coated with antibody against **fibrinogen** and are mixed with patient **serum.** Macroscopic agglutination indicates degradation products. This is a **nonspecific test** that will be **abnormal** when either **fibrin degradation products or fibrinogen degradation products are present** (DIC and primary fibrinogenolysis). In many institutions, this assay has been discontinued and the D-Dimer Assay is sufficiently sensitive to rule out the presence of DIC and venous thrombosis.

B. D-Dimer Assay: Latex particles are coated with antibody against **D-dimer.** Highly **specific** measurement for **fibrin degradation products**; does **not** detect fibrinogen degradation products. Abnormal result indicates a clot has formed, been stabilized by factor XIIIa, and is being lysed by plasmin (abnormal in **DIC**, but normal in primary fibrinogenolysis).

XIII. ANTICOAGULANT THERAPIES

A. Unfractionated Heparin Therapy

1. Treatment of choice to **prevent extension of existing clots** due to acute thrombotic events (e.g., venous and arterial thrombosis, pulmonary embolism, thrombophlebitis, and acute myocardial infarction)
2. Therapy involves a bolus of **heparin**, followed by continuous infusion.
3. **Antithrombin** must be present with levels of 40–60% of normal for heparin to work.
4. The **antithrombin/heparin** complex **inhibits serine proteases**, including XIIa, XIa, IXa, Xa, IIa, and kallikrein. **Inhibition is immediate.**
5. It **inhibits** the conversion of fibrinogen to fibrin, platelet aggregation, and activation of factor XIII.
6. Heparin activity can be immediately **reversed by** administration of **protamine sulfate.**
7. Monitor with the anti-FXa chromogenic assay. This method can be used to assay all heparinoids to include UFH and all of the low-molecular-weight heparinoids. **When using both the aPTT and the anti-FXa the** therapeutic range is approximately 0.3–0.7 units/mL. The aPTT range is reported in seconds and should be correlated against the anti-FXa quantitative units. The aPTT cannot be used to monitor the low-molecular-weight heparins.
8. Daily **platelet counts** should be performed on heparinized patients to **monitor for heparin-induced thrombocytopenia** (HIT). If detected, heparin therapy is immediately halted and different anticoagulant therapies are considered.

B. Warfarin (Coumadin®/Coumarin) Therapy

1. This oral anticoagulant is prescribed on an outpatient basis to prevent extension of existing clots and recurrence of thrombotic events, and prophylactically it is often prescribed postsurgery to prevent thrombosis.
2. **Vitamin K antagonist**
3. Warfarin inhibits liver synthesis of functional prothrombin group factors II, VII, IX, and X. Factor VII is affected first (short half-life) and to the greatest extent.

4. Overlap with heparin therapy is common, because full anticoagulant action of warfarin is not achieved for 4–5 days. Warfarin is often used for **up to 6 months** or longer.
5. **Monitor** with **PT** and **INR;** INR therapeutic range is 2.0–3.0 for most conditions. If INR is higher with serious bleeding, **vitamin K** can be administered to **reverse affects. Many institutions only report the INR.**

C. Other Medications Used in Hemostasis

1. **Low-molecular-weight heparin** (LMWH) (e.g., enoxaparin sodium, dalteparin, nadroparin, tinzaparin, and fondaparinux), subcutaneous injection, requires antithrombin to work
   a. Fixed dose response reduces the need for laboratory monitoring.
   b. Lower risk of heparin-induced thrombocytopenia (HIT)
   c. It is mainly an anti-Xa inhibitor; anti-IIa response is reduced.
   d. If monitoring is needed, perform anti-Xa assay.
   e. The therapeutic range for LMWHs is 0.5–1.0 u/mL.
2. **Direct thrombin inhibitor** (e.g., argatroban, bivalirudin, and dabigatran) inactivates thrombin only; does not require presence of antithrombin to work
   a. Used in place of unfractionated or low-molecular-weight heparin when HIT suspected
   b. These medications will prolong the PT, aPTT, and thrombin time.
3. **Fibrinolytic therapy:** Tissue plasminogen activator, streptokinase or urokinase, can be used to **lyse existing clots** and reestablish vascular perfusion.
   a. These medications convert plasminogen to plasmin.
   b. Plasmin destroys the fibrin clot, factors I, V, and VIII.
   c. Affected tests include PT, aPTT, thrombin time, fibrinogen, FDP, and D-dimer (also bleeding time because of low fibrinogen)
4. **Direct Oral Anticoagulants (DOACs)** (Pradaxa®, Boehringer Ingelheim), as a prophylactic agent after hip and knee replacement surgery, are becoming the first oral alternative to coumadin anticoagulation. It is an anti-IIa inhibitor.
   a. **Anti-Xa direct oral anticoagulants** have also become available for stroke prevention, treatment, and prophylaxis of venous thromboembolism: rivaroxaban (Xarelto®, Bayer Pharma AG and Janssen Pharmaceuticals), apixaban (Eliquis®, Bristol Myers Squibb), and edoxaban (Savaysa® in US, Lixiana® in EU, Diachii Sankyo).
   b. Patients on DOACs have no known dietary restrictions (although rivaroxaban absorption is increased with food intake). DOACs have predictable pharmacodynamics and pharmacokinetics, and, unlike oral vitamin K antagonists, these drugs do not require routine continuous monitoring.
   c. If monitoring is required, specific calibrated assays for the anti-IIa and the anti-Xa assays are necessary to quantify the drug levels.
5. **Antiplatelet medications** (e.g., aspirin, Plavix®, cangrelor, ticagrelor, and eptifibatide) are all used to inhibit platelet function. Nonsteroidal anti-inflammatory drugs (NSAIDS) may be used in conjunction with other anticoagulant therapies to prevent recurrence of thrombotic events.

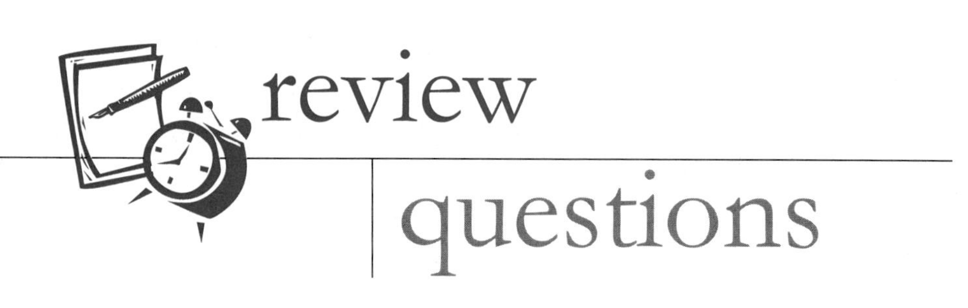

INSTRUCTIONS Each of the questions or incomplete statements that follow are comprised of four suggested responses. Select the *best* answer or completion statement in each case.

Principles of Coagulation

1. The hemorrhagic problems associated with scurvy are due to a deficiency of ________, which is a cofactor required for collagen synthesis.
   A. vitamin C
   B. prothrombin
   C. vitamin K
   D. protein C

2. The normal reference range of platelets counts is approximately: (____ $\times 10^9$/L)
   A. 25–50
   B. 150–400
   C. 200–500
   D. 2000–4000

3. Which of the following is a cause of thrombocytopenia?
   A. Hemophilia A
   B. Postsplenectomy
   C. Dysfibrinogemia
   D. Aplastic anemia

4. Platelets interacting with and binding to other platelets is referred to as
   A. Adhesion
   B. Aggregation
   C. Release
   D. Retraction

5. In platelet aggregation studies, certain aggregating agents induce a biphasic aggregation curve. This second phase of aggregation is directly related to
   A. Formation of fibrin
   B. Changes in platelet shape
   C. Release of endogenous ADP
   D. Release of platelet factor 3

6. A platelet aggregation agent that characteristically yields a biphasic curve when used in optimal concentration is
   A. Arachidonic acid
   B. Collagen
   C. Epinephrine
   D. Ristocetin

7. The platelet aggregation pattern drawn below is characteristic of the aggregating agent
   A. ADP
   B. Collagen
   C. Ristocetin
   D. Thrombin

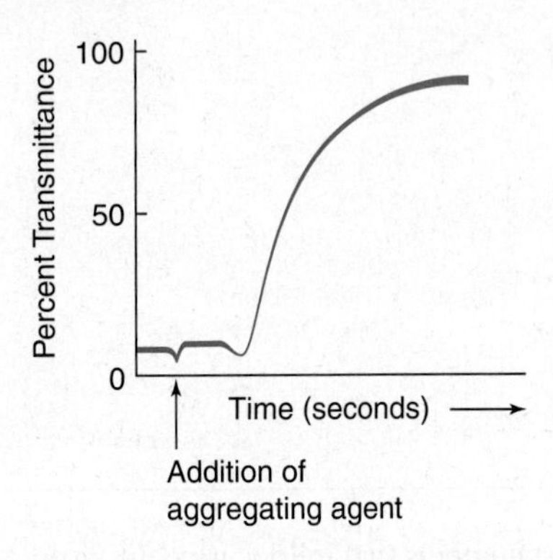

8. The operating principle of a photo-optic platelet aggregometer is best described as
   A. Aggregation on a foreign surface: Platelet aggregation is directly proportional to the difference in platelet counts performed before and after platelet-rich plasma is passed through a column of glass beads.
   B. Change in optical density: As platelets aggregate, the optical density of the platelet-rich plasma decreases.
   C. Electrical impedance: Platelet aggregates are counted as they pass through an aperture, temporarily interrupting the flow of current between two electrodes.
   D. Pulse editing: Editing electronically generated pulses can differentiate the number of free platelets versus platelet aggregates.

9. Of the following therapeutic agents, those considered to be antiplatelet medications are:
   A. Aspirin and Plavix®
   B. Coumadin® and heparin
   C. Heparin and protamine sulfate
   D. Tissue plasminogen activator and streptokinase

10. A potent inhibitor of platelet aggregation released by endothelial cells is
   A. Epinephrine
   B. Prostacyclin
   C. Ristocetin
   D. Thromboxane A_2

11. The reference value for mean platelet volume (MPV) is approximately
   A. 2–4 fL
   B. 5–7 fL
   C. 8–10 fL
   D. 11–14 fL

12. The platelet parameter PDW refers to the
   A. Average platelet volume
   B. Cell weight versus density
   C. Capacity to adhere to foreign surfaces
   D. Variation in platelet cell size

13. A normal histogram showing platelet size distribution is best described as
   A. Bimodal, nonskewed peaks
   B. Left-skewed single peak
   C. Right-skewed single peak
   D. Single peak, Gaussian distribution

14. Which of the following is the final normal maturation stage for platelets?
   A. Megakaryoblast
   B. Promegakaryocyte
   C. Thrombocyte
   D. Megakaryocyte

15. The recommended type of microscopy for the performance of manual platelet counts is
   A. Electron
   B. Dark field
   C. Light
   D. Phase contrast

16. The correct platelet count *expressed in SI units* is
   A. 178×10^9/L
   B. 178×10^3/L
   C. 356×10^9/cu. mm
   D. $712{,}000 \times 10^9$/L

17. The size threshold range used by electrical impedance methods to count particles as platelets is
    A. 0–10 fL
    B. 2–20 fL
    C. 15–40 fL
    D. 35–90 fL

18. In storage pool disease, platelets are primarily deficient in
    A. ADP
    B. Platelet factor 3
    C. Thrombasthenin
    D. Thromboxane A_2

19. The anticoagulant required for routine coagulation testing is
    A. Sodium heparin
    B. Sodium citrate
    C. Acid citrate dextrose
    D. Sodium fluoride

20. Which of the following is *not* synthesized in the liver?
    A. Factor VIII
    B. Plasminogen
    C. Protein C
    D. von Willebrand factor

21. When thrombin binds to thrombomodulin on the endothelial cell surface, thrombin can
    A. Activate the protein C pathway
    B. Activate factor V and factor VIII
    C. Convert fibrinogen to fibrin
    D. Stimulate platelet aggregation

22. The coagulation factors having a sex-linked recessive inheritance pattern are
    A. Factor V and factor VIII
    B. Factor VIII and factor IX
    C. Factor IX and factor X
    D. von Willebrand factor and factor VIII

23. Prekallikrein deficiency is associated with
    A. Prolonged aPTT that does not correct with a mixing study
    B. Autosomal dominant inheritance
    C. Increased risk of thrombosis
    D. Delayed bleeding at the incision site following surgery

24. Which of the following will cause the thrombin time to be prolonged?
    A. Factor VIII Deficiency
    B. Heparin
    C. von Willebrands disease
    D. Abnormal FV deficiency

25. The expected screening test results for a patient with a fibrin stabilizing factor deficiency are
    A. Prolonged prothrombin time
    B. Prolonged activated partial thromboplastin time
    C. Prolonged prothrombin time and activated partial thromboplastin time
    D. Normal prothrombin time and activated partial thromboplastin time

26. A patient on therapeutic warfarin will most likely have a(n)
    A. Normal PT/INR, increased aPTT, prolonged bleeding time, low platelet count
    B. Increased PT/INR, increased aPTT, normal bleeding time, normal platelet count
    C. Normal PT/INR, normal aPTT, normal bleeding time, normal platelet count
    D. Increased PT/INR, normal aPTT, prolonged bleeding time, low platelet count

27. The observation of a normal reptilase time and a prolonged thrombin time indicates which condition?
    A. Presence of fibrin degradation products
    B. Dysfibrinogenemia
    C. Hypoplasminogenemia
    D. Presence of heparin

28. von Willebrand factor is a
    A. Phospholipid required for multiple reactions in the coagulation sequence
    B. Plasma protein that binds platelets to exposed subendothelial collagen
    C. Plasma protein with procoagulant activity in the intrinsic coagulation system
    D. Platelet membrane glycoprotein that attaches the platelet to the injured vessel wall

29. Fibrin strands are cross-linked and the fibrin clot is stabilized by the activity of
    A. α_2-Antiplasmin
    B. Factor XIIIa
    C. Plasmin
    D. Thrombin

30. Which laboratory test is used to investigate a hypercoagulable state?
    A. Thrombin time
    B. Reptilase time
    C. APCR
    D. Euglobulin lysis

31. Which of the following enzymatically degrades the stabilized fibrin clot?
    A. Plasminogen
    B. Plasmin
    C. Prothrombin
    D. Thrombin

32. The activity of the lupus anticoagulant and anticardiolipin antibodies appears to be directed against
    A. Factor V
    B. Factor VIII
    C. Factor IX
    D. Phospholipid

33. In monitoring a patient on oral anticoagulant therapy, an INR of 1.3 was obtained. How would you interpret this result?
    A. The patient is adequately anticoagulated and should be tested again in 1 month.
    B. The patient is underanticoagulated and should be evaluated for a change in dietary habits.
    C. The patient is overanticoagulated and should receive a vitamin K injection.
    D. Data to determine the patient's status are insufficient.

34. The main regulatory protein of secondary hemostasis is
    A. Antithrombin
    B. Protein C
    C. α_2-Antiplasmin
    D. Tissue plasminogen activator

35. An advantage of the coagulation analyzers that use the electromechanical technology is that they
    A. Are more sensitive
    B. Are not affected by colored or hemolyzed plasma
    C. Do not need calibration
    D. Use a smaller sample size

36. Measurement of the time required for fibrin formation when thrombin is added to plasma evaluates the
    A. Fibrinogen concentration
    B. Prothrombin concentration
    C. Extrinsic clotting system
    D. Intrinsic clotting system

37. A fibrinogen assay is performed on the coagulation analyzer using the standard 1:10 dilution with Owren's buffer. The seconds obtained do not read on the standard curve. An alternate 1:20 dilution is performed and is 400 mg/dL when read off the curve. The concentration of fibrinogen to be reported in mg/dL is
    A. 160 mg/dL
    B. 200 mg/dL
    C. 400 mg/dL
    D. 800 mg/dL

38. Calculate the INR using the following data:

    Patient's PT 23.5 sec
    Mean normal PT 11.5 sec
    ISI 1.15

    A. 2.0
    B. 2.3
    C. 2.5
    D. 1.7

$$\text{INR} = \left[\frac{\text{Patient PT in sec}}{\text{Reference interval PT (geometric mean in sec:)}}\right]^{\text{ISI}}$$

39. A prolonged aPTT result is obtained on a patient diagnosed with acute disseminated intravascular coagulation (DIC). The patient has not yet been treated for this disorder. The most likely cause of the prolonged aPTT is
    A. In addition to DIC, the patient is deficient in a factor required for the extrinsic pathway.
    B. DIC is characterized by synthesis of less stable coagulation factors, which deteriorate rapidly in the circulation.
    C. Systemic activation of the coagulation system depletes some factors more rapidly than the liver can synthesize them.
    D. The patient has been misdiagnosed; a prolonged aPTT indicates that the problem is deficient, not excessive, coagulation.

40. Which laboratory test is decreased during a DIC event?
    A. Fibrinogen
    B. PT
    C. aPTT
    D. Antithrombin

41. Which of the following methods depends on cleavage of synthetic substrates by an active serine protease.
    A. Chromogenic
    B. Photo-optical
    C. Mechanical
    D. Immunodiffusion

42. Epsilon aminocaproic acid is the treatment of choice for
    A. von Willebrand disease
    B. Hemophilia A
    C. DIC with secondary fibrinolysis
    D. Primary fibrinogenolysis

43. A clot retraction defect is most likely due to
    A. Lack of platelet receptor glycoprotein Ib
    B. Lack of platelet receptor glycoprotein IIb/IIIa
    C. Insufficient ADP in dense bodies
    D. Absence of von Willebrand factor

44. Thrombocytosis is a characteristic of
    A. Disseminated intravascular coagulation
    B. Splenomegaly
    C. Polycythemia vera
    D. Idiopathic thrombocytopenic purpura

45. Given the following laboratory results, what is the appropriate reflex test?

PT	Normal
aPTT	Slightly prolonged
Platelet aggregation studies	Normal Normal
Collagen	Abnormal
ADP	
Ristocetin	

A. Ristocetin cofactor assay
B. D-dimer
C. PK screen
D. TT

46. A physician suspects a qualitative platelet defect in a young child. What may be the most useful screening test listed below?
A. PT
B. aPTT
C. PFA-100 EPI/COLL
D. TT

47. The coagulation factors referred to as "vitamin K-dependent" are
A. I, V, VIII, XIII
B. II, V, IX, XII
C. II, VII, IX, X
D. XI, XII, Fletcher, Fitzgerald

48. A patient on warfarin therapy will be deficient in a functional amount of
A. Fibrinogen and prothrombin
B. Stable and labile factors
C. Protein C and protein S
D. Fletcher and Fitzgerald factors

49. A 25-year-old male presents to his physician complaining of leg pain. The physician diagnoses a deep vein thrombosis (DVT) and wants to determine the cause of the thrombotic episode.

Which laboratory test may be used to investigate the hypercoagulable states?
A. PT
B. aPTT
C. APCR
D. Euglobulin lysis

50. An 85-year-old male with slurred speech and paralysis on the right side of the body is seen in the emergency department. A stat D-dimer is ordered and is very high. The physician suspects a thromboembolic event based on the D-dimer and needs to institute clot-dissolving therapy immediately. The most likely diagnosis and appropriate therapy for the patient is
A. Myocardial infarction; treat with aspirin
B. Pulmonary embolism; treat with warfarin
C. Deep vein thrombosis; treat with heparin
D. Stroke; treat with tissue plasminogen activator

51. Reversal of a heparin overdose can be achieved by administration of
A. Vitamin K
B. Protamine sulfate
C. Antithrombin
D. Warfarin

52. Which of the following best describes protein C?
A. Vitamin K-dependent inhibitor to clotting
B. Activator of factors V and VIII:C
C. Inhibitor of fibrinolysis
D. Synthesized by endothelial cells

53. The prothrombin time will detect deficiencies in the ________ pathway(s) when calcium and a tissue factor source such as rabbit brain are added to plasma.
A. Extrinsic
B. Extrinsic and common
C. Intrinsic
D. Intrinsic and common

54. A 65-year-old patient in the emergency department has a highly elevated PT/INR result and a suspected intracranial bleed. She is on oral blood thinners but the medications are not with her and she is unable to communicate. What medication would be suspected in this case?
    A. Plavix
    B. Aspirin
    C. Coumadin
    D. Enoxaparin

Specimen Acceptability

55. A specimen is received for a prothrombin time and activated partial thromboplastin time. The 5 mL tube has 2.5 mL of blood in it. Expected test results are would be
    A. PT and aPTT are both falsely short.
    B. PT and aPTT are both falsely long.
    C. PT and aPTT are both unaffected.
    D. PT is unaffected, and aPTT is falsely short.

56. A microtainer EDTA sample obtained during a fingerstick puncture is run on an automated cell counter, yielding a platelet count of $178 \times 10^9/L$. In the erythrocyte monolayer of the stained peripheral blood smear, an average of nine platelets per field is seen under 1000X magnification. Based on these data, you should
    A. Report the results because the platelet count and platelet estimate correlate.
    B. Recollect a specimen for a repeat platelet count because the platelet count and estimate do not correlate.
    C. Examine the periphery of the blood smear for clumping because the platelet count and estimate do not correlate.
    D. Rerun the platelet count on the available specimen to confirm the results.

57. The aPTT is a screening test for the laboratory evaluation of inherited and acquired deficiencies in which of the following?
    A. Extrinsic pathway of the coagulation cascade
    B. Intrinsic pathway of the coagulation cascade
    C. Platelets
    D. Vascular system

58. Laboratory tests requested on a patient scheduled for early morning surgery include a CBC with platelet count. An automated platelet count performed on the specimen is $57 \times 10^9/L$. In the monolayer area of the peripheral blood smear, there are approximately 12 platelets per oil immersion field, many of which are encircling neutrophils. Controls are in range. Based on this information, the best course of action is
    A. Report all the results because the instrument is functioning properly.
    B. Alert the physician immediately so cancellation of surgery can be considered.
    C. Thoroughly mix specimen and repeat platelet count; if results remain the same, report all results and indicate that platelet count has been confirmed by repeat testing.
    D. Have the specimen redrawn using 3.2% sodium citrate as the anticoagulant.

59. Phlebotomist Forgetful Frank collected a tube of blood for an aPTT on John Smith at 10:00 A.M. The blood was collected in a sodium citrate tube. At 4:30 P.M., Frank was getting ready to leave for the day when he discovered Mr. Smith's blood specimen on his blood collection tray. So before leaving, Frank delivered the tube of blood to the laboratory for testing. Which of the following best describes the expected results?
    A. Sodium citrate is a preservative as well as an anticoagulant, so the aPTT result should be accurate.
    B. An aPTT collected in sodium citrate will give falsely long results because some factors are unstable in this anticoagulant.
    C. A falsely prolonged aPTT may occur because some factors deteriorate rapidly at room temperature.
    D. Exposure of the plasma to erythrocytes for several hours has probably activated the factors, so the aPTT will be falsely short.

60. What is the most likely factor deficiency based on the following data?
    PT Normal
    aPTT Prolonged
    TT Normal
    A. FVII
    B. FII
    C. FIX
    D. FXIII

61. A sodium citrate tube is received in the laboratory for PT and aPTT testing. Results are as follows:

Prothrombin time	>100.0 sec (control 12.0 sec)
aPTT	>200.0 sec (control 32.0 sec)

A mixing study was performed and there was no correction of either the prolonged PT or the aPTT. What would be the likely coagulation abnormality to consider?
    A. Lupus inhibitor
    B. Factor XIII deficiency
    C. Hemophilia A
    D. Factor V Leiden

Case Studies

62. A 30-year-old female is admitted to the hospital with neurological symptoms. The following results are obtained:

Hemoglobin	60 g/L
Hematocrit	0.19 L/L
Platelet count	25×10^9/L
RBC morphology	Many schistocytes
ADAMTS-13	Markedly decreased

The most likely diagnosis for the patient is
    A. Thrombotic thrombocytopenic purpura
    B. Idiopathic thrombocytopenic purpura
    C. Hemolytic uremic syndrome
    D. von Willebrand disease

63. A 4-year-old child is seen in the emergency department with petechiae and a platelet count of 15×10^9/L. She has no previous history of bleeding problems. Three weeks earlier, she had chicken pox. The physician advises the parents to keep the child off the playground to avoid injury, and says the child will recover within 2–4 weeks with no further treatment. What condition does this child most likely have?
    A. Essential thrombocythemia
    B. Immune thrombocytopenic purpura (ITP)
    C. Thrombotic thrombocytopenic purpura
    D. Glanzmann thrombasthenia

64. Laboratory results on a 16-year-old female with frequent nosebleeds and severe menorrhagia are as follows:

Platelet count	250×10^9/L
PFA-100 EPI/COLL	>300.0 sec (reference range ≤ 80.0 sec)
Prothrombin time	13.0 sec (control 12.0 sec)
aPTT	75.0 sec (control 32.0 sec)
Platelet aggregation	Normal response to ADP, collagen, epinephrine; no response with ristocetin

These results are consistent with
    A. Christmas disease
    B. Hemophilia A
    C. Glanzmann thrombasthenia
    D. von Willebrand disease

65. Laboratory results on a 6-year-old female with petechiae and severe epistaxis are as follows:

Platelet count	145×10^9/L
PFA-100 assay	>prolonged closure time with both ADP/EPI collagen cartridges.
MPV	16.0 fL (reference range 8.0–10.0 fL)
Platelet aggregation	Normal response to ADP, collagen, epinephrine; no response with ristocetin
Prothrombin time	11.5 sec (control 12.0 sec)
aPTT	33.0 sec (control 32.0 sec)

These results are consistent with
    A. Bernard-Soulier syndrome
    B. von Willebrand disease
    C. Glanzmann thrombasthenia
    D. Ehlers-Danlos syndrome

66. A clot retraction defect is suspected in a newborn male experiencing severe bleeding following circumcision. This has happened in two previous male siblings. The following results are obtained:

Platelet count	320×10^9/L
PFA-100	Normal response
Platelet aggregation	Normal response to ristocetin; Normal response to ADP, collagen, epinephrine
Prothrombin time	12.0 sec (Normal range: 12.0–14.0 sec)
aPTT	51.0 sec (Normal range: 23.0–32.0 sec)

These results are characteristic of
    A. von Willebrand disease
    B. Glanzmann thrombasthenia
    C. Storage pool disease
    D. Hemophilia A or B

67. Results on a 35-year-old male presenting with sudden severe hemorrhagic problems are as follows:

Platelet count	225×10^9/L
PFA-100	Results in normal range
Prothrombin time	12.8 sec (control 12.0 sec)
aPTT	85.0 sec (control 32.0 sec)
aPTT 1:1 mixing study	65.0 sec

These clinical manifestations and laboratory results are consistent with

A. Lupus anticoagulant
B. von Willebrand disease
C. Hemophilia A
D. Factor VIII inhibitor

68. An 80-year-old man suffered a heart attack 1 month ago, and after the hospital stay he was discharged with instructions to follow an outpatient treatment plan. He arrives at the cardiology clinic today for lab work to monitor the treatment plan. The following results are obtained:

PT	52.0 sec (control 12.0 sec)
INR	5.5 (therapeutic range 2.0–3.0)
aPTT	50.0 sec (control 32.0 sec)

This patient is most likely on a

A. Nontherapeutic dose of low-molecular-weight heparinoid
B. Supratherapeutic dose of coumadin
C. Subtherapeutic dose of coumadin
D. Fibrinolytic agent such as tissue plasminogen activator

69. The following results are obtained on a 60-year-old male patient:

WBC	24.7×10^9/L
RBC	6.67×10^{12}/L
Hgb	200 g/L
Hct	0.61 L/L
Plt	79×10^9/L
PT	19.3 sec (control 12.0 sec)
aPTT	81.2 sec (control 32.0 sec)

The WBC, RBC, Hgb, Hct, and Plt were performed on blood collected in an evacuated tube containing EDTA. The PT and aPTT were performed on blood collected in an evacuated tube containing 3.2% sodium citrate. The standard collection procedure was followed, and all tests were performed within the appropriate time limits. Based on this information, the statement that best explains the prolonged coagulation test results is:

A. Coagulation reactions require platelet factor 3; availability of this component is insufficient when the platelet count is below 100×10^9/L.
B. The ratio of anticoagulant to blood is critical; the volume of anticoagulant must be decreased when the Hct is greater than 55%.
C. The PT and aPTT evaluate the extrinsic and intrinsic pathways, respectively; prolongation of both tests indicates a deficiency of a factor common to both systems.
D. Coagulation reactions are inhibited by a product released by leukocytes; this inhibitory activity becomes significant when the leukocyte count is greater than 20.0×10^9/L.

70. The following results are obtained on a 3-year-old boy with sudden severe hemorrhagic problems:

PFA-100	EPI/COLL: 75 sec. Closure time normal
Prothrombin time	13.0 sec (Normal range 12.0–14.0 sec)
aPTT	95.0 sec (Normal range: 32.0–36.0 sec)
aPTT 1:1 mixing study	35.0 sec
Platelet aggregation	Normal with ristocetin, ADP, collagen, and epinephrine

These clinical manifestations and laboratory results are consistent with

A. Aspirin therapy
B. von Willebrand disease
C. Hemophilia B
D. Lupus anticoagulant

71. Screening tests for a 46-year-old male patient admitted for minor surgery are as follow:

Platelet count	325×10^9/L
Bleeding time	4.5 min (reference range $\leq$ 8.0 min)
Prothrombin time	13.0 sec (control 12.0 sec)
aPTT	95.0 sec (control 32.0 sec)
aPTT 1:1 mixing study	32.0 sec

The patient has no clinical manifestations of a bleeding problem and has no personal or family history of bleeding problems, even following dental extraction. Several family members have been treated for deep vein thrombosis. Based on these laboratory results and the clinical history, the most likely cause of the prolonged aPTT is

A. Heparin present in the sample
B. Factor VIII deficiency
C. Factor XII deficiency
D. Factor XIII deficiency

72. A 25-year-old patient with a history of atrial fibrillation with a suspected DVT is admitted through the emergency room. She has trauma from an automobile accident with bleeding from the wounds that are not responding to blood component therapy. She is on a DOAC but she is not able to give them the medication information. Dabigatran presence can be excluded with which one of the following assays?

A. Normal PT
B. Abnormal aPTT
C. Normal D-dimer levels
D. Normal Anti-Xa

73. A 57-year-old man with prostate cancer is admitted to the intensive care unit with severe bleeding problems. The following laboratory results are obtained:
These laboratory results are consistent with

A. Primary fibrinogenolysis
B. DIC with secondary fibrinolysis
C. Factor II deficiency
D. Coumadin® therapy

Platelet count	Normal
Prothrombin time	Prolonged
aPTT	Prolonged
Fibrinogen	Decreased
Thrombin time	Prolonged
D-dimer	Negative
FDP	Positive
Antithrombin	Normal
RBC morphology	Schistocytes absent

74. A patient in the hospital for an acute myocardial infarction is placed on standard unfractionated heparin therapy and aspirin. Laboratory results are performed before instituting therapy and then daily for two days after. Results are as shown:

	Before Therapy	Day 2	Day 3
Prothrombin Time	Normal	Normal	Normal
aPTT	Normal	Prolonged	Prolonged
Platelet Count	$325 \times 10^9/L$	$160 \times 10^9/L$	$42 \times 10^9/L$

The most likely complication by Day 3 is
A. Disseminated intravascular coagulation
B. Primary fibrinogenolysis
C. Aspirin-induced thrombocytopenia
D. Heparin-induced thrombocytopenia

75. A 44-year-old female with known apixaban therapy requires emergency surgery. The best method to estimate the drug concentration would be:
A. PT
B. aPTT
C. Normal thrombin time
D. Anti-Xa chromogenic assay

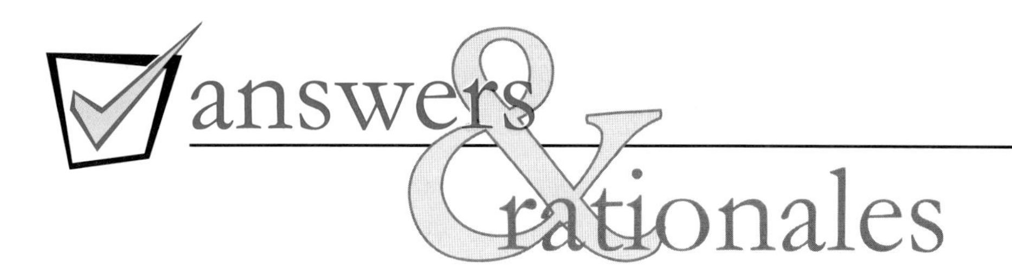

Principles of Coagulation

1.

A. Vascular integrity is influenced by vitamin C intake. In a deficiency or absence of vitamin C, collagen production is insufficient or abnormal. Vitamin C deficiency is associated with capillary fragility and the primary hemostasis bleeding symptoms of petechiae and mucosal bleeding.

2.

B. Normal platelet count reference interval is $150–400 \times 10^9$/L. Conditions that can cause elevated platelet counts may include a splenenectomy, hemorrhage, post-op surgery, myeproliferative syndromes. Those disorders that can cause decreased counts are aplastic anemia, megaloblastic anemia, acute leukemia, and myelodysplastic syndromes.

3.

C. Aplastic anemia occurs when the bone marrow fails to produce any of the three cell lines. Hemophiliacs have normal platelet counts. Erythropoietin is involved in the production of red blood cells. Dysfibrinogemia does not involve platelet counts.

4.

B. "Adhesion" refers to platelets interacting with something other than platelets. *In vivo* platelets adhere to collagen that is exposed when vessel damage occurs. "Aggregation" refers to attachment of platelets to other platelets. Release is the process by which platelet granule contents are secreted. Retraction describes one of the final steps in coagulation in which the fibrin-platelet plug contracts, restoring normal blood flow to the vessel.

5.

C. In platelet aggregation studies, the addition of the aggregating agent may induce an initial aggregation phase followed by a secondary wave. The initial phase is due to the interaction of the aggregating agent with the platelet. The second phase is due to release of nonmetabolic ADP from platelet granules, which promotes the additional wave of aggregation.

6.

C. Epinephrine is the only aggregating agent listed that typically gives a biphasic pattern. ADP and thrombin also give biphasic patterns when used in optimal concentrations. Arachidonic acid causes a rapid monophasic platelet aggregation. Collagen and ristocetin also induce monophasic aggregatory responses.

7.

B. Collagen is the only aggregating agent that includes a single-wave response preceded by a lag phase. During the lag phase, collagen stimulates platelets to release their granule contents. Endogenous ADP released from the platelets then initiates irreversible platelet aggregation.

8.

B. When an aggregating agent is added to an optically dense suspension of platelet-rich plasma (PRP), the platelets normally stick to each other, forming platelet aggregates. As additional platelets aggregate, the cell suspension becomes clearer and has a few large clumps of cells. At maximum aggregation, the specimen is relatively clear, allowing light transmission that is only partially obstructed by a few large platelet aggregates.

9.

A. Aspirin inhibits the enzyme cyclooxygenase in the prostaglandin pathway, preventing platelet aggregation. Plavix® (clopidogrel bisulfate) blocks the IIb/IIIa fibrinogen-binding platelet receptor, preventing platelet aggregation. Coumadin® and heparin inhibit clotting factors in secondary hemostasis. Protamine sulfate can be used to neutralize heparin. Tissue plasminogen activator and streptokinase are fibrinolytic system activators.

10.

B. Prostacyclin, also referred to as PGI_2, is the most potent inhibitor of platelet aggregation known. Injured endothelial cells release prostacyclin. Epinephrine and ristocetin are potent stimulators of platelet aggregation. Thromboxane A_2, generated by platelets via the prostaglandin pathway, also stimulates platelets to aggregate.

11.

C. The average volume of normal platelets is approximately 8–10 fL. This platelet parameter is equivalent to the erythrocyte parameter MCV (mean corpuscular volume). MPV is increased in the hereditary Bernard-Soulier syndrome and May-Hegglin anomaly, also in acquired disorders with increased need for platelet release from the bone marrow.

12.

D. PDW is an abbreviation for platelet distribution width. This parameter measures the uniformity of platelet size. It is the platelet equivalent of the red cell parameter RDW. It represents the coefficient of variation of the platelet population.

13.

C. A histogram showing platelet size distribution is made by plotting platelet size (*x* axis) versus number (*y* axis). The resulting curve is usually a single, right-skewed peak. This reflects a larger number of platelets in the lower size range with a "tail" of larger cells to the right of the majority.

14.

C. Platelets or thrombocytes are the mature form of megakaryocyte fragments in the peripheral blood. They play an important role in primary hemostasis by adherence to the ruptured vessel way at the site of an injury.

15.

D. Phase microscopy is currently recommended for manual platelet counts. This allows satisfactory discrimination between platelets and debris, a major problem in manual counts. Light microscopy may also be used; however, differentiating between platelets and debris is more difficult than with phase microscopy.

16.

A. Twenty microliters of blood (0.02 mL) added to 1.98 mL of diluting fluid gives a dilution of 1:100; the dilution factor is 100. The standard platelet counting area is the center mm^2 on both sides of the chamber. The standard formula for hemacytometer counts expressed in mm^3 is

$$\frac{\text{Total number cells counted} \times \text{Dilution factor}}{\text{Total area counted} \times \text{Depth}}$$

The correct equation for this problem is

$$\frac{356 \times 100}{2\ mm^2 \times 0.10\ mm} = 178{,}000$$
$$= 178 \times 10^3/mm^3$$

When expressed in SI units, the platelet count is $178 \times 10^9/L$ Answer A. Answer B is expressed in conventional units, not SI units.

17.

B. In the electrical impedance method for counting platelets, particles between 2 and 20 fL will be classified as platelets by the analyzer's computer. The normal average platelet volume is 10 fL. One dilution is used for counting and sizing of platelets and red blood cells. In the electrical impedance method, size thresholds differentiate the two.

18.

A. Platelets in storage pool disease are deficient in dense granules. The platelets in this disorder lack nonmetabolic ADP found in dense granules and normally released when the platelets are stimulated. This accounts for a poor response to aggregating agents.

19.

B. The Clinical and Laboratory Standards Institute (CLSI) recommends 3.2% (0.109 M) sodium citrate for coagulation testing. Sodium heparin is used for many chemistry tests, but will cause times that exceed linearity if used for coagulation tests. Acid citrate dextrose (ACD) is used for HLA phenotyping, DNA analysis, and paternity tests. Sodium fluoride is used for glucose testing.

20.

D. The liver produces most of the clotting factors as well as inhibitors to clotting. A patient with liver disease has impaired synthesis of these clotting factors and inhibitors. One of the few hemostatic proteins not produced by the liver is von Willebrand factor, which is produced by endothelial cells and megakaryocytes.

21.

A. Thrombomodulin, an endothelial cell receptor, has the ability to change the specificity of thrombin from a procoagulant to an anticoagulant. Once bound to thrombomodulin, thrombin has anticoagulant properties because of its activation of protein C. Protein C, along with its cofactor protein S, then exerts negative feedback on the clotting system by inactivating factor V and factor VIII.

22.

B. Factor VIII and factor IX are the sex-linked recessive hemostatic defects. von Willebrand factor deficiency and dysfibrinogenemia are inherited as autosomal dominant disorders. Factor V, factor X, and most of the other inherited hemostatic disorders have an autosomal recessive inheritance pattern.

23.

C. Prekallikrein (Fletcher factor) deficiency is one of the many autosomal recessive disorders. The aPTT will be prolonged and will correct with a mixing study because it is a factor deficiency. Because prekallikrein is an activator of the fibrinolytic system, prekallikrein-deficient patients cannot lyse clots efficiently and are prone to thrombosis. Fibrinolytic and anticoagulant therapies are indicated in patients who develop thrombosis. Delayed post operative bleeding at the incision site is characteristic of a factor XIII deficiency.

24.

B. The thrombin time is a test that measures fibrinogen. Thrombin reagent is added to undiluted patient plasma, and the time it takes for fibrinogen conversion to fibrin is measured. Anything that interferes with the ability of thrombin to convert fibrinogen to fibrin will prolong the test especially the presence of Heparin. Factor VIII cannot be measured by the thrombin time because it is part of the intrinsic system. The Factor V does not affect the thrombin time.

25.

D. Thrombin converts fibrinogen to the fibrin monomer. Fibrin monomers spontaneously polymerize to form the fibrin polymer. This is the endpoint of clot-based PT and aPTT tests. This fibrin polymer is unstable. Once activated, factor XIII, also known as fibrin-stabilizing factor, produces strong, covalent bonds to create a stable fibrin polymer. This occurs after the endpoint of the PT and aPTT has been reached. A factor XIII deficiency is suspected when delayed post-operative bleeding occurs at the incision site, and the deficiency can be confirmed with the 5 M urea clot solubility test.

26.

B. Warfarin is a vitamin K antagonist and affects liver synthesis of the prothrombin group factors II, VII, IX, and X. The factors are produced but are nonfunctional. Warfarin therapy is monitored with the prothrombin time (PT), which will detect nonfunctional II, VII, and X. The aPTT, though used to monitor heparin therapy, can detect nonfunctional II, IX, and X caused by warfarin therapy. Warfarin does not affect platelet function or quantity. Aspirin and other antiplatelet medications such as clopidogrel bisulfate (Plavix®) will affect platelet function and prolong the bleeding time.

27.

D. The Reptilase time (RT) is not affected by the presence of heparin, whereas the thrombin time (TT) is extremely sensitive to heparin. The Reptilase time is prolonged in both the TT and the RT. Presence of FDPs will prolong both the RT and the TT.

28.

B. von Willebrand factor (vWF) is a portion of the plasma protein known as the factor VIII/von Willebrand factor complex. Its function is to bind to platelet membrane glycoprotein Ib and form a bridge between the platelet and exposed subendothelial collagen. vWF is a carrier protein for factor VIII:C, but vWF does not have coagulant activity in secondary hemostasis as factor VIII:C does.

29.

B. Activated factor XIII is a transglutaminase that cross-links fibrin monomers between glutamine and lysine residues. Fibrin monomers that are not cross-linked lack the stability to maintain the hemostatic plug, as evidenced by the bleeding problems experienced by individuals deficient in factor XIII. Thrombin contributes to the formation of the fibrin clot, which is degraded by plasmin. Once the fibrin clot has been lysed and plasmin is free in circulation, α_2-antiplasmin quickly neutralizes plasmin.

30.

B. Activated Protein C Resistance (APCR), discovered in 1993, inhibits coagulation by degrading FVa and FVIIA. This is a mechanism that is recognized in familial thrombophilia. This disorder is one of the hypercoagulable states.

31.

B. Plasmin, the active form of plasminogen, is the enzyme responsible for degrading fibrin into several different fragments. The D-dimer test is abnormal when there is excessive fibrinolytic activity. Prothrombin is the inactive precursor of thrombin that cleaves fibrinogen to form fibrin, which is stabilized by the activity of factor XIII.

32.

D. The lupus anticoagulant was first discovered in patients with systemic lupus erythematosus. It is actually seen in more patients without SLE, but the original name remains. Lupus anticoagulant and anticardiolipin antibodies belong to the antiphospholipid antibody family. Their activity appears to be directed against the phospholipid portion of the prothrombinase complex (Xa-V-phospholipid-calcium). The antibodies are usually IgG, but can also be IgM. They are found in autoimmune disorders, neoplasms, and some infections. They can also be medication related and can be found in apparently normal individuals. Their presence is suspected when the patient is experiencing thrombosis and the aPTT is prolonged with no correction of the mixing study.

33.

B. The normal therapeutic range for anticoagulation with coumarin is an INR of 2–3. The subject, therefore, is under-anticoagulated. Dietary habits and dose levels should be considered. The patient should be reevaluated in 1 month.

34.

A. Antithrombin is the most important naturally occurring inhibitor to clotting and accounts for 80% of negative feedback in the coagulation cascade by inhibiting serine proteases. Protein C and its cofactor, protein S, inhibit cofactors V and VIII. α_2-Antiplasmin is responsible for neutralizing plasmin once the clot has been lysed. Tissue plasminogen activator activates the fibrinolytic system in response to clot formation.

35.

B. The electro-mechanical coagulation systems are not affected by hemolysis and lipemia such as the photo-optical methods may be influenced.

36.

A. When thrombin is added to patient plasma, fibrinogen is converted to fibrin. No factors above fibrinogen in the cascade are measured, including prothrombin. Both the thrombin time and fibrinogen test use thrombin reagent; both tests measure only one factor, fibrinogen.

37.

D. A 1:20 dilution is used when the time obtained on a patient sample is less than the shortest time used in preparation of the standard curve. A 1:20 dilution is diluted by a factor of 2 when compared to the usual 1:10 dilution. The value read off the curve must be multiplied by 2 to take into account the alternate dilution used.

$$400 \times 2 = 800 \text{ mg/dL}$$

38.

A. The PT seconds are dependent on the reagent or instrument used. Because of this, the World Health Organization recommends using the INR to monitor patients on stabilized Coumadin® therapy because it is *independent* of the reagent or instrument used. The INR is a means of standardizing the reporting of prothrombin times (PTs) worldwide. The INR is calculated by many instruments and laboratory information systems and can be calculated manually as follows:

$$\text{INR} = \left[\frac{\text{Patient PT in sec}}{\text{Reference interval PT (geometric mean in sec.)}}\right]^{\text{ISI}}$$

where

INR = the International Normalized Ratio

ISI = the International Sensitivity Index of the thromboplastin source. This value is determined by the manufacturer for each lot number of thromboplastin reagent. The closer to 1.00 the ISI, the more sensitive the thromboplastin reagent is in detecting factor deficiencies.

Patient PT = the prothrombin time in seconds for the patient.

Control PT is the geometric mean of the reference interval.

39.

C. As coagulation occurs *in vivo,* some factors are consumed just as they are when blood is allowed to clot in a test tube *in vitro.* The factors consumed during coagulation are I, II, V, VIII, and XIII. Results of laboratory procedures relying on one or more of these factors will be affected. All these factors except factor XIII contribute to the reactions evaluated in the aPTT procedure.

40.

A. The PT and aPTT are prolonged in DIC because of consumption of factors I, II, V, and VIII. Platelets are trapped in forming clots and are removed from circulation. The fibrinolytic system is activated by systemic intravascular coagulation; fibrin degradation products and fibrinogen degradation products are elevated. FDP and D-dimer tests will both be positive. Fibrinogen is decreased. The regulatory proteins antithrombin, protein C, and protein S are depleted trying to turn off systemic clotting.

41.

A. The proteolytic activity of antithrombin after activation to a serine protease can be assayed via methods that employ synthetic substrates. The cleavage of the synthetic substrate by an active serine protease will yield a chromogenic compound. Chromogenic methods can also be used to assay plasminogen, protein C, and heparin.

42.

D. Epsilon aminocaproic acid (EACA) is a specific inhibitor of plasmin and is used to turn off inappropriate lysing that occurs in primary fibrinogenolysis. Fibrinolysis seen in DIC is an appropriate body response to systemic clotting. If EACA is administered to a patient in DIC, clots that form will not be lysed, and this could be quickly fatal to the patient.

43.

B. Glanzmann thrombasthenia is a disorder characterized by absent or defective GP IIb/IIIa platelet receptors for fibrinogen binding and subsequent platelet aggregation. Clot retraction in these patients is abnormal due to the lack of the contractile protein actomyosin/thrombasthenin. Neither insufficient ADP in dense bodies, absence of von Willebrand factor, nor absence of the platelet receptor glycoprotein Ib affects clot retraction. Lack of glycoprotein Ib, the von Willebrand factor receptor site, causes the platelet adhesion defect seen in Bernard-Soulier disease.

44.

C. Polycythemia vera, a hemopoietic stem cell disorder characterized by excessive production of erythrocytic, granulocytic, and megakaryocytic cells in the bone marrow, is usually accompanied by thrombocytosis. ITP, DIC, and splenomegaly are all characterized by thrombocytopenia. In ITP, platelet destruction is mediated by immune mechanisms. Platelets are consumed in DIC and sequestered in an individual with an enlarged spleen.

45.

A. A normal response to ADP and collagen in platelet aggregation studies, and an abnormal ristocetin aggregation pattern, with a slightly prolonged aPTT, is indicative of the possibility of the presence of von Willebrands disease. An abnormal ristocetin cofactor assay could help to confirm this disorder.

46.

C. The PFA-100 test is a primary hemostasis screening test for platelet and vascular function. The prothrombin time and aPTT are secondary hemostasis screening tests and do not evaluate platelet function because platelet-poor plasma is used for testing. The thrombin time will screen for the presence of heparin and a number of issues involving fibrinogen levels and function.

47.

C. The prothrombin group factors II, VII, IX, and X are called vitamin K–dependent factors. Vitamin K is needed by the liver to synthesize functional circulating forms of these factors. In the absence of vitamin K, the liver synthesizes the prothrombin group factors, but they are nonfunctional because they lack the carboxyl (COOH) groups needed for binding to Ca^{2+} on phospholipid membranes. The oral anticoagulant warfarin is a vitamin K antagonist and causes liver synthesis of these nonfunctional factors.

48.

C. Vitamin K is required for liver synthesis of regulatory proteins C and S and functional clotting factors II, VII, IX, and X. A deficiency of vitamin K decreases the concentrations of these proteins and subsequently affects test results that measure one or more of them. Fibrinogen, Labile, Fletcher, and Fitzgerald factors do not require vitamin K for their synthesis.

49.

C. The most common hereditary thrombotic disorder, factor V Leiden, is caused by synthesis of an abnormal factor V molecule that is resistant to the inhibitory affects of protein C. The presence of factor V Leiden would be the most likely scenario in this instance.

50.

D. A high D-dimer level indicates the presence of a thrombus (deep vein thrombosis, pulmonary embolism) but is not useful in determining the location. If a thrombus breaks away and travels to the brain, a stroke occurs, causing the symptoms described in this patient. Tissue plasminogen activator will activate the fibrinolytic system to lyse the clot. It should be administered within hours of onset of symptoms to prevent irreversible brain damage. Because of the small window of treatment time, a D-dimer performed on a possible stroke patient should be done STAT. Aspirin, warfarin, and heparin can be administered to prevent the formation of new clots but will not lyse existing clots.

51.

B. A heparin overdose can result in hemorrhage. If bleeding becomes life threatening, protamine sulfate can be given. Heparin will dissociate from antithrombin if protamine sulfate is administered, because heparin has a higher affinity for protamine sulfate. Vitamin K, or prothrombin concentrates, can be administered in the management of bleeding for patients who overdose with warfarin, which is a synonym for Coumadin®.

52.

A. Protein C, a glycoprotein produced in the liver, is a potent inhibitor of coagulation. The activation of protein C, by the thrombin/thrombomodulin complex, will cause the inactivation of factors V and VIII:C. Protein C and its cofactor, protein S, are vitamin K–dependent proteins.

53.

B. The prothrombin time test measures the coagulant activity of the extrinsic and common pathway factors of I, II, V, VII, and X. The reagent used for the prothrombin time test contains calcium and tissue thromboplastin. Thromboplastin is an extract of tissue such as brain or placenta. The activated partial thromboplastin time test measures all coagulation factors present in the intrinsic and common pathways except factor XIII. Calcium, a phospholipid source, and an activating agent, such as kaolin, silica, or celite, are present in the reagents used for the activated partial thromboplastin time.

54.

C. The presence of an elevated PT/INR result in a subject on blood thinners with the presence of an intracranial bleed would make the physician suspect the presence of coumadin. The physician could confirm this with checking for decreased levels of FII, VII, and FX.

Specimen Acceptability

55.

B. A 9:1 ratio of blood to anticoagulant is needed for sodium citrate to bind all available calcium in the blood sample and prevent coagulation. When the 9:1 ratio is not maintained due to the tube not being full, excess sodium citrate present will bind reagent calcium in the test system. This will cause falsely prolonged PT and aPTT results.

56.

A. The results should be reported. A platelet estimate is obtained by multiplying the average number of platelets per oil immersion field (in an erythrocyte monolayer) by 20,000. This number is based on a normal erythrocyte count, which must be considered when comparing the platelet count and estimate. The estimate in this example is 180×10^9/L. This agrees with the platelet count.

57.

B. The aPTT is a screening method to detect deficiencies of coagulation factors in the intrinsic part of the coagulation assay which include FXII, FXI, FIX, and FVIII. It also can be used to screen for the presence of circulating inhibitors both specific and nonspecific.

58.

D. Platelets encircling neutrophils is a phenomenon referred to as platelet satellitosis. This "pseudothrombocytopenia" occurs when the blood of some individuals is anticoagulated with EDTA. Recollecting the specimen using sodium citrate often corrects this problem. If sodium citrate is used, the platelet count obtained must be multiplied by 1.1 for reporting purposes. Multiplying by 1.1 adds back the 10% loss of platelets seen when sodium citrate, with a 9:1 ratio of blood to anticoagulant, is used.

59.

C. Factors V and VIII are labile and deteriorate rapidly at room temperature. Blood for aPTT testing should be tested within 4 hours of draw. Sodium citrate is the appropriate anticoagulant for coagulation procedures.

60.

C. The most likely factor deficiency with a normal PT, abnormal aPTT, and a normal thrombin time would be the presence of a decreased FIX level. The thrombin time is of little value in this screen.

61.

A. The presence of elevated PT and aPTT with a failure to correct after a mixing study is performed usually indicates a nonspecific circulating inhibitor such as a lupus anticoagulant. Further testing for the presence and confirmation of this presence should be performed.

Case Studies

62.

A. With the severe anemia and many schistocytes, a microangiopathic hemolytic anemia should be considered (TTP, HUS). HUS is seen in children after a gastrointestinal infection, frequently caused by *E. coli* 0157:H7, and results in renal damage. TTP is seen in young adults and is more common in women than men. TTP causes neurological damage. Patients with TTP have unusually large multimers of von Willebrand factor because they have a deficiency of a metalloprotease, ADAMTS-13, responsible for breaking down the multimers. These large multimers of vWF bind strongly to platelets, causing platelet aggregation and thrombotic complications in multiple organs.

63.

C. Acute immune thrombocytopenic purpura is mainly seen in young children. A viral infection often precedes the onset of symptoms by several weeks. In 90% of patients with acute ITP, there is an increase in IgG immunoglobulin attached to the surface of the platelets. Spontaneous remission occurs in most patients within 2–6 weeks of the onset of the illness. A chronic form of ITP, believed to be a different disease, is seen in adults.

64.

D. The patient's platelet count is within the reference range, but the PFA-100 EPI/COLL screen is prolonged. This indicates a platelet function problem. The coagulation tests indicate a problem in the intrinsic clotting system (factors XII, XI, IX, VIII, Fitzgerald, and Fletcher). The one disorder in which both platelet function and the coagulant property of factor VIII:C are affected is von Willebrand disease. A synonym for von Willebrand factor is the ristocetin cofactor. In its absence, platelets will not aggregate with ristocetin. The platelet aggregation pattern confirms this diagnosis.

65.

A. Bernard-Soulier syndrome is a platelet adhesion defect that can be mistaken for von Willebrand disease. Platelets in this syndrome lack the glycoprotein Ib receptor, which is necessary for von Willebrand factor to attach to the platelet. Both disorders give identical platelet aggregation patterns. Bernard-Soulier syndrome is noted for giant platelets (note the increased MPV) and varying degrees of thrombocytopenia. Because von Willebrand factor is present in Bernard-Soulier syndrome, the aPTT is normal. However, the elevated levels of both of the PFA-100 cartridges are evident of a platelet functional defect.

66.

D. Because the platelet count is within the reference range, the normal PFA-100 results with normal closure times and normal platelet aggregations studies rule out a platelet disorder; the normal PT with a prolonged aPTT may be indicative of Hemophilia A or B. A good family history should be obtained since this has happened with other siblings.

67.

D. Failure of normal plasma to correct the aPTT indicates the presence of a circulating inhibitor. A factor VIII inhibitor is associated with hemorrhagic problems and would result in noncorrection of the mixing study. Hemophilia A and von Willebrand disease are both caused by factor deficiencies that would result in correction when a 1:1 mixing study is performed. The lupus anticoagulant is a circulating inhibitor that prolongs the aPTT with little or no correction of the mixing study, but it is associated with thrombosis, not severe hemorrhagic problems.

68.

B. Coumarin interferes with the function of vitamin K in the synthesis of prothrombin group factors II, VII, IX, and X. Tests that measure one or more of these factors will be prolonged. These factors are synthesized but are nonfunctional. Of the factors affected by coumarin, IX, X, and II are measured in the aPTT. Factors VII, X, and II are measured in the PT. The patient is on a supratherapeutic dose of coumarin, and the INR demonstrates this. Therapeutic range of INR should be between 2.0 and 3.0. The dose of Coumadin should be adjusted to bring the subject in therapeutic range.

69.

B. The required blood-to-anticoagulant ratio for coagulation testing is 9:1. If a volume of blood contains an elevated number of RBCs, generally considered to be a hematocrit greater than 55%, this ratio will be affected. Excess sodium citrate in the patient plasma, which acts as an anticoagulant by binding calcium ions, will bind the reagent calcium added back to the test plasma during the procedure. Falsely prolonged results are obtained. The specimen needs to be redrawn using less sodium citrate.

70.

C. Hemophilia B is inherited as a sex-linked recessive disorder of factor IX:C. Mothers are carriers who pass the disease on to male offspring. This disorder is strictly a secondary hemostasis defect, so tests for primary hemostasis such as the bleeding time and platelet aggregation studies are normal. Factor deficiencies correct when a 1:1 mixing study is performed; presence of heparin in the sample would result in little or no correction of the mixing study. Aspirin affects platelets in primary hemostasis.

71.

C. An abnormal aPTT that corrects with a 1:1 mixing study and a normal PT indicate a deficiency in the intrinsic coagulation pathway. Because factor XII is an activator of the fibrinolytic system, a deficiency can result in thrombosis. Factor IX deficiency causes bleeding into muscles and joints, not thrombosis. Factor XIII can be eliminated because it is not measured in the aPTT or PT, and a deficiency would cause a bleeding disorder.

72.

B. The prothrombin time is normal. The aPTT is more suitable for assessing dabigatran than the PT but should not be used to quantitate drug. The PT is more suitable for assessing Anti-Xa DOACs than aPTT, but should not be used to quantitate drug.

73.

A. Primary fibrinogenolysis is an unusual disorder in which the fibrinolytic system is activated in the absence of clot formation. Plasmin degrades factors V, VIII, and fibrinogen. The D-dimer test is positive if fibrin degradation products are present; they are absent in this disorder. The FDP test is positive in the presence of either fibrin degradation products *or* fibrinogen degradation products. Tests that are abnormal in DIC due to the systemic clotting are normal in primary fibrinogenolysis.

74.

D. Up to 5% of patients receiving unfractionated heparin therapy for more than 5 days develop an IgG antibody that can cause platelet activation, leading to thrombosis in the microvasculature. If this occurs, the platelet count drops quickly. Patients receiving heparin therapy should be monitored with daily platelet counts. Direct thrombin inhibitors such as lepirudin, bivalirudin, and argatroban can be used in place of heparin. Enoxaparin sodium, a low-molecular-weight heparin, is contraindicated as a treatment for heparin-induced thrombocytopenia. Aspirin therapy causes a qualitative, not quantitative, platelet defect.

75.

D. The anti-Xa chromogenic assay with a specific set of calibrators for apixaban is the method of choice for a patient on this DOAC. The presence and concentration of the apixaban needs to be known so the medical team can be aware of the time in which they can operate and the blood components to use to control the hemorrhaging.

answers & rationales

REFERENCES

McKenzie, S. B. (2019). *Clinical Laboratory Hematology,* 4th ed., in Press; Upper Saddle River, NJ: Pearson.

Rodak, B. F., Fritsma, G. A., and Doig, K. (2016). *Hematology Clinical Principles and Applications,* 6th ed. St. Louis: Elsevier.

McGlasson, D. L., Bessmer, D. S., and Neuhauser, T. S. (July 2001). Do We Still Need to Perform FDP Assays in Conjunction With D-Dimers? Supplement to the *Journal of Thrombosis and Haemostasis* (ISSN 0340-6245). Abstract P753.

Gosselin, R. C., et al. (2015). Effects of storage and thawing conditions on coagulation testing. *International Journal of Laboratory Hematology.* 37(4):551–559.

CHAPTER

4 Immunology and Serology

contents

I. INTRODUCTION TO IMMUNOLOGY

A. Definitions

1. Immunity is the process that occurs to defend the body against foreign organisms or molecules.
2. Immunity includes:
   a. Inflammation
   b. Complement activation
   c. Phagocytosis
   d. Antibody synthesis
   e. Effector T lymphocytes

B. Types of Immunity

1. **Innate** (nonspecific or natural)
   a. **Born with it**, do not need prior exposure
   b. The effectiveness of the immune response varies with age.
   c. **First line of defense:** Designed to keep microorganisms out
      1) **Physical barriers**, such as epithelial cells (intact skin), trapping of bacteria in mucus, etc.
      2) **Chemicals** secreted by cells and includes acidic pH of skin surface, complement, interferons, lysozymes, etc.
   d. **Second line of defense**
      1) **Phagocytosis:** The process of a white blood cell (WBC) engulfing bacteria
      2) **Inflammation:** Nonspecific response to tissue damage, or stimulating molecules, that includes
         a) Chemical (e.g., cytokine) release from damaged host cells
         b) Cellular movement, that is, chemotaxis
         c) Immune cells, such as macrophages, possess pattern recognizing receptors that bind pathogen-associated molecular patterns (PAMPs) and damage-associated molecular patterns (DAMPs)
         d) Elimination of foreign material
         e) Tissue repair
      3) **Complement system:** Enhances phagocytosis (i.e., opsonization), stimulates inflammatory response, and lyses foreign cells
2. **Adaptive** (specific or acquired)
   a. Acquired only after a specific challenge is encountered (primary exposure) and responds specifically to that challenge
   b. Two responses
      1) **Humoral-mediated immunity (HMI)**
         a) More important in protection against extracellular pathogens
         b) Antibody production by plasma cells
      2) **Cell-mediated immunity (CMI)**
         a) More important in protection against intracellular pathogens
         b) **Natural killer (NK) cells:** Rapid response to virus-infected cells and some activity against tumor cells

c) **T-helper cells**
d) **Cytotoxic T lymphocytes** (CTLs)
e) **Cytotoxins**

c. **Active immunity**
1) **Natural:** The host is exposed to foreign immunogen as a result of infection, and the host's immune cells manufacture specific products to eliminate foreign immunogen.
2) **Artificial:** Vaccination; immune system responds to an altered (noninfectious) organism or component of infectious agent
3) Active immunity generally endures for life.

d. **Passive immunity**
1) **Natural:** Maternal antibody crosses placenta to protect infant.
2) **Artificial:** Immune products from another animal injected into the host (e.g., pooled gamma-globulin)
3) Passive immunity short term; no memory cells produced

e. Antigens and immunogens
1) **Immunogen:** A substance capable of inducing an immune response
2) **Antigen:** A substance that specifically interacts with cells or substances of the immune system. Immunogens are also antigens, but not all antigens produce an immune response.
3) **Epitope:** The portion of a molecule (i.e., antigen) that binds to an antibody or T-cell receptor
4) **Thymic-dependent immunogens:** Molecules that require T-helper cells to stimulate antibody formation
5) **Thymic-independent immunogens:** Molecules that initiate antibody production without T-helper cells
6) Immunogenicity characteristics
   a) **Foreignness:** Must be recognized by the body as "nonself"
   b) **Size:** Greater than 10 kilodaltons
   c) **Chemical composition:** Proteins and large carbohydrates are the most immunogenic, whereas lipids and nucleic acids are weakly immunogenic.
   d) **Complexity:** The more complex a molecule, the more immunogenic it becomes.
   e) Route of entry into the host also determines immunogenicity.
   f) Dose of immunogen affects immunogenicity.
   g) **Degradability:** The immunogen needs to be degraded and presented to cells of the immune system.
7) A **hapten** is a low-molecular-weight molecule that alone is too small to stimulate an immune response but can combine with another molecule to induce a response.
8) **Adjuvant** is a compound that enhances an immune response. It is not immunogenic and cannot induce an antibody response alone.

f. **Antibody** (immunoglobulin [Ig] or gammaglobulin) is a protein that binds to antigens. There are five classes: **IgG, IgM, IgA, IgD**, and **IgE.** Antibodies primarily migrate in the beta and gamma regions during protein electrophoresis.
 1) Antibody monomers are composed of two heavy polypeptide chains and two light polypeptide chains.
  a) **Light chains**
   i) Two types: **kappa** and **lambda**
   ii) An antibody molecule will have only one type of light chain: kappa or lambda.
  b) **Heavy chains:** Immunoglobulin classes are defined by a unique heavy chain: IgM—mu (μ), IgG—gamma (γ), IgA—alpha (α), IgD—delta (Δ), IgE—epsilon (ε)
 2) Every heavy chain and light chain consists of one **variable domain** and one or more **constant domain.**
 3) The variable domain defines the **specificity** of an antibody. This portion of the molecule is referred to as the **fragment of antigen binding (Fab).**
 4) The **crystalline fragment (Fc)** of the antibody is located at the carboxy-terminus. It is responsible for the biologic activity of the molecule, including activating complement.
 5) Antibody heterogeneity
  a) **Isotypes**
   i) Variations between light and heavy chains
   ii) Defined by constant regions of all antibodies and kappa and lambda light chains
  b) **Allotypes**
   i) Species specific variations in the constant domains of heavy or light chains
   ii) Different alleles of heavy and light chains
  c) **Idiotypes**
   i) Variation in the variable region
   ii) A single clone of cells produces a single idiotype.
 6) **J (joining) chain:** Multiple monomers of IgM and IgA are linked by a J chain. One J chain is needed for each IgM or IgA molecule that is linked together.
 7) **Antibody classes**
  a) **IgG**
   i) **Predominant serum antibody,** approximately 75% of immunoglobulins in the blood
   ii) **Subclasses** include IgG1, IgG2, IgG3, and IgG4.
   iii) **Only immunoglobulin that crosses the placenta**
   iv) Produced in **secondary (anamnestic)** antibody response
   v) IgG1, IgG2, and IgG3 activate the classical complement pathway.

b) **IgM**
   i) **Five monomers** linked together by a J chain and interchain disulfide bonds
   ii) 10% of total serum immunoglobulins
   iii) **First antibody produced against an immunogen**
   iv) Produced in primary and, to a much lesser degree, secondary immune responses
   v) It is the **best activator of the classical pathway of complement**—only one molecule of IgM is required.
c) **IgA**
   i) **Serum and secretory forms:** Serum IgA is a single immunoglobulin molecule, whereas secretory IgA is a dimer held together by a J chain.
   ii) Two **subclasses:** IgA1 and IgA2
   iii) Accounts for 15–20% of total serum antibody
   iv) The functions of serum IgA are antigen clearance and immune regulation.
   v) The function of secretory IgA in mucous membranes is to block attachment of viruses, bacteria, and toxins to host cells.
d) **IgD**
   i) Primarily a cell membrane surface component of B lymphocytes acting as a receptor
   ii) Short half-life (2–3 days)
e) **IgE**
   i) **Responsible for allergic (type I hypersensitivity) reactions**
   ii) **The Fc portion of the antibody binds to receptors on mast cells and basophils.** Once attached to these cells, IgE binding an allergen triggers degranulation of the cell and release of allergic mediators such as histamine and leukotrienes.
   iii) Elevated IgE concentrations are often found during parasitic infections.

8) **Monoclonal antibodies**
   a) **Definition:** Identical antibodies that are produced from a single clone of plasma cells
   b) Found in individuals with the disease multiple myeloma
   c) Monoclonal antibodies are also produced by fusing an antigen-sensitized, splenic B lymphocyte with nonsecreting **myeloma cell**, thus creating an immortal cell line that secretes an antibody of a single idiotype.
9) Quantification of antibodies
   a) The purpose is to provide information about the functional immune status of an individual.
   b) IgG, IgM, and IgA are quantified using nephelometry, turbidimetry, and, less frequently, radial immunodiffusion.

II. THE IMMUNE SYSTEM

A. Myeloid Cells

1. Part of the nonspecific immune response
2. **Monocytes** and **macrophages**
   a. In the peripheral blood, this cell is a monocyte; in the tissue, it is a macrophage. Monocytes constitute 2–8% of the peripheral WBCs. Tissue macrophages include alveolar macrophage, Küppfer cells (liver), and astrocytes and microglia cells (nervous system).
   b. Functions
      1) **Phagocytosis of invaders**
      2) **Present immunogens to T-helper cells**, the first step in an adaptive immune response
      3) Release cytokines (monokines) that affect other cells' activities
   c. Macrophages have major histocompatibility complex (MHC) class II, complement, and antibody Fc receptors on their surface.
3. **Granulocytes**, also part of the nonspecific immune response
   a. **Neutrophils** (polymorphonuclear cells or PMNs)
      1) 40–60% of WBCs in circulation
      2) Function: Phagocytosis and contributes to inflammatory response
   b. **Eosinophils**
      1) 1–3% of circulating WBCs
      2) Mediate IgE allergic response
   c. **Basophils**
      1) 0–1.0% of circulating WBCs
      2) Has receptors for IgE and granules responsible for allergic reactions
4. **Lymphocytes**
   a. 20–40% of circulating WBCs
   b. **B lymphocytes (or B cells)**
      1) 20% of circulating lymphocytes
      2) Express surface molecules such as CD (cluster of differentiation) 19 and CD20.
      3) After birth, B cells mature in the bone marrow.
      4) B cells differentiate into either a plasma cell, whose role is to produce antibody, or a memory B cell.
   c. **T lymphocytes (or T cells)**
      1) 80% of circulating lymphocytes
      2) Express surface molecules such as CD2 and CD3
      3) **Functions**
         a. CTLs lyse host cells infected with viruses and tumor cells and also produce lymphokines.
         b. T cells stimulate (T-helper cells) or suppress (T-regulatory cells) other cells.

4) **T cell maturation**
   a. Pre–T cells begin in the bone marrow and fetal liver.
   b. T cells go to the thymus to mature.
5) **NK** cells are slightly larger than T or B cells and have cytoplasmic granules and are part of the innate immune response.

5. Other cells that assist in the immune response
   a. **Dendritic cells** present antigen to T cells.
   b. **Langerhans cells:** Dendritic cell found in the dermis and squamous epithelia
   c. **Mast cell:** Granulocyte resembling basophil that contains many chemicals that affect the immune response
   d. **Regulatory T (T-reg) cells:** These cells limit immune response preventing autoimmune disease and chronic inflammation

B. Cytokines

1. Soluble, small molecular weight proteins secreted by one cell type that affect (immunomodulate) other cells, for example, turn on genes in target cells (Table 4-1■)
2. **Interferons**
   a. Interferon-alpha (INF-α) and INF-β, examples of type I interferons, are antiviral proteins that inhibit viral replication and activate NK cells. They are produced by viral-infected cells.
   b. INF-γ, a type II interferon, has antiviral effects, activates macrophages and NK cells, and stimulates B cells to produce antibodies. It is produced by T-helper cells, type I.

TABLE 4-1 IMPORTANT CYTOKINES

Cytokine	Cellular Source	Primary Target
IL-1	Macrophages, B cells, fibroblasts, etc.	T cells, B cells, macrophages, endothelium, tissue cells
IL-2	T cells	T cells
IL-3	T cells	Stem cells
IL-4	T cells	B cells, T cells
IL-5	T cells	B cells
IL-6	T cells, B cells, fibroblasts, macrophages	B cells, hepatocytes
IL-7	Bone marrow, stromal cells	Pre–B cells, T cells
IL-8	Monocytes	Fibroblasts
IL-9	T cells	T cells, mast cells
IL-10	T cells	TH 1 cells
TNF	Macrophages, mast cells, lymphocytes	Macrophages, granulocytes, tissue cells
IFN-α	Leukocytes, epithelia, fibroblasts	Tissue cells
IFN-β	Fibroblasts, epithelia	Tissue cells, leukocytes
IFN-γ	T cells, NK cells, epithelia, fibroblasts	Leukocytes, tissue cells, TH 2 cells

3. **Tissue necrosis factors**
   a. Tumor necrosis factor-alpha (TNFα): Produced by macrophages, lymphocytes, and NK cells when encountering bacteria, viruses, tumor cells, toxins, and complement protein C5a
   b. TNFβ: Produced by CD4- and CD8-positive cells after exposure to a specific antigen
4. **Interleukins**
   a. **Interleukin 1** (IL-1) is produced by macrophages, B cells, and other cell types. IL-1 activates T-helper cells, increases the number of B cells, activates vascular endothelium, causes fever and acute-phase protein synthesis, and induces T cells to produce lymphokines.
   b. **IL-2** is produced by T-helper cells. IL-2 causes proliferation of activated T and B cells.
   c. **IL-3** is produced by activated T cells. IL-3 increases the number of mast cells in skin, spleen, and liver.
   d. **IL-4** is produced by activated T cells. IL-4 induces proliferation of T cells and class switching from IgM to IgG1 and IgE.
   e. Several other interleukins are known (Table 4-1).

C. Organs and Tissues of the Immune Cells

1. Primary lymph tissues of adults
   a. **Bone marrow:** Site where pre–B lymphocytes develop into mature B cells.
   b. **Thymus:** Site where pre–T lymphocytes develop into mature T cells.
2. Secondary lymphoid organs
   a. **Lymph nodes:** B cells migrate to the cortex and T cells to the paracortex.
      1) **Primary follicle:** Many small B cells
      2) **Secondary follicle:** After stimulation, primary follicle becomes a secondary follicle. The germinal center has small and large lymphocytes, blast cells, macrophages, and dendritic cells. The medulla contains plasma cells and large lymphocytes.
   b. **Spleen**
      1) Purpose: Filter blood
      2) Contains both T and B cells
   c. **Mucosal-associated lymphoid tissue** (MALT)
      1) Found in submucosa in gastrointestinal tract, respiratory tract, and urogenital tract
      2) These surfaces interact with the environment and can begin the immune response early.
      3) **Peyer's patch:** Specialized MALT found in the lower ileum

III. MAJOR HISTOCOMPATIBILITY COMPLEX

A. Human Leukocyte Antigens

1. Human leukocyte antigens (HLAs) are **cell surface markers** that allow immune cells to distinguish "self" from "nonself."
2. These antigens were first described on white blood cells (leukocytes) and are coded for by genes in the **MHC** located on chromosome six. A number of different alleles exist at each locus.

B. Three Classes of MHC Products

1. **Class I loci:** HLA-A, HLA-B, HLA-C, HLA-E, HLA-F, HLA-G, and HLA-J
   a. Molecules found on nearly every nucleated cell surface
   b. They present endogenous antigens, for example, from a virus infection.
   c. Antigen-presenting cells with MHC I molecules present antigens to CTLs.
2. **Class II:** Thirteen loci, including HLA-DM, HLA-DO, HLA-DP, HLA-DQ, and HLA-DR
   a. Molecules located on the surface of monocytes, macrophages, B cells, activated T cells, dendritic cells, Langerhans cells, and some epithelial cells
   b. Antigen-presenting cells with MHC II molecules present exogenous antigens to T-helper cells.
3. **Class III** products: Complement proteins, TNFα and β, and other proteins (e.g., heat shock protein) not associated with cell membrane surfaces

C. Nomenclature

1. HLA antigens are named according to the product expressed by the gene locus (capital letter) and the allele (number).
2. For example, HLA-A2; A is the locus and 2 is the allele.

D. Inheritance of HLA

1. **Haplotype:** Combination of inherited HLA alleles
2. Two haplotypes (one from each parent) are a genotype.
3. Because of the large number of alleles in the MHC, a person's HLA type is almost as unique as a fingerprint.

E. Clinical Significance

1. **Transplantation:** Transplants last longer if the HLA antigens from the recipient and the donor are closely matched.
2. **Platelet transfusion:** Although response to platelet transfusion is multifactorial, antibodies to class I HLA antigens are the primary cause of immune-mediated platelet transfusion refractoriness.
3. **Paternity testing:** HLA loci are polymorphic and recombination is rare. HLA inheritance patterns can exclude fathers with approximately 99% accuracy. However, because testing cannot include a father, DNA profiling is generally used in paternity cases.

4. **Diseases:** Not all individuals who have a particular HLA antigen have a disease, but many individuals with certain diseases express a particular HLA antigen. For example, HLA B-27 is associated with increased risk of ankylosing spondylitis.

IV. NONSPECIFIC IMMUNE RESPONSE

A. Nonspecific Immune Response: Cellular Mechanisms

1. Barrier, first line of defense: Skin and mucous membranes
2. **Polymorphonuclear neutrophils**
   a. Involved in nonspecific response by attachment to damaged epithelium, migration into tissues, chemotaxis, phagocytosis and digestion of target cells, increased metabolism, and degranulation
   b. Polymorphonuclear neutrophil defects
      1) **Chronic granulomatous disease:** Defect in oxidative pathway (respiratory pathway) phagocytes use to create hydrogen peroxide, which is used to kill bacteria
      2) **Myeloperoxidase deficiency:** Impaired production of toxic oxygen molecules (decrease respiratory burst) used by phagocytes to kill ingested bacteria
3. **Eosinophils**
   a. Granules contain acid phosphatase, peroxidase, histamines, and several other molecules.
   b. **Hypothesized functions**
      1) Clearing immune complexes
      2) Immunomodulation of innate and adaptive immunity
      3) Inflammatory disease such as asthma
      4) Protein in granules toxic to parasites
4. **Mediator cells**
   a. Mast cells, basophils, eosinophils, and platelets release substances that mediate immune reactions.
   b. The chemical mediators produce vascular dilation, increased vascular permeability, smooth muscle contraction, chemotaxins for phagocytes, and increased inflammatory response.
   c. **Mast cells** and **basophils** can degranulate when membrane-bound IgE binds an allergen or by nonimmunologic mechanisms such as surgical incisions, heat, and skin or mucous membrane infections.
   d. **Basophil function** is to amplify the reactions that start with the mast cell at the site of entry of the antigen. Their granules contain mediators (e.g., histamine and heparin) that play a role in anaphylactic reactions.
5. The mononuclear phagocyte system includes alveolar macrophages, splenic macrophages, Kupffer cells of the liver, etc.

B. Inflammation

1. Sequenced events following tissue damage that protect the host from foreign invaders and attempt to minimize tissue damage
2. **Increased vascular permeability**
   a. Upon injury, capillaries, arterioles, and venules dilate to **increase blood flow** to the site of the injury.
   b. Because of increased vascular permeability, fluid moves from circulation to the space around the injury, bringing fibrinogen and PMNs to the injury site.
3. **Migration of neutrophils**
   a. After the injury, **chemotaxins** and **endothelial activating factors** are released.
   b. PMNs adhere to activated **endothelial cells.**
   c. PMNs move between the endothelial cells to the site of tissue damage by a process called **diapedesis.**
   d. Chemicals are released and more PMNs are released from the storage pool, and the injury site is flooded with PMNs.
4. **Migration of mononuclear cells**
   a. Macrophages release IL-1, which attracts monocytes, macrophages, and lymphocytes to the injury site.
   b. About 4 hours after the injury, mononuclear cells migrate to the site of damage.
5. Cellular proliferation and repair: Fibroblasts help repair the damage and return the injury site to normal.

C. Chemical Mechanisms of the Nonspecific Immune Response

1. **Complement system:** Collection of serum proteins involved in lysis of cell membranes, mediation of inflammation, virus neutralization, enhancement of phagocytosis, and metabolism of immune complexes
   a. **Components are synthesized in the liver**, except C1, which is synthesized in the epithelial cells of the intestine.
   b. **Approximately 20 proteins are involved in three separate pathways of activation.** Many of the proteins have enzymatic activity splitting a substrate into two parts: a and b.
   c. Five proteins unique to the classical pathway: C1q, C1r, C1s, C4, and C2
   d. Three proteins unique to the alternative pathway: factor B, factor D, and properidin
   e. Six proteins common to both pathways: C3, C5, C6, C7, C8, and C9
   f. Activation of complement
      1) **Classical pathway:** Immune (antibody-antigen) complexes, require one IgM or two IgG molecules
      2) **Alternative pathway:** Antibody-independent, microbial components such as lipopolysaccharide, polysaccharide, teichoic acid, and peptidoglycan
      3) **Lectin pathway:** Binding of mannose-binding lectin to mannose residues on glycoproteins or carbohydrates on the surface of microorganisms

g. Outcome of complement activation
   1) **Anaphylatoxins:** C4a, C3a, and C5a cause basophils and mast cells to release histamine and also cause smooth muscle contraction and increased vascular permeability.
   2) **Immune adherence:** C3b adheres to immune complexes and surfaces of substances to facilitate clearing of these molecules.
   3) **Opsonization:** If C3b is attached to a cell, phagocytosis is enhanced.
   4) **Chemotaxis:** C5a is an anaphylatoxin and induces the migration of neutrophils and monocytes to the site.
   5) Cell lysis and virolysis of enveloped viruses through the formation of the **membrane attack complex** (MAC), components C5 through C9

h. **Control mechanisms**
   1) **C1 inhibitor** (C1INH) combines with C1r and C1s to block C1 activities. A deficiency in C1INH results in the syndrome **hereditary angioedema**, an autosomal dominant disease. The disease is characterized by unregulated classical pathway activation, resulting in vascular permeability and swollen mucous membranes in airways, which can become blocked.
   2) **Anaphylatoxin inactivator:** This compound removes a single amino acid from C4a, C3a, and C5a, rendering them useless as anaphylatoxins.
   3) **MAC inhibitors:** MAC is not formed because S protein binds to C5b-7 complex.
   4) **Complement receptor type I (CRI or CD35):** CRI binds C3b and C4b and inhibits the amplification loop.

i. **Complement deficiencies**
   1) Individuals can have **altered genes**, resulting in complement protein deficiencies (Table 4-2■).
   2) **Complement can be consumed** in infections and collagen vascular diseases.
   3) **C3 and C4 are measured to indicate consumption and follow disease states.**
   4) Total functional complement assay **(i..e., complement 50% hemolytic activitiy [CH50])** is used to measure the activity of the classical pathway.

TABLE 4-2 SELECTED COMPLEMENT DEFICIENCIES

Complement Deficiency	Significance
C3	Increased risk for overwhelming infections
C4 and C3	Indicate consumption with classical pathway activation
C1 (q, r, s), C4, and C2	Indicate collagen disease
C5, C6, and C7	Increased risk for *Neisseria meningitidis* infection

2. **Acute-phase reactants:** When injured, the body produces acute-phase reactants (proteins). They are nonspecific indicators of inflammation.
   a. **C-reactive protein (CRP)** concentration increases several hundred times after injury. CRP can activate the classical pathway of complement and can also bind to NK cells and monocytes, stimulating them to target tumor cells. CRP levels may also be increased during coronary heart disease.
   b. **Haptoglobin** removes free hemoglobin from circulation.
   c. **Fibrinogen** is found in increased quantities at the site of an injury; it is converted to fibrin to heal the injury.
   d. **α_1-Antitrypsin** is a family of serine protease inhibitors synthesized in the liver. Deficiency causes premature loss of elasticity in the lung and liver damage.
   e. **Ceruloplasmin** is the principal copper-transportation protein. It is vital in aerobic energy production, collagen formation, and protection against superoxide ions. Deficiency is called Wilson disease.
   f. **α_2-Macroglobulin** is a protease inhibitor. α_2-Macroglobulin and protease complexes are phagocytized by macrophages and fibroblasts.
   g. **Procalcitonin** is produced by many cell types and blood levels increase during inflammation and in particular bacterial sepsis.

V. ADAPTIVE IMMUNE RESPONSE

A. Antigen Recognition

1. **Antigen-presenting cells**
   a. **Monocytes/macrophages:** Phagocytic cells that process antigen and express it on the cell surface associated with MHC I or II molecules
   b. **Dendritic cells:** Phagocytic cells that process antigen and express it on the cell surface associated with MHC I or II molecules
   c. **B cells:** Nonphagocytic cells that attach to antigens in their native form, process antigens, and express them on their surface associated with MHC II molecules
2. **Antigen receptors**
   a. **B cell**
      1) The B cell antigen receptor is **monomeric IgM or IgD.**
      2) The B cell surface receptors have two identical antigen-binding pockets—the Fab portion of an antibody monomer.
   b. **T cells**
      1) The **T-cell receptor** consists of two nonidentical peptides; in close proximity is the co-receptor CD3.
      2) T cells recognize antigens that were processed by other cells.
      3) T-helper (TH) cells have **CD4** on their surface that interacts with MHC II on the antigen-presenting cell.
      4) **TH cell activation**
         a) Occurs when TH cells recognize an antigen
         b) Requires direct cell contact and cytokines such as IL-1 and IL-2
      5) CTLs have **CD8** on their surface, which interacts with MHC I on the antigen-presenting cell.

B. Cell-Mediated Immunity

1. **Mediated by TH 1 cells**, a subset of T-helper cells, that secrete cytokines that activate other cells involved in the response
2. **Monocytes and macrophages** are inflammatory reaction cells stimulated by cytokines from TH 1 cells.
3. **CTLs** are activated by cytokines from TH 1 cells and then destroy targets by cell-to-cell contact. The main function of CTLs is to destroy virus infected cells.
4. **NK cells**, because they kill target cells without being previously sensitized, are regarded as part of innate immunity, although NK cell activities are governed by cytokines and target cells missing MHC I.
5. **NK T cells** are of lymphoid lineage and share physical and functional characteristics of NK cells and T cells. Following activation, NK T cells produce a number of cytokines including IFN-γ and IL-2.

C. Humoral-Mediated Immunity

1. **B cell activation** begins when antigen binds to antibody on B cell surface and the antigen is internalized and linked to an MHC II molecule on the cell's surface.
2. **T and B cell interactions**
   a. B cell processes and presents the antigen, stimulating the TH 2 cell to produce cytokines.
   b. The **cytokines** stimulate the B cell to divide and differentiate into a memory B cell or a plasma cell that will synthesize antibody.
3. **Antibody diversity:** Antibodies can be produced that recognize an unlimited number of antigens, but there are a limited number of B cells. Antibody diversity is due to recombination events that occur during B cell maturation. **Plasma cells** produce antibodies with the same idiotype of the antibodies that were on the surface of the B cell that the plasma cell was derived from.
4. **Antibody production**
   a. Primary and secondary antibody responses
      1) **Primary antibody response:** Produced when host first encounters an antigen
         a) For about 5–7 days during the latent phase, no antibody is produced. During this time, the host is producing plasma cells that will secrete antibodies.
         b) **IgM** is the first antibody produced.
         c) Antibody production starts slowly, peaks, levels off, then declines.
      2) **Secondary (anamnestic) response:** Produced after the host has previously been exposed to an antigen
         a) Short latent phase (3–5 days)
         b) Higher antibody concentration
         c) IgG produced due to class switching
         d) IgG antibodies persist longer in circulation than IgM.
   b. **Antibody-dependent cell-mediated cytotoxicity (ADCC):** Cytolytic effector cells (e.g., NK cells and PMNs) can lyse antibody-coated target cells if there is direct contact.

VI. AUTOIMMUNE DISEASE

A. Definition

1. An autoimmune disease occurs when an individual produces antibodies or a T cell response to his/her own antigens.
2. There is a loss of self-tolerance.

B. Autoimmune Mechanisms

1. Antibody-cell surface component interaction
2. Formation of autoantigen-autoantibody complexes
3. Sensitization of T cells to self antigens
4. Genetic factors play a role in the development of autoimmune diseases. The presence of certain HLA types has been correlated with specific diseases (Table 4-3■).

C. Autoimmune Theories

1. **Forbidden-clone theory:** Burnet postulated that when an error in self-recognition occurs during fetal life and lymphocytes against an autoantigen are not destroyed, then autoantibodies are produced.
2. **Clonal anergy:** Clones developed during fetal life are not stimulated by low doses of antigens. The ability to produce antibodies against higher doses of antigens is still present.
3. **Sequestered-antigen theory:** Some antigens are hidden from the immune system during fetal development. When the tissue is damaged, the "hidden cells" are exposed to the immune system and antibodies are produced against these cells.
4. **Immunologic deficiency theory:** T-reg cells suppress antibody production by B cells. If T-reg cells exhibit decreased activity, then antibodies against autoantigens are produced.
5. **Molecular mimicry:** An individual can make antibodies or reactive T cells to an infectious agent that cross-react with self antigens.
6. **Polyclonal B cell activation:** A number of bacteria and viruses are known to nonspecifically stimulate B cells. If these B cells have activity against self antigens, an autoimmune disease can result.

TABLE 4-3 HLA TYPE AND ASSOCIATED DISEASES

HLA Type	Associated Diseases
HLA-B8	Graves disease and type 1 diabetes
HLA-B27	Ankylosing spondylitis
HLA-DR2	systemic lupus erythematosus (SLE), multiple sclerosis, Hashimoto disease, and myasthenia gravis
HLA-DR3	Sjögren syndrome, myasthenia gravis, SLE, Graves disease, and type 1 diabetes
HLA-DR4	Rheumatoid arthritis, type 1 diabetes, and pemphigus vulgaris

D. Diagnostic Tests for Non-Organ-Specific Autoimmune Diseases

1. **Antinuclear antibodies (ANAs)**
   a. Associated with **systemic lupus erythematosus** (SLE), mixed connective tissue disease, and rheumatoid arthritis (RA)
   b. Techniques used to detect ANA: Agglutination, indirect immunofluorescence, and enzyme immunoassay (EIA)
   c. Interpretation of indirect immunofluorescence results
      1) **Diffuse or homogeneous:** Evenly stains the nuclei and is associated with anti-DNA antibody and histones
      2) **Peripheral:** Stains the edge of the nuclei and is associated with anti-DNA antibody and anti-lamins (proteins found in the nuclear membrane) antibody
      3) **Speckled:** Numerous evenly distributed stained speckles within the nuclei associated with antibodies to extractable nuclear antigens—nuclear ribonucleoprotein (RNP) and anti-Smith (Sm)
      4) **Nucleolar:** Stains two or three large fluorescent areas within the nucleus and is associated with anti-RNP antibody
      5) **Centromere:** Stains as a discrete speckled pattern due to anti-centromere antibody
   d. **Autoantibodies and disease associations** (Table 4-4■)
2. **Rheumatoid factor**
   a. Rheumatoid factor (RF) is an anti-antibody, **typically IgM,** that binds to the Fc portion of abnormal IgG.
   b. RF is usually detected by **latex agglutination.** Patient serum is mixed with IgG-coated latex particles. Agglutination indicates the presence of RF.
   c. **Approximately 75% of patients with RA are positive for RF.** However, patients with chronic infections may also have RF.
   d. Also noted in chronic hepatitis, SLE, and syphilis

TABLE 4-4 AUTOANTIBODIES AND ASSOCIATED DISEASES

Autoantibody	Disease Associations
Centromere	CREST (calcinosis, Raynaud syndrome, esophageal hypomotility sclerodactyly, and telangectasia) syndrome
dsDNA	Found in SLE and low titers found in RA and Sjögren syndrome
Histone	Drug-induced SLE
Nuclear RNP	SLE and mixed connective tissue disease
Scl-70	Scleroderma (systemic sclerosis)
Sjögren syndrome A (SSA [Ro])	Sjögren syndrome and SLE
Sjögren syndrome B (SSB [LA])	Sjögren syndrome and SLE
Sm	Diagnostic for SLE (high specificity) if present but low sensitivity

3. **Cryoglobulins**
   a. Proteins that reversibly precipitate at 4°C
   b. Associated with autoimmune diseases such as vasculitis, glomerulonephritis, SLE, RA, and Sjögren syndrome

E. Non-Organ-Specific Autoimmune Diseases

1. **Systemic lupus erythematosus**
   a. Chronic, noninfectious inflammatory disease involving many organs
   b. Disease is **more likely to occur in women than men** and in African Americans than Caucasian Americans.
   c. **Tissue injury is caused by autoantibodies and immune complexes deposited in the tissues.** Depressed T-reg cell function allows production of antibodies against "self" antigens.
   d. **Severity of the disease varies.** Symptoms include fever, weight loss, malaise, weakness, arthritis, skin lesions, photosensitivity, butterfly rash (rash across the cheeks and bridge of the nose), renal disease, pericarditis, seizures, ocular changes, pancreatitis, and small-vessel vasculitis.
   e. **Laboratory findings** include the presence of several autoantibodies. ANA is generally positive but is not specific for SLE and serves as a screening test. However, a homogenous staining pattern is indicative of SLE. Autoantibodies with greater specificity but lower sensitivity are anti-dsDNA and anti-Sm.
2. **Rheumatoid arthritis**
   a. Chronic, noninfectious, systemic inflammatory disease that primarily involves the joints affecting over 2 million Americans
   b. Women are affected two to three times more often than men.
   c. The disease is **due to production of IgG or IgM antibodies** against IgG in the synovium. Immune complexes are deposited in the joints and occasionally other sites, which activate complement. The inflammatory response proceeds and damages the synovium. Immune complexes attract neutrophils and macrophages to the joint that degranulate and contribute to tissue destruction.
   d. **Symptoms** are highly variable and include fatigue, weight loss, weakness, mild fever, anorexia, morning stiffness, joint pain (that improves during the day), vasculitis, and rheumatoid nodules. Symptoms can resemble SLE.
   e. **Laboratory findings** include elevated erythrocytic sedimentation rate, elevated CRP, positive RF, cryoglobulins, and sometimes ANAs. Synovial fluid is cloudy, with a WBC count between 5,000 and 20,000/μL, elevated protein, poor mucin clot development, decreased complement, and positive RF.
3. **Sjögren syndrome**
   a. An inflammation of the salivary and lacrimal glands causing dryness of the mouth and eyes
   b. **Laboratory findings** include polyclonal hypergammaglobulinemia; autoantibodies against the salivary glands; and positive RF, ANA (speckled or diffuse pattern), anti-SSA, and anti-SSB.

4. **Autoimmune hemolytic anemia**
    a. Increased rate of red blood cell (RBC) destruction
    b. Results in a normocytic, normochromic anemia
    c. Autoantibody is directed against RBC antigens.
    d. **Laboratory findings** include positive direct antiglobulin test and sometimes cold agglutinins.

F. Organ-Specific Autoimmune Disease

1. Organ-specific autoimmune disease: Immunologic reactions take place in only one organ.
2. Autoimmune thyroiditis
    a. **Hashimoto disease**
        1) Humoral and cellular immunity are activated and destruction of normal thyroid tissue leads to hypothyroidism, loss of thyroid function, and low levels of thyroid hormones in the blood. The majority of the damage is due to cellular immunity.
        2) **Antithyroid antibodies** detected include antithyroglobulin and antithyroid peroxidase (anti-TPO). Anti-TPO antibodies likely do not contribute to thyroid damage. The anti-TPO antibody assay is regarded as superior to the antithyroglobulin antibody test for diagnosis.
    b. **Graves disease**
        1) The disease is characterized by hyperplasia and diffuses goiter caused by an autoantibody reacting with thyroid receptor on cells that overstimulates the thyroid gland. The autoantibody mimics the activity of thyroid-stimulating hormone (TSH). Approximately 75% of patients with Graves disease also have elevated anti-TPO antibodies.
        2) **Thyrotoxicosis results from overstimulation;** both free and total T_3 and T_4 are elevated, and TSH is decreased.
        3) Common findings: Exophthalmos (bulging eyes) and infiltrative dermopathy
3. **Myasthenia gravis**
    a. Neuromuscular disease in which the nerve synapses in muscles do not function normally
    b. Most patients exhibit **antibodies to acetylcholine receptors.** These autoantibodies block nerve impulses and can initiate damage to neurons.
    c. **Laboratory findings** include anti-acetylcholine receptor antibody, which has a specificity of nearly 100%.
4. **Multiple sclerosis (MS)**
    a. Considered a chronic progressive inflammatory disease with demyelinization of the nerves
    b. Studies suggest that certain viruses, in particular Epstein-Barr virus and human herpes virus 6, are associated with MS.
    c. Active lesions **(plaques)** contain CTLs, TH cells, and macrophages.

d. Most patients with MS have **increased IgG concentrations in the cerebrospinal fluid** (CSF).
e. The IgG index differentiates true increases due to production rather than increases in permeability of the blood-brain barrier.

$$\text{IgG index} = \frac{\text{IgG}_{\text{CSF}}/\text{albumin}_{\text{CSF}}}{\text{IgG}_{\text{serum}}/\text{albumin}_{\text{serum}}}$$

f. Reference range for IgG index is 0.0–0.77.
g. **Oligoclonal bands in CSF** on high-resolution electrophoresis are also indicative of MS, but patients with other conditions (SLE, viral meningitis, neurosyphilis, etc.) can have oligoclonal bands in the CSF.

5. **Type 1 diabetes**
   a. **Islet cell destruction in the pancreas** results in insulin-dependent or type 1 diabetes mellitus.
   b. **Autoantibodies and CTLs** reactive against pancreatic beta cells produce marked atrophy and fibrosis of the islet cells. This, in turn, causes insulin deficiency.
   c. Viruses can trigger autoantibody production by **molecular mimicry.** After outbreaks of mumps, measles, rubella, Coxsackie B virus, and infectious mononucleosis, new cases of type 1 diabetes appear in communities.
   d. HLA-DQ1.2 and HLA-DR2 decrease the risk of developing diabetes.
6. **Celiac disease**
   a. Autoimmune disease due to a hypersensitivity reaction to the cereal protein **gluten**
   b. Immune-dominant gluten peptides are modified by the enzyme transglutaminase 2 (TG2), leading to their binding to HLA-DQ2 or HLA-DQ8 molecules.
   c. CD4+ T cells recognize gluten peptides bound to HLA-DQ2.5 or HLA-DQ8 on the surface of antigen presenting cells, for example, dendritic cells and B cells. These T cells proliferate and produce cytokines such as IFN-γ, IL-2, and IL-21 triggering inflammation.
   d. **Mast cells** respond to nonimmunodominant gliadin fragments by releasing proinflammatory mediators.
   e. In addition, most patients produce antibodies directed against gluten peptides and TG2.
   f. The presence of TG2-specific antibodies in serum is the most specific and sensitive diagnostic marker of active celiac disease.

VII. HYPERSENSITIVITY

A. Definitions

1. **Hypersensitivity reaction:** Overreactive immune response to innocuous substances on reexposure that can result in tissue damage

2. Involve humoral- and cell-mediated responses
   a. Types I through III are humoral mediated and immediate.
   b. Type IV is cell mediated and delayed.
3. **Allergen:** Molecule that triggers a hypersensitivity reaction

B. Type I Hypersensitivity Reaction

1. Type I hypersensitivity (anaphylactic) reaction is classified as an **immediate hypersensitivity reaction** because it occurs within minutes after reexposure to an allergen. After the first (primary) exposure, basophils and **mast cells are sensitized with IgE.** Upon second exposure, IgE binds to a specific allergen and chemical mediators are released from those cells (degranulation), which causes allergic symptoms.
2. **Allergens and disease**
   a. The **magnitude of the allergic response** depends upon where the allergen enters the body. Individuals who exhibit symptoms are genetically predisposed to produce increased amounts of IgE to that allergin.
   b. Individuals can be **exposed to allergens** through the upper respiratory tract, absorption from the intestinal tract, and direct skin contact.
   c. **Allergic reactions occur in tissues with many mast cells:** Skin, nasal membranes, tongue, lungs, and gastrointestinal tract.
   d. Allergens contacting the nasal mucosa cause runny nose, itching eyes and nose, sneezing, and nasal congestion. Eosinophil levels in the blood stream and nasal secretions may be elevated, and IgE may be normal or elevated.
   e. **Allergens contacting the bronchus cause asthma.** Serum IgE levels are usually increased.
   f. Although food allergies are common, they are the least common form of type I hypersensitivity reactions. Symptoms include nausea, vomiting, cramps, abdominal pain, and diarrhea within 2 hours of ingesting the allergen.
   g. **Anaphylaxis** is the systemic form of type I hypersensitivity. It can be life threatening, causing shock or edema of the upper respiratory tract. Substances that can trigger this condition include peanuts; seafood; egg albumin; honeybee, wasp, or hornet stings; vaccines; penicillins; or sulfonamides.
3. **Mediators of symptoms**
   a. **Histamine**
      1) Causes contraction of bronchioles and smooth muscle of blood vessels
      2) Increases capillary permeability
      3) Increases mucus secretion in the airway
   b. **Prostaglandins** cause vasodilation and increased vascular permeability.
   c. **Leukotrienes** cause erythema and wheal formation, a red, elevated area on the skin. Leukotrienes have 30–1,000 times the ability of histamine to cause bronchospasms and also stimulate mucus secretion in the airways.

4. **Laboratory evaluation of allergies**
   a. **Total serum IgE levels**
      1) Historically, the radioimmunosorbent test was used to measure total IgE. Currently, solid-phase immunoassays are more common.
      2) These assays only detect circulating Ig. However, during allergic reactions, the majority is bound to mast cells and basophils.
   b. **Allergen-specific IgE:**
      1) Historically, the radioallergosorbent test was used to detect IgE against specific allergens.
      2) Today, immunoblot assays are used. Common allergens are separated electrophoretically and transferred to nitrocellulose. Patient serum is added to the strips, followed by a wash step and the addition of enzyme-labeled anti-human IgE.
5. **Treatment**
   a. Allergen avoidance and drug therapy
   b. Patients can undergo **immunotherapy (hyposensitization)**, commonly referred to as "allergy shots." Individuals receive injections of gradually increasing concentrations of the allergen to which they are allergic. Eventually, a state of **tolerance** to the allergen may develop.

C. Type II Hypersensitivity

1. Type II hypersensitivity (cytotoxic) reaction is due to **IgG or IgM antibodies directed against cell surface antigens.** It is also an example of an immediate hypersensitivity reaction.
2. Antibody-mediated tissue damage: PMNs bind to **antibody-sensitized cells** and destroy the cells by phagocytosis or ADCC reaction.
3. **Complement-mediated cell lysis:** Antibody-antigen complex on cell surface activates the classical complement pathway to cause cell lysis.
4. **Incompatible blood transfusion** is an example of this type of hypersensitivity reaction.
5. Damage to sensitized tissue cells causes inflammation, which, in turn, causes damage to normal tissue cells.

D. Type III Hypersensitivity

1. In type III hypersensitivity (immune complex) reactions, **immune complexes** are deposited on tissues, causing inflammation. This is another example of an immediate hypersensitivity reaction.
2. **Circulating immune complexes:** Large immune complexes are rapidly cleared by mononuclear phagocytes, but smaller immune complexes stay in circulation longer and can be deposited on tissue cells. The immune complexes can activate complement, which can lyse nearby (innocent bystander) cells. The immune complexes can also stimulate **degranulation of granulocytes**, which triggers inflammation and tissue damage.

3. The **heart valves and renal glomeruli** are two sites where immune complexes are often deposited.
4. **Examples**
    a. **Arthus reaction:** An allergen is injected intradermally.
    b. **Immune complex disorders (serum sickness):** Patients develop antibodies against heterologous serum proteins.
    c. **Glomerulonephritis:** Immune complexes are deposited on renal glomeruli, causing inflammation of the kidney and possibly renal failure.
    d. **Vasculitis:** Inflammation of the blood vessel walls

E. Type IV Hypersensitivity

1. Type IV hypersensitivity (cell-mediated) reactions are caused by soluble factors or lymphokines released by T cells; antibody and complement are not involved in this reaction. Recruitment and activation of the cells takes 24–72 hours; therefore, this reaction is also referred to as **delayed hypersensitivity.**
2. **Mechanism**
    a. **Lymphokines** are produced by activated T cells.
    b. These chemicals attract macrophages that become activated, causing them to degranulate.
    c. As more macrophages arrive at the site, ulceration and necrosis occur.
3. **Examples**
    a. **Tuberculin-type hypersensitivity:** Subcutaneous injection of tuberculosis antigen is used as a diagnostic skin test. Swelling occurring at the site within 24–72 hours indicates previous infection.
    b. **Contact sensitivity (dermatitis):** Allergens from poison ivy and poison oak cause sensitization, resulting in edema in the skin with the formation of microvesicles and itching on subsequent exposure. Most allergens causing delayed-type hypersensitivity reactions are haptens. For example, they must combine with fatty acids on the skin to be immunogenic.

VIII. IMMUNE DEFICIENCY

A. Primary Immune Deficiencies

1. Humoral immune deficiencies
    a. **Bruton X-linked agammaglobulinemia**
        1) A marked deficiency of all classes of immunoglobulins is detected after about 6 months of age.
        2) **Recurrent, life-threatening infections** occur with encapsulated bacteria, such as *Streptococcus pneumoniae* and *Haemophilus influenzae*, manifested as pneumonia, sinusitis, bronchitis, otitis, furunculosis, meningitis, and septicemia.
        3) A defect in a tyrosine kinase gene for a protein involved in signaling prevents pre–B cells from maturing. B cells are markedly decreased in number or absent.

b. **Hyper-IgM syndrome**
   1) X-linked genetic disease
   2) **Serum IgM is increased;** IgG and IgA are markedly decreased or absent.
   3) A defect in CD40 ligand on T-helper cells prevents class switching from IgM to IgG, IgA, or IgE.
   4) Affected individuals are prone to respiratory tract infections.
   5) Affected individuals often have autoantibodies to platelets, RBCs, and neutrophils.

c. **Selective IgA deficiency**
   1) This is the most common immunodeficiency disorder. Patients present with small amounts or absence of serum and secretory IgA. Because IgA is found in high concentration on mucous membranes, such as along the respiratory tract, these patients tend to suffer from multiple respiratory tract infections.
   2) Usually caused by a genetic defect, although the specific defect has not been identified, or by drugs (e.g., phenytoin and penicillin).
   3) Defect seems to be in the failure of B cells bearing IgA to differentiate into plasma cells.
   4) Anaphylaxis may result if IgA is administered to someone with this deficiency (i.e., blood transfusion).

d. **Ataxia-telangiectasia**
   1) Autosomal recessive disorder that presents with ataxia, telangiectasia, recurrent sinopulmonary infections, a high incidence of malignancy, and variable immune defects. Patients typically exhibit an IgA and sometimes IgE deficiency.
   2) It is not primarily an immunodeficiency but a defect in a kinase gene that regulates the cell cycle. B-and T-helper cells are affected.

2. **Cellular immune deficiencies**
   a. Because T cells are involved in both humoral- and cell-mediated responses, individuals with T-helper cell deficiencies can have a severe combined immunodeficiency (SCID), see below.
   b. **Congenital thymic hypoplasia (DiGeorge syndrome)**
      1) Symptoms include hypocalcemic tetany, due to underdevelopment of the thymus, and heart disease.
      2) Immune defect is variable, from slight decrease in T cells to no T cells in the bloodstream.
      3) Patients are very susceptible to opportunistic infections and have a poor prognosis.

3. **Severe combined immune deficiency**
   a. A group of diseases, with different causes, that affect T and B cell function, resulting in a suppression of humoral- and cell-mediated immune responses
   b. Defects in **adenosine deaminase** (ADA) or **purine nucleotide phosphorylase**
      1) Absence of these enzymes causes an accumulation of nucleotide metabolites in all cells, which is particularly toxic to T and B cells.

2) Very low number of T cells is present, and children often have an underdeveloped thymus, lack of tonsils or lymph nodes, hypogammaglobulinemia, and lymphopenia. Approximately 50% of SCID cases are due to ADA deficiency.

c. **Bare lymphocyte syndrome**

1) With an MHC class II deficiency, T-helper cells fail to develop. Patients present with hypogammaglobulinemia and no CMI response.
2) MHC class I deficiency is less severe. There is a loss of CTLs and response to intracellular pathogens.

d. **Wiskott-Aldrich syndrome**

1) Mutation in the gene, located on the X chromosome, that codes for the **Wiskott-Aldrich syndrome protein**, a protein involved with cytoskeletal reorganization necessary for delivering cytokines
2) The defect prevents T-helper cells from delivering lymphokines to B cells, macrophages, and other target cells.
3) Patients demonstrate eczema, thrombocytopenic purpura, and increased risk of infection, particularly encapsulated bacteria. Platelets are small and defective.

4. **Complement deficiencies**

a. Genetic deficiencies have been described for each of the complement proteins.
b. Homozygous deficiencies in any of the early components of the classical complement proteins result in an increase in immune complex diseases. A functioning alternative pathway maintains protection against bacterial infections.
c. Patients with defects in early alternative complement proteins, such as factor D and properdin, are susceptible to infections by *Neisseria meningitidis.*
d. Patients with a C3 defect have the most severe clinical manifestations.

B. Secondary Immune Deficiencies

1. Secondary immune deficiencies are due to an underlying cause.
2. Transient hypogammaglobulinemia of infancy presents as a decline in serum immunoglobulins during the first few months of life. Individuals eventually produce normal amounts of immunoglobulins.
3. **Malignancy**

a. Cancers can exert a suppressive effect on the immune system.
b. Impairment of antibody production is found in lymphomas, chronic lymphocytic leukemia, and multiple myeloma.

4. **Viral disease:** Certain viruses impair the function of the immune system.

a. Human immunodeficiency virus
b. Epstein-Barr virus
c. Cytomegalovirus

5. Nutritional deficiencies and defects: Malnutrition and protein-energy malnutrition syndromes (e.g., marasmus)

IX. HYPERGAMMAGLOBULINEMIA

A. Polyclonal Hypergammaglobulinemia

1. Tremendous amounts of several classes of immunoglobulins to several specific antigens are produced, resulting in a **broad spike in the gamma region on serum protein electrophoresis.**
2. **Infectious diseases:** Chronic antigenic stimulation from infectious organisms can create this condition.
3. **Inflammatory process:** Many acute-phase proteins are produced during inflammation and can cause a broadening of the alpha-2 peak in serum protein electrophoresis.
4. **Liver disease:** Because of a polyclonal increase in the gamma region and an increase in IgA, the depression between the gamma and the beta regions is absent. As a result, the beta and gamma regions form only one peak on serum protein electrophoresis—beta-gamma bridging, consistent with cirrhosis.

B. Monoclonal Hypergammaglobulinemia

1. Monoclonal hypergammaglobulinemia is a malignant transformation of a clone of B cells that produce identical antibodies. This causes a narrow peak on serum protein electrophoresis.
2. **Multiple myeloma**
   a. **Lymphoproliferative disease**, in which plasma cells produce a high concentration of myeloma (M) protein, which can be partial or complete immunoglobulin or light chains. The cause is unknown.
   b. Approximately 50% of patients with multiple myeloma have **Bence Jones protein** (light chain fragment) in their urine.
   c. **Symptoms:** Weakness, anorexia, weight loss, skeletal destruction (fractures), pain, anemia, renal insufficiency, and recurrent bacterial infections
   d. **Laboratory findings:** Monoclonal gammopathy and plasma cell infiltrate in bone marrow; hypercalemia from bone damage
   e. **Monoclonal immunoglobulins** (M proteins)
      1) Diagnostic of multiple myeloma, Waldenström macroglobulinemia, chronic lymphocytic leukemia, or lymphoma
      2) Immunoglobulin type determination is necessary for diagnosis and prognosis.
3. **Waldenström macroglobulinemia**
   a. **Uncontrolled proliferation of a clone of B cells** that synthesize a homogeneous IgM; cause unknown
   b. **Hyperviscosity of plasma** causes congestive heart failure, headache, dizziness, partial or total loss of vision, bleeding, and anemia.
   c. **Symptoms:** Weakness, fatigue, headache, and weight loss
   d. **Laboratory findings:** A spike in the beta or gamma region on serum protein electrophoresis, increased plasma viscosity, and abnormal accumulation of lymphoid cells in the bone marrow and tissues

4. **Primary amyloidosis**
   a. An amyloid protein is a nonstructural protein that becomes insoluble after an alteration in its secondary structure. In **amyloidosis**, these proteins accumulate in organs and tissue.
   b. **Monoclonal plasma cell disorder** in which abnormal immunoglobulin or Bence Jones protein or, less commonly, heavy chain fragment is produced.
   c. Insoluble proteins are deposited in some of the tissues: Skin, liver, nerves, heart, kidney, etc. This results in progressive loss of organ function.
   d. **Laboratory findings:** Frequent abnormalities of serum immunoglobulins and presence of Bence Jones proteins in the urine

X. TRANSPLANT IMMUNOLOGY

A. Types of Grafts

1. **Autograft:** Transfer of tissue from one site to another within an individual
2. **Isograft (syngraft):** Transfer of tissue between genetically identical individuals
3. **Allograft:** Transfer of tissue between two genetically nonidentical individuals of the same species
4. **Xenograft:** Transfer of tissue between two individuals of different species

B. Graft Acceptance and Rejection

1. Graft acceptance occurs when revascularization and healing lead to a repaired site in about 2 weeks.
2. **Two types of graft rejection**
   a. **First-set rejection:** The first time a graft is encountered, the immune system attacks and ultimately destroys (rejects) the nonself tissue. This occurs 10–14 days after transplantation.
   b. **Second-set rejection:** The second time nonself tissue with the same or similar antigens is encountered, it is rejected within 6 days.

C. Clinical Indications of Graft Rejection

1. **Hyperacute rejection** occurs within 24 hours of transplantation.
   a. The rejection is caused by a **preexisting antibody** to antigens on the grafted tissue. The tissue never becomes vascularized.
   b. **ABO blood group antibodies and MHC class I antibodies cause hyperacute rejection.** Donor and recipient must be of the same ABO blood type to avoid rejection. Hyperacute rejection is less commonly seen than acute or chronic.
   c. Crossmatches are performed on tissue transplants. Serum of the recipient is mixed with mononuclear donor cells, and the mixture is monitored for cytotoxicity.
2. **Acute rejection** occurs within weeks of transplantation. Rejection is usually due to a CMI response; histopathology reveals massive infiltration of lymphocytes and macrophages. Antibody to vessel walls activating complement can also trigger acute rejection.

3. **Chronic rejection** occurs months to years after transplantation; mechanisms of rejection include both HMI and CMI. Chronic rejection is characterized by progressive fibrosis and scarring of blood vessels due to proliferation of smooth muscle.

XI. TUMOR IMMUNOLOGY

A. Definitions

1. **Neoplasm:** An abnormal mass of tissue that results from the uncontrolled growth of normal cells even after the growth stimulus is removed
2. **Benign tumor:** Typically a mild and nonprogressive tumor that pushes aside normal tissue, but does not invade it, as the tumor expands
3. **Malignant tumor:** Generally consisting of poorly differentiated cells that grow rapidly and invade surrounding tissue, robbing the normal tissue of nutrients
4. **Metastatic tumor:** Secondary tumor derived from a malignant primary tumor

B. Tumor-Associated Antigens

1. **Tumor-specific peptides** are intracellular proteins expressed on the surface of a tumor due to interaction with MHC class I and class II molecules. This expression can be chemically induced.
2. **Virus-induced tumors:** Tumors caused by viruses usually have viral antigens on their surface. These cells are sometimes recognized as nonself by the immune system.
3. **Genome-encoded tumor antigens:** When **oncogenes** are deregulated, the protein product can lead to tumor formation. **Proto-oncogenes** are found in nearly all nucleated cells, from yeast to human, and are involved in cell growth. Alteration in gene expression or protein structure can initiate abnormal cell growth.
4. **Oncofetal antigens** are produced during fetal development but present in minute amounts after birth. However, they may become expressed after malignant transformation (e.g., α-fetoprotein [AFP] and carcinoembryonic antigen [CEA]).

C. Immunity to Tumors

1. **Natural immunity** to tumors occurs to a limited degree with macrophages and NK cells.
   a. **Macrophage-mediated cytotoxicity:** Occurs when macrophages come in close contact with tumor cells
   b. **NK cells:** Approximately 50% of tumors have mutations leading to decreased MHC class I products expressed on their surfaces; this may facilitate killing by NK cells
2. **Humoral-mediated immunity:** Antibodies can be produced to antigens found on the surface of tumor cells. The tumor cells can then be lysed by complement activation or ADCC reactions involving NK cells, PMNs, and macrophages. Antibody directed against tumor-associated antigens can lead to the destruction of cells with those antigens. However, that cell population can be replaced by other cancerous cells lacking that antigen.

3. **T cell-mediated immunity**
   a. Cytokines involved in tumor immunity
      1) IL-1 activates T cells, B cells, and NK cells and induces a fever.
      2) TNFα destroys tumor cells.
      3) INF-γ is produced by activated T cells and NK cells.
   b. CTLs can directly lyse tumor cells.

D. Tumor Markers

1. Tumor markers are glycoproteins found in small amounts in normal serum but elevated in certain types of cancers. They can be used to screen for cancer but more commonly are used to monitor therapeutic response or to determine tumor burden.
2. **Carcinoembryonic antigen**
   a. CEA levels are used in management of gastrointestinal tumors (colon cancer) and adenocarcinomas of the colon, pancreas, liver, and lung. It has the highest sensitivity among single markers for colorectal cancer.
   b. Can also be found in inflammatory bowel disease, ulcerative colitis, Crohn disease, polyps, tumors of the gastrointestinal tract, and cigarette smokers
   c. The **highest CEA levels** are found in **metastatic disease.**
3. **α-Fetoprotein**
   a. AFP is produced during embryonic and fetal development. AFP levels are high in patients with hepatocellular carcinoma, hepatoblastoma, and testicular and ovarian cancer.
   b. Can also be elevated in viral hepatitis, cirrhosis, and ulcerative colitis
   c. Important marker for **monitoring cancer therapy**
4. **Human chorionic gonadotropin** (HCG)
   a. Human chorionic gonadotropin is composed of two subunits: alpha and beta. HCG is found in serum and urine during pregnancy.
   b. HCG may be produced by neoplastic cells of testicular cancer and various other tumors. Levels are useful in evaluating patients with gestational trophoblastic disease, testicular tumors, and ovarian germ cell tumors.
5. **Prostate-specific antigen** (PSA)
   a. A glycoprotein that dissolves seminal gel formed after ejaculation
   b. Normal prostate tissue contains PSA, but it is present in low amounts in blood.
   c. Increased in prostate cancer, benign prostatic hyperplasia, and acute or chronic prostatitis
   d. PSA levels correlate with prostate size, stage of prostate cancer, and response to treatment. As men age, they commonly develop benign prostrate hyperplasia, which can produce elevated PSA levels.
   e. Used to **screen for prostate cancer** in conjunction with a digital rectal examination

6. Cancer antigen (CA)
   a. A number of serum proteins are used as cancer markers. CA72-4, CA19-9, and CA125 have been shown useful in the diagnosis and monitoring the progression of colorectal cancer.
   b. Elevated CA125 has been shown to be a diagnostic and prognostic biomarker associated with the presence of advanced-stage serous ovarian cancer.

XII. ANTIGEN-ANTIBODY REACTIONS

A. Antigen-Antibody Interaction

1. Forces that participate in antibody-antigen interaction
   a. **Electrostatic force or ionic bonding**
      1) Positively charged portions of one molecule are attracted to negatively charged portions of another molecule.
      2) This bonding is affected by the pH and ionic strength of the environment.
      3) Electrostatic force increases as the two molecules get closer together.
   b. **Hydrogen bonding**
      1) Hydrogen binds to an electronegative atom such as oxygen or nitrogen.
      2) A weak bond, but it contributes greatly to the antigen-antibody interaction
      3) Maximum binding strength occurs below 37°C.
   c. **Hydrophobic bonding**
      1) This is the attraction between **nonpolar groups.**
      2) The nonpolar groups tend to aggregate to reduce surface area, and this increases the strength of the bond.
   d. **Van der Waals force:** A weak, attractive force between an electron orbital of one atom and the nucleus of another atom
2. **Affinity**
   a. The strength of the interaction between a single antibody binding site and a single epitope
   b. The affinity constant describes whether the antigen-antibody complex is highly complementary, and therefore would bind readily, or not very complementary, and therefore would not bind readily.
3. **Avidity**
   a. The affinity for multivalent antigens and multiple antibodies to combine; the extent of binding capacity
   b. This is greater than the cumulative affinity constants for all antigen-antibody pairs.
4. Specificity and cross-reactivity
   a. **Specificity** refers to the antibody's greatest affinity for a particular antigen.
   b. **Cross-reactivity** occurs when the antibody combines with an antigen that is structurally similar to the immunogen that stimulated the antibody production or the antigen the antibody has the greatest affinity for (i.e., **heterophile antibodies**).

B. Immunoassays

1. Assays involving antibody-antigen reactions are called immunoassays.
2. **Examples**
   a. **Precipitation reaction:** Soluble antigen and soluble antibody react to form an insoluble product (precipitate), such as double gel diffusion, radial immunodiffusion, immunoelectrophoresis, immunofixation, nephelometry, and turbidimetry.
   b. **Agglutination reaction:** Soluble antibody reacts with insoluble antigen or soluble antigen reacts with insoluble antibody. Reactants are made insoluble by combining with latex particles, RBCs, dyes, or liposomes.
   c. **Labeled reaction:** A label producing a measurable end product is attached to an antibody or antigen. Labels include fluorochromes, enzymes, and chemiluminescent molecules.
   d. Testing serial dilutions of patient sera provides semiquantitative results (titer). A fourfold rise in titer between an acute and convalescent sample is considered clinically significant.

XIII. PRECIPITATION REACTIONS

A. Precipitation

1. **Zone of equivalence:** Maximum precipitation occurs when the concentrations of the antigen and antibody are about equal.
2. **Prozone** occurs when excess amount of **antibody** is present, and the antigen and antibody do not combine to form precipitates—the complexes remain soluble. This results in a false-negative result.
3. **Postzone** occurs when excess amount of **antigen** is present, and the antigen and antibody do not combine to form precipitates—the complexes remain soluble. This results in a false-negative result.

B. Types of Precipitation Reactions

1. **Fluid-phase precipitation:** Passive diffusion of soluble antigen and antibody
   a. **Turbidimetry** is the measurement of light transmitted through a suspension of particles. The formation of immune complexes decreases the amount of light passing through a suspension. The more immune complexes formed and the larger they are, the greater is the decrease in light able to pass through.
   b. **Nephelometry** is a direct measure of light scattered by particles suspended in solution. The scattering of light is proportional to the size and amount of immune complexes formed. **Nephelometry is more sensitive than turbidimetry.**
   c. **Flocculation** is the precipitation of fine particles in a confined space. The serologic tests for syphilis, Venereal Disease Research Laboratory (VDRL) and rapid plasma regain (RPR) are examples of flocculation tests.

2. **Precipitation reactions in agar gel**
   a. Antigen and antibody diffuse through the agar gel and precipitate when they reach the zone of equivalence. Molecular size determines the speed of travel through the gel.
   b. Precipitation reactions are used less frequently today than in the past.
   c. **Double immunodiffusion** (Ouchterlony technique)
      1) Antigen and antibody are placed in wells in the gel and diffuse toward each other. When optimum concentrations are met (at the zone of equivalence), a precipitate line forms.
      2) Can be used to determine if a specific antibody is present in serum
      3) Precipitant lines between adjacent wells of antigen can be reported as identity, partial identity, or nonidentity.
      4) **Common errors include** overfilling of wells, irregular well punching, unlevel incubation area, gel drying, increased room temperature, and antigen or antibody contamination by bacteria or fungi.
   d. **Countercurrent immunoelectrophoresis (CIE)**
      1) On an agar gel plate or slide, antigen is added to one well and antibody is added to another well. An electric current accelerates the movement of the antigen and antibody toward each other, resulting in precipitation sooner than if an electric current is not applied.
      2) CIE can be used to detect antibodies to infectious agents and microbial antigens. CIE has been replaced by easier-to-perform assays, such as agglutination tests.
   e. **Immunofixation electrophoresis**
      1) Serum, urine, or CSF is electrophoresed in a gel. Antiserum contained in a cellulose acetate strip is then placed on top of the electrophoresis gel. The antibodies diffuse into the electrophoresis gel and combine with the antigens, forming a precipitate.
      2) Detects the presence of an immunoglobulin in serum or urine
   f. **Rocket immunoelectrophoresis**
      1) Used to quantify antigens
      2) Antigens are electrophoresed in agar-containing antibody. A pH is selected so that the antibodies are immobile. The antibody and antigen combine to form precipitates in the shape of a "rocket."
      3) The height of the rocket is proportional to the concentration of antigen in the specimen.

XIV. AGGLUTINATION REACTIONS

A. General Information

1. **Definition:** Agglutination occurs when particles in suspension clump together due to antibody-antigen interaction, that is, formation of immune complexes.
2. IgM and IgG antibodies participate in agglutination reactions. Because IgM has more antigen-binding sites, it agglutinates more quickly.

3. **Comparison of agglutination and precipitation**
   a. Agglutination uses an antigen or antibody attached to a particle (insoluble), whereas precipitation uses soluble antigens and antibodies.
   b. Agglutination and precipitation reactions use antigens with at least two antigenic determinants **(epitopes).**
   c. In agglutination and precipitation reactions, antigen excess can result in a postzone reaction, whereas antibody excess can result in a prozone reaction.
   d. Agglutination reactions take minutes to hours, whereas precipitation reactions may take hours to days.
   e. Methods that utilize agglutination reactions are qualitative or semiquantitative, whereas precipitation methods give qualitative, semiquantitative, or quantitative results.

B. Classification of Agglutination Reactions

1. **Direct agglutination:** This method uses antigens naturally occurring on a particle to demonstrate agglutination (e.g., RBCs in type and crossmatch).
2. **Viral hemagglutination:** This is a naturally occurring process in which a virus (e.g., influenza virus) will agglutinate RBCs by binding to surface receptors.
3. **Passive and reverse passive agglutination**
   a. **Passive agglutination:** A technique in which soluble antigen is attached to a particle, producing agglutination with a specific soluble antibody
   b. **Reverse passive agglutination:** A technique in which an antibody is attached to a particle, producing agglutination with a specific soluble antigen
   c. Particles used include latex, gelatin, resin beads, and, less frequently, RBCs and *Staphylococcus aureus*.

XV. LABELED REACTIONS

A. Immunofluorescence

1. **Definition:** Antibodies labeled with a fluorescent dye are used to detect an antibody or antigen.
2. **Methods**
   a. **Direct immunofluorescence:** Conjugated (fluorescent-labeled) reagent antibody reacts with an antigen in a clinical sample to form an antigen-antibody complex.
   b. **Indirect immunofluorescent assays:** Antigen reacts with unlabeled antibody forming an antigen-antibody complex that is then complexed with a labeled antihuman antibody, creating an antibody-antigen-antibody "sandwich."
   c. **Biotin-avidin immunofluorescence:** This is an indirect assay in which the detection system is modified by using a biotin-labeled antibody followed by avidin-labeled fluorochrome. This extra step increases the specificity and sensitivity of the assay.
3. Commonly used **fluorochromes** include fluorescein isothiocyanate (FITC), R-phycoerythrin, quantum red, tetramethyl-rhodamine isothiocyanate, Texas red, phycocyanin, acridine orange, and propidium iodide.

4. **Antinuclear antibodies (ANAs):** Antibodies to nuclear antigens are present in many systemic autoimmune diseases, such as SLE, mixed connective tissue disease, and rheumatoid arthritis. This test is used as a screening test for diagnosing, developing a prognosis, and monitoring treatment of certain autoimmune diseases.
   a. **Indirect immunofluorescence for ANA screening.** Cultured cells on a microscope slide are incubated with patient serum. The cells are washed and then incubated with antihuman immunoglobulin conjugated with fluorescein. The slide is washed again and then viewed using a fluorescent microscope.
   b. **Enzyme-linked immunosorbent assays (ELISAs)** can also be used. This method can be semiautomated. However, ELISAs only allows detection of the antibodies and not pattern determination.

B. Enzyme-Linked Immunosorbant Assays

1. Enzyme-labeled reagents are used to detect antigens or antibodies.
2. Enzyme must be stable, specific, and cannot bind to antigen or antibody independently.
3. A colorless substrate is metabolized by the enzyme into a colored compound. The intensity of the color is directly proportional to the amount of enzyme present.

XVI. COMPLEMENT FIXATION

A. Principle

1. **Complement fixation** (CF) assays are sometimes used to detect antibody in patient sera. The serum is mixed with a specific known antigen. If antibody to the antigen is present, an immune complex forms. Complement is added, and if an immune complex is present, it will bind the complement.
2. When the antibody in patient serum and antigen combine, the complement present in the system combines with the antigen-antibody complexes and no free complement is available to cause lysis of the sensitized indicator RBCs. Therefore, **no hemolysis is a positive reaction**.
3. If antibody is absent, then complement is free to attach to the sensitized indicator RBCs and causes lysis. Therefore, **hemolysis is a negative reaction.**

B. Application

1. CF can be used to detect antibodies to viruses, *Rickettsia*, and fungi. Because IgM is efficient at binding complement, this assay works well for detecting IgM.
2. Although once the reference method for detecting many antibodies, it has largely been replaced by other methods that are easier to perform.

XVII. CELLULAR ASSAYS

A. Flow Cytometry

1. Flow cytometry can be combined with a cell sorter, **fluorescence-activated cell sorter.**

2. Can identify antigens on living cells
3. Cells in a sample are stained with specific fluorescent-labeled antibody that recognizes and binds to specific cell surface molecules.
4. LASER (light-amplified stimulated emitted radiation) light detects and counts stained cells.

B. Lymphocyte Subsets

1. **T-cell subsets**
   a. Enumeration of T cells is important in assessing immune response.
   b. Monoclonal antibodies are used in conjunction with flow cytometry to identify cell markers such as CD1, CD2, CD3, and CD4.
2. **B-cell subsets**
   a. **Classic test:** Labeled antibody to surface membrane immunoglobulin
   b. Monoclonal antibodies are now used in conjunction with flow cytometry to identify CD19 or CD20.
3. **Lymphocyte phenotyping in human immunodeficiency virus (HIV) infection**
   a. HIV kills T-helper cells, and the primary viral receptor for infection is CD4.
   b. CD4 and CD8 markers are monitored during HIV treatment. If the CD4 count falls below 200/μL, the patient is susceptible to opportunistic infections. The CD4/CD8 ratio is also a valuable prognosis marker. The reference value is ≥2.0.
4. Other cells identified by flow cytometry and monoclonal antibodies
   a. CD16 on NK cells, macrophages, and neutrophils
   b. CD34 on hematopoietic cells
   c. HLA-DR on B cells, monocytes, myeloid cells, and erythroid precursors
   d. Glycophorin A on erythroid cells
   e. CD14 on myelomonocytic cells
   f. CD41 on platelets and megakaryocytes

C. Assays to Assess Cell Function

1. **Lymphocyte transformation**
   a. Cells in vitro are challenged with antigens and then observed for transformation.
   b. Normal control cells are stimulated by the antigens while the patient's cells are observed for stimulation.
2. **Mixed-lymphocyte culture**
   a. Used to detect HLA-Dw on the surface of cells to ensure compatibility of donor cells with recipient cells
   b. This is critical for bone marrow transplants.
3. **Measurement of immune activation**
   a. All the events that lead to an immune response
   b. Measurement includes a WBC count with differential, immunoglobulin levels, and complement levels.

c. Signs of immune activation in the patient include swollen lymph nodes, fever, and malaise.
d. Cytokines (e.g., IL-2) are measured to detect immune disorders.

XVIII. STREPTOCOCCAL SEROLOGY

A. *Streptococcus pyogenes* (Group A Streptococci)

1. *S. pyogenes* causes pharyngitis, pyoderma, puerperal sepsis, and necrotizing fasciitis. It can also produce a toxin that results in scarlet fever.
2. **Post-streptococcal sequelae**
   a. Antibody-antigen complexes can lead to rheumatic fever and glomerulonephritis. Sequelae are often diagnosed by the antistreptolysin O (ASO), antihyaluronidase, anti-DNase B, or streptozyme (which measure five anti-streptococcal antibodies) tests.
   b. **Rheumatic fever**
      1) **Symptoms:** Carditis, chorea, erythema marginatum, polyarthritis, and/or subcutaneous nodules
      2) Occurs 3–4 weeks after infection
      3) **Mechanism:** M protein of *S. pyogenes* shares antigenic epitopes with proteins found in synovium, heart muscle, and heart valve, suggesting that the damage is from an autoimmune disease due to **molecular mimicry.**
      4) It is most commonly seen between 5 and 15 years of age, although it is rare in the United States because of rapid treatment of *S. pyogenes* infections.
   c. **Glomerulonephritis**
      1) **Symptoms:** Proteinuria, hematuria, hypertension, impaired renal function, and edema
      2) Occurs about 10 days after pharyngitis or 18–21 days after a skin infection
      3) **Mechanism:** Circulating antigen-antibody complexes are deposited on the glomerular basement membranes, where complement is activated resulting in damage to the membranes. Platelet aggregation and fibrin and fibrinogen buildup, causing capillary obstruction and impaired renal function.

B. Diagnostic Tests

1. Culture results yielding beta-hemolytic group A streptococci are most reliable; however, the sequelae are immunologically mediated and do not involve actively growing bacteria.
2. **ASO neutralization test**
   a. Streptolysin O is a hemolysin produced by most beta-hemolytic group A streptococci.
   b. Individuals with infection produce antibody to streptolysin O.
   c. The **classic ASO test** is a neutralization assay. Antibodies to streptolysin O prevent hemolysis.

   d. Serial dilutions of patient serum are prepared. The titer is the last tube with no hemolysis. The result is expressed in **Todd units**, the reciprocal of the original serum dilution (e.g., 1 : 8 = 8 Todd units).
   e. **Interpretation:** A fourfold increase in titer between acute and convalescent samples indicates a recent group A streptococcal infection.
   f. The ASO neutralization test is rarely performed in the United States; it has been replaced by other diagnostic methods.
3. **ASO rapid latex agglutination test**
   a. **Principle:** Latex particles coated with streptolysin O agglutinate when mixed with patient's serum containing ASO antibody.
   b. **Interpretation:** The following titers are considered indicative of a group A streptococcus infection: preschool children >85, school-age children >170, and adults >85.
4. **Streptozyme**
   a. Screening test produced by Wampole Laboratories (Cranbury, New Jersey) that detects antibodies to five *S. pyogenes* proteins: DNase B, hyaluronidase, NADase, streptokinase, and streptolysin O
   b. **Principle:** Streptozyme is a passive latex agglutination assay. Immunonephelometry assays are also available to detect these antibodies.
   c. **Interpretation:** A fourfold rise in titer between acute and convalescent sera is indicative of an infection.
5. **Anti-DNase B test**
   a. Anti-DNase B antibody peaks at 4–6 weeks after group A streptococcal infection and lasts for months.
   b. **Principle:** Today, most methods use latex agglutination or immunonephelometry.
   c. **Interpretation:** The following titers are considered indicative of a group A streptococcal infection: preschool children >60, school-age children >170, and adults >85.

XIX. SYPHILIS SEROLOGY

A. Causative Agent

1. *Treponema pallidum* subsp. *pallidum,* a spirochete
2. Transmitted by direct contact (including sexual contact) and across the placenta

B. Disease Stages

1. **Incubation period:** *T. pallidum* enters the body, reaches the bloodstream, and is disseminated to all organs. This early asymptomatic phase lasts 10 days to 10 weeks.
2. **Primary syphilis**
   a. The initial lesion is a painless, nonbleeding ulcer called a **chancre.**
   b. The chancre appears, on average, 2–3 weeks after the initial infection.

c. Within 1 week after the chancre appears, lymph nodes near the portal of entry enlarge, for example, the groin in sexually transmitted cases.
d. Antibodies are produced 1–4 weeks after the chancre appears.
e. Darkfield analysis of lesion demonstrates spirochetes.

3. **Secondary syphilis**
   a. Symptoms include skin rash, low-grade fever, malaise, pharyngitis, weight loss, arthralgia, and lymphadenopathy. Symptoms last 4–6 weeks.
   b. Spirochetes are present throughout the body during this stage.
   c. Ulcers develop on mucous membranes.
   d. Serologic tests are positive.
4. **Latent syphilis**
   a. Stage of syphilis with no signs or symptoms
   b. Nontreponemal and treponemal serologic tests are positive.
   c. **Early latent syphilis (**infection occurred within the past 12 months): One in four individuals relapses into secondary syphilis.
   d. **Late latent syphilis** (infection occurred more than 12 months ago): The patient is resistant to reinfection and to relapses.
5. **Tertiary syphilis**
   a. Symptoms occur 2–40 years after initial infection.
   b. **Gummas** (syphilis lesions due to hypersensitivity reaction to treponemal antigens) are found throughout the body.
   c. Syphilitic aortitis, aortic valve insufficiency, and thoracic aneurysm are possible.
   d. Neurosyphilis can cause blindness and senility.
6. **Congenital syphilis**
   a. ***Treponema pallidum* can cross the placenta** during any stage of the disease.
   b. **Infection of the fetus** causes late abortion, stillbirth, neonatal death, neonatal disease, or latent infection.
   c. The outcome depends on the stage of the mother's disease—primary or secondary syphilis causing the worst outcome—and the age of the fetus at time of infection.
   d. If the mother receives treatment during the first 4 months of pregnancy, congenital syphilis is usually avoided.
   e. Congenital syphilis presents in the neonate as diffuse maculopapular desquamatous rash (particularly around the mouth and on the palms and soles), hemolytic anemia, jaundice, hepatosplenomegaly, abnormal cartilage and bone involvement, and intellectual disability.
7. **Diagnosis:** Signs and symptoms, detection of spirochetes in lesion, and positive syphilis serology

C. Direct Detection

1. **Definitive diagnosis** of syphilis is made by detection of *T. pallidum* in CSF, umbilical cord, or skin or mucous membrane lesions—depending on the stage of the disease.

2. *Treponema pallidum* is detected using **darkfield microscopy or silver stain** of material from lesions. Material from the oral cavity should not be tested because *T. pallidum* cannot be differentiated from commensal spirochetes.
3. Direct fluorescent antibody-*T. pallidum* (**DFA-TP**) test: A fluorescence-labeled antibody is used to detect *T. pallidum* in lesions. The test is specific for pathogenic *Treponema* and can therefore be used on oral and rectal specimens, but it cannot distinguish among the causative agents of syphilis, yaws, pinta, and endemic syphilis.

D. Serologic Tests

1. **General principles**
   a. *Treponema pallidum* infection causes the host to produce nonspecific antibody, called **reagin**, and specific treponemal antibodies.
   b. The **nontreponemal antigen tests** detect reagin and are only used for screening because this antibody will cross-react with similar antigens present in SLE and other autoimmune diseases, pregnancy, and some chronic infections such as hepatitis. These conditions can result in biologic false positives.
      1) Examples of nontreponemal antigen tests include the VDRL, unheated serum reagin (USR), and RPR assays.
      2) The percentage of false positives in these tests is high (30–40%), so all reactive results must be confirmed using a test that detects antibodies specifically directed at *T. pallidum*, the so-called **treponemal antigen tests.**
   c. Treponemal antigen tests use *T. pallidum* cells as the antigen source. These assays are highly specific and include the *T. pallidum*-particulate agglutination (TP-PA), fluorescent treponemal antibody absorption (FTA-ABS), and microhemagglutination *T. pallidum* tests.
2. **VDRL test**
   a. This test measures the antibody (reagin) a patient has formed against cardiolipin, cholesterol, and lecithin.
   b. Serum samples are diluted to determine an antibody titer.
   c. **Tests are read microscopically for flocculation.** Results are reported as NR (nonreactive), WR (weak reactive), or R (reactive).
   d. The VDRL test is positive 1–3 weeks after the chancre appears.
   e. Mainly limited to use on CSF now, this is the only serologic test approved for testing CSF.
3. **USR test** is a modified VDRL test in which choline-chloride EDTA is added to the VDRL antigen. The addition of this compound allows serum that has not been heat inactivated to be tested.
4. **RPR test**
   a. **Macroscopic flocculation**
   b. The assay uses VDRL antigen with **charcoal particles.** The antigen is not attached to the charcoal as in latex agglutination assays. The charcoal is

trapped in the flocculation reaction, which allows the reaction to be seen macroscopically.

c. The test can be qualitative or semiquantitative. Dilutions are made to semiquantify the amount of antibody present. Because it is read macroscopically, it is the most commonly used nontreponemal antigen serologic assay.

5. **TP-PA test (Fujirebio Inc., Tokyo, Japan):** Treponemal antigen is combined with liposomes. If antibodies are present, a mat of agglutination forms in wells of a microtiter plate.
6. **FTA-ABS test**
   a. An indirect antibody test using the **Nichol's strain** of *T. pallidum* subsp. *pallidum* affixed into wells of microscope slides
   b. This test has been replaced by other assays and is no longer recommended by the Centers for Disease Control and Prevention (CDC).
7. **EIAs**
   a. The majority of the many commercially available assays use recombinant *T. pallidum* antigens.
   b. This method has the advantage of automation.

XX. *BORRELIA BURGDORFERI* SEROLOGY

A. *Borrelia burgdorferi*

1. Spirochete
2. Causes **Lyme disease**, also referred to as **Lyme borreliosis**

B. Transmission

1. The microorganism is transmitted to humans in the saliva of a **tick (*Ixodes*).**
2. Because ticks take days to feed, if a tick is removed within 24–36 hours, infection might be prevented.

C. Lyme Disease

1. **Early stage**
   a. A reddened area on the skin that occurs 2–32 days after being bitten by an infected tick
   b. The reddened area can develop into the classic target or "bull's eye" rash, called **erythema migrans.** The rash is present in about 60% of the cases.
2. **Late stage**
   a. The most common symptom of the late stage is arthritis affecting the knees, shoulders, and elbows.
   b. Approximately 15% of patients exhibit **aseptic meningitis**, facial nerve palsy, encephalitis, cranial neuritis, and radiculoneuritis.
   c. Approximately 8% of patients exhibit carditis.
   d. Chronic disease may present as a sclerotic or atrophic skin lesion or a lymphocytoma.

3. **Antibody response**
   a. The first antibody produced in Lyme disease is IgM, which is primarily directed against the outer surface protein **OspC** and **flagellin** subunits p41 (FlaB) and p37 (FlaA).
   b. Subsequently, in the late stage IgG antibody specific to a number of *B. burgdorferi* antigens is produced.
   c. Antibodies often persist for several years.

D. Diagnosis

1. Organisms can be cultured; however, this is time consuming and has only moderate sensitivity.
2. **Serology tests**
   a. Diagnosis can be made if a fourfold increase in titer is detected between an acute serum specimen and a specimen taken 6–8 weeks later (convalescent). A more rapid method is to detect IgM antibodies to *B. burgdorferi* antigens.
   b. Immunofluorescence and ELISAs are **screening methods.** Positive specimens should be confirmed by immunoblotting.
   c. **Immunoblot (western blot)**
      1) **Procedure**
         a) Antigens are electrophoretically separated on a polyacrylamide gel to form bands.
         b) The antigenic bands are transferred to an inert membrane filter (e.g., nitrocellulose) and then incubated with patient serum.
         c) After incubation, the membrane is washed and an enzyme-labeled antihuman antibody is added.
         d) Enzyme substrate is added to detect antigen-antibody reactions.
      2) **Results and interpretation**
         a) The **IgM** immunoblot is considered positive if two or more of the following protein bands are reactive: OspC, 39-KDa protein, and the 41-KDa protein.
         b) The **IgG** immunoblot is considered positive if five or more of the following protein bands are reactive: proteins of 18, 21 (OspC), 28, 30, 39, 41, 45, 58, 66, and 93 KDa.
         c) The immunoblot assay is considered a confirmatory test and should only be performed if a screening test is reactive.
         d) **EIA.** Commercial methods are based in indirect assays using antigen-coated plates and IgM capture assays.

XXI. RUBELLA SEROLOGY

A. Virus

1. Single-stranded **RNA** genome
2. Member of the family *Togaviridae*

B. Clinical Manifestations

1. **Rubella** (German measles)
   a. Mild, contagious disease characterized by an **erythematous maculopapular rash**
   b. This virus is spread by droplets through the upper respiratory tract.
   c. Patients may have a 1–5-day prodromal syndrome of malaise, headache, cold symptoms, low-grade fever, and swollen lymph glands at the back of the head.
   d. Complications include arthritis, encephalitis, and thrombocytopenic purpura.
2. **Congenital rubella**
   a. Infection of the mother during pregnancy can result in abortion, stillbirth, or birth defects.
   b. Typical birth defects that occur if the mother is infected during the first 8 weeks of pregnancy include congenital heart disease, cataracts, and neurosensory deafness.
   c. Mothers infected after 20–24 weeks of pregnancy rarely give birth to babies with birth defects.
   d. Babies born with congenital rubella syndrome exhibit thrombocytopenia, hepatitis, long-bone lesions, retinitis, encephalitis, interstitial pneumonitis, psychiatric disorders, thyroid disorders, and diabetes mellitus.

C. Immunologic Response

1. **Acute infections**
   a. As the rash fades, IgG and IgM antibodies can be detected.
   b. A blood specimen should be drawn when the symptoms start and another specimen 5–7 days later.
   c. If at least a fourfold rise in antibody titer is detected and clinical symptoms are present, then a diagnosis of rubella can be made.
   d. **IgG antibodies** offer **lifetime immunity,** whereas the **IgM antibodies disappear** at about 4–5 weeks after infection.
   e. Because of the widespread use of the rubella vaccine, infections in developed countries are rare.
2. **Congenital infections:** Diagnosis can be established if IgM antibodies are present in neonates that have a low birth weight or any symptom of congenital rubella.
3. Most rubella testing in the United States is done to determine a woman's immune status against rubella as part of a prenatal examination. The presence of IgG to rubella virus indicates immunity.

D. Diagnostic Tests

1. Test methods used include latex agglutination, passive hemagglutination, ELISA, and indirect immunofluorescence.
2. The **hemagglutination inhibition** test was once the standard test for the detection of rubella antibodies. It has been replaced by less technical demanding assays.

3. **ELISA:** Rubella-specific IgM is determined by either IgM-capture or indirect-IgM assays.
4. **Passive agglutination:** Latex particles coated with rubella virus are agglutinated by rubella IgG or IgM antibodies, if present.

XXII. EPSTEIN-BARR VIRUS SEROLOGY

A. EBV

1. **DNA virus**
2. Member of the **herpes virus group**
3. Transmission is through saliva.
4. Immunity lasts a lifetime; however, the virus causes latent infections, and persons infected remain carriers for life.
5. Serologic tests detect heterophile and virus-specific antibodies.

B. Diseases

1. **Infectious mononucleosis (IM)**
   a. A disease of the reticuloendothelial system
   b. Incubation period is 4–7 weeks.
   c. Onset may be acute or insidious with sore throat, fever, and lymphadenopathy.
   d. Common findings are **lymphocytosis**, with many **reactive (atypical) lymphocytes,** and enlarged cervical lymph nodes.
   e. Other signs include fever and malaise.
   f. The acute phase lasts 2 weeks and requires a long convalescence, up to 1–2 months.
   g. Individuals with infection have abnormal WBC differentials and sometimes abnormal liver function tests.
   h. Infections usually resolve in 4–6 weeks.
2. **Burkitt lymphoma**
   a. EBV is able to transform B cells into long-lived cells.
   b. Burkitt lymphoma is a **malignant neoplasm of B lymphocytes.**
   c. Found in restricted areas of Africa and New Guinea
   d. Primarily seen in children
3. **Nasopharyngeal carcinoma** is a nasopharyngeal squamous cell carcinoma found mainly in southern China.

C. Laboratory Tests

1. **Heterophile antibodie**s
   a. Heterophile antibodies produced in IM are not EBV specific and react with sheep, beef, ox, and horse RBCs. Approximately 80–85% of adult patients with IM will develop heterophile antibodies, whereas only 50% of children less than 12 years of age will produce heterophile antibodies.

b. **Paul-Bunnell presumptive test**
   1) **Principle:** Heterophile antibodies peak around 2–3 weeks after infection. Serial dilutions of serum are incubated with a 2% suspension of sheep RBCs. Agglutination is a positive reaction.
   2) **Results**
      a) The reference value is a titer of 28 or less.
      b) Titer of >56 is suggestive of IM.
   3) **Interpretation**
      a) The Paul-Bunnell test is a screening test to detect heterophile antibodies that is not specific to IM. The test is rarely used today.
      b) False-negative rate is 10–15%.

c. **Latex agglutination assays** (e.g., MonoSpot, Meridan Bioscience, Inc. Cincinnati, OH) using Paul-Bunnell antigen purified from bovine red cell membranes are available and demonstrate a high degree of sensitivity. However, the CDC does not recommend the test for routine use because of the large number of diseases that can cause false-positive results.

2. **EBV-specific tests**
   a. Most frequently used methods are based on EIA and chemiluminescence. Immunofluorescence is the reference method but is labor intensive.
   b. Can detect anti–viral capsid antigen (VCA), anti–early antigen/diffuse, (EA/d), anti–early antigen/restricted (EA/r), and anti–Epstein-Barr nuclear antigen (EBNA) antibodies
   c. **Interpretation:** VCA antibodies peak 3–4 weeks following infection, and IgM is not detectable in 12 weeks. High titer of IgM with IgG to VCA in the absence of antibodies to EBNA is generally sufficient to diagnosis a primary infection.

XXIII. VIRAL HEPATITIS SEROLOGY

A. Hepatitis Testing

1. Testing for antibodies and antigens in patient sera can determine the responsible virus, stage of infection, and immune status of the patient.
2. The most widely used test method is ELISA.

B. Hepatitis A

1. Hepatitis A virus (HAV): Member of the family *Picornaviridae*
2. **Epidemiology**
   a. Transmission by **fecal-oral route**
   b. Epidemics occur through fecal contamination of food or water.
3. **Clinical manifestations**
   a. Infections may be asymptomatic or symptomatic; **infections in children are usually asymptomatic.**
   b. Incubation period is 10–50 days.

c. **Symptomatic infections**
   1) **Symptoms** include fever, anorexia, vomiting, fatigue, abdominal pain, and malaise. Patient may become jaundiced. Symptoms are more severe in pregnant women.
   2) Recovery occurs in 2–4 weeks.
   3) Mortality rate is 0.1%, and chronic disease rarely occurs.
   4) Inactivated **vaccines**, first developed in 1995, are recommended for travelers, drug abusers, men who have sex with men, and children at 1 year of age.

d. **Laboratory tests**
   1) **Aspartate aminotransferase** (AST) and especially **alanine aminotransferase** (ALT) levels are increased and peak before jaundice occurs.
   2) Other findings include **hyperbilirubinemia**, decreased albumin, tea-colored urine, and pale-colored stools.
   3) Paired sera (acute collected at onset of symptoms and convalescent 3–4 weeks later) are analyzed for an increase in anti-HAV antibodies. Alternatively, a single acute sample with a higher titer of IgM compared to IgG is considered diagnostic of an acute infection.
   4) Anti-HAV antibodies are present at onset of symptoms and for years afterward.

C. Hepatitis B

1. Hepatitis B virus (HBV)
   a. Partially double-stranded DNA
   b. Member of the family *Hepadnaviridae*
2. **Epidemiology**
   a. The virus is transmitted via mucous membranes (e.g., sexual contact) or wounds contacting contaminated blood and body fluids, or parenterally. Parenteral infection occurs through transfusion of contaminated blood products, hemodialysis, intravenous drug use, contaminated needle sticks, tattooing, acupuncture, or ear piercing.
   b. **High-risk groups** for acquiring HBV infection include intravenous drug users, men who have sex with men, patients undergoing hemodialysis, and healthcare workers.
3. **Clinical manifestations**
   a. Incubation period is 50–180 days.
   b. **Symptoms** develop abruptly and include fever, anorexia, vomiting, fatigue, malaise, jaundice, and arthralgia.
   c. **Long clinical course:** Acute infection can last up to 6 months. Most patients recover within 6 months.
   d. Approximately 5% of patients with infections develop a chronic infection, in which the patient remains **hepatitis B surface antigen (HBsAg)** positive.

e. If chronic infections are active, severe damage to the liver occurs, which can result in liver cirrhosis or hepatocellular carcinoma.
f. All chronic carriers shed virus.
g. A recombinant HBV vaccine is recommended for healthcare workers. The Advisory Committee for Immunization Practices recommends routine vaccination for all children in the United States soon after birth and before hospital discharge.

4. **Laboratory tests**
   a. The **first marker that appears** at the end of the incubation period is HBsAg. The concentration of the surface antigen continues to rise and peaks about midway through the acute infection. Presence of this antigen indicates infectivity.
   b. Soon after HBsAg is detected in the blood, **heptatitis Be antigen** (HBeAg) appears. HBeAg peaks at about the same time as the surface antigen. HBeAg disappears about two-thirds of the way through the acute infection phase.
   c. The next marker to appear is **antibody to hepatitis B core** (anti-HBc), which begins to rise a couple weeks into the acute infection. Anti-HBc peaks at the end of the acute infection stage after HBsAg is no longer detectable and before **antibody to hepatitis B surface antigen** (anti-HBs) can be detected. This period is referred to as the "core window."
   d. The anti-HBc IgM antibody peaks a few weeks after the acute infection stage, and then disappears in about 6 months during recovery. Anti-HBc IgG will persist for several decades.
   e. **At the end of the acute stage, anti-HBe begins to rise** and peaks about 2–16 weeks later. The concentration of this antibody decreases slightly during a person's lifetime but never disappears.
   f. **The last marker to appear is anti-HBs.** It appears at the end of the acute stage and the beginning of the recovery stage. Its concentration peaks, then plateaus during recovery and never disappears. Presence of this antibody indicates immunity.
   g. **In chronic infections**, patients do not produce detectable levels of anti-HBs, and HBsAg persists. These patients become chronic carriers of the virus and are at risk for cirrhosis and hepatocellular carcinoma.

D. Hepatitis C

1. Hepatitis C virus (HCV)
   a. Single-stranded RNA virus
   b. Member of the family *Hepacivirus*
2. **Epidemiology**
   a. Parenteral transmission is most common.
   b. Sexual and perinatal transmission of the virus is less common.

3. **Symptoms**
   a. Causes either acute or chronic disease
   b. The **incubation period** is 2–26 weeks.
   c. **Acute infections** are asymptomatic or mild—nausea, vomiting, abdominal pain, fatigue, malaise, and jaundice.
   d. Approximately 50–80% of cases become chronic, with 25% leading to cirrhosis.
   e. About 20% of cirrhosis cases lead to cancer.
4. **Laboratory tests**
   a. Anti-HCV is diagnostic of HCV infection.
   b. Anti-HCV IgM does not distinguish between acute and chronic disease because both IgM and IgG antibodies are detectable for years.
   c. Third-generation EIA tests using recombinant viral antigen have the potential for false-positive results. All reactive samples should be confirmed with an HCV RNA assay.

E. Delta Hepatitis

1. Hepatitis D virus (HDV)
   a. Unclassified, single-stranded RNA subviral particle
   b. Requires HBsAg from HBV infection to replicate and infect the host
2. **Epidemiology**
   a. Occurs worldwide
   b. Transmission is via the parenteral and transmucosal routes.
3. **Symptoms**
   a. **Coinfection** occurs when patients acquire HBV and HDV infections simultaneously.
   b. **Superinfection** occurs in patients with an established HBV infection who acquire HDV infection; superinfections can progress to chronic HBV/HDV infection.
   c. Patients with **chronic** HBV/HDV infection have poor prognoses because of severe liver damage, inflammation, and cirrhosis.
   d. Vaccination against HBV also prevents HDV.
4. **Laboratory Tests**
   a. Only HBsAg positive patients are tested for HDV.
   b. **HDV-Ag** is the **first marker** to appear, detectable about 1–4 days before symptoms start.
   c. IgM anti-HDV appears next followed by low levels of IgG anti-HDV.
   d. The switch to high levels of IgG anti-HDV indicates past HDV infection.

XXIV. HUMAN IMMUNODEFICIENCY VIRUS SEROLOGY

A. Human Immunodeficiency Virus (HIV)

1. Member of the family *Retroviridae*
2. **HIV causes acquired immunodeficiency syndrome (AIDS).**

3. There are **two serogroups.** HIV-1 is the predominant strain, and it is found worldwide. HIV-2 is limited primarily to West Africa.
4. **HIV-1 has three subtypes:** M, N, and O. M is the major subtype.
5. HIV-1 is transmitted by unprotected sex, contaminated blood or blood products, contaminated needles, or perinatally.

B. HIV Replication

1. **HIV binds to the CD4 molecule** on T-helper cells, monocytes, macrophages, and other cells via viral gp120. Secondary receptors (co-receptors) are also important in viral binding. T-helper cells are the primary target.
2. The HIV envelope fuses with the host plasma membrane of the cell allowing the virus to enter. The viral RNA is then released.
3. The RNA is transcribed to a DNA:RNA hybrid by the activity of the viral enzyme **reverse transcriptase.** The RNA strand is removed, and a complementary DNA strand is added forming double-stranded DNA. Viral DNA is then inserted into the host cell's DNA by viral **integrase.**
4. The viral DNA is transcribed into mRNA, which is then translated into viral proteins. Mature viruses leave the host cell by budding.
5. The replication process kills the infected cell and gradually leads to a diminishing number of T-helper cells.

C. Immune Response and HIV

1. **Serologic effects**
   a. Antibodies to HIV generally appear about 12 weeks after infection. These are the first antibodies detected by ELISA and western blot assays.
   b. Neutralizing antibodies, antibodies able to interfere with infection of host cells, appear about 1 year after infection. Although these neutralizing antibodies can interfere with viral replication, they do not seem to play a major role in protection.
   c. HIV is able to escape the immune response by undergoing **antigenic variation.**
2. **Effect on T cells**
   a. As the disease progresses, there is a **depletion of CD4+ T-helper cells.** The immune deficiency worsens as more T-helper cells are killed by the virus.
   b. HIV compromises the immune response by destroying T-helper cells. These cells are key players in both humoral and cellular immune responses.
   c. **The ratio of CD4:CD8 cells is reduced from 2:1 (normal).**
3. **Additional effects**
   a. Decreased natural killer cell activity
   b. Defective chemotaxis in monocytes and macrophages
   c. Enhanced release of interleukin-1 and cachectin by monocytes

D. Symptoms

1. **Acute retroviral syndrome:** Initially, persons with infection (acute phase) will be asymptomatic or can have minor symptoms resembling infectious mononucleosis. The incubation period is 3–6 weeks. Very few people in this stage are diagnosed.
2. The virus continues to replicate rapidly in the lymphoid tissue. This stage is referred to as **clinical latency.** Patients remain asymptomatic as the virus replicates rapidly. Some virus is latent in resting T cells and is resistant to therapy.
3. As the number of T cells begins to decrease, the patient develops a number of infections caused by **opportunistic pathogens:** *Candida*, herpes simplex virus, cytomegalovirus, etc. This stage of HIV infection has sometimes been referred to as **AIDS-related complex.**
4. Final stage (full-blown AIDS) includes T cell depletion resulting in severe opportunistic infections and cancers, such as esophageal candidiasis, cryptococcosis, systemic cytomegalovirus and herpes simplex virus infections, *Pneumocystis jiroveci* pneumonia, and Kaposi's sarcoma (caused by human herpes virus 8).
5. CD4+ T cell counts and presence of a variety of opportunistic infections are used to stage the severity of the disease.

E. Laboratory Tests

1. EIA and chemiluminescent tests are used to detect antibodies to HIV antigens.
2. The CDC recommends that patients be screened with a HIV-1/-2 antibody p24 antigen combination test. In general, a nonreactive result needs no further testing. If, however, it is suspected that the patient might be in an early infection stage and has not formed antibodies, a nucleic acid amplification test (NAT) can be performed.
3. EIA reactive samples should be tested with an assay that differentiates HIV-1 antibodies from HIV-2 antibodies. Samples that are reactive should be considered positive for HIV antibodies.
4. Samples that are negative or indeterminate in the differentiating tests should be tested with an FDA-approved HIV-1 NAT.
5. Commercial assays are available that can detect HIV RNA and DNA in clinical specimens, primarily peripheral blood mononuclear cells.

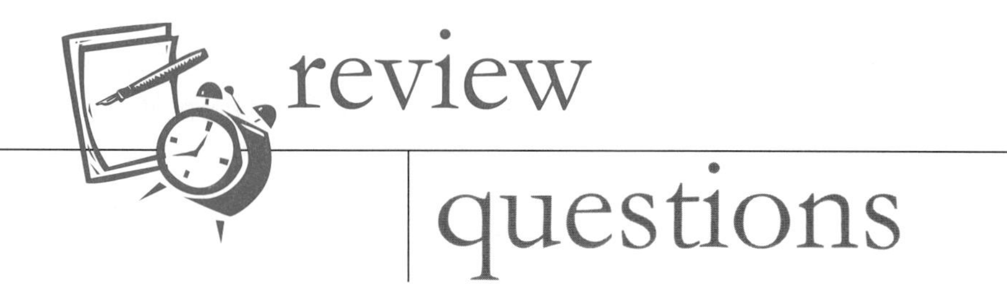

INSTRUCTIONS Each of the questions or incomplete statements that follows is comprised of four suggested responses. Select the *best* answer or completion statement in each case.

1. Color Plate 21■ depicts a monomeric immunoglobulin molecule. The portion of the molecule indicated by the dotted red circle and the red arrow is called the
   A. Fab fragment
   B. Fc fragment
   C. Heavy chain
   D. Hinge region

2. A hapten is
   A. Half of an immunoglobulin molecule
   B. A carrier molecule for an antigen that is not antigenic alone
   C. An immunoglobulin functional only in the presence of complement
   D. A determinant capable of stimulating an immune response only when bound to a carrier

3. Which of the following is characteristic of B cells?
   A. Phagocytic
   B. Participate in antibody-dependent cellular cytotoxicity (ADCC) reactions
   C. Contain surface immunoglobulins
   D. Secrete the C5 component of complement

4. A lymphokine is
   A. A soluble mediator produced by granulocytes and affecting lymphocytes
   B. A soluble mediator produced by lymphocytes
   C. A soluble mediator produced by plasma cells
   D. A molecule secreted by bacteria that lyses lymphocytes

5. For an antibody-coated antigen to be phagocytized by a monocyte or macrophage, what part of the antibody molecule binds to a receptor on the phagocytic cell?
   A. Fc region
   B. Fab region
   C. Hinge region
   D. Variable region

6. Cell-mediated immunity is primarily mediated by
   A. B cells
   B. T-helper cells
   C. Plasma cells
   D. Dendritic cells

7. Molecules that require T-helper cells to stimulate antibody formation
   A. Antigen
   B. Epitope
   C. Thymic-dependent immunogen
   D. Thymic-independent immunogen

8. Human leukocyte antigens (HLAs) are found on
   A. All nucleated cells
   B. Red blood cells only
   C. Solid tissue only
   D. White blood cells only

9. Which of the following is more likely to be diagnostic of an acute infection?
   A. A total acute antibody titer of 2 followed by a convalescent titer of 16
   B. A total acute antibody titer of 80 followed by a convalescent titer of 40
   C. A total antibody titer of 80
   D. An IgG antibody titer of 80

10. A young woman shows increased susceptibility to pyogenic infections. Upon testing, she shows a low level of C3. Which of the following statements is probably *true?*
    A. She has an autoimmune disease with continual antigen-antibody activity causing consumption of C3.
    B. She has DiGeorge syndrome.
    C. She has decreased production of C3.
    D. She may produce an inactive form of C2, a precursor of C3.

11. What is the predominant type of antibody found in the serum of neonates born after full-term gestation?
    A. Infant IgA
    B. Infant IgG
    C. Infant IgM
    D. Maternal IgG

12. An important part of the nonspecific immune response is(are)
    A. B cells
    B. Dendritic cells
    C. Polymorphonuclear cells (PMNs)
    D. Cytotoxic T lymphocytes (CTLs)

13. The major class of immunoglobulin found in adult human serum is
    A. IgA
    B. IgE
    C. IgG
    D. IgM

14. Which class of immunoglobulin possesses delta heavy chains?
    A. IgA
    B. IgD
    C. IgE
    D. IgG

15. Which class of immunoglobulin possesses 10 antigenic binding sites?
    A. IgA
    B. IgD
    C. IgG
    D. IgM

16. Color Plate 22■ represents a dimeric IgA molecule. The structure printed in red and indicated by the red arrow is called the
    A. J-piece
    B. Hinge region
    C. Heavy chain
    D. Light chain

17. Which class of immunoglobulin binds to basophils and mast cells to mediate immediate hypersensitivity reactions?
    A. IgA
    B. IgD
    C. IgE
    D. IgG

18. Type I hypersensitivity is
    A. Associated with complement-mediated cell lysis
    B. Due to immune complex deposition
    C. Mediated by activated macrophages
    D. An immediate allergic reaction

19. Elevated antithyroglobulin and antithyroid peroxidase are suggestive of
    A. Graves disease
    B. Hashimoto disease
    C. Myasthenia gravis
    D. Multiple sclerosis

20. Severe combined immunodeficiency (SCID) is an
    A. Immunodeficiency with decreased B cells and neutrophils
    B. Immunodeficiency with lymphocytopenia and eosinophilia
    C. Immunodeficiency with decreased or dysfunctional T and B cells
    D. Immunodeficiency with decreased lymphocytes and decreased complement concentration

21. An example of immune injury due to the deposition of antigen-antibody complexes is
    A. Acute glomerulonephritis
    B. Bee-sting allergy
    C. Contact dermatitis
    D. Penicillin allergy

22. The serologically detectable antibody produced in rheumatoid arthritis (RA) is primarily of the class
    A. IgA
    B. IgE
    C. IgG
    D. IgM

23. In bone marrow transplantation, immunocompetent cells in the donor marrow may recognize antigens in the recipient and respond to those antigens. This phenomenon is an example of
    A. Acute rejection
    B. Chronic rejection
    C. Graft-versus-host disease
    D. Hyperacute rejection

24. Multiple myeloma is a
    A. Lymphoproliferative disease of T cells
    B. Cancer of plasma cells characterized by increased antibody concentration
    C. Lymphoproliferative disease resulting in a decrease in antibody production
    D. Cancer of monocytes characterized by increased kappa and lambda chain synthesis

25. Which one of the following describes a direct immunofluorescent assay?
    A. Conjugated reagent antigen reacts with antibodies to form antigen-antibody complexes.
    B. Antigens react with unlabeled antibody-forming antigen-antibody complexes that attach to labeled antibodies.
    C. A dye is attached to a molecule, and it reacts with an immune complex to produce a color.
    D. Conjugated reagent antibody reacts with antigen to form antigen-antibody complexes.

26. In individuals allergic to pollen, hyposensitization protocols may be initiated. These individuals receive injections of
    A. Allergen
    B. Pooled human antisera
    C. Monoclonal antibody directed against human T cells
    D. Monoclonal antibody directed against human B cells

27. After exposure to antigen, the first antibodies that can be detected belong to the class
    A. IgA
    B. IgE
    C. IgG
    D. IgM

28. Corneal tissue may be transplanted successfully from one patient to another because
    A. The cornea is nonantigenic
    B. Corneal antigens do not activate T cells
    C. Anticorneal antibodies are easily suppressed
    D. The cornea occupies a privileged site not usually seen by the immune system

29. A kidney transplant from one identical twin to another is an example of a(n)
    A. Allograft
    B. Autograft
    C. Isograft
    D. Xenograft

30. In Bruton disease, measurement of serum immunoglobulins would show
    A. Elevated levels of IgE
    B. Elevated levels of IgG
    C. Normal levels of IgG and IgM but reduced levels of IgA
    D. The absence of all immunoglobulins

31. Diagnosis of group A streptococci (*Streptococcus pyogenes*) infection is indicated by the presence of
    A. Anti-protein A
    B. Anti-DNase B
    C. Anti-beta-toxin
    D. C-reactive protein (CRP)

32. A molecule found in human serum sometimes used as a tumor marker is
    A. Alpha-fetoprotein (AFP)
    B. HBsAg
    C. Biotin
    D. CD1

33. Which cell is the principal source of interleukin 2?
    A. B cell
    B. T cell
    C. Monocyte
    D. Plasma cell

34. The most specific and sensitive test for the diagnosis of celiac disease
    A. Anti-transglutaminase 2 (TG2) antibody
    B. Anti-acetylcholine receptor antibody
    C. Anti-Smith antibody
    D. Isolation of T cells reactive to pancreatic antigens

35. A major advantage of passive immunization compared to active immunization is that
    A. Antibody is available more quickly
    B. Antibody persists for the life of the recipient
    C. IgM is the predominant antibody class provided
    D. Oral administration can be used

36. The strength with which a multivalent antibody binds a multivalent antigen is termed the
    A. Affinity
    B. Avidity
    C. Reactivity
    D. Valence
37. How does the secondary humoral immune response differ from the primary response?
    A. The lag phase (the time between exposure to immunogen and production of antibody) is longer in the secondary immune response.
    B. IgM is the predominant antibody class produced in the secondary immune response.
    C. The antibody levels produced are higher in the secondary immune response.
    D. Cytotoxic T lymphocytes play an important role in the secondary response.
38. You would expect patients suffering from selective IgA deficiency to present with
    A. Food allergies
    B. Septicemias
    C. Recurrent yeast infections
    D. Recurrent respiratory tract infections
39. The type of immunity that follows the injection of an immunogen is termed
    A. Artificial active
    B. Natural active
    C. Artificial passive
    D. Innate
40. Patients born with an adenosine deaminase deficiency would likely suffer from
    A. Acquired immunodeficiency syndrome (AIDS)
    B. DiGeorge syndrome
    C. Severe combined immunodeficiency
    D. Wiskott-Aldrich syndrome
41. Innate immunity includes
    A. Anamnestic response
    B. Antibody production
    C. Cytotoxic T cell activity
    D. Phagocytosis by polymorphonuclear cells
42. The agglutination pattern shown in Color Plate 23■ was observed while performing an antibody titration. This agglutination pattern is an example of
    A. A prezone reaction
    B. A prozone reaction
    C. A postzone reaction
    D. Incomplete complement inactivation
43. The antibody most frequently present in systemic lupus erythematosus is directed against
    A. Surface antigens of bone marrow stem cells
    B. Surface antigens of renal cells
    C. Nuclear antigen
    D. Myelin
44. The rapid plasma reagin (RPR) assay for syphilis does not need to be read microscopically because the antigen is
    A. Cardiolipin
    B. Complexed with latex
    C. Complexed with charcoal
    D. Inactivated bacterial cells
45. The Venereal Disease Research Laboratory (VDRL) test for syphilis is classified as a(n)
    A. Agglutination reaction
    B. Flocculation reaction
    C. Hemagglutination reaction
    D. Precipitation reaction
46. One cause of a false-positive VDRL test is
    A. Brucellosis
    B. *Treponema pallidum* infection
    C. Rocky Mountain spotted fever
    D. Systemic lupus erythematosus

47. The portion of an antigen that binds to an antibody or T-cell receptor is called a(n)
    A. Allergin
    B. Avidin
    C. Epitope
    D. Valence

48. Identical antibodies produced from a single clone of plasma cells describes
    A. Reagin
    B. Cold agglutinins
    C. Heterophile antibodies
    D. Monoclonal antibodies

49. A 65-year-old male presents with a fractured wrist and complains of bone pain. A bone marrow aspirate reveals a large number of plasma cells. You should suspect
    A. A traumatic bone marrow aspirate collection
    B. Multiple myeloma
    C. Bare lymphocyte syndrome
    D. Hyper-IgM syndrome

50. What is the advantage of using immunofluoresence testing to diagnose systemic lupus erythematosus?
    A. High specificity
    B. Can identify staining patterns
    C. Does not require positive control
    D. Easy to interpret

51. The Fab portion of an antibody
    A. Binds T-cell receptor
    B. Consists of two light chains only
    C. Consists of two heavy chains only
    D. Contains the hypervariable region

52. In the enzyme-linked immunosorbent assay (ELISA), the visible reaction is due to a reaction between
    A. Enzyme and antibody
    B. Enzyme and substrate
    C. Fluorescent dye and antigen
    D. Latex particles and antibody

53. Elevated IgE levels are typically found in
    A. Type I hypersensitivity reactions
    B. Type II hypersensitivity reactions
    C. Type III hypersensitivity reactions
    D. Type IV hypersensitivity reactions

54. Loss of self-tolerance results in
    A. Autoimmune disease
    B. Graft-versus-host disease
    C. Immunodeficiency
    D. Tumors

55. A human cell with CD8 on its surface is most likely a
    A. B cell
    B. Monocyte
    C. T-helper cell
    D. Cytotoxic T cell

56. Which of the following statements about immunoglobulin light chains is *true?*
    A. Each immunoglobulin monomer has either one kappa or one lambda chain.
    B. There are two types: kappa and lambda.
    C. They consist of constant regions only.
    D. They form part of the Fc fragment.

57. Which of the following statements applies to the Fc fragment of an immunoglobulin molecule?
    A. It consists of the entire heavy chain.
    B. It contains the variable region of the heavy chain.
    C. It contains the antigen binding sites of the molecule.
    D. It is the region of the molecule that binds to receptors on various white blood cells.

58. Monoclonal antibodies are produced by
    A. Cultured T cells
    B. Human plasma cells
    C. Mouse plasma cells
    D. Hybridomas

59. Antibodies that bind to the same epitope are of the same
    A. Allotype
    B. Autotype
    C. Idiotype
    D. Isotype

60. Skin testing is a useful diagnostic tool in a number of disorders, such as tuberculosis. Which of the following statements about skin testing is *true?*
    A. A positive test depends on preformed antibody.
    B. Reactivity to a particular antigen may be transferred from one individual to another by sensitized lymphocytes.
    C. The intensity of the response correlates directly with the clinical activity of the disease.
    D. The maximum response will occur immediately.

61. The activity of natural killer (NK) cells
    A. Does not require previous exposure to an antigen
    B. Involves phagocytosis and killing of bacteria
    C. Requires interaction with cytotoxic T cells
    D. Requires interaction with B cells

62. Interaction between B-and T-helper cells involves
    A. MHC II molecule on B cell binding to MHC I molecule on the T cell
    B. MHC II molecule on B cell binding to CD3 on the T cell
    C. Foreign antigen on B cell binding to T-cell receptor
    D. CD3 molecule on B cell binding to T-cell receptor

63. Which of the following is a characteristic of T cells?
    A. Synthesize antibody
    B. Mature in the thymus
    C. Able to bind unprocessed antigen
    D. Primarily protect against extracellular parasites

64. The primary mechanism responsible for pathology in systemic lupus erythematosus is
    A. Allergic reaction to foreign molecules
    B. Antibodies directed against self antigens
    C. Polyclonal activation of cytotoxic T cells
    D. Lack of intracellular killing after neutrophil phagocytosis of bacteria

65. In the complement system
    A. A C3 deficiency would likely be asymptomatic
    B. Antibody is required for the activation of the lectin pathway
    C. C3b is an important opsonin
    D. C9 initiates the membrane attack complex

66. An autoimmune disease causing destruction of pancreatic cells can result in
    A. Hashimoto disease
    B. Multiple sclerosis
    C. Myasthenia gravis
    D. Type 1 diabetes

67. Two unrelated individuals receive the seasonal influenza vaccine. You would expect the two individuals to create antibodies to the immunogens in the vaccine of the same
    A. Allotype
    B. Autotype
    C. Heterotype
    D. Isotype

68. NK cells target altered host cells, such as tumor cells, based on
    A. Altered MHC I molecules on target cell
    B. Altered CD4 molecule on target cell
    C. Interleukin 3 released by target cell
    D. Complement proteins attached to target cell

69. Which of the following complement proteins is part of the membrane attack complex?
    A. C1
    B. C3
    C. C4
    D. C5

70. Which of the following is characteristic of contact dermatitis?
    A. Caused by preformed IgE antibody
    B. Characterized by infiltration of neutrophils into the site of the reaction
    C. The primary symptoms often occur in the respiratory tract.
    D. Usually due to a hapten

71. Which of the following statements about the test for C-reactive protein (CRP) is *true?*
    A. It correlates with neutrophil phagocytic function.
    B. It is an indicator of ongoing inflammation.
    C. It is diagnostic for rheumatic fever.
    D. Levels decrease during heart disease.

72. In the complement classical pathway,
    A. C3 is activated by binding C-reactive protein
    B. The sequence of activation is C1, C2, C3, C4
    C. C1q is activated by the presence of a single Fab region
    D. Activation by antibody requires one IgM or two IgG molecules

73. The alternative complement pathway
    A. Can be activated by bacterial capsule polysaccharides
    B. Uses C5b as a C3 convertase
    C. Bypasses steps C3 through C5 of the classical pathway
    D. Is inactivated by properdin

74. A cut on a person's finger becomes contaminated with the bacterium *Staphylococcus aureus.* The first response by the immune system consists of activity of
    A. B cells
    B. Monocytes
    C. Neutrophils
    D. T cells

75. Incompatible blood transfusions are examples of
    A. Type I hypersensitivity reactions
    B. Type II hypersensitivity reactions
    C. Type III hypersensitivity reactions
    D. Type IV hypersensitivity reactions

76. A soluble antigen and soluble antibody reacting to form an insoluble product describes
    A. Agglutination reactions
    B. Heterophile reactions
    C. Labeled reactions
    D. Precipitation reactions

77. Which of the following is an example of a treponemal antigen test used for the diagnosis of syphilis?
    A. CRP
    B. RPR
    C. VDRL
    D. TP-PA

78. A serum sample is positive for HBsAg. This result indicates that the person from whom the serum was taken
    A. Had a hepatitis B infection in the past but overcame the infection
    B. Has either active or chronic hepatitis B infection
    C. Was immunized recently against the hepatitis B virus (HBV)
    D. Is not infectious for the HBV

79. After adding sensitized sheep red blood cells in the complement fixation test, it is noted that all of the tubes exhibit hemolysis. What does this indicate?
    A. The patient serum was not heat inactivated.
    B. The sensitized red blood cells were unstable.
    C. The incubation temperature was too low.
    D. The patient serum lacked antibodies to the antigen in question.

80. The isotype of an immunoglobulin antibody
    A. Is defined by the heavy chain
    B. Is defined as different alleles of the same antibody type (e.g., IgG)
    C. Is constant for all immunoglobulins of an individual
    D. Is the variation within the variable region

81. A patient report states the presence of serum antibodies to OspC. What disease does the patient most likely have?
    A. Syphilis
    B. Strep throat
    C. Lyme disease
    D. Rubella

82. Identification of cells based on membrane molecules by flow cytometry involves
    A. Fluorescent-labeled antibody
    B. Enzyme-labeled antibody
    C. Peripheral blood cells first separated by Ficoll-Paque
    D. Complement proteins attaching to target cell

83. Hashimoto disease is an autoimmune disease primarily involving the
    A. Kidneys
    B. Liver
    C. Lungs
    D. Thyroid gland

84. Rheumatic fever sometimes occurs after group A streptococcal infections. In this condition, an autoimmune response attacks the endocardium and heart valves. This phenomenon is an example of
    A. Epitope spreading
    B. Molecular mimicry
    C. Polyclonal B cell activation
    D. Preferential activation of T-helper cells

85. "Superantigens" are toxins produced by some strains of *Staphylococcus aureus* and group A streptococci and cause damage by
    A. Molecular mimicry
    B. Polyclonal T cell activation
    C. Lysing white blood cells and platelets
    D. Lysing red blood cells

86. The first serologic marker to appear in patients with acute hepatitis B virus infection is
    A. Anti-HB
    B. Anti-HBc
    C. Anti-HBe
    D. HBsAg

87. A living donor is being sought for a child who requires a kidney transplant. The best odds of finding an MHC-compatible donor occur between the child and
   A. A sibling (brother or sister)
   B. An unrelated individual
   C. The child's father
   D. The child's mother

88. Cells that can act as antigen-presenting cells for exogenous antigens include
   A. All nucleated cells
   B. Endothelial cells
   C. B lymphocytes
   D. T lymphocytes

89. In patients with human immunodeficiency virus (HIV) infection, immune status can be monitored by measuring the ratio of
   A. CD3+ cells to CD8+ cells
   B. CD4+ cells to CD8+ cells
   C. Lymphocytes to monocytes
   D. T cells to B cells

90. Why does vaccination against hepatitis B virus (HBV) also prevent hepatitis D virus (HDV) infections?
   A. An immunogen from HBV in the vaccine is also associated with HDV.
   B. The HBV vaccine induces formation of heterophile antibodies that cross-react with HDV.
   C. The HBV vaccine stimulates liver cells to produce antiviral molecules active against all hepatitis viruses.
   D. HDV requires the host to be concurrently infected with HBV.

91. B lymphocytes and T lymphocytes are derived from
   A. Hematopoietic stem cells
   B. Macrophages or monocytes
   C. Mucosa-associated lymphoid tissue
   D. The fetal liver

92. A patient with suspected human immunodeficiency virus (HIV) infection has a reactive screening test. The secondary tests for anti-HIV-1 and anti-HIV-2 are both nonreactive. Which one of the following should be done?
   A. Repeat testing in 3 months
   B. Perform a western blot on the present sample
   C. Perform an HIV nucleic acid amplification test on the present sample
   D. Notify the primary care provider that the patient has an HIV infection

93. The primary target of human immunodeficiency virus
   A. B cells
   B. Pre–T cells
   C. CD4+ T cells
   D. CD8+ T cells

94. An antibody titration is depicted in Color Plate 24■. In this titration, a 0.2 mL aliquot of a patient's serum sample was added to 0.8 mL of saline, and this mixture was placed into tube #1. A 0.5 mL sample was removed from tube #1 and placed into tube #2, containing 0.5 mL of saline. This procedure was repeated through tube #10. The dilutions were assayed for antibody to an infectious agent. How should the antibody titer be reported?
   A. 256
   B. 512
   C. 640
   D. 1280

95. In a chemiluminescent immunologic assay, what is the signal detected?
   A. Light
   B. An electric signal
   C. A purple-colored compound
   D. A yellow-colored compound

96. A 28-year-old female complains to her family physician of abdominal pain, loss of appetite, and low-grade fever. Physical examination reveals abdominal tenderness and a low-grade fever. Her physician orders a hepatitis profile and obtains the results below.

Anti-HAV	Nonreactive
Anti-HBc	Reactive
Anti-HBs	Nonreactive
HBsAg	Reactive
HBeAg	Reactive
Anti-HCV	Nonreactive

Which of the following is the most likely conclusion?

A. Acute HAV infection
B. Acute HBV infection
C. Chronic HBV infection
D. Immunity to HBV due to past infection

97. An 11-year-old female presents with fever, sore throat, lethargy, and tender cervical lymphadenopathy. Relevant findings include splenomegaly and lymphocytosis, with many reactive lymphocytes. A heterophile antibody test was negative. Further laboratory results were as follows:

	IgG Titer	IgM Titer
Cytomegalovirus (CMV)	20	0
Epstein-Barr virus (EBV) VCA	0	80
Mono spot	0	0

What conclusion can be made concerning the diagnosis?

A. Acute CMV infection
B. Acute EBV infection
C. Chronic CMV infection
D. Chronic EBV infection

98. A male infant had been well until about 5 months of age, at which time he was diagnosed as having otitis media and bronchitis and was treated empirically. Over the next several months he presented with streptococcal pneumonia several times. At 10 months of age, a serum protein electrophoresis showed a virtual lack of gamma globulins. Quantitative serum levels were as follows: 75 mg/dL IgG and undetectable levels of IgM, IgA, and IgE. There were a normal number of T cells, and they exhibited normal mitogen stimulation.
What disease does this child most likely suffer from?

A. Combined immunodeficiency
B. DiGeorge syndrome
C. Iatrogenic immunodeficiency
D. X-linked agammaglobulinemia

99. A 33-year-old female presents to her primary care provider complaining of increased sweating and palpitations over a 3-month period. She has also lost 15 pounds. Examination reveals a swollen thyroid gland. Thyroid study reveals T3 of 4.8 nmol/L (reference range 0.8–2.4 nmol/L), T4 of 48 nmol/L (reference range 9–23 nmol/L), and thyroid-stimulating hormone 0.4 mU/L (reference range 0.4–5 mU/L). The patient likely has

A. Hashimoto disease
B. Addison disease
C. Circulating antibodies to thyroid peroxidase
D. Pituitary gland hyperactivity

100. A 38-year-old woman visited her physician because of fatigue, fever, and joint pain (proximal interphalangeal, wrist, and knee joints). She also noticed sensitivity to the sun and reported having a rash following recent exposure. Laboratory results included white blood cell count $5.5 \times 10^9/L$ (reference range $4.8–10.8 \times 10^9/L$) and red blood cell count $4.5 \times 10^{12}/L$ (reference range $4.0–5.4 \times 10^{12}/L$). Urinalysis results were within reference ranges, except for 4+ protein and 1+ red blood cells (RBCs) 0–3 hyaline casts/lpf and 0–1 RBC cast/lpf on microscopic examination. Which of the following tests would be most helpful in diagnosing this patient's condition?
    A. Anti-nuclear antibody
    B. α-Fetoprotein
    C. Anti-streptolysin O
    D. Hepatitis profile

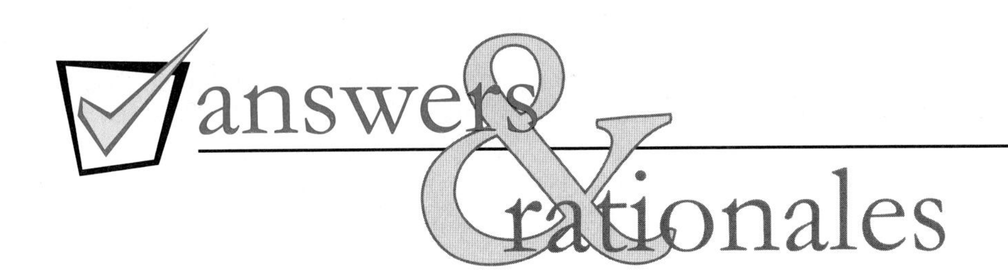

1.

A. The basic structure of all immunoglobulins is two light chains joined to two heavy chains by disulfide bonds. The amino terminus of both the heavy and light chains, together, constitutes the Fab fragment (fragment of antigen binding). The carboxy-terminus of the heavy chains constitutes the Fc fragment. The hinge region is the area at the center of the "Y," near the carboxy-terminus of the light chains.

2.

D. Haptens are substances that are not immunogenic by themselves. These molecules are not large or complex enough to stimulate the immune system. When bound to a carrier, they are capable of stimulating a specific immune response.

3.

C. B cells carry surface immunoglobulins that react to a specific antigen. The antigen can then be internalized processed and presented to an appropriate T-helper cell. B cells are not phagocytic, nor do they participate in antibody-dependent cellular cytotoxicity (ADCC) reactions. Complement proteins are secreted by hepatocytes.

4.

B. Lymphokines are soluble mediators of immune reactions. They are produced most often by T lymphocytes. Antibodies are produced by plasma cells.

5.

A. The Fc region of an IgG molecule fits into an Fc receptor (FcR) on macrophages and monocytes. The FcR binds to specific amino acid residues in the Fc region of the immunoglobulin. The variable region of immunoglobulin binds to the antigen.

6.

B. T-helper cells are the primary mediators of cell-mediated immunity (CMI). They secrete several different lymphokines that stimulate a number of other cells, such as cytotoxic T lymphocytes and monocytes. B cells differentiate into plasma cells during a humoral-mediated immune response. Dendritic cells are important antigen presenting cells (APCs), but they are not the primary mediators of a CMI response.

7.

C. An immunogen is a molecule that stimulates an immune response. Thymic-dependent immunogens require T cell interaction to stimulate B cells to differentiate into plasma cells that produce antibodies. As opposed to thymic-independent activation, when T cells are involved, the reaction produces memory T and B cells.

8.

A. Human leukocyte antigens (HLAs) are a group of antigens originally described on human white blood cells. It is now known that they are found on all nucleated cells of the body, including solid tissue cells. HLAs are not found on red blood cells.

9.

A. The most significant indicator of acute or recent infection is the presence of a rising antibody titer. A fourfold or greater rise in titer, from 2 to 16, is significant. Even relatively high antibody titers of IgG may indicate past infection. IgM is produced first following infections, so a high IgM titer is also suggestive of an acute infection.

10.

C. C3 may be decreased due to a genetic defect that causes deficient production. In certain autoimmune disorders, such as systemic lupus erythematosus (SLE), continual complement activation leads to low levels; however, susceptibility to pyogenic infections is not a feature of autoimmune diseases. DiGeorge syndrome is a deficiency in T cells, and complement protein C2 is not a precursor of C3.

11.

D. Antibody production is immunogen induced. Because the fetus develops in a sequestered site, it makes very little immunoglobulin. Maternal IgG crosses the placenta and is the primary antibody found in infant's circulation.

12.

C. Important parts of an animal's nonspecific immune response include phagocytosis, inflammation, and complement activation. B cells and cytotoxic T lymphocytes respond to specific antigens and are, therefore, involved in the adaptive, specific immune response. Dendritic cells are phagocytic, but their primary role is to present processed antigen to T cells. Polymorphonuclear cells are involved in phagocytosis.

13.

C. Immunoglobulin IgG is the predominant class of immunoglobulin found in serum. It accounts for approximately 80% of the total serum immunoglobulin. The reference range is 800–1600 mg/dL.

14.

B. The heavy chains divide human immunoglobulin molecules into separate classes and subclasses. The delta (Δ) heavy chain is found in IgD. The remaining classes IgA, IgE, IgG, and IgM correspond to α, ε, γ, and μ, respectively.

15.

D. The IgM molecule is a pentamer that contains 10 binding sites. However, the actual valence falls to five with larger antigen molecules, probably because of steric restrictions. IgA, IgG, IgD, and IgE monomers each has two antigenic binding sites.

16.

A. IgA is found in mucous secretions as a dimer stabilized by the J-piece. IgA is synthesized locally by plasma cells and dimerized intracellularly. IgM is also held together by a J-piece, but it exists as a pentamer.

17.

C. Mast cells and basophils have surface receptors (FcεRI) for the Fc portion of IgE. When IgE molecules, attached to the surface of mast cells and basophils, bind the allergen they are specific for, this triggers the cells to degranulate, producing the symptoms of immediate type I hypersensitivity. The main function of IgE appears to be the ability to trigger an immune response, thereby recruiting plasma factors and effector cells to areas of trauma or parasite infection.

18.

D. Type I hypersensitivity reactions occur immediately after second exposure to an allergen. On the first, or primary, exposure, IgE specific to the allergen is produced. The IgE binds to Fc receptors on the surface of basophils and mast cells. Immune complexes and complement are not involved in the response.

19.

B. Hashimoto disease is characterized by autoantibodies directed against thyroid antigens thyroglobulin and thyroid peroxidase. In Graves disease, T3 and T4 are elevated due to an autoantibody that mimics the activity of thyroid stimulating hormone (TSH). Patients with myasthenia gravis produce antibodies to acetylcholine receptors. Damage to the myelin sheath of nerve cells occurs in multiple sclerosis due to T cells and autoantibodies.

20.

C. SCID is defined as a condition in which adaptive immune responses (i.e., cell-mediated and humoral-mediated immune responses) do not occur because of a lack of T and B cell activity. A number of genetic defects can lead to this condition. Children born with SCID need to live in a sterile environment, and they have a short life expectancy.

21.

A. Acute glomerulonephritis is caused by the presence of a soluble circulating antigen (Ag) that provokes and combines with antibody (Ab). As these Ag-Ab complexes reach a critical size, they are deposited in the glomerular membranes of the kidney. Upon deposition, an acute inflammatory reaction occurs because of complement activation. Bee-sting and penicillin allergies are examples of IgE-mediated anaphylactic reactions. Contact dermatitis is mediated by T cells, not antibody.

22.

D. Rheumatoid factor (RF) is an immunoglobulin that reacts with antigenic determinants on an IgG molecule. Although they may be of several types, the one that is easily serologically detectable is IgM. This is because of the agglutination activity of the molecule. RF tests are commonly used in the diagnosis of rheumatoid arthritis.

23.

C. Bone marrow transplants by their nature contain immunologically competent cells: B cells and T cells in particular. Unless the transplanted marrow is HLA-matched perfectly to the donor, the immunocompetent cells in the transplant will recognize and react against the nonself HLAs of the recipient's tissues. This phenomenon is known as graft-versus-host disease, because the graft attempts to reject its host. Acute rejection, chronic rejection, and hyperacute rejection are examples of mechanisms a recipient's immune system uses to reject a graft.

24.

B. Plasma cells are normally end-stage cells; they live a few days and die. During multiple myeloma, plasma cells become cancerous and continue to secrete antibody. The cells also secrete excess light chains that can be found in the urine; these proteins are called Bence Jones proteins.

25.

D. In a direct immunofluorescence assay, a fluorescent molecule is linked to an antibody. This complex is often called a conjugate. Clinical material is fixed onto a microscope slide, and the conjugate is added. After a wash step, the slide is examined with a microscope using UV light. If antigen specific to antibody was present in the clinical specimen, fluorescence will be seen.

26.

A. Hyponsensitization, allergy injections, involves the administration of gradually increasing concentrations of an allergen. The goal is for the patient to become tolerant of the allergen and no longer exhibit an allergic response to the allergen. It is hypothesized that patients will ultimately develop high concentrations of IgG to the allergen, blocking IgE from binding and thereby preventing the allergic reaction.

27.

D. The first B cells to respond to antigen differentiate into plasma cells that produce IgM antibody. Later in the immune response, stimulated B cells undergo a phenomenon called "class switching" and begin to produce antibodies of the IgG, IgA, and IgE classes. High concentration of IgM in patient serum is indicative of a recent infection.

28.

D. Corneas are readily transplanted from one individual to another. This is because the cornea is nonvascularized and is a sequestered site. Thus, the immune system of the host does not "see" the cornea and recognize it as foreign.

29.

C. Identical twins have the same genetic makeup. Grafts between them would be isografts or syngeneic grafts. Autografts are transplantations from one site to another in the same individual. Xenograft refers to transplantation between different species. Transplantation between two nonidentical individuals of the same species is called an allograft.

30.

D. Bruton disease is a congenital form of agammaglobulinemia. It is a sex-linked phenomenon that affects males. Because B cells are not produced, affected males have levels of IgA, IgD, IgE, and IgM undetectable by routine assays. IgG may be absent or present at very low levels.

31.

B. The serologic diagnosis of group A streptococcal infection can be made by demonstrating anti-DNase B. The antistreptolysin O (ASO) assay can also be used; however, ASO response is poor in skin infections. C-reactive protein is an acute-phase protein indicating inflammation.

32.

A. α-Fetoprotein (AFP) and carcinoembryonic antigen are oncofetal antigens that become expressed after malignant transformation. Approximately 70% of patients with primary hepatoma have elevated levels of AFP. However, the major use of determining AFP levels is in monitoring patients undergoing cancer treatment.

33.

B. Interleukin 2 (IL-2) is a lymphokine produced by activated T-helper cells. IL-2 principally affects T cells, including the cell that released IL-2, acting on its target cells via the IL-2 receptor. This receptor is not present on resting cells.

34.

A. Celiac disease is characterized by antibody directed against transglutaminase 2 (TG2). There are also CD4+ T cells that bind to modified gluten proteins bound to human leukocyte antigens on the surface of antigen presenting cells. Anti-acetylcholine receptor antibody is seen in patients with myasthenia gravis. Anti-Smith antibody is a specific but low sensitivity test for systemic lupus erythematosus (SLE). Type 1 diabetes is characterized by T cells reactive to pancreatic antigens.

35.

A. In passive immunization, preformed antibody is delivered to the recipient, making the antibody available immediately. In active immunization, a period of days is required before antibody production occurs. Passive immunity is short-lived, in contrast to the possibly lifelong persistence of actively induced antibody. Because passive immunization involves the transfer of antibodies, the oral route cannot be used—antibodies are digested in the gastrointestinal tract. The antibodies administered by passive immunization consist largely of the IgG class.

36.

B. "Avidity" is used to describe the strength of binding between a multivalent antibody and multivalent antigen. "Affinity" describes the bond between a single antigenic determinant and an individual combining site. "Valence" refers to the number of antigenic determinants on an antigen.

37.

C. The secondary immune response is characterized by the predominance of IgG over IgM. In addition, because of the formation of memory cells following the primary response, the secondary response occurs much more quickly and strongly. This is the basis for immunization as a protection against various infectious diseases. Cytotoxic T lymphocytes are not involved in humoral immunity.

38.

D. IgA is present in high concentration on mucous membranes, such as lining the respiratory tract. This is the point of entry of most respiratory tract pathogens. Patients with deficiencies in certain complement proteins, such as C3 and C5, are more prone to septicemias. Patients with a defect in cell-mediated immunity would be expected to have increased risk of yeast infection.

39.

A. Active immunity follows exposure to an immunogen that stimulates the recipient to develop his or her own immune response. Vaccines are an example of artificial immunity in that the animal was exposed to the immunogen by the actions of a healthcare provider (unnatural). Surviving infections can result in natural active immunity. Protection is due to the formation of memory cells.

40.

C. An adenosine deaminase deficiency results in the accumulation of toxic metabolites in cells. Lymphocytes are most sensitive, thus resulting in the absence of these important immune cells. This results in severe combined immunodeficiency, where the individual cannot mount a cell-mediated immune response or a humoral-mediated immune response.

41.

D. Innate, or nonspecific, immunity refers to host defenses that are in general present at birth and do not require immunogen stimulation. Phagocytosis of bacteria by polymorphonuclear cells is an example. Cytotoxic T cell activity is part of the adaptive cell-mediated immune response, and antibody production is the mechanism of protection in the adaptive humoral-mediated immune response.

42.

B. Prozone occurs when an extremely high titer of antibody is present. In the first tubes of the titration, not enough antigen is present to allow for cross-linking and lattice formation. The antibody effectively blocks all the antigen sites present, so agglutination does not occur. Complement is not involved in antibody titration.

43.

C. Antinuclear antibody (ANA) is the most consistent feature of SLE. Although renal or nerve pathology may occur, that pathology is secondary to deposition of antigen-antibody complexes and subsequent activation of complement proteins. Bone marrow stems cells are not involved in the pathology of SLE.

44.

C. The rapid plasma reagin (RPR) and Venereal Disease Research Laboratory (VDRL) tests use a cardiolipin antigen. However, in the RPR test, charcoal particles are included with the antigen. When antibody in the patient sample combines with the antigen, the charcoal is trapped in the immune complex, allowing the reaction to be read macroscopically.

45.

B. The cardiolipin antigen is particulate, not soluble, in the VDRL test. However, the particles are too small to make macroscopic agglutinates when combined with antibody. This type of reaction is called a flocculation reaction and needs to be read with low-power microscopy.

46.

D. Patients with connective tissue disorders such as SLE may show a false-positive reaction in the VDRL test. Other causes of false positives include rheumatic fever, infectious mononucleosis, malaria, and pregnancy. *Treponema pallidum* subsp. *pallidum* is the causative agent of syphilis.

47.

C. Antigens can have multiple epitopes. Each epitope can be unique, binding an antibody with a different idiotype. "Valence" refers to the number of epitopes on an antigen.

48.

D. Monoclonal antibodies are derived from a single clone of plasma cells. Plasma cells are fused with a cancerous myeloma cell. Reagin has two meanings: it can refer to the antibody produced during syphilis or it can refer to IgE. Cold agglutinins are antibodies that agglutinate in cold temperatures (e.g., 4°C). Heterophile antibodies are antibodies produced following exposure to an immunogen that are able to bind a similar but different molecule.

49.

B. Multiple myeloma occurs more frequently in men than women and has an average age of onset of 70 years. The disease is characterized by an increase in plasma cells. These abnormal plasma cells, unlike normal plasma cells, divide and spread to the bone marrow. This results in lytic bone lesions, bone pain, and increased risk for fractures.

50.

B. Testing for ANAs is commonly performed by the immunofluorescence method—using fluorescein-conjugated antihuman antibody to detect patient antibody bound to nuclear components of test cells. These assays are very sensitive but in general have a low specificity. However, a homogenous pattern suggests SLE. Disadvantages include the need for a dark room and fluorescent microscope and expertise in evaluating the stained slides.

51.

D. The Fab portion of an antibody contains the hypervariable region. This portion of the molecule has a variable sequence of amino acids that affects the three-dimensional structure of the molecule and, therefore, determines the specificity (idiotype) of the antibody. This region contains the amino terminal portion of the two light chains and the two heavy chains.

52.

B. The indicator system in an ELISA test consists of an enzyme and its substrate. If the enzyme-labeled antibody has complexed with the immobilized antigen, the addition of substrate will produce a colored end product. Alkaline phosphatase is an enzyme frequently used in ELISA tests. Latex particles, fluorescent dyes, and red blood cells are not used in ELISA tests but in other test methodologies.

53.

A. Elevated IgE levels are found in type I hypersensitivity reactions. The antibody binds via the Fc portion of the molecule to Fc receptors on mast cells and basophils. When the attached antibody binds its specific allergen, the cell degranulates.

54.

A. The immune system recognizes host cells as self and is tolerant to antigens on those cells. The loss of tolerance will result in an autoimmune disease in which the immune system mounts an immune response against self cells. Graft-versus-host disease occurs when a bone marrow graft is incompatible with the host tissue and attacks the host.

55.

D. The CD8 molecule is found primarily on cytotoxic T cells, also called cytotoxic T lymphocytes. T-helper cells possess CD4 on their surface, as do several other cell types. CD3 is a marker found on most T cells.

56.

B. Light chains are of two distinct types: kappa and lambda. Either type may combine with any of the heavy chains, but in any one molecule, only one type of light chain is found. Therefor, each immunoglobulin monomer contains two light chains, either kappa or lambda. They extend into the Fab, or antigen-binding, site. This half of the chain is highly variable, whereas the carboxy-terminal portion of the molecule is a constant region.

57.

D. The Fc (crystalline) fragment of an immunoglobulin is produced by papain digestion of an immunoglobulin monomer. The Fc portion of antibodies binds to specific Fc receptors on the surface of some white blood cells. Only part of the heavy chain is found in the Fc fragment. The Fab fragment contains the antigen-combining sites of both the heavy chains and the light chains.

58.

D. A monoclonal antibody is produced by a single cell or clone. Plasma cells obtained from an immunized animal and subsequently fused with myeloma cells result in a hybrid myeloma or hybridoma that will indefinitely secrete a specific antibody. Hybridomas have been prepared from mouse and human plasma cells fused with myeloma cells. T cells do not produce antibodies.

59.

C. Idiotype of an antibody refers to the antigen specificity of the molecule. The isotype is the different classes and subclasses of antibodies (e.g., IgG, IgM, etc.). "Allotype" refers to different alleles of the same isotype. Genetically different individuals will produce antibodies of the same isotype, but they would have a different allotype.

60.

B. Skin testing is based upon the presence of T cells sensitized to antigen. Their activation produces a delayed hypersensitivity reaction, which reaches its peak in about 48 hours. There is no correlation of the amount of the reaction with clinical disease. If the sensitized T cells are transferred from one individual to another, the recipient individual will manifest the same delayed hypersensitivity as the donor.

61.

A. The natural killer (NK) cells destroy target cells through an extracellular nonphagocytic mechanism. NK cells are part of the host's innate resistance and, therefore, do not need previous exposure to an antigen to be active. They also do not need interaction with B or cytotoxic T cells.

62.

C. B cells have the ability to present antigen (immunogen) to T-helper cells. This interaction involves several surface molecules. The antigen is complexed with MHC II on the surface of the B cell. CD4 on the T cell interacts with MHC II, whereas T-cell receptor binds the antigen.

63.

B. T cells are produced in the bone marrow and mature in the thymus. Plasma cells, not T cells, produce antibody, and T cells can only react to antigen processed by an antigen-presenting cell. The cell-mediated immune response, which requires the activity of T cells, is primarily helpful in fighting against intracellular parasites.

64.

B. Antibodies directed against self antigens form immune complexes and activate complement. Circulating immune complexes, composed of nuclear antigen and antinuclear antibody, deposit in various organ systems, activate complement, and produce organ pathology. T cells are not directly involved in this process. Allergens, phagocytosis, and killing of ingested bacteria by neutrophils do not play a role in the pathogenic process.

65.

C. C3 is key to all three pathways. A decrease in this protein would likely lead to increase rate of infection and difficulty clearing immune complexes. The membrane attack complex is initiated by C5 binding to C4b2a3b on a cell membrane. Only the classical pathway requires antibody for activation. C3b receptors (complement receptor 1, CR1) are found on neutrophils and monocytes and add phagocytosis of C3b-coated bacteria and immune complexes.

66.

D. Destruction of the beta cells in the pancreas results in type 1 diabetes. An autoimmune response destroys the insulin-producing cells. The immune response is probably due to molecular mimicry. Cytotoxic T cells and antibodies directed against an infectious agent cross-react to the beta cells.

67.

D. Isotype is the class of antibody. Everyone receiving the vaccine would be expected to make IgG. Individuals would also make antibody of the same idiotype; this is what determines the specificity to the immunogens in the vaccine.

68.

A. NK cells target cells for destruction based on altered or absent MHC I molecules. Approximately 50% of tumor cells have mutations in the gene coding for MHC I molecules. NK cells are part of the innate immune response and do not need prior exposure to a molecule to respond.

69.

D. The membrane attack complex forms following the binding of C5b to a biologic membrane. The complex is formed by the sequential addition of C6, C7, C8, and C9. When C5b–C8 forms a complex with C9, a tubule is formed that bridges the cell membrane.

70.

D. Contact dermatitis is a cell-mediated hypersensitivity reaction. The offending substance is typically a hapten that combines with a carrier molecule on the skin surface. The hapten-carrier complex is recognized by T cells. IgE mediates immediate hypersensitivity reactions such as hay fever and some forms of asthma.

71.

B. CRP is an acute-phase reactant. Although it is elevated in inflammation, its presence is not diagnostic for any one disease, such as rheumatic fever. It does not correlate with antibody levels or with neutrophil phagocytic function. CRP levels are sometimes elevated during heart disease.

72.

D. Complement attaches to the Fc portion of the antibody molecule. At least two Fc binding sites are required for C1q to attach. Therefore, activation requires two IgG molecules or a single molecule of IgM, which is a pentamer. The C proteins were named in order of discovery. The correct reaction sequence is C1, C4, C2, C3. As the last step of this reaction sequence, C3 is split into C3a and C3b.

73.

A. The alternative pathway for complement activation is a nonspecific defense mechanism, in that it does not require the presence of antibody for activation. It can be activated by a variety of substances, including complex polysaccharides found in bacterial capsules and cell walls. These materials activate C3 directly. Properdin protein stabilizes some of the active complement proteins, and C4b2a is a C3 convertase.

74.

C. The first response to invading bacteria is mounted by the innate immune system. The innate immune system, although it lacks the specificity of the adaptive immune system, is nonetheless effective at handling many invading bacteria. The first response by the innate immune system consists of an influx of neutrophils into the tissue invaded by bacteria. Monocytes and macrophages, although they are phagocytic cells and part of the innate immune system, play only a minor role in the initial response to bacterial invasion.

75.

B. Incompatible blood transfusions are examples of a type II hypersensitivity reaction. These reactions are characterized as the antigen being a part of a cell. Antibody binds to the antigen, complement is activated, and the red blood cells are lysed.

76.

D. Precipitation reactions involve both soluble antigens and antibodies. These reactions are typically detected in agarose gels. With agglutination reactions, one of the reactants is soluble and the other is insoluble. A reactant is made insoluble by combining with a carrier particle such as latex beads.

77.

D. The *Treponema pallidum*-particulate antigen (TP-PA) test is currently the most commonly used confirmatory serologic test for syphilis. *Treponema pallidum* subsp. *pallidum*, the causative agent of syphilis, is the source of the antigen. The rapid plasma reagin (RPR) and Venereal Disease Research Laboratory (VDRL) are diagnostic tests for syphilis that use nontreponemal antigen. C-reactive protein (CRP) is not involved in syphilis testing.

78.

B. Hepatitis B surface antigen (HBsAg) is a marker for active or chronic infection by the hepatitis B virus; it indicates ongoing viral replication. A person positive for this marker is infectious. If the person had overcome a past infection, he or she would have antibody to the surface antigen (anti-HBs) but not the surface antigen. Immunization causes formation of anti-HBs antibody, and the surface antigen would not be present in serum.

79.

D. The first step in the complement fixation test, the test system, involves the reaction of antibody in the patient's serum to the corresponding antigen in the presence of guinea pig complement. If antibody-antigen binding occurs, complement will bind to the immune complexes. The second step is the addition of sensitized sheep red blood cells (the indicator system). If complement bound to the immune complexes in the first step, it is not available to lyse the sensitized red blood cells. If antibody was not present in the patient sample, complement will not bind to the immune complexes, and it will be free to lyse the sensitized cells. Therefore, hemolysis indicates no antibody was present.

80.

A. The isotype of an antibody is determined by which heavy chain is present. The term "idiotype" refers to the variable region of an immunoglobulin molecule. The variable region is the portion of immunoglobulin that binds antigen. Every immunoglobulin with a given antigenic specificity has a single idiotype.

81.

C. IgM antibody to OspC is an important early marker in the diagnosis of Lyme disease. This antibody, along with several others, is often detected by western blot. Antibodies to p35, p39, and the flagellin subunits p37 and p41 are also useful in diagnosing this disease.

82.

A. In order to identify cells in a mixed population by flow cytometry, the cells are first stained with fluorescent-labeled antibody. These antibodies are directed against known markers (molecules) on the plasma membrane. For example, CD3 is a T-cell co-receptor found on T-helper cells and cytotoxic T cells.

83.

D. Hashimoto disease is a type of thyroiditis due to an autoimmune disease. Patients produce autoantibodies and T cells that respond to thyroid antigens. This results in inflammation and swelling of the thyroid gland (goiter). The autoantibody blocks the uptake of iodine, which results in a decrease in the production of thyroid hormones (hypothyroidism).

84.

B. Group A streptococci contain antigenic determinants that are similar to antigenic determinants found on heart valve tissue in some individuals. The immune response occurring during the course of a group A streptococcal infection may be extensive enough to include an immune-mediated attack on the heart valves—rheumatic heart disease. "Molecular mimicry" is the term given to this phenomenon, whereby an immune response directed against one antigen may be extended to include activity against closely related antigens.

85.

B. Some strains of *Staphylococcus aureus* and group A streptococci produce toxins that have the properties of "superantigens." Superantigens react with T cells directly without processing by an antigen presenting cell. These toxins can stimulate many T cells, rather than only those T cells bearing T cell receptors specific for the bacterial toxins. The result is a massive T-cell response, leading to the release of cytokines and resulting in disease entities known as toxic shock syndrome (in the case of *S. aureus* infection) and toxic shock–like syndrome in the case of group A streptococci.

86.

D. HBsAg is the first serologic marker occurring in patients with hepatitis B virus infection. The antigen appears about 3–5 weeks before symptoms appear. About 2–4 weeks later, anti-HBc, primarily of the IgM class, begins to appear.

87.

A. Because the human leukocyte antigen (HLA) system is extremely polymorphic, the odds are greatly against finding an HLA-compatible donor in unrelated individuals. The genes coding for HLA antigens are inherited from one's parents and are expressed co-dominantly. Between an offspring and either parent, there is, statistically, a 25% chance of an HLA match. Between siblings, there is a 50% chance of an HLA match.

88.

C. Exogenous antigens are nonself antigens derived from infectious agents or immunizing preparations. Exogenous antigens are processed for presentation to specific T cells by specialized cells collectively referred to as antigen-presenting cells (APCs). APCs for exogenous antigens include B cells, macrophages, monocytes, and dendritic cells. B cells are not phagocytic, so they bind and internalize molecules not intact bacteria or viruses.

89.

B. Human immunodeficiency virus (HIV) preferentially infects T-helper cells, which are positive for the surface marker CD4. As the infection progresses, the number of CD4+ cells in the peripheral bloodstream decrease. CD8 is a marker found on another subset of T cells, cytotoxic T cells. The reference ratio of CD4:CD8 cells is 2:1. A decrease in the ratio indicates a decline in immune function.

90.

D. HDV requires HBsAg produced by HBV-infected cells. HDV, therefore, requires the host to be concurrently infected with HBV. The HBV vaccine prevents HBV infection and also HDV infection.

91.

A. Stem cells of the bone marrow give rise to both T and B cells, as well as other cells in the bloodstream. Macrophages and monocytes also arise from hematopoietic stem cells, but they do not differentiate into lymphocytes. Mucosa-associated lymphoid tissue contains mature lymphocytes, particularly B cells, but is not the source of lymphocytes. The fetal liver is a maturation site for B lymphocytes during fetal life but is not the source of those lymphocytes.

92.

C. Serum samples reactive on screening tests and negative on secondary HIV tests should be followed up by nucleic acid amplification test for HIV. The current screening tests are combination assays that detect both anti-HIV antibody and the viral protein p24. These patients could have a recent infection and have not yet produced antibodies. It generally takes about 12 weeks before detectable levels of antibody are present.

93.

C. HIV uses CD4 as a receptor for binding to target cells. While CD4 is found on other cells, for example, monocytes and macrophages, HIV preferentially infects T-helper cells. Initially, HIV is likely to encounter monocytes and macrophages and can use these cells to travel to various body sites including lymph nodes.

94.

C. The titer of this assay is the reciprocal of the highest dilution demonstrating the desired result, in this case tube #8. The dilution is determined as shown below.

Dilution for tube #1: 0.2 mL serum in a total volume of 1.0 mL = 1:5 dilution.

Dilutions in succeeding tubes: 0.5 mL diluted serum in a total volume of 1.0 mL = 1:2 dilution.

The dilutions in the series of tubes are as follows:

Tube #1, 1:5; tube #2, 1:10; tube #3, 1:20; tube #4, 1:40; tube #5, 1:80; tube #6, 1:160; tube #7, 1:320; tube #8, 1:640; tube #9, 1:1280; tube #10, 1:2560

The reciprocal of the dilution in tube #8 (1:640) is 640.

95.

A. In chemiluminescent assays, light is the end product. These assays require special instruments, luminometers, to measure the light emitted in the reaction. Chemicals used to generate light include luminol and luciferase.

96.

C. The presence of HBsAg indicates viral replication and that the patient is infectious; this marker can be seen in both acute and chronic infections. The lack of anti-HBs indicates that the patient is not immune to the infection. The presence of anti-HBc and HBeAg with HBsAg indicates a chronic infection.

97.

B. The symptoms of fever, lymphocytosis, and lymphadenopathy suggest EBV or CMV infection and lymphoma or leukemia. Heterophile antibodies become positive later than antibodies to viral core antigen (VCA) of EBV. In addition, only about 50% of children less than 12 years of age form heterophile antibodies following EBV infection. The IgM titer of 80 for EBV is consistent with acute EBV infection.

98.

D. The case history is typical of a child with X-linked agammaglobulinemia. He presented with chronic and recurrent infections beginning at 5 months of age, when transplacentally acquired IgG had declined. Normal IgG serum level is about 800–1200 mg/dL. The infant had normal T cell function, which rules out combined immunodeficiency and DiGeorge syndrome. "Iatrogenic immunodeficiency" refers to an immunodeficiency following therapy prescribed by a physician.

99.

C. Graves disease is due to an autoantibody bound to a thyroid receptor resulting in thyroid hyperactivity. This results in elevated T3 and T4 levels. Because the antibody functions like thyroid-stimulating hormone (TSH), the pituitary gland secretes less TSH, so levels are low. Approximately 75% of patients with Graves disease have antithyroid peroxidase antibodies.

100.

A. The presence of arthritis is suggestive of a number of autoimmune diseases. Protein, RBCs, and casts in the urine are indicative of kidney inflammation. These signs and symptoms along with the rash on the face are characteristic of SLE. A commonly used sensitive screening test for SLE is the ANA test. The ANA, however, is not specific for SLE. If the ANA were positive, additional autoantibody tests specific for SLE (e.g., anti-Smith) should be performed.

REFERENCES

Male, D., Brostoff, J., Roth, D. B., and Roitt, I. (2012). *Immunology*, 8th ed. Philadelphia: Elsevier.

Carroll, K. C., et al. (Eds.) (2019). *Manual of Clinical Microbiology*, 12th ed. Washington, DC: ASM Press.

Murray, P. R., Rosenthal, K. S., and Pfaller, M. A. (2015). *Medical Microbiology*, 8th ed. Philadelphia: Elsevier.

Stevens, C. D., and Miller, L. E. (2017). *Clinical Immunology & Serology*, 4th ed. Philadelphia: F. A. Davis.

Turgeon, M. L. (2018). *Immunology and Serology in Laboratory Medicine*, 6th ed. Philadelphia: Elsevier.

CHAPTER

5 Immunohematology

contents

I. OVERVIEW

A. Definition: Immunohematology is the study of blood group antigens and antibodies, human leukocyte antigens (HLAs) and antibodies, pretransfusion testing, identification of unexpected alloantibodies, immune hemolysis, autoantibodies, drugs, blood collection, blood components, cryopreservation of blood, transfusion-transmitted viruses, tissue banking and organ transplantation, blood transfusion practice, safety, quality assessment, records, blood inventory management, and blood usage review.

B. Immune System

1. **Acquired immunity** is a **specific response** of the immune system in which antibodies specific to a particular immunogen or antigen are produced. **Plasma cells** produce **antibodies.**
2. **Innate immunity** is a **nonspecific reaction** of the immune system that attacks all invaders in a similar manner. It includes physical and biochemical barriers and cells such as leukocytes, including neutrophils, monocytes/macrophages, and natural killer cells. Physical barriers include intact skin, mucous membranes, etc. Bactericidal enzymes are also biochemical barriers.

C. Antigen Characteristics

1. **Antigens** are substances that **combine with** an **antibody**. An **antigen** that causes a **specific immune response** is an **immunogen.** Immunogens are made of protein, carbohydrates, and combinations of both. Antigens are found on the surface of platelets and **white blood cells (WbCs) as well as red blood cells (RBCs)**. Some immunogens produce a greater response than others.
2. There are **23 RBC antigen systems** containing over 200 RBC antigens. RBC antigens are inherited and are composed of proteins, glycoproteins, and glycolipids.
3. **HLAs**
   a. Present on **leukocytes** and **tissue cells**
   b. **Genes** that encode the **HLAs** are part of the **major histocompatibility complex** (MHC).
   c. The **MHC** is on chromosome 6 and is divided into **Class I, II,** and **III.**
      1) **Class I** includes loci A, B, and C.
      2) **Class II** includes loci DR, DP, and DQ.
      3) **Class III** includes complement proteins.
   d. Immune response to transfused incompatible HLA antigens cause fever and chills. This is known as a febrile, nonhemolytic transfusion reaction.
   e. **HLAs** must be matched for **organ, tissue, bone marrow,** and **stem cell transplant** between donors and recipients. If the recipient is not matched correctly, a severe **graft-versus-host disease** results.
   f. **HLA test applications** include paternity testing, organ and tissue transplantation, bone marrow and stem cell transplantation, and platelet matching.

4. **Platelet antigens**
   a. Membranes have **protein antigens**.
   b. **Platelet antibodies** occur less frequently in the general population because of less antigen variability.
   c. Antibodies reacting with platelets may be ABO, HLA, or platelet specific.
   d. **Diseases:** Neonatal alloimmune thrombocytopenia and posttransfusion purpura

D. Antibody Characteristics

1. **Molecular structure**
   a. Each molecule has **two heavy** chains and **two light** chains.
   b. The **heavy chain** is responsible for the immunoglobulin **class specificity**. There are five classes of human antibodies: IgM, IgG, IgA, IgE, and IgD.
   c. The **antibody binding site** is found in the **variable region** of the heavy and light chains.
2. **IgM antibodies**
   a. Composed of five basic immunoglobulin units (pentamer)
   b. Can directly bind with RBCs and produce agglutination
   c. Can activate complement
   d. Cannot cross the placenta because of large size of molecule
   e. React optimally at room temperature and below
   f. Except in the case of the ABO blood group system, typically clinically insignificant
3. **IgG antibodies**
   a. Single immunoglobulin unit
   b. Cannot visibly agglutinate RBCs
   c. Cannot activate complement unless two molecules are present (i.e., IgG3)
   d. Can cross the placenta
   e. React optimally at 37°C
   f. Typically clinically significant; capable of causing transfusion reactions or hemolytic disease of the newborn (HDN)

E. Antigen–Antibody Interactions

1. Follow the law of mass action
2. Reversible
3. Antigen–antibody complex formed
4. Properties that influence antigen–antibody interactions are as follows:
   a. Antigen fits into antibody binding site (variable region)
   b. Size of antigen
   c. Shape of antigen
   d. Charge of antigen
5. **Antigen–antibody complexes** are held together by electrostatic charges, hydrogen bonding, hydrophobic bonding, and Van der Waals forces.

F. Antigen–Antibody Reactions *In Vivo*

1. **Transfusions** can lead to antigen–antibody complex formation and complement activation *in vivo*, if wrong blood type is transfused.
2. Transfusion of foreign antigens (RBC, HLA, and platelet) into a recipient can cause an immune response and antibody formation in the recipient (**alloantibodies**).
3. Antigen–antibody complexes are removed by the reticuloendothelial system: spleen, liver, and lymph nodes.

G. Antigen–Antibody Reaction *In Vitro*

1. Reactions are detected by **agglutination** or **hemolysis**.
2. Some antigen–antibody complexes require two stages for detection: **sensitization** and **lattice** formation.
    a. **Sensitization:** Antibody attaches to antigen but does not produce visible agglutination or hemolysis.
        1) **Factors affecting first stage of agglutination**
            a) **Serum-to-cell ratio:** This is the amount of antibody compared to the number of cells in solution. Increased amount of serum equals an increase in the number of antibodies in the solution.
            b) **Reaction temperature:** This is the temperature at which the antibody reacts best; most clinically important antibodies react best at **37°C**.
            c) **Incubation time:** This is the time allowed for the antibody to attach to the antigen. This reaction occurs by chance. Times will vary according to the antibody and media used *in vitro* (i.e., albumin, LISS—low-ionic-strength saline).
            d) **pH:** The optimal pH for *in vitro* reactions is 7.
    b. **Lattice formation:** Random collisions of antibody-coated RBCs link antibodies together to form visual agglutination.
        1) **Factors affecting visual agglutination**
            a) **Reaction temperature**
            b) **Incubation time**
            c) **pH**
            d) **Repelling negative charges:** In normal saline, RBCs have a net negative charge that repels other RBCs in solution. This charge inhibits agglutination.
3. **Antigen and antibody agglutination**
    a. **Zone of equivalence:** Antigen and antibody concentrations produce maximum agglutination.
    b. **Prozone (antibody excess):** Too much antibody compared with antigen concentration
    c. **Post-zone (antigen excess):** Too much antigen compared with antibody concentration

4. **Grading agglutination reactions**
   a. To standardize the strength of agglutination reactions:
      1) **4+ RBC button** is solid with a clear supernatant.
      2) **3+ RBC button** breaks into several large clumps, with a clear supernatant.
      3) **2+ RBC button** breaks into many medium-sized clumps, with a clear supernatant.
      4) **1+ RBC button** breaks into many medium- and small-sized clumps, with background having many free RBCs (appears cloudy).
      5) **$+^{w}$ RBC button** breaks into many clumps, barely or not visible macroscopically, with many RBCs in the background (use microscope to see clumps).
      6) **0 = no agglutinated RBCs**
5. **Hemolysis** is another indication of antibody–antigen reactions and is caused by **complement activation**. The supernatant appears clear red, with a smaller or nonexistent RBC button.

II. GENETICS

A. Definitions

1. **Chromosomes:** Structures that carry genetic information encoded on double-stranded DNA
2. **Mitosis:** Process of cell division that results in the same number of chromosomes in the new and parent cells
3. **Meiosis:** Process of cell division that occurs in gametes resulting in one-half the chromosomes in each new cell
4. **Blood group systems:** Groups of related RBC antigens inherited according to Mendelian genetics
5. **Phenotype:** Physical, observable expression of inherited traits; detectable products
6. **Genotype:** Inherited genes; actual genetic makeup
7. **Pedigree chart:** Visual map that displays a family history and can display inheritance patterns for individual traits
8. **Gene:** Smallest unit of inheritance
9. **Genetic locus:** Site on chromosome where specific genes are located
10. **Alleles:** Alternative forms of a gene
11. **Antithetical:** Opposite form of a gene, different allele
12. **Polymorphic:** Having two or more possible alleles at a locus
13. **Codominant:** Equal expression of both alleles in the phenotype
14. **Recessive:** Same allele must be inherited from both parents to be expressed, homozygous
15. **Dominant:** Only one allele must be inherited for it to be expressed; gene product always present
16. **Autosomal:** Genes expressed with equal frequency in males and females, on non-sex chromosome

17. **Sex-linked dominant:** Carried on the X chromosome; no father-to-son transmission; will be expressed if passed from father to daughter or from mother to son
18. **Sex-linked recessive:** It is carried on the X chromosome. Males inherit it from carrier mothers; traits are exhibited most commonly in males (e.g., hemophilia A). Females can exhibit the trait but must inherit it from both carrier mother and affected father.

B. Mendelian Inheritance Principles

1. **Law of independent segregation:** Two members of a single gene pair passed from one generation to the next in separate gametes
2. **Law of independent assortment:** Traits inherited from different chromosomes expressed separately and discretely
3. **Inheritance patterns:** The inheritance of blood group antigens (e.g., A, B, O) can be predicted using a **Punnett square.** Punnett squares have one parent's genotype on the top and the other parent's genotype on the side. See Table 5-1■.
4. Each box in a Punnett square represents a possible genotype for an offspring. An offspring from these particular parents would have a 25% chance of inheriting any one of the four possible variants. Punnett squares are useful for understanding inheritance of blood groups and ramifications of **heterozygosity** or **homozygosity.**
5. **Homozygous:** Individual inherits **identical alleles** at the same gene locus from both parents.
6. **Heterozygous:** Individual inherits **different alleles** at the same gene locus from each parent.
7. **Dosage effect:** Agglutination reactions are generally stronger for homozygous cells than heterozygous cells.
8. **Cis:** Genes are inherited on the **same** chromosome.
9. **Trans:** Genes are inherited on **separate** chromosomes. Genes inherited in transposition can weaken the trait's expression.
10. **Linkage and haplotypes**
    a. **Linked genes:** Genes that are close together on a chromosome and inherited as one unit. The law of independent assortment does **not** hold with linked genes.
    b. **Haplotype:** Set of genes inherited via one of the two parental gametes
    c. **Amorphs:** Genes that do not produce a detectable product

TABLE 5-1 PUNNETT SQUARE

		Mother's Genotype	
		A	**B**
Father's	**B**	AB	BB
Genotype	**O**	AO	BO

11. **Population genetics:** Statistical calculation to determine the prevalence of antigens in specific populations
    a. **Phenotype calculations:** Determine the frequency of an antigen in a population
    b. If a person has **multiple antibodies**, determine the **percentage of compatible units**; the **frequency for each antibody must be multiplied.** For example, if the individual antigen probabilities in the population are:

    30% E-positive, then it is 70% E-negative = 0.70

    78% M-positive, then it is 22% M-negative = 0.22

    80% c-positive, then it is 20% c-negative = 0.20

    Prediction of percentage of compatible units = the product of the individual probabilities or 0.70 × 0.22 × 0.20 = 0.03 or 3% if units are randomly chosen from inventory.
12. **Parentage testing: HLA antigens follow Mendelian genetics** principles and can be used to determine the parents of offspring. HLA genes are polymorphic with many alleles possible at each locus. The more alleles, the less likely it is to find two identical individuals. Parentage testing works on the principle of excluding falsely accused individuals using statistics.

III. ABO AND H BLOOD GROUP SYSTEMS AND SECRETOR STATUS

A. Landsteiner's Rule: If an individual has the antigen, that individual will not have the antibody. This is a universal law and has few exceptions.

B. Antigens of the ABO system
1. Found on **RBCs, lymphocytes, platelets, tissue cells, and bone marrow**
2. These antigens can be secreted by tissue cells if the appropriate genes are present.
3. **Glycolipid** or **glycoprotein**
4. **Developed *in utero*** at 5–6 weeks of gestation
5. **Full expression** of ABO antigens occurs between **2 and 4 years of age.**
6. **Frequencies:** See Table 5-2■.

TABLE 5-2 FREQUENCIES OF ABO ANTIGENS

Blood Type	Caucasian American, Frequency (%)	African American, Frequency (%)
O	45	49
A	40	27
B	11	20
AB	4	4

C. Inheritance and Development of A, B, and H Antigens

1. The **H antigen** is the building block for the **A and B antigens.** There are two alleles in the *H* gene: *H* and *h*. The ***H* allele is found in 99.99% of the world's population**, and *h* is a rare amorph allele.
2. The **H antigen** acts as the **acceptor molecule** for the two **sugars** that make up the A and B antigens.
3. The **A blood type** is the H antigen with **N-acetylgalactosamine** attached.
4. The **B blood type** is the H antigen with **D-galactose** attached.
5. The **O blood type** is the H antigen with **no additional sugar** attached.

D. ABO Subgroups

1. **Subgroups differ** in the **amount of** the **antigen expressed** on the RBCs. Subgroup A_1 possesses both A and A_1 antigens on the RBC surface. Subgroup A_2 only expresses A antigen.
2. **Blood group A** has two major subgroups, **A_1 and A_2. Eighty percent** of group A people are **A_1,** and **20%** of group A people are **A_2**.
3. People with subgroups of the A antigen can produce antibodies against A_1 antigen.
4. Subgroups of A include **A_1, A_2, A_3, A_x, A_m, A_{el},** and **A_{bantu}**.
5. **Subgroups of A** can be **detected with polyclonal Anti-A,B**. This is produced by group O individuals only. Anti-A,B will agglutinate A subgroups because it has specificity for both A and B antigens but cannot be separated into anti-A and anti-B. Anti-A_1 lectin recognizes A_1 but not the other A subgroups.
6. Subgroup **A_3** characteristically produces a mixed-field reaction with polyclonal anti-A and polyclonal anti-A,B.
7. If weak subgroups of A in recipients are not detected, there is no harm in a person with the subgroup receiving type O blood. However, if the person with the **weak subgroup of A donates blood** that is **transfused to a person with group O, intravascular hemolysis** may result.

E. A and B Antigens Are Codominant Traits:

If the **allele** is **present,** the **antigen** will be **expressed. *O* is an amorph allele** that produces no transferase to add sugars to the H determinant site.

F. Anti-A and Anti-B:

These antibodies are produced by humans, who **lack the corresponding antigen**, as a result of exposure to naturally occurring substances that resemble A and B antigens.

G. Anti-A and Anti-B Are IgM Antibodies:

This means they **activate complement** and cause **visible RBC agglutination**. They may cause **hemolysis** at room temperature.

H. Routine ABO Grouping

1. **Forward type:** Person's **RBCs** are mixed with reagent Anti-A and Anti-B.
2. **Reverse type:** Person's **serum** is mixed with reagent A_1 and B RBCs.

3. **ABO discrepancies occur when the forward and reverse groupings do not agree.**
   a. **Problems with forward grouping** (extra antigen present, weak antigens) could be caused by acquired B phenotype, polyagglutination, rouleaux, and ABO subgroups, transfusion of non-type specific blood, and bone marrow or stem cell transplants.
   b. **Problems with reverse grouping** (unexpected antibodies or weak/missing antibodies) could be seen in individuals with A subgroups with anti-A_1, cold alloantibodies, cold autoantibodies, and rouleaux, and in a newborn or elderly person.

I. Bombay (O_h) Phenotype

1. Person inherits ***hh* genotype**.
2. **Types as an O** (forward and reverse); has **alloanti-H** capable of activating complement and causing a hemolytic transfusion reaction
3. These people can **only** be **transfused with Bombay group blood.** Blood may be collected and frozen as autologous or from siblings who are also Bombay phenotype.

J. Secretor Status

1. Two alleles: ***Se*** and ***se***
2. People who inherit ***Se*** are **secretors** and are capable of expressing A, B and H antigens in their secretions.
3. A, B, and H antigens, appropriate to the individual's ABO group, are found in saliva, urine, tears, bile, amniotic fluid, breast milk, exudate, and digestive fluids of secretors (*Se*).

IV. Rh BLOOD GROUPS

A. Rh Blood Group System

1. Controlled by two genes *RHD* and *RHCE*. ***RHD*** controls **D expression; no d allele. *RHCE*** controls **C, c, E, e expression**.
2. Rh antigens are proteins.
3. **Rh terminology**
   a. The most common individual antigens are named in the **Fisher-Race** terminology, **D, C, c, E, e, C^w, G, etc.**
   b. **Haplotypes** are often expressed in a modified **Wiener** terminology such as **R_1R_1 for CDe/CDe**.
4. **Phenotype:** RBC antigens identified with specific antisera; **Genotype:** genes present on a person's chromosomes
5. **Rh system antigens**
   a. **D antigen: Most immunogenic** of Rh antigens
   b. **Weak D or Mosaic D**
      1) Weak D occurs when **D** is **weakly expressed due to genetic, positional effect, or missing portion of D mosaic. Weak D** must be **detected** by an **IAT** (indirect antiglobulin test).

2) **Genetic cause:** Weaker expression of the ***cDe*** **haplotype** may fail to react by direct agglutination testing, but it will **react strongly** by the **IAT**.
3) **Position effect:** Occurs when the **C antigen** is inherited **trans** to the **D antigen. This weak D** may be detected **without** carrying the test to the antiglobulin phase.
4) **Partial D:** Occurs when only **part** of the **D antigen** is inherited. There are multiple epitopes that make up the D antigen. A partial-D individual **lacks one or more** of these **epitopes** and is capable of **making antibody** to the epitopes that s(he) lacks. Partial-D individuals are usually detected because the antigen reacts strongly with monoclonal reagents. A partial D is suspected when a seemingly D-positive person makes anti-D after transfusion with D-positive blood.
5) **Weakly reactive D** means a person **is D-positive.** AABB *Standards for Blood Banks and Transfusion Services* state that all **Rh-negative donor units** must be **tested for weak D**, and those units that test **positive** must be **identified as D-positive**. However, **weak-D recipients** are **transfused with D-negative** blood.

c. **Other Rh system antigens**
1) **f or ce:** If *c* and *e* are present on the same haplotype, f antigen is expressed.
2) **Ce or** $\mathbf{rh_i}$**:** *C* and *e* are inherited as a haplotype made by D-positive individuals who make anti-C.
3) $\mathbf{C^w}$**:** Low-frequency antigen
4) **V or** $\mathbf{ce^s}$**:** 30% prevalence in African-Americans
5) **G:** In test tube appears to be anti-D and anti-C
6) **Rh:29:** Antibody to Rh:29 is the antibody to the high-frequency Rh antigen made by Rh_{null} people.

d. **Unusual phenotypes**
1) **D deletion:** No reaction occurs when tested with anti-E, anti-e, anti-C, and anti-c. **Written as D – –.**
2) $\mathbf{Rh_{null}}$ **phenotype:** This appears to have no Rh antigens. The membranes of their RBCs are abnormal, and the RBCs have a shortened life span. This can result from inheriting two nonfunctional *RHCE* alleles along with the dual deletion of the *RHD* alleles. Rh_{null} phenotype can also result from inheriting two recessive regulator alleles at the *RHAG* locus. The latter individuals pass on normal *RHD* and *RHCE* alleles to their children.

6. **Rh antibodies**

a. Produced in humans after exposure to Rh antigen through **pregnancy or transfusions**
b. **IgG antibody**; Rh antibodies generally do not activate complement.
c. Optimal reaction temperature: **37°C**
d. Reaction phase: **AHG** (antihuman globulin)
e. **Agglutination enhancement** occurs with LISS, enzymes, and PEG (polyethylene glycol).

f. Stronger reactivity of antibody with cells from homozygous individuals is shown with anti-C, anti-c, anti-E, and anti-e (dosage).
g. C and e, and E and c are usually found together.
h. These antibodies produce **hemolytic transfusion reactions (HTRs)**. Antibodies may not be currently detectable, but the person should always receive **antigen-negative blood** if they have a history of Rh antibodies.
i. Rh antibodies can cause **hemolytic disease of the newborn (HDN)**, because they can cross the placenta. **Rh immune globulin** (RhIG) administered after delivery (within 72 hours) can **protect** a woman **from making anti-D**.

V. OTHER BLOOD GROUP SYSTEMS

A. Kell Blood Group System

1. Abbreviation: **K**
2. Antibody class: **IgG**
3. Optimal reaction temperature: **37°C**
4. Reaction phase: **AHG**
5. Enzyme treatment: **No effect**
6. **Antigens:** K (Kell), k (Cellano), Kp^a, Kp^b, Kp^c, Js^a, Js^b, and Ku; **common Kell** system antigens **k, Kp^b, and Js^b**
7. **Allelic pairs:** Include K and k, Kp^a and Kp^b, Js^a and Js^b
8. **K is very immunogenic.** Although the K antigen is found in only about 9% of the population, **anti-K** is encountered quite frequently and can **cause HTR** and **HDN**.
9. **$Kell_{null}$:** This is also known as **K_0**. It occurs when **RBCs lack** the **Kell antigens** but **have** the **Kx antigen**.
10. The **Kx antigen** is produced by a gene located on a **different chromosome** than the Kell system genes. This antigen is inherited independently from the Kell antigens; the Kx antigen structure appears to be required for the expression of the Kell system antigens. **K_{null}** individuals have **increased** amounts of **Kx**.
11. **McLeod phenotype**
    a. Individuals who have an **alteration** of the **allele-producing *Kx*** on the X chromosome **lack Kx** on the red blood cells and have greatly **decreased expression of Kell antigens**.
    b. These individuals have decreased RBC survival as well as RBC morphologic and functional abnormalities.

B. Duffy Blood Group System

1. Abbreviation: **Fy**
2. Antibody class: **IgG**
3. Optimal reaction temperature: **37°C**
4. Reaction phase: **AHG**
5. Enzyme treatment: **Destroys Fy^a and Fy^b**

6. Clinically significant:
   a. **Anti-Fy^a** and **anti-Fy^b** can **cause HTR** and **HDN**.
   b. The Fy(*a*−*b*−) phenotype is more resistant to malarial infection by *Plasmodium vivax*.
7. **Antigens:** Fy^a, Fy^b
8. **Four phenotypes:** Fy(*a*+*b*−); Fy(*a*−*b*+); Fy(*a*+*b*+); Fy(*a*−*b*−)
9. **Alleles:** *Fy^a*, *Fy^b*, and *Fy* (silent allele)
10. Commonly show dosage effect: Weak antibodies react more strongly with homozygous cells.

C. Kidd Blood Group System

1. Abbreviation: **Jk**
2. Antibody class: **IgG**
3. Optimal reaction temperature: **37°C**
4. Reaction phase: **AHG**
5. Enzyme treatment: **Enhances agglutination**
6. Clinically significant: Associated with **HTR** and **mild HDN**
7. **Antigens:** Jk^a, Jk^b, Jk3
8. **Four phenotypes:** Jk(*a*+*b*−); Jk(*a*−*b*+); Jk(*a*+*b*+); Jk(*a*−*b*−)
9. **Alleles:** ***Jk^a*** codes for Jk^a and Jk3; ***Jk^b*** codes for Jk^b and Jk3.
10. **Show dosage effect:** Weak antibodies agglutinate homozygous cells more strongly than heterozygous cells.
11. These antibodies **bind complement.**
12. These **antibodies deteriorate in storage**, declining quickly to below the detectable level in human serum, and commonly **cause delayed HTR** (DHTR).

D. Lutheran Blood Group System

1. Abbreviation: **Lu**
2. Antibody class: **Lu^a IgM; Lu^b IgG**
3. Optimal reaction temperature: **Lu^a 4°C; Lu^b 37°C**
4. Reaction phase: **Lu^a room temperature; Lu^b AHG**
5. Enzyme treatment: **Variable effect**
6. Clinically significant:
   a. No clinical significance. **Anti-Lu^a** can be present without prior transfusion or pregnancy.
   b. **Anti-Lu^b** is rare and associated with HTR and HDN.
7. **Antigens:** 18 total, including Au^a and Au^b
8. **Alleles:** *Lu^a*, *Lu^b*

E. Lewis Blood Group System

1. Abbreviation: **Le**
2. Antibody class: **IgM**
3. Optimal reaction temperature: **Most often 4°C, sometimes 37°C**

4. Reaction phase: **Room temperature, 37°C,** and **AHG**
5. Enzyme treatment: **Enhanced agglutination**
6. Clinically significant: **No**
7. Produced by tissue cells and secreted into fluids. The antigens are adsorbed onto the RBC membranes.
8. May take 6 years to fully develop these antigens.
9. **Genetics: If *Le* gene is inherited, Le^a is adsorbed onto RBCs—Le(a+b−). Le^a** is the only antigen that can be **secreted** by a **nonsecretor**.
10. **If *Se* gene is also inherited, Le^b is adsorbed onto the RBC—Le(a−b+).**
11. Bombay phenotypes are Le^a positive if they inherit the *Le* gene.
12. Cells type as Le(*a*+*b*+), transiently during first years of life, Le(*a*+*b*−), Le(*a*−*b*+), Le(*a*−*b*−).
13. Lewis antibodies are sometimes formed during pregnancy but weaken and disappear after delivery.

F. I Blood Group System

1. Abbreviation: **I**
2. Antibody class: **IgM**
3. Optimal reaction temperature: **4°C**
4. Reaction phase: **Immediate spin (IS)** and **occasionally 37°C**
5. Enzyme treatment: **Enhanced agglutination**
6. Clinically significant: **No**
7. It can be a bothersome antibody, masking the reactions of a clinically significant alloantibody. May need to prewarm cell suspension and reagent or do cold autoabsorption to find clinically significant alloantibodies.
8. Strong anti-I is associated with *Mycoplasma pneumoniae* infection.

G. P Blood Group System

1. Abbreviation: $\mathbf{P_1}$
2. Antibody class: **IgM (anti-$\mathbf{P_1}$)**
3. Optimal reaction temperature: **4°C**
4. Reaction phase: **IS, 37°C** and **AHG**
5. Enzyme treatment: **Enhanced agglutination**
6. Clinically significant:
   a. Anti-P_1 is not clinically significant.
   b. Anti-$\mathbf{P_1 + P + P^k}$ is an **IgG clinically significant** antibody.
7. **Phenotypes:** P_1, P_2, p, $P_1{}^k$, $P_2{}^k$, and Luke
8. **Alleles:** P_1, P, P^k, and p
9. Anti-P_1 can be neutralized by soluble P_1 reagent.
10. **Autoanti-P is Donath-Landsteiner antibody.** Naturally occurring biphasic antibody associated with paroxysmal cold hemoglobinuria. It binds to the antigen on the patient's RBCs in the cold and fixes complement. The RBCs are hemolyzed when the temperature reaches 37°C.

11. Patients with **autoanti-P** may require a **blood warmer for transfusion.**
12. Anti-PP_1P^k is found in individuals of the p phenotype. It is clinically significant and associated with spontaneous abortions. Need compatible blood from other p phenotype individuals.

H. MNS Blood Group System

1. **M and N antigens**
   a. Abbreviation: **MN**
   b. Antibody class: **IgM**
   c. Optimal reaction temperature: **4** or **37°C**
   d. Reaction phase: **IS, 37°C,** or **AHG**
   e. Enzyme treatment: **Destroys antigens**
   f. Clinically significant: **No**
   g. **Antigens:** M and N associated with **glycophorin A**
2. **S and s antigens**
   a. Abbreviation: **Ss**
   b. Antibody class: **IgG**
   c. Optimal reaction temperature: **37°C**
   d. Reaction phase: **AHG**
   e. Enzyme treatment: **Variable effect**
   f. Clinically significant: **Yes**
   g. **Antigens:** S, s, and U associated with **glycophorin B**
3. Anti-M
   a. It is **clinically significant** if **IgG; IgM** antibody is **not** clinically significant.
   b. Demonstrates dosage effect
4. Anti-N is very rare.
5. Anti-S, anti-s, and anti-U
   a. **Clinically significant**, causing **HTR** and **HDN**
   b. Anti-U is rare and occurs in people with S−s−U−.

I. Miscellaneous Blood Group Systems

1. **Diego:** Di^a, Di^b, Wr^a, Wr^b; Di^b and Wr^b are high-incidence antigens.
2. **Cartwright:** Yt^a and Yt^b; Yt^a is a high-incidence antigen.
3. **XG:** Xg^a antigen has a higher incidence in females than in males.
4. **Scianna:** Sc1, Sc2, and Sc3; Sc1 and Sc3 are high-incidence antigens.
5. **Dombrock:** Do^a, Do^b, Gy^a, Hy, and Jo^a; Gy^a, Hy, and Jo^a are high-incidence antigens.
6. **Colton:** Co^a, Co^b, and Co3; Co^a is a high-incidence antigen.
7. **Chido/Rodgers:** Ch^a and Rg^a are both high-incidence antigens.
8. **Gerbich:** Ge2, Ge3, and Ge4 are high-incidence antigens.
9. **Cromer:** Cr^a and several others are high-incidence antigens.
10. **Knops:** Kn^a, McC^a, Sl1, and Yk^a are high-incidence antigens.
11. **Cost:** Cs^a and Cs^b; Cs^a is a high-incidence antigen.

12. **Vel:** Vel is a high-incidence antigen. Anti-Vel is a hemolytic, clinically significant antibody.
13. **John Milton Hagen:** JMH is a high-incidence antigen.
14. **Sid:** Sd^a is a high-incidence antigen.

VI. BLOOD BANK REAGENTS AND METHODS

A. Principle of Blood Bank Tests

Ag + Ab ↔ Ag-Ab reaction (immune complex)

B. Routine Blood Bank Testing Procedures

1. **ABO/Rh typing**
   a. Detects **A, B,** and **D antigens**
   b. **Source of antigens:** Patient's RBCs (forward grouping/typing); reagent RBCs (reverse grouping)
   c. **Source of antibodies:** Reagent anti-A, anti-B, and anti-D (forward grouping/typing); patient's serum (reverse grouping)
2. **Antibody screen**
   a. Detects specific **antibodies to RBC antigens**
   b. **Source of antigens:** Reagent antibody screening cells
   c. **Source of antibodies:** Patient's serum
3. **Antibody identification**
   a. Identifies antibodies to RBC antigens
   b. **Source of antigens:** Reagent antibody panel cells (10–20 cells)
   c. **Source of antibodies:** Patient's serum
4. **Crossmatch**
   a. Determines **compatibility** of **donor RBCs** with **recipient**
   b. **Source of antigens:** Donor cells
   c. **Source of antibodies:** Recipient's serum

C. Types of Blood Bank Reagents

1. **Reagent RBCs** possess **known antigens** and are treated to prolong their shelf life.
2. **Antisera** contain known **antibodies** against specific RBC antigens.
3. **Antiglobulin reagents** contain poly- or monospecific **antibodies** against human antibodies.
4. **Potentiators** are solutions that **enhance** the **formation of antigen–antibody complexes**.

D. Regulation of Reagent Production

1. Blood bank reagents are licensed by the Center for Biologics Evaluation and Research of the Food and Drug Administration (FDA).
2. FDA specifies potency and specificity of reagents before production.

TABLE 5-3 ABO ANTISERA REACTIONS

	Anti-A Reagent	Anti-B Reagent
Type A	+	0
Type B	0	+
Type AB	+	+
Type O	0	0

E. Reagent Antisera
1. **Polyclonal: Many B cell clones** produce antibodies against antigens.
2. **Monoclonal: A single B cell clone** produces antibody against a single epitope on an antigen.
   a. **Advantages:** Endless production, exactly the same antibody in each batch, no human/animal sources, no contamination
   b. **Disadvantages:** Single specificity; may not react with all portions of RBC antigen
3. **Blended monoclonal:** Reduces disadvantages of single clone
4. **ABO antisera**
   a. **Anti-A** and **Anti-B reagents** are used to determine if patient is A, B, AB, or O. See Table 5-3■.
   b. **Anti-A reagent** is colored with a **blue dye; Anti-B reagent** is colored with a **yellow dye.**
   c. Suspension of **patient's cells** is added to antisera.
   d. Agglutination is read at immediate spin. These antibodies are **IgM** and react best at room temperature or 4°C.
5. **D typing**
   a. These are **important antigens** to detect because **antibody–antigen reactions *in vivo* cause HTR and HDN**.
   b. Two types of reagents:
      1) **High protein:** Older reagent; need to run an Rh control with this reagent because the protein in the diluent may cause false positive reactions in patients with autoantibodies or abnormal serum proteins.
      2) **Low-protein monoclonal:** Rh control is usually not required. Only need to perform a control when patient has abnormal serum proteins.
6. **Antiglobulin reagents**
   a. **Polyspecific:** Detects both anti-IgG and anti-C3b or C3d; used often in direct antiglobulin tests (DAT)
   b. **Monoclonal:** This may be used to differentiate between antibodies to IgG and complement C3. Monospecific (antihuman IgG) reagents are typically employed for tests requiring an antiglobulin phase of testing.
7. **Reagent RBCs**
   a. **IgG-coated control cells (Check cells):** *AABB Standards for Blood Banks and Transfusion Services* require a control to **ensure antiglobulin reagent reactivity**

in each negative antiglobulin test tube. Check cells are prepared by attaching an IgG antibody to RBCs (sensitized RBCs).

b. **A_1 and B cells for reverse grouping:** These are used to **confirm forward typing** results. These cells **detect ABO antibodies**. Landsteiner's law: If the **patient's RBCs have an antigen**, they do **not** have the antibody in the serum.

c. **Antibody screening cells:** These are used to **detect antibodies present in a patient's serum**. Antibodies must be detected before patients are transfused to prevent hemolytic transfusion reactions and/or death. Each set of screening cells has two or three antigenically different RBC reagent cells. The **antigens of each cell are known** and printed on an **antigram** included with each set.

d. **Antibody panel cells:** Antibody identification procedures use a **panel of RBCs** whose **antigens** are **known**. The panel consists of 10 to 20 vials of RBCs. Every panel has an antigenic profile that lists all of the known antigens on each vial of RBCs.

e. **Other methods for antigen–antibody reaction detection**
   1) **Gel technology:** This technique uses **dextran acrylamide gel** combined with reagents or diluent. Anti-IgG cards are used for DATs and IATs.
   2) **Microplate methods:** The traditional tube method is adapted to the microtiter plate, in which **smaller volumes of serum and cells are used**, and it is read on an automated photometric instrument. The cell buttons are resuspended by tapping the sides of the plate.
   3) **Solid-phase adherence methods**
      a) **RBC screening cells where antigens** are **bound to surface** of microtiter plates.
      b) Add patient's serum.
      c) Antigen captures IgG molecules.
      d) Plates washed.
      e) Add indicator cells (anti-IgG-coated RBCs, Fc portion of IgG bound to RBC), antibody on indicator cells bind to patient antibody.
      f) **Negative** = RBC button; **Positive** = RBCs (indicator cells) dense mat of RBCs on the bottom of the wells.
   4) **Indirect antiglobulin test (IAT)**
      a) Purpose of the **IAT** is to **detect *in vitro* sensitization of RBCs**.
      b) In this procedure, reagent RBCs are mixed with patient's serum, then incubated at 37°C to allow IgG antibodies to attach to the RBCs. The solution is then washed to remove unbound proteins. **AHG is added to detect *in vitro* sensitization of RBCs.**
      c) **False positive tests** result from RBCs being agglutinated before the washing step (cold agglutinin), improper RBC suspension, dirty glassware, and overcentrifugation.
      d) **False negative tests** result from poor washing of RBCs, testing being delayed, loss of reagent activity, no AHG added, or use of an improper RBC suspension.

5) **Potentiating media (antibody enhancers)**
   a) **Definition:** Reagents added to the *in vitro* antiglobulin test to **enhance antigen–antibody complex formation**
   b) **LISS** increases antibody uptake of antigen by reducing the ionic strength and lowering the zeta potential.
   c) **Bovine albumin** (22 or 30%) allows sensitized RBCs to come close together to form agglutination lattices.
   d) **PEG additive** concentrates antibodies and reduces water and allows greater antibody uptake.
   e) **Proteolytic enzymes: Papain, ficin**, and **bromelin** are used. **Enzymes remove certain structures** from the RBC and **enhance** the **access of antibodies** to otherwise less prominent structures on the RBC. Antibodies that are **enhanced** include **Rh, Kidd,** and **Le** blood group systems. The following **antigens** are **destroyed** by the enzymes: **M, N, S, Xg^{a}, Fy^{a},** and **Fy^{b}.**

VII. DIRECT ANTIGLOBULIN TESTING

A. Direct Antiglobulin Test (DAT)

1. RBCs may combine with antibodies without agglutinating.
2. **Antihuman globulin (AHG)** is an *in vitro* reagent used to **agglutinate RBCs with antibodies attached** to them (sensitized RBCs).
3. Direct antiglobulin test
   a. **Detects IgG and/or complement proteins attached to RBCs** in autoimmune hemolytic anemia, HDN, a drug-related mechanism, or a transfusion reaction
   b. Indicates **immune-mediated** *in vivo* RBC destruction (antibodies attached to RBCs ***in vivo***)
   c. **Procedure**
      1) Patient's RBCs are washed three times with normal saline to remove unbound proteins.
      2) Polyspecific AHG is then added.
      3) Agglutination indicates that the patient has antibodies or complement proteins attached to RBCs.
   d. **Specimen of choice:** EDTA negates the *in vitro* activation of complement.

VIII. IDENTIFICATION OF UNEXPECTED ALLOANTIBODIES

A. Detection of Atypical and Unexpected Antibodies

1. Antibodies other than ABO in a person's blood
2. **Antibody screen**
   a. **Purpose:** To detect antibodies in patients requiring transfusions, pregnant women, blood and blood product donors, and patients with suspected transfusion reactions

b. **Screening cells:** Two to three different group O cells with known antigens included in an antigram.

c. **Procedure**
   1) Mix known RBCs with patient's serum.
   2) Add potentiator and incubate at 37°C.
   3) Spin and read results (if applicable to potentiator).
   4) Wash three times with saline.
   5) Add AHG, spin, and then read results.
   6) Read all negative results macroscopically (some facilities read all negative results microscopically).
   7) Add IgG-coated control cells (check cells) to all tubes with a negative reaction at AHG. Check cells must agglutinate or the test must be repeated.
   8) Spin and read for agglutination.

d. **Results:** Any **agglutination** at any phase of testing indicates an atypical or unexpected antibody.

e. **Autocontrol:** Use patient's serum and patient's RBCs. Autocontrol is used to detect **autoantibodies.** Often performed in conjunction with the antibody screen and is tested in all phases.

f. **Potentiators** are used to **enhance antibody detection**.

g. **Patient history:** A patient's transfusion and antibody history should be researched at that institution before transfusing the patient.

3. **Antibody identification**
   a. **Antibody panel:** Type **O cells with known antigens**; usually 10–20 bottles of different cells with known antigens
   b. **Purpose:** To **identify alloantibodies** detected in patient's serum

4. **Panel interpretation**
   a. **Autocontrol** determines if antibody is autoantibody or alloantibody.
   b. **Phases:** The **reaction phase** of the antibody is **important**. It will determine if the antibody is IgG or IgM. **Room temperature** reactions usually indicate an **IgM** antibody. Reactions at 37°C and/or AHG usually indicate an IgG antibody.
   c. **Reaction strength**
      1) **Single-strength** reactions usually indicate a **single antibody**.
      2) **Various-strength** reactions usually indicate **multiple antibodies or dosage**.
   d. **Ruling out**
      1) **Negative reaction (0)** indicates that the antibody(ies) does(do) not react with any antigen on that RBC. However, if that cell is heterozygous for an antigen, antibody may be showing dosage or reduced reaction strength. For antibodies that show dosage, rule out must be done using homozygous cells.
      2) **Positive reaction (+)** should **never** be used at any phase of testing to rule out! Always **use** this in **identification**.

e. Determining the **antibody specificity**
   1) **Single antibody:** If there is only one antibody, the reactions will match the antigen pattern on the antigram.
   2) **Multiple antibodies:** If there is more than one antibody, the reactions are difficult to match with a single antigen pattern on the antigram. Multiple antibodies may react with varying strengths.

f. **Rule of Three**
   1) Are there **three cells** with **positive reactions** from the panel cells?
   2) Are there **three cells** with **negative reactions** from the panel cells?
   3) If the answers to both of the two previous questions are yes, then there is a **95% probability** that the **antibody is correctly identified.**
   4) **Facilities may use a rule of two particularly for low-frequency antibodies that may not be present on even one cell line of a panel.**

g. **Phenotype patient**
   1) This is required to confirm antibody identification. If the patient is negative for the antigen, an antibody is possible.
   2) In the patient who has not been recently transfused, when his(her) RBCs are positive for the antigen, the antibody to that antigen is usually not produced.

5. **Multiple antibody resolution**
   a. May need to perform more tests to identify antibodies.
   b. Selected cells can be used to complete identification; use rule of three. Individual cells from a second panel can be used.
   c. Additional technique
      1) **One-stage enzyme:** Incubate patient's serum, enzyme, and RBCs.
      2) **Two-stage enzyme:** Pretreat panel or screening cells with enzymes, wash, and perform IAT without additional enhancements.

B. Antibodies to High-Frequency Antigens

1. **Definition:** Antibodies produced against antigens that occur in at least 98% of the population
2. When interpreting panels, the presence of an antibody to a high-frequency antigen is suspected when:
   a. the autocontrol is negative.
   b. reactions occur with most or all panel cells with AHG.
   c. reaction strength in all panel cells is the same.
3. **Additional testing:** Under the **rule of three**, there must be at least three positive and three negative cells. Choose cells from other panels that lack various high-incidence antigens.
4. **Clues for identification of antibodies to high-frequency antigens**
   a. I, H, P, P_1, and $P + P_1 + P^k$ produce **room temperature or cold** reactions.
   b. Lu^b, Ch, Rg, Cs^a, Kn^a, McC^a, Sl^a, and JMH produce weak and varying reactions with **AHG**.

C. Antibodies to Low-Frequency Antigens

1. If the **antibody screen** is **negative** and the **crossmatch** is **positive**, suspect antibodies to low-frequency antigens.
2. **Low-frequency antigens** include Lu^a, C^w, Kp^a, Wr^a, V, Bg^a, VS, and Co^b.
3. Crossmatching further units will usually result in compatibility.
4. If the antibody is found in a pregnant woman, test the father's RBCs with the mother's serum to determine if the fetus is in danger of HDN.

D. Enhancing Weak IgG Antibodies

1. If weak reactions are encountered that do not fit the pattern of a known antigen, repeat panel using different potentiators, increase incubation time, and/or increase serum-to-cell ratio.

E. Alloantibodies

1. Cold antibodies that react at 4°C and/or room temperature are usually not clinically significant. These antibodies can hide a clinically significant alloantibody.
2. Prewarmed techniques or adsorption of cold antibody can help detect any alloantibodies present. If the cold antibody reacts at 37°C, it may be clinically significant.

F. Autoantibodies

1. Can be detected by a **positive DAT** or **positive autocontrol**
2. Can be produced in response to drug effects, cold autoimmune disease, pneumonia, warm autoimmune disease, infectious mononucleosis, etc.

G. Cold Panels

1. Cold panels are done to **identify "cold" antibodies.**
2. **Antibody panels** are **performed** with the incubation at **4°C** instead of 37°C.
3. Because **most cold autoantibodies** are either **anti-I, anti-H, or anti-IH**, an abbreviated or "mini" cold panel can be performed.
   a. Select cells for panel: Use screening cells (type O), an autocontrol, cord blood, or i-positive cells from a commercial panel, and type specific cells for the patient (e.g., A cells for type A, B cells for type B).
   b. Add two drops of patient's serum to cells and incubate at 4°C for 20 minutes.
   c. Centrifuge, resuspend, and grade reactions after incubation.
   d. Interpretation: See Table 5-4■.

TABLE 5-4 INTERPRETATION OF ANTIBODY PANEL TO IDENTIFY COLD ANTIBODIES

	Screening Cell I	Screening Cell II	Autocontrol	Group O Cord	Type Specific
Anti-I	3+	3+	3+	0	4+
Anti-IH	3+	3+	3+	1+	2+
Anti-H	3+	3+	2+	2+	2+

H. Avoiding Cold Antibodies

1. Use IgG antihuman globulin.
2. Skip the immediate spin or room temperature phase.
3. Use 22% albumin instead of LISS.
4. **Use prewarmed technique.**
   a. Using 2–5% cell suspensions, place one drop of each panel cell and one drop of patient's cells into their respectively labeled tubes and incubate at 37°C for 10 minutes.
   b. Simultaneously, warm patient's serum at 37°C for 10 minutes.
   c. Add prewarmed serum to prewarmed panel cells and incubate at 37°C for 30 minutes.
   d. Wash three times in saline prewarmed to 37°C.
   e. Add AHG, spin, read, and grade reactions.
   f. Interpret reactions.
   g. Add IgG-coated control cells to negative tubes.

I. Adsorption Techniques

1. If the patient was not transfused in last 3 months, an autoadsorption can be performed.
2. If the patient was transfused within the past 3 months, use allogeneic cells lacking the same antigens as the patient for adsorption.
3. **Cold autoadsorption**
   a. Incubate patient's serum and cells at 4°C for 30–60 minutes.
   b. Remove serum and use serum for panel to test for alloantibody.
4. **Warm autoadsorption**
   a. Incubate patient's serum and cells at 37°C for 30–60 minutes.
   b. Remove serum and use serum in panel to test for alloantibody.

J. Elution

1. IgG that attaches to RBCs *in vivo* can be removed by elution (*in vitro*).
2. **Three types of elution techniques**
   a. **Intact RBC antibody removal** uses buffers to remove the antibody from the RBC without destroying the RBC.
   b. **Digitonin** releases the antibody by destroying the RBCs.
   c. **Lui freeze-thaw** is used to **remove IgM antibodies** (usually anti-A or B) present on newborn RBCs.
3. Once antibody releases, the last wash and the eluate supernatant are tested on a panel.
4. The last wash panel should be negative, and the eluate supernatant should reveal alloantibodies.

IX. PRETRANSFUSION TESTING

A. Compatibility Testing

1. Entails recipient identification, specimen collection and handling, review of patient's transfusion services records, ABO/Rh typing, antibody screen, antibody identification, ABO/Rh confirmation on donor units, crossmatching, screening donor units for antigens for which a recipient has an antibody(ies) in his(her) serum, and the transfusion.
2. **Definitions**
   a. **Full (complete) crossmatch:** Testing donor cells with recipient serum; carried through all phases and check cells
   b. **Compatible crossmatch:** No agglutination or hemolysis at any phase of testing performed
   c. **Incompatible crossmatch:** Agglutination or hemolysis at any phase of testing performed
   d. **Immediate-spin crossmatch:** Performed only at room temperature; IS is done with donor cells and recipient serum. It is designed to **detect ABO incompatibility**. It is appropriate to perform IS, if recipient's current and historic antibody screening is negative.
   e. **Electronic crossmatch:** Recipient ABO/Rh is tested in duplicate and results are entered into a validated blood bank computer system. The computer searches for the recipient's transfusion history . If the recipient has not been transfused in the last 3 months and his(her) antibody screen, both current and historic, is negative, blood for the recipient is issued without any additional testing.
3. **Purpose of crossmatch**
   a. To prevent transfusion of incompatible RBCs
   b. To maximize RBC life after transfusion
4. **Limitation of crossmatches**
   a. Does not guarantee normal RBC cell survival *in vivo*
   b. Does not detect transfusion-transmitted bacteria, viruses, or parasites
   c. Does not detect allergic reactions
   d. Does not detect WBC antigens
   e. Will not prevent antibody production to foreign antigens present on donor's RBCs
   f. Does not prevent delayed transfusion reactions
5. **Procedure**
   a. Blood sample: Acceptable blood collection tubes are plain red top (no anti-coagulant), yellow top (acid citrate dextrose or ACD, Formula B), purple top (EDTA), and blue top (citrate).
      1) Hemolyzed specimens are not acceptable.
      2) Specimens must be no older than 72 hours for patients transfused or pregnant within the last 3 months.

3) AABB *Standards for Blood Banks and Transfusion Services* state that the following information must be on the tube:
   a) Patient first and last name; must match name on armband
   b) Unique identifying number on patient sample and requisition
   c) Date of collection
   d) Signature or initials of phlebotomist
4) The patient must be able to state his(her) name and/or be identified by name band on arm before the tube can be drawn. Information on the tube must match information on the requisition.

6. **AABB standards** require **comparison** of **current** blood bank **workup with other** blood bank **tests performed** on the same patient **within 12 months** (including blood type, typing problems, allo- or autoantibodies, transfusion reactions, or special requirements).
7. AABB standards states that the **ABO** typing must be **repeated** on all units received into the blood bank, and **Rh** must be **tested** on all **Rh-negative** units.
8. **AABB standards for crossmatches**
   a. Use recipient serum and donor cells (segment taken from the bag of the unit to be transfused).
   b. **IS crossmatch:** This is used when the recipient has no history of alloantibodies and current antibody screen is negative. The donor cells and recipient serum or plasma are added to a tube. This tube is spun, and the reaction is graded. If **negative**, the recipient is transfused with this unit of blood. If **positive**, the crossmatch must be carried out as an antiglobulin crossmatch: IS, 37°C incubation, and AHG phases.
   c. **Antiglobulin crossmatch:** This is performed when a history of an alloantibody or the detection of one in the current antibody screen warrants an antiglobulin crossmatch. **AHG crossmatch** involves IS phase, addition of potentiator, 37°C incubation phase, three washes, antiglobulin phase, and finally IgG-coated control cells.
   d. **Electronic crossmatch:** AABB standards require
      1) Validated computer system
      2) Validated studies submitted to FDA
      3) Two identical ABO typings on recipient
      4) ABO on current sample
      5) ABO typing by two laboratorians or on two different samples
      6) Computer has donor unit information: product name, ABO and Rh, unique number, and interpretation of ABO confirmation test.
      7) Computer system contains recipient ABO and Rh.
      8) Computer alert for ABO incompatibilities
      9) Method to verify the correct entry of all data
      10) Advantages: Increased time efficiency, decreased sample volume requirement for patients needing numerous crossmatches
      11) Better inventory management

9. Tagging, inspecting, and issuing blood products
   a. **Every unit to be transfused is tagged.** The tag must contain the patient's full name, unique identification numbers, name of product, donor number, expiration date, ABO and Rh of unit, crossmatch interpretation, and identification of person doing testing or selecting unit.
   b. **Inspecting the unit:** Each unit must be inspected for expiration date, ABO and Rh, discoloration, clots, and bacterial contamination before release for transfusion.
   c. **Issuing:** Person taking the unit must have a request form that has the patient's full name, unique number, and product needed. Both persons issuing and receiving the unit must record their initials or sign that they have checked the unit tag against the request form and record the date and time. If RBCs are not stored in a monitored refrigerator or transfused within 30 minutes of issue, the unit must be returned to the blood bank.
10. **Incompatible crossmatches**
    a. Causes for an **incompatible IS crossmatch:** Wrong patient identification, wrong sample identification, cold alloantibody, presence of anti-A_1, or a cold autoantibody
    b. Causes for an **incompatible AHG crossmatch:** Alloantibody or autoantibody in patient's serum
11. **Emergency release of uncrossmatched blood**
    a. **Emergency release** must be **signed by physician** requesting blood.
    b. Unit must be tagged just like when performing a crossmatch. **Note that the blood** is an emergency release and **not crossmatched.**
    c. Must have full patient name and unique identification number, donor unit number, ABO and Rh, and expiration date on tag, requisition, and transfusion services records.
    d. **Segments** are **removed** from the unit before issuing so the blood can be **crossmatched after the release of the unit.**
    e. Name of the person issuing the unit must be on the requisition and transfusion services records.
12. **Massive transfusion**
    a. **Definition:** Total blood volume replacement within 24 hours (approximately 10–12 units)
    b. Each facility has a policy on when a new recipient sample is needed and if crossmatching is necessary.
13. **Maximum surgical blood order schedule (MSBOS):** Procedures are performed according to the patient's surgery. Choices include type and screen, crossmatch for two units, crossmatch for four units, or crossmatch for six units.
14. **Crossmatching autologous units**
    a. Blood is **pre-donated by recipient for** use during or after **recipient's own surgery.**

b. The blood must be transfused to intended patient; it **cannot be given to anyone else**.
c. Testing for infectious diseases is not required.
d. **IS crossmatch** is performed before issuing blood for transfusion.

15. **Crossmatching infants less than 4 months old**
    a. Newborns develop antibodies by 4–6 months of age. At less than 4 months of age, any antibodies in the reverse grouping or antibody screen are of maternal origin. **Pretransfusion testing** is only **ABO** (forward grouping) and **Rh**.
    b. If alloantibodies are detected in the mother's or infant's serum, the infant is transfused with units negative for the corresponding antigens.
16. **Pretransfusion testing** for fresh-frozen plasma (FFP), platelets, cryoprecipitate, plateletpheresis, and granulocyte concentrates is **ABO grouping**. These products are preferably ABO group specific or compatible.

X. HEMOLYTIC DISEASES OF THE NEWBORN

A. Etiology

1. In HDN or erythroblastosis fetalis, **maternal IgG antibodies cross the placenta** and **destroy the baby's RBCs**, which demonstrate the antigen specific for that antibody. Hemoglobin from lysed RBCs is metabolized into unconjugated bilirubin. The mother metabolizes the unconjugated bilirubin into conjugated bilirubin, and it is excreted into the small intestines. The fetus becomes anemic as RBC destruction continues. Cardiac failure and/or hydrops fetalis may result from anemia. After birth, unconjugated bilirubin that was previously metabolized by the mother now accumulates in the baby's circulation. The infant is unable to metabolize and excrete the bilirubin because its liver is not functioning at full capacity. The buildup of bilirubin leads to jaundice and can cause deafness, intellectual disability, **kernicterus** (bilirubin accumulation causes brain damage), or death.

B. Rh Hemolytic Disease of the Newborn

1. Most severe
2. D-negative mother develops antibodies during her first pregnancy with D-positive baby or after transfusion with D-positive RBCs. If the baby's RBCs are D-positive, the mother's anti-D antibodies attack the fetus of subsequent pregnancies.
3. **Laboratory results on newborn:** Positive **DAT**, increased **serum bilirubin**
4. Exchange transfusion may be needed to avoid kernicterus.
5. **Rh immune globulin (RhIG)** administered to the mother **provides passive anti-D** to prevent an Rh-negative woman from making anti-D. The passive antibodies attach to Rh-positive fetal RBCs that may enter the maternal circulation before the mother's immune system recognizes the fetal D antigen as foreign. The mother is **not alloimmunized** and does not produce antibodies against D antigen.

C. ABO Hemolytic Disease

1. Most common form of HDN; babies with A or B blood type born to O mother; usually mild disease
2. Usually not treated by transfusion
3. Infants are treated by **phototherapy** to **break down excess bilirubin.**
4. May require transfusion weeks to months after birth in rare cases

D. HDN Caused by Other IgG Antibodies (Kidd, Kell, etc.)

1. **Any IgG antibody** that can cross the placenta can cause HDN.
2. May be severe and require intrauterine or exchange transfusion
3. **Antibody titration**
   a. Used to predict severity of HDN
   b. Titer needs to be determined as soon as possible in pregnancy.
   c. Repeat titers on positive mothers at 16 and 22 weeks, and then every 1–4 weeks until delivery.
   d. A twofold rise in titer indicates a serious situation, and invasive procedures or an exchange transfusion may be necessary.
4. **Amniocentesis** performed
   a. Bilirubin in the amniotic fluid is measured at 450 nm rather than at 540 nm like hemoglobin. A comparison of the absorbance will correspond the lysis of RBCs (hemoglobin) and the conversion to bilirubin.

E. Laboratory Testing for Predicting Hemolytic Disease of the Newborn

1. ABO and D on mother prior to delivery
2. Antibody screen on mother; infants do not produce antibodies.
3. Amniocentesis may be used periodically to monitor hemolytic severity during pregnancy.

F. Suspected Cases of Hemolytic Disease of the Newborn

1. **Cord blood** of infants, born to **D-negative mothers** and in suspected cases of HDN, must be tested for the following:
   a. ABO
   b. D
   c. DAT

G. Prevention of Hemolytic Disease of the Newborn

1. **Prenatal Rh immune globulin (RhIG)** should be administered to **D-negative women at 28 weeks** (300 μg) and **at childbirth.**
2. One vial of RhIG should be administered to D-negative women after any potential risk of fetal–maternal bleed (i.e., abortions, ectopic pregnancies, amniocenteses, chorionic villus sampling, percutaneous umbilical blood sampling, intrauterine transfusions, and abdominal trauma).

3. **Postpartum administration**
   a. **D-negative women** who give birth to a **D-positive infant** need a 300-μg dose of **RhIG within 72 hours of delivery**.
   b. One **300-μg dose** of RhIG will **neutralize** up to 15 mL RBCs (30 mL whole blood) of **feto maternal hemorrhage**. If the feto-maternal hemorrhage is >15 mL RBCs, more than one dose is required to neutralize the RBCs.
4. **Fetal screen (rosette test):** A suspension of RBCs taken from the mother is incubated with anti-D. Anti-D binds to Rh-positive fetal RBCs, if present in the maternal circulation. After washing, D-positive indicator cells are added that bind to the anti-D on the fetal cells, forming a rosette around the sensitized Rh-positive fetal RBCs. This is a **screening method** to **detect fetomaternal bleeds >15 mL**. If the fetal screen is positive, a Kleihauer-Betke test is required to quantify the amount of bleed that has occurred.
5. **Kleihauer-Betke (KB) acid elution** is used to **determine** the **amount of a fetomaternal hemorrhage**. Principle: RBCs containing fetal hemoglobin are resistant to acid elution. A blood smear from the mother is made, dipped in an acid buffer, and then stained. The buffer lyses the mother's cells (ghost cells) but not the fetal cells. Pink fetal cells are counted. Results are reported as percent of fetal cells (# fetal cells ÷ total cells counted). The amount, in milliliters (mL), of fetal blood in maternal circulation equals the % fetal cells × 50. Divide the mL of cells by 30 to determine the number of Rh immune globulin doses needed. *Note:* Flow cytometry assays have been developed that can replace the traditional Kleihauer-Betke test.

H. Exchange Transfusions

1. Selection of blood for exchange transfusion
   a. Infant cells must be tested for ABO and D. ABO group of RBCs chosen for transfusion must be compatible with mother's ABO group. Group O blood is typically used.
   b. Mother's blood is used for antibody screen.
   c. Units must be antigen negative for all antibodies in mother's blood.
2. FFP is used to reconstitute packed RBCs to a hematocrit of approximately 40–50%. Group AB FFP is typically used.
3. Any blood products to be transfused must be hemoglobin S negative, cytomegalovirus (CMV) negative, and irradiated.

XI. BLOOD COLLECTION

A. Donor Selection

1. Registration questions include full name, address, home and work phone numbers, date of birth, sex, date of last donation, written consent, photo identification, ethnicity (optional), and intended use of donation.
2. Educational material is distributed to the donor. The donor must read material, and if the prospective donor shows symptoms of an infectious disease, the donor is excluded from donation.

3. Current **donor history questions include** the following:
    a. Have you ever donated or attempted to donate blood using a different (or another) name here or anywhere else?
    b. In the past 8 weeks, have you given blood, plasma, or platelets here or anywhere else?
    c. Have you for any reason been deferred or refused as a blood donor or told not to donate blood?
    d. Are you feeling well and healthy today?
    e. In the past 12 months, have you been under a doctor's care or had a major illness or surgery?
    f. Have you ever had chest pain, heart disease, recent or severe respiratory disease?
    g. Have you ever had cancer, a blood disease, or a bleeding problem?
    h. Have you ever had yellow jaundice, liver disease, viral hepatitis, or a positive test for hepatitis?
    i. Have you ever had malaria, Chagas disease, or babesiosis?
    j. Have you ever taken etretinate (Tegison) for psoriasis?
    k. In the past 3 years, have you taken acitretin (Soriatane)?
    l. In the past 3 days, have you taken piroxicam (Feldene), aspirin, or anything that has aspirin in it?
    m. In the past month, have you taken isotretinoin (Accutane) or finasteride (Proscar or Propecia)?
    n. In the past 4 weeks, have you taken any pills or medications?
    o. In the past 12 months, have you been given rabies shots?
    p. Female donors: In the past 6 weeks, have you been pregnant or are you pregnant now?
    q. In the past 3 years, have you been outside the United States or Canada?
    r. Have you ever received human pituitary-derived growth hormone?
    s. Have you received a dura mater (or brain covering) graft?
    t. Have you or any of your blood relatives ever had Creutzfeldt-Jakob disease or have you ever been told that your family is at an increased risk for Creutzfeldt-Jakob disease?
    u. In the past 12 months, have you had close contact with a person with yellow jaundice or viral hepatitis, or have you been given hepatitis B immune globulin (HBIG)?
    v. In the past 12 months, have you taken (snorted) cocaine through your nose?
    w. In the past 12 months, have you received blood or had an organ or a tissue transplant or graft?
    x. In the past 12 months, have you had a tattoo applied, ear or skin piercing, acupuncture, accidental needlestick, or come in contact with someone else's blood?
    y. In the past 12 months, have you had a positive test for syphilis?
    z. In the past 12 months, have you had or been treated for syphilis or gonorrhea?

aa. In the past 12 months, have you given money or drugs to anyone to have sex with you?
bb. At any time since 1977, have you taken money or drugs for sex?
cc. In the past 12 months, have you had sex, even once with anyone who has taken money or drugs for sex?
dd. Have you ever used a needle, even once, to take drugs that were not prescribed for you by a doctor?
ee. In the past 12 months, have you had sex, even once, with anyone who has used a needle to take drugs not prescribed by a doctor?
ff. Male donors: Have you had sex with another male, even once, since 1977?
gg. Female donors: In the past 12 months, have you had sex with a male who has had sex with another male, even once, since 1977?
hh. Have you ever taken clotting factor concentrates for a bleeding problem such as hemophilia?
ii. In the past 12 months, have you had sex, even once, with anyone who has taken clotting factor concentrates for a bleeding problem such as hemophilia?
jj. Do you have acquired immunodeficiency syndrome (AIDS) or have you had a positive test for the human immunodeficiency virus (HIV) virus?
kk. In the past 12 months, have you had sex, even once, with anyone who has AIDS or has had a positive test for the HIV virus?
ll. Are you giving blood because you want to be tested for HIV or the AIDS virus?
mm. Do you understand that if you have the AIDS virus, you can give it to someone else even though you may feel well and have a negative AIDS test?
nn. Were you born in, or have you lived in, or have you traveled to any African country since 1977?
oo. When you traveled there, did you receive a blood transfusion or any other medical treatment with a product made from blood?
pp. Have you had sexual contact with anyone who was born in or lived in any African country since 1977?
qq. In the past 12 months, have you been in jail or prison?
rr. From 1980 to present, have you spent more than 3 months in Europe?
ss. Have you read and understood all the donor information presented to you, and have all your questions been answered?

4. Examples of **donor deferrals:** See Table 5-5■.
5. All **donors** must pass a **physical exam** with the following criteria:
   a. Appear to be in good health
   b. 38% hematocrit (minimum)
   c. 12.5 g/dL hemoglobin (minimum)
   d. Body temperature must be below 99.5°F (37.5°C).
   e. Blood pressure must be below or equal to 180/100 mm Hg.
   f. Pulse must be between 50 and 100 bpm and regular.
   g. Weight must be a minimum of 110 pounds.

TABLE 5-5 POSSIBLE REASONS FOR CURRENT DONOR DEFERRALS		
a.	Hepatitis B IgG	12 months
b.	Tattoo/piercing	12 months
c.	Exposure to blood	12 months
d.	Sexual contact with a person at high risk for HIV	12 months
e.	Imprisonment (>72 hours)	12 months
f.	Postblood transfusion	12 months
g.	Rape victim	12 months
h.	Aspirin and aspirin-containing drugs	72 hours
i.	Human pituitary growth hormone injection	indefinite
j.	Sexual contact with anyone who used a needle to take illegal drugs	indefinite
k.	Taken clotting factors	indefinite
l.	AIDS or HIV positive	indefinite
m.	Males having sex with other males	indefinite
n.	Had viral hepatitis	indefinite
o.	Positive hepatitis B surface antigen (HBsAg)	indefinite
p.	Positive hepatitis B core (HBc)	indefinite
q.	Positive Human T-cell leukemia virus (HTLV)-I or HTLV-II	indefinite
r.	History of Creutzfeldt-Jakob disease	indefinite
s.	History of Chagas disease or babesiosis	indefinite

6. **Confidential unit exclusion** (optional)
   a. This is used to give **donors** a way to indicate if this **unit** should be **used for transfusion or discarded**. The most common way to accomplish this is to give the donor **two bar-coded labels**: One states that the blood is OK to use and the other states that the blood should not be used. The donor chooses the label and applies it to his/her records. Once the label is pulled from the backing, the only way of knowing which label is on the records is to scan the bar code.
7. **Informed consent:** The donor must sign a form that allows blood to be collected and used for transfusion.

B. Phlebotomy
1. **Identification** is a crucial step. The donor must be identified before phlebotomy can be done.
2. **Bag labeling:** The bag, attached satellite bags, sample tubes, and donor registration must have the same unique identification number. The labels consist of letters and bar codes.
3. **Postdonation care:** After donating, donors are urged to avoid alcohol and smoking immediately, drink lots of fluid for the next 3 days, and be aware that dizziness and fainting can occur a few hours after donation.

C. Special Blood Collection

1. **Autologous donation:** A donation of blood given by a person to be used for transfusions on themselves at a later date. There are four types—preoperative, intraoperative hemodilution, intraoperative collection, and postoperative collection.
   a. **Advantages:** No diseases transmitted, no alloantibodies formed, no transfusion reactions possible, especially good for patients with existing alloantibodies for whom it may be difficult to find compatible units
   b. **Disadvantages:** High waste amount (unused if surgery postponed), adverse donor reactions, and increased cost
2. **Preoperative collection**
   a. Blood is drawn and stored before surgery.
   b. Used for stable patients having a surgery that may require a transfusion
   c. Process begins with a physician's order.
   d. Patients must sign informed consent.
   e. Not asked detailed questions about high-risk behavior
   f. Facility makes policy regarding patient's health, age, weight, etc. Hemoglobin should not be below 11 g/dL or hematocrit below 33%.
   g. Blood not drawn sooner than every 72 hours and not drawn within 72 hours of surgery.
   h. Patient's name, transfusion facility, unique patient identification number, expiration date, and "For Autologous Use Only" or "Autologous Donor" tag is on the bag.
   i. ABO and D must be performed at the collecting facility. These tests must be repeated if the transfusing facility is different from the collecting facility.
   j. If transfused outside of the facility, HBsAg, anti-HBc, hepatitis C antibody, HIV 1/2 antigen and antibody, and serologic testing for syphilis must be performed before shipping.
   k. If the donor is positive for any of the above, physician's permission is required to use the unit, and a biohazard sticker is attached to the unit before shipping.
   l. An autologous unit cannot be used for allogeneic transfusion; if it is not used by the donor, it must be discarded.
3. **Intraoperative hemodilution (acute normovolemic hemodilution)**
   a. One to two units of the patient's blood are removed at the beginning of surgery and replaced by volume expanders.
   b. Units must be labeled with patient's name, unique identification number, date and time of phlebotomy, and "For Autologous Use Only."
   c. This blood can be stored at room temperature for up to 8 hours or at 1–6°C for 24 hours.
4. **Intraoperative collection (intraoperative salvage)**
   a. Blood lost into the abdominal cavity is collected by an instrument. It is washed with saline and transferred back into patient. Blood should not be used if blood will be contaminated with bacteria, as in peritonitis.

5. **Postoperative collection**
   a. Collect blood from surgical drains and deliver into sterile containers.
   b. Collected blood must be transfused within 6 hours.
6. **Directed donations**
   a. Patients choose their own donors.
   b. All AABB Standards for donation apply to directed donations.
   c. Policies about switching units from directed donation to general donor pool vary among institutions.
7. **Hemapheresis**
   a. **Leukapheresis:** Only WBCs removed from donor blood
   b. **Plateletpheresis:** Only platelets removed from donor blood
   c. **Plasmapheresis:** Only plasma removed from donor blood
   d. **RBC pheresis:** Only RBCs removed from donor
   e. **Apheresis instrument:** An electronic instrument that takes blood from a donor, separates the desired component, and returns the remaining components to the donor. (Process takes from 20 minutes to 2 hours.)
   f. All AABB Standards for donation apply to apheresis donors also. However, frequency of donation and additional testing are different for the three types of apheresis:
      1) **Plateletpheresis:** Platelet count of 150,000/μL; 48 hours required between donations, up to 24 times/year
      2) **Leukapheresis:** Not more than twice a week, 24 times/year
      3) **Plasmapheresis:** Every 4 weeks; total protein, IgG, and IgM monitored
      4) **RBC pheresis:** Every 16 weeks
8. **Therapeutic phlebotomy**
   a. One unit of blood is removed from a patient in a specified time interval.
   b. This is done to treat patients with polycythemia, hemochromatosis, and porphyria.

XII. BLOOD COMPONENTS: PREPARATION, STORAGE, AND SHIPMENT

A. Definitions

1. **Whole blood:** Blood collected from donors contains all cellular and liquid elements.
2. **Components:** Parts of blood used for treating patients, including RBCs, plasma, platelets, and cryoprecipitated antihemophiliac factor
3. **Hemotherapy:** Use blood or blood components to treat a disease in a patient

B. Blood Collection Bag

1. It is a **closed system** consisting of main bag with needle, tubing, and up to four satellite bags attached. The entire system is **sterile**.
2. **Standard phlebotomy** = 450 mL ± 45 mL or 500 mL ± 50mL

C. Anticoagulant Preservative Solutions

1. **Standard volume:** 63 mL for 450 mL collections or 70 mL for 500 mL collections
2. If an autologous unit is drawn on a patient weighing less than 110 pounds, the anticoagulant must be reduced.
   a. Reduced Volume Factor (A) = weight of patient ÷ 110 lb.
   A × 70 mL = amount of anticoagulant needed (B)
   70 − B = amount of anticoagulant to remove
   A × 500 mL = amount of blood to collect
   b. Example: 90-lb donor
   90 lbs ÷ 110 lbs = 0.81 = A
   0.81 × 70 mL = 56.7 mL = B
   70 mL − 56.7 mL = 13.3 mL of anticoagulant to be removed from bag
   0.81 × 500 mL = 405 mL of blood to be collected
3. **Types of anticoagulants and preservatives**
   a. **Adenine:** Used in ATP synthesis
   b. **Citrate:** Chelates calcium to prevent coagulation
   c. **CPD:** Citrate-phosphate-dextrose
   d. **CP2D:** Citrate-phosphate-2-dextrose
   e. **CPDA-1:** Citrate-phosphate dextrose adenine-1
   f. **Dextrose (glucose):** Sugar to support RBC life
   g. **Sodium bisphosphate:** Buffer to prevent decreased pH
4. **Storage**
   a. **Shelf life:** This is the length of storage time the blood unit can have that yields at least 75% of original RBCs still in recipient's circulation 24 hours after transfusion. Remember, blood is still "alive" when it is in a blood bag.
   b. Glucose, ATP, 2,3-BPG (also known as 2,3-diphosphoglycerate; 2,3-DPG), and pH decrease as RBCs are stored. After cells are transfused, ATP and 2,3-BPG levels are restored in about 24 hours.
   c. Substances that increase during storage are metabolic end products such as potassium, hydrogen ions, etc.
5. **Additive solutions**
   a. AS-1 contains mannitol.
   b. AS-3 contains citrate and phosphate.
   c. AS-5 contains mannitol.
   d. These must be added within 72 hours of collection.
   e. Usually, an additive solution is added to RBCs after plasma is removed.
   f. Additives extend the shelf life to **42 days** and reduce RBC viscosity during transfusion.
6. **Rejuvenation solution**
   a. Contains phosphate, inosine, pyruvate, and adenine
   b. Its purpose is to restore 2,3-BPG and ATP levels before freezing or transfusing a unit.
   c. May be necessary for autologous or rare units

d. RBCs can be rejuvenated up to 3 days past the expiration date and can then be frozen for future use.
e. RBCs can be rejuvenated, stored up to 24 hours at 1–6°C, and transfused. The cells must be washed before transfusion to remove the inosine.

7. **Blood component preparation**
   a. Whole blood is centrifuged and can be separated into RBCs, platelets, FFP, and cryoprecipitated antihemophiliac factor.
   b. **Process:** Whole blood bag is centrifuged; plasma is removed into a satellite bag. If platelets are to be prepared from whole blood, two spins are required. The first centrifugation will be a “soft” spin, leaving platelets suspended in the plasma layer. If platelets will not be produced, a single “hard” spin (increased time and rotations per minute) will be performed.
   c. AS-1 is put into RBC bag (if additive solution is used).
   d. RBC bag is sealed and removed from system.
   e. Plasma bag is centrifuged to sediment platelets (“hard” spin).
   f. Plasma is separated into FFP bag, leaving platelets with 40 to 70 mL of plasma in platelet bag.
   g. Platelet bag is sealed off and cut.
   h. Plasma is either frozen to make FFP within 8 hours of collection or frozen and later thawed in refrigerated conditions to make cryoprecipitate and cryo-poor plasma.
8. **Storage temperature and expiration dates for components**
   a. **Whole blood:** Storage 1–6°C; expires with CPD, CP2D anticoagulants in 21 days, with CPDA-1 anticoagulant in 35 days, with Adsol (AS-1, AS-3, or AS-5) in 42 days
   b. **RBCs:** Storage 1–6°C; expires with CPD, CP2D anticoagulants in 21 days, with CPDA-1 in 35 days, with AS-1, AS-3, and AS-5 in 42 days
   c. **Platelets:** Storage 20–24°C with rotation, expires in 5 days
   d. **FFP:** Storage −18°C, expires in 1 year; storage −65°C, expires in 7 years
   e. **Cryoprecipitate:** Storage −18°C, expires in 1 year
   f. **RBCs (frozen):** Storage −65°C, expires in 10 years
   g. **RBCs (deglycerolized, washed):** Storage 1–6°C, expires in 24 hours after thawing (deglycerolization)
   h. **RBCs (irradiated):** Storage 1–6°C, expires in 28 days or on originally assigned outdate, whichever comes first
   i. **Platelets (pooled):** Storage 20–24°C, expires in 4 hours after pooling
   j. **Cryoprecipitate (pooled):** Storage 20–24°C, expires 4 hours after pooling
   k. **FFP (thawed):** Storage 1–6°C, expires in 24 hours
   l. **Plateletpheresis:** Storage 20–24°C, expires in 5 days
   m. **Granulocyte pheresis:** Storage 20–24°C, expires in 24 hours

D. Storage and Transportation

1. FDA requirements and AABB Standards define calibration and maintenance procedures, storage temperature limits, and monitoring parameters for equipment used to store blood products.
2. **All refrigerators, freezers, and platelet incubators must have the following:**
   a. Recording device that monitors the temperature at least every 4 hours
   b. Audible alarm that ensure response 24 hours a day
   c. Regular alarm check
   d. Power failure and alarm activation emergency procedure
   e. Emergency power backup (continuous power source for alarms)
   f. Calibrated thermometer that is checked against referenced thermometer
   g. Written procedures for all the above
3. **Transportation**
   a. Temperature for **RBCs** of **1–10°C** is required during transport. A predetermined amount of wet ice in plastic bags is placed on top of the blood units to maintain the temperature for 24 hours.
   b. RBCs are packed in cardboard boxes with a styrofoam box inside. The ice is double-bagged and weighs approximately 9 pounds.
   c. Frozen components are shipped on dry ice. These should be well wrapped because dry ice evaporates, and space in the box for movement should be allowed.
   d. **Platelets** are shipped at **room temperature**. Platelets can survive without agitation for a maximum of 24 hours.
   e. When component shipments are received, observe and record the temperature and appearance of units. If temperature is out of range, units must be evaluated before transfusion. Institutions have policies for determination of the disposition of the units. All problems and dispositions must be documented and stored with transfusion services records.

E. Administration of Blood Components

1. Positive identification of patient, sample, and crossmatched unit
2. Only **normal saline** should be infused with blood components.
3. A standard **170-micron filter** must be used with all blood components. **Leukoreduction filters** may be used to reduce the number of leukocytes transfused with RBCs.
4. The maximum transfusion time allowed for one unit to be transfused is **4 hours.** If the unit cannot be completely infused within 4 hours, the unit should be divided into two satellite bags and transfused as two separate units.
5. Documentation and accurate recordkeeping are vital.

XIII. BLOOD COMPONENT THERAPY

A. Whole Blood

1. Infrequently used but can be useful in treating actively bleeding patients, patients who have lost at least 25% of their blood volume, or patients requiring exchange transfusions
2. When whole blood is not available, reconstituted whole blood (RBCs mixed with thawed type ABO FFP from a different donor) may be used.

B. RBCs

1. Used in patients undergoing chemotherapy or radiation therapy, trauma patients, and patients who underwent surgery, patients on dialysis, premature infants, and patients with sickle cell anemia
2. **Transfusing one unit** usually **increases** the patient's **hemoglobin** approximately **1 g/dL** and the **hematocrit by 3%.**

C. Leukocyte-Reduced RBCs

1. Used in patients who are chronically transfused or patients having known febrile transfusion reactions but commonly used for other patients.
2. The standard 170-micron filter does not remove leukocytes. A special filter is required for bedside filtration. Leukoreduction (filtration) can also occur in the manufacturing process, which typically occurs within 72 hours from the time of collection.
3. AABB Standards for **leukocyte reduction** states that **85% of RBCs must remain** and **leukocytes** must be **reduced to less than 5×10^6 WBC/unit.**

D. Frozen RBCs

1. **Method:** RBCs are frozen by first adding **glycerol** to prevent cell hydration and the formation of ice crystals that can cause cell lysis (40% weight per volume).
2. The unit is transferred to a polyolefin or polyvinyl chloride bag, and then the bag is placed in a metal or cardboard canister.
3. **Initial** freezing temp is **−80°C**, then for **long-term storage at −65°C for 10 years.**

E. Deglycerolized RBCs

1. Frozen RBCs are thawed, and then the glycerol must be removed.
2. **Deglycerolization:** Glycerol is removed from the RBCs by washing the cells with a series of saline solutions of decreasing osmolality.
3. Deglycerolization involves entering the bag, so the **deglycerolized RBCs expire in 24 hours.**

F. Washed RBCs

1. Used for patients who have a reaction to plasma proteins (allergic, febrile, and/or anaphylactic)

2. Used in infant or intrauterine transfusions
3. 10–20% of RBCs are lost in the process of washing the RBC unit with normal saline.

G. Irradiated RBCs

1. **T cells** can cause **graft-versus-host disease**, with 90% of cases being fatal.
2. Gamma irradiation **prevents T cell proliferation**.
3. AABB Standards require irradiation of cellular components (RBCs and platelets), if a donor is a blood relative of the intended recipient or donor unit is HLA matched for recipient. Recommended minimum dose of **gamma irradiation** is **25 Gy** (2500 rads).
4. Used for intrauterine transfusions, immunodeficient recipient, premature infants, patients receiving chemotherapy and radiation, and bone marrow or progenitor cells transplant patients

H. Platelets

1. **Purpose:** Used to **control or prevent bleeding**
2. Not indicated in patients with idiopathic thrombocytopenia
3. Indicated in patients with chemotherapy, post-bone marrow transplant patients, or patients experiencing postoperative bleeding
4. **Transfused platelets** have a **life span** of **3 to 4 days**.
5. **No crossmatch necessary**, but ABO type-specific preferred
6. **Platelet concentrates**
   a. Prepared from whole blood unit
   b. **Contain approximately 5.5 $\times$ 10^{10} platelets/unit**
   c. **Raise patient's platelet count by 5000 μL/unit after transfusion**
7. **Pooled platelets**
   a. Procedure is to choose one platelet bag of those to be pooled and empty content of other bags into it.
   b. Usual platelet order is **6–10 units**.
   c. **Opening the unit reduces** the **shelf life** of the bag **to 4 hours**. Platelets should be pooled immediately before transfusion.
8. **Plateletpheresis**
   a. HLA-matched patients who receive numerous platelet transfusions can develop antibodies to the class I HLA antigens on platelets. These patients require HLA matching before transfusion. If platelets to be transfused are not HLA matched, the platelets will not last 5 days in the patient's circulation.
   b. **Plateletpheresis packs contain approximately 3 $\times$ 10^{11} platelets per unit.**
9. **Leukocyte-reduced platelets**
   a. Filters can reduce the number of leukocytes in a bag while being transfused.
   b. Specific apheresis instruments can reduce leukocyte numbers during collection.

I. Fresh-Frozen Plasma

1. **Purpose:** To **replace coagulation factors** in the patient
2. Indicated in the following:
   a. Bleeding patients who require factors II, V, VII, IX, and X
   b. Abnormal coagulation due to massive transfusion
   c. Patients on anticoagulants who are bleeding or require surgery
   d. Treatment of thrombotic thrombocytopenic purpura (TTP) and hemolytic uremic syndrome (HUS)
   e. Patients with liver disease to prevent or correct bleeding
   f. Antithrombin III deficiencies
   g. Disseminated intravascular coagulation (DIC) when fibrinogen is >100 mg/dL
3. **Thawing**
   a. Thawed in water bath at **30–37°C** for **30–45 minutes** before transfusion
   b. Unit should be placed in watertight container before immersing in water bath to keep ports clean and prevent contamination.
   c. Water baths with agitators are preferred because the unit thaws faster.
   d. FDA-approved microwaves can also be used.

J. Cryoprecipitated Antihemophilic Factor (Cryoprecipitate)

1. Insoluble precipitate is formed when FFP is thawed between 1 and 6°C. It contains factor VIII, fibrinogen, factor XIII, and von Willebrand factor.
2. It is used for patients with **factor XIII deficiency, von Willebrand disease, and fibrinogen deficiency, and as a fibrin sealant**. *Note:* Patients with factor VIII deficiency are routinely treated with factor VIII concentrates.
3. Each unit must contain at least **150 mg/dL of fibrinogen** and **80 IU of factor VIII**.
4. **Pooled cryoprecipitate**
   a. Like platelets, cryoprecipitate is pooled into one bag before transfusion.
   b. Units are thawed in a similar fashion to FFP before pooling.
   c. Cryoprecipitate must be given within **4 hours** after pooling.
   d. **Formula** for figuring **factor VIII** in cryoprecipitate:

$$\#\text{of units} = \frac{\text{plasma volume} \times (\text{desired level \%} - \text{initial level \%})}{80\,\text{IU/bag}}$$

   e. Fibrin glue from cryoprecipitate: 1–2 units of cryoprecipitate are mixed with thrombin and applied topically to the bleeding area.

K. Granulocyte Pheresis

1. **Granulocyte transfusions** are rare and limited to **septic infants**.
2. The pheresis bag contains $>1.0 \times 10^{10}$ granulocytes, platelets, and 20–50 mL of RBCs.
3. The cells deteriorate rapidly and must be **transfused within 24 hours** of collection.

4. Store at 20–24°C with no agitation until transfused.
5. **Crossmatching** is **required** because of RBC contamination.

L. Labeling

1. Must conform with Title 21 of the **Code of Federal Regulations** (CFR), specifically 21 CFR 606.120 and 606.121, as well as **FDA** current thinking as described in "Guidance for Industry: Recognition and Use of a Standard for Uniform Blood and Blood Component Container Labels" (9/22/2006). In addition, facilities accredited by AABB must have implemented **ISBT 128 labeling systems** by May 1, 2008, in accordance with the "United States Industry Consensus Standard for the Uniform Labeling of Blood and Blood Components Using ISBT 128" (November 2005).
2. Current **labeling requirements include** proper name, unique number, amount of blood collected, amount and type of anticoagulant, volume of component, expiration date, storage temperature, ABO/D type, reference to the "Circular of Information for the Use of Human Blood and Blood Components," warning regarding infectious agents, prescription requirements, donor classification, and FDA license number if applicable.
3. Other products must be labeled as follows:
   a. **Irradiated components** must have name of the facility performing the irradiation.
   b. **Pooled components** must include final volume, unique number assigned to the pool, time of expiration, and name of facility preparing the pooled component.
   c. **Autologous units** must be labeled: "For Autologous Use Only."
4. "Circular of Information for the Use of Human Blood and Blood Components": Guidelines that provide a description of each component, indications and contraindications for use, and information of dosage, administration, storage, side effects, and hazards

XIV. TRANSFUSION THERAPY

A. Emergency Transfusions

1. Rapid loss of blood can result in hemorrhagic shock.
   a. **Symptoms:** Hypotension, tachycardia, pallor, cyanosis, cold clammy skin, oliguria, decreased hematocrit, decreased central venous pressure, central nervous system depression, and metabolic shock
2. **Priorities in acute blood loss**
   a. Replace and maintain blood volume.
   b. Make sure oxygen-carrying capacity is adequate.
   c. Maintain coagulation system integrity.
   d. Correct metabolic imbalances.
   e. Maintain colloid osmotic pressure.

3. **Massive transfusion:** Replacement of a person's entire blood volume (approximately 10 units) within 24 hours
4. **Emergency transfusions** result from trauma (gunshot wounds, stabbings, vehicular accidents, etc.) and surgical needs.
5. **Emergency release of blood:** It is preferable to transfuse type-specific blood. If time is not available to type the patient, **type O, D-negative** blood is **transfused into women of childbearing age. Type O, D-positive blood** is transfused into **men**. Physician must request emergency release indicating that no crossmatch is performed before the blood is transfused. The **crossmatch** is **performed during or following the transfusion**.

B. Neonatal and Pediatric Transfusions

1. Smaller blood volume than adults
2. Premature infants may need transfusion to offset the effect of hemoglobin F in their system. Hemoglobin F does not release oxygen readily.
3. **Iatrogenic blood loss** (blood taken from the neonate or infant for laboratory tests) causes the neonate or infant to develop an anemia that may be severe enough to transfuse.
4. Neonates and infants do not tolerate hypothermia well, so blood warmers may be used.
5. Washed or fresh blood is preferred for neonates or infants because of the liver's inability to metabolize citrate anticoagulants and potassium, which leaks from RBCs in donor units over time.
6. Transfusions are given in small volumes in multiple packs taken from a normal size blood unit.
7. Infants do not form antibodies for the first 4 months, so no crossmatch is necessary.
8. **Transfuse** CMV-negative and/or leukoreduced blood.

C. Transplantation

1. **Liver transplant patients** require large amounts of blood products (on average 20 units of RBCs, 25 units of FFP, 17 units of platelets, and 5 units of cryoprecipitate) because the liver produces many coagulation factors and cholesterol for RBC membranes.
2. **ABO compatibility is important in kidney, liver, and heart transplants**. It is not important in bone, heart valves, skin, and corneal transplants.
3. **Progenitor cell transplants**
   a. **Allogeneic or autologous**
   b. Derived from bone marrow or umbilical cord blood
   c. Transfusion support with leukocyte-reduced products to prevent alloimmunization and a greater chance of rejection
   d. **Conditions treated:** Severe combined immunodeficiency disease, Wiskott-Aldrich syndrome, aplastic anemia, Fanconi anemia, thalassemia, sickle cell

disease, acute leukemia, CML, lymphoma, myelodysplastic/myeloproliferative disorders, multiple myeloma, neuroblastoma, breast cancer, ovarian cancer, and testicular cancer

D. Therapeutic Hemapheresis

1. Replacement of blood from a patient to improve a patient's health
2. Conditions indicated for therapeutic exchanges: Multiple myeloma, Waldenström macroglobulinemia, hyperleukocytosis, TTP/HUS, sickle cell anemia, myasthenia gravis, and acute Guillain-Barré syndrome

E. Oncology

1. Chemotherapy drugs kill all cells that are undergoing mitosis: Stem cells, gastrointestinal epithelial cells, and hair follicles.
2. Action of chemotherapy drugs:
   a. Stopping DNA replication
   b. Interfering with mRNA production

F. Chronic Renal Disease

1. Patients being treated with dialysis have an increased uremic (blood urea nitrogen or BUN) content in blood that alters the RBC shape and causes the cells to be removed from circulation by the spleen.
2. Dialysis itself mechanically destroys RBCs.
3. Nonfunctioning kidneys do not produce erythropoietin to stimulate RBC production.
4. The use of transfusions in patients receiving dialysis has been dramatically reduced since erythropoietin therapy was initiated.

G. Sickle Cell Anemia

1. An abnormal hemoglobin (e.g., Hgb S) causes cells to "sickle" and to be removed from circulation, resulting in a lowered hematocrit.
2. Because these patients require many transfusions, phenotypically matched units are preferred.
3. Severe cases may be treated by bone marrow transplants.

H. Thalassemia

1. Decreased synthesis of the α- and β-globin chains
2. Hemolytic anemia results
3. Transfusion support necessary

I. Aplastic Anemia

1. Blood transfusion support is usually needed until bone marrow transplant can occur.

XV. TRANSFUSION REACTIONS

A. Types of Transfusion Reactions

1. Transfusion reactions are an adverse physiologic reaction to the infusion of blood.
   a. **Hemolytic:** This is a reaction that destroys the transfused blood cells *in vivo*. Large amounts of free hemoglobin are released into the blood and can cause systemic damage.
   b. **Nonhemolytic:** Febrile and allergic
2. **Acute reactions** occur rapidly, within hours of transfusion.
3. **Delayed reactions** occur days or weeks after transfusion.
4. **Immune-mediated transfusion reactions** are due to RBC or HLA antigens and antigen–antibody reactions.
5. Transfusion reactions can also be caused by bacteria, viruses, or parasitic organisms.

B. Hemolytic Transfusion Reactions

1. May be acute or delayed
   a. **Intravascular** reactions are usually acute, whereas **extravascular** reactions are usually delayed.
   b. Symptoms are variable; they may not be correlated with type of hemolysis.
2. **Mechanism**
   a. **Antibody binding** to RBCs
      1) **Intravascular hemolysis:** IgM antibodies activate the classical pathway of complement that lyses RBCs intravascularly. The lysis releases hemoglobin and RBC remnants into the blood. The excess hemoglobin binds to haptoglobin. Haptoglobin can bind a limited amount of hemoglobin, so the excess hemoglobin is found in the blood and urine.
      2) **Extravascular hemolysis:** Antibody-coated RBCs are removed from circulation by the liver and spleen. The cells lyse when sequestered and, subsequently, bilirubin is released into the blood. Antibodies responsible for this type of hemolysis do not activate the complement cascade or only partially activate it.
   b. **Anaphylatoxins** cause hypotension by triggering serotonin and histamine release.
   c. **Cytokine activation:** Sensitized RBCs are cleared from the blood by phagocytes. The phagocytes release cytokines that cause fever, hypotension, and activation of T and B cells.
   d. **Coagulation activation:** Antigen–antibody–complement complexes activate the clotting system and cause DIC.
   e. Renal failure is caused by systemic hypotension, reactive renal vasoconstriction, and intravascular thrombi.

C. Acute and Delayed Hemolytic Transfusion Reactions

1. **Acute hemolytic transfusion reactions**
   a. **Clinical signs/symptoms:** Severe, rapid onset, fever, chills, flushing, pain at site of infusion, tachycardia, hemoglobinemia, hemoglobinuria, hypotension
   b. **Major sequelae:** DIC, renal failure, irreversible shock, death
   c. **Mechanisms:** Antigen–antibody reaction activates complement or coats RBCs (i.e., ABO incompatible blood and antibodies to Vel or PP_1P^k antigens)
   d. **Occurrence:** 1:25,000 transfusions
   e. **Most common cause:** Identification error in patient, unit, and/or specimen
   f. **Diagnostic laboratory tests:** Elevated plasma-free hemoglobin, elevated bilirubin (6 hours posttransfusion), decreased haptoglobin, and positive DAT
2. **Delayed hemolytic transfusion reactions**
   a. Usually less severe than acute hemolytic transfusion reaction and dependent on the concentration of antibody in the blood rather than the type of antibody
   b. **Clinical signs:** 5–7 days posttransfusion, fever, mild jaundice
   c. **Major sequelae:** Usually none. However, antibodies in the Kidd system can cause major delayed hemolysis.
   d. **Causes:** Alloantibodies to Rh, Duffy, and Kidd antigens; patient with low concentration of alloantibody experiences anamnestic response when reexposed to RBC antigen
   e. **Occurrence:** 1:2,500 transfusions
   f. **Diagnostic laboratory tests:** Positive DAT, positive posttransfusion antibody screen, and decreased hemoglobin and hematocrit

D. Causes of Non-Immune-Mediated Mechanisms of RBC Destruction

1. Transfusion of hemolyzed units
2. Malfunctioning or unregulated blood warming units
3. Improper thawing and deglycerolization of a frozen RBC unit
4. Physical destruction by needles, valves, or equipment
5. RBC defects
6. Administration of drugs and/or non-isotonic solutions with blood unit

E. Immune-Mediated Nonhemolytic Transfusion Reaction

1. **Clinical signs**
   a. Fever with temperature increase 1°C over baseline temperature 8–24 hours posttransfusion
   b. Nausea, vomiting, headache, and back pain
2. **Causes:** HLA antibody in recipient to donor antigens; cytokines in blood products containing WBCs and platelets
3. **Occurrence**
   a. Common in patients with multiple pregnancies and transfusions
   b. Multiple exposures to HLA antigens
   c. Common in women
   d. 1:200 donor units transfused

F. Allergic Transfusion Reactions

1. **Urticarial reactions**
   a. Clinical signs: Wheals, hives, itching
   b. Sequelae: None
   c. Causes: Recipient forms antibodies to foreign proteins in donor plasma
   d. Occurs in 1–3% of recipients
2. **Anaphylactic reactions**
   a. Clinical signs: Rapid onset, severe wheezing and cough, and bronchospasms
   b. Sequelae: Syncope, shock, death
   c. Cause: Genetic IgA deficiency
   d. Occurs very rarely

G. Transfusion-Associated Graft-versus-Host Disease

1. Clinical signs: 3–30 days posttransfusion, fever, erythematous maculopapular rash, abnormal liver function
2. Sequelae: Sepsis, hemorrhage, 90% mortality rate
3. Cause: Transfused T cells react against recipient
4. Occurs rarely

H. Bacterial Contamination of Blood Products

1. Bacterial contamination usually occurs during phlebotomy or during thawing of frozen blood components.
2. Bacteria (*Yersinia enterocolitica*, most common) multiply in the bag during storage. Pan Genera Detection (Verax Biomedical) tests for antigens from both gram-positive (teichoic acid) and gram-negative (lipopolysaccharide) bacteria
3. Bacterial endotoxins can be present in the blood unit and cause symptoms similar to hemolytic transfusion reactions.
4. Two percent of units are contaminated.
5. Workup: Blood cultures drawn from patient; Gram stain and culture of the unit
6. Person issuing unit needs to check for discoloration, clots, cloudiness, or hemolysis before unit is released.

I. Circulatory Overload

1. Too much blood in a patient's vascular system caused by transfusing a unit too fast; most often occurs in children and elderly patients
2. Symptoms: Dyspnea, severe headache, peripheral edema, and signs of congestive heart failure occurring after transfusion; can be fatal

J. Other Complications

1. **Hemosiderosis:** This condition, which is characterized by the deposition of the iron-containing pigment hemosiderin in organs such as the liver and spleen, occurs in patients who have received multiple transfusions, especially those with hemolytic anemias.

2. **Citrate overload:** Massive transfusions introduce large amounts of citrate into the body. Citrate binds ionized calcium, but it can be alleviated by calcium chloride or calcium gluconate injections.

K. Transfusion Protocol and Suspected Transfusion Reaction Workup

1. Transfusionist checks and rechecks all paperwork, requisition, and blood bag tag before beginning the transfusion to ensure there were no clerical errors made.
2. Vital signs (blood pressure, temperature, respiration, and pulse) are taken before beginning and every 15 minutes for the first hour and then hourly until the transfusion is completed.
3. If a reaction is suspected:
   a. Stop the transfusion.
   b. Notify the physician and the laboratory.
   c. Physician evaluates the patient.
   d. Draw EDTA and red top tubes, and collect first voided urine for laboratory testing according to institutional policy.
4. **Laboratory responsibilities**
   a. Check all samples, requisition, histories, and bags for identical patient identification. **Clerical errors** are responsible for most transfusion reactions.
   b. Examine pretransfusion and posttransfusion patient samples for hemolysis.
   c. Perform **DAT** on posttransfusion patient sample. If the posttransfusion sample is positive, the DAT is then performed on the pretransfusion sample.
   d. If clerical errors are eliminated and pre- and posttransfusion patient samples show no hemolysis and have negative DAT, the workup is considered to be not indicative of a hemolytic transfusion reaction.
   e. If any positive DAT or hemolysis is found in posttransfusion samples that was not present in pretransfusion samples, further testing is required. Repeat ABO and D on pretransfusion patient sample, posttransfusion patient sample, and segments from the bag; repeat antibody screen and crossmatch on old and new patient samples. Other tests may include hemoglobin, hematocrit, haptoglobin, urine hemoglobin, and bilirubin.
5. **Transfusion reaction workup records**
   a. Must be retained in transfusion services indefinitely
   b. Bacterial contamination and transmitted diseases are reported to blood collection facility.
   c. Fatalities are reported to FDA's Office of Compliance, Center for Biologics Evaluation and Research, within 24 hours.

XVI. TRANSFUSION-TRANSMITTED DISEASES

A. Donor Infectious Disease Testing (Test and Date Testing Started)

1. HBsAg (before 1980)
2. HBc antibody (1986)
3. Hepatitis C virus (HCV) antibody (1990); HCV nucleic acid amplification test (NAT) testing (1999 under investigational new drug [IND]/licensed in 2002)

4. HIV-1/2 antibody (HIV-1: 1985; HIV-2: 1992)
5. HIV-1 p24 antigen (1996, discontinued 2002); HIV-1 NAT testing (1999 under IND/licensed in 2002)
6. HTLV-I/II antibody (1997)
7. Syphilis (before 1980)
8. CMV (only performed on small portion of inventory; CMV negative blood needed for premature infants, intrauterine transfusion, and immunocompromised recipients)
9. *Trypanosoma cruzi* antibody/Chagas disease (2007/currently not mandated)
10. West Nile virus NAT testing (2003 under IND/license 2007)
11. Zika virus (test development in progress)

B. Look-Back Studies

1. FDA requires **notification** of patients who received units from donors who subsequently tested positive for HIV-1/2 or HCV.
   a. Identify any blood products previously donated by a donor currently testing positive.
   b. Identify all blood products donated by that donor 12 months before the last negative screening test.
   c. Notify facilities that received units involved in the look-back investigation.
   d. Trace to patients and notify patients of potential exposure.

XVII. SAFETY AND QUALITY ASSURANCE

A. FDA Regulations

1. Mandate adherence to **Current Good Manufacturing Practice**
   a. Write standard operating procedures.
   b. Follow standard operating procedures.
   c. Record and document all work.
   d. Qualify personnel by training and education.
   e. Design and build proper facilities and equipment.
   f. Clean by following a housekeeping schedule.
   g. Validate equipment, personnel, processes, etc.
   h. Perform preventive maintenance on facilities and equipment.
   i. Control for quality.
   j. Audit for compliance with all the above.

B. Records

1. **Good recordkeeping**
   a. Use permanent ink on documents.
   b. Record data on proper form.
   c. **No white-out correction fluid** is permitted; cross out mistake and have person making correction date and initial it.
   d. No ditto marks used.
   e. Record "broken, closed, or not in use" when appropriate.

2. **Retention (indefinite)**
   a. Donor's identification information, medical history, physical exam, consent, and interpretations for disease markers
   b. Information on blood and components from an outside source, including numeric or alphanumeric identification on old unit and identification of the collecting facility, needs to be retained. However, the information from an intermediate facility may be used, if the intermediate facility retains the unit number and identification number of the collecting facility.
   c. Identification of facilities that carry out any part of the preparation of blood components and the functions they perform
   d. Final disposition of each unit of blood or blood component
   e. Notification to donors of permanent deferral
   f. Records of prospective donors who have been placed on surveillance or indefinitely deferred for the protection of the potential recipient
   g. Notification to transfusing facilities of previous receipt of units from donors subsequently found to be confirmed positive for HIV and (HTLV-1)
   h. Difficulty in blood typing, clinically significant antibodies, and adverse reactions to transfusions
   i. Notification to recipients of potential exposure to disease transmissible by blood
   j. Names, signatures, initials, or identification codes and inclusive dates of employment of those authorized to sign or review reports and records
3. **Retention (minimum of 10 years)**
   a. Donor's ABO, D, difficulty in blood typing, severe adverse reactions to donation, and apheresis procedure clinical record
   b. Records of blood component inspection before issue
   c. Patient's ABO and D type, interpretation of compatibility testing, and therapeutic procedures, including phlebotomy, apheresis, and transfusion
   d. All superseded procedures, manuals, and publications
   e. Control testing of components, reagents, and equipment
   f. Proficiency testing surveys, including dates, performed tests, observed results, interpretations, identification of personnel carrying out the tests, and any appropriate corrective actions taken
   g. Documentation of staff qualifications, training, and competency testing
   h. Quality systems audits and internal assessment records

C. Document Control

1. Must be complete, organized, appropriately stored, retrievable, and secure

D. Personnel Qualifications

1. Job descriptions with specific job duties are required.
2. Selection criteria for an employee must be developed.

3. Training must be provided during new employee orientation and whenever procedures change or if an employee performs poorly.
4. Competency assessment means evaluating the skill on a level of knowledge of an employee. This is accomplished through performance observation; written tests; review of results, records, or worksheets; and/or testing unknown samples (i.e., proficiency).

E. Supplier Qualifications

1. Evaluate products and services received from a supplier to see if established criteria are met.

F. Validation

1. Validation ensures that products or services will meet established criteria for a high degree of quality assurance.
2. All blood bank information systems must be validated before being put into use.

G. Federal, State, and Local Safety Regulations

1. FDA
   a. **Biologics Control Act of 1902**
      1) Licensing of manufacturers and products
      2) Labeling
      3) Facility inspections
      4) Suspension or revoking license
      5) Penalties for violation
   b. The Act was expanded in 1944 and implemented under the Public Health Service Act.
2. Occupational Safety and Health Administration (OSHA)
   a. **Occupational Safety and Health Act**
      1) Ensures a safe and healthy workplace
      2) Act enforced by OSHA
   b. Employers must inform employees about OSHA regulations and post OSHA literature that informs employees about their right to know.
   c. Updates to OSHA are published annually in the Code of Federal Regulations (CFR).
3. **Centers for Disease Control and Prevention (CDC)**
   a. CDC introduced universal precautions in 1987 to decrease risks of bloodborne pathogen exposure. Currently, these safety practices are referred to as **standard precautions**.
   b. In 1991, **OSHA** published the final standard on bloodborne pathogens. This regulation requires the following:
      1) Hazard-free workplace
      2) Provision of education and training to staff
      3) Evaluation of potential risks
      4) Evaluation of positions for potential risks

5) Posting of signs and use of labels
6) Implementation of standard precautions for handling biohazardous substances
7) Provision of personal protective equipment (PPE), such as gloves, fluid-resistant laboratory coats, and splash shields, at no cost to the employee
8) Provision of free hepatitis B vaccine to at-risk staff
9) Provision of free HBIG for any exposures to employee

XVIII. BLOOD USAGE REVIEW

A. Peer Review: Mandated by The Joint Commission Standards (for accreditation), CFR (for Medicare reimbursement), most states (for Medicaid reimbursement), College of American Pathologists (for accreditation), and AABB (for accreditation)

1. The Joint Commission requires the medical staff to review blood usage quarterly for the following:
   a. Appropriateness of transfusions for blood and blood products
   b. Evaluation of transfusion reactions
   c. Development and implementation of policies and procedures for blood product distribution, handling, use, and administration
   d. Adequacy of transfusion services to meet the needs of patients
   e. Blood product ordering practices
2. **Hospital transfusion practice** is usually monitored by the Hospital Transfusion Committee. This committee reviews the following:
   a. Statistical data (retrospectively, i.e., data collected over a specified period of time)
   b. Physician ordering patterns
   c. Concurrent review

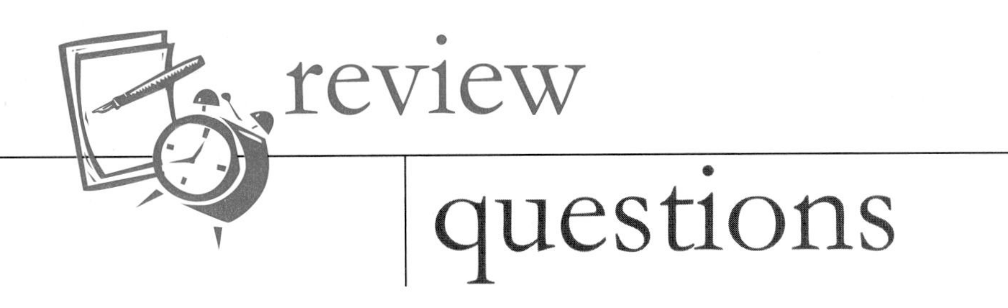

INSTRUCTIONS Each of the questions or incomplete statements that follows is comprised of four suggested responses. Select the *best* answer or completion statement in each case.

Blood Collection, Preservation, Processing, Component Preparation, and Quality Control

1. A woman wants to donate blood. Her physical examination reveals the following: weight—110 lbs, pulse—73 bpm, blood pressure—125/75 mm Hg, hematocrit—35%. Which of the following exclusions applies to the prospective donor?
   A. Pulse too high
   B. Weight too low
   C. Hematocrit too low
   D. Blood pressure too low

2. A potential donor has no exclusions, but she weighs only 87 pounds. What is the allowable amount of blood (including samples) that can be drawn?
   A. 367 mL
   B. 378 mL
   C. 415 mL
   D. 473 mL

3. A donor at a blood drive becomes sweaty and agitated during the donation. She appears pale and limp. What is the best course of action for this situation?
   A. Continue the donation
   B. Withdraw the needle, lift her feet, and administer ammonia
   C. Discontinue donation and provide a paper bag
   D. Call ambulance

4. How much anticoagulant would need to be removed from a 450 mL blood bag if a donor weighed 94 pounds?
   A. 9 mL
   B. 10 mL
   C. 12 mL
   D. 15 mL

5. Which of the following donors would be deferred indefinitely?
   A. History of syphilis
   B. History of gonorrhea
   C. Accutane® treatment
   D. Recipient of human growth hormone
6. Which of the following viruses resides exclusively in leukocytes?
   A. Cytomegalovirus (CMV)
   B. Human immunodeficient virus (HIV)
   C. Hepatitis B virus (HBV)
   D. Hepatitis C virus (HCV)
7. A 47-year-old women donated a unit of blood at a church blood drive. She meets all the physical criteria to donate, but she takes a blood thinner and B_{12} injections. Is she an acceptable donor?
   A. No, due to blood thinner
   B. No, due to B_{12} injections
   C. Yes, for platelets only
   D. Yes, red cells only
8. Which of the following best describes what must be done with a unit of blood drawn from a donor who is found to be at high risk of contracting acquired immune deficiency syndrome (AIDS)?
   A. Hold unit in quarantine until donor diagnosis is clarified.
   B. Use the blood for research dealing with AIDS.
   C. Properly dispose of unit by autoclaving or incineration.
   D. Use the plasma and destroy the red blood cells.
9. Which of the following is *least* likely to transmit hepatitis?
   A. Cryoprecipitate
   B. RBC
   C. Plasma protein fraction (PPF)
   D. Platelets
10. A pooled serum product from 16 donors has a repeatedly positive nucleic acid test (NAT) for HCV. The next action that should be taken is to:
    A. permanently exclude all the donors in the pool.
    B. test each donor in the pool for HCV.
    C. label all the donors as HCV positive.
    D. confirm the positive using a recombinant immunoblot assay.
11. Although cryoprecipitate has primarily been used for treatment of hypofibrinogenemia and hemophilia A, it contains other blood proteins useful in the treatment of coagulopathies. Which of the following is *not* found in cryoprecipitate?
    A. Fibronectin
    B. Factor XIII
    C. Factor VIII:vW
    D. Antithrombin III
12. Even though it is properly collected and stored, which of the following will fresh-frozen plasma (FFP) *not* provide?
    A. Factor V
    B. Factor VIII
    C. Factor IX
    D. Platelets
13. Blood needs to be prepared for intrauterine transfusion of a fetus with severe hemolytic disease of the newborn (HDN). The red blood cell unit selected is compatible with the mother's serum and has been leukodepleted. An additional step that must be taken before transfusion is to:
    A. add pooled platelets and fresh-frozen plasma.
    B. check that the RBC group is consistent with the father's.
    C. irradiate the RBCs before infusion.
    D. test the RBC unit with the neonate's eluate.

14. The addition of adenine in an anticoagulant-preservative formulation aids in which of the following?
   A. Maintaining ATP levels for red cell viability
   B. Maintaining platelet function in stored blood
   C. Reducing the plasma K^+ levels during storage
   D. Maintaining 2,3-BPG levels for oxygen release to the tissues

15. The pilot tubes for donor unit #3276 break in the centrifuge. What should be done to resolve this issue?
   A. Label the blood using the donor's previous records.
   B. Discard the unit because processing procedures cannot be performed.
   C. Discard the RBCs and salvage the plasma for fractionation.
   D. Remove sufficient segments to complete donor processing procedures.

Use the following information to answer questions 16 and 17.

A satellite bag containing 250 mL of fresh plasma is selected for quality control of cryoprecipitate production. Cryoprecipitate is prepared according to standard operating procedures. The final product has a total volume of 10 mL. The factor VIII assays are 1 IU/mL before and 9 IU/mL after preparation.

---

16. What is the percent yield of factor VIII in the final cryoprecipitate?
   A. 11%
   B. 25%
   C. 36%
   D. 80%

17. Does this product meet AABB Standards for cryoprecipitate production?
   A. Yes
   B. No; the percent recovery is too low.
   C. No; the final factor VIII level is too low.
   D. Data are insufficient to calculate.

18. What should be done with a unit of RBCs that was irradiated twice?
   A. Change expiration date and then issue the unit.
   B. Note on unit that it has been irradiated twice.
   C. Discard the unit.
   D. Issue immediately.

19. What is the expiration date/time of pooled cryoprecipitate?
   A. 30 minutes
   B. 2 hours
   C. 4 hours
   D. 8 hours

20. Which of the following is most accurate regarding platelet apheresis criteria?
   A. The minimum platelet count must be 3.0×10^{11}, pH must be ≥ 6.0.
   B. The minimum platelet count must be 3.0×10^{10}, pH must be ≤ 6.2.
   C. The minimum platelet count must be 3.0×10^{11}, pH must be ≥ 6.2.
   D. The minimum platelet count must be 5.5×10^{10}, pH must be ≤ 6.0.

21. Which of the following lists the correct shelf life?
   A. Frozen RBCs at −65°C = 7 years
   B. Fresh frozen plasma (FFP) at −18°C = 1 year
   C. Fresh frozen plasma (FFP) at −65°C = 1 year
   D. Platelets at 6°C = 5 days

22. When 2,3-BPG levels drop in stored blood, which of the following occurs as a result?
    A. RBC K^+ increases.
    B. RBC ability to release O_2 decreases.
    C. Plasma hemoglobin is stabilized.
    D. ATP synthesis increases.

23. The last unit of autologous blood for an elective surgery patient should be collected no later than ________________ hours before surgery.
    A. 24
    B. 36
    C. 48
    D. 72

24. For which of the following patients would autologous donation *not* be advisable?
    A. Patients with an antibody against a high-incidence antigen
    B. Patients with uncompensated anemia
    C. Open heart surgery patients
    D. Patients with multiple antibodies

25. What marker is the first to appear in hepatitis B virus infection?
    A. HBsAg
    B. Anti-HBc IgM
    C. Anti-HBs IgG
    D. Anti-HBc IgG

26. Biochemical changes occur during the shelf life of stored blood. Which of the following is a result of this "storage lesion"?
    A. Increase in pH
    B. Increase in plasma K^+
    C. Increase in plasma Na^+
    D. Decrease in plasma hemoglobin

27. It has been determined that a patient has posttransfusion hepatitis and received blood from eight donors. There is nothing to indicate that these donors may have been likely to transmit hepatitis. What action must be taken initially?
    A. Defer all donors indefinitely from further donations.
    B. Repeat all hepatitis testing on a fresh sample from each donor.
    C. Notify the donor center that collected the blood.
    D. Interview all implicated donors.

28. The temperature range for maintaining RBCs and whole blood during shipping is:
    A. 0–4°C
    B. 1–6°C
    C. 1–10°C
    D. 5–15°C

29. Platelets play an important role in maintaining hemostasis. One unit of donor platelets derived from whole blood should yield ________________ platelets.
    A. 5.5×10^6
    A. 5×10^8
    A. 5.5×10^{10}
    A. 5×10^{11}

30. Which component is recommended for patients with anti-IgA antibodies?
    A. Packed RBCs
    B. Washed RBCs
    C. Fresh plasma
    D. Leukoreduced RBCs

31. During preparation of platelet concentrate, the hermetic seal of the primary bag is broken. The red blood cells:
    A. must be discarded.
    B. may be labeled with a 21-day expiration date if collected in CPD.
    C. must be labeled with a 24-hour expiration date.
    D. may be glycerolized within 6 days and stored frozen.

32. The transfusion services' procedure manual must be:
    A. revised annually.
    B. revised after publication of each new edition of the AABB Standards.
    C. reviewed prior to a scheduled inspection.
    D. reviewed annually by an authorized individual.

33. Previous records of patients' ABO and Rh types must be immediately available for comparison with current test results for:
    A. 6 months.
    B. 12 months.
    C. 10 years.
    D. indefinitely.

34. Which of the following weak D donor units should be labeled Rh-positive?
    A. Weak D due to transmissible genes
    B. Weak D as position effect
    C. Weak partial D
    D. All choices are appropriate.

35. In order to meet the current AABB Standards for leukocyte reduction to prevent human leukocyte antigen (HLA) alloimmunization or CMV transmission, the donor unit must retain at least __________ of the original RBCs and leukocytes must be reduced to less than __________.
    A. 85%, 5×10^8
    A. 80%, 5×10^6
    A. 75%, 5×10^5
    A. 70%, 5×10^4

36. Which of the following tests is *not* performed during donor processing?
    A. ABO and Rh grouping
    B. HbsAg
    C. HIV-1-Ag
    D. HBsAb

37. A 70-kg man has a platelet count of 15,000/μL, and there are no complicating factors such as fever or HLA sensitization. If he is given a platelet pool of six units, what would you expect his posttransfusion count to be?
    A. 21,000–27,000/μL
    B. 25,000–35,000/μL
    C. 45,000–75,000/μL
    D. 75,000–125,000/μL

38. Which of the following tests on donor RBCs must be repeated by the transfusing facility when the blood was collected and processed by a different facility?
    A. Confirmation of ABO group and Rh type of blood labeled D-negative
    B. Confirmation of ABO group and Rh type
    C. Weak D on D-negatives
    D. Antibody screening

INSTRUCTIONS: Each numbered group of incomplete statements (questions 39–63) is followed by four suggested responses. Select the *best* answer or completion statement in each case. Lettered responses may be used once, more than once, or not at all.

For the following components prepared from whole blood (questions 39–43), indicate the required storage temperature.

---

39. Red blood cells, liquid
40. Red blood cells, frozen
41. Fresh-frozen plasma
42. Cryoprecipitate

43. Platelet concentrate
    A. 1–6°C
    B. 20–24°C
    C. −18°C or colder
    D. −65°C or colder

For the following components prepared from whole blood (questions 44–48), indicate the shelf life.

44. Red blood cells in citrate phosphate dextrose adenine-1 (CPDA-1)
45. Fresh-frozen plasma
46. Cryoprecipitate
47. Fresh-frozen plasma, thawed
48. Platelet concentrate in PL-732 bags (with agitation)
    A. 24 hours
    B. 5 days
    C. 35 days
    D. 1 year

Using the specified anticoagulant/preservative (questions 49–52), indicate the allowable shelf life for blood for transfusion therapy.

49. Citrate phosphate dextrose (CPD)
50. Citrate phosphate dextrose adenine (CPDA-1)
51. AS-1 (Adsol®)
52. EDTA
    A. 21 days
    B. 35 days
    C. 42 days
    D. Not an approved anticoagulant

For the following situations (questions 53–59), indicate whether the individual volunteering to donate blood for allogeneic transfusion should be accepted or deferred. Assume results of the physical examination to be acceptable unless noted.

53. A 65-year-old man whose birthday is tomorrow
54. A 45-year-old woman who donated a unit during a holiday appeal 54 days ago
55. A 50-year-old man who had sex with another man in 1980
56. A 25-year-old man who says he had yellow jaundice right after he was born
57. An 18-year-old with poison ivy on his hands and face
58. A woman who had a baby 2 months ago
59. A 35-year-old runner (pulse 46 bpm)
    A. Defer temporarily
    B. Defer for 12 months
    C. Defer indefinitely
    D. Accept

For the following patients (questions 60–63), indicate the component of choice for transfusion therapy.

60. Patients with warm autoimmune hemolytic anemia (AIHA) due to α-methyldopa (Aldomet®) with hemoglobin of 8.5 g/dL or above
61. Patients requiring transfusion with RBCs that will not transmit cytomegalovirus (CMV)
62. Patients with normovolemic anemia

63. Patients who are thrombocytopenic secondary to the treatment of acute leukemia
    A. Platelet concentrate
    B. RBC
    C. Leukocyte-reduced RBCs
    D. Transfusion not indicated

Blood Groups, Genetics, Serology

64. Most blood group antibodies are of which of the following immunoglobulin classes?
    A. IgA and IgD
    B. IgA and IgM
    C. IgE and IgD
    D. IgG and IgM

65. The following family study is performed:

Mother	Father	Child 1	Child 2
K+ k+	K− k+	K+ k−	K− k+

All other indications are that these children are both the products of this mating. Possible explanations for these results would include which of the following?
    A. A dominant inhibitor gene has been passed to child 1.
    B. Father has one *k* gene and one K^0 gene.
    C. Father has the McLeod phenotype.
    D. Mother has a *cis-Kk* gene.

66. Which of the following blood groups reacts *least* strongly with an anti-H produced in an A_1B individual?
    A. Group O
    B. Group A_2B
    C. Group A_2
    D. Group A_1

67. How many genes encode the following Rh antigens: D, C, E, c, e?
    A. One
    B. Two
    C. Three
    D. Four

Use the following information to answer questions 68 and 69.

A patient arrives in the obstetrics clinic 3 months pregnant. This is her first pregnancy, and she has never been transfused. Her prenatal screen includes the following results:

Cell Typing Results		Serum Typing Results	
Anti-A	Anti-B	A_1 cells	B cells
0	0	4+	4+

	Screening Cell I	Screening Cell II	Autocontrol
IS	4+	4+	0
37°C LISS	4+	4+	0
AHG	4+	4+	0
Check Cells			√

68. The test results could be due to:
    A. cold autoantibody.
    B. inheritance of *sese* genes.
    C. inheritance of *hh* genes.
    D. Rouleaux.

69. If the patient's RBCs were tested against anti-H lectin and did not react, this person would be identified as a(an):
    A. acquired B.
    B. O_h phenotype.
    C. secretor.
    D. subgroup of A.

70. If a person has the genetic makeup *Hh*, *AO*, *LeLe*, *sese*, which of the following substance will be found in the secretions?
    A. A substance
    B. H substance
    C. Le^a substance
    D. Le^a substance

71. The following results were obtained when typing a patient's blood sample.

Cell Typing Results		Serum Typing Results	
Anti-A	Anti-B	A_1 cells	B cells
4+	2+	0	4+

The laboratory scientist suspects that this is a case of an acquired B antigen. Which of the following would support this suspicion?
   A. A positive autocontrol test
   B. Secretor studies show that the patient is a nonsecretor.
   C. A patient diagnosis of leukemia
   D. The patient's RBCs give a negative result with a monoclonal anti-B reagent lacking the ES-4 clone.

72. Which antibody binds to RBCs at cold temperatures and causes lysis as the temperature rises through movement in peripheral circulation?
   A. Auto anti-P
   B. Anti-H
   C. Anti-I
   D. Auto non-specific antibody

73. Which of the following sugars must be present on a precursor substance for A and B antigenic activity to be expressed?
   A. D-Galactose
   B. N-Acetylgalactosamine
   C. Glucose
   D. L-Fucose

74. An antigen–antibody reaction alone does not cause hemolysis. Which of the following is required for RBC lysis?
   A. Albumin
   B. Complement
   C. Glucose-6-phosphate dehydrogenase (G6PD)
   D. Antihuman globulin (AHG)

75. A Caucasian American female's RBCs gave the following reactions upon phenotyping: D+ C+ E− c+ e+. Which of the following is the most probable Rh genotype?
   A. *DCe/Dce*
   B. *DCe/dce*
   C. *DCe/DcE*
   D. *Dce/dCe*

76. An African American patient has the following Rh phenotype: D+ C+ E+ c+ e+. Which of the following genotypes is the *least* probable?
   A. *DCE/dce*
   B. *DCe/DcE*
   C. *DCe/dcE*
   D. *DcE/dCe*

77. An individual of the *dce/dce* genotype given *dCe/dce* blood has an antibody response that appears to be anti-C plus anti-D. What is the most likely explanation for this?
   A. The antibody is anti-G.
   B. The antibody is anti-partial D.
   C. The antibody is anti-Cw.
   D. The reactions were read incorrectly.

78. If a patient has the Rh genotype *DCe/DCe* and receives a unit of RBCs from a *DCe/dce* individual, what Rh antibody might the patient develop?
   A. Anti-C
   B. Anti-c
   C. Anti-d
   D. Anti-E

Use the following information to answer questions 79–81.

The following results were obtained when testing the individuals below:

	Anti-					Test for
	D	C	E	c	E	Weak D
Husband	0	+	0	+	+	+
Wife	0	0	0	+	+	0
Infant	+	0	0	+	+	N/A

79. What percentage of this couple's offspring can be expected to be D-negative?
   A. 0%
   B. 25%
   C. 50%
   D. 75%

80. Which of the following conclusions regarding the family typing is most likely?
   A. The husband is not the infant's father.
   B. The husband is proved to be the infant's father.
   C. The husband cannot be excluded from being the infant's father.
   D. The D typing on the infant is a false positive.

81. Which, if any, of the three individuals below, can make anti-D?
   A. Husband
   B. Husband and wife
   C. Wife
   D. Child

82. What is the primary difference between weak D and partial D individuals?
   A. Weak D phenotype results from decreased epitopes of D antigens.
   B. Partial D phenotypes can make antibodies to D antigens.
   C. Partial D phenotype results from decrease expression of D antigens.
   D. Weak D phenotypes should be categorized as D negative.

83. An antibody screen is positive in the AHG phase in all three screen cells. The autocontrol is negative. What is the most likely explanation for these results?
   A. Auto antibody
   B. Cold antibody
   C. Excess protein
   D. Alloantibody(ies)

84. A victim of an auto accident arrives in the emergency department (ED) as a transfer from a hospital in a rural area. The patient has been in that facility for several weeks and has received several units of RBCs during that time. The ED resident orders two units of RBCs for transfusion. The sample sent to transfusion services is centrifuged and the cell–serum interface is not discernable. A subsequent sample produces the same appearance. You would suspect that the patient has:
   A. autoimmune hemolytic anemia.
   B. Anti-Fy^a.
   C. Anti-Jk^a.
   D. paroxysmal nocturnal hemoglobinuria.

85. Which of the following is a characteristic of the Xg^a blood group system?
   A. The Xg^a antigen has a higher frequency in women than in men.
   B. The Xg^a antigen has a higher frequency in men than in women.
   C. The Xg^a antigen is enhanced by enzymes.
   D. Anti-Xg^a is usually a saline-reacting antibody.

86. Testing on a patient sample needs to be done with a rarely used antiserum. The appropriate steps to take in using this antiserum include following the manufacturer's procedure and:
    A. performing a cell panel to be sure that the antiserum is performing correctly.
    B. performing the testing on screen cells.
    C. testing in duplicate to ensure the repeatability of the results.
    D. testing a cell that is negative for the antigen and one that is heterozygous for the antigen.

87. Which of the following is a characteristic of Kidd system antibodies?
    A. Usually IgM antibodies
    B. Corresponding antigens are destroyed by enzymes.
    C. Usually strong and stable during storage
    D. Often implicated in delayed hemolytic transfusion reactions

88. Which procedure would help to distinguish between anti-c and Fy^b in a mixed antibody panel?
    A. Increase the pH of the serum.
    B. Use a thiol reagent (e.g., dithiothreitol).
    C. Run a cold "mini" panel.
    D. Run an enzyme panel.

89. What is the primary difference between a patient with anti-S and a patient with anti-M?
    A. Anti-S is never clinically significant.
    B. Anti-S is similar to anti-M as both are naturally occurring.
    C. Anti-S requires patient to receive antigen-negative blood.
    D. Anti-S is cold-reacting and anti-M reacts at body temperature.

90. Which of the following statements is *not* true about anti-U?
    A. Is clinically significant
    B. Is only found in African American individuals
    C. Only occurs in S−s− individuals
    D. Only occurs in Fy(a−b−) individuals

91. A patient had an anti-E identified in his serum 5 years ago. His antibody screening test is now negative. To obtain suitable blood for transfusion, what is the best procedure to use?
    A. Type the patient for the E antigen as an added part to the crossmatch procedure.
    B. Type the donor units for the E antigen and crossmatch the E-negative units.
    C. Crossmatch donors with the patient's serum and release the compatible units for transfusion.
    D. Perform the crossmatch with enzyme-treated donor cells, because enzyme-treated RBCs react better with Rh antibodies.

92. A patient's RBCs are being typed for the Fy^a antigen. Which of the following is the proper cell type of choice for a positive control of the anti-Fy^a reagent?
    A. Fy(a+ b−)
    B. Fy(a+ b+)
    C. Fy(a−b+)
    D. Fy(a−b−)

93. What should be done if HDN is caused by anti-K?
    A. Give prophylactic immune globulin.
    B. Monitor mother's antibody titer.
    C. K is a low-frequency antigen so not likely an issue.
    D. Neutralize the antibody.

Refer to red cell panel chart 1 to answer questions 94–96.

RED CELL PANEL CHART 1

	Rh					MNSs				P	LEWIS		LUTHERAN		KELL				DUFFY		KIDD						
Cell #	D	C	E	c	E	M	N	S	s	P_1	Le^a	Le^b	Lu^a	Lu^b	K	k	Kp^a	Js^a	Fy^a	Fy^b	Jk^a	Jk^b	Xg^a	IS	37	AHG	CkC
1	0	+	0	+	+	+	+	+	0	0	+	0	0	+	0	+	0	0	+	+	+	+	+	0	0	0	√
2	+	+	0	0	+	0	+	0	+	+	0	+	+	+	0	+	0	0	+	+	+	+	+	0	0	0	√
3	+	+	0	0	+	0	+	0	+	+	0	+	0	0	0	+	0	0	0	+	+	0	+	0	0	0	√
4	+	0	+	+	0	+	0	+	0	+	+	0	0	+	+	+	0	0	0	+	+	0	+	0	0	4+	
5	0	0	+	+	+	0	+	0	+	+	+	0	0	+	0	+	0	0	+	0	0	+	0	0	0	3+	
6	0	0	0	+	+	+	0	0	+	+	0	+	0	+	0	+	0	0	+	0	+	+	0	0	0	0	√
7	0	0	0	+	+	+	+	0	+	+	0	0	0	+	+	0	0	0	+	+	+	+	+	0	0	2+	
8	0	0	0	+	+	+	+	0	+	+	0	+	0	+	0	+	0	+	0	0	+	+	0	0	0	0	√
9	0	0	+	+	+	+	0	+	0	0	0	+	0	+	0	+	0	0	0	+	0	+	0	0	0	3+	
10	0	0	0	+	+	+	0	+	+	0	0	+	+	+	0	+	0	0	+	0	+	0	0	0	0	0	√
11	/	/	/	/	/	/	/	/	/	/	/	/	/	/	/	/	/	/	/	/	/	/	/	0	0	0	√
A/C																								0	0	0	√

94. Which of the following antibodies would require additional testing in order to be ruled out?
    A. Anti-E, anti-K, anti-Kp^a, anti-Js^a, anti-Jk^b
    B. Anti-E, anti-S, anti-Le^b, anti-K, anti-Kp^a, anti-Fy^a
    C. Anti-E, anti-S, anti-Le^a, anti-K, anti-Kp^a, anti-Js^a, anti-Fy^a, anti-Jk^a
    D. Anti-E, anti-Le^a, anti-K, anti-Kp^a, anti-Js^a, anti-Fy^b, anti-Jk^a, anti-Jk^b

95. The most likely antibody(ies) in the patient's serum is(are):
    A. anti-S and anti-E.
    B. anti-E and anti-K.
    C. anti-Fy^b showing dosage.
    D. anti-K, anti-Js^a, and anti-Le^a.

96. From the cells in panel chart 2, choose a selected cell panel to help identify the antibody(ies) in the patient described in question 95.
    A. 1, 2, 5, 9, 10
    B. 2, 6, 7, 10
    C. 1, 4, 7
    D. 2, 3, 4, 6, 9

RED CELL PANEL CHART 2

	Rh					MNSs				P	LEWIS		LUTHERAN		KELL				DUFFY		KIDD		
Cell #	D	C	E	C	e	M	N	S	s	P_1	Le^a	Le^b	Lu^a	Lu^b	K	k	Kp^a	Js^a	Fy^a	Fy^b	Jk^a	Jk^b	Xg^a
1	0	+	0	+	+	+	+	+	0	0	+	0	0	+	0	+	0	0	0	+	0	+	+
2	+	+	0	0	+	0	+	0	+	+	0	+	+	+	0	+	0	0	+	+	+	+	+
3	+	+	0	0	+	0	+	0	+	+	0	+	0	0	0	+	0	0	0	+	+	0	+
4	+	0	+	+	0	+	0	0	+	+	0	+	0	+	0	+	0	0	+	0	+	0	+
5	0	0	+	+	+	0	+	0	+	+	+	0	0	+	0	+	0	0	+	0	0	+	0
6	0	0	0	+	+	+	0	0	+	+	0	+	0	+	0	+	0	0	+	0	+	+	0
7	0	0	0	+	+	+	+	0	+	+	0	0	0	+	+	0	0	0	+	0	+	0	+
8	0	0	0	+	+	+	+	+	0	+	0	+	0	+	0	+	0	0	0	0	0	+	0
9	0	0	+	+	+	+	0	+	0	0	0	+	0	+	0	+	0	0	0	+	0	+	0
10	0	0	0	+	+	+	0	+	+	0	0	+	+	+	0	+	0	0	+	0	+	0	0

97. Often when trying to identify a mixture of antibodies, it is useful to neutralize one of the known antibodies. Which one of the following antibodies is neutralizable?
    A. Anti-D
    B. Anti-Jk^a
    C. Anti-Le^a
    D. Anti-M

98. Which of the following antibodies does *not* match the others in terms of optimal reactive temperature?
    A. Anti-Fy^a
    B. Anti-Jk^b
    C. Anti-N
    D. Anti-U

99. A recently transfused patient's serum has a positive antibody screen. The panel performed at immediate spin (IS), in low-ionic-strength saline (LISS) at 37°C, and at AHG shows a strong anti-Fy^a and a weak possible anti-C. To confirm the anti-C, you would perform an:
    A. elution.
    B. absorption.
    C. antigen typing.
    D. enzyme panel.

100. The antiglobulin test does not require washing or the addition of IgG-coated cells in which of the following antibody detection methods?
    A. Solid-phase RBC adherence assays
    B. Gel test
    C. Affinity column technology
    D. Polyethylene glycol technique

101. Which set of antibodies could you possibly find in a patient with no history of transfusion or pregnancy?
    A. Anti-I, anti-s, anti-P_1
    B. Anti-Le^b, anti-A_1, anti-D
    C. Anti-M, anti-c, anti-B
    D. Anti-P_1, anti-Le^a, anti-I

102. Lymphocytotoxicity testing can be used to detect the presence of antibodies to:
    A. Wr^a and Wr^b.
    B. HLA antigens.
    C. Bg^a, Bg^b, and Bg^c.
    D. JMH antigen.

103. In which of the following instances can mixed-field agglutination be observed?
    A. Direct antiglobulin test (DAT) result of patient undergoing delayed hemolytic transfusion reaction
    B. Indirect antiglobulin test (IAT) result of patient who has anti-Le^a
    C. DAT result of patient on high doses of α-methyldopa
    D. Typing result with anti-A of patient who is A_2 subgroup

104. The antibody produced during the secondary response to a foreign antigen is usually
    A. IgM.
    B. a product of T lymphocytes.
    C. produced a month or more after the second stimulus.
    D. present at a higher titer than after a primary response.

105. Which of the following causes ABO reverse typing discrepancies?
    A. Acquired B antigen in a group A person
    B. IgM alloantibody at IS
    C. Bone marrow transplant recipient
    D. Polyagglutinable RBCs

106. A group A, D-negative obstetric patient with anti-D (titer 256) is carrying a fetus who needs an intrauterine transfusion. Which of the following units should be chosen?
    A. Group A, D-negative RBC
    B. Group A, D-negative whole blood
    C. Group O, D-negative RBC
    D. Group O, D-negative whole blood

107. Which of the following is generally detected with the antiglobulin phase of testing?
A. Anti-Jk^a
B. Anti-M
C. Anti-P_1
D. Anti-I

108. Which of the blood group systems is associated with antibodies that are generally IgM?
A. Rh
B. Duffy
C. Kell
D. Lewis

109. Some antigens that are primarily found on white blood cells can occur on erythrocytes. Which of the following are the RBC equivalents of HLAs?
A. Le^a, Le^b
B. Bg^a, Bg^b, Bg^c
C. Kp^a, Kp^b, Kp^c
D. Do^a, Do^b

110. The following phenotypes resulted from blood typing a mother, 6-month-old baby, and alleged father in a case of paternity testing.

	ABO	Rh	HLA
Mother	A	ce	A2, A29, B12, B17
Baby	O	ce	A2, A3, B12, B15
Alleged Father	A	DCce	A3, A9, B5, B27

Which of the following statements is true? The alleged father:
A. is excluded by the ABO system.
B. is excluded by the Rh system.
C. is excluded by the HLA system.
D. cannot be ruled out.

INSTRUCTIONS: Each numbered group of incomplete statements (questions 111–123) is followed by four suggested responses. Select the *best* answer in each case. Lettered responses may be used once, more than once, or not at all.

Eight blood samples are received in the laboratory for ABO grouping. For each patient (questions 111–118), indicate the most likely cell and serum reactions selected from the lettered reaction matrix.

111. A patient with an acquired antigen due to infection with gram-negative bacteria
112. A patient with multiple myeloma
113. A newborn
114. An A_2 individual making an anti-A_1
115. A patient with antibodies to acriflavin (a yellow dye)
116. A patient who is immunodeficient
117. A patient with an unexpected IgM antibody in his serum
118. A patient with cold hemagglutinin disease (CHD)

	Cell Typing Results		Serum Typing Results		
	Anti-A	Anti-B	A_1 cells	B cells	O cells
A.	+	+	+	+	+
B.	+	0	+	+	0
C.	+	+	0	+	0
D.	0	+	0	0	0

For the following items (questions 119–123), select the answer that most closely corresponds to the description.

119. Found predominantly in Caucasian Americans

120. Associated with weak Kell system antigenic expression
121. Associated with the presence of chronic granulomatous disease
122. Linked with MN
123. A rare allele of *M* and *N*
   A. McLeod phenotype
   B. M^g
   C. Kp^a
   D. Ss

Antibody Identification, Transfusion Therapy, Transfusion Reactions

For questions 124–132, refer to RBC panel chart 3.

124. The ethnicity of the donor of cell #3 is most likely of which descent?
   A. African American
   B. Inuit or Yupik
   C. Asian
   D. Caucasian American
125. The donor of cell #5 is homozygous for which combination of the following genes?
   A. Ce, P_1, M, s, k, Jk^a, Fy^a, Le^b
   B. Ce, P_1, s, k, Jk^a, Fy^a, Le^b
   C. Ce, s, k, Jk^a, Fy^a, Le^b,P_1
   D. Ce, s, k, Jk^a, Fy^a
126. After testing a patient's serum with the panel, one observes there are no reactions at IS or 37°C with cells #1–8. There is a 1+ AHG reaction with cells #1 and #6 and a 3+ AHG reaction with cells #4 and #5. All other cells, #2, #3, #7, and #8, are negative at AHG. Which of the following statements is *true*?
   A. Anti-Fy^a appears to be present.
   B. Anti-Fy^a is present as well as an antibody that is reacting with an undetermined antigen on Cells #4 and #5.
   C. Ficin will enhance the reactions of the antibody(ies) present.
   D. Anti-Fy^a is present but can be ignored because most people are Fy(a−b−).
127. The serum of a patient tested with the reagent RBC panel using an LISS additive demonstrates 3+ reactivity with cells #1–8 at the antiglobulin phase. The autocontrol is negative. This pattern of reactivity is most likely due to:
   A. rouleaux formation.
   B. warm autoantibody.
   C. alloantibody directed against a high-frequency antigen.
   D. antibody directed against a preservative present in LISS.
128. A patient's serum reacts with all the panel cells except cell #7 in the antiglobulin phase only. Which of the following techniques would be most helpful at this point?
   A. Treat the panel cells with a proteolytic enzyme and repeat the panel with untreated serum.
   B. Treat the panel cells with dithiothreitol (DTT) and repeat the panel with untreated serum.
   C. Treat the patient's serum with DTT and repeat the panel with treated serum.
   D. Treat the patient's serum with a proteolytic enzyme and repeat the panel with treated serum.

RED CELL PANEL CHART 3																				
Cell #	D	C	E	c	e	M	N	P_1	S	s	K	k	Jk^a	Jk^b	Fy^a	Fy^b	Lu^a	Le^a	Le^b	Xg^a
1	+	+	0	+	+	+	+	+	0	+	+	+	0	+	+	+	0	0	+	0
2	+	+	0	0	+	0	+	0	+	+	0	+	0	+	0	+	0	0	+	+
3	+	+	0	+	+	+	0	+	+	0	0	+	+	+	0	0	0	+	0	+
4	+	0	+	+	0	+	+	0	+	0	0	+	+	0	+	0	0	0	+	0
5	0	+	0	0	+	+	+	+	0	+	0	+	+	0	+	0	0	0	+	0
6	0	0	+	+	0	+	0	+	+	+	0	+	0	+	+	+	0	0	0	0
7	0	0	0	+	+	0	+	+	+	0	+	0	+	+	0	+	+	0	+	+
8	0	0	0	+	+	+	+	0	+	+	0	+	+	0	0	+	0	+	0	+

In addition to the RBC panel chart 3, use the following information to answer questions 129–132.

The patient is group A, D-negative and has not been recently transfused. Cells #5, #6, and #7 are negative in all phases with this patient's serum. The autocontrol is negative. Other cell results are as follows:

CELL #	IS	37°C LISS	AHG
1	0	1+	4+
2	0	1+	4+
3	2+	1+	4+
4	0	1+	4+
8	2+	0	0

129. From the reactions given, it appears that there is(are):
   A. one antibody reacting.
   B. one antibody reacting that shows dosage.
   C. "cold" and "warm" antibodies reacting.
   D. two "warm" antibodies reacting.

130. The antibody that reacts at IS is most likely:
   A. anti-D.
   B. anti-P_1.
   C. anti-Le^a.
   D. anti-Le^b.

131. The antibody that reacts at 37°C and with AHG is:
   A. anti-C.
   B. anti-D.
   C. anti-CD.
   D. anti-K.

132. What should be done to increase the probability that an antibody identification is correct?
   A. Make an eluate.
   B. Do saliva testing.
   C. Run an additional panel.
   D. Type the patient's cells for the corresponding antigens.

133. The following results were obtained upon testing a specimen of a patient, being admitted after a car accident, who had no recent history of transfusion or medical problems.
   ABO group: A
   Rh type: D-positive
   Antibody screening test: Positive, one screening cell only
   Direct antiglobulin test: Negative
   Antibody identification: Anti-K identified; 3 K+ cells that reacted with the patient serum and 3 K− cells that did not react with the patient serum were on the panel.
   Patient's cell phenotyping: K+

What is the most likely cause of the discrepant results?

A. Failure to read panel at antiglobulin phase
B. Failure to use positive and negative controls with anti-K
C. Panel cell reactions interpreted incorrectly
D. Patient has circulating donor cells that are K+

134. False negative results at the antiglobulin phase of an antibody screening test are most likely due to:

A. excessive washing of the red cells.
B. inadequate washing of the red cells.
C. warm autoantibody present in the patient's serum.
D. failure to allow the blood to clot properly.

135. What is the process of removing an antibody from the RBC membrane called?

A. Absorption
B. Adsorption
C. Elution
D. Immunization

136. At the end of an antiglobulin test, IgG-coated control cells are added to the negative tests and centrifuged. What does it mean if no agglutination occurs?

A. Test is valid.
B. Antiglobulin reagent was working properly.
C. Cells were not washed thoroughly.
D. Control cells are contaminated.

137. The crossmatch is performed using:

A. donor's serum and recipient's RBCs.
B. donor's RBCs and recipient's serum.
C. donor's serum and reagent red cells.
D. recipient's serum and reagent red cells.

138. A male trauma victim whose blood type is group AB, D-negative has a negative antibody screening test. He has been transfused with both of the group AB, D-negative units in inventory within the last hour. He is now in surgery and expected to need large amounts of blood. Of the following available units in inventory, which type should be given next?

A. 30 units of group O, D-positive
B. 26 units of group A, D-positive
C. 10 units of group O, D-negative
D. 5 units of group A, D-negative

139. Which of the following will the crossmatch do?

A. Prevent immunization
B. Prevent delayed transfusion reactions
C. Guarantee normal survival of the RBCs
D. Frequently verify donor ABO compatibility

140. Given that a patient's antibody screening test is negative, which of the following may cause a false positive result in a compatibility test?

A. Incorrect ABO typing of the donor or patient
B. An alloantibody against a low-frequency antigen on the donor cells
C. Prior coating of IgG antibody on the donor cells
D. Centrifuging for 15 sec

141. Which of the following will be incompatible in the crossmatch?

	Donor	Recipient
A.	Group A, D-negative	Group A, D-positive
B.	Group O, D-positive	Group A, D-positive
C.	Group AB, D-positive	Group A, D-positive
D.	Group A, D-positive	Group A, D-negative

142. A resident physician hand-delivers a blood sample, drawn by the attending physician, for pretransfusion testing from a patient who is difficult to draw. The sample is unlabeled. One should:
   A. discard the sample and request that the resident obtain a new sample, adhering to proper guidelines for labeling.
   B. label the specimen with the information the resident provides.
   C. label the specimen with information from the accompanying transfusion request form.
   D. request the sample be returned to the nursing station to be labeled.

143. A specimen of blood is received in transfusion services with request slips initialed by the phlebotomist. The tube has the patient's first and last name and medical records identification number on the label. What else must be on the tube label as required by AABB Standards?
   A. Patient's room number
   B. Date of phlebotomy
   C. Initials of phlebotomist
   D. Attending physician's name

144. A physician calls transfusion services and wants an additional unit of RBC crossmatched for a patient. Several specimens from that patient are identified that have been drawn over the past month. Which of the following available samples is the oldest acceptable specimen that may be used for crossmatching?
   A. 1 day old
   B. 4 days old
   C. 1 week old
   D. 1 month old

145. A patient has a hematocrit level of 21%. The surgeon wants to raise the hematocrit to 30% before surgery. How many units of RBCs need to be administered to this patient to raise the hemoglobin to the required level?
   A. 1
   B. 2
   C. 3
   D. 4

146. A patient with an anti-K and an anti-Jk^a in her plasma needs two units of RBC for surgery. How many group-specific units would need to be screened to find two units of RBC? The frequency of Jk(a+) is 77%; the K+ frequency is 10%.
   A. 6
   B. 10
   C. 20
   D. 36

Use the following information to answer questions 147 and 148.

Following childbirth, a female is bleeding because of disseminated intravascular coagulation (DIC). The attending physician orders cryoprecipitate for fibrinogen replacement. The freezer inventory contains the following cryoprecipitate: 6 bags Group A, 8 bags Group O, 6 bags Group AB, 12 bags Group B.

---

147. How many bags (units) should be thawed and pooled to provide 2 g of fibrinogen?
   A. 2
   B. 4
   C. 8
   D. 10

148. The patient types as group A. Which cryoprecipitate units would most appropriately be used to treat this patient?
   A. Group A only
   B. Group AB only
   C. Group A and group O
   D. Group A and group AB

149. If 98% of the RBCs are viable in a unit of blood at the time of transfusion, what percentage of RBCs will remain viable 28 days posttransfusion?
   A. 10%
   B. 30%
   C. 50%
   D. 70%

150. What is the component of choice for someone who needs an RBC transfusion when there is a history of febrile transfusion reactions?
   A. RBCs less than 5 days old
   B. Leukocyte-reduced RBCs
   C. RBCs 30 to 35 days old
   D. Frozen RBCs that have been thawed and deglycerolized

151. Which of the following is the component of choice when a physician is concerned about restoring or maintaining oxygen-carrying capacity?
   A. Albumin
   B. Cryoprecipitate
   C. Whole blood
   D. RBCs

152. The serum of a patient contains an antibody that reacts with all random donor cells and panel cells that have been tested. The best possibility to find compatible blood would be to test:
   A. grandparents.
   B. parents.
   C. siblings.
   D. spouse.

Use the following information to answer questions 153 and 154.

A resident physician on the trauma team runs a pretransfusion blood sample from a male trauma victim to transfusion services and wants six units of blood to be issued immediately. He indicates that he is willing to sign for uncrossmatched blood. He also indicates that he wants six units ready at all times. The patient has been admitted to this institution previously for a gastrointestinal bleed.

153. The resident says the victim has a donor card in his wallet indicating a group B, D-positive blood type. What should be done immediately?
   A. Issue six units of uncrossmatched group B, D-positive whole blood.
   B. Check patient and donor records to confirm the blood type, and then issue six units of uncrossmatched group B, D-positive blood.
   C. Withhold blood until ABO and compatibility testing are completed.
   D. Issue six units of uncrossmatched group O RBCs.

154. What should be the next step in the work-up of this emergency department patient?
   A. Prepare six units uncrossmatched group B, D-positive whole blood.
   B. Check blood bank records for any previous patient information.
   C. Type and screen the patient sample.
   D. Prepare six more units of uncrossmatched group O blood.

155. Four units of fresh-frozen plasma have been ordered to correct factor V deficiency in a group O patient. One should thaw and issue ______________ plasma.
A. group O only
B. group O and/or group A
C. group O and/or group AB
D. any blood group available

156. Which of the following is acceptable to be given intravenously with a blood transfusion?
A. 5% dextrose in water
B. Physiologic saline
C. Ringer's solution
D. Potassium chloride in saline

157. Hemolytic transfusion reactions are the most serious type of reactions to blood transfusion. The majority of hemolytic transfusion reactions are caused by ______________ errors.
A. blood typing
B. antibody identification
C. clerical
D. crossmatching

158. What type of transfusion reaction is often diagnosed by a positive DAT and a gradual drop in the patient's hemoglobin level?
A. Anaphylactic
B. Febrile
C. Delayed hemolytic
D. Acute hemolytic

159. What antibody is labile both in stored serum and the patient's plasma and is a frequent cause of delayed hemolytic transfusion reactions?
A. Anti-A
B. Anti-D
C. Anti-Jk^a
D. Anti-K

160. Anaphylactic/anaphylactoid transfusion reactions:
A. are IgD mediated.
B. occur only in IgE-deficient patients.
C. are common when patients have a positive DAT.
D. are associated with medications/antimicrobial therapy.

161. A transfusion of which of the following is least likely to transmit HIV, HCV, or HBV?
A. Pooled plasma, solvent/detergent treated
B. Cryoprecipitate
C. Leukocyte-reduced RBCs
D. Platelets

Use the following information to answer questions 162–164.

A transfusion reaction is reported by the nursing unit on a patient. The nurse reports that the patient had chills, fever, and back pain within a few minutes of starting the unit. The nurse asks what s/he should do.

162. You tell the nurse to immediately:
A. collect posttransfusion blood samples.
B. monitor the pulse and blood pressure.
C. discontinue the unit, keep the intravenous (IV) line open.
D. page the patient's physician for instructions.

163. Which of the following directives would *not* be included in the additional activities you would request the nurse to do?
   A. Return the unit to transfusion services.
   B. Obtain a posttransfusion blood sample in EDTA.
   C. Obtain a posttransfusion urine sample.
   D. Obtain a fresh unit from transfusion services for immediate infusion.

164. All paperwork checks on this transfusion reaction are OK. The pretransfusion sample has straw-colored plasma. The posttransfusion sample has red-tinged plasma. This is indicative of a(an):
   A. uncomplicated transfusion.
   B. intravascular transfusion reaction.
   C. error in which drugs have been infused with the blood.
   D. febrile transfusion reaction.

165. Whether a transfusion is from a random donor or from an autologous donation, the rate of reaction is actually the same. Which of the following sign or symptom is helpful in differentiating hypovolemia from a vasovagal response?
   A. Decrease in oxygen saturation
   B. Pallor
   C. Decrease in blood pressure
   D. Decrease in heart rate

166. Which of the following is appropriate with regard to blood component transfusion protocols?
   A. Obtain full set of vital signs pretransfusion, then at 15 minutes after transfusion initiation, and then hourly until complete.
   B. Always premedicate to prevent fever and allergic reactions.
   C. Obtain full set of vitals 24 hours after transfusion is completed.
   D. Premedicate for fever and allergic reactions if it is the patient's first transfusion.

167. Which of the following would *not* cause a positive hemagglutination reaction in the crossmatch?
   A. Incorrect ABO grouping of the donor
   B. Unexpected antibodies in the recipient serum
   C. A positive DAT on the recipient red cells
   D. A positive DAT on the donor red cells

168. Which of the following blood types necessitates that a separate Rh control tube be set up when using a monoclonal anti-D reagent?
   A. Group O, D-positive
   B. Group A, D-positive
   C. Group B, D-positive
   D. Group AB, D-positive

169. Six units of blood were ordered STAT for a young female patient who has the following tube typing results (the tube typing procedure uses a washed RBC suspension with monoclonal reagents). The physician has just called requesting emergency release of two units of RBCs.

Cell Typing Results				Serum Typing Results	
Anti-A	Anti-B	Anti-D	Rh control	A_1 cells	B cells
2+	4+	3+	2+	4+	4+

Which of the following should be done first?
   A. Perform a DAT on the patient's red cells.
   B. Tell the physician that no blood can be released until a full work-up has been done.
   C. Begin the antibody screening test.
   D. Select two units of group O, D-negative RBCs for emergency release.

170. Referring to the tube typing results in question 169, the most probable cause of the patient's positive Rh control test is that the patient has:
   A. a positive DAT result with anti-IgG.
   B. a cold autoantibody.
   C. leukemia.
   D. multiple myeloma.

171. A patient experiences severe rigors and goes into shock after receiving part of a unit of RBCs. The patient's temperature, which was 37.5°C pretransfusion, is now 40.0°C. Which of the following is the most likely type of reaction?
   A. Hemolytic
   B. Anaphylactic
   C. Septic
   D. Embolic

172. Referring to the reaction described in question 171, the incidence of this type of reaction is highest with which of the following components?
   A. RBC
   B. FFP
   C. Cryoprecipitate
   D. Platelets

173. The serum of a patient transfused 2 weeks ago reacts 3+ on IS and 1+ in the AHG phase of testing with all reagent RBCs except for the *ii* cell. The autocontrol reacts similarly to the panel cells. In order to crossmatch this patient, one should:
   A. use autoadsorbed serum.
   B. use the prewarmed technique.
   C. identify the antibody and obtain blood from the rare donor file.
   D. use a LISS additive.

INSTRUCTIONS: Each numbered set of test results or conditions (questions 174–184) is followed by four or five lettered responses. Select the *best* answer in each case. Lettered responses may be used once, more than once, or not at all.

Six units of blood from volunteer donors are tested for ABO group, Rh type, and unexpected antibodies. For each set of test results (questions 174–179), indicate the final disposition of the donated unit. Assume additional FDA required testing is nonreactive, unless noted.

	Cell Typing Results			Serum Typing Results		
	Anti-A	Anti-B	Anti-D	A_1 cells	A_2 cells	B cells
174.	0	0	3+	4+	3+	4+
175.	0	0	0	4+	4+	4+
	Weak D test = 3+, DAT = 0					
176.	0	0	0	4+	4+	4+
	Weak D test = 1+, DAT = 1+					
177.	0	0	3+	2+	0	4+
178.	0	0	3+	0	0	4+
179.	0	0	3+	4+	4+	4+
	Antibody screen = positive Antibody identification = anti-Fy^a					

A. Label group O, D-positive
B. Label group O, D-negative
C. Label the RBC group O, D-positive; do not use the plasma
D. Perform additional testing
E. Discard the unit

For the following conditions (questions 180–184), select the blood component of choice for treatment.

180. von Willebrand disease
181. Hypofibrinogenemia
182. Factor V deficiency
183. Liver disease
184. Hemorrhagic episode during intensive chemotherapy
    A. Platelet concentrate
    B. RBC
    C. Cryoprecipitate
    D. Fresh-frozen plasma

Hemolytic Disease (Hemolytic Disease of the Newborn, Immune Hemolytic Anemia)

185. Which of the following would not be included when routine testing is performed early in a pregnancy?
    A. ABO and Rh testing
    B. Antibody screening
    C. Amniocentesis
    D. Weak D testing on apparent Rh-negative patients

186. In which of the following blood group systems may the red blood cell typing change during pregnancy?
    A. P
    B. MNS
    C. Lewis
    D. Duffy

187. Which of the following is *not* considered a useful predictor of hemolytic disease of the newborn (HDN) during the gestational period?
    A. Anti-A
    B. Anti-D
    C. Anti-Fy^a
    D. Anti-U

188. Which is the class of immunoglobulin uniquely associated with HDN?
    A. IgA
    B. IgD
    C. IgE
    D. IgG

189. A neonate with a positive direct antiglobulin test (DAT) indicates that there was an incompatibility between a mother and her fetus. The system that is most commonly associated with an incompatibility is:
    A. ABO.
    B. Rh.
    C. Kell.
    D. Kidd.

190. The cord blood of an infant of a D-negative mother with anti-D, titer 2048, is submitted to the laboratory along with a sample of maternal blood with a request to select blood for possible exchange transfusion. The neonate appears to be D-negative. The weak D status cannot be determined because the DAT result is positive (4+). What is the most likely explanation for this?
    A. Wharton's jelly contaminated the sample.
    B. The baby has ABO HDN.
    C. The baby has a "blocked D" antigen.
    D. A different antibody is causing the positive DAT.

191. A newborn is group O, D-positive and has a 3+ DAT. The mother's antibody screening test is negative. Assuming the antibody detection test is valid, one should consider HDN due to an antibody directed against:
    A. Fy^b antigen.
    B. K antigen.
    C. low-incidence antigen.
    D. A or B antigen.

192. The most conclusive way to demonstrate the antibody that is causing a positive DAT in a newborn is to perform an antibody:
    A. titration using the mother's serum.
    B. panel using the mother's serum.
    C. panel using an eluate from the mother's RBCs.
    D. panel using an eluate from the baby's RBCs.

193. Which two of the following conditions are the most serious immediate consequences of HDN?
    A. Anemia and a positive DAT
    B. Hyperbilirubinemia and anemia
    C. Hyperbilirubinemia and jaundice
    D. Hyperbilirubinemia and kernicterus

194. A premature infant with hydrops fetalis and a bilirubin of 20 mg/dL is referred to an intensive care unit. The neonatologist wants to perform an exchange transfusion to correct anemia and prevent kernicterus. No blood specimen from the mother is available. The infant's serum has a positive antibody screen. The DAT is 4+. What would be the best approach in this situation?
    A. Identify the antibody in the serum and crossmatch blood negative for the offending antigen, using the serum in a crossmatch.
    B. Issue group O, D-negative blood for the exchange.
    C. Refuse to issue blood for exchange until a sample can be obtained from the mother.
    D. Identify the antibody in the serum and eluate and crossmatch blood negative for the offending antigen, using both the serum and eluate in a crossmatch.

195. Which of the following is *not* true of an exchange transfusion when an infant is suffering from HDN?
    A. Removes unconjugated bilirubin
    B. Reduces the amount of incompatible antibody in the baby's circulation
    C. Removes antibody-coated RBCs
    D. Provides RBCs of the baby's type

196. A massive fetomaternal hemorrhage in a D-negative woman who had a D-positive infant should be suspected if the:
    A. infant is premature.
    B. infant has a positive acid elution slide test.
    C. mother requires a transfusion following childbirth.
    D. weak D test on the maternal blood shows a mixed-field reaction microscopically.

197. A D-negative woman who received antepartum RhIG gave birth to a D-positive infant and received one vial of RhIG the same day. Because of postpartum hemorrhage, her physician ordered two units of RBCs for her 2 days later. The antibody screening test was positive, but the crossmatches were both compatible. The most likely cause for the positive antibody screening test was the presence of a(an):
    A. clinically significant anti-K.
    B. actively acquired anti-D.
    C. passively acquired anti-D.
    D. Rh antibody other than anti-D.

198. What is the principle of the Kleihauer-Betke stain?
   A. Fetal hemoglobin is more resistant to alkaline buffer than adult hemoglobin.
   B. Adult hemoglobin is more resistant to alkaline buffer than fetal hemoglobin.
   C. Fetal hemoglobin is more resistant to erythrosin and hematoxylin staining than adult hemoglobin.
   D. Adult hemoglobin is more soluble in acid buffer than fetal hemoglobin.

199. Which of the following antibodies present in an obstetric patient who has received multiple transfusions would be most likely to cause HDN in her infant?
   A. Anti-Le^a
   B. Anti-c
   C. Anti-P_1
   D. Anti-K

Use the following information to answer questions 200 and 201.

A Kleihauer-Betke acid elution stain for postpartum fetomaternal hemorrhage (FMH) is reported to be 2.1%.

200. What is the total volume of FMH?
   A. 16.5 mL
   B. 33 mL
   C. 56 mL
   D. 105 mL

201. With this amount of FMH, how many vials of a standard dose of RhIG should be administered to the mother within 72 hours of childbirth? (Presume the infant to be D-positive.)
   A. 2
   B. 3
   C. 4
   D. 5

Use the following information to answer questions 202–205.

A 64-year-old female is seen in the emergency department with a hemoglobin value of 8.9 g/dL. The resident sends a request for two units of packed red cells. She types as group O, D-positive using monoclonal antisera. Her ABO group and Rh type match previous records. She has not been transfused in the past 5 years. However, her antibody screen produces the following results:

	Screen Cell I	**Screen Cell II**	**Screen Cell III**	**Autocontrol**
IS	0	0	0	0
37°C LISS	0	0	0	0
AHG	4+	4+	4+	4+
CC	NT*	NT	NT	NT

*NT = not tested

202. What is the most likely cause for these results?
   A. Polyagglutination
   B. Rouleaux
   C. Transfusion reaction
   D. Warm autoantibody

203. To demonstrate whether the antibody(ies) has/have become attached this patient's RBCs *in vivo*, which of the following tests would be most useful?
   A. Direct antiglobulin test (DAT)
   B. Complement fixation test
   C. Elution procedure
   D. Indirect antiglobulin test

204. How would you identify the antibody(ies) on this woman's cells?
 A. Autoabsorption followed by a panel on the absorbed serum
 B. Elution followed by a panel on the eluate
 C. Enzyme-treated panel on her serum
 D. Perform a panel on the serum.

205. What is the best treatment for this woman's anemia?
 A. Transfusion with packed red cells
 B. Infusion of fresh-frozen plasma
 C. Steroid administration
 D. Plasma exchange

206. The specificity of the antibody in warm autoimmune hemolytic anemia (WAIHA) is most often associated with which of the following blood group systems?
 A. ABO
 B. Kell
 C. Kidd
 D. Rh

207. What is the most important consideration in patients suffering from life-threatening anemia and whose serum contains warm autoantibodies?
 A. Determine the specificity of the autoantibody.
 B. Determine the immunoglobulin class of the autoantibody.
 C. Exclude the presence of alloantibody(ies).
 D. Avoid transfusion.

208. The serum and eluate from a male patient with a 3+ DAT on α-methyldopa therapy demonstrates anti-e specificity. The patient denies knowledge of having received blood transfusions. To determine whether the anti-e is an auto- or alloantibody, one should:
 A. type the patient's RBCs with a low-protein anti-e reagent.
 B. adsorb the serum with the patient's RBCs.
 C. adsorb the eluate with R_2R_2 RBCs.
 D. adsorb the eluate with rr RBCs.

209. A patient has a 2+mixed-field DAT with anti-IgG. He was transfused 1 week ago with two units of RBCs during surgery. His eluate would most likely contain:
 A. no antibody.
 B. autoantibody.
 C. alloantibody.
 D. drug-related antibody.

210. An incompatible donor unit has a positive DAT. What should be done with the unit?
 A. Wash the donor cells and retest.
 B. Antigen type the unit.
 C. Use saline replacement and retest.
 D. Discard the unit.

211. Screening cells, major crossmatch, and patient autocontrol are positive in all phases. Identify the problem.
 A. Specific cold alloantibody
 B. Specific cold auto antibody
 C. Mixture of cold and warm alloantibodies
 D. Nonspecific autoantibody or excess protein

212. How is cold hemagglutinin disease (CHD) different from paroxysmal cold hemoglobinuria (PCH)?
   A. PCH is a common form of cold autoimmune anemia whereas CHD is rare.
   B. PCH is a warm autoimmune hemolytic anemia.
   C. The antibody in PCH is an IgG antibody unlike the IgM antibody in CHD.
   D. The antibody in PCH is an IgM antibody while an IgG antibody is common in CHD.

213. If during a Donath-Landsteiner test there is hemolysis in both the test and control tubes at the conclusion of the test, this indicates that the test is:
   A. positive.
   B. negative.
   C. invalid.
   D. false negative.

214. A patient has a positive DAT due to cephalosporin therapy and a negative antibody screening test result. Two units of RBCs have been ordered. In order to crossmatch this patient, one should crossmatch with:
   A. the eluate from the patient's RBCs and donor cells.
   B. autoadsorbed patient's serum and
   C. untreated donor cells.
   D. untreated patient's serum and untreated donor cells.
   E. cephalosporin-treated donor cells and untreated patient's serum.

215. A patient with drug-induced hemolytic anemia has the following DAT results:
   Polyspecific AHG = 3+
   Anti-IgG = 3+
   Anti-C3d = 0
   Which of the following drugs is most likely to be the cause?
   A. Phenacetin
   B. Quinidine
   C. Penicillin
   D. Tolmetin

216. A patient with cold hemagglutinin disease (CHD) has a positive DAT when tested with a polyspecific AHG. Which of the following would most likely be detected on her RBCs?
   A. IgM
   B. IgG
   C. IgA
   D. C3

217. A patient's preoperative antibody screening test is negative, but the autocontrol is positive. A DAT performed on his RBCs is 2+ with anti-IgG. His last transfusion was 9 months ago, and he has a negative drug history. Which of the following would most likely be present in his eluate?
   A. No antibody
   B. Alloantibody
   C. Alloantibody and autoantibody
   D. Autoantibody

218. A patient with WAIHA has a history of an anti-Jk^a in her autoabsorbed serum, and an anti-e in her eluate. Her autoabsorbed serum today is not showing anti-Jk^a on prewarmed panel, but the eluate is still showing anti-e. What blood would be selected for crossmatching packed red cells today?
    A. e-Negative
    B. Jk(a−)
    C. Jk(a−) and e-negative
    D. No screening is necessary because all transfused cells will be destroyed anyway.

INSTRUCTIONS: The numbered group of incomplete statements (questions 219–226) is followed by four suggested responses. Select the *best* answer in each case. Lettered responses may be used once, more than once, or not at all.

For the following situations (questions 219–226), indicate whether the women are candidates for Rh immune globulin (RhIG) prophylaxis. Assume that D-negative mothers have a negative test for weak D and a nonreactive antibody screening test unless noted.

219. Mother D-negative; infant weak D
220. Mother weak D (strong); infant D-positive
221. Mother D-negative; twin #1 D-negative, twin #2 D-positive
222. Mother D-negative with anti-Fy^a; infant D-positive
223. Mother group O, D-negative; infant group A, DAT = 2+, monoclonal anti-D-negative at immediate spin, weak D test not performed
224. Mother D-negative, with anti-D, titer 2, history of RhIG injection post-amniocentesis procedure at 30 weeks; infant D-positive
225. Female D-negative; miscarriage at 11 weeks
226. Mother D-negative; infant D-positive; rosette test = 1−2 rosettes per field
    A. Yes, 50-μg dose
    B. Yes, 300-μg dose
    C. Yes, additional testing necessary to determine dose.
    D. RhIG is not indicated.

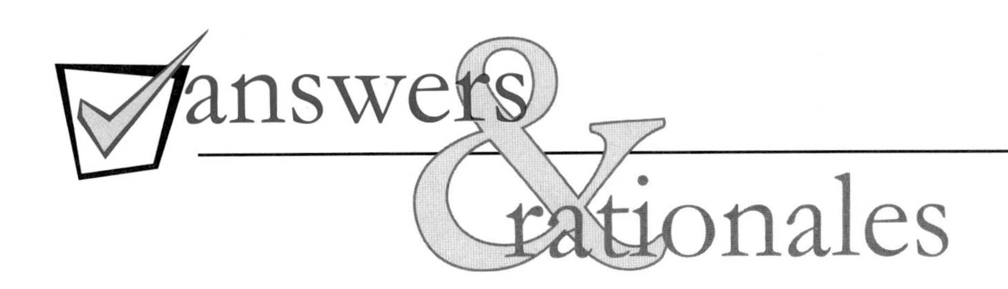

Blood Collection, Preservation, Processing, Component Preparation, and Quality Control

1\.

C. Some potential donors are rejected to protect the recipient, and others are rejected to protect themselves. In this case, the woman meets the criteria except that her hematocrit is too low, and the loss of a unit of blood may have a detrimental effect on her. The minimum acceptable hematocrit is 38%.

2\.

C. Donors are allowed to donate no more than 10.5 mL/kg of their body weight. This amount includes the samples used for testing drawn at the time of collection. The calculation for an 87-lb donor is

$$87 \text{ lbs} \div 2.2 \text{ lbs/kg} = 39.5 \text{ kg},$$
$$39.5 \text{ kg} \times 10.5 \text{ mL/kg} = 415.2 \text{ mL}.$$

If less than 300 mL is to be collected, the anticoagulant must be reduced proportionately.

3\.

B. The patient has had a syncopal episode or fainted. Remove the needle, position her feet above her head, and administer ammonia. Removal of the needle is for safety sake. Putting her feet above her head will bring more blood (oxygen) to the head region. The ammonia will arouse her to her senses. A cool towel will help to reduce the pallor and aid her in recovering her awareness of her surroundings. A cool drink will serve a similar purpose.

4\.

A. To calculate the amount of anticoagulant to remove when a donor weighs less than 110 pounds, divide donor weight by 110 lbs × 450 mL; divide the result by 100 × 14 (volume anticoagulant needed); then subtract that number from 63 mL (standard anticoagulant volume in 450 mL bag). This is the volume of anticoagulant to remove.

5\.

D. Recipients of human growth hormone are deferred indefinitely because of the risk of transmission of Creutzfeldt-Jakob disease. Recipients of recombinant growth hormone incur no deferral. A history of either syphilis or gonorrhea causes a deferral of 12 months from completion of treatment. Accutane®, a drug used to treat acne, may be a teratogen and requires a 1-month deferral after receipt of the last dose.

6.

A. Of the viruses listed, CMV is the only one that resides exclusively in leukocytes. Although CMV transmission is not a problem for most patients, it can cause serious disease in low-birth-weight neonates of CMV-negative mothers and immunocompromised patients. These patients should be transfused with CMV seronegative or leukocyte-reduced cellular components.

7.

D. Donors who have ingested blood thinners within 36 hours of donation need not be excluded from red blood cell (RBC) donation. The platelets prepared from such donors should be labeled and may be used in a multiple pool prepared for adult transfusion. Because aspirin affects platelet function, a single unit of platelet concentrate from this donor should not be used for platelet therapy for infants and neonates. This donor should not be the sole source of platelets and, therefore, would be temporarily deferred as a plateletpheresis donor.

8.

C. Under no circumstances should any blood component from a high-risk donor be released from the donor center to a transfusion unit. Donors in high-risk groups for AIDS must be deferred from donating. If high-risk activity becomes known retrospective to blood donation (such as in the self-exclusion process), the blood components from the donation must be retrieved and destroyed.

9.

C. Plasma protein fraction (PPF) and albumin preparations (5 and 20%) provide colloid replacement and volume expansion with virtually no risk of viral transmission. These are pooled products and are pasteurized by heating to 60°C for 10 hours. Other products, such as clotting factor concentrates, are usually treated by solvent-detergent method to inactivate viruses with lipid envelopes such as HBV, HCV, HIV, and human T-cell lymphotropic virus-1.

10.

B. It is acceptable according to FDA and AABB *Standards for Blood Banks and Transfusion Services* to screen donors for infectious diseases in pools of 16 to 24 donor sera. If a donor pool is positive for HCV, all individual donors making up the pool are tested individually using the same nucleic acid test (NAT) to find the positive donor. When that donor is identified, s/he is excluded from donating henceforth and all components from that donation are retrieved and destroyed.

11.

D. Cryoprecipitate provides the only known concentrated source of fibronectin, useful in the phagocytic removal of bacteria and aggregates by the reticuloendothelial system. It also contains factors VIII:C, VIII:vW, and XIII. Antithrombin III (AT III), necessary to prevent a thromboembolic disorder, is depleted in DIC and liver disease. Transfusion sources of AT III are fresh frozen plasma FFP and commercial concentrates, but AT III is not present in cryoprecipitate.

12.

D. FFP contains all the plasma clotting factors. FFP's primary use is for patients with clotting factor deficiencies for which no concentrate is available and patients who present multiple factor deficiencies such as in liver disease. Platelets are cellular elements, not a plasma clotting factor, and they must be maintained at 20–24°C with continuous gentle agitation to maintain their viability.

13.

C. The AABB Standards require that when a patient is likely at risk for graft-versus-host disease (GVHD), all cellular blood components must be irradiated before transfusion. This includes components for patients who are immunodeficient or immunocompromised, such as a patient on immunosuppressive therapy and a fetus who receives intrauterine transfusion. Irradiation of RBCs for exchange transfusion is not required by the AABB Standards, although many hospital transfusion services do so. Immunocompetent individuals require irradiated components if they are to receive cellular components from someone who may be homozygous for a shared HLA haplotype, such as a blood relative or an HLA-matched donor. Gamma irradiation of cellular components is the *only* way to prevent transfusion-associated GVHD that occurs when immunocompetent donor T cells survive in the patient's circulation and mount an immune response against the host cells. A minimum of 25 Gy delivered to the midplane of the container and at least 15 Gy to all other areas will prevent GVHD.

14.

A. The limiting criterion for *in vitro* storage of blood is the survival in the recipient of at least 75% of the transfused RBCs for at least 24 hours after transfusion. Additional adenine in an anticoagulant-preservative formulation provides a substrate for the continued generation of ATP *in vitro*. The overall effect is improved viability.

15.

D. Donor blood may not be labeled according to test results obtained from previous donations. Several segments removed from the donor unit will provide sufficient sample for all required testing but will limit the number of segments available for crossmatching. After centrifugation, the plasma may be removed from the segments and clotted with calcium chloride or a similar commercial product for use in test procedures requiring serum. Alternatively, institutions with sterile connecting devices may attach a small bag and remove an aliquot sufficient for testing.

16–17.

(16:C, 17:A) *In vitro* recovery of factor VIII must be assayed monthly to ensure proper control of conditions during cryoprecipitate production. A minimum of 80 international units (IU) per container must be present in the final product. One international unit is defined as the clotting activity of 1 mL of fresh plasma. The total number of factor VIII units is calculated from the following formula:

$$\text{Factor VIII (IU/mL)} \times \text{volume (mL)} = \text{Total IU Factor VIII}$$

In this case, $9\ \text{IU/mL} \times 10\ \text{mL} = 90\ \text{IU}$ per container in the final product. This exceeds the required 80 IU/container and so meets AABB *Standards*.

Although there is no existing standard for percent recovery of factor VIII during production, this information may be helpful in monitoring various stages of production when the monthly quality control assays fall below the acceptable standard. Recovery can be calculated by the following formula:

$$\frac{\text{Post (F VIII IU/mL} \times \text{volume mL)}}{\text{Pre (F VIII IU/mL} \times \text{volume mL)}} \times 100 = \text{\% Factor VIII recovery}$$

In this instance,

$$\frac{9\ \text{IU/mL} \times 10\ \text{mL}}{1\ \text{IU/mL} \times 250\ \text{mL}} \times 100 = 36\%\ \text{Factor VIII recovery}$$

18.

C. Discard the unit. The unit will have potassium accumulation related to the irradiation process and breakdown of cells. Although RBC units must be discarded, platelets can be issued if irradiated twice.

19.

C. Cryoprecipitate pooled in an open system has an expiration time of 4 hours. If the cryoprecipitate is pooled through a sterile closed system, the expiration time is extended by 2 hours so it will expire in 6 hours from completed pooling.

20.

C. A single donor unit of apheresis platelets must have a minimum platelet count of 3.0×10^{11}. The unit pH must be 6.2 or higher throughout the processing and storage of the unit. Additional plasma can be added to raise the pH.

21.

B. Frozen RBCs are good for 10 years at −65°C. FFP and cryoprecipitate are good for 1 year at −18 to −65°C. FFP can be stored for 7 years at −65°C. Platelets are good for 5 days at 20 to 22°C.

22.

B. A low RBC concentration of 2,3-BPG increases RBC affinity for O_2, causing less O_2 to be released to the tissues. As blood is stored, 2,3-BPG levels fall. Once the blood is transfused, red cells regenerate 2,3-BPG and ATP, which are fully restored in about 24 hours. Other metabolic changes that occur as blood is stored are an increase in plasma K^+ as red cells leak K^+, an increase in plasma hemoglobin, and a decrease in ATP.

23.

D. Autologous blood should not be drawn later than 72 hours prior to surgery. The reason is to allow time for adequate volume repletion. However, the medical director may decrease this time if the patient's condition warrants it.

24.

B. Preoperative autologous donation is commonly done for orthopedic surgery, radical prostatectomy, and open heart surgery. Patients with uncompensated anemia and hemoglobin levels below 11.0 g/dL are unable to donate because they do not have sufficient RBCs to maintain oxygen-carrying capacity after the donation. Because it is difficult to find donors for patients with multiple antibodies or an antibody to a high-incidence antigen, these individuals, if anemic, may be given supplemental iron and allowed to donate once their hemoglobin levels are above 11.0 g/dL. Their cells can also be frozen for later use.

25.

A. Anti HBs antibody indicates that an individual has developed immunity or been vaccinated for HBV. Anti-HBc IgM occurs in the early stage of infection. Anti-HBC IgG occurs as a secondary or anamnestic response and can persist for years postinfection. HBs antigen is not associated with immunity but rather with infection and is the first marker to appear.

26.

B. RBCs continue to metabolize, albeit at a slower rate, during storage at 1–6°C. Decreased ATP levels result in loss of RBC viability. Plasma hemoglobin, ammonia, and K^+ levels increase, whereas plasma Na^+ and pH and 2,3-BPG levels decrease. These biochemical changes are collectively referred to as the "storage lesion" of blood.

27.

C. Because the patient received eight units of blood and none of the donors has been implicated in other cases of hepatitis, none of these donors would be deferred. The donor center should be immediately notified so it can enter in each donor's record that s/he has been implicated in a case of transfusion-transmitted hepatitis. After a second implication, the donor would be indefinitely deferred. If only one donor had been implicated, s/he would have been indefinitely deferred.

28.

C. RBCs and whole blood must be stored between 1 and 6°C in a monitored refrigerator with a recording thermometer and audible alarm system. During transportation between collection and transfusion facilities, blood must be packed in well-insulated containers designed to maintain a temperature range of 1–10°C. Wet ice in a leak-proof plastic bag is placed on top of the blood. The amount of ice to be used is dictated by the transportation time, the number of units packed, and the ambient outside temperature.

29.

C. In addition to the minimum number of platelets that should be present, 5.5×10^{10}, the pH of the unit must be 6.2 or higher in at least 75% of the units. The units should be assayed at the end of the allowable storage period. A donor who has taken aspirin should not be the sole donor of platelets for a patient. Aspirin has an adverse effect on platelet aggregation.

30.

B. Patients with anti-IgA antibodies should not receive any plasma products as they may contain IgA. Washed or deglycerolized RBCs can be used as the plasma is removed during the washing process.

31.

C. RBCs expire 24 hours from the time the hermetic seal is broken, provided they are maintained at 1–6°C during the storage period. The new expiration date and time must be placed on the label and in the appropriate records. An open system exposes the blood to possible bacterial contamination. Blood may be frozen for up to 6 days after collection when maintained at 1–6°C in a closed system. If the seal is inadvertently broken on a rare unit during component preparation, the RBCs may be salvaged by glycerolization and freezing, providing this is accomplished within the 24-hour restriction.

32.

D. The AABB Standards require that an authorized individual (such as a supervisor or medical director) review the standard operating procedures (SOPs), policies, and process annually and document the review. The SOPs should be reviewed and revised as needed to reflect the techniques used by the laboratory. It is prudent to conduct a review before a scheduled inspection and following publication of each new edition of AABB Standards to ensure conformance with new requirements.

33.

B. Previous ABO and Rh records of patients must be retained for 10 years and be immediately available for 12 months as a check to confirm the identity of the current pretransfusion sample. Records of unexpected antibodies identified in the serum of intended recipients and of serious adverse reactions to blood components must be retained indefinitely. Consulting records may prevent a delayed hemolytic transfusion reaction when the antibody is no longer demonstrable.

34.

D. In the United States, the weak D test is performed routinely when a donor appears to be Rh-negative, and all weak D donor units are labeled Rh-positive. Weak D units are much less immunogenic than normal D units. In many countries, neither donors nor recipients are tested for weak D.

35.

B. In order to meet the current AABB Standards for leukocyte reduction to prevent HLA alloimmunization or CMV transmission, the donor unit must retain at least 80% of the original RBCs, and the leukocytes must be reduced to less than 5×10^6. Leukocyte reduction might also prevent febrile reactions in two ways: (1) By reducing the number of leukocytes in the component to a low enough level, one can prevent febrile reactions when patients have leukocyte antibodies. (2) Cytokines are also known to cause febrile reactions. If prestorage leukocyte reduction is done, cytokine generation should be prevented.

36.

D. ABO grouping must be determined by doing both cell and serum grouping. The Rh type must be determined by direct agglutination with anti-D; if negative, the test is incubated and converted to the antiglobulin test to detect weak D phenotypes. Performing an antibody screening test on the serum or plasma of a donor is required when the donor has a history of transfusion or pregnancy. For practical purposes, most donor centers screen all donors for clinically significant antibodies. The absence of hepatitis B surface antigen (HBsAg) and HIV must be confirmed using a method currently licensed by the FDA. The test for hepatitis B surface antibody (HBsAb) is not required.

37.

C. In the average-size adult (70 kg), a unit of platelet concentrate should raise the platelet count by 5000–10,000/μL if there are no other complicating factors to cause decreased survival. Complicating factors include fever, sepsis, disseminated intravascular coagulation (DIC), and HLA sensitization. One apheresis platelet unit is equivalent to 6–8 units of pooled platelet concentrate and has the advantage of decreased donor exposure.

38.

A. The ABO group on all units and the Rh type on all D-negative units must be repeated by the transfusing facility for units of RBCs or whole blood collected and processed at another facility. This is generally accomplished by repeating the cell grouping only. To save time and reagent cost, it is convenient to test units labeled group O with anti-A,B only. Confirmatory testing for weak D is not required. The Rh type of units labeled D-positive need not be confirmed. Repeat antibody screening and viral testing are not required.

39–43.

(39:A, 40:D, 41:C, 42:C, 43:B) The storage temperature for whole blood, modified whole blood, RBCs, including leukocyte-reduced and deglycerolized products, is between 1 and 6°C. This range may be extended to 10°C during brief periods of transport. RBCs are frozen in a glycerol solution. These units must be stored at −65°C or lower. Fresh-frozen plasma (FFP) and cryoprecipitate are stored at −18°C or colder with a 1-year expiration. Although this temperature meets AABB Standards, optimal storage temperature is −30°C or below. In fact, FFP expiration may be extended to 7 years if kept at −65°C or lower. Frozen storage at low temperatures maintains optimum levels of the labile coagulation factors V and VIII in FFP and VIII in cryoprecipitate. Plasma should be frozen within 8 hours of collection when collected in citrate-phosphate-dextrose (CPD) or CPDA-1. Platelet concentrates are stored at room temperature (20–24°C). They need to be agitated during storage.

44–48.

(44:C, 45:D, 46:D, 47:A, 48:B) Whole blood and RBCs may be stored up to 35 days when collected in CPDA-1, as long as the hermetic seal remains unbroken. Adenine added to the anticoagulant increases the viability of the cells. Cells stored only in CPD have a shorter allowable storage of 21 days. Addition of adsol solution extends expiration of RBCs to 42 days. FFP and cryoprecipitate expire 12 months from the date of collection if stored at −18°C or colder. The expiration time for these components is based on the deterioration of the labile factor VIII. Units stored beyond 12 months may have reduced levels of factor VIII unless stored at much lower temperatures. FFP is approved for 7-year storage if kept at −65°C or lower. Once thawed, FFP expires in 24 hours when stored at 1–6°C. The type of plastic used in the manufacture of the bag affects the allowable storage time for platelets. The older type of bag (polyvinylchloride) does not allow as effective gas exchange as the newer types of plastic. Platelet concentrates, prepared in PL-732 bags and stored at 20–24°C with agitation, expire 5 days from the date and time of collection.

49–52.

(49:A, 50:B, 51:C, 52:D) Blood cells continue to metabolize *in vitro*. Plasma glucose and ATP are depleted. Intermediary metabolites are generated. These may interfere with the production of energy via glycolysis. This results in a gradual loss of RBC viability. Storage at lowered temperatures (1–6°C) slows metabolism. ACD and CPD solutions contain sufficient glucose to support RBC viability for 21 days. CPDA-1 also contains adenine, which extends the shelf life to 35 days. Adenine maintains viability by ATP regeneration. RBCs prepared with additive solutions such as AS-1 have a shelf life of 42 days. EDTA is not an approved solution for the storage of blood for transfusion.

53–59.

(53:D, 54:A, 55:C, 56:D, 57:D, 58:D, 59:D) Donors may be accepted after age 17 years of age, provided all results of the physical examination are normal. There is no upper age limit. Elderly donors may participate in a blood program at the discretion of the local blood bank physician. Many senior citizens obtain written permission from their personal physicians and present approval at the time of donation. The interval between donations of blood for allogeneic transfusion is 8 weeks or 56 days. This time period is designed to protect the health of the donor. Exceptions at the discretion of the blood bank and personal physician may be made if the blood is intended for autologous use. A man who had a history of sex with another man after 1977 must be indefinitely deferred because of the possibility of transmitting HIV. A history of jaundice in the first days of life is indicative of hemolytic disease of the newborn and is not a cause for deferral. A mild skin rash caused by acne, poison ivy, psoriasis, or other allergies is not a cause for donor deferral, as long as the disorder does not extend into the antecubital area at the venipuncture site. Final acceptance or deferral may be made at the phlebotomist's discretion, dependent upon whether the arm can be properly prepared to maintain sterility of the product without undue discomfort to the donor. A woman who has been pregnant is deferred until 6 weeks following conclusion of the pregnancy unless her blood is needed for her infant and the donation is physician approved. The acceptable limits of the physical examination include the following:

Temperature: 37.5°C (99.5°F) or less
Pulse: 50–100 bpm
Blood pressure: systolic ≤ 180 mm Hg, diastolic ≤ 100 mm Hg

Runners or other athletes may be accepted when the pulse rate is less than 50 bpm, as long as no irregularity in beats is detected. These parameters are incorporated in the AABB Standards for the safety of the donor and are in general use by all blood-collecting facilities. For donor suitability, the FDA and AABB require only that the hemoglobin level be no less than 12.5 g/dL (with no sex differentiation) and that the temperature and blood pressure be within reference ranges as determined by a qualified physician or by persons under his or her supervision.

60–63.

(60:D, 61:C, 62:B, 63:A) Patients with warm AIHA secondary to α-methyldopa respond rapidly following cessation of the drug. They can usually be managed without transfusion. The direct antiglobulin test (DAT) might not revert to negative for up to 6 months or even longer. Leukocyte-reduced blood components ($\leq 5 \times 10^6$) are indicated in order to avoid repeated febrile episodes, CMV transmission, and alloimmunization to leukocytes. Leukocytes can be removed by filtration, centrifugation, or washing. Currently, the preferred and most efficient method is filtration with commercially available adsorption filters capable of reducing leukocytes to the required level. Patients with normovolemic anemia should be transfused with RBCs, which provide the RBCs needed to correct the anemia in the smallest volume. These patients may not be able to tolerate whole blood because of the volume increase. It is not necessary to use leukocyte-reduced RBC for patients with normovolemic anemia. Thrombocytopenia means there is a lack of platelets. Often platelet counts drop in acute leukemia and during the subsequent treatment. Platelet counts below 20,000/µL are not uncommon under the circumstances, and the patient is considered to have severe thrombocytopenia. Leukocyte-reduced platelets will lower the chance of alloimmunization and are routinely given prophylactically to people with leukemia.

Blood Groups, Genetics, Serology

64.

D. The body makes five different classes of immunoglobulins: IgA, IgD, IgE, IgG, and IgM. IgG makes up about 80% of the total serum immunoglobulin. Although IgA is more abundant than IgM (13% versus 6%), IgM is more common as a blood group antibody.

65.

B. From his phenotype, the father appears to be homozygous *kk* genetically. However, he is actually K^0k and has passed the K^0 gene to child 1. The K^0 gene at the *Kell* locus does not appear to result in the formation of any Kell system antigens. Child 1 has the genotype K^0K, having received the *K* gene from the mother, and has a phenotype expressing on the K antigen. Child 2 can have either the genotype *kk* or K^0k, with the mother contributing a *k* gene and the father either K^0 or *k*. The McLeod phenotype would result in weakened expression of K or k antigens. There has been no *cis-Kk* gene discovered, nor any dominant inhibitor gene that represses the expression of Kell system genes.

66.

D. All RBCs contain some amount of H substance. The only exception is the very rare O_h (Bombay) individual because these persons lack the *H* gene that codes for H substance. Group O cells contain the most H substance, and A_1B cells contain the least amount of H substance. The order of decreasing reactivity with anti-H is: O $> A_2 > A_2B > B > A_1 > A_1B$.

67.

B. Two genes control Rh antigen activity. *RHD* controls the expression of D antigen, and *RHCE* determines the C, E, c, and e antigens. *RHD* is absent or inactive in D-negative individuals. Alleles of *RHCE* are *RHCe, RHcE,* and *RHce*. The RH is often dropped (e.g., *CE, Ce, cE, ce*).

68.

C. This individual does not have a cold autoantibody, as demonstrated by the negative autocontrol at all phases of testing. Being a nonsecretor does not affect the ABO or Rh typing, nor will it cause the appearance of unexpected antibodies in the patient's plasma. Rouleaux is ruled out because reactions are still seen with antihuman globulin (AHG) after all of the patient serum or plasma has been washed away. Of the choices given, the most likely is that the patient is a Bombay phenotype individual, having inherited one *h* gene from each parent. The only other possibility is that the patient is a group O with a strong unexpected antibody or antibodies in his/her serum; however, that was not one of the choices given as an answer.

69.

B. Bombay (O_h) individuals' RBCs not only lack A and B substances but also lack H substance. People with blood type Bombay are genetically *hh* and, therefore, are unable to produce the precursor H substance upon which the A and B transferases act to produce A and B substances. In their serum, they will have anti-A, anti-B, anti-A,B, and an equally strong anti-H, which will react with normal group O cells. Neither O nor O_h RBCs react with anti-A,B or anti-A_1 lectin. However, O_h RBCs give a negative reaction with anti-H lectin, whereas O cells are positive, allowing differentiation of the two.

70.

C. The *Le* gene codes for a enzyme, L-fucosyl transferase, which attaches fucose to the subterminal sugar on the type 1 precursor substance producing Le^a substance. This occurs independently of the ABH secretor status. For Le^b as well as ABH substances to be present in the secretions, both the *Se* gene and the *Le* gene must be present. The *Se* gene produces a transferase that attaches a fucose to the terminal sugar on precursor substance, forming H substance in the secretions. Type 1H and type 2H are the precursors for A and B substance. The *Le* gene can act upon type 1H as well to form Le^b substance; therefore, a nonsecretor who has a *Le* gene will only secrete Le^a, whereas a secretor will secrete a little Le^a and a lot of cell lysis Le^b substance.

71.

D. Monoclonal reagents containing the ES-4 clone react well with acquired B RBCs and those lacking that clone do not react. Most human anti-B will react but not the individual's own anti-B. Acquired B antigens are often associated with carcinoma of the colon, gram-negative infection, and intestinal obstructions. Also, B substance will not be found in the saliva of a person with an acquired B antigen if the patient is an ABH secretor. Acquired B occurs in group A people when microbial enzymes deacetylate the A determinant sugar (N-acetylgalactosamine) so that it resembles the B sugar (D-galactose).

72.

A. Paroxysmal cold hemoglobinuria (PCH) is complement dependent and is facilitated by the IgG (Donath-Landsteiner antibodies) antibodies that bind P antigen in colder temperatures. Lyses occur due to complement-mediated hemolysis when cells move through circulation to warmer central locations. This biphasic reaction is indicative of PCH.

73.

D. The sugar L-fucose is attached to the terminal sugar of precursor substance by a fucosyl transferase. The fucosyl transferase coded by the *H* gene adds fucose to the precursor substance on RBCs. The fucosyl transferase encoded by the *Se* gene adds fucose to the precursor substance in the same configuration in the secretions. In both cases, the resulting configuration is called H substance. Without H substance present, the sugars giving A or B antigenic activity cannot attach.

74.

B. The complement cascade has many functions in the body associated with immunity and inflammation. The last stages of the complement cascade ultimately lead to cell lysis, such as hemolysis. IgM is the immunoglobulin that most readily activates complement. The IgG immunoglobulins can activate complement to a lesser extent. IgG3 activates complement more efficiently than the other IgG subclasses. Although G6PD deficiency can result in hemolysis in the presence of fava beans and certain drugs, the enzyme itself does not lyse RBCs. Albumin and AHG serum can be used in blood bank testing and do not harm RBCs.

75.

B. The answer is based on gene frequencies. The genes that code for the haplotypes *DCe* and *dce* are high in the Caucasian American population. A *DCe/dce* genotype has a frequency of approximately 31.1% in the general Caucasian American population. The other two possible choices among the answers that would fit the typing results are *DCe/Dce* and *Dce/dCe* and have frequencies of approximately 3.4 and 0.2%, respectively. *DCe/DcE* is incorrect because the typing does not indicate that the E antigen is present.

76.

C. All these genotypes have a low frequency in the African American population. *DCe/dcE* is the rarest, with a frequency of <0.1%. *DCe/DcE* is the most frequent, with an occurrence of 3.7%.

77.

A. RBCs that have either the C or D antigen also have the G antigen. When anti-G is made, it is capable of reacting with the G antigen on both C-positive and D-positive RBCs, therefore appearing to be anti-C plus anti-D. In the stated case, the immunizing RBCs were D-negative and C-positive. Therefore, what appears to be a combination of anti-D and anti-C is anti-G or a combination of anti-C and anti-G.

78.

B. The unit from the *DCe/dce* donor has the c antigen that the patient lacks. This antigen is a good immunogen. Although this patient can form the anti-E antibody, the donor cells lack the E antigen. Thus, the donor cells cannot stimulate the production of anti-E. Remember, "d" simply implies the absence of D and is not an antigen.

79.

C. Fifty percent of the children can be expected to be D-positive (*DCe/dce*) and 50% can be expected to be D-negative (*dce/dce*). The following chart clearly illustrates how the percentages were determined. The mother can pass on only *dce* haplotype, whereas the father can pass on *DCe* or *dce*.

	Father	
Mother	***DCe***	***dce***
dce	*DCe/dce*	*dce/dce*
dce	*DCe/dce*	*dce/dce*

80.

C. The husband's genotype is most likely *Dce/dCe*. He is weak D because of position effect and has a normal *D* gene. The *C* in trans position to a normal *D* gene often causes a weakened expression of D antigen. The infant has inherited the father's normal *D* gene but does not have *C* in trans position and therefore has a normal D antigen expression. Thus, the husband is not excluded and is probably the father.

81.

C. The wife is *dce/dce* and, lacking the D antigen, can make anti-D. The child is D+ and therefore cannot make anti-D. The husband, although being weak D, has passed a normal D antigen to the child. This indicates that the husband's "weak D" antigen is not the result of a partial D, and therefore he cannot make anti-D.

82.

B. Occasionally, people whose blood type as D positive make an apparent anti-D. The D antigen is made up of several epitopes or antigenic determinants. Those individuals missing one or more of these epitopes are called partial D. When individuals lack one or more of these epitopes, they can make an antibody, after appropriate stimulation, against the epitope or epitopes that they lack. All of these antibodies to D epitopes will react with "normal" D-positive cells that have all of the epitopes on the D antigen. Therefore, a D-positive or weak-D person appears to make an anti-D.

83.

D. High-frequency alloantibodies or multiple antibodies may cause all three cell lines to react positively. The negative autocontrol rules out autoantibodies. The reaction only with AHG is indicative of IgG so cold antibodies or IgM antibodies are not likely.

84.

C. Anti-Jk^a often declines in the serum to below detectable levels. Therefore, when a patient has been transfused and makes anti-Jk^a and then is not transfused again for a long time, the subsequent antibody screen may not reveal the presence of the anti-Jk^a. An intravascular delayed transfusion reaction is characteristic of the Kidd antibodies because, after a second stimulation, there is a slow rise in the antibody titer that activates complement very well. In the case presented, the antibody has been missed, and he received Jk(a+) cells at some point during his stay in the other hospital. This caused a severe delayed hemolytic transfusion reaction with intravascular hemolysis.

85.

A. The Xg^a antigen is produced by a gene on the X chromosome. Because women inherit two X chromosomes, there is a higher incidence of the antigen in females. The antibody is usually detected by an antiglobulin test, and the antigenic activity is depressed by enzymes.

86.

D. To ensure that an antiserum is reacting properly, positive and negative controls must be tested. The antiserum must be tested against a cell that is negative for the corresponding antigen to ensure that no interfering substances are present that will cause false positives. It must also be tested against a cell positive for the corresponding antigen. A heterozygous cell is used to determine whether or not the antiserum will be reactive with the smaller number of antigen sites on the RBCs seen in heterozygotes. For example, when using anti-K, you would test a *kk* (K−k+) cell and a *Kk* (K+k+) cell.

87.

D. Kidd antibodies are often weak and deteriorate during storage. They are usually IgG, AHG reactive only, and complement dependent. Reactions are enhanced when enzyme-treated panel cells are used. Kidd antibodies also show dosage effect, and the titer may drop to undetectable levels after the primary response. For this reason, they are often implicated in delayed hemolytic transfusion reactions when there is no previous record of the presence of the antibody. A Kidd antibody rarely occurs singly in a patient's serum but is often seen accompanying other antibodies.

88.

D. Enzymes denature the Fy^a and Fy^b antigens and render panel cells Fy(a−b−). Therefore, anti-Fy^a and anti-Fy^b will not react with enzyme-treated RBCs. These Duffy antibodies are clinically significant. They can cause hemolytic transfusion reactions and mild hemolytic disease of the newborn (HDN). They are usually IgG antibodies and are best detected by the AHG technique. Rh antibodies will react strongly with enzyme-treated cells.

89.

C. Both anti-S and anti-M are common and can occur naturally. Anti-S can be produced through immune stimulation. Anti-S can react at body temperature and be clinically significant. Patients with anti-S must receive antigen-negative blood, but patients with anti-M are crossmatch-compatible at 37°C.

90.

D. Anti-U is a clinically significant IgG antibody causing hemolytic transfusion reactions and HDN. All Caucasian Americans appear to be U+ , because no U negatives have been found. About 99% of African Americans are U+ and 1% are U−. Those people who are U− are also S−s− and lack the entire Ss sialoglycoprotein (glycophorin B) except for very rare genetic mutations.

91.

B. Although the patient's antibody screening is negative at this time, previous records show that the patient had an anti-E. Anti-E is a significant IgG antibody; only blood negative for the E antigen should be transfused to the patient. Failure to give E-negative blood could result in a serious delayed transfusion reaction due to an anamnestic response.

92.

B. For control purposes, the cell should have the weakest expression of the antigen in question; that would be an Fy(a+b+) cell. A weaker cell from a heterozygote is used because a weak antiserum might detect an antigen from a homozygote but not from a heterozygote (dosage effect). If this should happen, then RBCs might be mistyped as Fy(a−) when in fact the cells are Fy(a+).

93.

B. Most antibodies in the Kell system are RBC stimulated. They are generally IgG antibodies and usually detected in AHG phase testing. Because of their nature, they have been implicated in both transfusion reactions and HDN. The other choices are usually IgM antibodies that cannot cross the placenta and are rarely involved in transfusion reactions. In the case of HDN, the mother's antibody titer should be monitored. Additionally, fetal monitoring is critical, specifically bilirubin levels in the amniotic fluid to determine if intervention is required.

94.

A. Antibodies can be ruled out using only one cell that is homozygously antigen positive and nonreactive at all phases of testing with the patient serum. Preferably, two or three cells that are positive for the antigen and nonreactive with the patient serum increase confidence. Antibodies in the Duffy, Kidd, and MNSs systems often show dosage effect. Because there are more antigenic sites on homozygous cells than on heterozygous cells, these antibodies react more strongly with homozygous cells [cells with 2 "doses" of the antigen, such as Jk(a+b−)] than with cells that carry a single "dose" of the antigen [such as Jk(a+b+)]. These antibodies can be ruled out only using homozygous cells that are positive for the antigen and do not react with the patient serum. Of the answers available, "**A**" is the best choice. Additional antibodies may not be ruled out when a standard of three cells that are positive for the antigen and nonreactive with the patient serum is used.

95.

B. The most likely combination of antibodies is anti-E plus anti-K. More than one antibody is likely because the reactions seen are of varying strengths. The panel cells that did not react with the patient serum are all lacking the E and K antigens. The E antigen is present on cells #4, #5, and #9. The K antigen is present on cells #4 and #7. Note that cell #4 has the E and K antigens and reacts 4+ with AHG. Cells #5 and #9 have the E antigen but not the K antigen, and both cells react 3+ with AHG. Cell #7 has the K antigen but not the E antigen and reacts 2+ with AHG. Therefore, the anti-E is stronger than the anti-K, and when both antigens are present the reaction is stronger than a reaction with one antibody alone.

96.

C. Cells #1, #4, and #7 are the cells from this panel that will be helpful in confirming the antibodies, anti-E and anti-K, and ruling out the other possible antibodies. Cell #1 is E- and K-negative and should not react with the patient's serum. However, cell #1 is also S+s−, Le(a+), Jk(a−b+), and Fy(a−b+) and can help to rule out all of the other possible antibodies. Cell #4 is E+, K−, S−, s+, Le(a−), Jk(b−), and Fy(b−). This cell can help confirm the presence of anti-E. Cell #7 is E−, S−, Le(a−), K+, Jk(b−), and Fy(b−). This cell can help confirm the presence of anti-K.

97.

C. Anti-Le^a, -Le^b, and -P_1 may all be neutralized by commercially available soluble substances. Le^a and Le^b are not RBC antigens but are plasma substances that are absorbed onto RBCs in the circulation. Soluble antigens are more available to the antibodies and can attach to soluble antibodies more readily than particulate antigens. Thus, the plasma (soluble) Le^a and Le^b can be used to bind to the soluble antibodies, leaving no antibody to react with the particulate antigen on the RBCs. Soluble P_1 can be obtained from several sources and can be used in the same way to preferentially bind the anti-P_1, leaving no anti-P_1 to react with the particulate P_1 antigen on the RBCs.

98.

C. Anti-N is the only antibody listed that is generally a room-temperature saline agglutinin. The remaining choices, anti-Fy^a, anti-Jk^b, and anti-U, are best detected in the AHG phase of testing. Remember, this is where these antibodies are optimally reactive; it does not mean they will never react at other phases of testing. Some antibodies just don't read the books!

99.

D. The Fy^a antigen is destroyed by enzyme treatment. Therefore, the anti-Fy^a seen in the initial panel will not react in an enzyme-treated panel. Enzyme-treated cells react extremely well with antibodies of the Rh system. Because the second antibody is suspected of being a weak anti-C, the antibody will react more strongly with an enzyme-treated panel than it did in the initial LISS panel. Although one cannot rule out antibodies to Duffy system, MNSs system, or Xg^a using an enzyme-treated panel, all other major blood group system antibodies present in the patient's serum should react in this medium. An elution removes antibody from the RBCs; in our scenario, the antibody is seen in the serum. Absorption of the anti-Fy^a from the patient serum could be useful; however, finding cells that lack all of the antigens lacked by the patient to avoid missing an alloantibody is a difficult and time-consuming task. Additionally, absorption will unavoidably dilute the patient's serum slightly and may dilute the weak second antibody to a point where it cannot be identified. Antigen typing the patient's cells is useful in determining whether or not the patient can form anti-C and anti-Fy^a, but it will not exclude any other antibodies nor confirm the presence of any specific antibody.

100.

B. Solid-phase RBC adherence assays, the gel test, and affinity column technology are all third-generation antibody detection methods. They have equal or greater sensitivity for clinically significant antibodies than first- and second-generation techniques. In general, they have the following advantages: less hands-on time, smaller sample size, improved safety, and stable end-points, and they can be automated. In the gel test, the AHG test does not require washing or the addition of IgG-coated cells, because unbound globulins are trapped in the viscous barrier at the top of the gel column. Upon centrifugation, the anti-IgG in the column traps RBCs that have been coated with IgG during the incubation period. In affinity column technology, the viscous barrier traps unbound IgG, but *Staphylococcus aureus* derived protein A and protein G are in the column instead of anti-IgG and react with the Fc portion of IgG-coated RBCs. The other two techniques (solid-phase RBC adherence and polyethylene glycol) require a washing step.

101.

D. The three antibodies, anti-P_1, anti-Le^a, and anti-I, are most often non-RBC-stimulated IgM antibodies. All of these antibodies can also, however, be stimulated by exposure to RBCs carrying the corresponding antigen. Each of the other answers has at least one antibody that will be formed only due to exposure, either through transfusion or pregnancy, to the corresponding RBC antigen.

102.

B. Lymphocytotoxicity testing is performed by adding patient mononuclear leukocytes to wells containing sera that have antibodies to various HLA antigens and then adding guinea pig complement and indicator dye. The cells that take up the dye have had their cell membranes perforated by the action of the antigen–antibody reaction and complement, indicating that they carry the HLA antigen corresponding to the antibody in the well. Although the antibodies to Bg system antigens are antibodies to HLA antigens, the Bg terminology is only used for the remnant HLA antigens found on RBCs. The Wright system and JMH antigens are RBC antigens and are not related to the HLA system.

103.

A. Mixed-field agglutination refers to an agglutination pattern where there are two distinct cell populations, one agglutinated and one not. The appearance is clumps of cells among many unagglutinated cells. In a delayed hemolytic transfusion reaction, surviving donor cells will be coated with patient antibody and the patient's own cells will not, yielding a mixed-field DAT result. Other examples of mixed-field agglutination are seen in patients who have been transfused with blood of another ABO group, in patients with Lutheran antibodies, and in D-negative mothers with D-positive infants where there was a large fetomaternal bleed. Also, A_3 subgroup RBCs may demonstrate a mixed-field reaction with anti-A.

104.

D. The first antibody to become detectable in a primary immune response to a foreign blood group antigen is IgM followed by IgG, usually detectable from less than a week to several months after second exposure. After secondary exposure to the antigen, the antibody titer usually increases rapidly within several days. Antibodies are produced by plasma cells. The antibody produced by the plasma cells in the secondary response is IgG. Plasma cells are the terminal differentiation of the B lymphocytes.

105.

B. These antibodies will cause discrepancies on reverse typing. Note that the reverse typing utilizes the patient's plasma (where the antibodies would be) in combination with reagent (known antigens) red cells. Whereas, forward typing uses reagent antisera (known antibodies) and patient RBCs (unknown antigens).

106.

C. Blood for intrauterine transfusion should be group O, D-negative (because the fetus's blood group is unknown) and negative for the antigen corresponding to any other IgG antibody in the maternal serum. It should be recently drawn and administered as RBC (Hct 75–85%) to minimize the chance of volume overload. It should be irradiated, CMV safe, and known to lack hemoglobin S.

107.

A. Anti-Jk^a is an IgG antibody and is nearly always detected in the AHG phase. Rarely, it can be detected at the 37°C phase of testing. Anti-M, anti-P_1, and anti-I are generally IgM antibodies and react at room temperature and below by direct agglutination.

108.

D. Lewis system antibodies are generally IgM. Antibodies in the Rh, Duffy, and Kell systems are generally IgG. There may be rare IgM exceptions.

109.

B. Bg antibodies react with the RBC equivalents of HLA antigens. Bg^a corresponds with HLA-B7, Bg^b with HLA-B17, and Bg^c with HLA-A28. These antibodies can be frustrating in that few panel cells will react and the Bg type of panel cells is often not listed.

110.

C. There is no ABO exclusion. Although the alleged father and mother are group A, they could both be heterozygous (*AO*) with the baby inheriting the *O* gene from each parent. The child appears to be of the Rh genotype *dce/dce*. One of these haplotypes is inherited from the mother. It is feasible for the alleged father to be *DCe/dce*. He could then contribute the second haplotype. The baby can inherit the *A2B12* haplotype from the mother. Although *A3* can come from the alleged father, *B15* cannot and therefore there is a direct HLA exclusion.

111–118.

(111:C, 112:A, 113:D, 114:B, 115:C, 116:D, 117:A, 118:A) Discrepancies in ABO blood grouping may occur for numerous reasons. Any discrepancy between cell and serum grouping must be resolved before blood is identified as belonging to a particular ABO group. The presence of an acquired B antigen on cells that are normally group A can be found in some disorders, where gram-negative bacteria have entered the circulation. The serum will contain an anti-B, which will not agglutinate the patient's own cells that have the acquired B antigen. The RBC reaction with anti-B reagent may be weaker than usual. Protein abnormalities of the serum such as are present in multiple myeloma may cause the presence of what appear to be additional antibodies. The rouleaux of the RBCs caused by the excess globulin may appear to be agglutination. Saline replacement of the serum and resuspension of the cells will usually resolve the problem in the serum grouping. Washed RBCs should be used for the cell grouping. Infants do not begin making antibodies until they are 3 to 6 months of age. Newborns therefore will not demonstrate the expected antibody(ies) on reverse grouping. The antibody that is present is probably IgG from the mother that has crossed the placenta. An A_2 individual has the ability to make an antibody that agglutinates A_1 red cells. This anti-A_1 will cause a serum grouping discrepancy, but the antibody is almost always naturally occurring and clinically insignificant. A patient's serum may have antibodies to the yellow dye used to color anti-B reagents. If serum or plasma suspended RBCs are used in the cell grouping, a false positive reaction may occur. Using washed cells will eliminate the problem. Patients who are immunodeficient may have such depressed immunoglobulins that their serum does not react with the expected A and B reagent RBCs. An unexpected IgM antibody in the serum will react at room temperature and may interfere with ABO typing. Reverse grouping cells carry all of the normal RBC antigens. Therefore, they can react at room temperature with anti-M, anti-N, anti-P_1, etc. O cells may also react if they carry the antigen corresponding to the antibody in the patient's serum. Thus, a patient with anti-M in his serum could react with both reverse grouping cells and the O cells if all were positive for the M antigen. A patient with cold hemagglutinin disease (CHD) may have a discrepancy affecting both cell and serum groupings. The RBCs should be washed with warm saline before typing; the serum and reagent A and B cells should be prewarmed before mixing and testing and converted to the antiglobulin test if necessary.

119–123.

(119:C, 120:A, 121:A, 122:D, 123:B) The Kell system has a number of antigens, among which is Kp^a (Penney). This antigen has not been reported in African Americans. The corresponding antibody is very rare because so few individuals have the antigen that stimulates its production. When it is present, it is not a serious problem because Kp(a−) blood is easily found. The McLeod phenotype is one in which all the Kell-associated antigens are expressed only weakly. McLeod cells are missing a precursor substance called Kx. Kx is coded for by a gene present on the X chromosome. Some of the male children afflicted with chronic granulomatous disease are of the McLeod phenotype, but exactly how the two are associated is not clear. The locus *Ss* is closely linked with the locus *MN*, and they are considered part of the same blood group system. M^g (Gilfeather) is a rare allele in the MN system. When the antigen M^g is present, it can cause typing difficulties because it will not react with either anti-M or anti-N. Because the antigens MN are well developed at birth, they were often used in paternity testing. The presence of an M^gM or M^gN combination can look like a homozygous *M* or *N*, leading to a second-order (indirect) exclusion unless the RBCs are tested with anti-M^g. The presence of the antigen M^g antigen on the RBCs of the alleged father and child practically proves paternity. Currently, most paternity testing is done by DNA analysis, not by RBC antigen testing.

Antibody Identification, Transfusion Therapy, Transfusion Reactions

124.

A. The ethnicity of this donor is probably African American. This origin can be determined by looking at the Duffy (Fy) phenotype. About 70% of African Americans are Fy(a−b−). This phenotype is extremely rare in Caucasian American.

125.

D. Donor 5 is homozygous for the following genes: *Ce, s, k,* Jk^a, Fy^a, because the corresponding antigen is produced, and the antithetical antigen is not being produced by an allele (e.g., C+c− implies homozygosity: *CC*). The donor cannot be homozygous for *M,* because its allele is producing N antigen. There is no way to tell whether P_1 is homozygous, because it lacks a codominant allele, and P_1 does not show dosage. There is no Le^b gene. The antigen is produced by the action of the *Le* gene on type 1 H. The Lewis genes are *Le* and the amorph *le,* and dosage is not observed.

126.

A. Anti-Fy^a can be identified by eliminating specificities where the corresponding antigens appear on the panel cells that do not react. The differences in the strength of reactivity can be explained by the fact that the Duffy antigens show dosage effect (react stronger with cells from homozygotes). Cells #1 and #6 are from Fy^a heterozygotes [Fy(a+b+)]. Cells #4 and #5 are from Fy^a homozygotes [Fy(a+b−)]. When eliminating an antibody specificity known to show dosage effect, it is best to have a negative reaction with a panel cell from a donor who is homozygous for the corresponding gene. Fy^a and Fy^b antigens are destroyed by enzymes. Although the Fy(a−b−) type is common in African Americans, the frequency of Fy^a in Caucasian Americans is about 66%. Anti-E and anti-s should be ruled out with Fy(a−) cells from individuals who are homozygous for *E* and *s* (in other words, E+e− and S−s+).

127.

C. Serum must be present to cause rouleaux formation; it should not occur in the AHG phase of testing when the rouleaux-producing properties have been removed by washing. Warm and cold autoantibodies result in a positive autocontrol, usually equal in strength to reactivity observed with reagent red cells. Antibodies directed against preservatives in potentiating media should also react in the autocontrol. When the autocontrol is nonreactive and all panel cells are uniformly positive, one should suspect the presence of an alloantibody directed against a "public," or high-frequency, antigen. A selected panel of RBCs, each lacking a different high-frequency antigen, should be tested until a compatible cell is found. The patient's RBCs may be typed for a variety of high-frequency antigens. If such an antigen is found to be missing on the RBCs, the corresponding serum antibody is likely that specificity.

128.

B. Cell #7 is negative for the high-frequency antigen k (Cellano). Many other specificities cannot be ruled out because there is only one negative reaction. Treating the panel cells with DTT destroys Kell system antigens. If no reactions are seen when the panel is repeated with DTT-treated cells, then many other clinically significant antibodies can be ruled out, and the presence of anti-k would be supported. If the patient has not recently been transfused, his cells should be typed with anti-k and would be expected to be k-negative. Proteolytic enzymes neither destroy Kell system antigens nor enhance their reactions with Kell system antibodies. Treating serum with DTT will destroy IgM antibodies by cleaving disulfide bonds of the pentamer and would not be helpful because anti-k is generally IgG.

129.

C. From the presence of positive reactions taking place at two different temperatures, it appears that there are two different antibodies reacting. There is a cold antibody reacting with cells #3 and #8 at immediate spin (IS) and a warm antibody reacting with cells #1, #2, #3, and #4. It is unlikely that the cold antibody is carrying over to a warmer phase, because there is no 37°C reaction with cell #8.

130.

C. Anti-Le^a, -Le^b, and -P_1 are antibodies that react at IS (room temperature or below). Of these, P_1 and Le^b antigens are present on cell #7, which shows negative reactivity. This makes these specificities unlikely to be present in the patient's serum. Le^a antigen is present on cells #3 and #8, both of which show a positive IS reaction. Anti-D is usually IgG and reacts best at 37°C and AHG phases of testing.

131.

B. All the antibodies listed react at warm temperatures. The K antigen is present only on cells #1 and #7 and is absent from cells #2, #3, and #4 that reacted at 37°C and AHG phases of testing. Also, Anti-K and anti-k do not usually react without the addition of AHG. Anti-C and anti-D may react at 37°C without AHG, but usually only if albumin or enzymes are used as potentiators. Anti-C and anti-D are often found together. In this instance, however, there would be a positive reaction with cell #5 if anti-C were present as well as anti-D.

132.

D. A patient's RBCs should be negative for the antigen corresponding to the antibody identified as long as the autocontrol is also negative. In this case, one already knows that the patient is group A, D-negative. A standard approach has been to require three antigen-positive cells that react and three antigen-negative cells that do not react for each antibody identified to establish probability that the antibody(ies) has (have) been correctly identified. There are only two Le(a+) donor cells on this panel. The anti-Le^a reacts only at IS and the anti-D does not. Presumably, the screening cells have an additional Le(a+) cell. Because this antibody appears to be clinically insignificant, many would simply ignore it by eliminating the IS. At any rate, it would certainly not be necessary to run another panel.

133.

B. The patient's positive antibody screening test is consistent with an anti-K, and this is what was identified in the antibody identification. Three K antigen-positive and three K antigen-negative cells were tested and reacted appropriately. The antibody identification could have been misinterpreted, but it seems unlikely. The panel must have been read at the AHG phase of testing, because most examples of anti-K do not react at any other phase of testing. Positive and negative control cells (K+k+ and K−k+) should be tested with the anti-K at the same time as the patient's cells to be certain of the specificity of the anti-K antiserum. There is no indication that this has been done, and the patient's phenotype should not be K+. If the patient had circulating K+ donor cells, the K typing would have shown a mixed-field reaction, which has not been indicated.

134.

B. Although there are many potential sources for error in performing an indirect antiglobulin test, the most common error leading to a false negative reaction is the failure to wash the RBCs adequately before the addition of AHG reagent. Traces of free human globulin can neutralize the AHG reagent. Red cells known to be coated with IgG antibody (Coombs' control cells, check cells) are added to all negative tests. Agglutination of these control cells confirms that AHG was present in the system and that proper washing procedures were performed.

135.

C. Elution is a process in which bound antibody is released from RBCs. The eluate produced can then be further tested to identify the specificity of the antibody. Some elution methods use temperature, chemicals, or manipulation of the pH to dissociate antibodies from red cells.

136.

C. If the antiglobulin test was performed properly and the antiglobulin reagent is working properly, the IgG-coated control RBCs should be agglutinated; thus, this test is invalid. Unagglutinated cells after the addition of the control cells might mean that the cells were not washed well and that the antiglobulin reagent has been neutralized or that the antiglobulin reagent may have been omitted. The test must be repeated if this happens.

137.

B. The crossmatch is performed by testing the serum of the recipient with a suspension of the donor's RBCs. The serum and RBCs are usually tested at the IS phase to detect ABO mismatches, if the patient has no history of having unexpected antibodies in his/her serum and the current antibody screen is negative. Additional testing is done at 37°C and antiglobulin phases to detect the presence of clinically significant antibodies, if the patient has a positive antibody screen or a history of ever having an unexpected antibody in his/her serum. Because clinically significant antibodies (other than anti-A and anti-B) are almost always detected during the antibody screening test, AABB Standards sanctions performing only the IS crossmatch (for ABO compatibility) when the patient has a negative antibody screening test. An antiglobulin crossmatch *must be performed* when a patient has a positive antibody screening test because of a clinically significant antibody, or if the patient has a history of a clinically significant antibody. Compatible units must also be phenotyped for the corresponding antigen and shown to be negative. When an antiglobulin crossmatch is performed, potentiating media such as albumin, polyethylene glycol, or LISS may be added to the test system to enhance sensitivity and/or decrease incubation time.

138.

B. A group AB individual can receive RBCs from donors of all ABO groups. Because the patient does not have anti-D, it would be best to next select group A, D-positive units because the need for large amounts of blood is anticipated. These units should be given as RBCs, because the plasma has anti-B. If necessary, the patient may be later switched to group O, D-positive RBCs. It would not be wise to deplete the D negative supply, because D-negative women of child-bearing age may need blood and should not be exposed to the D antigen. The decision to transfuse D-positive blood to a D-negative patient must be approved by the physician in charge of the transfusion service.

139.

D. The crossmatch, which is the recipient's serum with the donor's cells, will reveal only if the patient has a detectable antibody against some antigen on the donor cells. In the presence of a negative antibody screening test, an incompatible crossmatch at the IS phase will most likely be due to an ABO mismatch between the recipient's serum and the donor's cells. For this reason, AABB Standards mandate performing only the IS crossmatch when the patient has a negative antibody screening test and no history of clinically significant antibodies. The crossmatch will not guarantee *in vivo* response to the transfused RBCs. Also, it will not detect all ABO typing errors, and it will not detect most Rh typing errors.

140.

C. A false positive crossmatch could occur if the donor has a positive DAT. A DAT should be done on the donor cells and, if positive, the unit should be removed from inventory. Another possible cause of a false positive crossmatch could be contaminants in dirty glassware causing clumping of RBCs. The other responses are true positives. If a strong incompatibility is immediately present, one should check the ABO type of the patient and the donor. If the antibody screening test was negative, one might suspect an antibody against a low-incidence antigen on the donor's cells.

141.

C. The crossmatch consists of testing donor cells with recipient serum. A group A individual will have anti-B in his/her serum, which will agglutinate AB cells. D-positive cells given to a D-negative person may cause antibody stimulation, but there will not be a visible reaction without a preformed antibody.

142.

A. The most critical step to ensuring safe transfusion is obtaining a properly labeled blood sample from the correct patient. Transfusion accidents due to ABO mismatches are usually the result of a patient receiving the wrong blood. The identity of the patient must be verified, both verbally and by comparison of the wristband with the transfusion request form. Blood tubes must be labeled properly at the bedside with the full name, another acceptable identifier such as the medical record number, and the date.

143.

B. Sufficient information for unique identification of the patient (including two independent identifiers) and the date of sample collection must be on the label. The phlebotomist's signature or initials must appear on either the tube of blood or on the request slips. It is not necessary for both to be signed. The physician's name, the patient's room number, and the time of the phlebotomy may be helpful but are not required by AABB Standards.

144.

A. According to AABB Standards, specimens used for antibody screening and crossmatching must be less than 3 days old if the patient has been transfused or pregnant within the past 3 months. Either serum or plasma may be used. The specimen must be labeled properly at the bedside at the time of collection. Specimens are required to be retained for only 7 days posttransfusion.

145.

B. In general, one unit of RBCs should raise a patient's hemoglobin by 1 g/dL and hematocrit by 3%. In this instance, a 9% rise is required, so three units would need to be given. This rule is true for patients of average size. A very large or heavy individual with an expanded blood volume may require additional units to attain the same level. Conversely, a pediatric patient may require fewer.

146.

B. The percentage of compatible blood is obtained by multiplying the frequencies of antigen negative. In this instance, one wants to find Jk(a−), K− blood. The incidence of Jk(a+) blood is 77%; therefore, the incidence of Jk(a−) blood is 23%. Likewise, K+ incidence is 10%; K− would be 90%. Multiply these two frequencies together to get the frequency for Jk(a−), K− units: $0.23 \times 0.90 = 0.21$, or an incidence of 21 units in 100. Divide 2 by this figure because 2 units are needed: $2 \div 0.21 = 9.5$, or 10 units must be screened to find 2 compatible units.

147.

C. Cryoprecipitate provides a source of fibrinogen and fibronectin in addition to factors VIII and XIII. This component is indicated for use in bleeding disorders associated with hypofibrinogenemia, such as DIC, when excessive fibrinogen consumption is occurring. Each unit contains an average of 250 mg of fibrinogen or 0.25 g. The AABB Standards require a minimum of 150 mg per individual collection. The amount of pooled product to administer is calculated by the formula:

$$\frac{\text{Total grams desired}}{0.25\,\text{g/unit}} = \text{Total number of cryoprecipitate units to administer}$$

For example,

$$\frac{2\,\text{g}}{0.25\,\text{g/unit}} = 8\,\text{units}$$

148.

D. Plasma compatible with the recipient's ABO group is preferred when large volumes are transfused. Both group O and group B plasma contain anti-A that can cause a positive direct antiglobulin test (DAT) when infused into either group A or AB recipients. Compatibility testing is not required before cryoprecipitate administration. Plasma compatibility is not as important with cryoprecipitate as with platelet concentrates. Approximately 10 mL of plasma is in a cryoprecipitate unit and 50 mL in a single platelet concentrate.

149.

D. Approximately 1% of transfused red cells are cleared daily from the circulation of a recipient. The clearance rate may be increased in patients with autoimmune hemolytic anemia, pernicious anemia, aplastic anemia, hemorrhage, splenomegaly, and fever. Transfused cells survive normally in patients with anemia because of intrinsic RBC enzyme defects, spherocytosis, and paroxysmal nocturnal hemoglobinuria.

150.

B. Febrile reactions are brought about by the interaction of antibodies in the recipient directed against antigens on donor leukocytes or by cytokines secreted by leukocytes. The antigens involved are both the HLA and granulocyte-specific antigens. Leukocyte-reduced RBCs are the component of choice for a patient with repeated febrile transfusion reactions. Although frozen RBCs that have been thawed and deglycerolized are considered leukocyte reduced, the cost and time involved in preparation make them an unpractical choice.

151.

D. RBCs are the component of choice to maintain or restore oxygen-carrying capacity. This component has the least effect on blood volume and the maximum effect on the oxygen-carrying capacity of all the products available for transfusion. In some patients, increasing the total blood volume more than what is absolutely necessary could have a detrimental effect. Examples are patients with chronic anemia or congestive heart failure.

152.

C. Children inherit half their genetic characteristics from each parent. Because the parents' antigen composition is not identical (a situation only found in identical twins), the child cannot be totally compatible with either parent. Siblings, however, have access to the same genetic material from each parent and so may have identical genes and antigens. A spouse genetically would be equivalent to a random donor.

153.

D. Because time is of the essence when a trauma victim is severely hemorrhaging, transfusion services personnel must respond promptly. Group-specific blood may not be issued on the basis of previous patient or donor records. If the situation is so urgent as to preclude performing an ABO and Rh typing, or when a blood sample cannot be obtained, group O RBCs may be issued. The decision as to whether group O, D-positive or O, D-negative RBCs should be used will depend upon inventory and the age and sex of the trauma victim. Transfusion services located in a trauma center should have a written procedures manual with well-defined criteria. All staff must be familiar with these guidelines.

154.

B. The first step in any pretransfusion workup is to check the blood bank records for previous information on the patient. This information must match the ABO group and Rh type on the sample obtained currently. This helps to ensure that patients are not given the wrong blood type. A mismatch may indicate that the wrong patient was drawn or the label was incorrectly applied. After the initial release of six units of uncrossmatched group O blood, there should be ample time to at least check records and obtain an ABO group and Rh type on the patient sample before more blood is required.

155.

D. Large volumes of transfused plasma should be ABO compatible with the recipient's RBCs. Isoagglutinins present in the plasma will attach to the corresponding antigen on the patient's red cells *in vivo* and cause a positive DAT and perhaps hemolysis. Plasma of any blood group can be given to a group O patient, because his/her RBCs will not be agglutinated by anti-A or anti-B in donor plasma.

156.

B. Physiologic saline is the only generally acceptable solution that is allowed to be added to blood or blood components. Ringer's solution causes small clots to develop in anticoagulated blood, and 5% dextrose causes hemolysis. Other solutions and medication should not be added to blood unless they have been proven safe and are sanctioned by the FDA.

157.

C. The majority of deaths due to hemolytic transfusion reactions are caused by clerical errors, not laboratory errors. Patients, blood samples, and laboratory records, if misidentified, can lead to the wrong ABO type blood being administered to the patient. These deaths most often occur in areas of high stress, such as in emergency departments and surgical suites.

158.

C. A delayed hemolytic transfusion reaction is generally the result of a patient's second exposure to an antigen present on donor RBCs. The patient at some time previously had been exposed to the antigen, and this is his/her anamnestic response. This reaction usually occurs from 3 to 14 days after transfusion and is accompanied by extravascular RBC destruction. Often the patient is asymptomatic. The DAT is usually positive in a delayed hemolytic reaction, because the reaction is extravascular and coated cells are present in the peripheral circulation. An acute hemolytic transfusion reaction is usually intravascular, and the coated cells are destroyed by complement, leaving the DAT negative or at most weakly positive. Anaphylactic and febrile reactions do not involve RBC antibodies and do not cause a positive DAT.

159.

C. Kidd antibodies are generally IgG, complement dependent, and warm reacting. However, they are usually weak and labile. Because of this, they may go undetected in pretransfusion testing and the patient may inadvertently be transfused with antigen-positive blood, leading to a delayed transfusion reaction.

160.

D. Anaphylactic reactions are IgE mediated, although similar in presentation anaphylactoid reactions may not be IgE mediated. IgA-mediated reactions can occur in IgA deficient patients. Anaphylactic reactions most commonly occur due to previous exposure to stimulating agents such as medications specifically antimicrobial therapy.

161.

A. Viral inactivation methods such as the use of a solvent/detergent combination have eliminated the risk of transmission of viruses with a lipid envelope in clotting factor concentrates. This method has been applied to group-specific frozen plasma. Pooled plasma, solvent/detergent-treated is much safer than the other components listed from the standpoint of HIV, HBV, and HCV, because the process destroys lipid-enveloped viruses. It does not destroy non-lipid-enveloped viruses such as parvovirus B19. However, it has been withdrawn from the market in the United States and is not currently being used. Another approach to safety is "FFP-Donor Retested," which means that the FFP (fresh-frozen plasma) has been held for 90 days or more and released only after the donor has been retested negative for infectious disease markers. It is not a pooled product. The retesting should show that the donor was not in an infectious window period when the plasma was drawn.

162.

C. The transfusion of the unit should be stopped, and the transfusionist should keep the patient's IV line open with physiologic saline in case medications must be given quickly to counteract the transfusion reaction. The unit must then be returned to transfusion services along with all of the transfusion set and any attached IVs, such as any physiologic saline that was being infused along with the unit. The patient's physician should be notified, but after the transfusion is discontinued and the new IV of physiologic saline has been hung. Monitoring pulse and blood pressure is a good idea but is not an immediate necessity.

163.

D. Returning the unit to the blood bank and obtaining posttransfusion blood and urine samples is required by AABB Standards. No more blood or blood products should be transfused into the patient until the reaction has been investigated. If the patient has an antibody that caused the transfusion reaction, any RBC units transfused must be negative for the corresponding antigen.

164.

B. Red-tinged plasma is indicative of hemolysis. When this is seen in the posttransfusion sample but not in the pretransfusion sample, it is evidence that an intravascular hemolytic transfusion reaction has occurred. The antibody attached to antigen on the patient's RBCs, and the resulting antigen–antibody complex activated the complement cascade. This resulted in hemolysis of the coated RBCs in the patient's vascular system. Other likely laboratory findings in this situation include hemoglobinuria and decreased plasma haptoglobin. Although intravascular hemolysis can be seen in situations where a drug has been administered with the blood, there are several possible causes of an intravascular hemolytic transfusion reaction. In the scenario given, there is no evidence that would suggest any particular cause.

165.

D. In vasovagal reactions, both heart rate and blood pressure decrease. Hypovolemia shows a decreased blood pressure but an elevated heart rate. The heart rate increases in hypovolemia as a compensatory response to the decreased blood pressure.

166.

A. Premedication may be desirable but it may mask potential reactions and is not required or consistently recommended. Close monitoring of vitals is critical during the entire infusion to ensure any changes are noted immediately and the transfusion is halted to reduce severe effects of transfusion. Immediate transfusion reactions can result in anaphylaxis, which can be life threatening.

167.

C. The crossmatch is performed using the recipient's serum and the donor's RBCs. Therefore, a positive DAT on the recipient's cells will not affect the crossmatch results. A positive reaction may be obtained when the recipient has an antibody directed against a corresponding antigen on the donor's RBCs. If this is a low-frequency antigen, the crossmatch may be incompatible and the antibody screening result negative. A positive reaction may also indicate that the donor's RBCs are coated with human globulin. This can be confirmed by performing a DAT on the donor's red cells. Units of blood demonstrating a positive DAT should be returned to the collecting facility.

168.

D. Monoclonal anti-D reagents are low-protein reagents, therefore, a negative reaction with anti-A and/or anti-B (also low-protein) serves as a control. When the patient appears to be group AB, D-positive, it is necessary to set up a separate control. A drop of the patient's cell suspension with his/her own serum (autocontrol) or with 6–8% albumin makes a suitable control.

169.

D. Both the ABO grouping and Rh typing are in question. Because the transfusion need is urgent, group O, D-negative donor units should be selected initially for this young woman of childbearing age. They should be transfused, if necessary, before the problem has been resolved or crossmatching performed. In some cases, the risk of withholding transfusion is far greater than the risk of a transfusion reaction in a patient with an unresolved antibody problem. The physician must sign an emergency release form indicating that the clinical situation was such to warrant the release of blood.

170.

B. The patient most likely has a potent cold autoagglutinin. The antibody screening test and crossmatches with group O, D-negative donor units should be set up as soon as possible by prewarmed technique. In the past, when Rh typing was primarily done with high-protein reagents, an Rh control, containing all the potentiating ingredients found in the Rh reagent except for the anti-D, were tested in parallel. The most likely cause of a positive Rh control with a high-protein reagent is a strongly positive DAT result. This would not be the cause in this case because monoclonal anti-D is a low-protein reagent. The usual cause of false positive reactions with low-protein reagents is a potent cold autoagglutinin. A single wash may not remove all the antibody from the patient's RBCs. The cells should be washed with warm saline; and if they are still autoagglutinated, antibody can be removed by 45°C heat elution or treatment with a sulfhydryl reagent such as DTT, which destroys IgM antibodies. Because washed RBCs were used when performing the patients blood typing, multiple myeloma could not be the cause of the false positive, because the abnormal protein causing the pseudo-agglutination (rouleaux) would have been washed away.

171.

C. Although rigors and shock may be caused by hemolytic or anaphylactic reactions, bacterial sepsis is the most likely cause in this case. The sudden rise of the patient's temperature from normal to 40°C or above is typical of such an infection. Bacterial sepsis is an important cause of transfusion reactions, with about one-fourth of these reactions resulting in death.

172.

D. The incidence of bacterial sepsis is highest with platelet components. It is higher with pooled platelets than platelets collected by apheresis. Pooled platelets usually involve six or more donations from different donors, multiplying the chance of contamination. Most bacteria grow better at room temperature (the normal storage temperature for platelets) than refrigerator temperature. Sepsis from RBCs is usually due to *Yersinai enterocolitica,* which grows well at refrigerator temperature.

173.

B. The reactions are most likely all caused by the cold autoagglutinin anti-I. The I antigen is not present on *ii* cells. Autoadsorption of the patient's serum with his/her own cells should not be performed following recent transfusion. Alloantibody may be adsorbed onto circulating donor RBCs, resulting in false negative reactions with repeat testing of the autoadsorbed serum and reagent red cells. The weak reactions in the AHG phase of testing are most likely due to complement being bound at room temperature by the cold autoantibody reacting with the anti-C3d in polyspecific AHG reagent. A prewarmed technique, in which the donor's cells and patient's serum are warmed separately to 37°C before combining, is commonly used to eliminate interference from cold agglutinins. Many transfusion services use an anti-IgG monospecific AHG reagent, instead of a polyspecific reagent that contains anti-IgG and anti-C3d, in order to avoid such problems, but the prewarmed crossmatch should eliminate complement from being bound. Because the patient was recently transfused, there is a slight possibility that the reactions with AHG could be caused by a high-incidence alloantibody causing delayed hemolysis. Such an antibody would still react by a prewarmed technique.

174–179.

(174:A, 175:A, 176:E, 177:D, 178:D, 179:C) The ABO group and Rh type must be determined by the blood-collecting facility with every donation. The unit must be labeled using the interpretation of current testing, not with previous donor records from repeat donors. When the IS reaction of the donor RBCs is positive with anti-D (with a negative Rh control), the unit may be labeled D-positive. If the RBCs fail to agglutinate anti-D directly, the test must be incubated and converted to the antiglobulin test to detect weak D phenotype. All units tested with anti-D that are IS negative but are found to be weak D-positive must be labeled D-positive to avoid sensitizing an intended D-negative recipient to the D antigen. A DAT should be performed as a control along with the weak D test. For the test to be valid, the DAT must be negative. If the donor is DAT-positive, the weak D status cannot be interpreted because the donor's RBCs are coated with antibody before the incubation with anti-D. DAT-positive units of blood should be discarded. Two different test methods, a cell grouping and a serum grouping, must be used for ABO grouping; the results of these methods must be in agreement before a label is applied to the unit. Although testing the RBCs with anti-A,B and testing the serum with A_2 red cells is not required, many collecting facilities incorporate these additional reagents to detect discrepancies due to subgroups of A or B. When the cell and serum groupings are not in agreement, additional testing to resolve the discrepancy is required. Weak or missing red-cell reactions with anti-A,B or anti-A, or both, accompanied by serum reactions with A_1 cells, but not A_2 cells, are an indication that the donor may be a subgroup of A with anti-A_1. Extended incubation of the cell grouping, testing with additional A_1 cells, A_2 cells, and anti-A_1 lectin, and adsorption/elution/titration/secretor studies are techniques used to resolve discrepancies due to subgroups. Donor units found to contain unexpected antibodies should be processed into RBCs with small amounts of plasma. They should be labeled to indicate the antibody specificity. It is helpful to attach a tie tag with this information to the unit. Transfusing large amounts of antibody containing plasma (such as anti-Fy^a) into a Fy(a+) recipient may cause decreased RBC survival and, therefore, is not used for individual transfusion to patients. Plasma from units with antibodies may be salvaged for reagent use or source plasma.

180–184.

(180:C, 181:C, 182:D, 183:D, 184:A) There are three parts to the factor VIII molecule: F VIII:C, F VIII:Ag, and F VIII:vW. Individuals manifesting the X-linked (gene carried on the X chromosome) disorder known as hemophilia A are deficient in F VIII:C. The clinical severity, resulting in hemorrhage either spontaneously or following trauma, depends on the level of F VIII:C present. Deficiency in F VIII:vW is known as von Willebrand disease. It is not X-linked and is the most common inherited coagulopathy. Deficiency in F VIII:vW results in impaired platelet adhesion and aggregation, leading to prolonged bleeding. Cryoprecipitate contains both F VIII:C and F VIII:vW and may be used for treatment of these disorders, although it is not the preferred treatment. F VIII concentrates have become safer with improved viral inactivation processes, and some now have therapeutic amounts of F VIII:vW as well. Cryoprecipitate also contains an average of 250 mg of fibrinogen per unit, as well as factor XIII and fibronectin, and currently it is primarily used to treat hypofibrinogenemia. Although factor V deficiency is rare, it can present severe manifestations leading to hemarthrosis. Treatment of choice is FFP because F V is a labile factor not found in cryoprecipitate. FFP can be used to correct the factor deficiencies found in liver disease (factors II, VII, IX, and X). Because all these are stable factors, the plasma need not be fresh even though FFP is commonly used. Platelet concentrates are used to correct thrombocytopenia following chemotherapy. Fresh whole blood is seldom available. Specific components are instead provided to give the patient exactly what is needed and conserve blood resources.

Hemolytic Disease (Hemolytic Disease of the Newborn, Immune Hemolytic Anemia)

185.

C. ABO testing, Rh testing (for weak D when applicable), and antibody screening should all be performed early in a pregnancy. Amniocentesis should be done only when clinically indicated. Furthermore, amniocentesis generally is not done before the third trimester, although in recent years the procedure has been done as early as 14 weeks.

186.

C. The Lewis typings of a pregnant woman may appear to be Le(a−b−), even though the original typing may have been Le(a−b+). When women are pregnant, they have an increased plasma volume and increased amount of lipoprotein in relation to RBC mass. Because Lewis antigens are adsorbed onto RBCs and lipoprotein from plasma, the dilutional effect and greater lipoprotein mass would lead to less adsorption of Le^b onto RBCs. After the pregnancy, the woman will return to her original type.

187.

A. Prenatal testing for all pregnant women should include ABO, Rh, and antibody screening to exclude the presence of unexpected antibodies with the potential for causing HDN. The presence of an unexpected antibody does not indicate that the infant will be affected. Testing the RBCs of the father, to determine whether the corresponding antigen is expressed and, if so, whether he is a homozygote or heterozygote, should indicate the probability for the presence of the antigen on infant cells. ABO-HDN is not predictable until postpartum, when the blood type of the infant is determined.

188.

D. IgG is the only immunoglobulin that is transported across the placenta. It does not cross the placenta because of low molecular weight or simple diffusion, as evidenced by higher concentrations of antibody present in cord than in maternal serum. IgG molecules are actively transported via the Fc portion beginning in the second trimester. Therefore, potentially any IgG blood group antibody produced by the mother could cause HDN, if the fetus possesses a well-developed corresponding antigen. The disease varies widely in severity, being dependent on multiple factors.

189.

A. Although the ABO system is most often implicated in fetomaternal incompatibilities, it very rarely causes clinical symptoms. ABO-HDN generally occurs when group O mothers have group A or B children. Although Rh-HDN can be prevented, there is no prevention for ABO-HDN, and generally there is none needed because exchange transfusion is rarely necessary.

190.

C. When D+ RBCs are sufficiently coated with antibody, leaving no or few remaining sites to react with D antiserum, the cells are referred to as having a "blocked D" and may react weakly or not at all with a low-protein anti-D reagent. One may suspect this phenomenon, confirmed by elution of anti-D from the RBCs when the DAT is strongly positive. Enough antibody may be removed either with a gentle heat elution (45°C) or using chloroquine diphosphate to permit accurate D typing of the coated RBCs.

191.

C. Given that all prenatal and neonatal testing is valid, one should consider an antibody against a low-incidence antigen. The low-incidence antigen was of paternal origin, and it stimulated the mother to form an IgG antibody. To prove this theory, an eluate from the baby's cells should be tested with the father's cells. Also, the mother's serum and the baby's eluate could be tested with a panel of cells positive for various low-incidence antigens to identify the specificity of the antibody.

192.

D. An antibody panel performed on an eluate made from the baby's RBCs is the most conclusive way to identify positively the antibody causing the positive DAT. This would be especially helpful in a case where the mother has several antibodies that could cause HDN. However, RBCs for transfusion in the neonatal period should be negative for any antigen corresponding to any IgG antibody that crossed the placenta.

193.

B. During the first few hours of life, the primary risk to a baby with HDN is heart failure caused by severe anemia. After the first 24 hours, in which the anemia can be compensated, the highest risk to the infant comes from hyperbilirubinemia. Kernicterus, which is brought on by hyperbilirubinemia (generally >18 mg/dL of unconjugated bilirubin) in a full-term infant in the first days of life, can cause irreversible brain damage. Depending on the severity of the hyperbilirubinemia, one or more exchange transfusions may be needed.

194.

D. A positive DAT on the infant's RBCs indicates that IgG antibody has crossed the placenta and coated the neonate's RBCs. Identification of the antibody in the maternal serum and elution of the same antibody from the infant's RBCs confirms the specificity of the offending antibody. In lieu of a maternal blood sample, the identity of the antibody may be confirmed by testing the infant's eluate and serum. The eluate contains the antibody(ies) responsible for the clinical HDN; the serum may contain additional maternal antibody(ies) directed against antigens absent on the infant's cells but present on the donor's cells. Blood compatible with both serum and eluate should be prepared for exchange transfusion.

195.

D. Providing blood of the baby's type is exactly what one does not want to do. This would defeat the purpose of the exchange transfusion. For example, if a D+ infant was suffering from HDN because of an anti-D, the transfusion of D-positive cells would allow transfused cells to be coated with anti-D. The transfused cells would then be removed from the circulation by the reticuloendothelial system and would have decreased survival.

196.

D. A mixed-field weak D test on maternal blood indicates the presence of D-positive baby cells circulating with the mother's D-negative cells, suggestive of a large fetomaternal hemorrhage. If a mother does demonstrate a positive weak D test when previously it was negative, a Kleihauer-Betke acid elution test should be done on the mother's RBCs. This test is used to quantify the amount of the fetal blood that has entered the mother's circulation. The results of the test will determine how many vials of Rh immune globulin should be administered to the patient. One vial will protect against approximately 30 mL of fetal blood (or 15 mL of red cells) that have entered the mother's circulation. A more sensitive method to identify fetomaternal hemorrhage than the test for weak D is the rosette test. A maternal RBC suspension is incubated with human anti-D, allowing antibody to coat D+ fetal cells. D+ indicator cells are added that bind to the coated D+ cells, forming rosettes. This is a qualitative test and must also be followed by a quantitative test, such as the Kleihauer-Betke acid elution test.

197.

C. The most likely cause for the positive antibody screening test is the presence of a passively acquired anti-D. Because the mother received antepartum Rh immune globulin (RhIG), anti-D from that injection may still be present at childbirth. Because antepartum RhIG was given, it is unlikely that active immunization has occurred. Passively acquired anti-D rarely has an antiglobulin titer above 4 and should be entirely IgG. When in doubt about whether anti-D is passive or represents active immunization, it is always better to administer RhIG at the appropriate time. The crossmatches are compatible because D-negative RBCs would have been chosen for transfusion.

198.

D. The Kleihauer-Betke acid elution stain is used to quantify the amount of fetal cells present in the maternal circulation postpartum to calculate the correct dose of RhIG to administer. Adult hemoglobin is soluble in acid buffer, whereas fetal hemoglobin is resistant to acid elution. A thin blood smear is subjected to acid elution, pH 3.2, and then is stained with erythrosin B and Harris hematoxylin. Normal adult cells appear as pale ghosts microscopically; fetal cells are bright pink. The number of fetal cells in 2000 maternal cells is calculated. The volume of fetal hemorrhage is calculated as follows:

$$\frac{\text{Number of fetal cells}}{\text{Number of maternal cells}} \times \frac{\text{material blood volume}}{\text{(estimate 5000 mL)}} = \text{fetal bleed}$$

This is equivalent to: Fetal cells expressed as a percentage of maternal cells × 50 = mL of fetal whole blood. One vial of a standard 300-μg dose protects the D-negative mother against sensitization to the D antigen for a 30-mL bleed. Therefore, the fetal hemorrhage volume is divided by 30 to determine the number of vials.

199.

B. Neither anti-P_1 nor anti-Le^a is likely to cause HDN. They are almost exclusively IgM antibodies (cannot cross the placenta), and the corresponding antigens are not well developed on neonatal RBCs. Both anti-K and anti-c are almost exclusively IgG antibodies and are capable of causing serious HDN. However, the K antigen has a much lower frequency (<10%) in the population than the c antigen (>80%), so the infant is much more likely to be c+.

200.

D. The Kleihauer-Betke (KB) acid elution stain is used to estimate the amount of fetal RBCs present in the circulation of a D-negative mother postpartum. Failure to quantify the fetomaternal hemorrhage (FMH) may result in the administration of insufficient Rh immune globulin. Sensitization to the Rh antigen may occur, leading to HDN in subsequent pregnancies. The fetal bleed is calculated using the formula: KB% × 50 = milliliters fetal blood present or 2.1 × 50 = 105 mL.

201.

C. One standard dose of RhIG (300 μg) protects the mother from a 30-mL bleed. Because the precision of a Kleihauer-Betke stain is poor, a margin of safety is employed to prevent RhIG prophylaxis failure. The total bleed in milliliters is divided by the level of protection in one dose (30 mL). For decimals less than five, round down and add one dose (e.g., 3.4 rounds down to 3 + 1 = 4 vials total dose); for decimals five or greater, round up and add one dose (e.g., 3.6 rounds up to 4 + 1 = 5 vials total dose).

Example:

$$\frac{\text{65 mL bleed}}{\text{30 mL}} = 2.2\text{; give 3 vials RhIG}$$

202.

D. A positive autocontrol reacting at the antiglobulin phase of testing indicates that the patient has a positive DAT. All screening cells react at the same strength at the same phase of testing as the autocontrol. This indicates the presence of a warm (IgG) autoantibody, both on the patient's cells and in her serum. This patient's serum would be expected to react 4+ at AHG with all cells tested. Polyagglutinable cells will not react in the autocontrol, because the patient will lack the antibody corresponding to the antigen causing the polyagglutination. Rouleaux will not be present in the antiglobulin phase because all of the serum proteins are washed away before the AHG is added. A transfusion reaction may demonstrate a positive autocontrol and/or antibody screen; however, the reaction will be mixed field, because the patient's cells will not react with her alloantibody but the donor cells will react with the patient's antibody.

203.

A. The DAT is the easiest and the quickest way to detect *in vivo* sensitization of RBCs. The indirect antiglobulin test is used to detect *in vitro* sensitization of RBCs and is most commonly used in antibody detection tests and crossmatching. Uses of the DAT include investigation of HDN, autoimmune hemolytic anemia, transfusion reactions, and drug-induced sensitization of RBCs.

204.

B. The only method that can be used to identify an antibody coating RBCs is to perform an elution on those cells and then test the eluate against a panel. Autoabsorption of the patient's serum and then a panel on the autoabsorbed serum would be the method of choice for the identification of alloantibodies in her serum because she has not been recently transfused. Any panel on her serum would simply react with all panel cells tested because of the presence of the autoantibody.

205.

C. Most patients having warm autoimmune hemolytic anemia (WAIHA) respond well to steroids, which decrease the autoantibody production. Transfusing these individuals usually will cause the autoantibody to be produced in greater amounts. Transfusion in these cases is often counterproductive because the donor cells are destroyed as quickly as the patient's own cells and the expected increment in hemoglobin from the transfusion does not occur. Because this woman needs more oxygen-carrying capacity, transfusion with FFP will not help her. Plasma exchange may remove antibody from her circulation but will not provide any oxygen-carrying capacity.

206.

D. Most antibodies in WAIHA have specificity that appears to be directed toward the Rh blood group system antigens. Sometimes, the antibody has a simple specificity; anti-e is the most common warm autoantibody of simple specificity. Usually the antibody has a broad specificity, reacting with RBCs of most Rh phenotypes except for rare phenotypes such as Rh_{null}. In addition, there are mimicking or relative specificities—for example, an apparent auto anti-e that can be adsorbed onto e-negative RBCs.

207.

C. Although it is best to avoid transfusing patients with warm autoantibodies, life-threatening anemia may develop, which necessitates them to receive blood. The primary concern in patients demonstrating serum warm autoantibody is to detect and identify the presence of underlying alloantibodies that may be masked by the reactions of the autoantibody. One must be certain to differentiate between auto- and alloantibodies. If the autoantibody appears to have a simple specificity such as anti-e, alloantibody identification can be accomplished by testing reagent RBCs that are e-negative and antigen positive for the alloantibodies to be excluded. Alternatively, when sufficient e-negative panel cells are not available to do a thorough rule out, warm autoadsorption of the serum with the untransfused patient's RBCs will remove autoantibody but not alloantibody. Alloantibodies will cause the transfused RBCs carrying the corresponding antigen to be removed from the recipient's circulation even more rapidly than the patient's own RBCs and will not provide the oxygen-carrying capacity the patient requires.

208.

A. Autoantibodies are directed against antigens present on the patient's own RBCs. The easiest way to determine whether the anti-e is auto or allo when the patient has not been recently transfused is to type the patient's RBCs with a low-protein anti-e reagent. A high-protein reagent should not be used, since a false positive reaction is likely to occur. The preparation of an eluate when patients have no history of recent transfusion is not necessary; it is presumed that the eluate contains only autoantibody.

209.

C. When a patient has been recently transfused, a mixed-field positive DAT may indicate the presence of clinically significant alloantibody attached to circulating donor's RBCs. A positive DAT may also reflect autoantibody attached to patients or donor's RBCs, either because of drug sensitivity or secondary to clinical disease, which is less likely in this case. It is important to obtain information, including diagnosis, clinical condition, medication history, and laboratory data such as hematocrit, bilirubin, haptoglobin, and reticulocyte count, both pre- and posttransfusion to determine whether a delayed hemolytic transfusion reaction (DHTR) has occurred. A DHTR commonly demonstrates a mixed-field DAT result.

210.

D. Discard the unit. The incompatible unit may have RBCs coated with antibody or complement or both. If the RBCs are sensitized, then there is a problem with the donor unit and may cause a problem for the patient if the cells lyse.

211.

D. Abnormal, excess, or nonspecific protein autoantibody would cause positive reaction in screen cells, crossmatch, and autocontrol. Alloantibodies are not associated with a positive autocontrol. Specific allo or auto antibodies would not typically cause reaction in all phases or all test formats.

212.

C. Paroxysmal cold hemoglobinuria (PCH) is the rarest form of cold autoimmune hemolytic anemia. It is characterized by an IgG antibody that usually exhibits anti-P specificity. The anti-P attaches to the RBC during exposure to cold and then activates complement when the patient rewarms, causing hemolysis. A diagnostic test used to aid in the identification of PCH is the Donath-Landsteiner test. CHD is usually caused by anti-I, which is IgM.

213.

C. The Donath-Landsteiner test is a diagnostic test for PCH. A characteristic of the antibody involved is that it will bind to RBCs at cold temperatures; at 37°C it will cause hemolysis. In the Donath-Landsteiner test, a tube with the patient's serum and test cells is incubated at 4°C whereas a control tube is incubated at 37°C. After the 4°C incubation, the tube is placed in the 37°C incubator. After incubation, the tubes are centrifuged and examined for hemolysis. If hemolysis is noted in the test and none in the control, the test is positive. If no hemolysis is noted in either tube, the test is negative, and if hemolysis is present in both tubes, the test is invalid.

214.

C. Cephalosporin antibodies will generally *not* react with RBCs unless the RBCs have been treated with the drug. The negative antibody screening test indicates that crossmatches will be similarly compatible. An eluate from the patient's RBCs would be expected to be nonreactive with untreated RBCs as well. An eluate would not be prepared unless the patient had been recently transfused and a DHTR was suspected.

215.

C. Of the drugs listed, only penicillin has the observed DAT profile. IgG alone is also generally seen when α-methyldopa and cephalosporin are the implicated drugs. When phenacetin, quinidine, and Tolmetin are the drugs in question, only C3 (complement) is usually detected on the patient's RBCs. Antibody in the patient's serum and/or eluate will not react with reagent cells unless the RBCs are first treated with penicillin. This occurs because the antibody produced by the patient reacts with epitopes found on the penicillin coating the RBCs.

216.

D. Although the cold autoagglutinin is generally IgM, complement is usually the only protein detected on the RBCs. The IgM antibody binds complement at lower temperatures in the extremities (such as fingers exposed to cold temperatures) and then dissociates when the RBCs circulate. The polyspecific AHG is not required to have anti-IgM but must have anti-IgG and anti-C3d.

217.

D. Autoantibody(ies) directed against self-antigens may attach to a patient's own RBCs *in vivo*, resulting in a positive DAT. A variety of elution techniques can remove this antibody from the RBCs for testing. When a patient has not been transfused recently (within 3 to 4 months), it may be presumed that only autoantibody is present in the eluate. If recently transfused, donor's cells may be present in the patient's circulation. Alloantibody may be attached to donor cells, and autoantibody may be attached to patient's or donor's cells. When this is the case, alloantibody and autoantibody could be recovered in the eluate.

218.

B. A patient with a history of having had anti-Jk^a in her serum must always be given Jk(a−) blood. Anti-Jk^a in the plasma often drops to below detectable levels of antibody in the absence of stimulus. However, if Jk(a+) cells were to be given to the patient, the antibody would quickly rebound to high levels and cause a delayed hemolytic transfusion reaction. It is difficult to procure e− blood because ~80% of the population is e+. Add that to the need for Jk(a−) blood and the likelihood of finding suitable units drops further. It is much more important to avoid transfusing against the alloantibody, anti-Jk^a, than the autoantibody. The autoantibody will destroy transfused cells at the same rate it is destroying the patient's RBCs; however, the alloantibody will destroy the transfused cells more rapidly.

219–226.

(219:B, 220:D, 221:B, 222:B, 223:B, 224:B, 225:A, 226:C) Mothers who are not candidates to receive RhIG are (1) D-positive, (2) D-negative giving birth to a D-negative infant, or (3) D-negative who have produced alloanti-D. For purposes of determining RhIG candidacy, the weak D phenotype is considered to be D-positive. If the mother is D-negative and has not made anti-D, she must receive RhIG when giving birth to a D-positive or weak D phenotype infant. When only one of the infants in a multiple birth is D-positive and the other(s) is (are) D-negative, the mother is a candidate for RhIG. The presence of antibodies other than anti-D in the pre- or postpartum serum does not preclude a D-negative woman from receiving RhIG. When the infant's RBCs are DAT+, it may be difficult to determine the correct Rh status. Because RhIG is a low-risk product, experts recommend a fail-safe approach and give RhIG when in doubt. Most obstetricians routinely inject RhIG at 28 weeks antenatally to prevent sensitization during a third-trimester fetal bleed. This injected anti-D is sometimes detectable postpartum but does not preclude additional administration of RhIG at childbirth. Whenever doubt exists as to the weak D status of the infant or the origin of the anti-D, postpartum RhIG should be administered. The preferred method for determining FMH is the rosette test, which is more sensitive than a microscopic weak D test. The rosette test will detect FMH of >10 mL. A positive test would show one or more rosettes per field when an enhancing medium is used. Additional testing must be performed to quantify the amount of FMH to prevent sensitization to the D antigen. The Kleihauer-Betke acid elution stain is the standard technique available to determine whether a bleed of more than 15 mL red cells (30 mL whole blood) occurred, necessitating additional 300-μg doses beyond the standard one-vial dose. Other methods include the enzyme-linked antiglobulin test and flow cytometry. The 50-μg dose of RhIG is used only when a female of 12-weeks' gestation or less suffers a miscarriage. It is not intended for administration postpartum or for injection antenatally, either at 28 weeks or after amniocentesis.

REFERENCES

AABB. (2018). *Standards for Blood Banks and Transfusion Services*, 31st ed. Bethesda, MD: American Association of Blood Banks.

Roback, J. D. (Ed.) (2011). *Technical Manual*, 17th ed. Bethesda, MD: American Association of Blood Banks.

Harmening, D. M. (2019). *Modern Blood Banking and Transfusion Practices*, 7th ed. Philadelphia: F. A. Davis.

Klein, H., and Anstee, D. (2014). *Mollison's Blood Transfusion in Clinical Medicine*, 12th ed. Hoboken, NJ: Wiley.

CHAPTER

6 Bacteriology

contents

I. AEROBIC GRAM-POSITIVE BACTERIA

A. Staphylococci and Similar Microorganisms

1. *Staphylococcus aureus*

a. Approximately 30% of the population carries *S. aureus* as resident biota, primarily in the nares.
b. Isolated from abscesses, wound infections, and carbuncles
c. Causes food poisoning (via enterotoxin), pneumonia, osteomyelitis, endocarditis, wounds, staphylococcal scalded skin syndrome, etc. *S. aureus* can produce a biofilm and readily colonizes foreign body implants like artificial joints and pins.
d. Produces enterotoxins and **toxic shock syndrome toxin-1** (TSST-1)
e. **Identifying characteristics**
   1) Gram-positive cocci arranged in clusters
   2) Colonies are opaque and smooth. *S. aureus* grows well on most media and is usually beta-hemolytic on sheep blood agar (SBA).
   3) Catalase and coagulase positive
   4) Latex agglutination assay detects clumping factor and protein A on the surface of *S. aureus*. Newer tests also have antibodies that detect the most clinically relevant polysaccharide capsular antigens 5 and 8.
   5) Extracellular staphylococcal coagulase converts fibrinogen to fibrin and is detected in the tube coagulase test. *S. aureus* is typically positive within 4 hours.
   6) Negative for ability to metabolize the substrate pyrrolidonyl-α-naphthylamide **(PYR)** and ornithine
   7) Staphylococci can tolerate the high salt concentration (7.5%) of **mannitol salt agar** (MSA).
      a) *S. aureus* ferments mannitol and produces yellow colonies on MSA.
      b) Most coagulase-negative staphylococci do not ferment mannitol and therefore produce red colonies.
   8) Penicillin resistance is due to **beta-lactamase** production. Methicillin-resistant *S. aureus* **(MRSA)** is resistant to β-lactam antibiotics because of production of altered penicillin-binding proteins. Rare strains of vancomycin-intermediate *S. aureus* **(VISA)** and vancomycin-resistant *S. aureus* **(VRSA)** have been reported. Vancomycin resistance is due to the VanA operon that alters the target of vancomycin in the cell wall. VISA occurs following overproduction of the target peptidoglycan precursors.

2. **Coagulase-negative staphylococci**

a. Coagulase-negative staphylococci are very common skin biota and are mostly nonpathogenic. However, they can cause disease in patients who are immunocompromised or neutropenic. This group of bacteria causes urinary tract infections (UTIs) and, due to biofilm production, is associated with infections of catheters, implants, and shunts.
b. Gram-positive cocci arranged in clusters

c. Colonies appear white to gray on blood agar and nonhemolytic.
d. Catalase positive and coagulase negative
e. Commonly encountered species
1) ***Staphylococcus epidermidis***—Most common species of coagulase-negative staphylococci, novobiocin susceptible
2) ***S. saprophyticus***—Significant only in UTIs, novobiocin resistant
3) ***S. lugdunensis***—Frequent cause of endocarditis, ferments manitol, PYR positive, and typically clumps in plasma (slide coagulase) because of the presence of clumping factor. *S. lugdunensis* is tube coagulase test negative.

3. ***Micrococcus***
a. *Micrococcus* spp. are **considered normal biota** of the skin and mucous membranes; they rarely cause infections.
b. On Gram stain, arranged in tetrads and appear larger than *Staphylococcus* spp., see Table 6-1 ■.
c. Colonies often appear yellow and nonhemolytic on SBA.

B. *Streptococcaceae* and Similar Microorganisms

1. **General Characteristics**
a. Catalase-negative, gram-positive cocci arranged in pairs and chains
b. Can be alpha- or beta-hemolytic, or nonhemolytic on SBA
c. Lancefield grouping is based on a cell wall antigen.

2. **Group A *Streptococcus* (*Streptococcus pyogenes*)**
a. Infections are spread by respiratory secretions, and some children may carry the bacteria in the respiratory tract without illness. However, *S. pyogenes* is always considered pathogenic.
b. Infections include **strep throat** (pharyngitis), impetigo, cellulitis, scarlet fever, pneumonia, otitis media (middle ear infections), and **necrotizing fasciitis**.
c. Sequelae include **rheumatic fever** and **post-streptococcal glomerulonephritis**.
d. Susceptible to **bacitracin** (A disk) and PYR positive, but often identified by serologic latex agglutination test
e. Colonies are pinpoint (<1 mm), translucent, and will show a large zone of beta-hemolysis.

TABLE 6-1 COMPARISON BETWEEN MICROCOCCI AND STAPHYLOCOCCI

	Micrococci	Staphylococci
Acid production from glucose under anaerobic conditions (fermentation)	O	+
Modified oxidase test	+	O
Bacitracin (0.04 unit disk)	S	R
O = negative, + = positive, R = resistant, S = sensitive		

f. Virulence factors include
   1) Cell wall **M protein** inhibits phagocytosis, and antibodies to M protein are protective.
   2) **Streptococcal pyrogenic exotoxin** (Spe A, Spe B, Spe C, and Spe F), formerly referred to as **erythrogenic toxin**, causes the rash seen in scarlet fever. These toxins act as superantigens interacting with macrophages and T-helper cells to stimulate a massive release of cytokines and are associated with streptococcal toxic shock syndrome (STSS).
   3) **Streptokinase** dissolves clots.
   4) **Hyaluronic acid** capsule inhibits phagocytosis.
   5) **Streptolysin O** and **streptolysin S** lyse erythrocytes, platelets, and neutrophils.
   6) Hyaluronidase hydrolyzes hyaluronic acid, an interstitial barrier, facilitating spread of the infection. Strains that produce a hyaluronic acid capsule will not produce hyaluronidase.

3. ***Streptococcus dysgalactiae* subsp. *equisimilis***
   a. These isolates typically express **Lancefield group C or G antigens** and form large beta-hemolytic colonies.
   b. The clinical spectrum of disease resembles *S. pyogenes* and includes pharyngitis, skin infections, necrotizing fasciitis, STSS, endocarditis, glomerulonephritis, and acute rheumatic fever.
4. **Group B *Streptococcus* (*S. agalactiae*)**
   a. **Normal biota** of the gastrointestinal tract of humans and animals
   b. Important cause of infections in OB/GYN patients; 25% of all females carry the bacteria as normal vaginal biota
   c. With **early onset infections**, neonates acquire infections during birth, resulting in sepsis and meningitis. Additionally, *S. agalactiae* can cause postpartum fever, osteomyelitis, and wound infections, as well as endocarditis, pneumonia, and pyelonephritis in patients who are immunocompromised.
   d. Colonies are medium-size (>1 mm), flat, creamy, and show small zones of beta-hemolysis. Some strains may be nonhemolytic.
   e. **CAMP test and hippurate hydrolysis positive, PYR negative**
   f. Unlike *S. pyogenes, S. agalactiae* is **resistant to bacitracin**. However, isolates are often identified by serologic latex agglutination. Many other beta-hemolytic streptococci are also resistant to bacitracin.
5. **Group D *Streptococcus***
   a. **Normal fecal and oral biota**
   b. These bacteria are associated with wound infections, UTIs, and abdominal abscesses. Isolation of group D streptococci in blood cultures is an indicator of colon cancer.
   c. Colonies are gray to white, translucent, round, and convex.
   d. Alpha-hemolytic or nonhemolytic, rarely beta-hemolytic
   e. They are **bile-esculin positive, negative for growth in 6.5% NaCl, and PYR negative**. Bacteria resistant to bile that possess the enzyme esculinase will hydrolyze esculin into esculetin and glucose. Esculetin will react with the ferric citrate in the medium to produce a dark color.

6. **Viridans streptococci**
   a. **Normal biota** of the oral cavity, respiratory tract, and gastrointestinal (GI) tract mucosa
   b. Major cause of bacterial **endocarditis** in people with damaged heart valves; also causes wound infections and brain abscesses
   c. May enter the blood after dental procedures
   d. Viridans *Streptococcus* spp. include *S. mutans* group, *S. salivarius* group, *S. anginosus* group, *S. bovis* group, and *S. mitis* group.
   e. Alpha-hemolytic, some strains nonhemolytic
   f. Optochin resistant and insoluble in bile; do not grow on bile-esculin medium
7. ***Streptococcus pneumoniae***
   a. **Normal upper respiratory tract biota but can cause:**
      1) **Lobar pneumonia** in the elderly and patients who are alcoholics
      2) **Otitis media** in infants and children
      3) **Meningitis**; however, a pediatric vaccine is available that has reduced the number of childhood meningitis cases
   b. *S. pneumoniae* is an important cause of community-acquired bacterial pneumonia. Sputum samples are often rust colored from blood.
   c. Gram-positive diplococci (cocci in pairs) that are **lancet or bullet shaped**, and alpha-hemolytic
   d. Grows on SBA with 5–10% CO_2, at 48 hours
   e. **Colony morphology**
      1) **Mucoid** strains produce a large polysaccharide capsule.
      2) **Umbilicated**, depressed centers caused by autolytic enzymes
      3) After 48 hours, colonies become nonviable.
   f. **Optochin** (O or P disks) will inhibit growth (zone of inhibition), and *S. pneumoniae* is bile (10% sodium deoxycholate) soluble.
8. ***Enterococcus***
   a. Most commonly encountered species are *E. faecalis* and *E. faecium.*
   b. **Identifying characteristics**
      1) **Bile-esculin positive**
      2) **Positive for growth in 6.5% NaCl**
      3) PYR positive
      4) Express Lancefield group D antigen
      5) Can be alpha-, beta-, or most commonly nonhemolytic
   c. **Vancomycin-resistant enterococci (VRE):** Resistance is due to altered peptidoglycan cross-link target, D-Ala-D-Ala to D-Ala-D-Lac or D-Ala-D-Ser. The vast majority of VRE isolated from humans are *E. faecium.* *E. gallinarum*, a less commonly isolated species, exhibits intrinsic low-level vancomycin resistance.
9. ***Gemella***
   a. *Gemella* spp. have been associated with a number of infections, including endocarditis, meningitis, brain abscesses, lung abscesses, and osteomyelitis.
   b. PYR and leucine aminopeptidase (LAP) positive, and bile-esculin negative

10. ***Leuconostoc***
    a. *Leuconostoc* spp. have been linked to osteomyelitis, ventriculitis, postsurgical endophthalmitis, and bacteremia in neonates.
    b. The *Leuconostoc* spp. are vancomycin resistant, and PYR, LAP, and catalase negative.
11. ***Aerococcus***
    a. Species of *Aerococcus* have been isolated from human specimens for many years. They are generally considered contaminants but have been infrequently associated with bacteremia and endocarditis.
    b. *Aerococcus urinae* and *A. sanguinicola* have been linked to UTIs, septicemias, and endocarditis.
12. ***Abiotrophia*** **and** ***Granulicatella***
    a. Formerly referred to as **nutritionally variant streptococci**; require vitamin B_6 (pyridoxal or pyridoxamine) for growth.
    b. Species include *A. defectiva, G. adiacens*, and *G. elegans.*
    c. These species are normal biota of the oral cavity and have been associated with endocarditis, ophthalmic infections, and infections of the central nervous system (CNS).

C. Aerobic Non-Spore-Forming Gram-Positive Bacilli

1. ***Listeria monocytogenes***
    a. Causes spontaneous abortion and meningitis in animals (e.g., sheep)
    b. Found in the environment (soil and water), and is normal biota of the vagina and intestines in humans
    c. *L. monocytogenes* causes a variety of infections in neonates, pregnant women, and patients who are immunocompromised. **Meningitis** is a common outcome of infection.
    d. **Identifying characteristics**
        1) *L. monocytogenes* grows on most media; colonies are small and white with a narrow zone of beta-hemolysis.
        2) Colonies closely resemble group B streptococci on SBA
        3) *L. monocytogenes* demonstrates both umbrella motility in semisolid media at room temperature and end-over-end (tumbling) motility in a wet mount.
        4) Hippurate hydrolysis, CAMP test, esculin, and catalase positive
2. ***Corynebacterium***
    a. ***Corynebacterium diphtheriae*** causes diphtheria.
        1) Diphtheria is characterized by a pseudomembrane formed by dead cells and exudate at the back of the throat.
        2) Bacterial toxin damages major organs, resulting in a high death rate.
            a) **Toxigenic *C. diphtheriae* strains** are infected with a bacteriophage that contains the gene for the diphtheria toxin.
            b) Nontoxigenic *C. diphtheriae* strains lack the bacteriophage gene and do not produce the diphtheria toxin.

3) Found only in humans
4) **Identifying characteristics**
   a) Gram stain: Diphtheroid morphology arranged in "picket fences" and can be very pleomorphic
   b) Staining with methylene blue will reveal metachromatic granules, which are red to purple intracellular granules. This characteristic is not unique to *C. diphtheriae.*
   c) Urease and pyrazidamidase negative, nitrate and catalase positive, and nonmotile
   d) The **Elek** test uses antitoxin to detect toxin production.
   e) Media
      i. **Cystine-tellurite:** *Corynebacterium* spp. form black colonies from hydrolysis of tellurite.
      ii. **Tinsdale's agar:** *Corynebacterium* spp. form brown to black colonies with halos from hydrolysis of tellurite.
      iii. **Loeffler agar** is a nonselective medium that supports growth and enhances pleomorphism and the formation of metachromatic granules. Most *Corynebacterium* spp. produce small, white to gray colonies.
      iv. *C. diphtheriae* will grow on SBA as small, white, dry colonies. Most strains are nonhemolytic.

b. ***Corynebacterium jeikeium***
   1) *C. jeikeium* is an important cause of **nosocomial infections** and produces infections after prosthetic device implants and infections in patients who are immunocompromised.
   2) Pyrazidamidase positive
   3) Resistant to many antimicrobial agents

c. ***Corynebacterium urealyticum***
   1) Cause UTIs
   2) Is rapid urease positive and grows very slowly

3. ***Arcanobacterium***
   a. Six species of *Arcanobacterium* have been named; one is generally regarded as being clinically significant: *A. haemolyticum.*
   b. The natural habitat of these organisms has not been confirmed, although *A. haemolyticum* has been associated with pharyngitis and wound and tissue infections.
   c. *A. haemolyticum* forms small beta-hemolytic colonies on SBA and are catalase negative and nonmotile.
   d. *A. haemolyticum* can be identified by the CAMP inhibition test. This bacterium produces phospholipase D, which inhibits the activity of the *S. aureus* beta-lysin. *Corynebacterium pseudotuberculosis* also exhibits this phenomenon.

4. ***Erysipelothrix rhusiopathiae***
   a. *E. rhusiopathiae* primarily infects animals. Humans generally become infected through contact with infected animals (occupational exposure) or rarely by consuming infected meat.

b. Human infections often result in cellulitis (erysipeloid lesions that can resemble erysipelas caused by *S. pyogenes*) but may also present as bacteremia or endocarditis.
c. **Identifying characteristics**
   1) Nonmotile, pleomorphic gram-positive bacilli
   2) Catalase negative
   3) Hydrogen sulfide positive

5. ***Rhodococcus***
   a. The most commonly isolated pathogen from this genus is *R. equi.* It can be found in soil and is a recognized cause of pulmonary disease in horses.
   b. In humans, most infections involve the lower respiratory tract and occur in individuals who are immunocompromised. Nearly two-thirds of infected patients are infected with the human immunodeficiency virus (HIV).
   c. Isolates typically form pink colonies.

6. ***Nocardia***
   a. Generally found in patients who are immunocompromised with chronic pulmonary disorders
   b. ***N. asteroides* is was believed to be a common clinical isolate, but new studies indicate that it is likely nonpathogenic**; other more clinically relevant species include *N. brasiliensis*, *N. nova*, and *N. farcinica.*
   c. **Identifying characteristics**
      1) **Pleomorphic, branching gram-positive bacilli** in chains that produce a beading arrangement, appear fungal-like
      2) **Partially acid-fast**, catalase positive, nonmotile
      3) Requires up to 6 weeks for growth
      4) Exudate contains masses of filamentous organisms with pus that resemble sulfur granules.

7. ***Streptomyces***
   a. A large number of *Streptomyces* spp. have been described. They are commonly found in the soil.
   b. **Actinomycotic mycetoma** is the clinical presentation most often seen in humans, and the most common isolate is *S. somaliensis.* Actinomycotic mycetoma is a chronic bacterial infection producing inflammation of the tissue, forming sinus tracts, and often lymphadenopathy.

D. Aerobic Spore-Forming Gram-Positive Bacilli

1. **General Characteristics of *Bacillus* spp.**
   a. **Bacterial spores** can survive adverse conditions for prolonged periods of time and are frequent contaminants of laboratory cultures.
   b. Spores can be central or terminally located.
   c. Most *Bacillus* spp. are nonpathogenic, and frequently only genus identification is necessary.
   d. ***B. anthracis*** (anthrax) and ***B. cereus*** (food poisoning and wounds) are pathogenic species.

e. *Bacillus* spp. form straight bacilli, with square ends (boxcar morphology) appearing in chains and singly.
f. The majority of the species will grow on SBA and phenylethyl alcohol (PEA) agar and are **catalase positive**.
g. Cultures form large, flat colonies.

2. ***Bacillus anthracis***
a. Causes anthrax, a zoonosis that is rare in the United States
b. Three clinical forms of anthrax
1) **Cutaneous anthrax:** Most common form worldwide, characterized by necrotic skin lesions called black eschars
2) **Pulmonary anthrax:** "Wool-sorter's disease," spread by inhalation of spores from sheep's wool
3) **Gastrointestinal anthrax:** Rarest form; follows ingestion of spores
c. *B. anthracis* is considered a **potential bioterrorism agent** and was used as such in a series of attacks in the United States in 2001.
d. It produces large, **nonhemolytic colonies** with filamentous projections, sometimes referred to as "Medusa-head" colonies.
e. *B. anthracis* typically does not grow on PEA agar at 24 hours.
f. **Preliminary testing by sentinel laboratories:** Typical colony morphology, gram-positive bacilli with spores, catalase positive, and nonmotile
g. Confirmatory testing (e.g., phage typing and nucleic acid amplification tests [NAATs]) is performed by a reference laboratory.

3. ***Bacillus cereus***
a. *B. cereus* is an important cause of **food poisoning** and occasionally wounds. It may also cause opportunistic eye, bone, and brain infections.
b. *B. cereus* and *B. subtilis* are also common **laboratory contaminants**.
c. Colony morphology: Large, flat, beta-hemolytic colonies with irregular edges
d. **Motile** and resistant to 10 μg of penicillin

II. AEROBIC GRAM-NEGATIVE BACTERIA

A. *Neisseria* and Similar Microorganisms

1. **Family *Neisseriaceae***
a. Includes the genera *Neisseria, Eikenella*, and *Kingella*, among several others.
b. Many species are normal biota of the upper respiratory tract of animals.
c. Kidney bean-shaped, gram-negative diplococci or coccobacilli
d. The *Neisseriaceae* are oxidase positive, fastidious, and grow best in 5–10% CO_2 at 37°C. The pathogenic species cannot tolerate cold; therefore, media must be at room temperature before plating.

2. ***Neisseria gonorrhoeae***
a. Humans are the only host for *N. gonorrhoeae*. It is fastidious and does not survive long outside the host. *N. gonorrhoeae* can be isolated from the urethra, cervix, anal canal, oropharynx, skin lesions, joints, and blood.

1) **In males**, it causes acute urethritis, which is characterized by a pus-containing urethral discharge and dysuria and can also cause prostatitis and epididymitis.
2) **In females**, it causes urethral infections and cervicitis. Infections can be asymptomatic or produce cervical discharge, fever, acute pain, and dysuria. *N. gonorrhoeae* can also cause pelvic inflammatory disease (PID), gonococcal arthritis, salpingitis, endometritis, and peritonitis.

b. **Neonates** can be infected during vaginal delivery, resulting in gonococcal ophthalmia neonatorum, which is a severe conjunctivitis leading to blindness. To prevent newborn conjunctivitis, antimicrobial eye drops (e.g., erythromycin) are administered to all infants at birth.

c. *N. gonorrhoeae* is not normal biota.

d. On direct Gram stain, *N. gonorrhoeae* often appears **intracellular in neutrophils**.

e. Must culture immediately, and clinical material must be free of lubricants and spermicides

1) *N. gonorrhoeae* is fastidious, requiring enriched media such as chocolate agar. **It does not grow on SBA**.
2) **Selective media** include modified Thayer-Martin, Martin-Lewis, New York City, and GC-Lect agars.
3) The bacteria require increased CO_2 with a humidified atmosphere.
4) Because of autolysis, gonococci cannot be incubated for prolonged times without subculturing.

f. Colonies are flat, smooth, and glistening gray or tan.

g. **Identifying characteristics**

1) Superoxol, catalase, oxidase, and glucose positive
2) Maltose, lactose, sucrose, DNase, and nitrate negative

h. Many clinical laboratories perform NAATs on clinical specimens. These assays are rapid, sensitive, and specific. A negative aspect is that if cultures are not performed, antimicrobial susceptibility testing is not an option.

i. Many strains are positive for beta-lactamase production. The recommended treatment for gonorrhea is a single dose of 250 mg of intramuscular ceftriaxone and 1 g of oral azithromycin.

3. ***Neisseria meningitidis***

a. Spread by respiratory droplets and may be normal biota of the nasopharynx

b. Causes meningococcal meningitis, meningococcemia, leading to disseminated intravascular coagulation, and Waterhouse-Friderichsen syndrome

c. Specimens: Cerebrospinal fluid (CSF), sputum, blood, and nasopharyngeal swabs

d. Colonies are flat, smooth, and gray to white on chocolate agar. *N. meningitidis* will grow on SBA incubated in increased (5%) CO_2 and produce bluish-gray colonies.

e. **Identifying characteristics**
   1) Catalase, oxidase, glucose, and maltose positive
   2) DNase and nitrate negative
f. Two vaccines are available: 1) protects against serogroups A, C, Y, and W-135 and 2) protects against serogroup B.

4. **Normal biota *Neisseria***
   a. Many *Neisseria* spp. are normal biota of the upper respiratory tract. Species include *N. elongata, N. mucosa, N. lactamica, N. cinerea, N. polysaccharea, N. flavescens, N. subflava*, and *N. sicca.*
   b. In rare cases, these organisms can cause meningitis, endocarditis, and other infections.
   c. Many species are not fastidious and will grow on most nutrient agars.
5. ***Moraxella catarrhalis***
   a. Member of the family *Moraxellaceae*
   b. Resembles *Neisseria* and is normal biota of the upper respiratory tract
   c. Causes otitis media, sinusitis, and respiratory tract infections including pneumonia
   d. Will grow on most nutrient agars
   e. **Identifying characteristics**
      1) Catalase, oxidase, DNase, nitrate, and butyrate esterase (tributyrin hydrolysis) positive
      2) Asaccharolytic, all carbohydrate tests are negative

B. *Enterobacteriaceae*

1. **General family characteristics**
   a. Most medically important family of gram-negative bacilli
   b. Most species are normal biota of the GI tract. *Salmonella, Shigella*, and *Yersinia* are not normal GI biota.
   c. Major cause of nosocomial infections
   d. Diseases include UTIs, gastroenteritis, septicemia, food poisoning, wound infections, peritonitis, pneumonia, and meningitis
   e. The family exhibits four **serologic characteristics**
      1) **O (somatic) antigen**—A cell wall antigen (heat stable)
      2) **K antigen**—Capsular antigen (heat labile)
      3) **H (flagellar) antigen**—Flagellar antigen (heat labile)
      4) **Vi antigen**—Capsular antigen of *Salmonella* Typhi (heat labile)
   f. *Enterobacteriaceae* are facultative anaerobes. They ferment glucose, are nitrate and catalase positive, and, with the exception of *Plesiomonas*, are oxidase negative.
   g. **Enteric media**
      1) **MacConkey (MAC) agar:** Lactose-positive colonies are pink/red, and lactose-negative colonies are colorless.
      2) **Eosin-methylene blue (EMB) agar:** Colonies of lactose fermenters have a dark center, and lactose nonfermenters are colorless. *E. coli* has a dark center and usually shows a green metallic sheen.

3) **Hektoen-enteric (HE) agar:** Lactose and/or sucrose fermenters form yellow/orange colonies. *Salmonella* colonies are green with black centers (H_2S positive), and *Shigella* colonies are green.
4) **Xylose-lysine-desoxycholate (XLD) agar:** Colonies of lactose and/or sucrose fermenters are yellow. *Salmonella* produce clear red colonies with black centers (H_2S), and *Shigella* also have clear colonies.
5) **Salmonella-Shigella (SS) agar:** Lactose fermenters produce red colonies; *Salmonella* colonies are colorless with black centers, and *Shigella* colonies are colorless.
6) **Bismuth sulfite agar:** *Salmonella* Typhi produces black colonies; lactose-fermenting colonies are yellow-orange.
7) **Brilliant green agar:** *Proteus* and *Salmonella* species produce red/pink colonies, whereas *Shigella* and most lactose fermenters will not grow.
8) **Selenite broth:** The broth is an enhancement medium for stool cultures. *Salmonella* growth is enhanced, whereas gram-positive and coliform (normal GI biota) bacteria are inhibited. It is no longer commonly used.

2. **Important genera**

a. ***Escherichia***

1) ***E. coli* is normal GI biota** and a very common clinical isolate.
2) *E. coli* causes UTIs, appendicitis, peritonitis, gallbladder infections, endocarditis, meningitis in newborns, gastroenteritis, and food poisoning.
3) **Identifying characteristics**
   a) **Triple sugar iron (TSI):** Acid over acid (A/A) and H_2S negative
   b) **MAC agar:** Pink/red colonies
   c) On **SBA**, colonies are shiny, opaque, off-white, 2–4 mm in diameter, and usually **beta-hemolytic**.
   d) **EMB agar:** Green metallic sheen colonies with dark centers
   e) **Indole**, methyl red (MR), motility, and *o*-nitrophenyl-β-D-galactopyranoside (ONPG) positive
   f) Voges-Proskauer (VP), citrate, and urease negative
4) **Enterohemorrhagic *E. coli* (EHEC)** causes hemorrhagic colitis and hemolytic uremic syndrome (HUS), leading to kidney failure in young children.
   a) Acquired by eating undercooked hamburger or other contaminated foods such as apple cider, basil, sprouts, etc.
   b) The principal virulence factor is Shiga toxin (Stx) 1 and 2. Many strains of Stx-producing *E. coli* belong to the serogroup O157:H7. However, several other serogroups have been reported that produce Stx-1 and/or Stx-2. *E. coli* O157:H7 is thought to cause over 80% of all cases of HUS in the United States
   c) Growth on **sorbitol-MacConkey (SMAC) agar:** Sorbitol replaces lactose in the medium. *E. coli* O157:H7 does not metabolize sorbitol; most other *E. coli* strains rapidly ferment sorbitol, producing pink

colonies on SMAC. *E. coli* O157:H7 colonies appear colorless on SMAC. Confirmatory testing is by detection of Stx-1 and Stx-2.

d) EHEC typically does not produce β-glucuronidase, which can hydrolyze a synthetic molecule 4-methyl-umbelliferyl-D-glucuronide (*MUG*). Therefore, EHEC isolates are MUG negative.

5) Other strains of *E. coli* causing human intestinal infections
   a) **Enterotoxigenic *E. coli* (ETEC)** produces severe epidemic diarrhea, mainly from drinking contaminated water. It is an important cause of "traveller's diarrhea."
   b) **Enteroinvasive *E. coli* (EIEC)** causes bloody diarrhea by invading the intestinal epithelium. Infections resemble shigellosis.
   c) **Enteropathogenic *E. coli* (EPEC)** causes watery diarrhea.

b. ***Shigella***
   1) Causes shigellosis, a form of bacterial dysentery, characterized by abdominal pain, fever, and diarrhea
   2) Infections are most severe in children and the elderly. Can result in HUS. Outbreaks are known to occur in daycare centers and nursing homes.
   3) Highly pathogenic; Less than 50 bacteria can cause disease
   4) Causes food poisoning by direct fecal contamination from infected humans
   5) **Four serogroups based on O antigens**
      a) ***S. dysenteriae* (serogroup A)** produces an enterotoxin, which affects the large intestines, and a neurotoxin that may result in paralysis. *S. dysenteriae* is mannitol and ONPG negative.
      b) ***S. flexneri* (serogroup B)** produces a mild diarrhea. It is mannitol positive and ONPG negative.
      c) ***S. boydii* (serogroup C)** produces a mild diarrhea. *S. boydii* is mannitol positive and ONPG negative. It is difficult to biochemically distinguish *S. flexneri* from *S. boydi*.
      d) ***S. sonnei* (serogroup D)** produces a mild diarrhea. It is the most common cause of shigellosis in the United States. *S. sonnei* is mannitol and ONPG positive. It is a delayed lactose fermenter.
   6) **Identifying characteristics**
      a) TSI: Alkaline over acid (K/A)
      b) H_2S, VP, motility, citrate, urease, and lactose negative
      c) MR positive

c. ***Klebsiella***
   1) *Klebsiella* spp. typically cause UTIs and pneumonia. Many infections are nosocomial, and individuals who are diabetics and alcoholics are prone to infections.
   2) The most common species isolated is ***K. pneumoniae* (*K. pneumoniae* subsp. *pneumoniae*).**
   3) *Klebsiella pneumoniae* carbapenemase is an example of an extended-spectrum beta-lactamase.

4) **Identifying characteristics**
   a) **TSI:** A/A with gas
   b) On MAC agar, the pink colonies are very mucoid because of capsule production.
   c) *Klebsiella* spp. are H_2S and MR negative and nonmotile. Except for *K. oxytoca* the *Klebsiella* are indole negative.
   d) *Klebsiella* (*Enterobacter*) *aerogenes* is arginine negative and lysine positive.
   e) VP, citrate, and lactose positive
5) ***Klebsiella* (*Calymmatobacterium*) *granulomatis***
   a) The causative agent of **granuloma inguinale**, a sexually transmitted disease
   b) **Identification**
      i. Does not Gram stain or grow on laboratory media
      ii. In clinical specimens Wright or Giemsa stained, Donovan bodies may be seen. Donovan bodies are intracellular pleomorphic bipolar staining bacterial cells.

d. ***Enterobacter***
1) The genus includes about 12 species. They are found in soil, water, and dairy products.
2) *E. cloacae* is the most common species isolated. *Enterobacter* spp. are occasional clinical isolates that have been linked to respiratory tract infections and wounds and isolated from blood.
3) **Identifying characteristics**
   a) H_2S, MR, and indole negative
   b) VP and citrate positive
   c) All species except *E. taylorae* are lactose positive.
   d) *E. cloacae* is arginine positive and lysine negative.

e. ***Cronobacter***
1) A multispecies complex formerly referred to as *Enterobacter sakazakii*. The natural habitat for *Cronobacter* is not known; although it has been found in wastewater.
2) *Cronobacter* has been found in a variety of dry foods, **including powdered infant formula**, skimmed milk powder, herbal teas, and starches. Illnesses are rare, but they are frequently lethal for infants.
3) Isolates produce a yellow pigment.

f. ***Serratia***
1) Causes opportunistic infections in patients undergoing chemotherapy and patients who are immunocompromised
2) ***S. marcescens* is the most common clinical isolate.**
3) **Identifying characteristics**
   a) DNase, gelatinase, and lipase positive, unique among the enterics
   b) VP and citrate positive
   c) ONPG positive but a delayed lactose fermenter
   d) Some strains produce a red pigment, which is enhanced with room temperature incubation.

g. ***Salmonella***

1) **The genus contains two species, *S. enterica* and *S. bongori*,** with over 2500 serotypes. Most serotypes are pathogenic to humans and cause moderate to severe gastroenteritis. The majority of human cases of salmonellosis are due to serotypes belonging to the species *S. enterica*, which includes the serotype *S.* Typhi.
2) **There are many animal reservoirs.**
3) Transmitted through contaminated water and undercooked food, especially poultry
4) *Salmonella* Typhi causes **typhoid fever**, the most severe form of salmonellosis, which is characterized by a septicemia followed by a GI tract infection. Humans are the only reservoir for *S.* Typhi; infections are spread via the fecal-oral route.
5) Most human infections in the United States are caused by serotypes *Salmonella* Enteritidis and *Salmonella* Typhimurium.
6) *Salmonella* isolated from stool cultures form lactose-negative and H_2S-positive colonies on enteric media.
7) **Identifying characteristics**
    a) H_2S, motility, and citrate positive
    b) Indole, urease, and lactose negative
    c) Colonies on HE agar are green with black centers.
    d) *Salmonella* Typhi and some strains of *Salmonella* Cholerasuis possess a polysaccharide capsule referred to as Vi antigen. Unlike other *Salmonella* isolates, *Salmonella* Typhi does not produce gas from glucose.

h. ***Proteus***

1) Four species are recognized. ***Proteus vulgaris*** and ***P. mirabilis*** are the **most common** isolates.
2) **Identifying characteristics**
    a) *P. vulgaris* and *P. mirabilis* are typically H_2S positive.
    b) *P. mirabilis* and many strains of *P. vulgaris* exhibit swarming motility on SBA.
    c) All species are urease, tryptophan deaminase (TDA), and phenylalanine deaminase (PDA) positive.
    d) ONPG and therefore lactose negative
    e) *P. mirabilis* is indole negative; *P. vulgaris* is indole positive.

i. ***Yersinia***

1) Three pathogenic species of *Yersinia*
    a) ***Y. pestis* causes plague**; it is endemic to the southwestern United States. Small animals (e.g., rodents) are natural reservoirs, and the bacteria are transmitted by fleas. *Y. pestis* is considered a potential bioterrorism agent.
    b) ***Y. enterocolitica* causes enterocolitis** in humans; it is acquired by drinking contaminated water or by eating contaminated meat. Isolates are urease, sucrose, and ONPG positive but a delayed lactose fermenter. Therefore, colonies are colorless on MAC at 18 hours, but A/A on TSI.
    c) ***Y. pseudotuberculosis* is a rare cause of lymphadenitis in children.**

2) Small coccobacilli
3) **Cefsulodin-irgasan-novobiocin (CIN) medium** is a selective and differential medium for isolation of *Y. enterocolitica*. Colonies of *Yersinia* will ferment mannitol and absorb the dye, neutral red, producing clear colonies with a pink center. *Aeromonas* spp. will also grow on this medium and form colonies with pink centers.
4) All species except *Y. pestis* are nonmotile at 37°C but motile at 25°C. *Y. pestis* is nonmotile at both temperatures.
5) Presumptive identification of *Y. pestis* is based on isolation of the bacterium from respiratory tract, blood, or lymph nodes with the following characteristics: pinpoint colonies on SBA after 24 hours incubation, gram-negative bacilli, oxidase and urease negative, and catalase positive. Growth may be better at 28°C than 35°C. Confirmatory testing is performed by a regional reference laboratory.

j. ***Edwardsiella***
1) *E. tarda* is the most common isolate. It is primarily a fish pathogen rarely associated with opportunistic infections in humans.
2) **Resembles *Salmonella***, H_2S positive, and ONPG negative
3) Unlike *Salmonella, E. tarda* is indole positive and citrate negative.

k. ***Citrobacter***
1) *C. freundii* is the most common species isolated.
2) *C. freundii* resembles *E. coli* on MAC but can be differentiated because of being H_2S positive and indole negative.

l. ***Morganella***
1) *M. morganii* is the only species.
2) Indole positive, VP and citrate negative
3) PDA and TDA positive

m. ***Providencia***
1) There are five species of *Providencia*, and four have been isolated from humans. The most common isolate is probably *P. rettgeri*.
2) PDA, TDA, indole, and citrate positive and VP negative

n. ***Plesiomonas shigelloides***
1) Acquired by eating undercooked seafood
2) *P. shigelloides* is primarily associated with a self-limiting gastroenteritis. Treatment is required only in patients who are immunocompromised or other severe cases.
3) Only member of the family *Enterobacteriaceae* oxidase positive

3. **Less frequently isolated genera**
a. *Cedecea*
b. *Ewingella*
c. *Erwinia*
d. Kluyvera
e. *Tatumella*

C. *Haemophilis* and Similar Organisms

1. **General characteristics**
   a. Most species are normal upper respiratory tract biota.
   b. Some *Haemophilus* spp. are members of the **HACEK** (***H****aemophilus,* ***A****ggregatibacter aphrophilus, Aggregatibacter actinomycetemcomitans,* ***C****ardiobacterium hominis,* ***E****ikenella corrodens*, and ***K****ingella*) group. Members of this group are fastidious (i.e., require complex nutrients for growth) and important causes of endocarditis. They typically inhabit the oral cavity of humans.
   c. Pleomorphic gram-negative coccobacilli ranging from very small to filamentous
   d. **Growth requirements** include hemin (X factor), which is released from hemoglobin, and/or nicotine adenine dinucleotide (NAD, V factor), which is a heat-labile compound; see Table 6-2 ■.
   e. *Haemophilus* spp. do not grow on SBA because of NADase in the agar (NADase inactivates NAD) but will grow on horse or rabbit blood agar, which contains no NADase. Chocolate agar is routinely used for culture.
   f. Grows at 35–37°C with 5–10% CO_2 and is susceptible to drying and temperature changes
   g. Colony morphology: Smooth, round, flat, opaque, and tan on chocolate agar
   h. **Satellitism:** *Haemophilus* spp. can grow around colonies of *S. aureus* growing on an SBA plate. *S. aureus* releases NAD. Therefore, *Haemophilus* will grow near the *S. aureus* colonies, forming tiny clear pinpoint colonies.
   i. Nonmotile, catalase and oxidase positive
2. **Clinically relevant species**
   a. ***Haemophilus influenzae***
      1) **Six capsular serotypes, a–f, and eight biotypes, I–VIII**
      2) *H. influenzae* type b was a major cause of meningitis in children. The widespread use of the *H. influenzae* type b (Hib) **vaccine** has greatly reduced childhood meningitis and other invasive diseases caused by this serotype.

TABLE 6-2 IDENTIFICATION OF *HAEMOPHILUS* SPP

	Requires		β-Hemolysis on	
	X Factor	**V Factor**	**Horse Blood**	**ALA***
H. influenzae	+	+	–	–
H. ducreyi	|		–	–
H. aegyptius	+	+	–	–
H. haemolyticus	+	+	+	–
H. parainfluenzae	–	+	–	+
H. paraphrophilus	–	+	–	+

**Aminolevulinic acid (ALA) is converted to porphyrin, + = positive, – = negative*

3) Serotypes other than b are frequent cause of respiratory tract infections, including acute sinusitis, chronic bronchitis, and pneumonia. Otitis media with effusion (middle ear infections) and sinusitis are often caused by nontypeable strains, those lacking a capsule.
4) ***H. influenzae* isolates should be tested for beta-lactamase.**
5) This species can be isolated from a variety of specimens, including blood, sputum, CSF, and eye swabs.
6) Specific detection of Hib capsular antigen is by latex agglutination.

b. ***Haemophilus aegyptius***
1) **Causes pinkeye, a very contagious conjunctivitis**
2) Similar to *H. influenzae* with the exception of being sucrose positive

c. ***Haemophilus influenzae* biogroup aegyptius**
1) Causes a conjunctivitis, followed by invasive disease known as Brazilian purpuric fever
2) It resembles *H. influenzae* biotype III in that it is indole negative, urease positive, and ornithine decarboxylase negative.

d. ***Haemophilus ducreyi***
1) **Causes genital ulcers, a sexually transmitted disease**
2) Produces chancroids and buboes (swollen lymph nodes)
3) Chocolate agar with vancomycin inhibits normal biota and contaminants and is used to recover *H. ducreyi.*

3. ***Kingella***

a. *K. kingae* is the most clinically relevant species. It colonizes the throat of children. *K. oralis* has been isolated from the mouth of adults.
b. *K. kingae* shows a predilection for infections of the bones and joints in children. Infections in adults are generally limited to those who are immunocompromised.
c. *K. kingae* is best isolated from joints and bones in blood culture media. *Kingella* will grow on sheep blood, chocolate, and modified Thayer-Martin agars. They will not grow on MAC agar.
d. *K. kingae* forms short coccobacilli, white to beige large colonies on SBA is oxidase positive and does not grow on MAC agar.
e. *K. denitrificans* can be confused with *Neisseria gonorrhoeae* because it will produce acid from glucose and does not grow on MAC agar. Unlike *N. gonorrhoeae*, however, *K. denitrificans* is nitrate reduction positive and forms coccobacilli compared to diplococci.

D. Nonfermentative Gram-Negative Bacilli

1. **General characteristics**

a. Found in water, soil, food, and plants, and a few are normal biota of humans
b. Approximately 20% of all gram-negative bacilli isolates are nonfermentative gram-negative bacilli (NFB).

c. **General characteristics of NFB**
   1) Most species are obligate aerobes.
   2) They do not metabolize carbohydrates under anaerobic conditions (fermentation).
   3) Most are oxidase positive.
   4) **TSI:** K/no change
   5) Grow on SBA but varied growth on MAC

2. ***Pseudomonas aeruginosa***
   a. ***P. aeruginosa* is the most important NFB.** It is a common clinical isolate that can infect humans, animals, plants, and fish.
   b. *P. aeruginosa* is a member of the ***Pseudomonas* fluorescent group** along with *P. fluoresceins* and *P. putida*. All members of the fluorescent group produce **fluorescein (pyoverdin)**, a yellow pigment that fluoresces. Growth on **cetrimide agar** enhances fluorescein production.
   c. It causes eye (in contact lens wearers) and ear infections and is responsible for "swimmer's ear," which is an external otitis.
   d. Lower respiratory tract infections in patients with **cystic fibrosis** (CF) are common and potentially severe.
   e. Causes burn wound infections
   f. Important pathogen in individuals who are immunocompromised
   g. *P. aeruginosa* is resistant to a number of disinfectants and has been responsible for serious **nosocomial (healthcare-associated) infections.** It is especially associated with hospital environments and equipment, whirlpools, and swimming pools.
   h. **Identifying characteristics**
      1) Oxidase positive
      2) Motile
      3) Lactose negative
      4) Oxidizes glucose
      5) **Colony morphology**
         a) Large, irregular colonies with a grapelike odor and metallic sheen on SBA
         b) **β-hemolytic** colonies with a feathery edge on SBA
         c) **Mucoid colonies (due to a capsule) when isolated from patients with CF**
         d) **Pigment:** Only *P. aeruginosa* produces **pyocyanin**, a blue pigment. Pyocyanin mixes with fluorescein to produce a blue-green color.
   i. **Very resistant to antimicrobial agents,** the aminoglycosides and carbapenams are often used for treatment.

3. ***Stenotrophomonas maltophilia***
   a. Acquired as transient biota from hospitals
   b. Causes pneumonia, UTIs, wound infections

c. **Identifying characteristics**
   1) Oxidase negative
   2) *S. maltophila* is one of the only nonfermentative, gram-negative bacillus that is oxidase negative and maltose positive.
   3) Resistant to most antimicrobials

4. ***Burkholderia cepacia***
   a. *B. cepacia* causes healthcare-associated infections and is also an important respiratory tract pathogen in patients with CF; second most common cause to *P. aeruginosa.*
   b. It was formerly called *Pseudomonas cepacia.* Enhanced growth on ***P. cepacia* (PC) agar** that inhibits *P. aeruginosa*
   c. Colony morphology: Colorless or yellow on nutrient agar
   d. Oxidase and lactose positive

5. ***Burkholderia mallei***
   a. Causes **glanders**, a highly contagious disease of livestock, particularly among horses, mules, and donkeys
   b. *B. mallei* can be transmitted to humans by animal contact. The bacterium is also considered a **potential bioterrorism agent.**
   c. *B. mallei* grows on MAC agar, is oxidase variable and **nonmotile**, reduces nitrate to nitrite without gas, and oxidizes glucose.

6. ***Burkholderia pseudomallei***
   a. Causes **melioidosis**, a disease of humans and animals endemic to Southeast Asia and northern Australia
   b. *B. pseudomallei* is found in soil, and infections are acquired through the skin or by inhalation.
   c. *B. pseudomallei* grows on MAC agar, is oxidase positive and **motile**, and oxidizes several sugars, including glucose and lactose.

7. ***Acinetobacter***
   a. Obligate aerobic, coccobacillus found as normal biota of the GI and respiratory tracts
   b. *Acinetobacter* spp. are important causes of healthcare-associated infections, most often *Acinetobacter baumanii-calcoaceticus* complex (ABC organisms). **Isolates tend to be multidrug resistant.**
   c. These bacteria are especially important in the intensive care setting, causing bacteremia, pneumonia/ventilator-associated pneumonia, meningitis, urinary tract infections, central venous catheter-related infections, and wound infections.
   d. *Acinetobacter* spp. grow on most media and may resemble enterics on MAC and EMB agars. Some species, such as *A. baumanii*, produce acid from glucose aerobically (saccharolytic group), whereas others are asacchrolytic.
   e. **Identifying characteristics**
      1) Nonmotile and oxidase negative
      2) Nitrate negative and catalase positive

8. ***Alcaligenes***
   a. Habitat like *Pseudomonas* spp. *Alcaligenes faecalis* is the more clinically relevant species.
   b. Opportunistic pathogen, asacchrolytic

E. Miscellaneous Gram-Negative Bacilli

1. ***Francisella***
   a. *F. tularensis* causes **tularemia** and is a **potential agent of bioterrorism.**
   b. **The bacteria are carried by wild animals**, including deer, rabbits, beavers, and squirrels.
   c. Humans may acquire the infection by skinning animals or eating undercooked game, or from animal bites and the bite of deerflies or ticks.
   d. Intracellular bacteria that resist phagocytosis
   e. *F. tularensis* causes skin ulcers at the site of inoculation and can cause infections of the lymph nodes, eyes, lungs, and GI system.
   f. Biosafety level 3 is required when handling the organism or suspect specimens.
   g. **Identifying characteristics**
      1) Faintly staining coccobacilli
      2) The medium of choice is glucose-cystine blood agar.
      3) Colony morphology: Small and grayish
      4) Agglutination and direct fluorescent antibody tests are used to confirm the identification.
2. ***Brucella***
   a. **Causes brucellosis, also known as undulant fever**
   b. Normal gastrointestinal biota of animals
   c. Humans usually acquire the infection by drinking contaminated milk or by aerosols from slaughterhouse exposure. The incubation period is 1–3 weeks.
   d. Four species infect humans: *B. melitenis, B. abortus, B. suis*, and *B. canis. B. melitenis* causes the most severe infections. *Brucella* has been considered a **potential bioterrorism agent.**
   e. Facultative intracellular parasite
   f. Biosafety level 3 organism
   g. Isolated from blood and **bone marrow**
   h. **Identifying characteristics**
      1) They are fastidious organisms but will grow on Brucella, buffered charcoal yeast extract (BCYE), and modified Thayer-Martin agars, and require 10% CO_2 in humidified air and 3–4 weeks for growth. Isolation in automated blood culture monitoring systems is recommended.
      2) Strict aerobe
      3) Oxidase and catalase positive
      4) Slide agglutination in antisera can be used for presumptive diagnosis of brucellosis. Further testing is not performed in most clinical laboratories.
      5) Serologic testing of patient sera is the primary method for diagnosing brucellosis.

3. ***Bordetella***
   a. ***B. pertussis* causes pertussis.**
   b. It inhabits the mucous membranes of the respiratory tract of humans.
   c. Three stages of pertussis (whooping cough)
      1) **Catarrhal:** General flulike symptoms
      2) **Paroxysmal:** Repetitive coughing episodes
      3) **Convalescent:** Recovery phase
   d. **Nasopharyngeal swabs** are recommended for diagnosis. *B. pertussis* grows on **Bordet-Gengou** (potato infusion) and **Regan-Lowe agar**s (charcoal-horse blood agar). Media are often made selective by adding cephalexin. However, polymerase chain reaction (PCR) is generally used for diagnosis. Swabs for PCR can be transmitted to the laboratory for testing without a transport medium.
   e. Other species
      1) ***B. parapertussis*** causes mild respiratory infections in humans.
      2) ***B. bronchiseptica*** causes kennel cough in dogs and is an infrequent cause of respiratory infections in humans.
   f. **Identifying characteristics**
      1) *B. pertussis* colonies are small and smooth; they resemble mercury droplets and are beta-hemolytic.
      2) Gram stain shows minute, poorly stained coccobacilli, single or in pairs.
      3) Most species will grow on MAC agar except *B. pertussis.*
      4) *B. pertussis* is urease negative, whereas all other species are urease positive.
4. ***Actinobacillus***
   a. ***Actinobacillus*** spp. are found mostly as oral biota of animals.
   b. **Infections are caused by animal bites**, which can result in cellulitis.
   c. *Actinobacillus* spp. grow well on SBA and chocolate agar but will not grow on MAC agar. They produce colonies that show starlike centers.
   d. Most species are catalase and glucose positive.
5. ***Pasteurella***
   a. ***Pasteurella*** spp. are normal respiratory/GI biota of animals. Humans acquire the bacteria from animal bites (cats and dogs) or by inhalation of dried animal feces.
   b. Causes **cellulitis** but can progress into osteomyelitis, meningitis, joint infections, and pneumonia
   c. ***Pasteurella multocida* causes most human infections.**
   d. **Identifying characteristics**
      1) Grows well on nonselective agars but not MAC
      2) Oxidase, catalase, indole, and nitrate positive
      3) Nonmotile, pleomorphic, gram-negative coccobacilli that may show bipolar staining
      4) Very susceptible to penicillin
6. ***Eikenella corrodens***
   a. **Normal biota of the mouth and upper respiratory tract**
   b. *E. corrodens* causes abscesses of the oral cavity and human bite wound infections. It is a member of the HACEK group and has been associated with endocarditis.

c. Approximately 50% of the strains **corrode or pit the agar surface.**
d. Requires hemin (factor X) for growth, unless 5–10% CO_2 is present
e. Produces a bleachlike odor

7. ***Legionella***
   a. First discovered in 1976 as the cause of pneumonia in people attending an American Legion convention in Philadelphia
   b. *Legionella* spp. are aquatic organisms that may be found in various water systems, including humidifiers, whirlpools, and air conditioning chillers. They are resistant to commonly used concentrations of chlorine.
   c. **Most human infections are caused by *L. pneumophila* serogroup 1.**
   d. Causes **legionellosis**, which can be asymptomatic or mild to severe pneumonia. Legionnaires disease, a primary pneumonia, is the severe form of legionellosis. **Pontiac fever** is a mild form, characterized by flulike symptoms.
   e. The urine antigen test is the most common laboratory assay used for the diagnosis of legionellosis.
   f. Specimens from the lower respiratory tract, lung biopsy, bronchial wash, expectorated sputum, etc. are sometimes used for cultures for the diagnosis of the pneumonic form of the disease.
   g. **Identifying characteristics**
      1) On a Gram stain, *Legionella* spp. appear as thin, poorly staining gram-negative bacilli. It is better to use 0.1% basic fuchsin as the counterstain instead of safranin.
      2) *Legionella* spp. **require L-cysteine for growth.** They will grow on **BCYE agar** but not on SBA. However, some species will grow on Brucella blood agar, a medium more nutritious than SBA. They can produce tiny colonies on chocolate agar.
      3) They are asacchrolytic, and most biochemical tests are negative.
      4) Most species will **autofluoresce** when exposed to ultraviolet light, including *L. pneumophila.*
      5) Other identifying tests: Direct fluorescent antibody test, urine antigen test, and nucleic acid probes
8. ***Chromobacterium***
   a. *Chromobacterium violaceum* is found in water and soil.
   b. Produces a purple or violet pigment on nutrient agar
   c. Causes wound infections acquired from contaminated soil or water
9. ***Gardnerella vaginalis***
   a. *Gardnerella* are very small gram-variable coccobacilli. They differ from *Lactobacillus* spp., which are large gram-positive bacilli.
   b. In low numbers, *G. vaginalis* is considered normal vaginal biota.
   c. *G. vaginalis* is associated with **bacterial vaginosis (BV)**, UTIs, PID, and postpartum sepsis and may infect the newborn. *G. vaginalis* probably does not cause BV, but its presence is indicative of the condition.

d. Presence of **clue cells**, epithelial cells with numerous bacteria attached, is suggestive of BV.
e. Catalase negative
f. Amsel and Nugent scoring systems are used to diagnose BV. Cultures alone are too sensitive (false positive results). Approximately 50–60% of women who do not meet the criteria for BV are culture positive for *G. vaginalis*.

10. ***Bartonella***
a. Oxidase-negative, gram-negative, curved bacilli
b. *Bartonella quintana*
1) Agent of **trench fever**
2) Also causes growth of neoplastic blood vessels in various parts of the body (bacillary angiomatosis) and other infections such as endocarditis
3) Spread by human lice
c. *B. henselae*: Causes **cat-scratch disease** and also bacillary peliosis hepatitis and bacillary angiomatosis.

11. ***Cardiobacterium hominis***
a. Found as normal biota in humans in the upper respiratory tract and possibly the gastrointestinal and genital tracts
b. It is a member of the HACEK group and is mainly associated with endocarditis
c. In Gram stains, *C. hominis* appears as short chains, pairs, or rosettes of irregularly staining bacilli with bulbous ends.
d. *C. hominis* requires CO_2 for initial isolation and can be recovered on SBA, although growth is enhanced in media containing yeast extract. It is oxidase positive, catalase negative, and weakly indole positive.

12. ***Streptobacillus moniliformis***
a. Found as normal oral biota in rats and other rodents
b. Infections following animal bites results in a disease called **rat-bite fever.**
c. Ingestion of contaminated food or water results in **Haverhill fever.**
d. The bacteria are best isolated from blood, synovial fluid, and abscess material.
e. *S. moniliformis* is a nonmotile, facultative, gram-negative pleomorphic bacillus. It grows on media enriched with SBA (15% is optimal) incubated in a CO_2 incubator.

F. *Vibrio* and Similar Microorganisms

1. **General characteristics**
a. Most are indole positive, and all are oxidase positive except *V. metschnikovii.*
b. Some species cause GI disease.

2. ***Vibrio***
a. The genus contains about 30 species that are inhabitants of marine water.
b. All species are **halophilic** (salt loving) except *V. cholerae* and *V. mimicus.*
c. **Thiosulfate-citrate-bile salt sucrose (TCBS) agar** is a selective and differential (based on sucrose fermentation) medium that supports the growth

of most species and is particularly useful for isolating *V. cholerae* and *V. parahaemolyticus*. *V. cholerae* is sucrose positive and will produce yellow colonies on TCBS agar, whereas *V. parahaemolyticus* is sucrose negative.

d. Most laboratories use biochemical testing to presumptively identify species and then confirm with slide agglutination with antisera against somatic O antigens.

e. ***Vibrio cholerae***
   1) ***V. cholerae* O1** serologic group causes cholera, characterized by severe watery diarrhea with flecks of mucus sometimes referred to as "**rice-water**" stool.
   2) **Serogroups non-O1** generally cause a mild choleralike illness. Serogroup O139 produces severe disease similar to *V. cholerae* O1.
   3) *V. cholerae* O1 is subdivided into three serotypes: Inaba, Ogawa, and Hikojima.
   4) *V. cholerae* O1 has two biotypes: classical and El Tor.
   5) Cholera infections are acquired by ingestion of undercooked seafood or contaminated drinking water. Cases can also be acquired via the fecal-oral route. Cholera is endemic to Southeast Asia, Africa, and South America.
   6) Important virulence mechanisms of *V. cholerae* include **cholera toxin** (choleragen, an enterotoxin), motility, pili, and mucinase.
   7) Symptoms seen in cholera are caused by the enterotoxin that alters ion transport of intestinal mucosa, resulting in a massive release of water.
   8) In addition to causing cholera, *V. cholerae* can also cause bacteremia, wound infections, and otitis media.

f. ***Vibrio parahaemolyticus***
   1) Causes a mild to moderate choleralike diarrhea disease
   2) Acquired by eating raw shellfish
   3) Important cause of food poisoning in Asia, particularly in Japan and Taiwan

g. ***Vibrio vulnificus***
   1) Highly virulent, causing septicemia after ingestion of undercooked seafood, notably raw oysters
   2) Causes a rapidly progressive wound infection that can result in a septicemia after exposure to marine water

h. ***Vibrio alginolyticus***
   1) Very common in marine environment
   2) Suspected causes of otitis media and wound infections

3. ***Aeromonas***
   a. **Found in fresh and salt water**
   b. Infects humans and fish
   c. Causes cellulitis and diarrhea
   d. Clinically important species include *A. hydrophilia* complex, *A. caviae* complex, and *A. veronii* biovar sobria.

e. Generally cause a self-limiting infection not usually requiring treatment; however, wound infections may require antimicrobial therapy.
f. *A. hydrophila* is typically beta-hemolytic and oxidase, citrate, indole, VP, and ONPG positive.

4. ***Campylobacter***
   a. *Campylobacter* spp. are a major cause of food poisoning, causing gastroenteritis, diarrhea, and septic arthritis.
   b. Infection is acquired by eating undercooked contaminated poultry or other meat products. Dogs and cats can also be reservoirs.
   c. ***C. jejuni*** causes most infections in this genus.
   d. Part of routine stool culture work-ups
   e. **Identifying characteristics**
      1) Curved bacilli that may appear S-shaped or spiral on Gram stain
      2) **Most species are microaerophilic.**
      3) A number of **selective media (**e.g., charcoal cefoperzone deoxycholate agar and Campy-colistin vancomycin amphotericin B) are available for the isolation of *C. jejuni* and *C. coli* from stool specimens.
      4) ***C. jejuni*** **grows at 42°C but will grow slowly at 37°C.** Stool specimens for the recovery of *C. jejuni* should be incubated at 42°C.
      5) They do not oxidize or ferment carbohydrates, and most human isolates are catalase and oxidase positive.
      6) On wet mount, they will show darting motility.
      7) Resistance to cephalothin and sensitivity to nalidixic acid has been used in the past for identification of *C. jejuni* and *C. coli*; however, because of variability in the sensitivity pattern, disk identification tests are no longer recommended.
      8) *C. fetus* is a rare cause of extraintestinal infections and does not grow at 42°C.

5. ***Helicobacter pylori***
   a. *H. pylori* causes peptic and duodenal ulcers and has been linked to stomach cancer.
   b. Oxidase, rapid urease, and catalase positive
   c. The microorganism can be **isolated from gastric biopsy** on SBA, Brucella, and Skirrow's agars incubated microaerophilically. Selective media for enteric *Campylobacter* are **not** recommended.
   d. Other methods to determine *H. pylori* colonization include fecal antigen detection, urea breath test, and demonstration of urease activity in stomach biopsy material.

III. MYCOBACTERIA

A. General Characteristics

1. Cause **tuberculosis** (TB) and other diseases
2. Mycobacteria are slender, nonmotile, nonspore-forming, obligate aerobes.
3. There are about 50 species of *Mycobacterium*, 14 of which are pathogenic to humans.

4. It is necessary to decontaminate samples containing normal biota before culturing, and sputum must also be digested. Specimens from normally sterile sites (e.g., CSF and blood) do not require decontamination.
5. Mycobacteria resist Gram staining because of a high concentration of mycolic acids (long-chain fatty acids) in their cell wall that prevent penetration of crystal violet and safranin.
6. Mycobacteria are **acid-fast** and are referred to as **acid-fast bacilli** (AFB). The primary stain in the acid-fast stain is **carbol fuchsin.** The Ziehl-Neelsen stain requires heating during the staining step, whereas the Kinyoun's stain does not. They can also be stained by the fluorescent **auromine-rhodamine stain.**
7. **Specimens**
   a. **Lower respiratory tract:** Sputum and bronchial washings, usually three to five samples, are collected early in the morning on different days.
   b. **Urine:** Three to five different morning voids
   c. Blood and bone marrow
   d. Tissue and body fluids
8. Centers for Disease Control and Prevention direct smear acid-fast evaluation and reporting criteria; see Table 6-3 ■.
9. **Digestion and decontamination of sputum samples**
   a. The mycobacteria are slightly more resistant to acids and alkalis than contaminating bacteria making up the normal biota. Therefore, mild treatments, such as 2% NaOH with *N*-acetyl-L-cysteine (NALC), are effective. Only specimens containing normal biota, such as sputum that contains bacteria from the oral cavity, need to be decontaminated.
   b. NALC is a mucolytic agent that liquefies mucus in respiratory specimens, releasing mycobacteria.
   c. NaOH increases the pH to a level that is antibacterial.
10. **Solid media**
    a. **Lowenstein-Jensen** (LJ) contains egg components for growth and malachite green to slightly inhibit growth of normal biota.
    b. **Lowenstein-Jensen-Gruft** is made selective by the addition of penicillin and naladixic acid. It is also supplemented with RNA.

TABLE 6-3 REPORTING CRITERIA FOR AFB ON DIRECT SMEAR

Report	Fuchsin Stain (×1000)
No AFB seen	0
Doubtful, repeat	1–2/300fields
1+	1–9/100fields
2+	1–9/10fields
3+	1–9/field
4+	>9/field

c. **Middlebrook medium** can be broth (7H9) or agar based (7H10 or 7H11) and contains 2% glycerol to support the growth of *M. avium* complex (MAC). These media generally exhibit growth several days before egg-based media. Antimicrobials can be added to make the media selective for mycobacteria.

11. **Liquid media**
   a. **Middlebrook 7H9 broth** is often used to maintain stock cultures and prepare isolates for biochemical tests.
   b. *Mycobacterium* growth index tube **(MGIT®)** by Becton Dickinson (Franklin Lakes, New Jersey) contains a modified 7H9 broth. The large amount of oxygen in the broth quenches fluorescence of a fluorchrome. As mycobacteria grow, they consume the oxygen, and the fluorchrome will fluoresce when exposed to ultraviolet light.
   c. Several automated, continuous monitoring systems are available.
12. **Runyon groups**
   a. Except for members of the *M. tuberculosis* complex, the mycobacteria can be placed into groups according to their growth rate and photoreactivity. However, due to variability in the criteria among *Mycobacterium* spp., Runyon classification is rarely used.
   b. **Growth rate:** Rapid growers produce colonies on solid media within 1 week. Most common pathogens are slow growers, and weakly pathogenic species are rapid growers.
   c. **Photoreactivity**
      1) **Photochromogens** produce yellow to orange pigment only when exposed to light.
      2) **Scotochromogens** produce yellow to orange pigment in the light and in the dark.
      3) **Nonchromogens** (nonpigmented) do not produce pigment.
   d. Members of Runyon **group 1** are slow growers and photochromogens. **Group 2** members are slow growers and scotochromogens. Mycobacteria that are slow growers and nonchromogens belong to **group 3. Group 4** contains the rapidly growing mycobacteria.
13. Biochemical tests for the identification of the mycobacteria
   a. Due to the slow growth rate of many mycobacterial species, many laboratories have begun using matrix-assisted laser desorption/ionization time of flight (MALDI-TOF) for the identification of mycobacteria by protein analysis. In addition, many mycobacteria can be identified by high-pressure liquid chromatography of cell wall lipids.
   b. **Catalase:** All mycobacteria typically produce catalase; however, different forms of catalase can be differentiated in the laboratory.
      1) **Heat-sensitive catalase:** A suspension of a *Mycobacterium* sp. is heated at 68°C for 20 minutes. A 1:1 mixture of 30% hydrogen peroxide and 10% Tween 80 is added; after 5 minutes, the suspension is observed for bubbles. Members of the *M. tuberculosis* complex, including *M. tuberculosis* and *M. bovis*, are negative.

2) **Semiquantitative catalase:** A 1 mL aliquot of a mixture of hydrogen peroxide and Tween 80 is added to a 2-week-old culture deep of mycobacteria. After 5 minutes, the height of the column of bubbles is measured. Members of the *M. tuberculosis* complex produce columns of bubbles <45 mm.

c. **Nitrate**

1) In the test for nitrate reductase, $NaNO_3$ is added to a heavy suspension of mycobacteria. The suspension is incubated for 2 hours at 35°C, and then nitrate reagents (HCl, sulfanilamide, and *N*-naphthylenediamine dihydrochloride) are added. Formation of a pink color is a positive reaction.

2) *M. tuberculosis* and *M. kansasii* are nitrate reductase positive, and most other *Mycobacterium* spp. are negative.

d. **Niacin**

1) Niacin (nicotinic acid) is a precursor in the synthesis of NAD. Although all mycobacteria produce niacin, some species produce an excess amount that is excreted from the cell. Niacin accumulates in the medium and is detected by reacting with a cyanogen halide.

2) *M. tuberculosis* is one of the few species positive for the accumulation of niacin.

e. **Growth on MAC agar**

1) MAC agar without crystal violet is inoculated with a 7-day broth culture of the test organism. This is not the same formulation used for gram-negative bacilli.

2) *M. fortuitum* and *M. chelonei* are the only mycobacteria able to grow on MAC agar in 5 days.

f. Susceptibility to thiophene-2-carboxylic acid hydrazide (T2H): differentiates *M. bovis* (susceptible) from most other species (resistant).

g. Arylsulfatase

1) Bacteria are added to a broth containing tripotassium phenolphthalein disulfate and incubated for 3 days.

2) If the bacteria produced arylsulfatase, the substrate will be cleaved releasing phenolphthalein, which will turn pink or red after the addition of 1M sodium carbonate.

3) *Mycobacterium xenopi* is positive while *M. tuberculosis* isolates remain colorless (negative).

14. **Nucleic acid assays**

a. Because of their slowly growing nature, rapid and specific direct nucleic acid assays are used commonly in clinical laboratories for the identification of the mycobacteria.

b. The Amplified *Mycobacterium tuberculosis* Direct (Hologic Gen-Probe Inc., San Diego, California) and the Xpert MTB/RIF (Cepheid, Sunnyvale, California) are two direct nucleic acid amplification commercial assays for the *Mycobacterium tuberculosis* complex., *Mycobacterium avium* complex, *M. avium, M. intracellularae, M. kansasii*, and *M. gordonae*. The assays are highly specific and takes less than 2 hours. They are approved for use on culture isolates.

B. Clinically Important *Mycobacterium*

1. ***Mycobacterium tuberculosis***
   a. Causes **tuberculosis**, a chronic primarily lower respiratory tract disease
   b. Spread by person-to-person contact via infected droplets, dust, etc.
   c. Only a few bacteria are necessary to cause disease.
   d. **Primary tuberculosis**
      1) Infection begins in the middle or lower areas of the lungs.
      2) The bacteria can spread to the lymphatic system, CNS, and heart.
      3) Macrophages phagocytize the bacteria and form multinucleated cells, which are eventually surrounded by fibroid cells. Together the cells form granulomatous lesions called **tubercles**, which can be seen on chest X-rays. The lesions can calcify, at which point they are called "**ghon complexes.**" While the bacteria are contained within the granulomas, the patient is typically asymptomatic. This stage of the disease is called a **latent infection.**
      4) Primary TB may not lead to active TB in people with healthy immune systems.
   e. **Reactivation or secondary tuberculosis**
      1) Occurs in people who have had latent TB
      2) Reactivation, because of alteration in the cell-mediated immune response, can be triggered by poor nutrition, alcoholism, or hormonal factors associated with pregnancy and diabetes.
      3) Treatment requires long-term combination therapy, which can last up to 24 months. The four first-line drugs are isoniazid, rifampin, ethambutol, and pyrazinamide.
   f. **Multidrug-resistant *M. tuberculosis*** (MDR-TB) is defined as simultaneous resistance to isoniazid and rifampin.
   g. **Extremely-drug-resistant *M. tuberculosis*** (XDR-TB) is defined as resistance to any fluoroquinolone, and at least one of three injectable second-line drugs (capreomycin, kanamycin, and amikacin), in addition to isoniazid and rifampicin.
   h. **Purified protein derivative (PPD):** Skin test that determines exposure to *M. tuberculosis*
      1) Antigen is composed of heat-killed, filtered, ammonium sulfate precipitated protein from *M. tuberculosis.*
      2) Injected intradermally and is examined at 48 hours for swelling (induration)
      3) A positive skin test indicates previous exposure to the bacteria but not necessarily active disease.
   i. **Gamma-interferon release assays** (IFGRAs)
      1) Is a blood test based on the release of interferon gamma from T cells exposed to *M. tuberculosis* antigen.
      2) The test does not produce a false-positive result in patients who have received the tuberculosis vaccine. However, like the PPD skin test, the IFGRAs cannot distinguish between current and past infections.
   j. Colonies on LJ medium appear nonpigmented (tan or **buff**), dry, heaped, and granular in 14–21 days at 37°C.

k. Acid-fast stain often shows ropelike formations (cording) from broth culture.
l. Niacin and nitrate positive, *p*-nitro-α-acetylamino-β-hydroxypropiophenone **(NAP)** susceptible

2. ***Mycobacterium leprae***
   a. Agent of **Hansen disease** (leprosy)
   b. **Cannot be grown on artificial media**
   c. Diagnosis is based on characteristic skin lesions and visualizing AFB in lesions.
3. ***M. avium*** complex
   a. *M. avium* and *M. intracellulare* are difficult to distinguish and are referred to as *M. avium* complex.
   b. *M. avium* complex can cause disseminated disease in patients who are immunocompromised, such as patients with HIV infection, producing lung infections, lymphadenitis, and intestinal infections.
   c. Members of the complex are slowly growing nonchromogens.
4. ***M. kansasii***
   a. ***M. kansasii*** causes pulmonary infections and is the most commonly isolated photochromogen in the United States. It has been isolated from tap water around the world.
   b. It causes a lung disease that resembles classic TB and rarely disseminates, except in patients with severe immunosuppression.
   c. It is a slow grower and is nitrate and catalase positive.
5. ***Mycobacterium scrofulaceum*** causes cervical lymphadenitis and other types of infections predominantly in children. It is a slowly growing scotochromogen.
6. ***Mycobacterium ulcerans, M. marinum***, and ***M. haemophilium*** have all been implicated in skin infections. Their predilection for surface areas and body extremities is related to their optimal growth temperature range of 30–32°C. *M. haemophilium* requires ferric ammonium citrate or hemin for growth and can be grown on chocolate agar.
7. ***Mycobacterium bovis*** is responsible for a zoonosis, producing pulmonary infections primarily in cattle and occasionally in humans. *M. bovis* is a non-chromogen like *M. tuberculosis*, but it is nitrate and niacin negative and sensitive to T2H.
8. *M. fortuitum, M. chelonae*, and *M. abscessus* may cause abscesses, osteomyelitis, wound and lung infections; however, they are weakly virulent. These species are among the rapidly growing mycobacteria.
9. *Mycobacterium gordonae* is found in freshwater, including tap water, and is rarely pathogenic. It is a slowly growing scotochromogen often isolated as a contaminant.

IV. ANAEROBIC BACTERIA

A. General Characteristics

1. Anaerobic bacteria (i.e., obligate anaerobes) comprise most normal biota of the mucous membranes.

2. Suspect anaerobic bacteria in the following situations:
   a. Foul odor (from gas production) and necrotic tissue
   b. Anaerobic body sites, abscesses, and wounds
   c. Surgical specimens
3. **Definitions**
   a. **Obligate anaerobe:** Bacterium that cannot use oxygen for metabolism and oxygen is lethal to the microorganism
   b. **Aerotolerant anaerobe:** Bacterium that cannot use oxygen but can grow in its presence
   c. **Facultative anaerobe:** Bacterium that will use oxygen if it is present and can grow, albeit more slowly, without oxygen
   d. **Obligate aerobe:** Bacterium that requires oxygen at concentrations found in room air, about 20%
   e. **Microaerophile:** Bacterium that requires oxygen at concentrations of 5–10%
   f. **Capnophile:** Bacterium that requires increased concentration of CO_2

B. Anaerobic Media

1. Media contain supplements that enhance anaerobic growth. Vitamin K is added to enhance the growth of *Prevotella* and *Porphyromonas*, and hemin is an added enrichment for *Bacteroides* and *Prevotella.*
2. **Centers for Disease Control and Prevention (CDC) anaerobic blood agar:** For general growth of all anaerobes
3. **Bacteroides bile esculin (BBE) agar:** Selective and differential medium used to culture and presumptively identify *Bacteroides fragilis*
4. **Kanamycin-vancomycin laked sheep blood (KVLB) agar:** Enriched selective medium for isolation of slowly growing anaerobes such as *Prevotella* and *Bacteroides*, laked blood enhances pigment formation
5. **Phenylethyl alcohol (PEA) agar:** Enriched and selective medium used to grow most anaerobes, including *Clostridium* and *Bacteroides*; inhibits the growth of facultative, anaerobic, gram-negative bacilli (e.g., *Enterobacteriaceae*)
6. **Columbia-colistin-naladixic agar with 5% sheep blood:** Inhibits gram-negative organisms and is used to grow most gram-positive anaerobes and facultative anaerobes
7. **Egg yolk agar** is used to detect proteolytic enzymes (lipase and lecithinase) produced by *Clostridium.* **Lecithinase** activity produces an opaque zone from the cleavage of lecithin releasing insoluble fats (diglyceride). **Lipase** cleaves lipids, releasing glycerol, which floats to the top of the medium producing a blue-green sheen (mother-of-pearl) on the agar surface.
8. **Broths** with **reducing agents**, such as thioglycolate and cooked (or chopped) meat, can be used to grow anaerobic bacteria. Sometimes **resazurin**, an oxidation-reduction indicator, is added. The indicator is pink in the presence of oxygen and colorless when reduced.

9. Solid media must be placed in **anaerobic conditions** in order for obligate anaerobes to grow.
   a. Commonly used systems include anaerobic GasPak jars and bags and anaerobic hoods. In the presence of **palladium**, a catalyst, the following reaction occurs:

$$2H_2 + O_2 \rightarrow 2H_2O_2$$

   b. An oxidation-reduction indicator (E_h) must be used to determine if anaerobic conditions have been met. **Methylene blue** is the most commonly used oxidation-reduction indicator. When anaerobic conditions are achieved, the methylene blue indicator will turn from blue (oxidized) to white, indicating reduction.
10. **Aerotolerance testing:** Before attempting to identify a possible anaerobic bacterium, it first must be demonstrated to be an obligate anaerobe. A colony is inoculated to an anaerobic blood agar plate, which is incubated anaerobically, and to a chocolate agar plate incubated under conditions of increased CO_2. Isolates growing only on the plate incubated anaerobically are obligate anaerobes.

C. Gram Stain Morphology

1. *Bacteroides, Prevotella*, and *Porphyromonas*: Pale, pleomorphic gram-negative coccobacilli with bipolar staining
2. *Fusobacterium*: Long, thin, filamentous gram-negative bacilli with tapered ends arranged end to end, sometimes curved
3. *Actinomyces*: Branching gram-positive bacilli
4. *Clostridium*: Large gram-positive bacilli, spore location (terminal, central, or subterminal) is important in species identification

D. Biochemical Reactions

1. Important anaerobic biochemical tests include catalase, auto-fluorescence, nitrate, urease, bile sensitivity, carbohydrate fermentation, and indole.
2. Antimicrobial susceptibility disks can also be used to help identify anaerobes.

E. Anaerobic Gram-Negative Bacilli

1. ***Bacteroides fragilis***
   a. ***B. fragilis* is a nonpigmented bacillus responsible for most anaerobic infections**, and many isolates are becoming more resistant to antimicrobial agents.
   b. **Major normal biota of the colon**
   c. Causes infections by gaining entry into normally sterile body sites, especially after surgery, trauma, or disease
   d. **Important virulence mechanisms** include a capsule that stimulates inflammatory reactions and promotes antiphagocytosis and endotoxin which can also stimulate inflammation.

e. **Identifying characteristics**
   1) Nonmotile gram-negative bacilli with rounded ends and may be pleomorphic
   2) Nonhemolytic on anaerobic blood agar
   3) Biochemistry: **Growth in 20% bile**, catalase positive, lipase negative lecithinase negative, and gelatinase negative
   4) Produces brown to black colonies on BBE agar
   5) *B. fragilis* is resistant to penicillin, kanamycin, and vancomycin and susceptible to rifampin.

2. ***Prevotella melaninogenica***
   a. **Pigmented saccharolytic gram-negative bacilli**
   b. Normal biota of the oropharynx, nose, and GI and urogenital tracts
   c. Causes head, neck, and lower respiratory tract infections
   d. **Identifying characteristics**
      1) Young colonies appear tan and exhibit brick-red fluorescence under ultraviolet (UV) light. Older colonies are brown to black. It may take up to 3 weeks to see a brown to black pigment.
      2) Biochemistry: Ferments glucose and many other carbohydrates and is inhibited by 20% bile
      3) Susceptible to rifampin and resistant to kanamycin

3. ***Porphyromonas***
   a. **Asaccharolytic** or weak fermenters, pigmented colonies, gram-negative bacilli
   b. Normal biota of the oropharynx, nose, and GI and urogenital tracts
   c. Causes infections of the head, neck, oral cavity, and urogenital tract
   d. **Identifying characteristics**
      1) Brick red fluorescence under UV light
      2) *Porphyromonas* spp. will not grow on KVLB agar and are inhibited by bile, vancomycin, penicillin, and rifampin. However, they are resistant to kanamycin.

4. ***Fusobacterium***
   a. Asaccharolytic or weak fermenters, nonpigmented colonies, fusiform gram-negative bacilli
   b. **Normal biota of the upper respiratory and GI tracts**
   c. *Fusobacterium* spp. cause pulmonary, blood, sinus, and dental infections in addition to brain abscesses. Many infections are associated with metastatic conditions.
   d. Two important species are ***F. nucleatum*** (causes serious pulmonary infections) and ***F. necrophorum*** (lung and liver abscesses, and arthritis). *F. nucleatum* is the more common isolate, but *F. necrophorum* causes more serious infections.
   e. **Identifying characteristics**
      1) Colony morphology: Opalescent with speckles
      2) Indole and lipase positive, nitrate and catalase negative

3) Relatively biochemically inactive
4) Inhibited by kanamycin and colistin, resistant to vancomycin

F. Anaerobic Gram-Positive Spore-Forming Bacilli

1. **General characteristics of the *Clostridium* and *Clostridioides* species**
    a. Some species are normal GI biota of humans and animals, and others are found in soil, water, and dust.
    b. Most species are anaerobic; a few are aerotolerant.
    c. Large gram-positive bacilli; some species appear gram-negative
    d. Catalase negative
    e. Most *Clostridium* species are motile; nonmotile species include *C. perfringens, C. ramosum*, and *C. inocuum*.
    f. Produce a variety of exotoxins
2. ***Clostridium perfringens***
    a. *C. perfringens* is the most important pathogens in the genus. It causes **gas gangrene (myonecrosis)**, postabortion sepsis, abdominal infections, and enterocolitis.
    b. Major cause of **food poisoning** (from meats and gravy), resulting in a mild to moderate diarrhea without vomiting
    c. Bacteria are acquired through puncture wound or by ingestion. *C. perfringens* is normal biota of the GI tract and can spread from this site following trauma.
    d. *C. perfringens* is also normal biota of the female genital tract and can cause postpartum and postabortion infections.
    e. Patients who are diabetic with circulatory disorders are more prone to infection.
    f. *C. perfringens* secretes enzymes and exotoxins that cause severe tissue damage. Species are subdivided into types based on exotoxins produced. All types produce alpha-toxin (lecithinase).
    g. **Identifying characteristics**
        1) Produces a **double zone of beta-hemolysis on SBA** incubated anaerobically
        2) *C. perfringens* exhibits a positive (enhanced hemolysis) **reverse CAMP test.** In this assay, *Streptococcus agalactiae* (group B streptococci) is substituted for *Staphylococcus aureus* in the standard CAMP test.
        3) Positive for **lecithinase** and glucose, lactose, maltose, and fructose fermentation
        4) Spores are subterminal but difficult to induce.
        5) **Nonmotile**
        6) Nagler test: Antilecithinase antibody is swabbed onto half of an egg yolk agar plate. The isolate is inoculated onto both halves of the plate. *C. perfringens* produces lecithinase, which will produce an opaque zone on the half of the plate without the antibody. The antibody will neutralize lecithinase, preventing the opaque zone from forming. This test is not performed much today.

3. ***Clostridium tetani***
   a. Causes **tetanus**
   b. *C. tetani* produces **tetanospasmin**, a neurotoxin that affects the anterior horn cells of the spinal cord, resulting in involuntary muscle contractions. Contractions begin with the neck and jaw ("**lock jaw**") and progress to a backward arching of the back muscles.
   c. Bacteria and spores gain entry into the host by puncture wounds contaminated with soil, or by wounds, which may include gunshots, burns, or animal bites. The bacteria produce little necrosis.
   d. **Treatment and prevention:** Antitoxin and vaccine (DTaP: diphtheria, tetanus, and acellular pertussistrivalent vaccine) booster every 5 years
   e. **Identifying characteristics**
      1) Gram-positive bacilli with round/terminal spores that resemble drumsticks
      2) Gelatinase, indole and motility positive, lecithinase and lipase negative
      3) Generally not cultured; diagnosis made by signs and symptoms and toxin detection
4. ***Clostridium botulinum***
   a. Causes **botulism**
   b. **Botulism toxin** is a neurotoxin that binds to the synapse of nerve fibers, resulting in acute (flaccid) paralysis and death. Of the seven toxogenic types, types A, B, E, and F are associated with human botulism.
   c. **Foodborne botulism** is usually acquired by ingestions of spoiled, home-canned foods and fermented fish in which the spores are not destroyed.
   d. **Infant botulism** is the most common type of botulism, 73% of cases in the United States in 2016. Bacteria are ingested and grow in the infant GI tract and can cause a rapidly fatal infection. Honey can contain botulinum spores and should not be given to children less than 12 months old.
   e. **Wound botulism** occurs if bacterial spores enter a wound and germinate.
   f. **Identifying characteristics**
      1) Lipase, lecithinase, glucose, and motility positive
      2) Spores are oval/subterminal and resemble tennis rackets.
5. ***Clostridioides* (*Clostridium*) *difficile***
   a. Causes antibiotic-associated pseudomembranous colitis and diarrhea, also referred to as *C. difficile*-associate disease
   b. *C. difficile* is normal GI biota in a small percentage of the population, and as many as 30% of hospitalized patients may carry the bacteria. It is a significant cause of healthcare-associated infections.
   c. High carriage rate in the intestines of patients who have received broad-spectrum antimicrobial agents that have eliminated the normal intestinal biota
   d. **Produces enterotoxin A and/or cytotoxin B:** Infections can be diagnosed by detecting either toxin in the stool. The toxins can be detected using various immunologic methods, including enzyme immunoassay.
   e. NAATs of stool samples are a stand-alone test (does not require confirmation) and are commonly used for diagnosis.

f. **Identifying characteristics**
   1) Because *C. difficile* can be normal biota, stool cultures can sometimes be too sensitive; they are time consuming and not frequently performed. Cultures for *C. difficile* should only be performed on watery or unformed stools. It is also important to test isolates for toxin production. Cycloserine-cefoxitin-fructose agar (CCFA) is used for isolating *C. difficile* from stool specimens. *C. difficile* is weakly fructose positive. Despite being fructose positive, the colonies are yellow. In reduced (i.e., anaerobic) conditions, the pH indicator turns yellow at a pH of about 5.3. The product will also fluoresce yellow-green.
   2) Lecithinase, lipase, and indol negative, and positive for motility and glucose and fructose fermentation
   3) Spores are oval and subterminal.

6. **Other *Clostridium* spp.** are infrequently associated with infections.
   a. *C. septicum*, normal biota of the gastrointestinal tract, indicates colon cancer when isolated in blood cultures. This is a characteristic associated with the *Streptococcus bovis* group as well.
   b. *C. septicum*, along with *C. perfringens*, is a member of the histotoxic group and is occasionally linked to gas gangrene.

G. Anaerobic Nonspore-Forming Gram-Positive Bacilli

1. **Anaerobic *Actinomyces***
   a. Normal biota of animal and human mucous membranes
   b. ***A. israelii***, which causes abdomen and chest infections and pelvic actinomycosis in women with intrauterine devices, is the most common pathogen.
   c. **Identifying characteristics**
      1) Exudate contains sulfur granules—dense clumps of bacteria.
      2) Gram-positive bacilli with a beaded appearance, often filamentous
      3) Colony morphology: Smooth to molar toothlike
2. ***Cutibacterium* and *Propionibacterium***
   a. Species include *Cutibacterium (Propionibacterium) acnes* and *P. propionicus*
   b. Often called anaerobic diphtheroids
   c. Normal biota of the skin, mouth, and GI tract
   d. Rarely pathogenic
   e. Catalase and indole positive
3. ***Mobiluncus***
   a. Associated with **BV**, PID, and abdominal infections
   b. Curved bacilli
   c. Motile, catalase and indole negative
   d. Inhibited by vancomycin
4. ***Lactobacillus***
   a. *Lactobacillus* is normal biota of the GI and female genital tracts. This organism helps to maintain an acidic environment in the vagina. If the population of lactobacilli decreases, the risk of BV increases.
   b. Rarely pathogenic

c. Lactobacilli are generally aerotolerant anaerobes that will form small alpha-hemolytic colonies on SBA.
d. Catalase negative and nonmotile bacilli

5. *Bifidobacterium*: Mostly nonpathogenic normal oral and intestinal biota
6. *Eubacterium*: Mostly nonpathogenic normal oral and intestinal biota
7. *Eggerthella*: Part of the normal human intestinal microbiome. *E. lenta* has recently been identified in bacteremia, generally in older patients.

H. Anaerobic Gram-Positive and Gram-Negative Cocci

1. General characteristics of anaerobic cocci
   a. Normal biota of the intestines, female genital tract, oral cavity, and respiratory tract
   b. Weak pathogens, associated with polymicrobial liver and brain abscesses and wound infections
2. **Anaerobic gram-positive cocci**
   a. ***Peptococcus***, the only species is *P. niger*
      1) Catalase positive
      2) Produces olive-green colonies that become black
   b. *Peptostreptococcus*
      1) *Peptostreptococcus* is the most common gram-positive anaerobic coccus isolated in the clinical laboratory.
      2) ***P. anaerobius*** is inhibited by **sodium polyanethole sulfonate** (SPS).
   c. ***Finegoldia magna***, formerly *Peptostreptococcus magnus*
   d. ***Peptoniphilus asaccharolytica***, formerly *Peptostreptococcus asaccharolyticus*
3. **Anaerobic gram-negative cocci**
   a. ***Veillonella***
   b. **Identifying characteristics**
      1) Small, gram-negative cocci
      2) Reduces nitrate to nitrite, does not ferment any carbohydrates
      3) Inhibited by kanamycin and colistin but resistant to vancomycin

V. *CHLAMYDIA, RICKETTSIA, MYCOPLASMA*, AND SIMILAR ORGANISMS

A. *Chlamydia* and *Chlamydophila*

1. **Obligate intracellular parasites**
2. Formerly believed to be energy parasites, gene sequencing has identified the ability to produce some ATP via substrate-level phosphorylation. The bacteria require glucose-6-phosphate from the host cell.
3. Contain both DNA and RNA and are susceptible to antimicrobial agents
4. **Diagnosis**
   a. **Cytological methods:** Detect chlamydia inclusions in epithelial cells
   b. **Cell cultures** are required to grow the bacteria and are rarely performed today
   c. **NAATs** are the most common diagnostic method.
   d. **Serology:** Antibody to lipopolysaccharide and outer membrane protein antigens

5. Three important species
   a. ***Chlamydia trachomatis***
      1) Causes lymphogranuloma venereum, trachoma, urethritis, conjunctivitis, and infant pneumonia
      2) **Trachoma is the leading cause of blindness in the world.**
      3) **No animal vectors:** It is spread by human-to-human contact.
      4) **Diagnosis:** Enzyme immunoassays and NAATs
   b. ***Chlamydophila* (*Chlamydia*) *pneumoniae***
      1) Mild respiratory tract infections producing flulike symptoms, may also cause Guillain-Barré syndrome
      2) No animal vectors; it is spread by human-to-human contact.
      3) **Diagnosis** is best made by using NAATs.
      4) **Serology:** Detection of antibodies by micro-immunofluorescence in serum is also a common mode of diagnosis.
   c. ***Chlamydiophila (Chlamydia) psittaci***
      1) Causes **psittacosis** (ornithosis) or parrot fever, a disease of parrots, parakeets, cockatiels, and other birds such as turkeys and chickens
      2) Humans get infections by the inhalation of bird fecal dust; infections are uncommon in the United States.
      3) **Incubation period 1–2 weeks:** Chills, fever, malaise, can progress to pneumonia, which can be fatal
      4) Occupational hazard to farmers, pet shop employees, and bird owners
      5) Diagnose by serology

B. *Rickettsia* and Similar Genera

1. *Rickettsia* and *Ehrlichia* are **obligate intracellular parasites** requiring nucleotides and other metabolic building blocks from host cells.
2. **Infections are generally spread by insect vectors** (ticks, mites, and lice).
3. Diagnosis is often made by clinical symptoms, patient history, and serology. Immunohistology and polymerase chain reaction assays are also available.
4. Weil-Felix serologic test utilizes *Proteus* antigens. This assay is nonspecific and is not used much today.
5. Direct microscopic examination for *Rickettsia* organisms is possible using stains such as Giemsa, Machiavello, or Gimenez. The Gimenez stain is recommended, which colors the organisms a brilliant red against a green background.
6. The bacteria can be grown in embryonated eggs and cell cultures. However, cultures require a biosafety level 3 laboratory, and, for safety concerns, cultures are not recommended.
7. **Clinically important species**
   a. ***R. rickettsii*** causes Rocky Mountain spotted fever (RMSF) and is the most important species in the United States. It is a member of the spotted fever group and is carried by ticks. RMSF is a very serious disease; death rates are approximately 25%.

b. *R. prowazekii* causes typhus, also called epidemic or louse-borne typhus; it is carried by human lice. Squirrels are also reservoirs. Brill-Zinsser disease is a reactivation of the original infection.
c. ***R. typhi*** causes endemic or murine typhus. It is transmitted by fleas.
d. ***Coxiella burnetii*** causes Q fever. It is transmitted by inhalation, contact with fomites, and ingestion of contaminated milk.
e. ***Ehrlichia chaffeensis*** causes ehrlichiosis or human monocytic ehrlichiosis. It is transmitted by ticks and is endemic to the United States.
f. ***Anaplasma (Ehrlichia) phagocytophilum*** causes human granulocytic anaplasmosis.
g. *Orienta (Rickettsia) tsutsugamushi* causes scrub typhus, a disease found primarily in the Asian continent.

C. *Mycoplasma* and *Ureaplasma*

1. Smallest free-living organisms, about the size of a large virus and beyond the resolution of light microscopes
2. They lack a cell wall, making them pleomorphic and resistant to all antibiotics that inhibit cell wall synthesis (e.g., beta-lactams).
3. They contain both RNA and DNA and can self-replicate.
4. Infections can be diagnosed by serology, and this is probably the most common method of diagnosing *Mycoplasma pneumoniae* infection.
5. When attempting to recover mycoplasmata or perform NAATs a number of clinical specimens can be submitted. If swabs are used, the site should be vigorously sampled because the bacteria are primarily cell associated.
6. Many species of *Mycoplasma* and *Ureaplasma* grow on special laboratory media, including **SP4 and A8 agars and Shepard's 10 B broth.** *U. urealyticum* produces a strong alkaline pH because of the activity of **urease.** Some species will also grow on chocolate agar. Some species produce fried egg colony morphology (e.g., *M. hominis*).
7. **Clinically important species**

a. ***M. pneumoniae***
   1) Causes tracheobronchitis and community-acquired primary atypical (walking) pneumonia, resulting in a dry, nonproductive cough
   2) Spread by direct respiratory contact
   3) Mostly seen in teenagers and young adults; lacks a seasonal distribution

b. ***M. hominis***
   1) Opportunistic pathogen linked to PID in sexually active adults
   2) May cause infant meningitis and postpartum fever

c. ***Ureaplasma urealyticum***
   1) Causes urethritis and may cause other genital tract infections
   2) Requires urea

VI. SPIROCHETES

A. Genera Causing Human Disease: *Treponema, Leptospira*, and *Borrelia*

1. Spirochetes are long, slender, helically curved bacilli that cannot usually be seen on Gram stain.
2. Special stains such as silver and Giemsa will stain spirochetes, silver for all spirochetes and Giemsa only for *Borrelia.*
3. Spirochetes can be observed by **darkfield** or **phase-contrast microscopy.**

B. *Treponema pallidum* subsp. *pallidum*

1. Causes **syphilis**
2. Transmitted by sexual contact, direct blood transmission, or transplacentally (congenital syphilis)
3. **Stages of syphilis**
   a. **Primary:** Chancre at the site of inoculation
   b. **Secondary:** Skin rash and lesions on oral mucosa
   c. **Latent:** Absence of clinical symptoms
   d. **Tertiary:** CNS disorders (neurosyphilis), aneurysms, and skin, liver, and bone disorders
4. **Congenital syphilis** occurs when a fetus is infected *in utero.* The outcome is often quite severe. Infection can result in stillbirth and birth defects such as malformed bones and cartilage, anemia, jaundice, and hepatosplenomegaly. Up to 40% of babies born to women with untreated syphilis may be stillborn, or die from the infection soon after birth.
5. ***T. pallidum* cannot be cultured on artificial media.** The bacteria exhibit corkscrew motility when seen by darkfield microscopy on material taken from lesions.
6. **Generally diagnosed by serology**
   a. **Nontreponemal antigen tests** include the Venereal Disease Research Laboratory **(VDRL)** and rapid plasma reagin **(RPR)** tests, which detect antibodies to cardiolipin in a complex of cardiolipin-lecithin-cholesterol and are nonspecific. These antibodies are sometimes referred to as **reagin.** Biologic false positives are caused by Lyme disease, various viruses, autoimmune disorders (e.g., systemic lupus erythematosus), and pregnancy.
   b. **Treponemal antigen tests** include the fluorescent treponemal antibody absorption **(FTA-ABS)** test and the *Treponema pallidum*-particulate antigen **(TP-PA)** test, which are specific and confirmatory.
   c. The treponemal antigen tests are more specific, have fewer false-positive results than the nontreponemal tests. Both nontreponemal and treponemal assays are sensitive in secondary syphilis. After successful treatment, the antibody titer of nontreponemal tests typically declines, while the antibody titer in treponemal tests remain relatively high.
7. Other clinically important species include *T. pallidum* subsp. *pertenue* (yaws), *T. pallidum* subsp. *endemicum* (endemic syphilis), and *T. carateum* (pinta). These agents are rare in the United States.

C. *Borrelia*

1. ***Borrelia recurrentis***
   a. *B. recurrentis* causes **epidemic relapsing fever**, which is characterized by recurrent high fever, chills, muscle pain, and headache. Other *Borrelia* spp. cause **endemic relapsing fever** transmitted by arthropods such as ticks (tickborne relapsing fever).
   b. Humans are the only known reservoir for *B. recurrentis*; bacteria are transmitted by body lice (Louse-borne relapsing fever).
   c. *Borrelia* spp. are difficult to culture, and serologic tests are insensitive.
   d. **Diagnosis** is based on observing bacteria in the peripheral bloodstream via the Giemsa or silver stains, or by darkfield microscopy. Due to low bacterial numbers, it can be difficult to diagnose infections by staining.
2. ***Borrelia burgdorferi***
   a. Causes **Lyme disease**, also known as Lyme borreliosis
   b. ***B. burgdorferi* is the most common tickborne disease in the United States.** It is transmitted by the deer tick (*Ixodes damninii*).
   c. **Stages of Lyme disease**
      1) **Early localized (stage I):** A rash at the bite site **(erythema migrans)** produces a characteristic "bull's eye" pattern in about 60% of the patients.
      2) **Early disseminated (stage II):** Bacteria enter the bloodstream (producing flulike symptoms) and then can go to the bones, joints (arthritis), CNS (meningitis, paralysis), or heart (palpitations, carditis). Patients present with fatigue, malaise, arthralgia, myalgia, and headaches.
      3) **Late stage (stage III):** This stage is characterized by chronic arthritis and acrodermatitis that can continue for years.
   d. **Diagnosis**
      1) Serologic tests are sensitive in diagnosing Lyme disease. **Western immunoblotting** is considered the most accurate method for antibody detection. EIA and immunofluorescent assays are generally used as screening tests.
      2) Difficult to culture and too few bacteria to detect by direct microscopy

D. *Leptospira*

1. *L. interrogans* causes leptospirosis (Weil's disease).
2. **Zoonosis of rodents, dogs, and cattle**
3. **Humans acquire the infection by contact with contaminated animal urine.**
4. The infection can produce fever, kidney, liver, and CNS involvement.
5. **Diagnosis of leptospirosis**
   a. Direct examination via darkfield microscopy, or with silver stain
   b. Microorganisms can be recovered in cultures. Blood is the most sensitive specimen during early infections. Urine should be cultured after the second week. Media include Ellinghausen-McCullough-Johnson-Harris and Fletcher's.
   c. Most cases are diagnosed by serology, although methods vary in sensitivity.

VII. ANTIMICROBIAL AGENTS AND ANTIMICROBIAL SUSCEPTIBILITY TESTING

A. Definitions

1. An **antibiotic** is a molecule produced by microorganisms that inhibits the growth of other microorganisms. Antibiotics can also be synthetic.
2. **Cidal:** Kills microorganisms (e.g., bactericidal compound kills bacteria)
3. **Static:** Inhibits the growth of microorganisms (e.g., bacteriostatic compound inhibits bacterial growth)
4. **Synergy:** When two or more antimicrobials are used and the combined effect is greater than what would be expected for the simple additive effect of the agents

B. Spectrum of Action

1. Narrow-spectrum antimicrobial agent: Limited range of action
2. Broad-spectrum antimicrobial agent: Active against a wide range of bacteria

C. Classes of Antimicrobial Agents and Their Mode of Action

1. **Beta-lactam antibiotics** inhibit cell wall synthesis (e.g., penicillins, cephalosporins, monobactams, and carbapenems). They are the most used class of antibacterial agents. The class cephalosporin contains a large number of agents categorized as **narrow spectrum** (first generation), **intermediate spectrum** (second generation), **broad spectrum** (third generation), **broad spectrum** (fourth generation), and **extended spectrum** (fifth generation). The **carbapenems**, for example, imipenem, meropenem, and ertapenem, are regarded as having the broadest spectrum among the beta-lactam antibiotics. They are resistant to many beta-lactamases.
2. **Beta-lactamase inhibitors:** Bacteria can exhibit resistance to the beta-lactam antibiotics by producing an enzyme **(beta-lactamase)** that cleaves the beta-lactam ring, inactivating the antibiotic. Beta-lactamase inhibitors can be given with a beta-lactam antibiotic to provide effective treatment. Clavulanic acid, sulbactam, tazobactam, avibactam, and RPX7009 are examples of beta-lactamase inhibitors.
3. **Aminoglycosides** inhibit protein synthesis at the 30S ribosomal subunit and are active against gram-negative and gram-positive bacteria (e.g., gentamicin, tobramycin, and netilmicin). Tobramycin is bactericidal, whereas the others are bacteristatic. They have no activity against obligate anaerobes. Because of potential toxicity, dosage should be monitored using peak and trough values in peripheral blood.
4. **Tetracyclines** inhibit protein synthesis at the 30S ribosomal subunit (e.g., doxycycline and minocycline). They are active against gram-positive and gram-negative bacteria and *Mycoplasma* and *Chlamydia*. Increased resistance has limited their use.
5. **Chloramphenicol** inhibits protein synthesis by binding to the 50S ribosomal subunit. It is broad spectrum and used to treat serious gram-negative infections such as meningitis. Risk of bone marrow toxicity, aplastic anemia (bone marrow suppression), limits use to serious infections.

6. **Macrolides** inhibit protein synthesis by targeting the 50S ribosomal subunit (e.g., azithromycin, erythromycin, and clarithromycin).
7. **Ketolides** semi-synthetic macrolides that inhibit protein synthesis by targeting the 50S ribosomal subunit (e.g., telithromycin).
8. **Oxazolidinones** inhibit protein synthesis by targeting the 50S ribosomal subunit (e.g., linezolid).
9. **Sulfonamides** inhibit folic acid synthesis by forming nonfunctional analogs of folic acid.
10. **Glycopeptides** inhibit cell wall formation by inhibiting peptidoglycan synthesis; vancomycin is the only glycopeptide approved for use in the United States. Vancomycin-resistant enterococci, vancomycin-intermediate *S. aureus*, and vancomycin-resistant *S. aureus* have been isolated.
11. **Quinolones** inhibit DNA activity by inactivating DNA gyrase. Newer agents are known as fluoroquinolones (e.g., ciprofloxacin and levofloxacin).
12. **Polymyxins** disrupt plasma membranes; they are used to treat infections caused by gram-negative bacteria (e.g., polymyxin B and polymyxin E).
13. **Nitrofurantoin** inhibits bacterial enzymes; nitrofurantoin is used to treat UTIs.

D. Antimicrobial Susceptibility Testing

1. Bacterial infections can sometimes be treated once the identification has been confirmed, for example, *S. pyogenes* and penicillin (i.e., empirical treatment). However, because drug resistance is variable among most bacterial species, testing must be done to determine which agent is the best to use. Bacteria can exhibit a resistance phenotype from an altered permeability to the drug, efflux pumps that eliminate the drug, enzymatic inactivation of the drug, altered metabolic pathway that bypasses reaction inhibited by the drug, or an altered target.
2. **Dilution tests**
   a. In these assays, bacteria are exposed to different concentrations of antimicrobial agents. The smallest concentration that inhibits growth of the bacteria is recorded; this value is the **minimal inhibitory concentration** (MIC).
   b. **Broth dilutions:** Dilutions of the antimicrobial agents are prepared in broth. The assays are generally performed in microtiter plates.
   c. **Agar dilutions:** Dilutions of the antimicrobial agents are prepared in agar. Bacteria are inoculated onto the agar plates.
   d. **The minimum bactericidal concentration** (MBC) of an antimicrobial agent is defined as the lowest concentration of an antimicrobial agent that kills at least 99.9% of the bacteria in the original inoculum. This can be determined by first performing a broth dilution test and then subculturing the tubes without visible growth to agar media without antimicrobial agents. The sample taken from the tube with the lowest concentration of antimicrobial agent showing no growth on the agar media is representative of the MBC.

3. **Disk diffusion**
   a. Also referred to as the **Kirby-Bauer sensitivity test**
   b. **Standardization**
      1) **Mueller-Hinton agar (MHA),** 4 mm thick in Petri dish at a pH 7.2–7.4, is required. In the case of fastidious microorganisms (e.g., *Streptococcus pneumoniae*), MHA with 5% sheep red blood cells is used. For *influenzae, Haemophilus* test medium (HTM) is used. HTM is Mueller-Hinton base supplemented with hematin, NAD, and yeast extract.
      2) **Bacterial inoculum,** 10^8 colony forming units/mL, which is equal to a McFarland #0.5 turbidity standard
      3) MHA plates are incubated for 18 hours at 35°C in ambient air. Both HTM and MHA with sheep red blood cells are incubated in 5–7% CO_2 for 18–20 hours.
   c. After incubation, the **diameters of the zones of inhibition** are measured. The zone sizes are compared to standard interpretation charts, and the results are reported as **sensitive (S), intermediate (I), or resistant (R).**
   d. **Quality control organisms** vary depending on the susceptibility test and antimicrobials used.
   e. **Detection of MRSA**
      1) Methicillin is no longer available in the United States, so when referring to MRSA it is actually oxacillin or nafcillin resistance that is being discussed.
      2) Because populations of MRSA are often heteroresistant (some cells sensitive and much fewer resistant), testing procedures should be modified to be sensitive for the detection of MRSA.
      3) **Cefoxitin** is a more powerful inducer of oxacillin resistance and can be used in disk diffusion assays. The procedure is the same as for routine disk diffusion except that interpretive criteria are changed: for *S. aureus*, zones of ≤21 mm are reported as oxacillin resistant and results ≥22 mm are reported as sensitive.
      4) In broth dilution tests with oxacillin, *S. aureus* isolates with MICs ≤2 μg/mL are considered sensitive and results ≥4 μg/mL are resistant.
4. **Gradient diffusion**
   a. **Etest®** (AB Biodisk) provides quantitative antimicrobial susceptibility testing results.
   b. Procedure
      1) A bacterial suspension equal to a McFarland #0.5 turbidity standard is prepared.
      2) The bacteria are lawned onto a Mueller-Hinton agar plate and the Etest strips are placed on top of the agar. Each strip contains a different antimicrobial agent.
      3) After incubation, the bacteria produce an elliptical zone of inhibition around the strip. The MIC is read from a scale on the strip where the zone of inhibition crosses the strip.

5. Miscellaneous assays
   a. **Beta-lactamase** is an enzyme that confers resistance to penicillin and some of the semisynthetic penicillins (e.g., ampicillin). Several methods are available for detecting the presence of beta-lactamase. Some *Enterobacteriaceae* can produce an **extended-spectrum beta-lactamase** (ESBL). These enzymes inactivate the broad and extended spectrum cephalosporins such as ceftriaxone, cefotaxime, and ceftaroline, in addition to the monobactam aztreonam. *N. gonorrhoeae, N. meningitidis, H. influenzae*, and *Pasteurella* spp. should be tested for beta-lactamase production.
   b. **Detecting ESBLs:** test bacteria against drugs that detect ESBL, in decreasing order of sensitivity: cefpodoxime, ceftazidime, cefotaxime, ceftriaxone, aztreonam. Detection can be difficult because bacteria may only have moderate reductions in sensitivity to carbapenems.
   c. **Detecting carbapenemases:** Bacteria producing carbapenemases are resistant to most beta-lactam antibiotics including carbapenem. The enzyme was first detected in *K. pneumoniae* and was subsequently found in other *Klebsiella* spp., *E. coli*, and *Enterobacter* spp. This led to the phrase, carbapenemase-producing *Enterobacteriaceae.*
      1) Detecting carbapenemases in *Enterobacteriaceae* is a two-step approach—a screening process using carbapenems followed by a confirmation test to detect the presence of a carbapenemase in isolates that tests nonsusceptible to the carbapenems.
      2) **Modified carbapenem inactivation method (mCIM):** The test organism is incubated in water or tryptic soy broth with a filter paper disk containing a carbapenem for 4 hours. If the organism produces a carbapenemase, the carbapenem will be hydrolyzed. The disk is then placed on a lawn of growth of a carbapenem-sensitive control organism. Growth of the control organism up to the disk, indicates the presence of a carbapenemase in the test organism. The Clinical and Laboratory Standard Institute recommends this method as a confirmation test.
      3) **Carba NP test:** In this colorimetric assay, test bacteria are lysed and incubated with a solution of imipenem, zinc sulfate, and phenol red. Carbapenemase production is indicated by a pH change due to the hydrolysis of imipenem. This assay offers poor detection of OXY-48-like carbapenemase producers.
      4) **Modified Hodge Test:** The assay is based on the inactivation of a carbapenem by carbapenemase-producing *Enterobacteriaceae* that enables a carbapenem-susceptible indicator strain to grow toward a carbapenem-containing disk. While generally considered the reference method, the modified Hodge test is not performed much today due to long turn-around time and low sensitivity and specificity for certain carbapenemases.
      5) **PCR assays:** The Xpert Carba-R (Cepheid, Sunnyvale, California) is a PCR method that detects the five major families of carbapenem-resistance genes.

d. The **D-zone test** is used to detect the presence of **inducible clindamycin resistance** by erythromycin. Even though clindamycin and erythromycin are in different classes, the mechanisms of resistance are similar. A plate is inoculated as for a disk diffusion assay. A 15-µg erythromycin disk is placed 15 to 20 mm from a 2-µg clindamycin disk. After incubation, the plate is examined for a flattening of the zone of inhibition around the clindamycin disk, resembling the letter D, indicating the presence of inducible resistance to clindamycin.

VIII. PROCEDURES AND IDENTIFICATION OF BACTERIA

A. Plating Procedures

1. **General information**
   a. The clinical specimen and the suspected pathogens will determine the selection of the primary plating media.
   b. The media used will vary among laboratories because of local pathogens and personal preference of the laboratorians.
   c. Clinical specimens should be transported to the clinical microbiology laboratory as soon after collection as possible. Some specimens, such as those collected on swabs, require a transport medium to maintain viability of pathogens present.
   d. Specimens can be deemed unacceptable if they are not properly labeled, in transit too long, not placed in appropriate transport medium, or of insufficient quantity or quality.
2. **Clinical specimens**
   a. **Blood**
      1) Blood is normally sterile.
      2) Definitions and characteristics
         a) **Bacteremia:** Bacteria in the blood
         b) **Septicemia:** Bacteria increasing in numbers in the blood causing harm to the patient
         c) When drawing blood cultures, avoid skin contamination and collect sample, if possible, before antimicrobial therapy.
         d) Bacteria are in highest numbers in the blood just before fever spikes. It is important to collect several specimens at different times for greatest potential of bacterial yield (sensitivity). **The volume of blood collected has the greatest effect on isolation of bacteria.**
         e) Drawing multiple samples increases sensitivity. In acute sepsis, two samples should be drawn one immediately after the other from two different sites. Collection of 10–20 mL per culture for adults is recommended.
      3) **Cultures**
         a) Blood culture systems utilize bottles containing liquid media.
         b) Generally, two bottles are inoculated: one for aerobes and one for obligate anaerobes. However, because of the reported decrease in the

incidence of anaerobic bacteremias, a number of hospitals have stopped using anaerobic bottles.

c) Most aerobic bottles contain 5–10% CO_2.

d) Blood culture bottles often contain sodium polyanethol sulfonate **(SPS)**, an anticoagulant that also inhibits complement and inactivates neutrophils. SPS has been shown to inhibit the growth of some bacteria.

e) Several semi-automated continuous monitoring systems are available. These instruments combine an incubator with a monitoring system to identify potentially positive samples.

b. **Cerebrospinal fluid**

1) CSF surrounds the brain and spinal cord and carries nutrients and waste; it is normally sterile.
2) Meningitis is an inflammation of the meninges.
3) Encephalitis is an inflammation of the brain.
4) The most common isolates found in CSF are *Neisseria meningitidis, Streptococcus pneumoniae, Streptococcus agalactiae, E. coli, S. aureus*, and *Listeria monocytogenes.*
5) Diagnoses are made by a direct Gram stain and culturing on SBA, MAC, and chocolate agars.

c. **Throat**

1) ***S. pyogenes*** (group A *Streptococcus*) is the most important pathogen isolated in throat cultures; group B streptococci, group C streptococci, group G streptococci, and *Arcanobacterium* spp. might also be clinically significant. Screening for other pathogens may occur upon request.
2) Alpha-hemolytic streptococci viridans group, *Neisseria* spp., *Corynebacterium* spp., and coagulase-negative staphylococci make up the majority of the normal oral biota.
3) Culture on SBA and other media as needed by special request

d. **Sputum**

1) Used to diagnose lower respiratory tract infections (e.g., pneumonia)
2) The lower respiratory tract is normally sterile. However, sputum from the lungs acquires normal biota passing through the oral cavity.
3) A **direct Gram stain** is performed to determine the quality of the specimen. Acceptable specimens are cultured on sheep blood, MAC, and chocolate agars.
4) Several methods are used to determine specimen acceptability. Typically, squamous epithelial cells are an indication of contamination with oral biota, whereas polymorphonuclear cells (PMNs) indicate a quality specimen. A general rule for an acceptable specimen might be <10 squamous epithelial cells and >25 PMNs/low-power field. This does not pertain to neutropenic or atypical pneumonia samples, which often have nonpurulent sputum. Two commonly used scoring systems are the Bartlett's Q-score and the Murray-Washington method.

5) Common significant sputum isolates
   a) *S. pneumoniae* is an important cause of community-acquired pneumonia, and it is the most common cause of pneumonia in geriatric patients.
   b) *K. pneumoniae* is associated with healthcare-associated pneumonia and pneumonia in patients who are alcoholics.
   c) *S. aureus* causes community-acquired and healthcare-associated pneumonia, usually secondary to another infection or predisposing factor.
   d) *P. aeruginosa* causes healthcare-associated and severe pneumonia in patients with CF.
   e) *H. influenzae* causes infection in infants, children, and patients who are immunosuppressed. The incidence of infections has decreased since routine use of the Hib vaccine.
   f) *L. pneumophila* primarily infects middle-aged males. *Legionella* spp. will not grow on routinely used media (i.e., SBA, chocolate, and MAC).
   g) *M. pneumoniae* causes primary atypical pneumonia, which is mostly seen in young adults. *Mycoplasma* will not grow on routinely used media.

e. **Urine**
   1) Urine is normally sterile.
   2) **Bacteriuria** is bacteria in the urine, but it may not indicate a UTI.
   3) Calibrated loops are used to determine colony counts on media.
   4) Urine specimens are generally plated onto SBA and MAC or EMB.
   5) Common significant urine isolates include *E. coli, Klebsiella* spp., *Enterobacter* spp., *Proteus* spp., *S. aureus, Staphylococcus saprophyticus, Enterococcus* spp., *P. aeruginosa*, and yeast.

f. **Stool**
   1) Feces contain many species of anaerobic and facultative anaerobic normal biota.
   2) Bacteria causing gastroenteritis include *Shigella* spp., *Salmonella, Campylobacter jejuni, E. coli* (e.g., O157:H7), *Yersinia enterocolitica, Clostridioides difficile*, and *Vibrio* spp.
   3) Plating protocols vary widely but in general include selective and differential media for the isolation and screening of specific pathogens.
   4) Direct NAAT, such as the Filmarray™ (Biofire), has replaced routine stool culture is some laboratories.
   5) Rotavirus is an important cause of diarrhea in young children.

g. **Genital tract**
   1) Laboratorians commonly test for *N. gonorrhoeae* and *C. trachomatis.*
   2) The cervix is typically a sterile site. The vagina contains normal biota that changes with age. *Lactobacillus* spp. are the predominant biota during childbearing years. Earlier and late in life, staphylococci and corynebacteria predominate.

3) Types of genital tract infections
   a) **Cervicitis** and **urethritis** usually caused by *N. gonorrhoeae* and *C. trachomatis*
   b) **BV**, or nonspecific vaginitis, is due to overgrowth of some species of normal vaginal biota, most likely *Mobiluncus*. There is a corresponding decrease in lactobacilli. *Gardnerella vaginalis* is considered normal vaginal microbiota and may only be an indicator of BV.
   c) **PID** is a complication of infection caused by *N. gonorrhoeae* or *C. trachomatis* involving the endometrium or fallopian tubes.
   d) **Prostatitis** is usually caused by enterics.
   e) **Genital warts,** caused by the human papillomavirus, is the most common sexually transmitted disease.
   f) Genital herpes is primarily caused by herpes simplex virus 1, and a few cases are associated with herpes simplex virus 2.
4) Plating protocols for *N. gonorrhoeae* include using specific **selective media** (e.g., modified Thayer-Martin).
5) Molecular techniques are commonly used for detecting both *N. gonorrhoeae* and *C. trachomatis*.

h. **Wounds/abscesses**
   1) Superficial skin infections: *S. aureus* and *S. pyogenes*
   2) Folliculitis (hair follicle infection): *S. aureus* and *P. aeruginosa*
   3) Boils, bedsores, etc.: *S. aureus*
   4) Impetigo: *S. pyogenes* and *S. aureus*
   5) Erysipelis: *S. pyogenes* and less commonly *Erysipelothrix rhusiopathiae*
   6) Deep and surgical wounds and abscesses: Anaerobes from normal body sites

B. Biochemical Identification of Bacteria

1. **Gram stain**
   a. Bacteria can be placed into one of two groups, gram-positive or gram-negative, based on difference in their cell wall. Gram-positive bacteria have a thick layer of peptidoglycan, while gram-negative bacteria have a thin layer of peptidoglycan and an outer membrane.
   b. Gram-positive bacteria retain the primary stain, crystal violet and appear blue. Gram-negative bacteria decolorize, retain the counterstain safranin, and appear pink.
2. **Catalase test**
   a. The enzyme catalase produces water and oxygen from hydrogen peroxide (H_2O_2). Several drops of H_2O_2 are added to a bacterial smear on a microscope slide.
   b. If catalase is present, water and oxygen (bubbles) will form. Staphylococci are positive and streptococci are negative.
3. **Coagulase test**
   a. **Clumping factor (slide coagulase):** Formerly slide coagulase tests used rabbit plasma. Clumping indicates a positive reaction and identification of *S. aureus*. However, *S. lugdunensis* and *S. schleiferi* can also produce positive results.

Newer tests are based on latex agglutination and detect protein A in the cell wall and have higher sensitivity and specificity for *S. aureus*.

b. The **tube coagulase test** uses rabbit plasma like the slide method, but it is incubated at 37°C for up to 24 hours. *S. aureus* is positive. *S. intermedius* and *S. hyicus* are animal pathogens that are also positive. Tests must be checked at 4 hours for clot formation. Some strains produce staphylokinase, which can dissolve the clot, producing a false negative result.

4. **PYR test**
   a. This test detects the enzyme L-pyrrolidonyl arylamidase. A colony is placed on filter paper with the substrate pyrrolidonyl-α-naphthylamide (PYR).
   b. A red color after the addition of *p*-dimethylaminocinnamaldehyde (DMACA) is a positive PYR test. *S. pyogenes* and *Enterococcus* spp. are typically positive. The PYR test can also be used to differentiate *S. aureus* (negative) from *S. lugdunensis* and *S. schleiferi*, both of which are positive.
5. **Bile solubility test**
   a. Colonies of *Streptococcus pneumoniae* are soluble in sodium deoxycholate (bile).
   b. In the presence of bile at 37°C, the colonies autolyze within 30 minutes, and disappear from the agar surface.
6. **Hippurate hydrolysis test**
   a. The hippurate hydrolysis test detects the bacterial enzyme hippuricase, which hydrolyzes hippurate to glycine and benzoic acid.
   b. A positive hippurate will give a purple color after the addition of ninhydrin.
   c. Group B streptococci are hippurate positive, whereas most other beta-hemolytic streptococci are negative. In addition, the test can be used to differentiate *C. jejuni* (positive) from most other *Campylobacter* spp.
7. **Oxidase test**
   a. The oxidase test detects cytochrome oxidase that is used in the electron transport system. Several drops of oxidase reagent (tetramethyl-*p*-phenylenediamine dihydrochloride) are placed on filter paper containing bacterial colonies or directly on plate colonies.
   b. Colonies should be taken from nonselective, nondifferential media. Media with a high concentration of glucose can inhibit oxidase activity.
   c. A positive oxidase test is indicated by a purple color within 10 to 20 seconds.
8. **Indole test**
   a. The indole test detects the bacterial enzyme **tryptophanase.** Tryptophan is broken down by tryptophanase into pyruvic acid, ammonia, and indole.
   b. Indole is detected by an aldehyde indicator (Ehrlich's reagent), yielding a red color, or Kovac's reagent, yielding a bright pink color. The Ehrlich method is more sensitive but requires an extraction step with xylene.
   c. A **spot indole test**, using DMACA, has been shown to be more sensitive in detecting indole activity. The presence of a blue to blue-green color is positive. Colonies from media containing dyes (e.g., EMB and MAC) should not be tested because of the risk of a false positive result.

9. **Urease test**
   a. Urease breaks down urea to form ammonia (NH_3). Organisms are inoculated onto a urea agar slant and incubated at 35°C for 18–24 hours.
   b. A positive urease test is indicated by a bright pink color.
10. **Triple sugar iron agar (TSI)**
    a. TSI will show the pattern of glucose, lactose, and sucrose fermentation, in addition to H_2S and gas production.
    b. **Phenol red** is the pH indicator. The color of uninoculated medium is reddish-orange, yellow is acid, and red is alkaline.
    c. **Alkaline slant/alkaline deep (K/K):** Nonfermenter, not *Enterobacteriaceae*
    d. **Alkaline slant/acid deep (K/A):** Nonlactose and nonsucrose fermenter, glucose fermenter
    e. **Acid slant/acid deep (A/A):** Lactose and/or sucrose fermenter, and glucose fermenter
    f. **Black deep, production of H_2S gas:** Test system detects enzymes that produce hydrogen sulfide (H_2S) from sulfur-containing molecules in the medium. H_2S reacts with iron salts in the medium to form a black precipitate composed of ferrous sulfide.
11. **IMViC** (indole, methyl red, Voges-Proskauer, and citrate)
    a. **Indole:** Bacteria positive for indole produce tryptophanase, which breaks down tryptophan to pyruvic acid, ammonia, and indole. A pink color is a positive reaction, see above.
    b. **Methyl red (MR):** MR is a pH indicator; it is yellow at an acid pH, indicating glucose fermentation. Red is negative.
    c. **Voges-Proskauer (VP):** A positive VP reaction detects the metabolism of glucose to acetyl-methyl-carbinol (acetoin). Alpha-naphthol followed by 40% KOH is used to detect acetoin. Red is positive, and yellow is negative. Bacteria are usually MR or VP positive.
    d. **Citrate:** This test determines if citrate is used as a sole carbon source. Blue is positive and green is negative.
12. **ONPG (*o*-nitrophenyl-β-D-galactopyranoside)**
    a. This test detects the presence of β-galactosidase, an enzyme that cleaves ONPG and lactose. This test is useful in detecting delayed (late) lactose fermenters that lack, or are deficient in, beta-galactoside permease.
    b. Yellow is a positive reaction, indicating the ability to ferment lactose.
13. **Amino acid degradation test**
    a. A positive test detects bacterial enzymes that break down various amino acids. The color of positive and negative reactions depends on the pH indicator used.
    b. **Deaminase reaction:** Detects the ability of an organism to remove the amino group from specific amino acids
    c. **Decarboxylation reaction:** Detects the ability of bacteria to remove the carboxyl group from a specific amino acid
    d. **Examples** include tryptophan (tryptophan deaminase), lysine (lysine decarboxylase), and ornithine (ornithine dihydrolase).

14. **Carbohydrate fermentation test**
    a. A positive test detects the ability of bacteria to produce organic acids by the fermentation of various carbohydrates.
    b. Positive and negative reactions depend on the pH indicators used. Tubed media are inoculated and overlayed with sterile mineral oil to produce an anaerobic environment.
15. **Nitrate reduction test**
    a. A positive test determines the ability of an organism to reduce nitrate (NO_3) to nitrite (NO_2) and nitrogen gas (N_2).
    b. After the addition of the reagents (*N,N*-dimethyl-α-naphthylamine and sulfanilic acid), a pink color is positive for reduction of NO_3 to NO_2. A colorless reaction requires the addition of zinc dust to confirm a negative result. Development of a pink color after adding zinc indicates a true negative. Remaining colorless after adding the addition of zinc indicates that NO_3 was completely reduced to N_2, a positive result for nitrate reduction.

C. Multitest Systems

1. Most biochemical testing is performed using multitest methodologies.
2. Examples
    a. Analytical Profile Index (API; bioMérieux Clinical Diagnostics)
    b. Enterotube II (Becton Dickinson)
    c. Micro-ID (Remel)
    d. Vitek (bioMérieux Clinical Diagnostics), semiautomated, identification, and minimal inhibitory concentration combination plates available
    e. Microscan (Beckman Coulter) semiautomated, identification, and minimal inhibitory concentration combination plates available

D. MIDI, Inc. Identification Systems

1. The Sherlock Microbial Identification System (MIDI, Inc., Newark, Delaware) identifies the fatty acid composition of the bacterial cell wall as determined by gas chromatography.
2. The fatty acids in mycobacteria have a larger molecular weight and are identified via high-performance liquid chromatography in the Sherlock Mycobacteria Identification System.

E. Matrix-Assisted Laser Desorption/Ionization time of flight mass spectrometry

1. Biomolecules in the specimen are vaporized and ionized by a laser. The ions are separated by their molecular weight in a gas phase.
2. Ions with smaller m/z (mass-to-charge) ratio (lighter ions) and more highly charged move faster through the drift space and reach the detector sooner. Consequently, the **time of ion flight** differs according to the m/z value of the ion.
3. The instrument determines the m/z of biologic molecules, like proteins, and produces spectra of the molecules within minutes. This provides a unique protein spectral fingerprint. A computer then compares the unknown spectra to a database of protein spectra from known organisms.

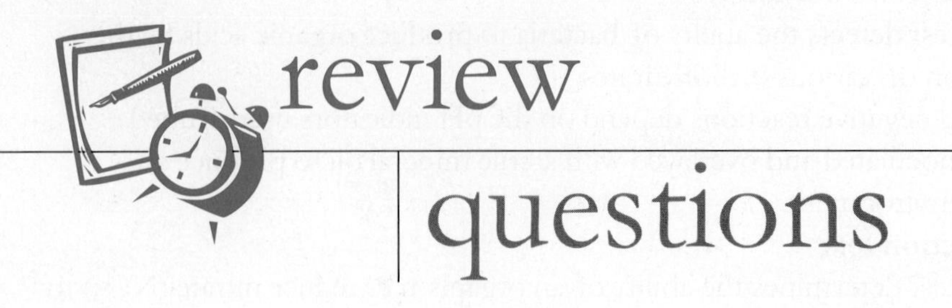

INSTRUCTIONS Each of the questions or incomplete statements that follow is comprised of four suggested responses. Select the *best* answer or completion statement in each case.

Aerobic Gram-Positive Bacteria

1. A test for the hydrolysis of esculin in the presence of bile is especially useful in identifying species of the genus
   A. *Abiotrophia*
   B. *Corynebacterium*
   C. *Enterococcus*
   D. *Staphylococcus*

2. The organism associated with a disease characterized by the presence of a pseudomembrane in the throat and the production of an exotoxin that is absorbed into the bloodstream with a lethal effect is
   A. *Arcanobacterium haemolyticum*
   B. *Staphylococcus aureus*
   C. *Streptococcus pyogenes*
   D. *Corynebacterium diphtheriae*

3. Although not common pathogens, *Aerococcus* spp. are noted for causing urinary tract infections and
   A. Pneumonia
   B. Endocarditis
   C. Wounds
   D. Gastritis

4. *Abiotrophia*, formerly known as nutritionally variant streptococci (NVS), will not grow on routine blood or chocolate agars because they are deficient in
   A. Hemin
   B. Pyridoxal
   C. Vitamin B_{12}
   D. Thiophene-2-carboxylic hydrazide

5. Exfoliatin produced by *Staphylococcus aureus* is responsible for causing
   A. Enterocolitis
   B. Toxic shock syndrome
   C. Scalded skin syndrome
   D. Staphylococcal pneumonia

6. A gram-positive rod sometimes associated with pharyngitis
   A. *Arcanobacterium haemolyticum*
   B. *Bacillus cereus*
   C. *Corynebacterium urealyticum*
   D. *Erysipelothrix rhusiopathiae*
7. A gram-positive coccus that is catalase positive, lysostaphin resistant, and modified oxidase positive is best identified as a member of the genus
   A. *Micrococcus*
   B. *Lactococcus*
   C. *Pediococcus*
   D. *Staphylococcus*
8. *Nocardia brasiliensis* infections in humans characteristically produce
   A. Carbuncles
   B. Draining cutaneous sinuses
   C. Septic shock
   D. Serous effusions
9. *Erysipelothrix* infections in humans characteristically produce
   A. Pathology at the point of entrance of the organism
   B. Central nervous system pathology
   C. Pathology in the lower respiratory tract
   D. The formation of abscesses in visceral organs
10. The soil inhabitant, *Streptomyces*, is associated with
    A. Erysipeloid
    B. Thrush
    C. Actinomycotic mycetoma
    D. Anthrax
11. *Staphylococcus saprophyticus*, a recognized pathogen, is a cause of
    A. Furuncles
    B. Impetigo
    C. Otitis media
    D. Urinary tract infections
12. Color Plate 25 ■ shows the Gram stain of a blood culture on a 23-year-old woman who presented with fever and flulike symptoms in her ninth month of pregnancy. The isolate on sheep blood agar (SBA) produced small, translucent beta-hemolytic colonies. Which of the following is the most likely etiologic agent in this case?
    A. *Listeria monocytogenes*
    B. *Propionibacterium acnes*
    C. *Streptococcus agalactiae*
    D. *Streptococcus pyogenes*
13. The etiologic agent most commonly associated with septicemia and meningitis of newborns is
    A. *Streptococcus agalactiae*
    B. *Streptococcus bovis* group
    C. *Streptococcus pneumoniae*
    D. *Streptococcus pyogenes*
14. Which of the following is the most commonly isolated species of *Bacillus* in opportunistic infections such as bacteremia, posttraumatic infections of the eye, and endocarditis?
    A. *B. circulans*
    B. *B. cereus*
    C. *B. licheniformis*
    D. *B. subtilis*
15. Loeffler's serum medium is recommended for the cultivation of
    A. *Abiotrophia* sp.
    B. *Corynebacterium diphtheriae*
    C. *Leuconostoc* sp.
    D. *Streptococcus agalactiae*

16. On Tinsdale agar, colonies of *Corynebacterium diphtheriae* are characterized by the observance of
    A. Liquefaction of the agar surrounding the colonies on the medium
    B. Opalescent colonies with a white precipitate in the surrounding agar
    C. Black colonies on the culture medium surrounded by brown halos
    D. Pitting of the agar medium surrounding the colonies

17. Precipitates of diphtheria toxin and antitoxin formed in agar gels are an *in vitro* means for detecting toxigenic strains of *Corynebacterium diphtheriae*. The name of this test procedure is the
    A. D-test
    B. Elek test
    C. Nagler test
    D. Modified Hodge test

18. The etiologic agent of the disease erysipelas is
    A. *Staphylococcus aureus*
    B. *Streptobacillus moniliformis*
    C. *Streptococcus agalactiae*
    D. *Streptococcus pyogenes*

19. *Staphylococcus aureus*, when present, could most likely be recovered from a stool sample if the primary plating medium included
    A. Bismuth sulfite
    B. Phenylethyl alcohol
    C. Thiosulfate-citrate-bile salts sucrose
    D. Xylose-lysine-deoxycholate

20. A common member of the normal biota of the upper respiratory tract is
    A. *Corynebacterium jeikeium*
    B. *Lactobacillus*
    C. *Staphylococcus epidermidis*
    D. Viridans streptococcus

21. Streptococci obtain all their energy from the fermentation of sugars to
    A. Formic acid
    B. Lactic acid
    C. Succinic acid
    D. Valeric acid

22. Streptococci are unable to synthesize the enzyme
    A. Catalase
    B. Kinase
    C. Hyaluronidase
    D. Lipase

23. The beta-hemolysis produced by group A *Streptococcus* seen on the surface of a SBA plate incubated aerobically is primarily the result of streptolysin
    A. H
    B. M
    C. O
    D. S

24. A sputum culture yields moderate growth of gram-negative diplococci forming tan colonies that are tributyrin hydrolysis positive. You should suspect
    A. *Actinomyces* sp.
    B. *Bacillus* sp.
    C. *Moraxella* sp.
    D. *Rhodococcus* sp.

25. The production of H_2S is one characteristic used to differentiate which of the aerobic gram-positive bacilli?
    A. *Corynebacterium*
    B. *Erysipelothrix*
    C. *Lactobacillus*
    D. *Nocardia*

26. Growth in a 48-hour semisolid agar stab culture at room temperature reveals lateral filamentous growth away from the stab near the top of the medium. This observation is most characteristic of which organism?
    A. *Rhodococcus* sp.
    B. *Corynebacterium urealyticum*
    C. *Enterococcus faecalis*
    D. *Listeria monocytogenes*

27. This bacterium, pathogenic for swine, horses, and cattle, is also known to cause disease in compromised human hosts. When grown on culture media, it produces pale pink colonies that help to presumptively identify it as
    A. *Arcanobacterium hemolyticum*
    B. *Actinomyces naeslundii*
    C. *Gardnerella vaginalis*
    D. *Rhodococcus equi*

28. Most common cause of pneumonia in elderly patients
    A. *Chlamydophila pneumoniae*
    B. *Klebsiella pneumoniae*
    C. *Mycoplasma pneumoniae*
    D. *Streptococcus pneumoniae*

29. *Nocardia* can be differentiated from *Actinomyces* based on
    A. *Nocardia* being an obligate anaerobe
    B. The partial-acid fast staining reaction of *Actinomyces*
    C. The production of sulfur granules in cases of nocardiosis
    D. *Nocardia* being catalase positive

30. *Enterococcus faecium* is characteristically
    A. Inhibited by the presence of bile in culture media
    B. Able to grow in the presence of high concentrations of salt
    C. L-pyrolidonyl-α-naphthylamide (PYR) negative
    D. Beta-hemolytic

31. A negative PYR test is demonstrated by
    A. *Enterococcus faecalis*
    B. *Enterococcus faecium*
    C. *Streptococcus pyogenes*
    D. Viridans streptococci

32. A Gram stain of a sputum specimen from a patient with a suspected case of lobar pneumonia reveals many white blood cells and many gram-positive cocci, which are primarily in pairs. Which of the following statements would be appropriate, given these findings?
    A. A PYR test should be performed on the culture isolate.
    B. An Elek test should be performed on the culture isolate.
    C. An optochin test should be performed on the culture isolate.
    D. A hippurate hydrolysis test should be performed on the culture isolate.

33. A child presented in August at the pediatric clinic with a superficial skin infection of the neck. The large, itchy lesions were cultured, and the diagnosis of impetigo was made. One of the etiologic agents of this clinical condition is
    A. *Erysipelothrix rhusiopathiae*
    B. *Corynebacterium diphtheriae*
    C. *Staphylococcus saprophyticus*
    D. *Streptococcus pyogenes*

34. An identifying characteristic of *Staphylococcus aureus* is
    A. DNase negative
    B. Coagulase negative
    C. Mannitol fermentation positive
    D. Growth inhibition in presence of increased salt

35. Which of the following organisms is able to hydrolyze sodium hippurate to benzoic acid and glycine?
    A. *Streptococcus agalactiae*
    B. *Streptococcus pneumoniae*
    C. *Listeria monocytogenes*
    D. *Enterococcus faecalis*

36. Which of the following is characteristic of *Listeria monocytogenes*?
    A. CAMP test positive
    B. Catalase negative
    C. Esculin hydrolysis negative
    D. Motile at 37°C

37. Which of the following is associated with *Staphylococcus aureus*?
    A. Exotoxin production causing scarlet fever
    B. Coagulase production converts fibrinogen to fibrin.
    C. Produces a superantigen that triggers rheumatic fever
    D. Isolates are typically beta-lactamase negative.

38. Which of the following is a characteristic of most staphylococci that would help in their isolation from clinical specimens?
    A. Bile resistance
    B. Growth at 55°C
    C. High salt tolerance
    D. Resistance to novobiocin

39. Which of the following species of *Bacillus* is nonmotile?
    A. *B. cereus*
    B. *B. subtilis*
    C. *B. anthracis*
    D. *B. thuringiensis*

40. Which one of the following diseases involves erythrogenic toxin?
    A. Cutaneous anthrax
    B. Diphtheria
    C. Impetigo
    D. Scarlet fever

41. Cultures of the posterior pharynx are most commonly submitted to the clinical laboratory for the detection of
    A. *Corynebacterium diphtheriae*
    B. *Staphylococcus aureus*
    C. *Streptococcus pneumoniae*
    D. *Streptococcus pyogenes*

42. *Streptococcus sanguis*, a viridans streptococcus, is most commonly associated with which of the following clinical conditions?
    A. Otitis media
    B. Pharyngitis
    C. Relapsing fever
    D. Subacute bacterial endocarditis

43. Rust-colored sputum in cases of lobar pneumonia is common of which of the following possible etiologic agents?
    A. *Corynebacterium jeikeium*
    B. *Staphylococcus aureus*
    C. *Streptococcus pneumoniae*
    D. *Streptococcus pyogenes*

44. A urine culture from a 23-year-old female grew a catalase-positive gram-positive coccus (>100,000 cfu/mL), which would most likely be
    A. *Staphylococcus saprophyticus*
    B. *Enterococcus faecalis*
    C. *Streptococcus bovis* group
    D. *Streptococcus* viridans

45. Cystine-tellurite blood agar plates are recommended for the isolation of
    A. *Corynebacterium diphtheriae*
    B. *Streptococcus agalaciae*
    C. *Streptococcus pyogenes*
    D. Group D streptococci

46. The pulmonary form of anthrax is known as
    A. Valley fever
    B. Walking pneumonia
    C. Farmers' lung
    D. Woolsorters' disease

47. Pleomorphic gram-positive bacilli in a Gram stain best describes
    A. *Bacillus anthracis*
    B. *Bacillus subtilis*
    C. *Listeria monocytogenes*
    D. *Corynebacterium pseudodiphtheriticum*
48. An aerobic gram-positive rod known to cause bacteremia in hospitalized, patients who are immunocompromised is
    A. *Bacillus anthracis*
    B. *Corynebacterium jeikeium*
    C. *Corynebacterium ulcerans*
    D. *Corynebacterium urealyticum*
49. A patient on immunosuppressive therapy undergoing a bone marrow transplant de veloped a pulmonary abscess with symptoms of neurologic involvement. A brain abscess was detected by magnetic resonance imaging, and aspirated material grew an aerobic, filamentous, branching gram-positive organism, which stained weakly acid-fast. The most likely etiologic agent in this case would be
    A. *Actinomyces israelii*
    B. *Nocardia* sp.
    C. *Mycobacterium tuberculosis*
    D. *Propionibacterium acnes*
50. Which of the following is catalase negative?
    A. *Bacillus*
    B. *Corynebacterium*
    C. *Leuconostoc*
    D. *Listeria*
51. Colonies of *Listeria monocytogenes* on an SBA plate most closely resemble colonies of
    A. *Corynebacterium diphtheriae*
    B. *Streptococcus agalactiae*
    C. *Streptococcus bovis* group
    D. *Rhodococcus equi*
52. The most common etiologic agent of infections associated with the surgical insertion of prosthetic devices such as artificial heart valves and cerebrospinal fluid shunts is
    A. *Corynebacterium urealyticum*
    B. *Staphylococcus capitis*
    C. *Staphylococcus epidermidis*
    D. *Streptococcus mutans*
53. The description of "Medusa head" colonies on solid agar is most characteristic of
    A. *Bacillus anthracis*
    B. *Enterococcus faecalis*
    C. *Staphylococcus saprophyticus*
    D. *Streptococcus agalactiae*
54. Which of the following is most likely to be isolated in cultures from the anterior nares of healthcare workers?
    A. *Bacillus cereus*
    B. *Streptococcus pneumoniae*
    C. *Staphylococcus aureus*
    D. *Staphylococcus saprophyticus*
55. Ethylhydrocupreine HCl susceptibility is a presumptive test for the identification of
    A. Viridans streptococci
    B. *Streptococcus pyogenes*
    C. *Streptococcus agalactiae*
    D. *Streptococcus pneumoniae*
56. Solubility in the presence of sodium desoxycholate is characteristic of
    A. *Enterococcus faecalis*
    B. *Streptococcus agalactiae*
    C. *Streptococcus mutans*
    D. *Streptococcus pneumoniae*

57. Family members attending a picnic became ill about 2 hours after eating. The illness was characterized by rapid onset of violent vomiting but no fever. The most likely bacterial cause of such symptoms would be food poisoning due to
    A. *Enterococcus faecium*
    B. *Bacillus subtilis*
    C. *Staphylococcus aureus*
    D. *Listeria monocytogenes*

58. The novobiocin susceptibility test is used for the identification of
    A. *Corynebacterium diphtheriae*
    B. *Streptococcus pyogenes*
    C. *Streptococcus pneumoniae*
    D. *Staphylococcus saprophyticus*

59. Tellurite reduction is used for the presumptive identification of
    A. *Bacillus anthracis*
    B. *Corynebacterium diphtheriae*
    C. *Erysipelothrix rhusiopathiae*
    D. *Staphylococcus saprophyticus*

60. The etiologic agent of the majority of adult joint infections is
    A. *Abiotrophia* sp.
    B. *Leuconostoc* sp.
    C. *Staphylococcus aureus*
    D. *Streptococcus pneumoniae*

61. Which of the following is associated with infections in humans often linked to deli meats and improperly pasteurized dairy products?
    A. *Bacillus subtilis*
    B. *Listeria monocytogenes*
    C. *Leuconostoc* sp.
    D. *Streptococcus agalactiae*

62. *Bacillus cereus* has been implicated as the etiologic agent in cases of
    A. Food poisoning
    B. Impetigo
    C. Pelvic inflammatory disease
    D. Toxic shock syndrome

63. The causative agent of "malignant pustule" is
    A. *Bacillus anthracis*
    B. *Corynebacterium ulcerans*
    C. *Erysipelothrix rhusiopathiae*
    D. *Listeria monocytogenes*

64. An infant was hospitalized with a severe, tender erythema. The child's epidermis was loose, and large areas of skin could be peeled off. The condition described is most consistent with a clinical syndrome associated with
    A. *Streptococcus pyogenes*
    B. *Staphylococcus aureus*
    C. *Bacillus anthracis*
    D. *Erysipelothrix rhusiopathiae*

65. A catalase-negative gram-positive coccus is isolated from a urine sample of a hospitalized patient. The bacterium produced a black pigment on bile-esculin agar and formed acid from glucose in the presence of 6.5% NaCl. What is the most likely identification of this bacterium?
    A. *Abiotrophia* sp.
    B. *Enterococcus faecalis*
    C. Group B streptococci
    D. Group D streptococci

Aerobic Gram-Negative Bacteria

66. Generally, vancomycin is active against gram-positive bacteria. However, which of the following is more likely to exhibit resistance?
    A. *Staphylococcus epidermidis*
    B. *Streptococcus pyogenes*
    C. *Enterococcus gallinarum*
    D. *Bacillus subtilis*

67. The majority of clinical isolates of *Klebsiella* are
    A. *K. ozaenae*
    B. *K. pneumoniae*
    C. *K. aerogenes*
    D. *K. oxytoca*

68. The enterotoxins of both *Vibrio cholerae* O1 and noninvasive (toxigenic) strains of *E. coli* produce serious diarrhea by what mechanism?
    A. Stimulation of adenylate cyclase, which gives rise to excessive fluid secretion by the cells of the small intestine
    B. Penetration of the bowel mucosa
    C. Stimulation of colicin production
    D. Elaboration of a dermonecrotizing toxin

69. Colonies of *Neisseria* sp. turn color when a redox reagent is applied. The color change is indicative of the activity of the bacterial enzyme
    A. Beta-galactosidase
    B. Urease
    C. Cytochrome oxidase
    D. Phenylalanine deaminase

70. Which of the following is true of *Shigella sonnei*?
    A. Large numbers of organisms must be ingested to produce disease.
    B. H_2S positive
    C. Produces red colonies on Salmonella-Shigella agar after 18 hours of incubation
    D. The organism is a delayed lactose fermenter.

71. An environmental sampling study of respiratory therapy equipment produced cultures of a yellow, nonfermentative (at 48 hours), gram-negative bacillus from several of the nebulizers, which would most likely be species of
    A. *Chryseobacterium*
    B. *Pseudomonas*
    C. *Alcaligenes*
    D. *Moraxella*

72. The characteristics of being lactose negative, citrate negative, urease negative, lysine decarboxylase negative, and nonmotile best describe which organism?
    A. *Proteus vulgaris*
    B. *Yersinia pestis*
    C. *Salmonella enterica*
    D. *Shigella dysenteriae*

73. A fermentative gram-negative bacillus that is oxidase positive, motile, and grows well on MacConkey agar is
    A. *Aeromonas hydrophila*
    B. *Pseudomonas aeruginosa*
    C. *Stenotrophomonas maltophilia*
    D. *Yersinia enterocolitica*

74. Fecal cultures are inoculated on thiosulfate-citrate-bile salts-sucrose agar specifically for the isolation of
    A. *Shigella*
    B. *Vibrio*
    C. *Campylobacter*
    D. *Salmonella*

75. The K antigen of the family *Enterobacteriaceae* is
    A. Heat labile
    B. The somatic antigen
    C. Located on the flagellum
    D. The antigen used to group *Shigella*

76. The causative agent of melioidosis is
    A. *Burkholderia cepacia*
    B. *Burkholderia pseudomallei*
    C. *Moraxella catarrhalis*
    D. *Stenotrophomonas maltophilia*

77. Which microorganism will grow only on culture media supplemented with either cysteine or cystine?
    A. *Actinobacillus lignieresii*
    B. *Bartonella bacilliformis*
    C. *Francisella tularensis*
    D. *Kingella kingae*

78. A test that could be used to screen for enterohemorrhagic *E. coli*
A. ONPG
B. MUG
C. Motility
D. Growth at 42°C

79. An example of an oxidase-positive, glucose nonfermenting organism is
A. *Aeromonas hydrophila*
B. *Escherichia coli*
C. *Klebsiella pneumoniae*
D. *Pseudomonas aeruginosa*

80. A nonlactose fermenter is isolated from a stool specimen. A biochemical multitest assay identifies the isolate as *Shigella* sp. Subsequently, the isolate demonstrates agglutination in *Shigella* group B antisera. Which of the following is most likely
A. The isolate is *Shigella sonnei.*
B. The isolate is *Shigella flexneri.*
C. The isolate should be reported as *Shigella* species.
D. Antisera test should be repeated.

81. The species of *Vibrio* closely associated with rapidly progressing wound infections seen in patients with underlying liver disease is
A. *V. alginolyticus*
B. *V. cholerae*
C. *V. vulnificus*
D. *V. parahaemolyticus*

82. Severe disseminated intravascular coagulation often complicates cases of septicemia caused by
A. *Acinetobacter* sp.
B. *Moraxella* sp.
C. *Neisseria gonorrhoeae*
D. *Neisseria meningitidis*

83. The *Haemophilus influenzae* vaccine protects against which serotype?
A. Serotype a
B. Serotype b
C. Serotype c
D. Serotype d

84. *Salmonella* Typhi exhibits a characteristic biochemical pattern, which differentiates it from the other salmonellae. Which of the following is characteristic of *S.* Typhi?
A. Large amounts of H_2S are produced in TSI agar.
B. Agglutination in Vi grouping serum
C. Citrate positive
D. Produces gas from glucose fermentation

85. The sexually acquired disease characterized by genital ulcers and tender inguinal lymphadenopathy, which is caused by a small, gram-negative bacillus, is known as
A. Chancroid
B. Bacterial vaginosis
C. Syphilis
D. Trachoma

86. Which of the following diseases is most likely to be acquired from a hot tub or whirlpool?
A. Q fever
B. Erysipelas
C. *Acinetobacter* cellulitis
D. *Pseudomonas* dermatitis

87. *Campylobacter* spp. are associated most frequently with cases of
A. Osteomyelitis
B. Gastroenteritis
C. Endocarditis
D. Appendicitis

88. An organism occasionally misidentified as an enteric pathogen because some isolates produce H_2S is
   A. *Burkholderia cepacia*
   B. *Burkholderia pseudomallei*
   C. *Pseudomonas putida*
   D. *Citrobacter freundii*

89. The etiologic agent of whooping cough is
   A. *Bordetella pertussis*
   B. *Brucella suis*
   C. *Francisella tularensis*
   D. *Haemophilus ducreyi*

90. An important characteristic of *Neisseria gonorrhoeae* or the infection it produces is
   A. A Gram stain of the organism reveals gram-negative bacilli.
   B. Asymptomatic infections are common in females.
   C. It produces disease in humans and domestic animals.
   D. The bacteria survive long periods outside the host's body.

91. A physician orders a urea breath test; she must suspect an infection caused by
   A. *Citrobacter freundii*
   B. *Campylobacter jejuni*
   C. *Providencia rettgeri*
   D. *Helicobacter pylori*

92. A gram-negative, "kidney bean" cellular morphology is a distinguishing characteristic of
   A. *Neisseria meningitidis*
   B. *Yersinia pestis*
   C. *Bartonella* spp.
   D. *Actinobacter* spp.

93. Which of the following nonfermenters is rarely isolated in the United States?
   A. *Pseudomonas aeruginosa*
   B. *Stenotrophomonas maltophilia*
   C. *Burkholderia mallei*
   D. *Burkholderia cepacia*

94. Erythromycin eye drops are routinely administered to infants to prevent infections caused by
   A. *E. coli*
   B. *Haemophilus influenzae*
   C. *Pseudomonas aeruginosa*
   D. *Neisseria gonorrhoeae*

95. *Neisseria lactamica* closely resembles *Neisseria meningitidis* but can be differentiated from it by its ability to metabolize
   A. Maltose
   B. Lactose
   C. Glucose
   D. Sucrose

96. A causative agent of the form of conjunctivitis known as pinkeye is
   A. *Haemophilus aegyptius*
   B. *Moraxella lacunata*
   C. *Chlamydia trachomatis*
   D. *Klebsiella ozaenae*

97. *Cronobacter* spp. have frequently been linked to
   A. Infections in infants due to contaminated formula
   B. Pneumonia in coal miners
   C. Wound infections associated with marine water
   D. Wound infections following contact with dogs

98. *Acinetobacter baumannii*
   A. Requires cysteine
   B. Is oxidase negative
   C. Ferments glucose
   D. Does not grow on MacConkey agar

99. *Legionella pneumophila* is the etiologic agent of both Legionnaires disease and
   A. Swine fever
   B. Pontiac fever
   C. Rift Valley fever
   D. San Joaquin Valley fever

100. In suspected cases of brucellosis, what is the most sensitive specimen to submit for culture?
   A. Bone marrow
   B. Nasopharyngeal swab
   C. Sputum
   D. Stool

101. Hemolytic uremic syndrome is a complication after infection with
   A. *E. coli* O157:H7
   B. *Salmonella* Typhi
   C. *Vibrio cholerae* O1
   D. *Yersinia enterocolitica*

102. Identify the fermentative agent that may infect reptiles and fish as well as humans when they are exposed to contaminated soil or water.
   A. *Aeromonas*
   B. *Chromobacterium*
   C. *Chryseobacterium*
   D. *Enterobacter*

103. *Campylobacter jejuni* is
   A. Nonmotile
   B. Oxidase negative
   C. Hippurate hydrolysis positive
   D. A gram-negative coccobacillus

104. Which of the following has a negative oxidase test?
   A. *Aeromonas*
   B. *Chryseobacterium*
   C. *Rahnella*
   D. *Vibrio*

105. Which of the following is *true* of *Neisseria gonorrhoeae*?
   A. Adversely affected by fatty acids in clinical specimens
   B. Rapid growth on sheep blood agar
   C. Ferments glucose and maltose
   D. ONPG positive

106. The method of serogrouping *Shigella* used in the clinical laboratory is based on
   A. Vi antigen
   B. H antigens
   C. K antigens
   D. O antigens

107. The symptom of diffuse, watery diarrhea that produces a relatively clear stool containing mucus flecks is suggestive of an infection caused by
   A. Enterohemorrhagic *E. coli*
   B. *Shigella dysenteriae*
   C. *Vibrio cholerae*
   D. *Yersinia enterocolitica*

108. An example of a halophilic microorganism is
   A. *Morganella morganii*
   B. *Plesiomonas shigelloides*
   C. *Vibrio parahaemolyticus*
   D. *Yersinia pestis*

109. Which of the following statements is true of *Brucella*?
   A. They are strictly human pathogens.
   B. They are nonfastidious and grow on most nonselective laboratory media.
   C. The risk of accidental laboratory infection is no greater than with any other organism.
   D. Slide agglutination in antisera is a commonly used screening test for identification.

110. Infection of the gastric mucosa leading to gastritis or peptic ulcers is most commonly associated with
   A. *Campylobacter jejuni*
   B. *Helicobacter pylori*
   C. *Salmonella* Typhi
   D. *Shigella sonnei*

111. Which of the following describes *Acinetobacter* sp.?
   A. Commonly susceptible to most antimicrobials
   B. Generally gram-negative cocci morphology
   C. Oxidase positive
   D. Infections associated with use of medical devices

112. Explosive watery diarrhea with severe abdominal pain after eating raw shellfish is most characteristic of infection caused by
   A. *Campylobacter jejuni*
   B. *Helicobacter pylori*
   C. *Shigella dysenteriae*
   D. *Vibrio parahemolyticus*

113. An unheated suspension of *Salmonella* Typhi typically produces agglutination of Vi antisera. After heating the same suspension, agglutination will occur in which grouping sera?
   A. A
   B. B
   C. C_1
   D. D

114. The species of *Campylobacter* noted to produce septicemia, septic arthritis, meningitis, jaundice with hepatomegaly, and thrombophlebitis in debilitated patients is
   A. *C. coli*
   B. *C. fetus*
   C. *C. laris*
   D. *C. sputorum*

115. *Shigella sonnei* is differentiated from other *Shigella* sp. by
   A. A positive ONPG
   B. A positive phenylalanine deaminase reaction
   C. Its negative oxidase reaction
   D. Its ability to demonstrate motility at 22°C

116. A positive Voges-Proskauer reaction is characteristic of
   A. *Enterobacter aerogenes*
   B. *Escherichia coli*
   C. *Proteus vulgaris*
   D. *Providencia rettgeri*

117. Which of the following is true regarding *Vibrio cholerae*?
   A. It is halophilic.
   B. It is nonmotile.
   C. Forms clear colonies on TCBS agar
   D. Produces a potent exotoxin causing severe diarrhea

118. The classic toxigenic strains of which serogroup are implicated in epidemic infections of *Vibrio cholerae*?
   A. O1
   B. O2
   C. O3
   D. O4

119. *Brucella* spp. are
   A. The etiologic agents of relapsing fever
   B. Small spiral organisms
   C. Primarily a cause of endogenous human infections
   D. Intracellular pathogens

120. Which of the following reactions is typical for *E. coli*?
   A. Beta-hemolytic on sheep blood agar
   B. Colorless colonies on MacConkey agar
   C. Colorless colonies on xylose-lysine-desoxycholate agar
   D. Green colonies with black centers on Hektoen-enteric agar

121. *Yersinia pestis* is characteristically
   A. Urease negative
   B. Hydrogen sulfide positive
   C. Motile at 20–25°C
   D. Oxidase positive

122. Lack of motility is characteristic of
A. *Enterobacter cloacae*
B. *Klebsiella oxytoca*
C. *Morganella morganii*
D. *Providencia stuartii*

123. In cases of legionellosis
A. Person-to-person transmission is common
B. Farm animals are important animal reservoirs
C. Patients can present with a self-limited nonpneumonic febrile illness
D. Specimens may be cold enriched to enhance recovery of the organism

124. A pathology report signifies the finding of Donovan bodies in a lymph node biopsy from the groin of a 28-year-old male. The physician calls the laboratory requesting culture confirmation of the suspected infectious agent. You should inform the physician that
A. A urethral swab should be collected.
B. A lymph node aspirate should be collected.
C. A blood culture should be ordered.
D. The causative agent cannot be cultured on routine laboratory media.

125. A blood culture of a patient with endocarditis yields *Aggregatibacter aphrophilus.* What is the likely source of this patient's infection?
A. Endogenous from the oral cavity
B. Aerosol inhalation associated bird contact
C. Puncture wound contaminated with soil
D. Wound following rat bite

126. *Kingella kingae* is most noted for causing
A. Urinary tract infections associated with bladder catheters
B. Pneumonia in the elderly
C. Bone and joint infections in children
D. It is strictly a nonpathogen

127. Isolation of *Neisseria gonorrhoeae*
A. Is enhanced by cold enrichment
B. Requires incubation under increased CO_2
C. From contaminated sites is made easier by the use of cefsulodin-irgasan-novobiocin (CIN) agar
D. Is not affected if clinical specimen is refrigerated before culturing

128. A positive indole reaction is characteristic of
A. *Escherichia coli*
B. *Proteus mirabilis*
C. *Salmonella* Choleraesuis
D. *Serratia marcescens*

129. Which one of the following organisms would produce a yellow slant and a yellow butt on TSI agar after incubating 18 hours?
A. *Escherichia coli*
B. *Proteus mirabilis*
C. *Salmonella* Typhimurium
D. *Shigella sonnei*

130. Pyocyanin is characteristically produced by
A. *Pseudomonas aeruginosa*
B. *Pseudomonas fluorescens*
C. *Shewanella putrefaciens*
D. *Stenotrophomonas maltophillia*

131. Color Plate 26 ■ shows the Gram stain of cerebrospinal fluid from a 1-year-old girl suspected of having meningitis. After 24 hours of growth, small tan colonies were isolated on chocolate agar incubated in CO_2. Sheep blood agar also incubated in CO_2 had no growth. Which of the following organisms should be suspected?
A. *Brucella canis*
B. *Bordetella parapertussis*
C. *Haemophilus influenzae*
D. *Neisseria meningitidis*

132. Which of the following is *true* concerning *Campylobacter jejuni*?
   A. Catalase negative
   B. Isolated best at 24°C
   C. Commonly found in ocean water
   D. A leading cause of bacterial diarrhea worldwide

133. Of the following microorganisms, which one will turn a dark purple when tetramethyl-*p*-phenylenediamine hydrochloride is applied?
   A. *Acinetobacter baumannii*
   B. *Stenotrophomonas maltophilia*
   C. *Moraxella catarrhalis*
   D. *Yersinia enterocolitica*

134. *Cardiobacterium hominis* has been recovered as an etiologic agent from cases of endocarditis. An identifying characteristic of the organism is
   A. Positive oxidase
   B. Requires a microaerophilic environment for growth
   C. Growth on MacConkey agar
   D. Inability to grow on sheep blood agar

135. *Vibrio vulnificus* is a well-established human pathogen that is known to cause
   A. Gastroenteritis
   B. Pneumonia
   C. Pyelonephritis
   D. Wound infections

136. Which of the following organisms produce a positive phenylalanine deaminase reaction?
   A. *Citrobacter freundii*
   B. *Klebsiella pneumoniae*
   C. *Providendia stuartii*
   D. *Yersinia enterocolitica*

137. All members of the *Pseudomonas* fluorescent group are noted for producing
   A. Pyomelanin
   B. Pyocyanin
   C. Pyoverdin
   D. Pyorubrin

138. Which of the following organisms is unable to grow on MacConkey agar?
   A. *Bordetella bronchiseptica*
   B. *Burkholderia cepacia*
   C. *Kingella denitrificans*
   D. *Plesiomonas shigelloides*

139. Which of the following is true of *Haemophilus* spp.?
   A. Obligate parasites
   B. Grow well on sheep blood agar
   C. Small gram-negative diplococci
   D. Many are found as normal biota in the gastrointestinal tract.

140. *Legionella pneumophila*
   A. Infections are most often acquired from environmental sources.
   B. Metabolizes a number of carbohydrates
   C. Stains easily as gram-negative bacilli
   D. Does not autofluoresce

141. Which of the following is the optimal clinical specimen for the recovery of *Legionella pneumophila*?
   A. Stool
   B. Blood
   C. Bronchial washings
   D. Nasopharyngeal swab

142. Which of the following is true for the diagnosis of *Bordetella pertussis* infection?
   A. Most strains grow well on MacConkey agar.
   B. Cultures are the common mode of diagnosing infections.
   C. Throat washes are recommended for isolation.
   D. Swabs for PCR analysis can be transported dry.

143. Production of a yellow pigment on nutrient or sheep blood agar is characteristic of which of the following members of the family Enterobacteriaceae?
   A. *Enterobacter aerogenes*
   B. *Citrobacter freundii*
   C. *Cronobacter sakazakii*
   D. *Klebsiella oxytoca*

144. A gram-negative bacillus was recovered from the urine of a child with a history of recurrent urinary tract infections. The organism was oxidase negative, lactose negative, urease positive, and motile. The most likely identification of this agent would be
   A. *Escherichia coli*
   B. *Klebsiella pneumoniae*
   C. *Proteus mirabilis*
   D. *Pseudomonas aeruginosa*

145. *Acinetobacter baumannii* complex is characteristically
   A. Motile
   B. Oxidase positive
   C. Sensitive to penicillin
   D. Able to grow on MacConkey agar

146. Which of the following is characteristic of *Eikenella corrodens*?
   A. It is a gram-negative diplobacillus.
   B. Most isolates require both hemin and NAD.
   C. It is found in the mouth and upper respiratory tract of humans.
   D. It is often found in pure culture when recovered from infections.

147. Which of the following species of *Pasteurella* is associated with human infections following cat bites?
   A. *P. avium*
   B. *P. canis*
   C. *P. multocida*
   D. *P. stomatis*

148. Which of the following *Legionella* spp. is positive for hippurate hydrolysis?
   A. *L. micdadei*
   B. *L. longbeachae*
   C. *L. gormanii*
   D. *L. pneumophila*

149. Which of the following is characteristic of *Haemophilus aegyptius*?
   A. Is also referred to as *Haemophilus influenzae* biogroup *aegytius*
   B. Requires X and V factor
   C. Requires X factor only
   D. Aminolevulinic acid positive

150. *Kingella denitrificans* can be differentiated from *Neisseria gonorrhoeae* because it is
   A. Able to grow on Thayer-Martin agar
   B. Able to reduce nitrate
   C. Oxidase positive
   D. Glucose positive

151. Which member of the family *Enterobacteriaceae* is oxidase positive?
   A. *Cronobacter*
   B. *Ewingella*
   C. *Plesiomonas*
   D. *Vibrio*

152. In the past, povidone iodine, tincture of iodine prep pads and swabs, and other disinfectants have been recalled because of microbial contamination. The most likely organism to be isolated in these cases is
   A. *Bordetella bronchiseptica*
   B. *Klebsiella pneumoniae*
   C. *Pseudomonas aeruginosa*
   D. *Serratia marcescens*

153. Foodborne outbreaks of brucellosis are most commonly associated with eating
   A. Raw shellfish
   B. Imported cheese
   C. Contaminated potato salad
   D. Improperly cooked hamburger

154. *Serratia* spp. are unique in the family *Enterobacteriaceae* because of their ability to produce extracellular hydrolytic enzymes. Which of the following is produced by *Serratia* species?
   A. DNase
   B. Hyaluronidase
   C. Kinase
   D. NADase

155. *Haemophilus ducreyi* is the causative agent of
   A. Chancroid
   B. Lymphogranuloma venereum
   C. Trachoma
   D. Whooping cough

156. The optimal specimen for the recovery of *Bordetella pertussis* is
   A. Anterior nares swab
   B. Blood
   C. Expectorated sputum
   D. Nasopharyngeal swab

157. Which of the following is the most common indicator of bacterial vaginosis?
   A. *Eikenella*
   B. *Capnocytophaga*
   C. *Gardnerella*
   D. *Listeria*

158. Blood cultures are recommended for the recovery of which of the following microorganisms?
   A. *Acinetobacter baumannii-calcoaceticus* complex
   B. *Brucella canis*
   C. *Chlamydia trachomatis*
   D. *Yersinia enterocolitica*

159. *Yersinia pseudotuberculosis* is known to manifest commonly as which of the following clinical conditions?
   A. Epiglottitis
   B. Hepatitis
   C. Mesenteric lymphadenitis
   D. Pseudomembranous colitis

160. Cefsulodin-irgasan-novobiocin (CIN) agar is recommended for the recovery of
   A. *Brucella suis*
   B. *Cardiobacterium hominis*
   C. *Rhodococcus equi*
   D. *Yersinia enterocolitica*

161. Why are cultures for *Gardnerella vaginalis* not recommended?
   A. The bacteria grow so slowly that results take too long to be relevant.
   B. Isolation of the bacteria may not be clinically significant.
   C. It is unsafe to grow this bacterium.
   D. The bacteria do not grow on artificial media.

162. Buffered charcoal yeast extract agar is the recommended medium for the recovery of
   A. *Hafnia alvei*
   B. *Legionella pneumophila*
   C. *Neisseria meningitidis*
   D. *Vibrio cholerae*

163. Swimmer's ear, a form of external otitis is commonly caused by
   A. *Acinetobacter baumannii-calcoaceticus* complex
   B. *Bordetella bronchiseptica*
   C. *Haemophilus influenzae*
   D. *Pseudomonas aeruginosa*

164. A number of vacationers who have traveled outside the United States have had their vacations interrupted by a case of "traveler's diarrhea," which is commonly associated with which etiologic agent?
   A. *Aeromonas hydrophila*
   B. *Escherichia coli*
   C. *Proteus mirabilis*
   D. *Vibrio parahemolyticus*

165. On Gram stain, a morphology that resembles "seagull wings" is most characteristic of
   A. *Campylobacter jejuni*
   B. *Neisseria gonorrhoeae*
   C. *Plesiomonas shigelloides*
   D. *Yersinia pseudotuberculosis*

166. The flattened adjacent sides of the cellular appearance of which microorganism are said to resemble kidney beans?
   A. *Aeromonas hydrophila*
   B. *Campylobacter jejuni*
   C. *Neisseria gonorrhoeae*
   D. *Pasteurella multocida*

167. Bacteria-producing clear colonies with black centers on Hektoen-enteric agar were isolated from a stool culture from a patient with diarrhea. Which of the following is true?
   A. The bacteria are lactose fermenters.
   B. Colony morphology is suggestive of *Salmonella.*
   C. Colony morphology is suggestive of *Shigella.*
   D. Colony morphology is suggestive of *Yersinia enterocolitica.*

168. Which of the *Neisseria* spp. produces acid from glucose but not from maltose, lactose, or sucrose?
   A. *Neisseria gonorrhoeae*
   B. *Neisseria lactamica*
   C. *Neisseria meningitidis*
   D. *Neisseria sicca*

169. Which of the *Neisseria* spp. produces acid from glucose and maltose but not sucrose or lactose?
   A. *Neisseria gonorrhoeae*
   B. *Neisseria lactamica*
   C. *Neisseria meningitidis*
   D. *Neisseria sicca*

170. The causative agent of the septicemic, hemolytic disease known as Oroya fever is
   A. *Bartonella bacilliformis*
   B. *Burkholderia mallei*
   C. *Haemophilus aegyptius*
   D. *Yersinia pestis*

171. The "nonpathogenic" *Neisseria* spp. are generally regarded as normal microbiota of the
   A. Skin
   B. Upper respiratory tract
   C. Gastrointestinal tract
   D. Urinary tract

172. Lack of motility is a characteristic of
   A. *Enterobacter*
   B. *Klebsiella*
   C. *Salmonella*
   D. *Serratia*

173. Violet-colored colonies are typically produced by
   A. *Chromobacterium violaceum*
   B. *Chryseobacterium meningosepticum*
   C. *Pseudomonas aeruginosa*
   D. *Serratia marcescens*

174. Which of the following is true of *Pasteurella multocida*?
   A. Most common human infections occur in soft tissues, bones, and joints.
   B. Humans harbor the organism as part of their normal biota.
   C. It grows well on MacConkey agar.
   D. Isolates are typically penicillin resistant.

175. Pus was aspirated from an empyema. A Gram stain of the aspirated material showed many white blood cells and numerous gram-negative bacilli. The culture grew many colonies producing a soluble green pigment. The most likely etiologic agent in this case would be
   A. *Chromobacterium violaceum*
   B. *Legionella pneumophila*
   C. *Pseudomonas aeruginosa*
   D. *Serratia marcescens*

176. Which of the following is correct for *Aeromonas hydrophila* complex?
   A. Beta-hemolytic
   B. Forms clear colonies on cefsulodin-irgasan-novobiocin (CIN) medium
   C. Member of the family Enterobacteriaceae
   D. Oxidase negative

177. *Edwardsiella tarda* is occasionally isolated in stool specimens and can biochemically be confused with
   A. *Salmonella*
   B. Enterohemorraghic *E. coli*
   C. *Vibrio cholerae*
   D. *Yersinia enterocolitica*

178. The porphyrin test determines an organism's requirement for
   A. Cystiene
   B. Hemin
   C. NAD
   D. Thiol

179. Which of the following is an occasional cause of respiratory tract infections and is rapidly urea positive?
   A. *Bordetella bronchiseptica*
   B. *Brucella abortus*
   C. *Campylobacter fetus*
   D. *Escherichia coli*

180. The most common etiologic agent of community-acquired uncomplicated cases of cystitis is
   A. *Enterobacter aerogenes*
   B. *Escherichia coli*
   C. *Klebsiella pneumoniae*
   D. *Proteus vulgaris*

181. In a sinus culture, you notice small pinpoint colonies growing around medium white colonies on sheep blood agar. The small colonies are likely
   A. *Burkholderia pseudomallei*
   B. *Campylobacter jejuni*
   C. *Haemophilus influenzae*
   D. *Yersinia pestis*

182. Colonies that are said to resemble "droplets of mercury" are characteristic of
   A. *Bordetella pertussis*
   B. *Burkholderia cepacia*
   C. *Campylobacter jejuni*
   D. *Yersinia pestis*

183. When an epidemiologic survey for the detection of upper respiratory tract carriers of *Neisseria meningitidis* or *Bordetella pertussis* is being conducted, the optimal type of specimen to be obtained for culture is
   A. Anterior nares
   B. Buccal cavity
   C. Nasopharyngeal
   D. Throat

184. Chronic carriers, persons who remain infected with an organism for long periods often without symptoms, are typically associated with the dissemination of
   A. *Bordetella pertussis*
   B. *Campylobacter jejuni*
   C. *Salmonella* Typhi
   D. *Yersinia pestis*

185. Milk has classically been the primary food associated with the transmission of some diseases, especially for those diseases of cattle transmissible to humans, such as
A. Brucellosis
B. Glanders
C. Meliodosis
D. Pontiac fever

186. Association with faucet aerators and humidifiers used with ventilators in intensive care units is commonly a factor in outbreaks of infections with which of the following microorganisms?
A. *Klebsiella pneumoniae*
B. *Pseudomonas aeruginosa*
C. *Salmonella* spp.
D. *Serratia marcescens*

187. Which of the following is true of *Neisseria gonorrheae*?
A. Household pets are reservoirs
B. Initial infections in women are often asymptomatic.
C. Ferments glucose and maltose
D. Grows readily on sheep blood agar

188. The selective nature of Hektoen-enteric agar is due to the inclusion of which one of the following?
A. Bile salts
B. *Bis*-sodium metasulfate
C. Bromothymol blue
D. NaCl

189. For the selective isolation of *Vibrio* spp. the recommended agar is
A. Thiosulfate-citrate-bile salt-sucrose agar
B. Charcoal yeast extract agar
C. Mannitol salt agar
D. Tinsdale agar

190. When performing the oxidase test, which of the following would be appropriate?
A. The reagent used is *o*-nitrophenyl-β-D-galactopyranoside.
B. A nichrome wire loop should be used to acquire inoculum for testing.
C. Colonies from sheep blood agar can be used.
D. A positive colony turns dark purple after 30 seconds following application of the reagent.

191. The porphyrin test is most useful for the identification of which of the following?
A. *Campylobacter*
B. *Haemophilus*
C. *Moraxella*
D. *Neisseria*

192. A physician has requested a stool culture for enterohemorrhagic *E. coli*. Which one of the following would be the best screening medium?
A. MacConkey agar with lactose
B. MacConkey agar with sorbitol
C. Xylose-lysine-deoxycholate agar
D. Brilliant-green agar

193. Reptiles kept as pets are sometimes associated with the transmission of
A. *Campylobacter*
B. *Helicobacter*
C. *Salmonella*
D. *Vibrio*

194. A young man developed keratitis associated with the use of contact lenses that had been immersed in a contaminated cleaning solution. The most common bacterial etiologic agent in such cases is
A. *Chryseobacterium meningosepticum*
B. *Pseudomonas aeruginosa*
C. *Francisella tularensis*
D. *Escherichia coli*

195. Bacterium associated with gastric cancer
    A. *Campylobacter jejuni*
    B. *Helicobacter pylori*
    C. *Salmonella* Typhimurium
    D. *Yersinia enterocolitica*

196. New York City agar was developed for the isolation of
    A. *Bordetella pertussis*
    B. *Campylobacter fetus*
    C. *Haemophilus influenzae*
    D. *Neisseria gonorrhoeae*

197. Besides *Pseudomonas aeruginosa*, which of the following is an important cause of lower respiratory tract infections in patients with cystic fibrosis?
    A. *Actinobacillus actinomycetemcomitans*
    B. *Burkholdia cepacia*
    C. *Chryseobacterium meningosepticum*
    D. *Serratia marcescens*

198. *Eikenella corrodens* is an opportunistic pathogen, but it is most noted for causing
    A. Abscesses of the oral cavity
    B. Pneumonia
    C. Postsurgical wound infections
    D. Urinary tract infections

Mycobacteria

199. Mycobacteria have a large amount of a component in their cell wall that other bacteria lack. That component is
    A. Fatty acids
    B. Murein
    C. Sterols
    D. Teichoic acid

200. The species of *Mycobacterium* that would be most commonly associated with contamination of the hot water system in large institutions such as hospitals is
    A. *M. haemophilum*
    B. *M. marinum*
    C. *M. ulcerans*
    D. *M. xenopi*

201. *Mycobacterium fortuitum*, a rapidly growing *Mycobacterium*, grows on MacConkey agar in 5 days. Which other species of *Mycobacterium* is able to demonstrate growth within the same time period on MacConkey agar?
    A. *M. bovis*
    B. *M. chelonei*
    C. *M. kansasii*
    D. *M. tuberculosis*

202. A slowly growing, orange-pigmented, acid-fast bacillus was isolated from a cervical lymph node of a child with symptoms of cervical adenitis. The most likely etiologic agent in this case would be
    A. *Mycobacterium avium* complex
    B. *Mycobacterium chelonei*
    C. *Mycobacterium fortuitum*
    D. *Mycobacterium scrofulaceum*

203. When clinical specimens are processed for the recovery of *Mycobacterium tuberculosis*, the generally recommended method for digestion and decontamination of the sample is
    A. 6% NaOH
    B. HCl
    C. NALC-NaOH
    D. Trisodium phosphate

204. The etiologic agent of Hansen disease is
    A. *Mycobacterium bovis*
    B. *Mycobacterium fortuitum*
    C. *Mycobacterium leprae*
    D. *Mycobacterium tuberculosis*

205. The finding of five to six acid-fast bacilli per field (×800 to ×1000) in a carbol fuchsin smear of expectorated sputum should be reported as
    A. 1+
    B. 2+
    C. 3+
    D. 4+

206. Mycobacteria can be examined by using the
    A. Dieterle stain
    B. Gimenez stain
    C. Kinyoun stain
    D. Wright's stain

207. Which of the following is characteristic of *Mycobacterium kansasii*?
    A. Rapid growing
    B. Nonchromogenic
    C. Considered a laboratory contaminant
    D. Infections usually acquired by respiratory route

208. Which of the following mycobacteria has an optimal growth temperature 30–32°C?
    A. *M. avium* complex
    B. *M. bovis*
    C. *M. ulcerans*
    D. *M. xenopi*

209. Which one of the following drugs is considered as primary antimycobacterial therapy?
    A. Isoniazid
    B. Kanamycin
    C. Amikacin
    D. Ciprofloxacin

210. In the decontamination and digestion procedure for the isolation of mycobacteria from sputa samples, what is the role of NALC?
    A. Bactericidal for normal biota
    B. Liquefies mucus
    C. Growth stimulant
    D. Neutralizes pH to prevent damage to mycobacteria

211. Which one of the following tests would be appropriate in the diagnosis of a mycobacterial infection?
    A. Elek test
    B. CAMP test
    C. Nagler test
    D. PPD test

212. Which of the following *Mycobacterium* sp. is associated with livestock and causes a zoonosis?
    A. *M. bovis*
    B. *M. fortuitum*
    C. *M. gordonae*
    D. *M. xenopi*

213. Which of the following *Mycobacterium* is most noted for being associated with patients with acquired immunodeficiency syndrome?
    A. *M. avium* complex
    B. *M. marinum*
    C. *M. kansasii*
    D. *M. bovis*

214. Which of the following *Mycobacterium* produces an orange pigment and is most commonly recovered from water?
    A. *M. intracellulare*
    B. *M. gordonae*
    C. *M. asiaticum*
    D. *M. kansasii*

215. Which of the following *Mycobacterium* appears as buff-colored colonies after exposure to light and is niacin positive?
    A. *M. bovis*
    B. *M. scrofulaceum*
    C. *M. tuberculosis*
    D. *M. ulcerans*

216. The *Mycobacterium* that is the etiologic agent of "swimming pool granuloma" is
    A. *M. fortuitum*
    B. *M. kansasii*
    C. *M. marinum*
    D. *M. xenopi*

217. Susceptibility to thiophene-2-carboxylic acid hydrazide (T2H) is characteristic of which of the following mycobacteria?
    A. *M. avium* complex
    B. *M. bovis*
    C. *M. kansasii*
    D. *M. tuberculosis*

218. Which of the following is a fluorescent stain for mycobacteria?
    A. Auromine-rhodamine
    B. Calcofluor white
    C. Fluorescein isothiocyanate
    D. Ziehl-Neelsen

219. The most common photochromogenic *Mycobacterium* isolated in the United States is
    A. *M. bovis*
    B. *M. kansasii*
    C. *M. tuberculosis*
    D. *M. xenopi*

220. Skin cultures for the recovery of *Mycobacterium* spp. should be incubated at
    A. 22°C
    B. 30°C
    C. 35°C
    D. 42°C

221. The gamma-interferon release assays for diagnosing tuberculosis
    A. Can distinguish between current and past infections
    B. Is based on release of gamma interferon by T cells
    C. Produces a false-positive result in patients who have received the PPD skin test
    D. Produces a false-positive result in patients who have received the tuberculosis vaccine

222. Which of the following specimens is routinely decontaminated when trying to recover *Mycobacterium* spp.?
    A. Sputum
    B. Pleural fluid
    C. Lung biopsy
    D. Cerebrospinal fluid

223. Which of the following is *not* true of *Mycobacterium leprae*?
    A. Causes Hansen disease
    B. Difficult to grow *in vitro*
    C. Easily transmitted from person to person
    D. Usually grows in peripheral limbs of infected patients

Anaerobic Bacteria

224. The potentially lethal intoxication type of food poisoning often associated with improperly canned food is caused by
    A. *Bacteroides fragilis*
    B. *Clostridium botulinum*
    C. *Clostridium perfringens*
    D. *Clostridium septicum*

225. Which of the following is considered a zoonotic disease?
    A. Anthrax
    B. Botulism
    C. Myonecrosis
    D. Tetanus

226. An anaerobically incubated blood agar plate shows colonies surrounded by an inner zone of complete red cell lysis and an outer zone of incomplete cell lysis (double zone of beta-hemolysis). The most likely presumptive identification of this isolate would be
    A. *Clostridium perfringens*
    B. *Clostridium tetani*
    C. *Fusobacterium nucleatum*
    D. *Prevotella melaninogenica*

227. A cervical mucosal abscess specimen was sent to the laboratory for bacteriologic examination. The culture of this sample grew an anaerobic gram-negative bacillus that was inhibited by bile, produced a black pigment, and was negative for indole production and positive for glucose, sucrose, and lactose fermentation. This isolate would most likely be
    A. *Bacteroides fragilis*
    B. *Campylobacter ureolyticus*
    C. *Porphyromonas gingivalis*
    D. *Prevotella melaninogenica*

228. Which one of the following is true of *Clostridium tetani*?
   A. It produces rapid tissue necrosis.
   B. It is a gram-positive, nonspore-forming bacillus.
   C. Microorganisms commonly found in the microbiome of the intestinal tract.
   D. Disease is caused by an exotoxin acting on the central nervous system.

229. The characteristic colony morphology of *Actinomyces israelii* on solid agar resembles
   A. "Medusa head"
   B. A molar tooth
   C. A fried egg
   D. Ground glass

230. What is the predominant indigenous biota of the colon?
   A. Anaerobic, gram-negative, nonspore-forming bacteria
   B. Anaerobic, gram-positive, nonspore-forming bacteria
   C. Aerobic, gram-negative, nonspore-forming bacteria
   D. Aerobic, gram-positive, spore-forming bacteria

231. Obligate anaerobic, gram-negative bacilli, recovered from an abdominal wound, were found to be resistant to penicillin. Growth of this organism was not inhibited by bile. What is the most likely identification of this isolate?
   A. *Bacteroides fragilis*
   B. *Clostridium septicum*
   C. *Eubacterium lentum*
   D. *Fusobacterium nucleatum*

232. Which of the following is described as obligate anaerobic gram-positive cocci?
   A. *Capnocytophaga*
   B. *Peptostreptococcus*
   C. *Propionibacterium*
   D. *Veillonella*

233. Color Plate 27 ■ shows the filamentous gram-positive rod recovered from an aspirate of a closed chest abscess. It grew only under anaerobic conditions and was not acid-fast. What is the most likely presumptive identification of the isolate seen?
   A. *Actinomyces israelii*
   B. *Bacteroides fragilis*
   C. *Clostridium septicum*
   D. *Propionibacterium acnes*

234. Kanamycin-vancomycin laked-blood (KVLB) agar incubated anaerobically is primarily used for isolation of
   A. *Bacteroides fragilis*
   B. *Bifidobacterium dentium*
   C. *Clostridium perfringens*
   D. *Peptostreptococcus anaerobius*

235. The diagnosis of pseudomembranous colitis, *Clostridioides (Clostridium) difficle*-associated disease, is often made by
   A. Serology
   B. Culturing blood specimens
   C. Nucleic acid amplification test of stool sample
   D. Acid-fast stain of fecal material

236. The anaerobic, gram-negative, curved, motile bacilli associated with bacterial vaginosis belong to the genus
   A. *Actinomyces*
   B. *Bifidobacterium*
   C. *Lactobacillus*
   D. *Mobiluncus*

237. An infant was seen in the emergency department with symptoms of neuromuscular weakness and constipation. The diagnosis of infant botulism was confirmed by the demonstration of toxin in the child's stool. The child most likely contracted this disease by
   A. A scratch wound caused by a cat
   B. Ingestion of spores that germinated in the intestine
   C. A puncture wound with a contaminated household item
   D. Ingestion of preformed toxin found in a contaminated jar of pureed vegetables

238. The majority of the gram-positive, nonspore-forming, anaerobic bacilli isolated from clinical material will likely be
   A. *Bifidobacterium dentium*
   B. *Capnocytophagia ochracea*
   C. *Eubacterium limosum*
   D. *Cutibacterium (Propionibacterium) acnes*

239. Which of the following clostridia has a terminal spore that causes the cell to swell?
   A. *C. botulinum*
   B. *C. difficile*
   C. *C. perfringens*
   D. *C. tetani*

240. The gram-negative, anaerobic bacillus frequently implicated in serious clinical infections such as brain and lung abscesses is
   A. *Prevotella melaninogenica*
   B. *Eubacterium lentum*
   C. *Fusobacterium nucleatum*
   D. *Peptostreptococcus anaerobius*

241. Which one of the following is a nonspore-forming, gram-positive, anaerobic bacillus?
   A. *Clostridium*
   B. *Fusobacterium*
   C. *Propionibacterium*
   D. *Veillonella*

242. Which of the following statements is true of *Clostridium botulinum*?
   A. Infant botulism is the most common clinical form.
   B. Pathogenicity is related to a potent exotoxins destroying host tissue.
   C. Oval spores are located centrally.
   D. Of the seven toxogenic types, types C and D are associated with human botulism.

243. A tube of semisolid medium that contains resazurin appears pink. What does this indicate?
   A. Acid environment
   B. Alkaline environment
   C. Motility
   D. Presence of oxygen

244. Identify the *Fusobacterium* sp. considered to be the most frequent isolate recovered from clinical infections.
   A. *F. varium*
   B. *F. nucleatum*
   C. *F. mortiferum*
   D. *F. necrophorum*

245. Septicemia caused by which of the following is generally associated with an underlying malignancy?
   A. *Bifidobacterium dentium*
   B. *Clostridium septicum*
   C. *Eubacterium lentum*
   D. *Lactobacillus catenaforme*

246. Which of the following is the most potent bacterial exotoxin known?
   A. Botulinum toxin
   B. Erythrogenic toxin
   C. *C. difficile* toxin B
   D. *C. perfringens* alpha-toxin

247. Which of the following is most commonly recovered from cases of gas gangrene?
   A. *Clostridium bifermentans*
   B. *Clostridium perfringens*
   C. *Clostridium sordellii*
   D. *Clostridioides difficile*

248. Which of the following organisms is a gram-negative bacillus?
   A. *Eubacterium lentum*
   B. *Bifidobacterium dentium*
   C. *Propionibacterium acnes*
   D. *Porphyromonas* spp.

249. Which of the following statements is true of clostridia?
   A. Isolates typically will not grow on phenylethyl alcohol agar.
   B. Clinically significant clostridia are found in the normal biota of the colon and in the soil.
   C. Tetanus is caused by ingesting preformed toxin and can be prevented by boiling food prior to eating.
   D. *C. tetani* spores will form in the presence of oxygen; therefore, anaerobiosis in a wound is not required to cause tetanus.

250. Gram-positive bacilli with central spores are seen in the direct Gram stain of a tissue biopsy. After 24 hours of incubation, no growth is seen on the sheep blood agar plate incubated aerobically and the chocolate agar plate incubated in increased CO_2. Which of the following is the likely cause of the infection?
   A. *Bacillus*
   B. *Clostridium*
   C. *Lactobacillus*
   D. *Prevotella*

251. Small alpha-hemolytic colonies are seen on a sheep blood agar plate after 48 hours of incubation on a vaginal culture. This describes which of the following?
   A. *Bacteroides*
   B. *Clostridium*
   C. *Lactobacillus*
   D. *Porphyromonas*

252. Which of the following statements is true regarding *Clostridium perfringens*?
   A. There are five serologic types.
   B. Spores are terminally located.
   C. Alpha-toxin is produced by all strains.
   D. Spores are readily seen in laboratory media.

253. Which is a correct statement regarding *Clostridium tetani*?
   A. It is proteolytic.
   B. It is lecithinase positive.
   C. It is characteristically nonmotile.
   D. It produces terminal spores.

254. Which anaerobic, gram-negative rod can be presumptively identified by its Gram stain morphology and inhibition by bile and a 1-μg kanamycin disk?
   A. *Bacteroides fragilis*
   B. *Eubacterium lentum*
   C. *Fusobacterium nucleatum*
   D. *Porphyromonas gingivalis*

255. Which of the following tests is most appropriate for the presumptive identification of *Prevotella melaninogenica*?
   A. Sodium polyanethole sulfonate (SPS) sensitivity test
   B. Nagler test
   C. Cytotoxin assay
   D. Fluorescence test

256. Which of the following tests is most appropriate for the identification of *Clostridioides (Clostridium) difficile* isolates?
   A. SPS sensitivity test
   B. Nagler test
   C. Lecithinase positive
   D. Fluorescence on cycloserine-cefoxitin-fructose agar

257. Which of the following tests is most appropriate for the presumptive identification of *Clostridium perfringens*?
   A. SPS sensitivity test
   B. Reverse CAMP test
   C. Cytotoxin assay
   D. Esculin hydrolysis

258. Which of the following tests is most appropriate for the presumptive identification of *Peptostreptococcus anaerobius*?
   A. SPS disk
   B. Colistin disk
   C. Kanamycin disk
   D. Vancomycin disk

259. A curved appearance on Gram stain is characteristic of which of the following?
   A. *Actinomyces israelii*
   B. *Clostridium septicum*
   C. *Fusobacterium nucleatum*
   D. *Propionibacterium acnes*

260. Purulent material from a cerebral abscess was submitted to the laboratory for smear and culture. On direct Gram stain, gram-positive cocci in chains and gram-negative bacilli with pointed ends were seen. Plates incubated aerobically exhibited no growth at 24 hours. On the basis of the organisms seen on the smear, what is the most likely presumptive identification of the etiologic anaerobic agents?
   A. *Veillonella* sp. and *Clostridium* sp.
   B. *Eubacterium* sp. and *Veillonella* sp.
   C. *Peptostreptococcus* sp. and *Nocardia* sp.
   D. *Fusobacterium* sp. and *Peptostreptococcus* sp.

261. Which of the following is an important virulence factor of *Bacteroides fragilis*?
   A. Neurotoxin
   B. Exotoxins
   C. Polysaccharide capsule
   D. Protease

262. Which of the following is true of *Bacteroides fragilis*?
   A. Lipase and lecithinase positive
   B. Anaerobic gram-positive bacillus
   C. Commonly associated with intra-abdominal infections
   D. Among the most antimicrobial-sensitive anaerobic bacteria

263. Which of the following is a likely causative agent in aspiration pneumonia?
   A. *Lactobacillus* sp.
   B. *Mobiluncus* sp.
   C. *Porphyromonas* sp.
   D. *Clostridium* sp.

264. To ensure that anaerobic conditions have been achieved in anaerobic jars or chambers, an oxygen-sensitive indicator is employed, such as
   A. Bromcreosol purple
   B. Methylene blue
   C. Methyl red
   D. Phenol red

265. Egg yolk agar showing a precipitate in the medium surrounding the colony is positive for
   A. Lecithinase production
   B. Lipase production
   C. Protease activity
   D. Starch hydrolysis

266. After 72 hours of anaerobic incubation, small olive-green to black colonies are seen. A Gram stain reveals gram-positive cocci. What is the most likely identification of this organism?
   A. *Fingoldia magna*
   B. *Peptococcus niger*
   C. *Peptostreptococcus anaerobius*
   D. *Veillonella parvula*

267. Which of the following is an important cause of food poisoning?
   A. *Bacteroides fragilis*
   B. *Campylobacter ureolyticus*
   C. *Clostridium perfringens*
   D. *Clostridium histolyticum*

268. Which bacterium is part of the normal vaginal biota that helps resist the onset of bacterial vaginosis?
   A. *Peptostreptococcus* sp.
   B. *Peptococcus* sp.
   C. *Lactobacillus* sp.
   D. *Mobiluncus* sp.

Chlamydia, Rickettsia, and *Mycoplasma*

269. *Chlamydia trachomatis* causes which of the following?
   A. Rat-bite fever
   B. Inclusion conjunctivitis
   C. A skin disease found predominantly in tropical areas
   D. Zoonosis in birds and parrot fever in humans

270. Which one of the following microorganisms *cannot* be cultivated on artificial cell-free media?
   A. *Chlamydia trachomatis*
   B. *Mycoplasma hominis*
   C. *Mycoplasma pneumoniae*
   D. *Ureaplasma urealyticum*

271. An etiologic agent of primary atypical pneumonia is
   A. *Chlamydia trachomatis*
   B. *Chlamydiophila psittaci*
   C. *Mycoplasma pneumoniae*
   D. *Ureaplasma urealyticum*

272. The recommended medium for the recovery of *Mycoplasma pneumoniae* from clinical specimens is
   A. Charcoal yeast extract medium
   B. Fletcher semisolid medium
   C. Middlebrook
   D. SP4 agar

273. *Chlamydophila (Chlamydia) psittaci* infections in humans most commonly result after exposure to infected
   A. Amphibians
   B. Arthropods
   C. Avians
   D. Mammalians

274. Which of the following is *not* true of *Coxiella burnetii*?
   A. It is an obligate intracellular parasite.
   B. It is transmitted from animals to humans by inhalation.
   C. A rash appears first on the extremities and then on the trunk.
   D. Is the etiologic agent of Q fever, which may be acute or chronic

275. Which of the following is *true* about mycoplasmas?
   A. Resistant to penicillin
   B. Not able to survive extracellularly
   C. Easily stained using the Gram stain
   D. Grow on routine nonselective culture media

276. Corneal scrapings are useful for the diagnosis of infection caused by
   A. *Chlamydia trachomatis*
   B. *Ehrlichia chaffeensis*
   C. *Mycoplasma hominis*
   D. *Rickettsia prowazekii*

277. Which of the following *Mycoplasmataceae* has *not* been connected with human genital infections?
   A. *Mycoplasma genitalium*
   B. *Mycoplasma hominis*
   C. *Mycoplasma pneumoniae*
   D. *Ureaplasma urealyticum*

278. Which of the following is true about *Chlamydophila pneumoniae*?
   A. Common agent of lower gastrointestinal tract infection
   B. Humans become infected from animal reservoirs.
   C. Penicillin is an effective treatment.
   D. Serology is commonly used to diagnose infections.

279. What is the common method for confirmation of *Chlamydia trachomatis* in sexually transmitted infections?
   A. Cell culture
   B. Nonculture EIA methods
   C. DNA-amplification techniques
   D. Culture on modified Thayer-Martin agar

280. Colonies said to have the appearance of a "fried egg" are characteristic of
   A. *Ehrlichia chaffeensis*
   B. *Mycoplasma genitalium*
   C. *Mycoplasma hominis*
   D. *Ureaplasma urealyticum*

281. Human infection with the causative agent of Q fever is acquired commonly by
   A. Inhalation of infectious material
   B. The bite of a mite (chigger)
   C. The bite of a body louse
   D. The bite of the arthropod *Phlebotomus*

282. For nonspecific staining of *Rickettsia* the recommended stain is
   A. Gimenez stain
   B. Gomori silver stain
   C. Gram stain
   D. Kinyoun stain

283. Rocky Mountain spotted fever is transmitted by the bite of a tick infected with
   A. *Rickettsia akari*
   B. *Rickettsia conorii*
   C. *Rickettsia prowazekii*
   D. *Rickettsia rickettsii*

284. Transmission of the sylvatic form of typhus infection caused by *Rickettsia prowazekii* is associated with
   A. Bats
   B. Rabbits
   C. Raccoons
   D. Squirrels

285. The mild type of typhus fever that is caused by recrudescence of an initial attack of epidemic typhus is known as
   A. Brill-Zinsser disease
   B. Q fever
   C. São Paulo typhus
   D. Tsutsugamushi disease

286. The causative agent of endemic or murine typhus is
   A. *Rickettsia akari*
   B. *Rickettsia conorii*
   C. *Rickettsia prowazekii*
   D. *Rickettsia typhi*

287. For the detection or recovery of mycoplasmata.
   A. A Gram stain can be used.
   B. A swab can be used to gently remove material from the nasopharynx.
   C. A transport medium is not needed.
   D. Some species, such as *Mycoplasma hominis*, can be grown on SP4 agar.

288. A genital specimen is inoculated into 10 B broth. After overnight incubation, an alkaline reaction is noted without turbidity. What is the most likely explanation?
   A. pH change due to molecules in the clinical specimen
   B. Presence of *Mycoplasma genitalium*
   C. Presence of *Mycoplasma hominis*
   D. Presence of *Ureaplasma urealyticum*

Spirochetes

289. Detection of antibody against cardiolipin is useful for the diagnosis of which of the following diseases?
   A. Leptospirosis
   B. Lyme disease
   C. Relapsing fever
   D. Syphilis

290. During the first week of leptospirosis, the most reliable way to detect the presence of the causative agent is by the direct
   A. Culturing of blood
   B. Culturing of urine
   C. Examination of blood
   D. Examination of cerebrospinal fluid

291. Serious congenital infections are associated with
   A. *Borrelia burgdorferi*
   B. *Borrelia recurrentis*
   C. *Treponema pallidum* subsp. *pallidum*
   D. *Treponema pallidum* subsp. *pertenue*

292. A helicoidal, flexible organism was demonstrated in a blood smear. This motile organism was approximately 12 μm long, approximately 0.1 μm wide, and had semicircular hooked ends. The description of this organism corresponds most closely to the morphology of
   A. *Borrelia*
   B. *Leptonema*
   C. *Leptospira*
   D. *Treponema*

293. The etiologic agent of epidemic relapsing fever is *Borrelia recurrentis*, which is commonly transmitted by
   A. Fleas
   B. Lice
   C. Mosquitoes
   D. Ticks

294. Which of the following is true of serologic tests for diagnosing syphilis?
   A. False-positive tests are more frequent with the fluorescent treponemal antibody absorbance (FTA-ABS) test than with the rapid plasma reagin (RPR) assay.
   B. Inactivated *Treponema pallidum* serves as the antigen in the Venereal Disease Research Laboratory (VDRL) assay.
   C. The antibody titer in the *Treponema pallidum* antigen (TP-PA) test will decline if the patient is adequately treated.
   D. The tests are usually positive (high sensitivity) in secondary syphilis.

295. *Borrelia burgdorferi*, a spirochete transmitted by *Ixodes dammini* in the northeastern United States, is the etiologic agent of
   A. Lyme disease
   B. Rat-bite fever
   C. Relapsing fever
   D. Q fever

296. The axial fibrils of spirochetes most closely resemble which bacterial structure?
   A. Cytoplasmic membrane
   B. Flagellum
   C. Pilus
   D. Sporangium

297. Which of the following is true regarding spirochetes?
   A. Motility is via flagella.
   B. Spirochetes are gram positive.
   C. They are visualized best using dark field or phase optics.
   D. All human spirochete diseases are generally transmitted human to human.

298. A positive VDRL test for syphilis was reported on a young woman known to have hepatitis. When questioned by her physician, she denied sexual contact with any partner symptomatic for a sexually transmitted disease. Which of the following would be the appropriate next step for her physician?
   A. Treat her with penicillin
   B. Identify her sexual contacts for serologic testing
   C. Test her serum using a *Treponema pallidum*-particulate antigen assay
   D. Reassure her that it was a biologic false-positive caused by her liver disease

Antimicrobial Agents and Antimicrobial Susceptibility Testing

299. A suspension of the test organism for use in broth dilution and disk diffusion testing is adjusted to match the turbidity of a
   A. #0.5 McFarland standard
   B. #1.0 McFarland standard
   C. #2.0 McFarland standard
   D. #3.0 McFarland standard

300. When testing the antimicrobial susceptibility of *Haemophilus influenzae* strains by disk-agar diffusion, the recommended medium is
   A. Chocolate agar
   B. Charcoal yeast extract agar
   C. Mueller-Hinton base supplemented with 5% sheep blood
   D. Mueller-Hinton base supplemented with hematin, NAD, and yeast extract

301. The chemotherapeutic agents structurally similar to the vitamin *p*-aminobenzoic acid that act by inhibiting bacteria via inhibition of folic acid synthesis are
   A. Aminoglycosides
   B. Penicillins
   C. Macrolides
   D. Sulfonamides

302. Which of the following beta-lactam antibiotics is considered to have the broadest spectrum?
   A. Carbapenems
   B. Semi-synthetic penicillins
   C. First-generation cephalosporins
   D. Fifth-generation cephalosporins

303. Penicillin is active against bacteria by
   A. Inhibition of protein synthesis at the 30S ribosomal subunit
   B. Reduction of dihydrofolic acid
   C. Inhibition or peptidoglycan synthesis
   D. Inhibition of nucleic acid function

304. The minimum bactericidal concentration (MBC) of an antimicrobial agent is defined as the lowest concentration of that antimicrobial agent that kills at least _______ of the original inoculum.
   A. 95.5%
   B. 97%
   C. 99.9%
   D. 100%

305. Resistance to clindamycin can be induced *in vitro* by
   A. Ampicillin
   B. Erythromycin
   C. Gentamicin
   D. Penicillin

306. The term that denotes a situation in which the effect of two antimicrobial agents together is greater than the sum of the effects of either drug alone is
   A. Additivism
   B. Antagonism
   C. Sensitivity
   D. Synergism

307. Beta-lactamase-producing strains of *Haemophilus influenzae* are resistant to
   A. Chloramphenicol
   B. Erythromycin
   C. Ampicillin
   D. Trimethoprim sulfamethoxazole

308. The medium recommended by the Clinical and Laboratory Standards Institute for routine susceptibility testing of nonfastidious bacteria is
A. MacConkey agar
B. Middlebrook 7H10 agar
C. Mueller-Hinton agar
D. Trypticase soy agar

309. The pH of the agar used for the Kirby-Bauer test should be
A. 7.0–7.2
B. 7.2–7.4
C. 7.4–7.6
D. 7.6–7.8

310. Which drug known to be active against parasitic infections has importance as a therapeutic agent in cases of disease caused by anaerobic bacteria?
A. Isoniazid
B. Metronidazole
C. Rifampin
D. Trimethoprim

311. An example of a bactericidal antimicrobial agent is
A. Chloramphenicol
B. Erythromycin
C. Tetracycline
D. Tobramycin

312. The extended-spectrum beta-lactamases confer resistance to
A. Amikacin
B. Ceftriaxone
C. Erythromycin
D. Rifampin

313. Which of the following media should be used for *in vitro* susceptibility testing of *S. pneumoniae*?
A. Chocolate agar
B. Charcoal yeast extract agar
C. Mueller-Hinton base supplemented with 5% lysed horse blood
D. Mueller-Hinton base supplemented with 1% hemoglobin and 1% IsoVitaleX

314. Rapid testing for beta-lactamase production is recommended, before initiation of antimicrobial therapy, for isolates of
A. *Serratia marcescens*
B. *Haemophilus influenzae*
C. *Staphylococcus epidermidis*
D. *Streptococcus pyogenes*

315. The phenomenon of bacterial resistance to the bactericidal activity of penicillins and cephalosporins, with only inhibition of the organism's growth, is known as
A. High-level resistance
B. Intrinsic resistance
C. Inducible resistance
D. Tolerance

316. Bacteria producing carbapenemase would be expected to be resistant to
A. Aminoglycosides
B. Cephalosporins
C. Fluoroquinolones
D. Tetracyclines

317. Clavulanic acid is classified as a
A. Beta-lactam
B. Beta-lactamase inhibitor
C. Macrolide
D. Aminoglycoside

318. Which of the following antimicrobial agents acts by inhibiting cell wall synthesis?
A. Clindamycin
B. Gentamicin
C. Naladixic acid
D. Vancomycin

319. In the modified carbapenem inactivation method (mCIM) assay
   A. Growth of the control organism up to a carbapenem disk indicates carbapenemase production by the test organism.
   B. No growth of the control organism up to a carbapenem disk indicates carbapenemase production by the test organism.
   C. No growth of the control organism up to a carbapenem disk indicates carbapenemase production by the control organism.
   D. Growth of the control organism up to a carbapenem disk indicates a problem with the assay, and it should be repeated.

320. Which of the following antimicrobial agents acts by inhibiting protein synthesis?
   A. Gentamicin
   B. Methicillin
   C. Rifampin
   D. Ampicillin

321. Chloramphenicol is an important antimicrobial agent for the treatment of meningitis as well as several other serious infections. Unfortunately, chloramphenicol exhibits significant complications that limit its clinical usefulness. These effects include
   A. Allergic reactions and anaphylaxis
   B. Bone marrow suppression
   C. Significant gastrointestinal manifestations
   D. Photosensitivity

322. Which one of the following antimicrobial agents is recommended when screening for methicillin-resistant *Staphylococcus aureus*?
   A. Erythromycin
   B. Oxacillin
   C. Cefoxitin
   D. Azithromycin

Procedures and Biochemical Identification of Bacteria

323. Which of the following body sites is normally colonized by normal microbiota?
   A. Lungs
   B. Trachea
   C. Cervix
   D. Skin

324. During childbearing years, the normal biota of the vagina is predominantly
   A. *Enterococcus*
   B. *Lactobacillus*
   C. *Propionibacterium*
   D. Coagulase-negative *Staphylococcus*

325. The Microbial Identification (MIDI) system is based on
   A. Antibiograms
   B. Colony pigment on ChromAgar
   C. Fatty acid analysis
   D. Multiple biochemical tests

326. Which of the following is a correct statement regarding blood cultures?
   A. Collection of 5–10 mL per culture for adults is recommended.
   B. One blood culture collection is regarded as sufficient to detect most cases of bacteremia or septicemia.
   C. Volume of blood cultured is more critical than timing of culture.
   D. Blood drawn for culture may be allowed to clot.

327. In capnophilic incubators, carbon dioxide concentrations should be maintained between
   A. 1% and 5%
   B. 5% and 10%
   C. 10% and 15%
   D. 15% and 20%

328. The recommended anticoagulant for use when a body fluid or joint fluid that may clot is sent for microbiologic examination is
   A. Heparin
   B. Sodium polyethanol sulfonate (SPS)
   C. Sodium EDTA
   D. Sodium citrate

329. When performing an oxidase test
   A. Bacteria should be taken from media with a high glucose content.
   B. *Pseudomonas aeruginosa* can be used as a negative control.
   C. Plates incubated anaerobically should be exposed to room air for about 15 minutes before testing.
   D. Formation of a purple color after 1 minute is considered positive.

330. The majority of cases of laboratory-related infections are associated with
   A. Infectious aerosols
   B. Contamination of abraded skin
   C. Puncture wounds
   D. Person-to-person transmission

331. The quality of an expectorated sputum is evaluated based on the
   A. Amount of bacteria seen in a direct Gram stain
   B. Number of red blood cells in comparison to epithelial cells in a direct Gram stain
   C. Number of white blood cells in comparison to epithelial cells in a direct Gram stain
   D. Viscosity of the sample and macroscopic appearance of blood

332. Which of the following media is both selective and differential?
   A. Sheep blood agar
   B. Chocolate agar
   C. Mannitol salt agar
   D. Mueller-Hinton agar

333. In matrix-assisted laser desorption/ionization time of flight (MALDI-TOF) mass spectrometry, how are biomolecules separated?
   A. Mass
   B. Mass to charge ratio
   C. Number of charges on the molecules
   D. Time it takes for vaporization by a laser

334. It is generally most appropriate to perform a hippurate hydrolysis test to aid in the identification of
   A. *Enterobacteriaceae*
   B. Gram-negative cocci
   C. Gram-positive, spore-forming gram-positive bacilli
   D. Beta-hemolytic gram-positive cocci

335. Continuous blood culture systems that detect changes in headspace pressure in bottles are referred to as
   A. Fluorescence methods
   B. ^{14}C detection methods
   C. Colorimetry methods
   D. Manometric methods

336. In the catalase test, the formation of bubbles is due to
   A. Production of oxygen (O_2)
   B. Production of hydrogen gas (H_2)
   C. Breakdown of water
   D. Oxidation of hydrogen peroxide

337. Which of the following would be appropriate for positive and negative controls in the PYR test?
   A. *Staphylococcus aureus* and *Staphylococcus lugdunensis*
   B. *Streptococcus pyogenes* and *Staphylococcus lugdunensis*
   C. *Streptococcus pyogenes* and *Enterococcus faecalis*
   D. *Streptococcus pneumoniae* and alpha-hemolytic streptococci viridans group

Case Studies

338. A purulent aspirate of joint fluid from a 28-year-old female with joint pain was sent for microbiologic examination. The Gram stain of this sample revealed many polymorphonuclear cells with intracellular and extracellular gram-negative diplococci. Given the specimen type and microscopic findings, the appropriate selective medium for primary isolation would be
    A. Mannitol salt agar
    B. Potassium tellurite agar
    C. Modified Thayer-Martin agar
    D. Cefsulodin-irgasan-novobiocin

339. A 21-year-old sexually active woman came to the university student health service with a 2-day history of urinary frequency with urgency, dysuria, and hematuria. She had no history of prior urinary tract infection. Laboratory test showed a white blood cell count of $10 \times 10^9/L$. The urine sediment contained innumerable white cells. Cultures yielded more than 10^5 colony-forming units/mL of a lactose-fermenting gram-negative rod. The most likely etiologic agent in this case is
    A. *Escherichia coli*
    B. *Klebsiella pneumoniae*
    C. *Morganella morganii*
    D. *Proteus mirabilis*

340. A 36-year-old man was seen in the emergency department. He complained of fever and headache. He had returned 1 week previously from a 6-week visit to a village in India. Among the differential diagnoses was typhoid fever. What is the most critical laboratory test necessary to establish or eliminate the diagnosis?
    A. Blood cultures
    B. Sputum cultures
    C. Stool cultures
    D. Urine cultures

341. A 45-year-old man was seen in the emergency department with fever, chills, nausea, and myalgia. He reported that 2 days earlier he had eaten raw oysters at a popular seafood restaurant. On admission, he was febrile and had hemorrhagic, fluid-filled bullous lesions on his left leg. The patient had a history of diabetes mellitus, chronic hepatitis B, and heavy alcohol consumption. The patient, who had a temperature of 102.2°F, was admitted to the intensive care unit for presumed sepsis, and treatment was begun. A curved gram-negative rod was isolated from blood cultures drawn on admission and fluid from the bullous leg wound. On the third day, disseminated intravascular coagulation developed, and he died. The most likely etiologic agent in this case would be
    A. *Aeromonas hydrophila*
    B. *Plesiomonas shigelloides*
    C. *Vibrio vulnificus*
    D. *Yersinia enterocolitica*

342. Gram-positive rods were recovered from the chest fluid drawn from a teenager with right lower lobe pneumonia who lived on a dairy farm. At 24 hours, pinpoint colonies grew on sheep blood agar that showed faint zones of beta-hemolysis. The isolate was catalase negative and demonstrated a positive CAMP test. Which of the following is the most likely etiologic agent in this case?
    A. *Listeria monocytogenes*
    B. *Streptococcus agalactiae*
    C. *Arcanobacterium pyogenes*
    D. *Streptobacillus moniliformis*

343. A 3-year-old was brought to the emergency department by her parents. She had been febrile with a loss of appetite for the past 24 hours. Most recently, the parents noted that it was difficult to arouse her. She attended a daycare center, and her childhood immunizations were current. On examination, she demonstrated a positive Brudzinski sign indicative of meningeal irritation. Cultures of blood and cerebrospinal fluid (CSF) were sent to the laboratory. Her CSF was cloudy, and the Gram stain showed many polymorphonuclear cells containing gram-negative diplococci. The white blood cell count was 25×10^9/L, with 88% polymorphonuclear cells. The CSF protein was 100 mg/dL, and the glucose was 15 mg/dL. Cultures of the blood and CSF grew the same organism. The most likely etiologic agent in this case is
A. *Haemophilus influenzae*
B. *Listeria monocytogenes*
C. *Moraxella catarrhalis*
D. *Neisseria meningitidis*

344. A young woman complaining of the sudden onset of fever, vomiting, diarrhea, and rash was seen by her gynecologist. She was admitted to the hospital, where a culture of vaginal discharge grew many coagulase-positive staphylococci. The most likely diagnosis in this case would be
A. Kawasaki disease
B. Pelvic inflammatory disease
C. Scalded skin syndrome
D. Toxic shock syndrome

345. A 32-year-old male was seen in the emergency department with symptoms of lower right quadrant abdominal pain and diarrhea. A complete blood count showed a leukocytosis with an increased number of neutrophils. He was admitted, and a stool culture was obtained. The culture showed many gram-negative bacilli, which were oxidase negative, citrate negative, and indole negative. The triple sugar iron reaction was acid over acid, but there was no evidence of gas or H_2S production. The organism was positive for urease and ONPG and negative for phenylalanine. The characteristic symptomatology and the biochemical reactions confirmed that the etiologic agent was
A. *Salmonella* Paratyphi
B. *Shigella dysenteriae*
C. *Vibrio parahaemolyticus*
D. *Yersinia enterocolitica*

346. In August, a patient presented at a community hospital in New England with symptoms of a skin rash, headache, stiff neck, muscle aches, and swollen lymph nodes. A silver-stained biopsy of a skin lesion showed spirochetes. On the basis of the clinical syndrome and laboratory detection of a causative agent, the patient was diagnosed as having
A. Lyme disease
B. Plague
C. Rabbit fever
D. Relapsing fever

347. Several international participants in an Eco-Challenge adventure race in Borneo became ill with symptoms of chills, diarrhea, headaches, and eye infections. The racers hiked in the mountains and jungles, swam in rivers, and slogged through flooded streams for 2 weeks. Contact with contaminated water and soil during the race was highly associated with illness. What is the most likely etiologic agent in this case?
    A. *Borellia recurrentis*
    B. *Brucella canis*
    C. *Franciscella tularensis*
    D. *Leptospira interrogans*

348. An anemic patient was transfused with packed red blood cells. Approximately 1 hour after the transfusion began, the patient developed fever and hypotension consistent with endotoxic shock. The red blood cells had been stored at 4°C for approximately 21 days before their use. The organism most likely to be involved in this case is
    A. *Campylobacter fetus*
    B. *Neisseria meningitidis*
    C. *Pseudomonas aeruginosa*
    D. *Yersinia enterocolitica*

349. A college student got a summer job working at a marina. While repairing the outboard motor on a rental boat, he received several lacerations on his right forearm. No medical treatment was sought at the time of the injury, but after several weeks he noted that the lesions were not healing and he sought the opinion of his physician. A biopsy of one of the lesions revealed a cutaneous granulomatous condition. Given the history, which of the following microorganisms would most likely be the etiologic agent in this case?
    A. *Mycobacterium marinum*
    B. *Nocardia asteroides*
    C. *Pseudomonas aeruginosa*
    D. *Vibrio vulnificus*

350. A woman, who had recently returned from a vacation in Mexico, was admitted to the hospital. She was febrile and complained of flulike symptoms. Her case history revealed that she had eaten cheese that had been made from unpasteurized milk while on vacation. The most likely etiologic agent in this case would be
    A. *Bordetella pertussis*
    B. *Listeria monocytogenes*
    C. *Staphylococcus aureus*
    D. *Yersinia enterocolitica*

351. A 7-year-old female became ill with an intestinal illness after visiting a petting zoo featuring farm animals such as calves, lambs, and chickens. She had bloody diarrhea and went on to develop hemolytic uremic syndrome. The most likely etiologic agent in this case is
   A. *E. coli* 0157:H7
   B. *Shigella dysenteriae*
   C. *Vibrio cholerae* 01
   D. *Vibrio cholerae* non01

352. A middle-aged man with a history of smoking and drinking for over 40 years developed shortness of breath, fever, frontal headache, diarrhea, and cough. He worked in the produce section of a supermarket, which routinely misted the fresh greens. His medical history included a kidney transplant several years ago for which he remains on antirejection therapy. His sputum Gram stain showed numerous polymorphonuclear cells but rare microorganisms. An X-ray of his chest showed an infiltrate in the left lower lobe, and a diagnosis of atypical pneumonia was made. Which of the following is the most likely etiologic agent in this case?
   A. *Bordetella pertussis*
   B. *Klebsiella pneumoniae*
   C. *Legionella pneumophila*
   D. *Moraxella catarrhalis*

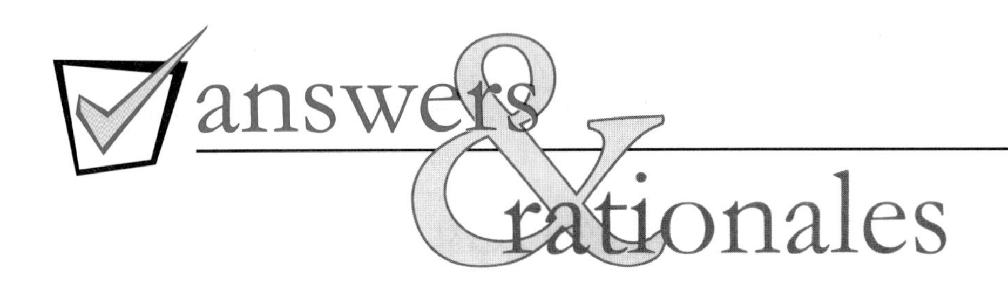

Aerobic Gram-Positive Bacteria

1.

C. *Enterococcus* and other group D streptococci can be presumptively identified based on their ability to hydrolyze esculin in the presence of 1–4% bile salts. The medium is made selective for enterococci by the addition of either sodium azide or 4% bile salts. Organisms able to grow on this medium and hydrolyze esculin produce esculetin, which reacts with an iron salt to form a black color in the agar.

2.

D. Strains of *C. diphtheriae* infected by a lysogenic bacteriophage produce an extremely potent exotoxin. Absorption of the toxin may cause a rapidly fatal hypertoxic disease characterized by myocarditis and neuritis. This disease most commonly affects children aged 1 to 10 years. Transmission is by contact with a human carrier or with contaminated fomites.

3.

B. *Aerococcus* spp. were first described in air and dust. Their normal habitat has not been established, but they can occur as a part of the normal biota of the human urinary tract and oral cavity. Some species have been noted to cause urinary tract infections, septicemias, and endocarditis.

4.

B. Nutritionally variant streptococci (NVS) are now termed *Abiotrophia*. These clinically significant microorganisms, which account for 5–6% of the cases of endocarditis, are frequently not able to be recovered because of insufficient quantities of vitamin B_6 (pyridoxal) in the culture medium. The routine use of a pyridoxal disk, a streak of *Staphylococcus*, or vitamin B_6–supplemented culture media is required for isolation.

5.

C. Scalded skin syndrome is a form of dermatitis produced by strains of *S. aureus* that elaborate exfoliative toxin. Two types of this toxin have been identified: exfoliation A and exfoliation B. This potent toxin acts by disturbing the adhesive forces between cells of the stratum granulosum, which causes the appearance of the clear, large, flaccid bullae and the skin to peel off. Infants and children are most commonly affected with this form of dermatitis, beginning about the face and trunk and subsequently spreading to the extremities.

6.

A. *A. haemolyticum* is an infrequent cause of pharyngitis. Symptoms can be mild to severe and resemble pharyngitis caused by *S. pyogenes*. *E. rhusiopathiae* produces a disease called erysipeloid.

7.

A. Staphylococci and micrococci are both catalase positive gram-positive cocci. Staphylococci are more clinically significant, so it is important to differentiate *Micrococcus* from *Staphylococcus*. Micrococci are modified oxidase positive, whereas staphylococci are negative.

8.

B. Nocardiosis is characterized by mycetoma or chronic suppurative infection. Draining sinus tracts in the subcutaneous tissue are a common manifestation of the disease. *Nocardia* spp. are soil saprophytes that may produce disease in humans either by the inhalation of contaminated material or through skin abrasions. Microscopic examination of pus from suspected cases will demonstrate partially acid-fast, gram-positive, branching filamentous or coccoid organism.

9.

A. Infection caused by *E. rhusiopathiae* in humans is primarily erysipeloid. Erysipeloid is usually the result of contact with an infected animal or contaminated animal product. The characteristic presentation is cutaneous spreading lesions of the fingers or hand that are raised and erythematous. Although generally confined to the skin, *E. rhusiopathiae* has been implicated in rare cases of endocarditis.

10.

C. *Streptomyces* causes the tissue infection mycetoma following implantation of the bacteria into a wound contaminated with soil. The infection is characterized by pus-draining sinus tracts. The bacteria are nonspore-forming gram-positive bacilli.

11.

D. The recovery rate of coagulase-negative *S. saprophyticus* from urinary tract infections in young females is second only to that of *E. coli*. The organism has a predilection for the epithelial cells of the urogenital tract and is often seen in large numbers adhering to these cells on Gram stain. Key to the identification of this coagulase-negative *Staphylococcus* is its resistance to novobiocin.

12.

A. The organism seen in Color Plate 25 ■ is *L. monocytogenes*. *Listeria* is an important animal and human pathogen that is known to cause abortion, meningitis, and septicemia in humans. This gram-positive rod is actively motile at room temperature (but not at 35°C), hydrolyzes esculin, produces catalase, and is oxidase negative. When recovered on sheep blood agar plates from clinical samples, it is often initially confused with group A or group B streptococci because of its beta-hemolysis.

13.

A. *S. agalactiae* (group B *Streptococcus*) is a principal cause of bacterial meningitis and septicemia in neonates. The organism, which is a part of the indigenous microbial biota of the vagina, is transmitted by the mother before birth, usually as the baby passes through the birth canal. Neonatal infection with group B streptococci may occur either as an early-onset disease (at birth) or as a delayed-onset syndrome that manifests itself weeks after birth.

14.

B. The vegetative cells and spores of *B. cereus* are widely distributed in the environment. The virulence mechanisms of *B. cereus* are an enterotoxin and a pyogenic toxin. Accidents in nature resulting in cuts or abrasions contaminated with soil or vegetation, intravenous drug abuse, ingestion of contaminated foods, and traumatic introduction into a normally sterile site through the use of contaminated medical equipment are associated with infection.

15.

B. The formation of the characteristic *C. diphtheriae* granules and cellular morphology seen in methylene blue stains is enhanced when the organism is grown on Loeffler's serum medium. Although this medium is primarily designed for the recovery of *C. diphtheriae* from clinical samples, it is not a differential medium. The agar slant, when inoculated, may demonstrate growth of corynebacteria within 8–24 hours.

16.

C. Tinsdale medium, for the primary isolation of *C. diphtheriae*, not only inhibits indigenous respiratory biota but differentiates colonies of *C. diphtheriae*. The potassium tellurite in the medium is taken up by colonies of *Corynebacterium*, causing them to appear black. Colonies of *C. diphtheriae* are presumptively identified when black colonies surrounded by a brown halo are seen on this agar medium. However, other corynebacteria and some staphylococci will produce a similar reaction.

17.

B. The Elek immunodiffusion test is recommended for detecting toxigenic strains of *C. diphtheriae*. In the test, diphtheria antitoxin is impregnated on a sterile filter paper strip, which is pressed onto the surface of an Elek agar plate. Test and control strains are then inoculated perpendicular to the strip on both sides and without touching the strip. A positive reaction by toxigenic strains produces a precipitin line at a 45-degree angle to the inoculum streak.

18.

D. Erysipelas results from person-to-person transmission of group A streptococci. Symptoms occur when nasopharyngeal infection spreads to the face. The rare complication of an upper respiratory infection with *S. pyogenes* is characterized by sensations of burning and tightness at the site of invasion. Erythema associated with this superficial cellulitis rapidly spreads with an advancing elevated margin. *E. rhusiopathiae* causes a similar disease referred to as erysipeloid.

19.

B. Phenylethyl alcohol (PEA) agar is a selective medium for the isolation of gram-positive cocci. Blood agar medium is supplemented with 0.15% PEA, which is inhibitory to most gram-negative aerobic bacilli. This medium is particularly helpful when a specimen containing gram-positive cocci is contaminated with a *Proteus* spp. due to the inhibition of swarming by PEA.

20.

D. Viridans streptococci are the most common normal biota in upper respiratory cultures. They are opportunistic pathogens with low virulence. Subacute endocarditis is seen in patients with previously damaged heart valves.

21.

B. Whether growing aerobically or anaerobically, streptococci obtain all their energy from the fermentation of sugars to lactic acid. Streptococci are all catalase negative and grow on conventional media such as sheep blood agar. Most are part of the normal biota of human skin, throat, and intestine but produce a wide variety of infections when introduced in tissues or blood.

22.

A. Organisms that synthesize the enzyme catalase are able to protect themselves from the killing effects of H_2O_2 by converting it to H_2O and O_2. Streptococci are unable to synthesize the heme prosthetic group for this enzyme and are catalase negative. Therefore, they grow better on blood-containing media because of the catalase-like activity of hemoglobin.

23.

D. Streptolysin S is primarily responsible for the beta-hemolysis seen on the surface of a sheep blood agar plate inoculated with a group A *Streptococcus*. Of the two hemolysins secreted by beta-hemolytic group A *Streptococcus*, streptolysin S is stable in the presence of atmospheric oxygen. Streptolysin O is inactivated in the presence of oxygen, and it is best demonstrated when the agar has been stabbed and subsurface hemolysis is revealed.

24.

C. *Moraxella catarrhalis* is a gram-negative diplococcus that resembles members of the genus *Neisseria*. It produces the enzyme butyrate esterase, which produces a positive tributyrin hydrolysis test. *M. catarrhalis* causes otitis sinusitis and lower respiratory tract infections.

25.

B. *Erysipelothrix rhusiopathiae* is a nonmotile, catalase-negative, gram-positive bacillus that often appears as long filaments. Unlike other aerobic gram-positive bacilli, this organism produces H_2S, which can be demonstrated in triple sugar iron agar. Erysipeloid, a skin disease of the hands usually associated with the handling of infected animals, is the human infection produced most commonly by this agent.

26.

D. *L. monocytogenes* is motile at room temperature. When inoculated into a semisolid medium, growth away from the stab is characteristic of motility. Motility is generally enhanced just below the agar surface, giving the growth pattern an "umbrella" appearance. *L. monocytogenes* is nonmotile at 35°C.

27.

D. *R. equi* is found in soil and commonly produces disease among livestock. These gram-positive bacilli can demonstrate primary mycelia and were formerly in the genus *Nocardia*. This species is characterized by its pink pigmentation on culture media and its inability to ferment carbohydrates.

28.

D. *S. pneumoniae* is the leading cause of pneumonia in elderly patients, particularly over the age of 60 years. It is an encapsulated, gram-positive, lancet-shaped diplococcus. There are approximately 90 types of pneumococci based on specific capsular antigens. Fastidious in its growth requirements, the organism on sheep blood agar produces characteristic alpha-hemolytic colonies, which are convex and often mucoid in appearance and bile soluble.

29.

D. Species of the genus *Nocardia* are ubiquitous in the soil and thus characteristically produce exogenous forms of infection as a result of inhalation of contaminated fomites or a traumatic incident with soil contamination. A diagnostic characteristic, depending on the species, is the acid fastness of the filamentous bacilli or coccoid forms. Unlike *Actinomyces* spp., which are catalase-negative, gram-positive, nonspore-forming anaerobic bacilli, *Nocardia* spp. are catalase-positive aerobic organisms. "Sulfur granules" are characteristic of actinomycotic pus and upon examination would reveal acid-fast branching filaments in the case of nocardiosis.

30.

B. *E. faecium* is an important agent of human infection. Their differentiation from other enterococcal strains is of importance because of their resistance to most clinically useful antimicrobial agents, including vancomycin. The ability to tolerate a high concentration of salt is characteristic of the clinically significant species of *Enterococcus*. *E. faecium* is PYR positive and is usually nonhemolytic.

31.

D. Viridans streptococci do not produce the enzyme pyroglutamyl aminopeptidase and, therefore, in the PYR test do not produce a positive or red color. The PYR test is used predominantly for the presumptive identification of group A streptococci and *Enterococcus*. *Micrococcus* and *Lactococcus* are known to produce a positive reaction as well, although the reaction may be delayed.

32.

C. *S. pneumoniae* is a leading cause of lobar pneumonia as well as other serious bacterial infections. The Gram stain smear of clinical specimens can provide a rapid presumptive diagnosis when the characteristic morphology and Gram reaction is observed. The optochin disk test can be performed to presumptively identify this organism. Optochin lyses pneumococci, producing a zone of inhibition around the disk.

33.

D. Bacteriologic cultures of a typical impetigo lesion may yield either a pure culture of *S. pyogenes* or a mixed culture of *S. pyogenes* and *S. aureus*. The thick crust form of impetigo, which is most commonly seen, is primarily caused by *S. pyogenes*. It is the bullous form of impetigo for which *S. aureus* is the etiologic agent. The route of infection is direct inoculation of the causative agents into abraded or otherwise compromised areas of the skin.

34.

C. Identifying characteristics of *S. aureus* include the production of the extracellular enzymes coagulase and DNase and its ability to grow in the presence of high salt concentrations. Differential and selective media, such as mannitol salt agar, have been developed for the recovery of this organism. Selective media and rapid identification tests are important for this widely recognized opportunistic pathogen.

35.

A. Group B streptococci (*Streptococcus agalactiae*), unlike other streptococci, can hydrolyze sodium hippurate to benzoic acid and glycine. If glycine is produced, the addition of ninhydrin to the medium will reduce the glycine to produce a purple color. The use of ninhydrin to detect glycine is a sensitive and rapid test of hippurate hydrolysis.

36.

A *L. monocytogenes* and *S. agalactiae* produce an extracellular factor known as the CAMP factor. The test is performed by making a streak of the test isolate perpendicular to a streak of *S. aureus*. A positive CAMP reaction is indicated by a zone of enhanced beta-hemolysis (arrowhead shape) at the point where the zone of hemolysis produced by *S. aureus* joins with that produced by the beta-hemolytic test isolate. Unlike *S. agalactiae, L. monocytogenes* is catalase positive.

37.

B. In the coagulase tube test, *S. aureus* forms a clot from enzyme activity converting fibrinogen to fibrin. Most isolates are beta-lactamase positive. Scarlet fever and rheumatic fever are caused by *S. pyogenes*.

38.

C. The physiology of staphylococci enables them to remain infectious in the environment longer than many other pathogenic bacteria. Staphylococci are somewhat heat resistant and can survive dry conditions. Their high salt tolerance enables strains to grow in salt-preserved foods and cause food poisoning. Staphylococci, however, cannot resist temperatures as high as 55°C for long periods, and they are not bile resistant. Most species are sensitive to novobiocin.

39.

C. Motility is a key test for the differentiation of *B. anthracis* from other species of *Bacillus*. Suspect *Bacillus* colonies are inoculated in a broth medium and allowed to grow to a visible turbidity. A sample of this actively growing culture should be examined using the hanging-drop technique for motility. *B. anthracis* is nonmotile and can therefore be easily differentiated from commonly encountered motile species.

40.

D. The rash of scarlet fever is a result of the action of streptococcal pyogenic exotoxin produced by group A streptococci. Because of the rapid diagnosis and treatment of group A streptococci infections, scarlet fever is rare in most developed countries. The other diseases listed do not involve an erythrogenic toxin.

41.

D. Cultures of the tonsillar fossae and posterior pharynx are most commonly obtained in suspected cases of streptococcal pharyngitis. *S. pyogenes* is most often associated with cases of pharyngitis but is also the agent of scarlet fever and erysipelas in addition to wound infections (e.g., necrotizing fasciitis). Rapid identification of this organism and prompt antimicrobial therapy are required to prevent sequelae (i.e., rheumatic fever and acute glomerulonephritis).

42.

D. Subacute bacterial endocarditis is an inflammation of the inside lining membrane of the heart, which most often is caused by a member of the viridans group of streptococci. *S. sanguis* is one of several species that may lodge in an abnormal heart or on valves damaged by previous infection. Viridans streptococci are normal inhabitants of the human upper respiratory tract.

43.

C. *S. pneumoniae* is most commonly associated with cases of lobar pneumonia. Patients characteristically produce blood-tinged, rust-colored sputum in which the characteristic gram-positive lancet-shaped diplococci can be found. *S. pneumoniae* forms alpha-hemolytic colonies when grown on SBA.

44.

A. *S. saprophyticus* is recognized as an etiologic agent of uncomplicated cystitis cases in young females. These nonhemolytic, coagulase-negative staphylococci closely resemble *S. epidermidis* on SBA. Identification of *S. saprophyticus* is facilitated by demonstrating its resistance to novobiocin.

45.

A. Clinical material sent to the laboratory for the recovery of *C. diphtheriae* should be inoculated onto cystine-tellurite agar plates or Tinsdale medium. On tellurite-containing media, colonies of this pathogen will appear dark-brown to black, which aids in their differentiation. Suspicious colonies should be further tested for their biochemical activity and toxin production.

46.

D. *B. anthracis* is the causative agent of woolsorters' disease or the pulmonary form of anthrax. The mode of infection is the inhalation of spores, usually during the performance of his/her occupation (sheep shearing or processing of animal hide or hair). Prompt diagnosis and treatment of this disease is needed because it is known to progress rapidly to a fatal form of septicemia.

47.

D. *C. pseudodiphtheriticum* is morphologically similar to all other members of the genus *Corynebacterium*. They are all gram-positive, nonspore-forming bacilli that are pleomorphic or form palisades ("picket fences"). These bacteria often stain irregularly and have a pleomorphic club-shaped appearance.

48.

B. *C. jeikeium* is a low-virulence organism resistant to multiple antimicrobials. Its multiple drug resistance allows it to remain in hospital environments, and it is often cultured from the skin of hospitalized patients. In compromised patients it has been implicated in cases of septicemia, wound infections, and endocarditis in association with intravenous catheter use.

49.

B. In patients who are immunocompromised, *Nocardia* spp. can cause invasive pulmonary infection and can often spread hematogenously throughout the body. Lesions in the brain are commonly associated with dissemination and have a poor prognosis. The organism is ubiquitous in nature, and infection is acquired by traumatic inoculation or inhalation.

50.

C. Of the genera listed, only *Leuconostoc* is catalase negative. *Leuconostoc* is vancomycin resistant and associated with infections in hospitalized patients. It has also been linked to septicemias in neonates.

51.

B. *L. monocytogenes* is a small, gram-positive bacillus that is actively motile at room temperature. When grown on sheep blood agar, this organism produces small, translucent beta-hemolytic colonies, which may be visually mistaken for beta-hemolytic streptococci. Biochemically, *L. monocytogenes* differs from streptococci because it possesses the enzyme catalase.

52.

C. *S. epidermidis* is a saprophytic microorganism found on the skin and mucous membranes of humans. This coagulase-negative *Staphylococcus* is seen frequently as a contaminant in blood cultures when improper venipuncture technique has been used. *S. epidermidis* has been implicated in serious human infections associated with the surgical insertion of prosthetic devices.

53.

A. *B. anthracis* is the etiologic agent of human anthrax that occurs in any of three forms: cutaneous, pulmonary, and gastrointestinal. On Gram stain, this organism appears as a large, spore-forming, gram-positive bacillus that characteristically grows in long chains. Colonies on agar plates are large and opaque with fingerlike projections referred to as "Medusa head" forms.

54.

C. Staphylococci colonize various skin and mucosal surfaces in humans. *S. aureus* is carried as transient biota in the anterior nares. *S. saprophyticus* is less likely found as normal biota and is associated with urinary tract infections. Hospital personnel may harbor resistant strains of *S. aureus*, and person-to-person contact is a substantial infection control concern. Cultures of the anterior nares are recommended when screening for carriers in the hospital environment.

55.

D. The susceptibility of alpha-hemolytic streptococcal isolates to optochin, or ethylhydrocupreine HCl, is a presumptive test for the differentiation of *S. pneumoniae* from viridans streptococci. Viridans streptococci are typically resistant to this agent and show no zone of inhibition or a zone of less than 10 mm with a 6-mm disk. *S. pneumoniae* characteristically is susceptible and produces a zone of inhibition greater than 14 mm.

56.

D. Solubility of *S. pneumoniae* colonies by surface-active agents, such as sodium desoxycholate, is a widely used presumptive identification procedure. When a 10% solution of this reagent is applied to test colonies, *S. pneumoniae* will be totally dissolved. Colonies of viridans streptococci typically remain intact when bile is applied.

57.

C. The ingestion of food contaminated with enterotoxin produced by *S. aureus* is the most likely cause of the disease in the case described. *S. aureus* multiplies rapidly in improperly stored food. Within a few hours, levels of 10^5 organisms per gram of food can be found. Enterotoxin is elaborated when the organism reaches stationary growth phase. Ingestion of small amounts of toxin results in a rapid onset (1–6 hours) of vomiting and diarrhea as a result of a neural response.

58.

D. Most strains of *S. saprophyticus* are resistant to novobiocin. This organism is frequently found in urine culture of young women and may be misidentified as *S. epidermidis*. A 5-μg disk is used in the test, and a zone of 16 mm or less determines resistance.

59.

B. On serum-cystine-sodium thiosulfate-tellurite medium (Tinsdale medium), *C. diphtheriae* is differentiated from other cornybacteria and other bacteria of the respiratory tract by its ability to produce black colonies surrounded by a brown-black halo after 48 hours of incubation. Growth factors needed by *C. diphtheriae* are provided by the addition of the serum. Potassium tellurite is inhibitory to many gram-positive and gram-negative bacteria, but corynebacteria are resistant.

60.

C. *S. aureus* is the predominant pathogen involved in joint infections of adults. Bacterial arthritis can occur following infection in other parts of the body or bacteremia. *S. pyogenes* and *Neisseria gonorrhoeae* each account for a significant number of adult infections, whereas *S. pneumoniae* and *Haemophilus influenzae* predominate in childhood infections.

61.

B. *L. monocytogenes* is a cause of human and bovine abortion. In humans, the mother's symptoms are usually mild, resembling the flu and causing a low-grade fever. The organism can be isolated from aborted fetuses as well as from the maternal placenta. When infection with this etiologic agent is detected early, appropriate therapy can be initiated, which may prevent the death of the fetus.

62.

A. *Bacillus* spp. are gram-positive, spore-forming bacilli widely found in the environment. *B. cereus* is of particular interest as an etiologic agent of human cases of food poisoning. This enterotoxin-producing microorganism is most commonly associated with cases of food poisoning following ingestion of reheated rice served at Asian restaurants.

63.

A. *B. anthracis* infects humans by three routes: respiratory, GI, and cutaneous. Malignant pustule is the name given to lesions seen in cutaneous anthrax in humans. The lesion is, however, neither malignant nor a pustule. The disease produces a localized abscess on the skin, which forms a characteristic black eschar surrounded by a red raised ring.

64.

B. Scalded skin syndrome is the dermatitis associated with the effects of the exfoliative toxin produced by strains of *S. aureus*. Exfoliatin acts in humans to disrupt the adhesive forces between cells of the stratum granulosum, creating large flaccid bullae. This syndrome occurs primarily in infants and children; the primary infection is usually unrelated to the areas where lesions appear.

65.

B. *E. faecalis* and *E. faecium* grow in the presence of bile, hydrolyze esculin, and produce acid from glucose in the presence of high salt concentration. These bacteria also express streptococcal group D antigen. The ability to tolerate high salt concentrations differentiates the enterococci from the group D streptococci like the *S. bovis* group.

Aerobic Gram-Negative Bacteria

66.

C. Vancomycin, a glycopeptide antibiotic, is often used to treat colitis. Most gram-positive bacteria are sensitive to this agent. However, *E. gallinarum* exhibits intrinsic drug resistance to vancomycin. Acquired vancomycin in other *Enterococcus* spp. (e.g., *E. faecalis* and *E. faecium*) was first reported in the year 2000. Rare cases of vancomycin-intermediate and vancomycin-resistant S. aureus have also been reported.

67.

B. *K. pneumoniae* is the species most frequently recovered from the vast majority of clinical cases. Members of the genus *Klebsiella* have a capsule and appear mucoid on cultures. This highly encapsulated organism can cause severe pneumonia, nosocomial infections of several types, infantile enteritis, and other extraintestinal infections.

68.

A. Enterotoxins are produced in the intestinal tract and primarily cause diarrhea. The heat-labile enterotoxin of *E. coli*, which resembles cholera toxin, acts to stimulate the enzyme adenylate cyclase. The stimulation of adenylate cyclase by the toxin increases the production of cyclic AMP, causing rapid gastrointestinal fluid loss. Diarrhea results following stimulation of the secretion of chloride ions by the cells lining the small intestine.

69.

C. The genus *Neisseria* contains organisms that possess cytochrome oxidase activity. Colonies can be identified by the development of a dark purple color following the application of tetramethyl-*p*-phenylenediamine dihydrochloride. The reaction relies on the property of the molecule to substitute for oxygen as an electron acceptor. In the presence of the enzyme and atmospheric oxygen, the molecule is oxidized to form indophenol blue.

70.

D. *Shigella* has a low-infecting dose and has been reported to cause outbreaks in daycare centers and can be spread to family members. *S. sonnei* is a delayed-lactose fermenter, producing acid from lactose after about 48 hours. After 18 hours of incubation on Salmonella-Shigella agar, colonies would be clear.

71.

A. *Chryseobacterium* spp. are ubiquitous in the environment and are especially associated with moist soil and water. *Chryseobacterium* (formerly *Flavobacterium*) *meningosepticum*, a known nosocomial pathogen, has been implicated in outbreaks of meningitis in hospitals and is associated with the use of contaminated respiratory therapy equipment. Adult human infections are rare; these opportunistic microorganisms occur primarily in patients who are immunocompromised.

72.

D. *S. dysenteriae*, the type species of the genus, is a causative agent of bacillary dysentery. Differential and selective media for the recovery of enteric pathogens from stool samples would demonstrate *Shigella* species as H_2S negative, non-lactose-fermenting, gram-negative bacilli. Further biochemical testing would generally show these organisms to be unable to use citrate as their sole carbon source, unable to decarboxylate the amino acid lysine, and urease negative.

73.

A. *A. hydrophila* is typically found in fresh water and has been implicated in human infections. Growth on MacConkey agar and a positive oxidase reaction are characteristic of this organism. A positive oxidase reaction differentiates this organism from all of the *Enterobacteriaceae*, except *Plesiomonas shigelloides*. On sheep blood agar, many strains of *Aeromonas* produce beta-hemolysis.

74.

B. A highly selective medium, thiosulfate-citrate-bile salt-sucrose (TCBS) is used for the isolation of *Vibrio* spp. Species able to ferment sucrose, such as *V. cholerae*, produce yellow colonies. Nonsucrose-fermenting organisms produce green colonies.

75.

A. The K (capsule) antigen surrounds the bacterial cell and masks the somatic antigens of the cell wall, which are used to group members of the family *Enterobacteriaceae*. These heat-labile antigens can be removed by heating a suspension of the culture at 100°C for 10–30 minutes. Antisera that contain K antibody can be used to demonstrate the presence of the capsular antigens.

76.

B. *B. pseudomallei* is the causative agent of melioidosis. The bacterium is found in soil and water in subtropical areas of Southeast Asia and Australia. Melioidosis exhibits several forms, from skin abscesses to abscess formation in internal organs.

77.

C. *F. tularensis* requires cysteine or cystine for growth. Glucose-cysteine with thiamine and cystine heart media are commercially available for suspected cases of tularemia. They both require the addition of 5% sheep or rabbit blood. Buffered charcoal yeast extract (BCYE) also supports the growth of *F. tularensis*, a medium generally used by clinical laboratories for growth of *Legionella* spp.

78.

B. Enterohemorrhagic *E. coli* (EHEC) is a lactose fermenter like most other *E. coli* strains. EHEC is typically MUG negative, which helps to differentiate it from other *E. coli* isolates. EHEC is also sorbitol fermentation negative, unlike other *E. coli* strains.

79.

D. *P. aeruginosa* is the most commonly encountered gram-negative species that is not a member of the family *Enterobacteriaceae*. It is ubiquitous in nature and is found in homes and hospitals. It is an opportunistic pathogen responsible for nosocomial infections.

80.

B. *S. flexneri* and *S. boydii* are difficult to distinguish biochemically. *S. flexneri* will agglutinate in *Shigella* group B antisera, while *S. boydii* agglutinates in group C antisera. Both species produce similar clinical manifestations of infection.

81.

C. *V. vulnificus* is implicated in wound infections and septicemia. The organism is found in brackish or salt water. Ingestion of contaminated water or seafood is the typical mode of transmission. Wound infections are associated with contamination at the site with organisms in water.

82.

D. The Waterhouse-Friderichsen syndrome of disseminated intravascular coagulation occurs in cases of fulminant meningococcemia—*N. meningitidis* septicemia. Invasion of the circulatory system by *N. meningitidis* may produce only a transient bacteremia or meningitis or may go on to cause a rapidly fatal infection. In cases of meningococcemia with intravascular coagulation, acute adrenal insufficiency due to hemorrhage into the adrenal gland may result.

83.

B. Before the development of an effective vaccine, the strain of *H. influenzae* implicated in the majority of cases of bacterial meningitis in children 1–6 years of age was serotype b. This serotype is surrounded by a weakly immunogenic polyribitol phosphate capsule. The widespread use of *H. influenzae* type b (Hib) vaccine, beginning in 1985, has significantly reduced the incidence of invasive *H. influenzae* type b disease.

84.

B. Unlike most other salmonellae, *Salmonella* Typhi produces only a small amount of hydrogen sulfide, produces no gas from glucose, is citrate negative, and possesses a capsular antigen (Vi). Identification of *Salmonella* Typhi, the etiologic agent of typhoid fever, may be delayed if laboratory scientists do not have a good appreciation of its atypical characteristics. It is also important to note that the bacilli appear in the patient's circulatory system several days before a stool culture will be positive.

85.

A. Chancroid or soft chancre is caused by *H. ducreyi*, a small, gram-negative coccobacillus. Painful genital lesions and painful swelling of the inguinal lymph nodes characterize the disease. The incubation period following contact with an infected person ranges from 1 to 5 days, after which the patient notes the painful, round, nonindurated primary lesion on the external genitalia. Signs of regional lymphadenitis appear in about one-half of the cases a few days after the appearance of the primary lesion.

86.

D. Pseudomonads are ubiquitous microorganisms generally associated with moist environments. Cases have been increasing as the popularity of health spas increases. In some cases the pattern of dermatitis caused by these organisms matches the areas covered by the individual's swimsuit. When not properly maintained, whirlpools create a favorable environment for the growth of these organisms.

87.

B. *C. jejuni* rivals *Salmonella* as the most common bacterial cause of diarrheal disease in humans. *Campylobacter* enterocolitis is characterized by fever, bloody diarrhea, and abdominal pain. Special selective culture media and incubation under a microaerophilic atmosphere at 42°C are required for the recovery of this organism from clinical samples.

88.

D. Screening procedures for the recovery of the enteric pathogen *Salmonella* rely heavily on differential media, which indicate lactose fermentation and the production of H_2S. Isolates of *C. freundii* recovered from stool samples on a medium such as Hektoen-enteric (HE) would resemble *Salmonella* in that the organism is not able to ferment lactose and does produce a significant amount of H_2S. However, unlike *Salmonella*, most strains of *C. freundii* will produce acid from sucrose, forming yellow colonies on HE agar. *C. freundii* isolates will typically ferment lactose.

89.

A. Whooping cough, or pertussis, is caused by *B. pertussis*, a minute, encapsulated, nonmotile, gram-negative, pleomorphic bacillus. The best identification method is the polymerase chain reaction. Regan-Lowe medium is recommended for the isolation of this agent.

90.

B. *N. gonorrhoeae* is a primary pathogen of the urogenital tract. It is an important cause of sexually transmitted diseases. Surface structures such as pili aid in attachment to mucosal epithelial cells and invasion of submucosa to produce infection.

91.

D. *H. pylori* produces urease and is rapidly urea positive. In the urea breath test, a patient is given an oral solution of radioactive urea. If *H. pylori* is present in large numbers in the stomach, radioactive carbon dioxide (CO_2) will be produced and absorbed into the bloodstream and exhaled from the lungs. About 30 minutes after administering the urea solution, the patient's breath is tested for radioactivity.

92.

A. *N. meningitidis* and *N. gonorrhoeae* are most commonly described as having a "kidney bean" cellular morphology. Occasionally, some *Moraxella* spp. will exhibit this morphology. These gram-negative diplococcal organisms appear with the paired cells having adjacent walls that are flattened.

93.

C. *B. cepacia* is the most common *Burkolderia* spp. in clinical specimens. *P. aeruginosa* is the most common gram-negative bacillus that is not in the family *Enterobacteriaceae* and *S. maltophilia* the second most common. *B. mallei* has not been isolated recently in the United States.

94.

D. Ophthalmia neonatorum, a form of conjunctivitis, is associated with *N. gonorrhoeae*. The infection is transmitted to the newborn by the mother as it passes through the birth canal. The use of an ophthalmic solution of erythromycin is recommended for the prevention of this form of conjunctivitis.

95.

B. *N. lactamica* is part of the normal nasopharyngeal biota of humans. In the laboratory, this agent may be mistakenly identified as *N. meningitidis*, an organism of significant pathogenicity. Differentiation of these two species is easily accomplished by demonstrating the fermentation of lactose or an ONPG (*o*-nitrophenyl-β-D-galactopyranoside)-positive test.

96.

A. *H. aegyptius* is a cause of "pinkeye" (conjunctivitis). This form of conjunctivitis is highly contagious and is frequently seen in children attending daycare centers. The agent is an aerobic gram-negative bacillus that is nonmotile and requires both hemin (X factor) and nicotine adenine dinucleotide (NAD, V factor) for growth. Other causes of conjunctivitis include *S. aureus, H. influenzae, S. pneumoniae*, and *Moraxella catarrhalis*.

97.

A. *Cronobacter* spp. can live in dry environments such as dry foods, powdered infant formula, powdered milk, herbal teas, and starches. It can cause serious infections in infants and the elderly. Infections have also been reported in patients who are immunocompromised.

98.

B. *Acinetobacter* spp. are opportunistic pathogens for humans and are important causes of nosocomial infections. They are oxidase negative and will grow on most laboratory media, including MacConkey agar. *Acinetobacter* spp. are nonfermenters, but *A. baumannii* can form pink to purple colonies on MacConkey agar that can be mistaken for lactose fermentation. Many strains of *A. baumannii* will oxidize glucose.

99.

B. Pontiac fever is caused by *L. pneumophila*, as is Legionnaires disease, but it is not as serious an infection. This febrile illness is characteristically self-limited and does not demonstrate significant pulmonary symptoms. The incubation period, unlike that for Legionnaires disease, is short, followed by symptoms of malaise, muscle aches, chills, fever, and headache.

100.

A. *Brucella* spp. are fastidious, gram-negative, coccobacillary organisms. They are predominantly animal pathogens, but occasionally produce disease in humans. The usual specimens for recovery of *Brucella* are blood and bone marrow, with the latter considered the more sensitive.

101.

A. *E. coli* O157:H7 produces a toxin similar to Shiga toxin produced by *Shigella dysenteriae*. It is most commonly transmitted by ingestion of undercooked ground beef or raw milk. Hemorrhagic colitis is characteristic of infection, but infection can also lead to hemolytic uremic syndrome resulting from toxin-mediated kidney damage.

102.

A. *Aeromonas* spp. are found in bodies of fresh water and salt water that can be flowing or stagnant and contaminated with sewage. These organisms are known as one of the animal pathogens that cause "red leg disease" in frogs. The largest number of human cases occur between May and November and seem to be highly associated with exposure to water or soil.

103.

C. *C. jejuni* are small, curved, motile gram-negative rods that are hippurate hydrolysis positive. They are found in the gastrointestinal tract of a variety of animals. Campy agar (a selective medium) is used for isolation from stool and is incubated at 42°C under microaerophilic conditions (10% CO_2, 5% O_2 with balance N_2).

104.

C. *Rahnella* is a member of the family *Enterobacteriaceae* and is oxidase negative. It has been isolated from a variety of clinical specimens such as wounds and blood cultures. *Aeromonas, Chryseobacterium*, and *Vibrio* are all oxidase positive.

105.

A. *N. gonorrhoeae* is the causative agent of gonorrhoea and is very sensitive to drying, temperature variations, and fatty acids in clinical material. *N. gonorrhoeae* will grow on chocolate agar but not sheep blood agar. Incubation under CO_2 is required for recovery, and selective media like Thayer-Martin are recommended.

106.

D. The most commonly used method for serogrouping *Shigella* is based on the somatic oligosaccharide or O antigens. The O antigens are also used to serogroup *E. coli* and *Salmonella.* Because *Shigella* spp. are nonmotile, the H or flagella antigens cannot be used; however, H antigens are used for *E. coli* and *Salmonella.* The capsule (K) antigens are used to serogroup *K. pneumoniae.*

107.

C. *V. cholerae* produces an exotoxin that causes infected individuals to lose massive amounts of fluids. Severe dehydration is usually the cause of death in untreated patients. Proper therapy begins with intravenous fluids to restore the patient's water volume and electrolyte balance. The microorganism does not invade the intestinal mucosa but is attached to the surface of enterocytes. The other bacteria listed produce toxins or invasive diseases that often produce inflammation resulting in bloody diarrhea.

108.

C. *V. parahaemolyticus* is classified as a halophilic *Vibrio* sp. requiring increased osmotic pressure, in the form of salt, for growth. This makes routine biochemical test media less than optimal because of their low NaCl content. Growth in the presence of 1% NaCl but no growth in media without the added Na^+ is the test for the differentiation of halophilic organisms. Marine water is the normal habitat of most *Vibrio* spp.

109.

D. *Brucella* spp. are hazardous, especially in aerosol-generating procedures. It is important for the laboratory to be notified whenever brucellosis is suspected. Isolates can be presumptively identified using antisera to bacterial antigens. Most laboratories send isolates to a reference laboratory for confirmation or definitive identification because they lack specialized media and containment facilities.

110.

B. *H. pylori* is found in the human gastric mucosa colonizing the mucous layer of the antrum and fundus but does not invade the epithelium. Approximately 50% of adults over the age of 60 years are infected, with the incidence of gastritis increasing with age. *H. pylori* has been cultured from feces and dental plaque, supporting the theory of a fecal-oral or oral-oral route of transmission.

111.

D. *Acinetobacter* is widely distributed in nature and commonly colonizes hospitalized patients. Infection occurs mainly in compromised hosts. They colonize medical devices and are important causes of healthcare-associated infections. Most human infections are due to *A. baumanii-calcoaceticus* complex. Its resistance to many of the commonly used antimicrobial agents limits the selection of therapeutic agents.

112.

D. *V. parahemolyticus* is found in brackish or salt water. The mode of transmission is the ingestion of contaminated water or seafood. *V. parahemolyticus* is halophilic.

113.

D. Organisms biochemically resembling *Salmonella* are typically tested using a polyvalent antiserum composed of antibodies against the commonly isolated strains, including antisera against the Vi antigen. The Vi antigen is a heat-labile capsular antigen associated with *Salmonella* Typhi. Heating a *Salmonella* Typhi suspension removes the Vi antigen, and the organism can now react with the somatic grouping antisera. *Salmonella* Typhi demonstrates a positive agglutination reaction in D-grouping sera.

114.

B. *C. fetus* subsp. *fetus* is occasionally implicated in human disease. This organism, unlike *C. jejuni*, is characterized as producing extraintestinal symptoms. Those persons most at risk of infection are those with preexisting disease who are in a debilitated condition.

115.

A. *S. sonnei* is a group D *Shigella* and is characterized by its ability to ferment lactose. *S. sonnei* is ONPG positive but is a delayed lactose fermenter. This is the most commonly isolated species of *Shigella* in the United States. The genus *Shigella* is characterized biochemically by being negative for citrate, urease, motility, and lysine decarboxylation.

116.

A. The Voges-Proskauer (VP) test is a broth test that detects the presence of acetoin from the metabolism of glucose in the medium. A red color indicates a positive reaction. The most common clinical isolates from the genera *Providencia, Escherichia, Salmonella*, and *Proteus* are generally VP negative, whereas most members of the genera *Klebsiella, Enterobacter*, and *Serratia* are positive. *Enterobacteriaceae* that are VP positive are typically methyl red negative.

117.

D. Pathogenic mechanisms of *V. cholerae* include adherence to enterocytes via pili, motility, enzymes such as protease and mucinase, and the production of an enterotoxin causing severe diarrhea. *V. cholerae* is one of the few *Vibrio* sp. that does not require salt. It is sucrose positive and will therefore produce yellow colonies on TCBS.

118.

A. Classic epidemic strains of *V. cholerae* are included in the antigenic O group 1. The Ogawa and Inaba strains are considered the predominant epidemic strains. The strain O139 has also been associated with outbreaks of cholera.

119.

D. *Brucella* spp. are small, gram-negative intracellular parasites implicated in zoonotic infection of humans. Brucellosis presents as an undulant febrile illness. In the United States, disease caused by *Brucella* sp. is mainly job related or involves food or animal associations, such as in hunters or those who drink raw milk.

120.

A. *E. coli* is a lactose-fermenting member of the family *Enterobacteriaceae*. Various selective and differential agars are available for the differentiation of lactose fermenters from those that do not degrade lactose. In some media, H_2S production may be demonstrated. Isolates of *E. coli* would produce yellow colonies at 24 hours on xylose-lysine-desoxycholate (XLD) agar. Non-lactose fermenters such as *Shigella* would produce red colonies on XLD agar. On MacConkey agar, lactose fermenters produce pink colonies; on Hektoen enteric agar, colonies would be orange. Most strains of *E. coli* are beta-hemolytic on sheep blood agar.

121.

A. *Y. pestis* is the causative agent of plague. The organism is endemic in rodents and is transmitted to humans by the rat flea. This oxidase-negative organism, unlike other *Yersinia* spp., is nonmotile at 20–25°C. It is also negative for H_2S and urease.

122.

B. Motility can be important in the identification of microorganisms. Of the *Enterobacteriaceae*, the genera *Klebsiella* and *Shigella* are characteristically nonmotile, as is *Tatumella*. Motility of the *Enterobacteriaceae* can normally be detected by the use of a semisolid motility medium, which is grossly observed for the determination of motility. The hanging-drop method is perhaps the most accurate means of detecting motility of nonfermentative microorganisms.

123.

C. Pneumonic legionellosis (Legionnaires disease) and the nonpneumonic illness known as Pontiac fever are the two clinical forms of disease caused by *L. pneumophila*. The optimal temperature for cultivation is 35°C, and cold enrichment is not appropriate. A urine antigen test is often used diagnostically, and erythromycin is the drug of choice for therapy.

124.

D. *K. granulomatis* is the etiologic agent of the sexually transmitted disease granuloma inguinale. It is a pleomorphic, gram-negative, encapsulated bacillus, although it does not Gram stain well. First seen as inclusions (Donovan bodies) in mononuclear cells from genital ulcers stained with the Giemsa or Wright stain, these organisms are extremely difficult to recover.

125.

A. *A. aphrophilus* is a member of the HACEK group. These agents are regarded as part of the normal microbiome of the oral cavity. They can gain access to the bloodstream and cause subacute bacterial endocarditis.

126.

C. *Kingella* spp. normally inhabit the oral cavity of humans. *K. kingae* is a leading cause of osteomyelitis and septic arthritis in children aged 6 to 36 months. The agents spread from the oral cavity via the bloodstream.

127.

B. *N. gonorrhoeae* is a fastidious organism requiring the addition of serum or blood to the culture media in order to grow. A selective medium such as modified Thayer-Martin or GC-Lect should be used for primary isolation, especially from sites that may be contaminated with normal biota. Collection and processing of specimens must be done under optimal conditions, because this organism is sensitive to drying and low temperatures.

128.

A. The indole reaction is a widely used method for differentiating lactose-positive *E. coli* from other members of the family *Enterobacteriaceae*. Organisms such as *E. coli*, which possess the enzyme tryptophanase, are able to metabolize the amino acid tryptophan with the production of indole, pyruvic acid, and ammonia.

129.

A. *E. coli* produces an acid over acid (A/A) reaction on TSI agar that indicates that glucose and either lactose or sucrose or both have been fermented. Bacteria that ferment lactose or sucrose produce large amounts of acid in the medium. The enteric pathogens *Salmonella* and *Shigella* can be ruled out when such a reaction is observed, because they are generally not able to use either lactose or sucrose within 18 hours.

130.

A. Pyocyanin is the nonfluorescent, blue-green, diffusible pigment produced by *P. aeruginosa*. It is the only bacterium able to produce this pigment. Pyocyanin mixes with the yellow pigment fluorescein to turn culture media green. Most *P. aeruginosa* strains can be identified presumptively by their characteristic grapelike odor, colony morphology, and blue-green pigment.

131.

C. Color Plate 26 ■ is a Gram stain of a cerebrospinal fluid specimen revealing many white blood cells. All of the bacteria listed are fastidious; however, *H. influenzae* would be expected to grow on chocolate agar but not sheep blood agar (SBA). *N. meningitidis*, also an important cause of meningitis, would be expected to grow on SBA incubated in CO_2. *B. parapertussis* and *Brucella* sp. would likely grow on both SBA and chocolate agar, and both are uncommon isolates.

132.

D. *C. jejuni* is an important human pathogen most commonly associated with cases of bloody diarrhea, fever, and abdominal pain in humans. Special handling of cultures suspected to contain this organism is required for optimal recovery. Cultures should be incubated at 42°C in a microaerophilic atmosphere and examined at 24 and 48 hours for spreading nonhemolytic colonies, which may be slightly pigmented.

133.

C. *M. catarrhalis* possesses the enzyme indophenol oxidase. When a 1% solution of tetramethyl-*p*-phenylenediamine (oxidase reagent) is applied to colonies of these organisms, the colonies turn a purple color, which rapidly darkens. The other species listed are oxidase negative.

134.

A. *C. hominis* is a rare pathogen that is recovered predominantly from cases of endocarditis. It is characterized as a fermentative, gram-negative bacillus that is nonmotile, catalase negative, oxidase positive, and weakly indole positive. *C. hominis* will grow on sheep blood agar, but growth is enhanced by the addition of yeast extract to media.

135.

D. *V. vulnificus* is a halophilic, lactose-fermenting organism. The isolate is associated with two distinct clinical conditions: primary septicemia and wound infection. Septicemia with this organism appears to be correlated in most cases with preexisting hepatic disease. Septicemia due to *V. vulnificus* characteristically produces a fulminant disease with a high mortality rate. Wound infection with this organism is usually associated with trauma and contact with a marine environment.

136.

C. Members of the tribe *Proteae* are characteristically positive for phenylalanine deaminase (PDA). This includes *Proteus vulgaris, P. stuartii*, and *M. morganii*. *Tatuella ptyseos* belongs to the family *Enterobacteriaceae* and is also PDA positive.

137.

C. The water-diffusible yellow pigment fluorescein (pyoverdin) is produced by members of the *Pseudomonas* fluorescent group, which includes *P. aeruginosa, P. fluorescens*, and *P. putida*. *P. aeruginosa* also produces pyocyanin, a blue pigment that combines with pyoverdin forming green-pigmented colonies. *P. aeruginosa* is the most clinically significant member of this group.

138.

C. *Kingella* spp. are gram-negative bacilli or coccobacilli that may appear in short chains. *K. denitrificans* can be isolated from the human upper respiratory tract, will grow on modified Thayer-Martin agar, and is oxidase-positive. The growth of this organism is inhibited by MacConkey agar, and growth is poor on TSI agar.

139.

A. *Haemophilus* spp. are obligate parasites of animals and are found primarily in the upper respiratory tract and oral cavity. Chocolate agar is the preferred culture medium for *Haemophilus*. Unlike 5% sheep blood agar, it provides both hemin (X factor) and NAD (V factor) required for growth. They appear as small gram-negative coccobacilli on Gram stain.

140.

A. *L. pneumophila* requires the use of special laboratory media for cultivation and does not stain well by the conventional Gram stain. Most *Legionella* spp. are motile, biochemically inert, and autofluoresce. The primary mode of transmission is by the airborne route, usually in association with an environmental source of bacteria.

141.

C. Tissue samples from the lower respiratory tract (lung biopsy) have the greatest yield of positive cultures for *L. pneumophila*. However, these specimens require invasive procedures and are not commonly performed. Cultures of lower respiratory tract specimens, such as bronchial wash and expectorated sputum, are appropriate for the isolation of *L. pneumophila*. The bacteria are seldom recovered from blood specimens.

142.

D. While cultures are considered nearly 100% specific, the diagnosis of pertussis, or whooping cough, is often made by polymerase chain reaction (PCR) assay. Nasopharyngeal swabs are recommended; they can be transported to the laboratory without a transport medium for PCR. Regan-Lowe, a charcoal-based medium, provides the best growth if cultures are attempted. Isolates will not grow on MacConkey agar.

143.

C. *C. sakazakii* produces a yellow pigment that aids in its presumptive identification. Some strains of *Enterobacter cowanii* are also pigmented. *C. sakazakii* is an occasional clinical isolate that has been linked to respiratory tract infections and wounds. It has been linked to powdered foods.

144.

C. *P. mirabilis* is commonly associated with urinary tract infections as well as infections in other parts of the body. It is a motile organism that characteristically swarms across the surface of sheep blood agar plates. Members of the genus *Proteus* are characteristically rapidly urea positive, lactose negative, and phenylalanine deaminase positive.

145.

D. *A. baumannii* is not able to reduce nitrate. This species will oxidize but not ferment glucose. *Acinetobacter* spp. are able to grow on MacConkey agar, and they are oxidase negative, nonmotile, and characteristically resistant to penicillin.

146.

C. *E. corrodens* is a facultatively anaerobic gram-negative bacillus that requires hemin in the culture medium to grow aerobically. This organism, which is a part of the normal indigenous oral microbiota of humans, is seldom found in pure culture. It is commonly associated with polymicrobial infections following bite or clenched-fist wounds. Infections of the face and neck may also involve this organism, which produces pitting of the agar on which it is isolated.

147.

C. In the genus *Pasteurella, P. multocida* is the species commonly recovered in clinical specimens. This gram-negative coccobacillus is a normal inhabitant of the oral cavity of domestic animals. Humans most often become infected from a bite or scratch of a cat or dog, which produces a rapidly progressing, painful, suppurative wound infection. Penicillin is an effective drug for the treatment of *Pasteurella* infections.

148.

D. *L. pneumophila* is able to hydrolyze hippurate. *L. pneumophila* will also autofluoresce. Although most of the studies done on legionellosis are based on this species, *L. pneumophila* is the species most often associated with human disease.

149.

B. *H. aegyptius* causes a contagious form of conjunctivitis. The bacterium requires both X and V factors and is therefore negative for delta-aminolevulinic acid (ALA). *H. influenzae* biogroup *aegytius* is a separate organism from *H. aegyptius.*

150.

B. *K. denitrificans* is most often associated with endocarditis. It is morphologically similar to *N. gonorrhoeae* both on Gram stain and colonies on culture media. Confusion is further compounded by its ability to grow on modified Thayer-Martin medium and its positive oxidase and glucose reaction. The ability of *K. denitrificans* to reduce nitrates is a key test for its differentiation from *N. gonorrhoeae.*

151.

C. *Plesiomonas* was previously in the family *Vibrionaceae.* Based on nucleic acid and antigenic studies, it was moved to the family *Enterobacteriaceae.* It is now the only member of the family *Enterobacteriaceae* that is oxidase positive.

152.

C. The recalls described illustrate the ubiquitous nature of *P. aeruginosa* in the environment and its resistance to many disinfectants. In addition, the bacterium has minimal nutritional requirements and the ability to tolerate a wide range of temperatures (4–42°C). *P. aeruginosa* is an opportunistic pathogen commonly associated with hospital-acquired infections.

153.

B. Ingestion of contaminated unpasteurized (raw) milk or cheese is one of the primary routes of infection. Brucellosis is found worldwide, and symptoms vary from asymptomatic to a debilitating systemic infection. Only four of the six species are typically pathogenic for humans: *B. abortus, B. melitensis, B. suis,* and *B. canis.*

154.

A. The production of DNase, lipase, and gelatinase differentiates the genus *Serratia* from other *Enterobacteriaceae. Serratia* spp., especially *S. marcescens,* have a close association with healthcare-associated infections. *Serratia* can produce severe infections such as septicemia and meningitis and are frequently difficult to eradicate because of the characteristic antimicrobial-resistant strains found in the hospital environment.

155.

A. *H. ducreyi* is the causative agent of chancroid, a serious sexually transmitted disease. The disease is more prevalent in the tropics than in temperate parts of the world. The bacteria produce buboes in the groin and can cause a septicemia.

156.

D. Posterior nasopharyngeal cultures are recommended for the recovery of *B. pertussis* in suspected cases of pertussis (whooping cough). Swabs of the nasopharynx are inoculated on the selective agar Regan-Lowe. Cephalexin is added to the culture medium to inhibit the growth of contaminating indigenous biota.

157.

C. *G. vaginalis* is associated with cases of bacterial vaginosis (BV) formerly called "nonspecific vaginitis." Although *G. vaginalis* is probably not involved in the pathogenesis of BV, its presence in high numbers is considered a presumptive diagnosis. These small, gram-negative bacilli are frequently seen in great numbers on the surface of epithelial cells ("clue cells") taken from the vagina.

158.

B. Cultures of blood and bone marrow are the recommended specimens for the isolation of *Brucella* spp. Inoculation of a blood culture bottle for a continuous monitoring system is the most sensitive recovery method. The lysis-centrifugation method (Isolator®, Wampole Laboratories) is more sensitive than a biphasic culture bottle.

159.

C. Mesenteric lymphadenitis is one of the common manifestations of human *Y. pseudotuberculosis* infections. Symptoms produced by this agent closely resemble those of acute appendicitis. This gram-negative coccobacillus grows well on routine culture media and has an optimal growth temperature of 25–30°C.

160.

D. Cefsulodin-irgasan-novobiocin (CIN) agar is recommended for the primary isolation of *Yersinia* and *Aeromonas. Y. enterocolitic* produces "bull's-eye" colonies at 48 hours; colonies show a dark red center surrounded by a translucent border. This is a selective and differential agar that suppresses the growth of normal fecal biota and differentiates colonies of *Y. enterocolitica.*

161.

B. *G. vaginalis* is associated with BV but cultures are not recommended for diagnosis. Many women carry *G. vaginalis* as normal vaginal biota; therefore, the isolation of the organism may not be clinically significant. The disease can be diagnosed by detecting "clue" cells, vaginal epithelial cells with gram-variable bacilli attached to their surface.

162.

B. *L. pneumophila*, the causative agent of Legionnaires disease, can be recovered from respiratory tract secretions. The bacterium is fastidious and, like *Francisella tularensis*, requires cysteine or cystine for growth. The culture medium most commonly recommended is BCYE agar, which is incubated in a moist chamber at 35°C. Growth on this medium may not be visible for 3–4 days, after which further identification procedures may be carried out.

163.

D. Swimmer's ear is a form of external otitis common to persons who swim and fail to completely dry their ear canals when leaving the water. The organism most commonly associated with this condition is *P. aeruginosa.* It is an organism known to be an opportunistic pathogen and one that favors a watery environment.

164.

B. Traveler's diarrhea is caused by strains of toxin-producing invasive or enteropathogenic *E. coli.* Enterotoxigenic *E. coli* can produce one or two exotoxins: one is heat stable and one is heat labile. Contaminated food products and water in foreign countries seem to be the major vehicle for human infection with these agents.

165.

A. Fresh isolates of *C. jejuni* on Gram stain characteristically reveal a "gull-wing" appearance. These gram-negative bacilli are motile with a typical darting pattern on wet mounts. They stain poorly using the Gram stain method, and it is recommended that carbol-fuchsin or basic fuchsin be substituted for the counterstain safranin.

166.

C. *N. gonorrhoeae* is said to resemble a kidney bean on Gram stain because of its characteristic gram-negative diplococcal morphology in which the adjacent sides are flattened. Typically, these organisms are found intracellularly when direct smears of clinical material are examined. Smears from the female genital tract must be interpreted with caution, however, because other normal biota microorganisms are morphologically similar.

167.

B. *Salmonella* is lactose fermentation negative and H_2S positive. On Hektoen-enteric medium, the bacteria will produce clear colonies with black centers. *Shigella* spp. are also lactose fermentation negative but are H_2S negative.

168.

A. *N. gonorrhoeae* is identified in the clinical laboratory by its ability to ferment only glucose. The diagnosis of the sexually transmitted disease caused by this agent can be definitively made only by the isolation and identification of *N. gonorrhoeae* in the clinical laboratory. Morphologically, all members of the genus are alike, and all are oxidase positive, which makes definitive identification procedures necessary. Nucleic acid amplification tests are used frequently to diagnose gonorrhea.

169.

C. *N. meningitidis* is a human pathogen most commonly associated with meningitis. These oxidase-positive, gram-negative diplococci are identified either by fermentation tests or serologic methods that use specific antisera. *N. meningitidis* ferments both glucose and maltose.

170.

A. *B. bacilliformis* is the causative agent of Oroya fever and verruga peruana. It is a pleomorphic, gram-negative rod that is an intracellular parasite of red blood cells and can be cultured from blood in the acute stage of the disease. The disease is rare and occurs primarily in South America.

171.

B. Many *Neisseria* spp. are found as normal microbiota in the upper respiratory tract and oral cavity of humans. Species other than *N. gonorrhoeae* and *N. meningitidis* are generally considered nonpathogenic. However, on rare cases these species have been linked to meningitis, endocarditis, and other infections.

172.

B. *Klebsiella* spp. are all nonmotile, which aids in their identification. *Klebsiella* spp. produce a capsule resulting in mucoid colonies. *Shigella*, another genus in the family *Enterobacteriaceae*, is also nonmotile.

173.

A. *C. violaceum* is a motile, gram-negative bacillus found in soil and water that can be pathogenic for humans. The production of a nonwater-soluble violet pigment by these organisms aids in their identification. *Chromobacterium* is catalase and oxidase positive and generally attacks carbohydrates fermentatively.

174.

A. *P. multocida* is the species in the genus most often encountered in the clinical laboratory. It is normal oral biota in animals but not humans. The mode of transmission generally involves traumatic inoculation of the organism through the skin, producing soft tissue infections such as cellulitis. It can also cause osteomyelitis and joint infections. *P. multocida* grows on sheep blood agar but not on MacConkey agar.

175.

C. *P. aeruginosa* has not only a characteristic grape-like odor but also a blue-green color. These oxidative, motile organisms are oxidase positive and are able to grow at 42°C. In humans, these opportunistic organisms cause many types of infections, but they are primarily associated with burn wound infections.

176.

A. *Aeromonas* can be differentiated from many other fermentative gram-negative bacilli, such as the *Enterobacteriaceae*, in that they are oxidase positive. Isolates are ONPG positive. On sheep blood agar medium, colonies are beta-hemolytic. *Aeromonas* spp. will grow on cefsulodin-irgasan-novobiocin (CIN) medium and form colonies with pink centers.

177.

A. *E. tarda* is a motile member of the family *Enterobacteriaceae*. These organisms are infrequently isolated in the clinical laboratory. Biochemically, they may initially resemble *Salmonella* in many ways, such as hydrogen sulfide production and the inability to ferment lactose.

178.

B. The porphyrin test is commonly used to test for the X factor (hemin) requirement of *Haemophilus* spp. A positive test result indicates that the organism possesses the enzymes to convert aminolevulinic acid (ALA) into porphyrins and, therefore, would not require hemin. If porphyrins are produced, this rapid test will show red fluorescence under UV light after a 4-hour incubation period.

179.

A. *B. bronchiseptica* in humans produces either a respiratory illness or wound infections. The organism is a part of the normal respiratory biota of laboratory animals such as rabbits and guinea pigs. *B. bronchiseptica* may cause problems for researchers because it can cause outbreaks of bronchopneumonia in experimental animals. It also causes kennel cough in canines.

180.

B. *E. coli* is frequently the etiologic agent of community-acquired cystitis. This agent can be easily recognized by its fermentation of lactose, negative citrate reaction, and positive indole test. On eosin methylene blue agar, *E. coli* produces characteristic dark colonies with a metallic sheen.

181.

C. "Satellitism" is the name given to the appearance of colonies of *H. influenzae* on sheep blood agar medium around colonies of organisms that provide an essential growth factor. *H. influenzae* requires both hemin and NAD. Colonies of some organisms, such as *Staphylococcus* and *Neisseria*, produce NAD, which diffuses into the surrounding agar and enables *H. influenzae* to grow deriving hemin from the red blood cells.

182.

A. *B. pertussis* is the etiologic agent of pertussis. On Bordet-Gengou or Regan-Lowe agars, the organism forms small, round colonies that resemble mercury droplets. A nasopharyngeal swab is recommended as the optimal specimen for the recovery of this agent.

183.

C. *N. meningitidis* is the etiologic agent of one form of inflammation of the meninges, known as epidemic cerebrospinal meningitis. Infection with *B. pertussis* produces the highly contagious respiratory infection pertussis. Both diseases are spread by droplet infection or fomites contaminated with respiratory secretions. The microorganisms are present in greatest numbers in the upper respiratory tract, and specimens for isolation and identification should be collected on nasopharyngeal swabs.

184.

C. *Salmonella* Typhi is commonly spread by chronic carriers. Without treatment, this enteric bacillus can be carried throughout a person's lifetime and is sequestered most often in the gallbladder. Carriers are usually asymptomatic, and the presence of the organism can be confirmed only by isolation and identification in the clinical laboratory.

185.

A. *Brucella* infects cattle and may be transmitted to humans by the ingestion of contaminated milk or other dairy products. Milk is able to support the growth of many clinically significant microorganisms, which may often be ingested in unpasteurized dairy products. Meliodosis and glanders are caused by *Burkholderia pseudomallei* and *B. mallei*, respectively. Pontiac fever is caused by *L. pneumoniae*. None of these is transmitted by milk.

186.

B. *P. aeruginosa* is a major cause of hospital-acquired infections. These opportunistic organisms are able to survive in moist environments for prolonged periods and may be transferred to patients who are immunocompromised. *Pseudomonas* infections in recent years have accounted for as much as 10% of nosocomial infections.

187.

B. *N. gonorrhoeae* is only found in humans. The bacteria are fragile and do not survive for long outside human hosts. Women are often asymptomatic when originally infected. The most commonly used nonselective medium for the isolation of *N. gonorrhoeae* is chocolate agar. Isolates typically do not grow on SBA. They only ferment glucose.

188.

A. Hektoen enteric agar was developed to improve the isolation of *Shigella* and *Salmonella* from stool specimens. The selective nature of this agar is due to bile salts. The medium also contains three carbohydrates—lactose, sucrose, and salicin—along with a pH indicator to detect carbohydrate fermentation. Fermentative organisms turn the medium yellow. Ferric ammonium citrate and sodium thiosulfate are included in the medium to detect H_2S production. H_2S-producing organisms appear as black-centered colonies.

189.

A. Thiosulfate-citrate-bile salt-sucrose (TCBS) agar is recommended for use in the selective isolation of *Vibrio* spp. associated with cholera, diarrhea, or food poisoning. The selective agent in this medium to inhibit gram-positive organisms is oxgall, a naturally occurring substance containing bile salts and sodium cholate. Sucrose is the carbohydrate in the medium. *V. cholerae* and *V. alginolyticus* ferment sucrose and appear as large yellow colonies. *V. parahemolyticus* is unable to ferment sucrose and exhibits colonies with blue to green centers.

190.

C. The oxidase test detects organisms that produce the enzyme cytochrome oxidase. A 1% solution of dimethyl- or tetra-methyl-*p*-phenylenediamine dihydrochloride is applied to filter paper, and the test organism is then rubbed into the impregnated area. Because Nichrome wire may cause a false-positive result, a platinum or plastic loop or wooden applicator stick should be used to pick the colony. The rapid development of a dark purple color in the area where the organism was inoculated is a positive oxidase test.

191.

B. Strains of *Haemophilus* able to synthesize heme are identified by the porphyrin test. Species such as *H. influenzae*, which require heme, would give a negative test result, whereas *H. parainfluenzae* would be positive. A red color is indicative of a positive reaction in this test.

192.

B. Enterohemorrhagic *E. coli* (EHEC) will ferment lactose and produce pink colonies on MacConkey agar with lactose. This is the typical result for most *E. coli* strains. However, EHEC does not ferment sorbitol at 18 hours, producing clear colonies on MacConkey agar with sorbitol. Clear colonies on this medium should be selected for further testing.

193.

C. Exotic pets such as iguanas, snakes, and turtles are known to carry *Salmonella*. Young children who do not practice good handwashing after touching family pets are particularly at risk for infection. Natural medicinal products made from snakes or other animals known to carry *Salmonella* have been implicated in cases of salmonellosis.

194.

B. Keratitis is a serious clinical condition that is characterized by inflammation of the cornea, which, if not appropriately treated, may lead to loss of vision. *P. aeruginosa* is the most common agent of bacterial keratitis associated with lens-cleaning solution. Pseudomonads are opportunistic pathogens that are commonly associated with contaminated fluids.

195.

B. *H. pylori* is implicated as an etiologic agent of gastritis and peptic ulcer disease. This organism can be demonstrated in gastric biopsy specimens. *H. pylori* has been identified as a carcinogen and linked to gastric carcinoma.

196.

D. New York City (NYC) medium was developed by the New York City Public Health Laboratory for the isolation of *N. gonorrhoeae*. It is a horse serum–based medium that is selective by the addition of colistin, vancomycin, and amphotericin B. Modified Thayer-Martin, another commonly used selective medium for *N. gonorrhoeae*, is chocolate based.

197.

B. Like *P. aeruginosa, B. cepacia* is a ubiquitous opportunistic organism. Although *P. aeruginosa* is by far the most important cause of lower respiratory tract infections in patients with cystic fibrosis, *B. cepacia* is also a significant cause of morbidity. Both of these bacteria are oxidase positive and will grow on MacConkey agar. *P. aeruginosa* typically produces a green discoloration of the medium it is grown on.

198.

A. *E. corrodens* can be normal biota of the oral cavity of humans. It is a weak pathogen that is associated with polymicrobial abscesses of the oral cavity. *E. corrodens* will grow on sheep blood and chocolate agars. Some strains will produce pitting of the agar.

Mycobacteria

199.

A. Mycobacteria characteristically possess a large amount of mycolic acids, long chain fatty acids, unlike gram-positive cocci and gram-negative bacteria. The high fatty acid content acts to protect these organisms from dehydration and the lethal effects of alkali, various germicides, alcohol, and acids. Thus, these bacteria do not stain well with the Gram stain, and an acid-fast staining technique must be used. Mycolic acids also permit the bacteria to survive inside macrophages.

200.

D. The optimal growth temperature of *M. xenopi* is 42°C, which enables its survival and replication as an environmental contaminant in hot water systems. Human infections caused by *M. xenopi* are rare. The majority of clinically significant *Mycobacterium* spp., those not known to cause cutaneous infections, have an optimal growth temperature of 37°C.

201.

B. Growth on MacConkey agar is a test used for differentiation of rapidly growing mycobacteria. The MacConkey agar used for mycobacteria identification is a different formulation than that used for enterics, in that crystal violet is omitted. A MacConkey agar plate is inoculated with a 7-day broth culture of the test organism. The inoculated plate is then incubated at 35°C. Plates are checked for growth at 5 days, and if no growth is detected, they are checked daily until day 11, at which time they are discarded as negative. *M. fortuitum* and *M. chelonei* are the only mycobacteria able to grow on MacConkey agar in 5 days.

202.

D. *M. scrofulaceum* is defined as a scotochromogen because of its ability to produce pigmentation in the dark. This slowly growing *Mycobacterium* is a cause of cervical adenitis and other types of infections predominantly in children. Therapy may require susceptibility studies that include the secondary drugs, because the organism is known in some cases to be resistant to isoniazid and streptomycin.

203.

C. The *N*-acetyl-L-cysteine-sodium hydroxide (NALC-NaOH) method is recommended because the addition of NALC allows the concentration of NaOH to be reduced to 2%. The NALC is a mucolytic agent that frees trapped organisms in the sample, and the NaOH acts as a decontaminant. The optimal treatment reduces the numbers of indigenous microorganisms present in the sample without significantly reducing the number of tubercle bacilli.

204.

C. Hansen disease (leprosy) is caused by *M. leprae.* Chronic skin lesions and sensory loss characterize this disease. Skin or biopsy specimens taken from within the margin of a lesion will demonstrate the causative agent. Cultures of this agent on artificial media, unlike other mycobacteria, have not been successful. Cultivation can be accomplished by injecting bacilli into the foot pads of mice or systemically into armadillos.

205.

C. The Centers for Disease Control and Prevention has adopted the diagnostic standards recommended by the American Thoracic Society as published in 1981. This is a method of reporting the number of acid fast bacilli (AFB) observed in fuchsin-stained smears of clinical material. Up to nine AFB per field should be reported as a positive, at 3+.

206.

C. Acid-fast bacilli can be demonstrated in stained smears of clinical material using the Ziehl-Neelsen or Kinyoun acid-fast stains. The Kinyoun carbolfuchsin method uses a higher concentration of phenol in the primary stain to accelerate the staining process. Therefore, unlike the Ziehl-Neelsen stain, the Kinyoun stain does not need to be heated.

207.

D. Members of the genus *Mycobacterium* are characterized as obligate aerobic bacilli that, because of the high fatty acid content of their cell wall, exhibit acid fastness when stained. Most species pathogenic for humans are slow-growing. *M. kansasii* is a slow-growing photochromogen most commonly transmitted via the respiratory route.

208.

C. *M. ulcerans* and *M. marinum* have both been implicated in skin infections. Their predilection for surface areas of the body is related to their optimal growth temperature range of 30–32°C. At body temperature (37°C) or higher, these organisms grow poorly, if at all.

209.

A. Rapid development of drug resistance is a concern in the treatment of tuberculosis. Patients are treated generally with a combination of at least two of the primary (first-line) drugs, such as isoniazid, rifampin, ethambutol, and pyrazinamide. Because of the slowly growing nature of the bacteria, they are innately resistant to a number of agents. Kanamycin, amikacin, and some fluoroquinolones are considered second-line drugs.

210.

B. NALC (*N*-acetyl-L-cysteine) is a mucolytic agent used in decontamination and digestion procedures for the recovery of mycobacteria. NALC liquefies mucus, releasing trapped bacteria. NaOH, between 2 and 4%, is frequently used as a bactericidal agent to prevent the overgrowth of normal biota in clinical specimens.

211.

D. A positive tuberculin skin test reaction is an example of a hypersensitivity reaction. Tuberculin preparations are prepared from culture filtrates, which are precipitated with trichloroacetic acid and are known as purified protein derivative (PPD). A positive test demonstrates an area of induration following an intradermal injection of PPD.

212.

A. *M. bovis* causes tuberculosis in cattle. This agent is an etiologic agent of tuberculosis in humans as well, and it must be differentiated from *M. tuberculosis* when recovered from clinical material. Unlike *M. tuberculosis, M. bovis* is negative for niacin production and nitrate reduction.

213.

A. The *M. avium* complex is sometimes referred to as *Mycobacterium avium-intracellulare* complex. These slowly growing bacilli are uncommon in immunocompetent individuals. These bacteria cause disseminated infections in patients with acquired immunodeficiency syndrome and are important causes of morbidity and mortality in these patients.

214.

B. *M. gordonae* has been recovered from water stills, faucets, and bodies of water in nature, which is why it has been called the "tap water scotochromogen." These organisms are not considered to be pathogenic for humans, but because they may be recovered as contaminants, their identification is recommended. Members of Runyon group II, they are slow growing and form yellow-orange colonies that do not depend on exposure to light.

215.

C. The human tubercle bacillus is *M. tuberculosis*. Growth of this well-known human pathogen appears in 2–3 weeks when incubated at 35°C. These niacin-positive mycobacteria form dry heaping colonies that are buff colored.

216.

C. *M. marinum* is the causative agent of "swimming pool granuloma." Typically, patients with abraded skin come in contact with water containing this agent and develop granulomatous skin lesions. Lesions generally occur on the extremities, because the skin temperature is close to the organism's optimal growth temperature of 30–32°C.

217.

B. *M. bovis* is susceptible to 5 μg/mL of thiophene-2-carboxylic acid hydrazide (T2H). This *Mycobacterium* is associated with cattle and is rarely isolated from humans in the United States. Growth occurs only at 35°C and is differentiated from other mycobacteria by its susceptibility to T2H.

218.

A. Auromine-rhodamine is a fluorescent stain used to visualize the mycobacteria. The bacteria retain the stain and will appear bright yellow against a black background. Because it is easier to see the bacilli, this stain is more sensitive than a fuschin-based stain (e.g., Ziehl-Neelsen). The calcofluor white stain is a fluorescent stain used to visualize fungi.

219.

B. *M. kansasii* is the most commonly isolated photochromogen in the United States. It is the second most commonly isolated nontuberculosis *Mycobacterium* sp. behind *M. avium* complex. *M. kansasii* produces chronic lung disease resembling classic tuberculosis.

220.

B. Skin cultures for the recovery of *Mycobacterium* spp. should be incubated at 30°C. The mycobacteria associated with these types of infections include *M. ulcerans, M. marinum*, and *M. haemophilium*. The optimal temperature for these slow growers is 30–32°C.

221.

B. In the gamma-interferon release assays (IFGRAs), a blood sample is collected, and the white blood cells are exposed to *M. tuberculosis* antigen. If the patient has a history of *M. tuberculosis* infection, T cells will release interferon gamma, which is generally detected by an enzyme immunoassay. While the test cannot distinguish current infection from past infection, it does not give a false-positive result in patients who have received the tuberculosis vaccine.

222.

A. The mycobacteria are only slightly more resistant to the decontamination procedures than other bacteria. Therefore, it is only appropriate to decontaminate specimens for mycobacteria that are contaminated with normal biota. Because sputum passes through the oral cavity, it contains a large amount of normal oral biota. The other specimens listed are typically sterile and lack normal biota.

223.

C. *M. leprae* is the causative agent of Hansen disease (leprosy). This bacterium cannot be grown on artificial media and requires laboratory animals for cultivation. The optimal temperature for *M. leprae* is lower than the core body temperature of 37°C; therefore, infections generally occur in the skin in the extremities. The bacteria are likely spread from nasal secretions and not the lesions; they are not highly contagious, as most people believe.

Anaerobic Bacteria

224.

B. Improperly home-canned foods, especially low-acid-content vegetables, cause the majority of the cases of foodborne botulism. The ubiquitous nature of *C. botulinum* enables the spores to contaminate a variety of foods. Contamination and subsequent germination under anaerobic conditions stimulate toxin formation. The patient becomes ill following the ingestion of food that contains nanograms of preformed toxin.

225.

A. Zoonotic diseases are diseases of animals that are transmissible to humans. *B. anthracis* is found in the environment. Anthrax is transmitted to humans by exposure to contaminated animal products such as cattle hides, goat hair, or wool. Wound botulism and tetanus are often linked to puncture wounds contaminated with soil. Myonecrosis, gas gangrene, can be endogenous from the gastrointestinal tract or, like botulism, from contaminated wounds.

226.

A. Isolates of the anaerobic, spore-forming bacillus *C. perfringens* characteristically produce a pattern of double zone beta-hemolysis on sheep blood agar plates incubated anaerobically. A Gram stain of such colonies should demonstrate a medium-sized gram-positive bacillus that does not contain spores. For further identification the isolate should be inoculated on an egg yolk agar plate to detect lecithinase production.

227.

D. *P. melaninogenica* was isolated from this cervical abscess. This anaerobic organism is part of the indigenous microbiota of the respiratory, gastrointestinal, and genitourinary tracts and is considered a significant human pathogen. The black pigment appears after several days when growing on laked blood agar plates. Prior to pigmentation, this isolate can be presumptively identified by its brick-red fluorescence under UV light. Pigmented *Porphyromonas* spp. are asaccharolytic.

228.

D. *C. tetani* is an obligate anaerobe. Spores are widespread in nature and cause disease by contaminating puncture wounds. The exotoxin, tetanospasmin, produced by this organism is one of the most powerful bacterial toxins known. The bacteria produce minimal tissue damage at the site of infection; the disease is an intoxication.

229.

B. The gram-positive, nonspore-forming, anaerobic bacillus *A. israelii* is a slowly growing organism that is considered to be an opportunistic pathogen. Colonies may not be visible before 5–7 days or longer. When colonies are seen, they appear white, opaque, lobate, irregular, and shiny and are described as resembling a molar tooth. Some *Actinomyces* sp. have a dry "crumbled" appearance. *A. israelii* is part of the indigenous biota of the human mouth, and a few *Actinomyces* spp. have been found to inhabit the vagina.

230.

A. The predominant indigenous biota of the human intestinal tract is anaerobic, gram-negative, nonspore-forming bacilli. *B. fragilis*, in particular, predominates in the fecal biota. Trauma involving the intestinal area or bowel surgery predisposes patients to an endogenous anaerobic infection. Although these organisms are present in large numbers, their routine identification in fecal cultures is of no diagnostic value.

231.

A. *Bacteroides fragilis*, the most commonly isolated anaerobe and a predominant part of the indigenous fecal biota in humans, is not inhibited by the presence of bile. Bile-esculin agar plates are used for the selection and presumptive identification of *B. fragilis*. Although not used as a component of selection media for *B. fragilis*, it is important to note that, in general, gram-negative, nonspore-forming, anaerobic bacilli are susceptible to penicillin. *B. fragilis* is an exception in that it is known to be resistant to penicillin.

232.

B. The second most commonly encountered group of anaerobes in human infections is the anaerobic, gram-positive cocci. They may account for one-fourth of all anaerobes isolated in clinical laboratories. Estimating their clinical significance, however, is often difficult. Important isolates include *Fingoldia magna* (formerly *Peptostreptococcus magnus*) and *Peptostreptococcus anaerobius*.

233.

A. The closed chest abscess described is characteristic of human actinomycosis, which is often caused by *A. israelii*, an anaerobic, gram-positive, nonspore-forming bacillus. The organism is not acid-fast, which helps to differentiate it from *Nocardia* spp. Actinomycotic pus characteristically shows "sulfur granules" or solid yellow particles made up of masses of the filamentous bacilli seen on the Gram stain in Color Plate 27 ■.

234.

A. Kanamycin-vancomycin laked blood (KVLB) agar is selective for the *Prevotella* and *Bacteroides* spp. Presumptive identification of *B. fragilis* can be accomplished utilizing its antimicrobial resistance pattern. *B. fragilis.* is resistant to vancomycin and kanamycin, unlike *Fusobacterium* spp., which are resistant to vancomycin but susceptible to kanamycin. A KVLB agar plate should be part of the primary plating media for anaerobic cultures.

235.

C. *C. difficile* is an important cause of a healthcare-associated infection called pseudomembranous colitis. Hospitalized patients treated with broad-spectrum antimicrobial agents become colonized when their normal intestinal biota is diminished. The most rapid and accurate diagnostic method is nucleic acid amplification test (NAAT) on stool specimens. Detecting toxin A and/or B by enzyme immunoassay is a rapid screening test, but positive results should be confirmed by NAAT.

236.

D. Although it has a gram-positive-like cell wall, *Mobiluncus* stains gram-variable to gram-negative. This curved and motile bacillus seems to contribute to the pathology of BV. A Gram stain of the discharge that is produced in this condition can be used for the detection of these distinctively curved organisms. The presence of "clue cells," gram-variable pleomorphic bacilli on vaginal epithelial cells, is diagnostic of BV.

237.

B. Infant botulism or "floppy infant" syndrome is seen in children up to 12 months of age. This infectious process begins with the ingestion of food contaminated with spores of *C. botulinum*. Following ingestion, viable spores are carried to the lower bowel, where they germinate and elaborate the powerful neurotoxin that produces the characteristic flaccid paralysis.

238.

D. *C. acnes* is the most frequently isolated of all the gram-positive, nonspore-forming, anaerobic bacilli. It is a part of the normal human bacterial biota and predominates on the surface of the body, but may also be recovered from the upper respiratory tract, intestines, and urogenital tract. This organism is a common contaminant of blood cultures because of its presence on the skin. Care in the preparation of the skin before venipuncture helps to eliminate confusion caused by the recovery of this anaerobic isolate.

239.

D. The spore of *C. tetani* is located terminally and is larger than the sporangium. Characteristically, when seen on Gram stain, the cells of *C. tetani* resemble a drumstick or tennis racket. Spores can be readily seen in late growth phase cultures incubated at 35°C.

240.

C. *Fusobacterium nucleatum*, a gram-negative, anaerobic bacillus, is part of the indigenous microbial biota of the respiratory, gastrointestinal, and genitourinary tracts. It is frequently implicated as the causative agent in metastatic suppurative infections such as brain abscesses. These pale-staining bacilli characteristically appear as long, thin bacilli with pointed ends.

241.

C. *Propionibacterium* spp. are nonspore-forming, anaerobic, gram-positive bacilli. *Clostridium* spp. typically form spores, although it is difficult to induce some species to form spores *in vitro*. *Veillonella* is a gram-negative coccus, and *Fusobacterium* is a gram-negative bacillus.

242.

A. *C. botulinum* is the causative agent of botulism, a disease produced by an exotoxin that acts on the central nervous system. Types A, B, E, and F are causes of human botulism; types C and D and less commonly types A and B are associated with disease in animals and birds. This anaerobic organism produces oval subterminal, spores that germinate in food products or less commonly in wounds.

243.

D. Resazurin is an E_h indicator used in anaerobic culture media. When the oxygen concentration is reduced, the resazurin indicator is colorless. A pink color in the medium indicates aeration and an unsuitable environment for the preservation of obligate anaerobic organisms.

244.

B. *F. nucleatum* is the most frequent clinical isolate within the genus *Fusobacterium*. These anaerobes are part of the indigenous biota of human mucous membranes, oral cavity, intestine, and urogenital tract. *F. necrophorum* is, however, much more virulent.

245.

B. *C. septicum* is isolated in the clinical laboratory in cases of serious or often fatal infections. Bacteremia is seen in association with an underlying malignancy. The most common types of cancer are colon or cecum, breast, and leukemia or lymphoma.

246.

A. Botulinal toxin is the most potent exotoxin known. When absorbed, this exotoxin produces the paralyzing disease botulism. Toxin acts in the body by blocking the release of acetylcholine in the neuromuscular junction of the peripheral nervous system, causing muscle paralysis.

247.

B. *C. perfringens* is the species most commonly associated with clostridial myonecrosis or gas gangrene. These soil and water saprophytes most frequently gain entrance to the human body through traumatic wounds. Once they have been introduced into injured tissue, the characteristic syndrome of myonecrosis due to the elaboration of exotoxins may occur. Other species involved with myonecrosis are *C. septicum, C. novyi, C. sordellii*, and *C. histolyticum.*

248.

D. *Eubacterium, Bifidobacterium*, and *Propionibacterium* are all anaerobic, gram-positive, nonspore-forming bacilli. This group of anaerobic microorganisms is difficult to identify in the clinical laboratory. These organisms are rarely isolated. *Porphyromonas* spp. are anaerobic, gram-negative bacilli.

249.

B. Clostridia bacteria and spores are widespread in the soil and intestinal track of animals. They will grow on phenylethyl alcohol agar, and many clostridia require anaerobic conditions for spore formation.

250.

B. Most *Clostridium* spp. are gram-positive, and they generally form spores. Because they are obligate anaerobes, they will not grow on sheep blood or chocolate agars incubated aerobically. *Bacillus* spp. also form spores, but they are facultative anaerobes and would therefore grow on media incubated aerobically. *Lactobacillus* is a nonspore-forming, gram-positive bacillus, and *Prevotella* is a gram-negative bacillus.

251.

C. *Lactobacillus* spp. are normal biota of the vagina and digestive tract and are rarely pathogenic. They are aerotolerant anaerobes and will produce alpha-hemolysis on sheep blood agar plates incubated aerobically. These organisms can also produce a green discoloration on chocolate agar.

252.

C. *C. perfringens* produces spores that are oval and central in location but that are rarely seen in foods or on laboratory cultures. This organism is divided into five types, A to E, based on the quantities and types of exotoxins produced. Type A is responsible for human cases of myonecrosis and food poisoning. Alpha-toxin or lecithinase is produced by all strains of *C. perfringens.*

253.

D. *C. tetani* is a strict anaerobe that is motile and produces terminal round spores. Biochemically, it does not utilize carbohydrates, with the rare exception of glucose. *C. tetani* is gelatinase and indole positive but is nonproteolytic and H_2S negative. The clinical manifestations of tetanus are the result of the release of a neurotoxic exotoxin.

254.

C. *F. nucleatum* characteristically appears on Gram stain as a gram-negative rod with pointed ends. Its growth is inhibited by a 1-μg kanamycin disk and the presence of bile. *Bacteroides fragilis* and the pigmented species *Prevotella* and *Porphyromonas* are not inhibited by kanamycin.

255.

D. *P. melaninogenica* can be rapidly presumptively identified on media containing laked blood with the use of an ultraviolet light source. This important anaerobic pathogen can be differentiated after 5–7 days' incubation by its black pigmentation. The use of ultraviolet light enables a more rapid differentiation because of the appearance of a brick red fluorescence before the pigment is demonstrated.

256.

D. The symptoms of *C. difficile* infection are toxin mediated. This organism is known to cause pseudomembranous colitis associated with the use of antimicrobial therapy. Cytotoxins can be directly detected in stools by enzyme immunoassays; however, nucleic acid amplification tests are recommended. While cultures are infrequently performed, isolates will fluoresce on cycloserine-cefoxitin-fructose agar.

257.

B. A reverse CAMP test aids in the identification of *C. perfringens.* In this test, a single straight streak of *S. agalactiae* is made down the center of the plate. Suspected *C. perfringens* isolates are inoculated at right angles to the *S. agalactiae* inoculum. After anaerobic incubation, *C. perfringens* will exhibit enhanced hemolysis at the intersection where the two species meet.

258.

A. The identification of *P. anaerobius* is made easier by the use of the sodium polyethanol sulfonate (SPS) disk. The test is performed by growing the organism in the presence of a disk impregnated with SPS. A zone of inhibition of 12–18 mm around the disk is considered sensitive and a presumptive identification of this organism.

259.

C. *F. nucleatum* is a thin gram-negative rod with pointed ends and a slightly curved appearance in fresh isolates. As the bacteria are subcultured, they may lose their curved appearance and appear as thin rods. *F. nucleatum* is found in human specimens and is considered clinically significant.

260.

D. Anaerobes are a major cause of brain abscess. *Peptostreptococcus* spp. are associated with human disease, usually in polymicrobial infections, and can be seen on a Gram stain of clinical material. The characteristic Gram stain morphology of *Fusobacterium* would enable a physician to make a presumptive identification of the presence of anaerobic biota in this clinical case.

261.

C. The *B. fragilis* capsule stimulates abscess formation and helps the bacteria evade phagocytosis. The capsule is a contributing factor to the pathology produced by this anaerobe. *B. fragilis* is the most common anaerobic gram-negative bacillus isolated in the clinical laboratory. It also produces endotoxin that, when in serum, can contribute to systemic inflammation.

262.

C. *B. fragilis* is among the most antimicrobial-resistant anaerobes. Beta-lactamase production is responsible for its resistance to the penicillins. This anaerobe is also resistant to first-generation cephalosporins and aminoglycosides.

263.

C. The common agents in cases of aspiration pneumonia are oral anaerobes, such as the black-pigmented *Prevotella* and *Porphyromonas*, and *Bacteroides*, fusobacteria, and anaerobic streptococci. These endogenous organisms, when in an abnormal site, possess virulence factors that enable them to produce disease. Often these are polymicrobic infections mixing anaerobes with aerobic or facultative organisms such as *Enterobactericeae* or *Staphylococcus aureus.*

264.

B. Methylene blue strips are the most commonly used oxidation-reduction (E_h) indicators. When anaerobic conditions are achieved, the methylene blue indicator will turn from blue (oxidized) to white, indicating reduction. Resazurin, another E_h indicator, is used in anaerobic transport systems and anaerobic culture media such as the prereduced anaerobically sterilized (PRAS) system. Resazurin when oxidized is pink; when reduced, the color fades to white, indicating anaerobiosis.

265.

A. An area of precipitate in the agar around the colonies indicates that the organism produced lecithinase. Lecithinase (alpha-toxin) cleaves lecithin in the medium, producing an insoluble product. *C. perfringens* is positive for lecithinase.

266.

B. *P. niger* produces a pigment that begins olive green and gradually becomes black. This is the only species in the genus. It is a weak pathogen sometimes found in polymicrobial infections.

267.

C. *C. perfringens* is one of the most important causes of foodborne diseases in the United States. The bacterial spores can survive cooking (typically found in meats and gravies), and upon cooling they germinate into vegetative cells. When the bacteria are ingested, they sporulate in the intestinal tract. The enterotoxin is a spore coat protein made in excess and released by the bacteria.

268.

C. *Lactobacillus* spp. are found as normal biota in the gastrointestinal and female genital tract. The bacteria produce acids from the metabolism of carbohydrates, resulting in an acid environment in the vagina. If the population of lactobacilli decreases, the vaginal pH will rise toward neutrality. This favors the growth of other bacteria, such as *Mobiluncus*, that can result in bacterial vaginosis.

Chlamydia, Rickettsia, and *Mycoplasma*

269.

B. *C. trachomatis* is the causative agent of inclusion conjunctivitis, trachoma, and genital tract infections, including lymphogranuloma venereum. Trachoma is a primary cause of blindness worldwide. The disease is preventable, but when it is not treated, the organism produces hypertrophy of the lymphoid follicles on the inner surface of the upper eyelid. This process causes the upper eyelid to evert (entropion), which ultimately leads to blindness.

270.

A. The *Chlamydia* and *Chlamydiophila* are obligate intracellular parasites. It was originally thought that they required ATP from their host cell. Recent studies have demonstrated that the chlamydiae can produce small amounts of ATP. As such, these bacteria cannot be grown on artificial media. They can be cultivated in cell cultures.

271.

C. *M. pneumoniae* causes primary atypical pneumonia. The pneumonia is atypical in that it is milder than the pneumonia caused by *S. pneumoniae.* Chest X-rays of patients with atypical pneumonia may show bilateral infiltrates, although physical examination reveals few chest findings.

272.

D. Provided that arginine is added for *Mycoplasma hominis*, SP4 agar or broth can be used for the growth of *M. pneumoniae* and *M. hominis. M. pneumoniae* is a slow-grower, so most infections are diagnosed by serologic assays. M. *pneumoniae* is an important respiratory tract pathogen of humans. It is found only in humans and is typically spread person to person.

273.

C. Human infections with *C. psittaci* (psittacosis) occur after exposure to infected birds and their droppings. A true zoonosis, psittacosis is a disease of birds that may be contracted by humans. The disease produced by this organism may be mild or fulminant, the latter of which has a high mortality rate. Clinical manifestations of the disease include severe headache, weakness, and mild pulmonary symptoms.

274.

C. Unlike rickettsial diseases, no rash occurs in *C. burnetti* infections. The organism is an obligate intracellular parasite that is able to survive for long periods in the environment. It causes a zoonosis and is transmitted to humans by inhalation and contact with fomites. Infections can also be acquired by ingestion of unpasteurized milk.

275.

A. Mycoplasmas are small, pleomorphic organisms that lack a cell wall and are best visualized by darkfield or phase microscopy or the Diene stain. Penicillin is not an effective treatment because of their absence of a cell wall, and isolation requires media supplemented with peptone, yeast extract, and serum. Species of the genus *Mycoplasma* are well-known human pathogens that cause a variety of infections.

276.

A. *C. trachomatis*, a leading cause of blindness, can be detected in corneal scrapings of suspected cases of trachoma and inclusion conjunctivitis. Clinical material can be tested using enzyme immunoassays (EIAs) or NAATs, historically they were cultured in McCoy cells. Trachoma is a chronic inflammatory process of the conjunctiva that results in corneal involvement.

277.

C. *M. hominis, M. genitalium*, and *U. urealyticum* have been linked to human genital infections. These species can also be isolated from asymptomatic sexually active adults. *M. pneumoniae* is primarily a respiratory tract pathogen.

278.

D. *C. pneumoniae* is an important cause of sporadic and epidemic lower respiratory tract disease characterized as atypical pneumonia. The organism is a human pathogen spread person to person. Most infections are diagnosed serologically. Tetracycline and erythromycin are effective treatments.

279.

C. PCR DNA amplification has been shown to be more sensitive than cell culture and nearly 100% specific for the detection of *C. trachomatis*. Suitable specimens for detection are cervical secretions and urine. When confirmation of *C. trachomatis* is needed, tissue culture remains the method of choice.

280.

C. *Mycoplasmas* are implicated in a variety of human infections. *M. pneumoniae*, in particular, is a clinically important respiratory tract pathogen. When grown on culture media, colonies, most notably *M. hominis*, are said to have a “fried egg” appearance because the central portion of the colony has grown into the agar and thus appears more dense and is slightly raised.

281.

A. Q fever is caused by infection with *C. burnetii*, which has unique characteristics. Unlike other rickettsiae, this organism is able to resist heat and drying for long periods and does not rely on an arthropod vector for transmission. Infectious fomites such as dust from contaminated cattle hides and fluids released during birth are considered the primary modes of infection.

282.

A. Direct microscopic examination for *Rickettsia* organisms is possible using such stains as Giemsa, Machiavello, or Gimenez. The recommended procedure is the nonspecific Gimenez stain, which colors the organisms a brilliant red against a green background. The staining technique calls for flooding a thin smear, which has been air dried, with a solution of carbol-fuchsin for 1–2 minutes. After washing with tap water, malachite green is added for 6–9 seconds before the final washing with tap water.

283.

D. Transovarian passage from generation to generation in ticks perpetuates *R. rickettsii* for several generations outside an animal host. A blood meal serves to reactivate the rickettsiae carried by the arthropod vector. Rodents and small mammals are the natural reservoirs for the rickettsiae that cause this form of spotted fever.

284.

D. Flying squirrels, *Glaucomys volans*, are associated with cases of the sylvatic form of typhus in the United States. The squirrel louse transmits the organism among the squirrel population. Humans contract the disease through association with infected squirrels. The disease is more common in the winter months, when squirrels seeking shelter enter dwellings.

285.

A. Humans who have had the classic form of typhus may remain infected with the causative agent *R. prowazekii*. Relapses or recrudescence of disease may occur in these persons years or decades after the initial attack. The latent form of infection is known as Brill-Zinsser disease and may serve as an interepidemic reservoir for epidemic typhus.

286.

D. Murine typhus is transmitted to humans by fleas infected with *R. typhi*. Prevalent in the southern United States, it is primarily a disease of rodents and is sometimes transmitted to humans. Control of disease outbreaks is related to rodent (rat) control and the related rat flea population. The symptoms of murine or endemic typhus are similar to those of the classic epidemic form seen in Europe.

287.

D. Because the mycoplasmata lack a cell wall, they will not Gram stain. Some species can be recovered by **vigorously** swabbing mucous membranes or other body sites like the throat. *M. hominis* grows readily on SP4 agar.

288.

D. 10 B broth is used with genital specimens to isolate *U. urealyticum*. The bacterium requires urea and produces a strong alkaline pH because of the activity of urease. The bacteria are slow growers and form tiny colonies. The broth will typically not appear turbid.

Spirochetes

289.

D. Cardiolipin is a tissue lipid produced as a by-product of treponemal infection. Nontreponemal tests for syphilis take advantage of antibodies made to cardiolipin. The most commonly used tests are the rapid plasma reagin (RPR) for serum and the Veneral Disease Research Laboratory (VDRL) for cerebrospinal fluid.

290.

A. *Leptospira* spp. are most reliably detected during the first week of illness by the direct culturing of a blood sample. The media of choice are Fletcher semisolid and Stuart liquid medium, both of which are supplemented with rabbit serum. One or two drops of the patient's blood are added to 5 mL of culture medium, which is incubated in the dark at 30°C or room temperature for up to 6 weeks. After the first week of disease and lasting for several months, the urine becomes the specimen of choice for isolation of the organism. Direct microscopic examination is not reliable for detection because of the low numbers of organisms normally present in body fluids.

291.

C. Syphilis is caused by *T. pallidum* subsp. *pallidum.* Congenital syphilis occurs when a pregnant woman has a septicemia, and the spirochetes cross the placenta and infect the fetus. Infection can affect fetal development and cause premature birth or fetal death, or the pregnancy may go to term. Following *in utero* infection, the infant is most often born with lesions characteristic of secondary syphilis; perinatal death is not an uncommon consequence of infection.

292.

C. The description given is characteristic of members of the genus *Leptospira.* Blood and other fluids, such as cerebrospinal fluid and urine, are examined by direct darkfield microscopy and stained preparations for the presence of these organisms in suspected cases of leptospirosis. The number of organisms present in clinical samples is low, and detection is difficult even when concentration methods are used. Culture and serologic tests are available for the diagnosis of disease produced by these organisms.

293.

B. The human body louse, *Pediculus humanus*, is the vector for *B. recurrentis.* Pathogenic species not only have specific vectors but also well-defined geographic distributions. Epidemic relapsing fever is found in Ethiopia, Sudan, and parts of South America.

294.

D. The antigen in the VDRL and RPR tests is cardiolipin; these are so called "nontreponemal" tests. The treponemal antigen tests, FTA-ABS and TP-PA, are more specific (fewer false-positive results) than the nontreponemal tests. After successful treatment, the antibody titer of nontreponemal tests typically declines, while the antibody titer in treponemal tests remains relatively high. Both nontreponemal and treponemal assays are sensitive in secondary syphilis.

295.

A. Lyme disease was first described in 1975 following an outbreak in Lyme, Connecticut. The etiologic agent, *B. burgdorferi*, is transmitted to humans by the tick vector *Ixodes dammini.* Clinically, the disease peaks in the summer and produces an epidemic inflammatory condition characterized by skin lesions, erythema, headache, myalgia, malaise, and lymphadenitis. Rat-bite fever is caused by *Spirillum minus.* Relapsing fever is caused by *Borrelia*, and Q fever is caused by *Coxiella burnetti.*

296.

B. The basic structure of spirochetes is an outer membrane, cytoplasmic membrane-peptidoglycan complex, cytoplasm, and axial fibrils. The fibrils are attached to the cytoplasmic membrane close to the ends of the cell, extending along the body under the outer membrane. The axial fibrils most closely resemble bacterial flagella and are associated with motility of the organism.

297.

C. Spirochetes are gram-negative, but most do not stain with the Gram stain. Silver impregnation can be used to visualize them in smears. The direct observation using darkfield or phase microscopy is recommended to view these delicate, coiled cells in body fluids or tissue sections. Treponemal diseases in humans are generally transmitted human to human, while borreliosis is transmitted by insect vectors. Spirochetes are motile by axial filaments.

298.

C. Infections other than syphilis can cause a positive VDRL result. The VDRL test detects an antibody that is not directed against *T. pallidum* antigens. It is a good screening test for syphilis, but it is not highly specific. Confirmation with a specific treponemal test, such as the TP-PA assay, is required.

Antimicrobial Agents and Antimicrobial Susceptibility Testing

299.

A. Standardization of the susceptibility testing procedure is essential for determining the susceptibility of an organism to antimicrobial agents. A #0.5 McFarland standard is used when adjusting the turbidity of the suspension of test organism. A #0.5 McFarland standard has a turbidity consistent with approximately 1.5×10^8 organisms/mL of broth or saline.

300.

D. Hemophilus Test Medium (Mueller-Hinton base supplemented with hematin, NAD, and yeast extract) is recommended for use in the disk-agar diffusion susceptibility testing procedure of *Haemophilus*. The testing of *Haemophilus* spp. requires supplemented media to support the growth of these fastidious organisms. *In vitro* growth of *H. influenzae* requires the presence of accessory growth factors: X factor (hemin) and V factor (NAD).

301.

D. Sulfonamides act to interfere with the ability of bacteria to use *p*-aminobenzoic acid, which is a part of the folic acid molecule, by competitive inhibition. These chemotherapeutic agents are bacteriostatic and not bactericidal. The drug sulfisoxazole is a member of this group and is used in the treatment of urinary tract infections, especially those caused by *E. coli*, which must synthesize folic acid for growth.

302.

A. Beta-lactam antibiotics inhibit cell wall synthesis. The carbapenems are regarded as having the broadest spectrum among this class of drugs. They exhibit resistance to most beta-lactamases. However, recently members of the family Enterobacteriaceae have been found to produce carbapenemases.

303.

C. Inhibitors of peptidoglycan synthesis such as penicillin act to inhibit cell wall development. Bacteria unable to produce peptidoglycan for their cell walls are subject to the effects of varying osmotic pressures. The peptidoglycan component of the cell wall protects the bacterium from lysis.

304.

C. The requirement of 99.9% killing defines the minimum bactericidal concentration (MBC) of an antimicrobial agent. The MBC test is an additional quantitative assessment of the killing effect of a drug on a specific patient isolate. This test, done to evaluate a drug's activity, is sometimes requested in cases of life-threatening infections.

305.

B. Even though clindamycin and erythromycin are in different classes, the mechanisms of resistance are similar. The presence of erythromycin can induce clindamycin resistance. The D-zone test is used to detect the presence of this inducible resistance.

306.

D. The therapeutic effect of antimicrobial therapy is often increased by the use of a combination of drugs. A combination of antimicrobials is said to be synergistic when the sum of their effects is greater than that derived from either drug when tested independently. A tenfold decrease in the number of viable cells from that obtained by the most effective drug in the combination is the definition of synergism. Synergistic combinations of antimicrobials are used primarily in the treatment of tuberculosis, enterococcal endocarditis, and certain gram-negative bacillus infections.

307.

C. Beta-lactamase production by strains of *H. influenzae* renders them resistant to the antibacterial effect of penicillin and ampicillin. It is recommended that rapid beta-lactamase testing be performed on isolates in life-threatening clinical infections such as meningitis. The rapid tests all rely on this enzyme's ability to act on a beta-lactamase ring and in turn produce a color change, which denotes a positive result due to the production of penicilloic acid.

308.

C. The recommended plating medium for use in both the disk diffusion and tube dilution susceptibility test procedures is Mueller-Hinton. Low in tetracycline and sulfonamide inhibitors, this medium has been found to show only slight batch-to-batch variability. For the susceptibility testing of fastidious organisms (e.g., *S. pneumoniae*), 5% lysed sheep blood should be added.

309.

B. The Kirby-Bauer or disk-agar diffusion susceptibility test requires that the pH of the agar be tested at room temperature to ensure an optimal range of 7.2–7.4 before use in the procedure. A sample of the Mueller-Hinton medium can be tested by macerating it in distilled water and testing with a pH meter electrode; a surface electrode is acceptable for direct testing. Another acceptable method is to allow the agar to solidify around the electrode of a pH meter and then obtain a reading.

310.

B. Metronidazole, a drug recommended for the treatment of amebic dysentery and trichomoniasis, is a synthetic compound that acts by inhibiting DNA synthesis. The use of this drug for treating anaerobic infections has gained emphasis in light of resistance patterns of many of the commonly recovered anaerobes. Metronidazole is consistently active against all gram-negative, anaerobic bacilli; is able to cross the blood-brain barrier; and is the only agent consistently bactericidal against susceptible isolates.

311.

D. Tobramycin, an aminoglycoside, is the only antimicrobial agent, of those listed, that is bactericidal. Bactericidal agents destroy the bacteria, whereas bacteriostatic drugs only arrest the growth of the microorganism when the drug is present. All aminoglycosides, with the exception of spectinomycin, are bactericidal in their activity.

312.

B. The extended spectrum beta-lactamases (ESBLs) confer resistance to the extended-spectrum cephalosporins such as ceftriaxone and cefotaxime. ESBLs cleave the antibiotic, inactivating it. So far, ESBLs have only been found in gram-negative bacteria.

313.

C. Most fastidious bacteria do not grow satisfactorily in standard *in vitro* susceptibility test systems that use unsupplemented media. For certain species, such as *H. influenzae, N. gonorrheae, S. pneumoniae,* and other *Streptococcus* species, modifications have been made to the standard Clinical and Laboratory Standards Institute (CLSI) methods. In the case of *S. pneumoniae,* current CLSI broth dilution test conditions include cation-supplemented Mueller-Hinton broth with 5% lysed horse blood.

314.

B. *H. influenzae* should be tested for beta-lactamase production. The test can be performed directly, and the methods are rapid and reliable for the detection of penicillin and ampicillin resistance. Rapid test methods, in general, rely on a color change to detect the presence of this enzyme. A pH indicator may be used to detect the penicilloic acid produced when the beta-lactam ring of penicillin is cleaved, or a color change can be observed when the beta-lactam ring of a chromogenic cephalosporin is hydrolyzed by the enzyme.

315.

D. Tolerance is described as the ability of certain strains of organisms to resist lethal concentrations of antimicrobial agents like penicillin. The growth of these organisms is only inhibited by these cidal drugs. This mechanism of bacterial resistance is attributed to a deficiency of cell wall autolysins.

316.

B. Carbapenemases are active against most beta-lactam antibiotics. This includes the penicillins, cephalosporins, and carbapenems. The carbapenem antibiotics have a broad spectrum of activity. The members of the family *Enterobacteriaceae* are the most significant producers of carbapenemases.

317.

B. Clavulanic acid is a beta-lactamase inhibitor. It can be administered with amoxicillin or ticarcillin and is effective in treating infections caused by beta-lactamase-producing bacteria such as staphylococci, *Klebsiella*, and *H. influenzae*. Sulbactam and tazobactam are also beta-lactamase inhibitors.

318.

D. Vancomycin, which acts to inhibit cell wall synthesis of susceptible bacteria, is produced by an actinomycete. The main activity of this drug is to inhibit peptidoglycan synthesis, but it also has an effect on other aspects of bacterial metabolism. Vancomycin is a bactericidal antibiotic.

319.

A. In the modified carbapenem inactivation method (mCIM) assay, the test organism is incubated with a disk containing a carbapenem. If the bacteria produce a carbapenemase, the enzyme will inactive the antibiotic. When the disk is placed on a lawn of carbapenem-sensitive control bacteria, the control bacteria will grow up to the disk.

320.

A. Gentamicin is a member of the aminoglycoside group of antibiotics. These drugs act on the 30S ribosomal subunit to inhibit protein synthesis. Gentamicin is particularly effective against a wide variety of gram-negative bacilli.

321.

B. Bone marrow toxicity is the major complication of chloramphenicol. Reversible bone marrow suppression with anemia, leukopenia, and thrombocytopenia occurs as a direct result of the agent on hematopoiesis. The second form of bone marrow toxicity is a rare but usually fatal aplastic anemia. The mechanism of this response is not known.

322.

C. Methicillin resistance is often an inducible characteristic. Cefoxitin is a more powerful inducer of methicillin, or oxacillin, resistance than oxacillin itself. Drug resistance can be detected in disk diffusion assays.

Procedures and Biochemical Identification of Bacteria

323.

D. Normal biota can offer the host protection against infections by providing competition to pathogenic bacteria. The trachea, lungs, and cervix are not typically colonized with bacterial biota. When diagnosing lower respiratory tract infections, procedures such as bronchoscopy or percutaneous transtracheal aspitate are used to obtain a specimen that is not contaminated by upper respiratory tract biota.

324.

B. The biota of the female genital tract changes with age and the associated effects of pH and estrogen concentration in the mucosa. *Lactobacillus* spp. are the predominant biota during childbearing years. Earlier and later in life, staphylococci and corynebacteria predominate.

325.

C. The MIDI system is based on the analysis of fatty acids in the cell wall of microorganisms. The bacteria are grown under standardized conditions, and the fatty acids are extracted. The *Mycobacterium* fatty acids are analyzed by high-performance liquid chromatography. Gas liquid chromatography is used for other bacteria and yeasts. Results are compared to a computerized database.

326.

C. Most commercially available blood culture media contain the anticoagulant SPS. Anticoagulation is important because certain bacteria do not survive well within clotted blood. Two to three blood cultures are recommended, and 10–20 mL of blood is recommended for adults.

327.

B. Incubation of inoculated bacteriologic culture media requires that attention be given to optimal temperature ranges, adequate moisture, and proper atmospheric conditions for growth. The optimal atmosphere for many clinically significant isolates is one that contains 5–10% carbon dioxide. Capnophilic environments may be obtained by using incubators equipped with a tank of carbon dioxide and a regulator. The portable Fyrite carbon dioxide gas analyzer may be used for the daily monitoring of capnophilic incubators.

328.

B. Microbiologic examination of body fluids is less effective when bacteria become trapped in clotted specimens. The most effective anticoagulant for use in the microbiology laboratory is SPS in a concentration of 0.025–0.05%. Fluids known to clot on standing should be transported to the laboratory in a sterile tube containing SPS. This polyanionic anticoagulant is also anticomplementary and antiphagocytic.

329.

C. The oxidase test determines the presence of the cytochrome C used in the respiration of oxygen via the electron transport chain. All oxidase positive bacteria are therefore aerobic. *P. aeruginosa* is oxidase positive. Media with a high glucose concentration can produce false negative results. Bacteria taken from media with dyes may cause aberrant results.

330.

A. Infectious aerosols put laboratory professionals at risk for acquiring many diseases. The handling of clinical specimens that require pipetting, centrifugation, or decanting may produce infectious aerosols. Bacteria frequently are present in greater numbers in aerosol droplets than in the liquid medium.

331.

C. Typically, squamous epithelial cells are an indication of contamination with oral microbiota, whereas polymorphonuclear cells indicate a quality specimen. Two commonly used scoring systems are the Bartlett's Q-score and the Murray-Washington method. Unacceptable specimens should not be cultured because they can give misleading results.

332.

C. Mannitol salt agar is highly selective and differential. It is used for the isolation and identification of staphylococcal species. The 7.5% concentration of sodium chloride results in inhibition of most bacteria other than staphylococci. Mannitol fermentation, as indicated by a change in the phenol red indicator, aids in the differentiation of staphylococcal species because most *S. aureus* isolates ferment mannitol (changing the color of the medium to yellow) and most coagulase-negative staphylococci are unable to ferment mannitol.

333.

B. The biomolecules in MALDI-TOF mass spectrometry are added to a solid matrix and vaporized by a laser. The molecules are then separated by the mass to charge (m/z) ratio, and their time of flight through the instrument is determined. This produces a unique protein spectrum for different species of bacteria.

334.

D. The hippurate hydrolysis can be useful to identify group B streptococci, which are positive. Group B streptococci are typically beta hemolytic. However, streptococci are generally identified by serotyping. *L. monocytogenes* and *C. jejuni* are also hippurate hydrolysis positive.

335.

D. Bacterial metabolism of carbohydrates in the culture media produces the by-product carbon dioxide, which is captured as head gas in sealed culture vials. Manometric systems measure the head space pressure. It is possible to detect bacterial metabolism in these systems within only a few hours of inoculation.

336.

A. In the catalase test, hydrogen peroxide is reduced to water and oxygen. The formation of oxygen produces the bubbles seen in a positive test. The catalase test is used to differentiate the staphylococci (positive) from the streptococci (negative).

337.

A. Pyrrolidonyl-α-naphthylamide (PYR) is the substrate. The test detects the presence of the enzyme L-pyrrolidonyl arylamidase. The PYR test helps differentiate *S. aureus* (positive) from *S. lugdunensis* (negative). *S. pyogenes* and many *Enterococcus* spp. are also PYR positive.

Case Studies

338.

C. Disseminated gonococcal infection produces symptoms of arthritis, especially in the major joints of the body. Samples of joint fluid from these patients should be inoculated to a selective medium for the isolation of *N. gonorrhoeae* in addition to nonselective media. Thayer-Martin agar has a chocolate agar base formulated to support the growth of fastidious *Neisseria* spp. while suppressing the growth of normal or indigenous biota by the addition of antimicrobial agents. Only about 50% of patients with gonococcal arthritis will have positive synovial fluid cultures.

339.

A. The anatomy of the female urethra allows bacteria from the perirectal region to reach the bladder easily. *E. coli* is the most common pathogen in uncomplicated community-acquired urinary tract infections. Other organisms are more prevalent in nosocomial or recurrent infections.

340.

A. *Salmonella* Typhi, the causative agent of typhoid fever, is commonly associated with invasion of the bloodstream. The presence of organisms is the result of an extravascular site of infection. The extravascular sites in the case of typhoid fever are the small intestine, the regional lymph nodes of the intestine, and the reticuloendothelial system. The bacteremic phase is seen before the organism can be recovered in stool.

341.

C. *V. vulnificus* is responsible for septicemia after consumption of contaminated raw oysters. Infections are most severe in patients with hepatic disease, hematopoietic disease, or chronic renal failure and those receiving immunosuppressive drugs. Mortality in patients with septicemia can be as high as 50% unless antimicrobial therapy is started rapidly.

342.

C. *A. pyogenes* has been reclassified several times. It was formerly a member of the genera *Corynebacterium* and *Actinomyces. A. pyogenes* is a well-known animal pathogen causing soft tissue infections in a wide variety of farm animals. Mode of transmission to humans is unknown, but most cases occur in a rural environment and include a history of abrasion or undetected wounds with animal exposure. *L. monocytogenes* is also a gram-positive bacillus that is CAMP positive; however, it is catalase positive.

343.

D. *N. meningitidis* is a leading cause of bacterial meningitis. Disease is transmitted by respiratory droplets among people in prolonged close contact, such as in daycare centers. Chemoprophylaxis with rifampin is appropriate for those in close contact with the patient: household members, daycare staff, and classmates. Routine use of the vaccine Hib has signficanttly reduced the incidence of invasive *H. influenzae* infections.

344.

D. *S. aureus* has been isolated from a majority of the reported cases of the clinical syndrome described—toxic shock syndrome. First reported in the late 1970s, the disease was linked to the use of a specific brand of tampons. Symptoms are associated with the production of a pyrogenic exotoxin (toxic shock syndrome toxin-1, TSST-1) by the coagulase-positive *S. aureus.*

345.

D. The etiologic agent in this case is *Y. enterocolitica.* Disease caused by this organism frequently mimics the symptoms of appendicitis, although it has been implicated in a variety of clinical illnesses such as bacteremia, cholecystitis, and mesenteric lymphadenitis. *Y. enterocolitica* grows slowly at 35°C and, unless in large numbers or pure culture, may be overlooked in the laboratory. A key finding for *Y. enterocolitica* is a positive urease.

346.

A. Lyme disease is an inflammatory disease seen predominantly in the northeast and mid-Atlantic United States during the summer months. The initial symptoms of this disease may be followed months later by more serious complications, such as meningoencephalitis, myocarditis, and arthritis of the large joints. The etiologic agent of this tick-borne disease is *B. burgdorferi.* The spirochetes causing Lyme disease have not been demonstrated in peripheral blood smears. An indirect immunofluorescence test and an ELISA test are available for the detection of specific antibody in the patient's serum. The western blot assay is often used for serologic confirmation.

347.

D. Human infections caused by *Leptospira* characteristically produce the clinical symptoms of fever, anemia, and jaundice. Weil disease is another name for leptospirosis. Infections result from contact with the urine or tissue of infected animals like rats and mice or from water contaminated with urine of these animals. Most infections resolve in about a week, but they can go on for much longer and can cause fatal kidney and liver damage.

348.

D. *Y. enterocolitica* causes a variety of infections. This organism is able to grow at refrigerator temperatures (4°C). Contamination of stored blood units is not visually detected because the organism is able to reproduce in red blood cells without causing lysis or a color change.

349.

A. *M. marinum* produces lesions on the skin or the extremities of humans. This species of *Mycobacterium* is a free-living organism found in salt or brackish water. Human infection characteristically follows trauma to the body in or around water.

350.

B. *L. monocytogenes* has been associated with human disease following the ingestion of unpasteurized dairy products. The organism is capable of replicating at refrigerator temperatures and is commonly found in low numbers in animal products. Listeriosis associated with contaminated food, in uncompromised patients, usually produces a self-limiting, nonspecific febrile illness.

351.

A. *E. coli* 0157:H7 is associated with hemolytic uremic syndrome. These strains produce verotoxin (also called Shiga toxin) and are associated with outbreaks of diarrheal disease following ingestion of undercooked hamburger at fast-food restaurants and contact with calves at petting zoos. Cattle infected with this strain serve as the reservoir, and humans become infected by eating products made from their meat or contaminated with their excretions.

352.

C. The clinical presentation suggests the etiologic agent is *L. pneumophila.* The Gram stain is not helpful in making the diagnosis because of the poor staining quality of this microorganism. Examination of the sputum using fluorescent antibody to *L. pneumophila* could provide a rapid positive identification.

REFERENCES

Tille, P. (2018). *Bailey and Scott's Diagnostic Microbiology*, 14th ed. Philadelphia: Mosby.

Mahon, C. R., and Lehman, D. C. (2019). *Textbook of Diagnostic Microbiology*, 6th ed. St. Louis: Saunders Elsevier.

Carroll, K. C., et al. (2019). *Manual of Clinical Microbiology*, 12th ed. Washington, DC: American Society for Microbiology Press.

Murray, P. R., Rosenthal, K. S., and Pfaller, M. A. (2015). *Medical Microbiology*, 8th ed. Philadelphia: Elsevier Mosby.

CHAPTER

7 Mycology

contents

I. INTRODUCTION AND GENERAL CHARACTERISTICS

A. Mycology Terms

1. **Molds:** Multicellular fungi
2. **Yeasts:** Single-cell fungi
3. **Mycosis:** Fungal infection
4. **Systemic mycosis:** Multiorgan infection caused by fungi
5. **Opportunistic mycosis:** Fungal disease that occurs primarily in patients who are immunocompromised
6. **Dimorphic fungi:** Fungi that show both a nonmold (e.g., yeast) and a mold phase
7. **Saprobe:** Organism capable of living on decaying organic material

B. Fungal Structure

1. **Hyphae** are long, branching filaments that come together to form the **mycelium.** There are two main types of hyphae.
   a. **Septate hyphae** have cellular separation or cross-walls. Septate hyphae range in diameter from 3 to 6 μm.
   b. **Sparsely septate (formerly aseptate) hyphae** contain few, if any, cellular separations. Sparsely septate hyphae range in diameter from 5 to 15 μm. **Coenocytic** also refers to hyphae lacking cross-walls.
   c. **Pseudohyphae** are a chain of cells formed by budding that resemble true hyphae. Pseudohyphae differ from true hyphae in that they are constricted at the septa, form branches that begin with septation, and have terminal cells smaller than other cells.
2. Hyphae are classified as **vegetative** or **aerial.**
   a. **Vegetative hyphae** function in food absorption and are the portion that extends below the agar surface or nutrient substrate.
   b. **Aerial hyphae** extend above the agar or nutrient substrate, and their function is to support reproductive structures called **conidia.**
3. Conidia are sporelike asexual reproductive structures not produced by cleavage, conjugation, or free-cell formation. Conidia are only formed by the **imperfect fungi.**
   a. Conidia morphology is important in fungal identification.
   b. Conidia classification is based on conidia morphologic development.
   c. **Microconidia** are single-celled, small conidia.
   d. **Macroconidia** are multicellular, large conidia.
4. Types of conidia
   a. **Arthroconidia** are conidia resulting from the fragmentation of hyphae into individual cells. Some fungi will have arthroconidia separated by normal **(disjunctor)** cells.
   b. **Blastoconidia:** Conidia that form as the result of budding
   c. **Chlamydoconidia** result from terminal cells in the hyphae that enlarge and have thick walls. These conidia can survive adverse environmental

conditions. Chlamydoconidia are found in molds, whereas similar structures **(chlamydospores)** are found in hyphae produced by some yeasts.

d. **Poroconidia:** Conidia formed by being pushed through a small pore in the parent cell

e. **Phialoconidia:** Tube-shaped conidia that can be branched

f. **Annelloconidia** are vase-shaped conidia; the remaining parent outer cell wall takes on a saw-toothed appearance as the conidia are released.

C. Sexual and Asexual Reproduction

1. **Sexual reproduction**
   a. Requires the formation of specialized fungal structures called **spores**
   b. Fungi that undergo sexual reproduction are termed **perfect fungi.**
   c. Types of spores
      1) **Ascospores:** Spores contained in a saclike structure
      2) **Basidiospores:** Spores contained in a club-shaped structure
      3) **Oospores:** Spores resulting from the fusion of cells from two different hyphae
      4) **Zygospores:** Spores resulting from the fusion of two identical hyphae
2. **Asexual reproduction**
   a. Asexual reproduction only involves division of the nucleus and cytoplasm.
   b. Fungi that undergo asexual reproduction are termed **imperfect fungi.**
   c. **Imperfect fungi are the only fungal group to produce conidia.**

II. CULTURE AND ISOLATION

A. Fungal Media

1. **Sabouraud dextrose agar (SDA)**
   a. General-purpose, nutritionally poor medium mildly selective for fungi, no longer commonly used; several different formulations available
   b. In one formulation, the agar has an acidic pH (5.6) that inhibits most bacteria. Modified SDA (Emmons) has a neutral pH and better supports the growth of fungi but is less inhibitory for bacteria.
2. **Sabouraud-brain heart infusion (SABHI) agar**
   a. A nonselective medium for isolation of all fungi
   b. Contains dextrose, peptone, and brain heart infusion
   c. Can be made selective for dimorphic fungi by the addition of **cyclohexamide, chloramphenicol**, and **gentamicin.** Cyclohexamide inhibits the saprophytic fungi and chloramphenicol inhibits many gram-positive and gram-negative bacteria, whereas gentamicin inhibits primarily gram-negative bacteria.
3. **Brain heart infusion with blood (BHIB) agar**
   a. Used to grow most fungi, especially those from sterile body sites
   b. Contains brain heart infusion and sheep red blood cells
   c. Can be made selective for dimorphic fungi by the addition of **cyclohexamide, chloramphenicol**, and **gentamicin**

4. **Selective agars** contain various antimicrobial agents that will enhance the growth of specific fungal pathogens and will inhibit bacteria and other undesired growth.
   a. **Inhibitory mold agar (IMA)**
      1) IMA is used to grow most fungal pathogens; it is especially formulated to recover the cyclohexamide-sensitive *Cryptococcus* spp.
      2) Contains gentamicin and chloramphenicol
   b. **Dermatophye test medium (DTM)**
      1) Used to isolate the dermatophytes
      2) DTM contains cyclohexamide and gentamicin and phenol red as a pH indicator.
5. **Differential agars** are used to enhance pigment development, conidia production, and mold-to-yeast phase transition.
   a. **Potato dextrose agar (PDA)**
      1) Used to enhance conidia development
      2) Enhances pigment development of *Trichophyton rubrum*
   b. **Bird seed (niger seed) and caffeic acid agars** are selective and differential media used to grow *Cryptococcus neoformans.* Due to the activity of **phenol oxidase,** *C. neoformans* forms black to brown colonies. Chloramphenicol can be added to make the media selective.
   c. **Cornmeal agar with Tween 80:** Used to differentiate *Candida* spp.
   d. **Agars containing rice, casein,** and **other nutrients** are used to differentiate *Trichophyton* spp.

B. Culture Considerations

1. **Fungal cultures are generally incubated at 30°C.**
2. Growth requires from several days to several weeks.
3. Cultures should be maintained in a high-humidity environment.
4. Several techniques are used to obtain culture material for slide preparation.
   a. **Tease mount method:** A dissecting needle is used to pull apart a fungal colony, which is placed on a slide. This method may damage fungal structure, especially conidia. It may take several attempts to obtain a specimen with intact conidia.
   b. **Cellophane tape method:** Cellophane tape is used to transfer aerial hyphae from the colony to a microscope slide for examination.
   c. The **slide culture method** uses a block of agar overlaid with a cover slip. Fungal colonies are grown on the side of the agar block. The cover slip is removed and used for microscopic examination. This method minimizes damage to the fungal structure.

C. Direct Examination Methods

1. **Saline wet mount** is used to view fungal elements, such as hyphae, conidia, and budding yeasts. It has limited use and is most commonly applicable for vaginal secretions to diagnose vaginitis.
2. **Lactophenol cotton blue wet mount** is used to stain and preserve fungal elements primarily in culture isolates.

3. **Potassium hydroxide (KOH)** is used to dissolve nonfungal materials in skin, nail, and hair samples.
4. **Gram stain** can be used to view yeasts.
5. **India ink** can be used to reveal capsules surrounding *C. neoformans* found in cerebrospinal fluid (CSF). However, due to low sensitivity, direct antigen detection assays have generally replaced the India ink wet mount.
6. **Calcofluor white stain** is a fluorochrome that stains chitin found in the cell wall of fungi. The stain is not absorbed by human tissue. The slide is viewed using an ultraviolet light. Fungi will appear white to blue to green depending on the wavelength of light. KOH can be added to clear the specimen of cellular debris.

III. BODY SITES AND POSSIBLE FUNGAL PATHOGENS

A. Blood: *Candida* spp., *Blastomyces dermatitidis, Histoplasma capsulatum*, and *C. neoformans*

B. Cerebrospinal Fluid: *C. neoformans, Candida* spp., *H. capsulatum*, and *Coccidioides immitis*

C. Hair: *Microsporum* and *Trichophyton*

D. Nails: *Aspergillus, Epidermophyton,* and *Trichophyton*

E. Skin: *Candida, Microsporum, Trichophyton, Epidermophyton*, and *B. dermatitidis*

F. Lungs: *Candida albicans, Aspergillus, Rhizopus, Penicillium, H. capsulatum, B. dermatitidis,* and *C. immitis*

G. Throat: *C. albicans* and *Geotrichum candidum*

H. Urine: *C. albicans* and *Candida glabrata*

I. Genital Tract: *C. albicans*

IV. YEASTS

A. Introduction

1. Yeasts are common causes of vaginitis and urinary tract infections (UTIs) in women and can cause a number of other diseases in individuals who are healthy or immunocompromised. In addition, yeast can cause newborn infections and meningitis. The most common cause of yeast infections is ***C. albicans.***
2. **Methods for identification**
   a. **Microscopic appearance**
      1) Saline wet mounts and Gram stains will show budding yeast.
      2) Yeasts are discovered in routine urinalysis.
      3) **India ink** preparations are used to show the capsule surrounding ***C. neoformans.***

b. **Culturing**

1) Yeasts are grown on SABHI at 22–30°C.
2) Yeasts will form cream-colored, mucoid to smooth colonies within several days. On blood agar, yeast colonies can resemble nonhemolytic *Staphylococcus* colonies.
3) **Cornmeal agar with Tween 80** is used to differentiate *Candida* spp. by enhancing the formation of fungal elements such as hyphae, pseudohyphae, and conidia.
4) ***C. albicans*** will show **chlamydospores** with clusters of blastoconidia along the hyphae.
5) ***Candida tropicalis*** typically produces long-branched pseudohyphae. Blastoconidia are produced singly or in short chains. This species does not produce chlamydospores.

c. **Germ tube production**

1) **Germ tubes** are hyphaelike extensions of young yeast cells showing parallel sides, are nonseptate (showing no cell wall division), and will not constrict at their point of origin. **Pseudohyphae** look like germ tubes but are septate and constricted at their point of origin.
2) Germ tube procedure: Yeasts are incubated with serum at 37°C for up to 3 hours and examined for germ tube production.
3) ***C. albicans*** is positive for germ tube production. ***C. tropicalis*** is used for the negative control; however, some strains can produce germ tubes if incubated over 3 hours.

d. **Carbohydrate assimilation test**

1) Assimilation tests determine the aerobic utilization of carbohydrates.
2) Agar slants containing various carbohydrates are inoculated with yeast suspended in saline. The medium contains the pH indicator bromcresol purple. The tubes are incubated at room temperature and read at 7 and 14 days. Use of the carbohydrates results in the formation of yellow colonies.
3) A number of commercially prepared tests based on carbohydrate utilization and enzyme hydrolysis are also available.

e. **Urease test**

1) Used to identify ***Cryptococcus* spp.**, which are urease **positive.**
2) ***C. albicans*** is used for the negative control.
3) A positive urease is indicated by formation of a pink to purple color.

f. **Chromagars** allow for the identification of several species of yeasts. The media contain a variety of substrates. The ability to metabolize different substrates results in the production of colonies of different colors.

B. Clinically Significant Yeasts

1. ***Candida albicans***

a. *C. albicans* is the most common yeast isolate and is the causative agent of candidiasis, a general term for *Candida* infections.

b. *C. albicans* is normal biota of the mucous membranes lining the respiratory, gastrointestinal, and female genital tracts. Most adult infections are

endogenous, whereas infants acquire infections from their mothers (**exogenous** infections).

c. **Types of candidiasis**
   1) Thrush (oral cavity)
   2) Vulvovaginitis (vagina)
   3) Onychomycosis (nail infections)
   4) Paronychomycosis (cuticle infections)

d. *C. albicans* can also cause systemic infections, including meningitis, UTIs, and heart and lung infections.

e. Predisposition to *Candida* infections includes burns, wounds, diabetes mellitus, antimicrobial therapy, pregnancy, leukemia, and immune problems.

f. **Culture characteristics**
   1) *C. albicans* grows on most fungal media as well as sheep blood, chocolate, and eosin-methylene blue agars.
   2) On cornmeal agar with Tween 80, isolates produce chlamydospores.
   3) **Biochemical tests**
      a) A positive germ tube can be a presumptive identification of *C. albicans*; however, not all strains are positive. *Candida dubliniensis* is also positive and will form chlamydospores.
      b) Except for *Candida krusei*, all *Candida* spp. are urease negative. Not all strains of *C. krusei* are urease positive.
      c) *Candida* spp. are inositol negative.

g. **Other clinically important species**: *C. glabrata, C. tropicalis, C. krusei, Candida parapsilosis*, etc.

2. ***Cryptococcus neoformans***

a. Causes cryptococcosis, which can produce a mild to moderate pulmonary infection; however, in patients who are immunocompromised, cryptococcosis can lead to systemic infections and meningitis. Cryptococcosis is also associated with prostate and tissue infections.

b. *C. neoformans* can be acquired by contact with bat, pigeon, or other bird droppings, in addition to contaminated vegetables, fruit, and milk.

c. **Identifying characteristics for direct specimens**
   1) On Gram stain, the yeasts appear in spherical form and are not of uniform size.
   2) Hematoxylin and eosin stains are used to show capsules in tissue.
   3) Direct antigen test for cryptococcal antigen: Performed on CSF and serum specimens

d. **Culture characteristics**
   1) Brown to black colonies on bird seed or caffeic acid agars
   2) Only forms blastoconidia
   3) **Biochemical tests**
      a) Positive for urease and phenol oxidase
      b) Inositol utilization positive
      c) Negative for nitrate reduction

3. ***Trichosporon***
    a. *Trichosporon beigelii* was the name formerly used for the species in the genus *Trichosporon* causing most human infections, but this species name is no longer valid. Species associated with human infections, including the human hair infection **white piedra** and rarely the systemic disease referred to as trichosporonosis, are referred to as *Trichosporon asahii, Trichosporon ovoides, Trichosporon inkin, Trichosporon mucoides, Trichosporon asteroides*, and *Trichosporon cutaneum.*
    b. *Trichosporon* spp. can be isolated from the soil, animals, and humans.
    c. **Culture characteristics**
        1) *Trichosporon* spp. form cream-colored, smooth colonies on solid media in about 1 week.
        2) Hyaline hyphae with blastoconidia and arthroconidia are produced.
        3) **Biochemical tests**
            a) Positive for urease
            b) Can assimilate some carbohydrates
4. ***Rhodotorula***
    a. *Rhodotorula* spp. are found in moist environments such as on shower curtains and toothbrushes. They have also been isolated from soil and dairy products. Although they have been associated with hospital-acquired infections, they are generally considered commensals or contaminants.
    b. *Rhodotorula* resemble the *Cryptococcus*, but they are inositol negative. Some species produce a pink pigment.
5. ***Geotrichum candidum*** is actually a mold that can be confused with yeast based on colony morphology. Microscopically, *G. candidum* forms true hyphae with rectangular **arthroconidia.** This fungus has been isolated from a number of clinical specimens, but its clinical significance is questionable.

V. OPPORTUNISTIC FUNGI

A. Introduction

1. Many fungi rarely cause disease in healthy individuals, but they can cause disease in individuals with medical conditions (e.g., diabetes) and in patients who are immunocompromised.
2. General characteristics of opportunistic fungi
    a. Most opportunistic fungi form colonies within several days (rapid growers).
    b. Humans generally acquire infections through inhalation of the conidia.
    c. Most opportunistic fungi live on organic matter **(saprophytic fungi)** found in the soil.
    d. **Laboratory identification**
        1) Opportunistic fungi are inhibited by many antimicrobial agents (e.g., cyclohexamide); therefore, media should not contain these substances when trying to isolate opportunistic fungi.
        2) Because they are frequent contaminants and are found in high numbers in the environment, opportunistic fungi **must be repeatedly isolated in patients** to be considered significant.

3) Identification is based on microscopic morphology. The hyphae are **hyaline** (lightly pigmented).

B. Clinically Significant Opportunistic Fungi

1. ***Aspergillus* spp.**
   a. Causes **aspergillosis**, which can affect the skin, heart, lungs, and central nervous system. Pulmonary aspergillosis affects the bronchi, lungs, or sinuses.
   b. ***Aspergillus fumigatus*** is the most common cause of aspergillosis. *Aspergillus niger* is an important cause of **otomycosis**, a superficial mycotic infection of the outer ear canal characterized by inflammation, pruritus, and scaling.
   c. **Identifying characteristics**
      1) **Colony morphology:** *Aspergillus* spp. form granular/fluffy or powdery growth within 2 days on SABHI. Pigmentation varies according to species.
      2) **Microscopic appearance: Hyphae are septate; conidiophores terminate in a large, spherical** vesicle bearing **phialides.**
   d. **Species identification** is based on colony appearance and microscopic characteristics. *Aspergillus* spp. have **septate hyaline hyphae.** Conidiophores arise from a **foot cell** and support a single **vesicle** at their tip. Flask-shaped phialides, in a single or double row, produce chains of **phialoconidia.**
      1) ***A. niger*** colonies are yellow to black with a yellow reverse.
      2) ***Aspergillus flavus*** colonies are green to brown with red-brown reverse.
      3) ***Aspergillus terreus*** colonies are green to yellow with yellow reverse.
      4) ***Aspergillus clavatus*** colonies are blue to green with white reverse.
      5) ***A. fumigatus*** colonies are green to gray with tan reverse.
2. **Zygomycetes**
   a. Members of the class Zygomycetes include the genera *Absidia, Mucor, Rhizomucor, Rhizopus*, and *Syncephalastrum.*
   b. Cause of infections is known as **zygomycoses** and **mucormycoses.**
      1) Produce allergic reactions in susceptible individuals
      2) Mucormycoses are uncommon in otherwise healthy individuals. Infections of the paranasal sinuses that can extend to the central nervous system (rhinocerebral) are probably the most common. Infections can rapidly progress to a fatal outcome in patients who are immunocompromised or in diabetics with ketoacidosis.
      3) Spores gain entry (e.g., via inhalation) into body sites and can cause infections in those areas.
      4) Some zygomycetes produce toxins that can cause gastrointestinal disturbances.
      5) Blood infections **(fungemia)** can lead to central nervous system disorders.
   c. **Identifying characteristics**
      1) **Colony morphology:** Growth after several days is dense; colonies show a cotton candy texture, and pigmentation ranges from white, to gray, to brown.
      2) **Microscopic appearance:** Hyaline hyphae are sparsely septate and are ribbonlike with thin walls.

3) Zygomycetes typically form **rhizoids**, which resemble tree roots and function in attachment and nutrient absorption.

d. **Species identification**

1) ***Absidia* spp.** exhibit branching **sporangiophores** between the **rhizoid** (rootlike hyphae). A slight swelling below the **columella** at the base of the **sporangia** is present.

2) ***Mucor* spp.:** Single or branching sporangiophores are present, but rhizoids are absent. No swelling is noted below the columella.

3) ***Rhizopus* spp.** produce unbranched sporangiophores that arise opposite rhizoids. No swelling is noted below the columella.

3. ***Fusarium***

a. *Fusarium* spp. are opportunistic fungi associated with a variety of clinical presentations, including mycetomas, keratitis, and systemic infections.

b. **Identifying characteristics**

1) **Colony morphology:** Initially *Fusarium* produces white, cottony colonies that quickly develop pink or violet centers.

2) **Microscopic appearance:** They form septate hyphae and two forms of conidiation: (1) conidiophores, with phialides producing large, sickle-shaped macroconidia with three to five septa; and (2) simple conidiophores, with small, oval conidia singularly or in clusters.

VI. CUTANEOUS AND SUPERFICIAL FUNGI

A. Introduction

1. **Superficial mycoses** are infections that involve the outer epithelial layers of the skin and top layers of the hair and nails.
2. **Cutaneous mycoses** involve deeper layers of the skin and more tissue.
3. **Dermatophyte** is the term used to group the various fungi that cause infections (dermatophytoses) of the skin, hair, and nails.

a. The dermatophytes are **keratinophilic** (i.e., able to metabolize keratin).

b. Dermatophytes contain three genera.

1) ***Trichophyton*:** Infects nails, hair, and skin

2) ***Epidermophyton*:** Infects skin and nails

3) ***Microsporum*:** Infects hair and skin

4. Superficial and cutaneous fungi are rarely invasive to other areas of the body.
5. Dermatophyte infection is termed **tinea.**
6. **Types of tinea infections and their causative agents**

a. **Tinea pedis** or **athlete's foot**: An infection of the spaces between the toes

1) Caused by *Trichophyton* spp. and *Epidermophyton* spp.

2) Characterized by itching and scaling

b. **Tinea corporis or ringworm:** An infection of smooth skin

1) Caused by *Microsporum* spp. and *Trichophyton* spp.

2) Characterized by circular patches of scaly skin

c. **Tinea unguium or onychomycosis:** An infection of the nails
   1) Caused by *Epidermophyton* spp. and *Trichophyton* spp.
   2) Characterized by discoloration, thickening, and progressive destruction of the nails

d. **Tinea capitis:** An infection of the scalp
   1) Caused by *Microsporum* spp. and *Trichophyton* spp.
   2) Characterized by circular bald patches on the scalp

e. **Tinea barbae or barber's itch:** An infection of beard hair
   1) Caused by *Microsporum* spp. and *Trichophyton* spp.
   2) Characterized by skin lesions

f. **Tinea cruris or jock itch:** An infection of the groin
   1) Caused by *Trichophyton* spp. and *Epidermophyton* spp.
   2) Characterized by itching and scaling of the groin area

7. Identification of the dermatophytes is primarily based on colony morphology and microscopic appearance. In some cases, it may be necessary to perform an *in vitro* **hair perforation test.** Sterile hair is infected with the isolated fungus and after incubation is examined microscopically for wedge-shaped perforations.

B. Characteristics of the Dermatophytes

1. ***Trichophyton***
   a. **Colony characteristics:** Two colony types will be seen between 7 and 10 days on SABHI at room temperature.
      1) **Buff granular colonies**, rose to tan colored, with a yellow, brown, or **red reverse**
      2) **White fluffy colonies** with a colorless to **yellow reverse**
   b. **Microscopic characteristics**
      1) **Macroconidia** are smooth/thin walled, pencil shaped, contain three to seven cells, and are few in number. See Figure 7-1■.
      2) **Microconidia** are round to club shaped in grapelike clusters and are few to numerous in number.

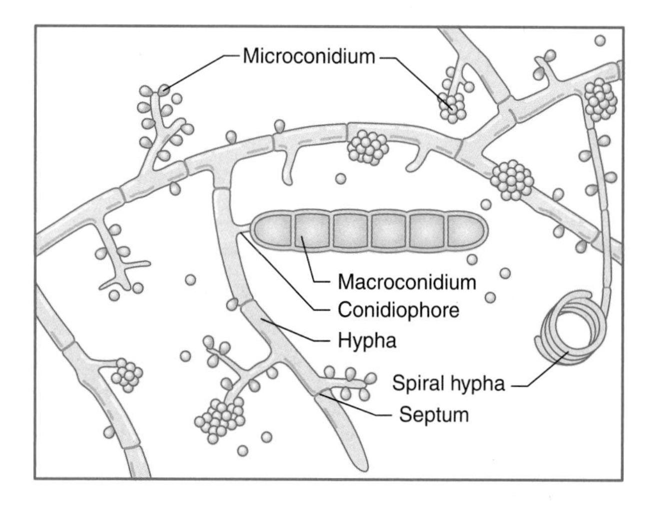

Figure 7-1 ■ *Trichophyton*

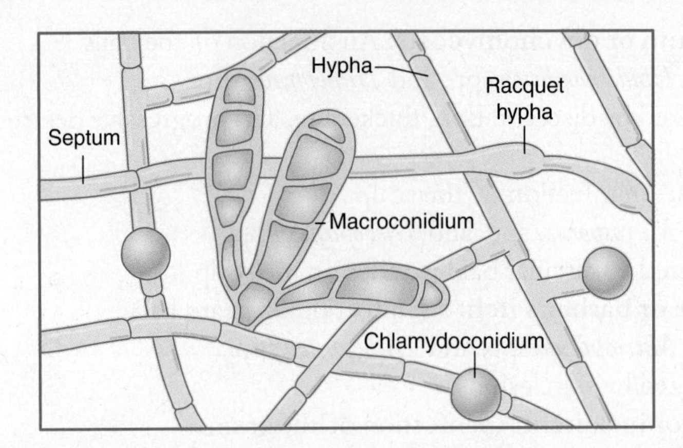

Figure 7-2 ■ *Epidermophyton*

c. Species identification
   1) ***Trichophyton mentagrophytes*** characteristically produces grapelike clusters of microconidia. Some strains produce numerous macroconidia. *T. mentagrophytes* is positive in the hair perforation test.
   2) ***Trichophyton rubrum*** produces few or numerous macroconidia; numerous club-shaped microconidia are borne singularly on the hyphae. *T. rubrum* forms deep red reverse on PDA. *T. rubrum* is negative in the hair perforation test.
   3) ***Trichophyton verrucosum*** produces only chlamydoconidia on SDA or PDA. On thiamine-enriched media, **elongated rat-tail macroconidia** are produced. *T. verrucosum* is negative in the hair perforation test.

2. ***Epidermophyton***
   a. **Culture characteristics:** On SABHI at room temperature, colonies will appear yellow with a tan reverse within 10 days.
   b. **Microscopic characteristics**
      1) **Macroconidia** are smooth/thin walled, club shaped, contain two to five cells, and are numerous in number. See Figure 7-2■.
      2) **Microconidia** are not present.
      3) *Epidermophyton floccosum* invades nails, and on KOH preparation chains of arthroconidia can be seen.
   c. At room temperature on SDA, *E. floccosum* forms khaki-yellow colonies with tan reverse.

3. ***Microsporum***
   a. **Colony morphology:** On SABHI at room temperature, colonies will be light tan, with a salmon-colored reverse. *Microsporum* spp. are very slow growers.
   b. **Microscopic characteristics**
      1) **Macroconidia** are rough/thin to thick walled, spindle shaped, contain 4–15 cells, and are numerous in number. See Figure 7-3■.
      2) **Microconidia** are club shaped, single, and few in number.
   c. Species identification
      1) ***Microsporum audouinii*** forms pectinate (comblike) septate hyphae with terminal chlamydoconidia often with pointed ends. Unlike

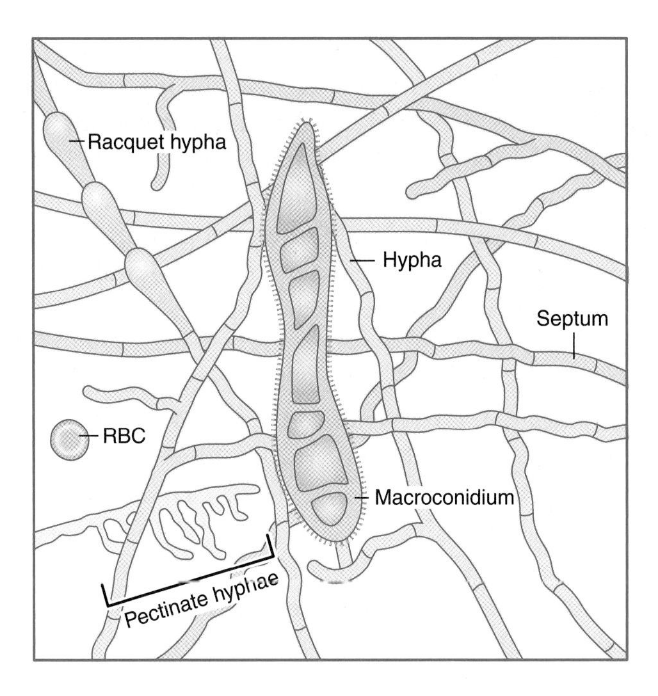

Figure 7-3 ■ *Microsporum*

other dermatophytes, this species grows poorly on rice grains. It is an **anthropophilic** (found in humans) species.

2) ***Microsporum canis*** forms numerous thick-walled, spindle-shaped macroconidia with tapered ends and 6–15 cells. It is a **zoophilic** species (found in animals).
3) ***Microsporum gypseum*** produces numerous thin-walled, elliptical macroconidia containing four to six cells. It is a **geophilic** species (found in the soil).

C. Superficial Mycoses

1. **Tinea (pityriasis) versicolor**
   a. Infection of the stratum corneum caused by lipophilic yeast belonging to the ***Malassezia furfur*** complex. Infection commonly occurs on the upper back, chest, shoulders, upper arms, and abdomen. There may be an association between the disease and excessive sweating.
   b. Diagnosis is made by KOH preparation of skin scrapings from the lesions that demonstrate characteristic yeastlike cells and hyphae (spaghetti and meatballs). Most lesions will fluoresce yellow under a Wood's lamp.
2. **Tinea nigra**
   a. Tinea nigra is characterized by the presence of brown to black nonscaly macules on the palms of the hands and less commonly the dorsa of the feet. Infections are most commonly caused by ***Hortaea werneckii***; synonyms are *Phaeoannellomyces werneckii, Exophiala werneckii*, and *Cladosporium werneckii.*
   b. The presence of numerous light brown, frequently branching septate hyphae and budding cells (some with septates) on KOH preparations is suggestive of infection.

3. **Black piedra**
   a. Black piedra is a fungal infection of the scalp hair and less frequently the beard, mustache, and axillary and pubic hairs. The disease is characterized by the presence of hard, dark nodules on the hair shaft. ***Piedra hortaea*** is the causative agent.
   b. Diagnosis can be made by submerging hair in a solution of 25% KOH or NaOH with 5% glycerol and heating. Microscopic examination will reveal compact masses of dark, septate hyphae and round to oval **asci** containing two to eight hyaline, aseptate banana-shaped **ascospores.**
4. **White piedra**
   a. White piedra is a fungal infection of facial, axillary, or genital hairs and less commonly the scalp. It is characterized by the presence of soft, white, yellowish, beige, or greenish nodules on the hair shaft. ***Trichosporon ovoides*** is the causative agent of scalp infections, whereas ***Trichosporon inkin*** causes most cases of pubic white piedra.
   b. Microscopic evaluation of hair treated in 10% KOH or 25% NaOH with 5% glycerol reveals intertwined hyaline septate hyphae breaking up into oval or rectangular **arthroconidia.** Culture characteristics of the *Trichosporon* spp. were previously discussed with the yeasts.

VII. SUBCUTANEOUS FUNGI

A. Introduction

1. Fungi causing subcutaneous mycoses can gain entry into the subcutaneous tissue via trauma to the skin.
2. Resulting subcutaneous lesions are characterized by being chronic, hard, crusted, and ulcerated.
3. Humans acquire the infections from vegetation contaminated with the fungi. The feet are commonly affected.
4. Subcutaneous mycoses are mainly caused by **dematiaceous fungi,** which is a group of slowly growing fungi found in the soil and vegetation. "Dematiaceous" refers to hyphae that appear darkly pigmented, olive green, brown, and black when viewed microscopically.

B. Subcutaneous Mycoses

1. **Mycetoma** is a granulomatous fungal or bacterial infection of the subcutaneous tissue causing cutaneous abscesses. Fungal mycetoma is called eumycetoma while the bacterial form is called actinomycetoma. Exudate from mycetomas will contain red, yellow, or black granules. Most eumycetoma infections are found in Africa. Causative agents include *Pseudoallescheria boydii, Exophiala, Acremonium*, and *Madurella.*
2. **Chromoblastomycosis** is a localized infection characterized by chronic, hard, or tumorlike lesions. Most infections involve the feet or lower legs. It is seen mostly in tropical areas. Most infections are caused by ***Fonsecaea pedrosoi.*** Other fungi causing chromoblastomycosis are *Phialophora, Cladosporium, Exophiala*, and *Wangiella.* The presence of **sclerotic bodies** (copper-colored fungal cells) in lesions is characteristic. Colonies are folded or heaped and are gray to black.

3. **Phaeohyphomycosis** is a superficial or subcutaneous infection that can become systemic. Resulting systemic infections can cause endocarditis and brain abscesses. Fungi causing phaeohyphomycosis include *Bipolaris, Curvularia*, and *Phialophora. Alternaria*, a dematiaceous fungus generally considered a saprophyte, has been associated with some cutaneous infections.
4. **Sporotrichosis** is a subcutaneous infection; lymph and pulmonary infections can also occur. Sporotrichosis is known as rose gardener's disease. Infections can come from rose thorns and contact with sphagnum moss. *Sporothrix schenckii*, the cause of sporotrichosis, is a **dimorphic** fungus. When grown on media with blood at 35°C, these fungi grow as small yeasts. When grown on SDA or PDA at room temperature, they are in the mold phase characterized by delicate hyphae and microconidia. Yeast cells may be seen in segmented neutrophils and are "cigar shaped."

VIII. SYSTEMIC FUNGI

A. Introduction

1. This fungal group is often acquired via inhalation and can disseminate to any of the body's organ systems.
2. Most systemic fungi are dimorphic, exhibiting a nonmold (e.g., yeast) parasitic phase at 35–37°C and a mold (or mycelial) saprobic phase at 25–30°C.
3. **Identifying characteristics**
   a. Identification is based on temperature and medium requirements and colony and microscopic morphology.
   b. Most systemic dimorphic fungi are very slow growers and require 3–7 weeks to grow.
   c. Because the **mold forms are highly infective**, slants are used for culture.
   d. Colonies are membranous and develop tan aerial mycelia.
   e. Conidia identification is necessary in species identification.
   f. **Conversion of dimorphic fungi from the mold to yeast phase is confirmation that the fungus in question is dimorphic.**
4. **Systemic dimorphic fungi**
   a. *Blastomyces dermatitidis* (blastomycosis)
   b. *Coccidioides immitis* (cocccidioidomycosis)
   c. *Histoplasma capsulatum* (histoplasmosis)
   d. *Paracoccidioides brasiliensis* (paracoccidioidomycosis)
   e. *Talaromyces (Penicillium) marneffei* (talaromycosis formerly penicilliosis)

B. Description of the Agents

1. ***Blastomyces dermatitidis***
   a. Blastomycosis is a respiratory infection that can affect the skin and bones. Infections are acquired by inhalation of conidia or hyphae and can be mild to chronic.
   b. The precise environmental location of this fungus is unknown. Outbreaks have occurred following contact with moist environments such as streams and rivers

and contact with decaying vegetation. Cases in the United States occur most frequently in the Ohio and Mississippi River basins. More cases occur in males than in females.

c. *B. dermatitidis* can be cultured from tissue or body fluids.

d. **Identifying characteristics**

1) **Microscopic appearance**

a) The **mold phase** is characterized by the presence of single smooth-walled, round to oval conidia at the ends of short conidiophores. The mold phase of *B. dermatitidis* can be confused with *Scedosporium apiospermum* or *Chrysosporium* spp. *S. apiospermum* causes **eumycetoma** and can infect the brain, bones, eyes, lungs, etc. *Chrysosporium* is commonly considered a contaminant.

b) **Yeast phase:** Large, round, thick-walled, budding yeasts with broad-based blastoconidia

2) **Culture**

a) At room temperature, initially a yeastlike colony develops, and over time the colony will become fluffy white to tan.

b) Conversion from the mold to yeast phase requires 4–6 days.

2. ***Coccidioides immitis***

a. Coccidioidomycosis (valley fever) is an infection of the lungs, bones, joints, skin, lymph nodes, central nervous system, and adrenal glands. Infections can be acute or chronic and self-limiting or requiring medications.

b. Most infections in the United States are in the semiarid southwest desert region (Lower Sonoran Life Zone). Infections are sometimes called desert or valley fever in the San Joaquin Valley of California, where many cases are diagnosed.

c. Infections are often acquired through spore inhalation from the environment. Activities that increase airborne dust, such as plowing and construction, can facilitate transmission.

d. **Identifying characteristics**

1) **Microscopic appearance**

a) Branching thick-walled, rectangular (barrel-shaped) **arthroconidia**

b) Tissue phase shows round, thick-walled **spherule** filled with small **endospores.** The tissue phase can only be grown under special conditions *in vitro.*

2) **Culture**

a) At 37°C on SABHI agar, colonies will appear moist and white and turn fluffy white in about a week.

b) **As with all mold phase fungi, always use a biological safety cabinet to prevent inhalation of spores.**

3. ***Histoplasma capsulatum***

a. Histoplasmosis can be a fatal pulmonary infection but can also affect the spleen, liver, kidneys, bone marrow, and heart.

b. Infection is acquired by spore inhalation from barns, chicken houses, and bat caves. *H. capsulatum* has been associated with **guano**, in particular from starlings and bats.
c. Most infections occur in the southern and Midwestern United States and along the Appalachian Mountains. The major risk factor for infection is environmental exposure.
d. **Identifying characteristics**
   1) **Microscopic appearance**
      a) The mold phase will show conidiophores at 90-degree angles to hyphae supporting smooth macroconidia (8–16 μm in diameter) with finlike edges **(tuberculate).** Microconidia are small (2–5 μm in diameter) and round to teardrop shaped.
      b) Yeasts appear as **small** single-budding cells that are unremarkable in morphology. In clinical specimens, yeasts are often found inside monocytes and macrophages.
   2) **Culture**
      a) On blood-containing media, the colonies are initially moist and develop tan aerial mycelia.
      b) Mature colonies are woolly and velvety and appear tan colored.

4. ***Paracoccidioides brasiliensis***
   a. Paracoccidioidomycosis is a chronic granulomatous disease of the lungs and skin that can spread to the liver and spleen.
   b. Mostly found in South America
   c. Acquired by spore inhalation or ingestion
   d. **Identifying characteristics**
      1) **Microscopic appearance**
         a) Yeast cells grown at 35–37°C are thick walled, with multiple budding yeast cells with very narrow necks.
         b) The mold phase exhibits mostly hyphae with intercalary and terminal chlamydoconidia.
      2) **Culture**
         a) When grown on blood-containing media at 35–37°C, the colonies are waxy, wrinkled, and cream to tan colored.
         b) When grown on SDA or PDA at room temperature, colonies are initially smooth. Colonies become tan with aerial mycelia.

5. ***Talaromyces marneffei***
   a. Typically spread by inhalation and affects the lungs. Infection can disseminate via the blood stream infecting other organs and producing a rash. Most cases occur in patients with acquired-immunodeficiency syndrome (AIDS) and other immunocompromised states.
   b. Located in southeast Asia, southern China, and eastern India

c. **Identifying characteristics**
   1) The **yeast cells** are oval and small (3–8 μm) and resemble *H. capsulatum.*
   2) At 22–30°C, structures typical of the genus *Penicillium* develop. Green aerial mycelium and reddish-brown hyphae are produced along with a red diffusible pigment.

6. ***Pneumocystis***
   a. *Pneumocystis* spp. are nonfilamentous (do not produce hyphae) fungi found in the **lower respiratory tract** of humans and other animals.
   b. Four species of *Pneumocystis* have been named; ***Pneumocystis jirovecii*** is the name currently given to the species that infects humans.
   c. In healthy individuals, infections are generally asymptomatic. However, in patients who are immunocompromised, such as those with AIDS, the infection can result in a serious or fatal pneumonia. *Pneumocystis* pneumonia remains an important opportunistic infection in patients with AIDS.
   d. **Diagnosis**
      1) *P. jirovecii* are found primarily in the **lungs.** Specimens used for the detection of this fungus include bronchoalveolar lavage, induced sputum, open lung biopsy, transbronchial aspirate, and nasopharyngeal aspirates.
      2) Diagnosed primarily with nucleic acid probes and amplification assays
      3) **Microscopic examination**
         a) **Stains**: Methanamine silver, periodic acid-Schiff, Giemsa, calcofluor white, etc.
         b) **Microscopic appearance:** Cysts (8 μm) contain several intracystic bodies, trophozoites (2–3 μm) with dark staining nuclei (depending on the stain).

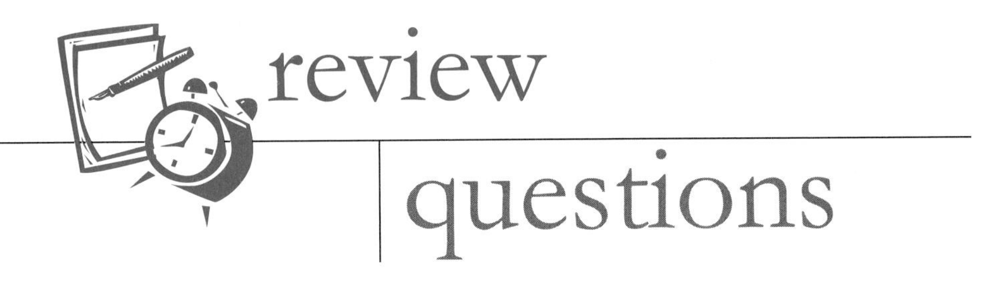

INSTRUCTIONS Each of the questions or incomplete statements that follow is comprised of four suggested responses. Select the *best* answer or completion statement in each case.

1. A bulldozer operator became ill while working on a new highway in the San Joaquin Valley. He developed chest pain, anorexia, headache and general malaise, and myalgia with fever. Chest X-ray showed pneumonic infiltrate and a single, well-defined nodule in the left lower lobe. His leukocyte count and sedimentation rate were slightly elevated. Although no fungus was seen in direct examination of a sputum specimen, processing included a culture on Sabouraud dextrose agar with chloramphenicol and cycloheximide. Within 3 days at 30°C, this culture produced moist, grayish growth, and white aerial mycelia began to develop (see Color Plate 28 ■). A lactophenol cotton blue wet mount of this organism is seen in Color Plate 29 ■. What is the most likely identification of this fungus?
   A. *Aspergillus fumigatus*
   B. *Blastomyces dermatitidis*
   C. *Coccidioides immitis*
   D. *Histoplasma capsulatum*

2. A 38-year-old male from Ohio presented to his physician with a mild influenzalike illness that included headache and malaise. His chest X-ray showed no infiltrates. His past medical history was unremarkable. He had no history of travel but reported recently cleaning the bell tower at his church, which was littered with bird excrement. The most likely agent causing his disease is
   A. *Aspergillus fumigatus*
   B. *Coccidioides immitis*
   C. *Candida albicans*
   D. *Histoplasma capsulatum*

3. A 44-year-old gardener pricked herself with a rose thorn. A subcutaneous infection characterized by the development of necrotic ulcers followed. The causative fungus was cultured as a small yeast form at 35°C (see Color Plate 30■) and as a mold at room temperature with delicate hyphae and conidia. This disease is
   A. Blastomycosis
   B. Chromomycosis
   C. Mycetoma
   D. Sporotrichosis
4. A yeastlike fungus was isolated from a sputum sample. No hyphae were produced on cornmeal agar with Tween 80. The isolate was negative for nitrate assimilation and positive for inositol assimilation and produced urease at 37°C. These findings are typical of
   A. *Candida krusei*
   B. *Cryptococcus terreus*
   C. *Cryptococcus neoformans*
   D. *Trichosporon beigelii*
5. A 24-year-old Vietnamese refugee was seen at a clinic in Houston. His chief complaints were weight loss and fever. A complete blood count confirmed he was suffering from anemia as well. Multiple skin lesions were present on his arms, some of them draining pus. Gram stain of the pus revealed what appeared to be yeastlike cells. A culture of the pus grew a green mold at 22°C, which produced a red soluble pigment (see Color Plate 31■). A lactophenol cotton blue wet mount of this organism is seen in Color Plate 32■. The causative agent in this case is
   A. *Aspergillus fumigatus*
   B. *Fusarium* sp.
   C. *Trichoderma* sp.
   D. *Talaromyces marneffei*
6. A section of a lymph node stained with the Gomori silver and hematoxylin and eosin stains is shown in Color Plate 33■. A lactophenol cotton blue wet mount of a mold that grew from this specimen is shown in Color Plate 34■. Large, one-celled, smooth to tuberculate macroconidia and smooth or echinulate microconidia are typical of mycelial phase growth of
   A. *Blastomyces dermatitidis*
   B. *Coccidioides immitis*
   C. *Histoplasma capsulatum*
   D. *Paracoccidioides brasiliensis*
7. Which of the following types of *Candida albicans* infection is commonly acquired from an exogenous source?
   A. Diaper rash
   B. Neonatal thrush
   C. Perianal infection
   D. Urinary tract infection
8. In a direct examination of a potassium hydroxide (KOH) wet mount of a nail specimen, *Epidermophyton floccosum* could be detected as
   A. Arthroconidia
   B. Blastoconidia
   C. Macroconidia
   D. Microconidia
9. The mold phase of the systemic fungus *Blastomyces dermatitidis* can be confused with
   A. *Scedosporium apiospermum*
   B. *Sporothrix schenckii*
   C. *Aspergillus* sp.
   D. *Penicillium notatum*
10. It is usually difficult or impossible to identify a fungal culture before it is mature. However, hyaline, septate hyphae, and a young conidiophore with a foot cell (see Color Plate 35■) and a swollen vesicle are excellent clues to the identification of
    A. *Acremonium*
    B. *Aspergillus*
    C. *Paecilomyces*
    D. *Penicillium*

11. Zygomycetes are rapidly growing, airborne saprobes. In clinical specimens, they
    A. Are common as normal, human microbiota
    B. Are found only as contaminants
    C. May be seen in a dimorphic tissue phase
    D. May be found as a cause of rapidly fatal infection

12. *Trichophyton rubrum* and *Trichophyton mentagrophytes* can be differentiated by the
    A. Consistently different appearance of their colonies
    B. Endothrix hair infection produced by *T. rubrum*
    C. Fluorescence of hairs infected with *T. rubrum*
    D. *In vitro* hair penetration by *T. mentagrophytes*

13. Broad, coenocytic hyphae found in tissue would be most typical of infection with
    A. *Aspergillus*
    B. *Blastomyces*
    C. *Microsporum*
    D. *Rhizopus*

14. A fungus infecting only skin and nails typically produces in culture
    A. Spindle-shaped, hyaline, echinulate macroconidia and microconidia
    B. Cylindrical or club-shaped, smooth, thin-walled macroconidia and microconidia
    C. Many microconidia in clusters or along the hyphae
    D. Large, thin-walled, club-shaped macroconidia without microconidia

15. The most useful finding for prompt, presumptive identification of *Candida albicans* is its
    A. Failure to assimilate sucrose
    B. "Feathering" on eosin methylene blue (EMB)
    C. Production of chlamydospores
    D. Production of germ tubes

16. Identify the dimorphic fungus that typically has a tissue phase in which the large mother cells have one to a dozen narrow-necked buds and a slowly growing mycelial form with intercalary chlamydoconidia and coiled hyphae.
    A. *Blastomyces dermatitidis*
    B. *Coccidioides immitis*
    C. *Histoplasma capsulatum*
    D. *Paracoccidioides brasiliensis*

17. Which of the following stains greatly enhances the visibility of fungi by binding to the cell walls, causing the fungi to fluoresce blue-white or apple green?
    A. Rhodamine-auramine
    B. Warthin-Starry
    C. Calcofluor white
    D. Periodic acid-Schiff

18. The formation of arthroconidia is an important characteristic in the identification of the following dimorphic fungi
    A. *Coccidioides*
    B. *Geotrichum*
    C. *Trichosporon*
    D. *Sporothrix*

19. A black pigment produced by colonies growing on bird seed agar is due to
    A. Urease
    B. Phenol oxidase
    C. Sucrose assimilation
    D. Arthroconidia production

20. Which of the following fungi pair contains examples of opportunistic pathogens?
    A. *Absidia* and *Mucor*
    B. *Histoplasma* and *Mucor*
    C. *Coccidioides* and *Absidia*
    D. *Coccidioides* and *Aspergillus*

21. Observation of hyaline or dematiaceous hyphae is an early clue in the identification of common, airborne fungi. Which of the following genera contains species found as dematiaceous contaminants?
    A. *Alternaria*
    B. *Aspergillus*
    C. *Fusarium*
    D. *Penicillium*

22. Which of the following fungi is most likely to be found as a common saprobe and as an agent of keratitis?
    A. *Exophiala*
    B. *Phialophora*
    C. *Fusarium*
    D. *Wamgiella*

23. The microscopic identification of *Pneumocystis jirovecii* is based on the detection of
    A. Arthroconidia in subcutaneous tissue biopsies
    B. Cysts and trophozoites in respiratory specimens
    C. Yeasts in respiratory specimens
    D. Tuberculate macroconidia in lung biopsies

24. Fungi that undergo asexual reproduction are termed
    A. Imperfect
    B. Perfect
    C. Aseptate
    D. Septate

25. Hyaline septate hyphae, branched or unbranched conidiophores, and multicelled banana-shaped conidia are characteristic of which of the following?
    A. *Fusarium*
    B. *Curvularia*
    C. *Acremonium*
    D. *Trichophyton*

26. Which of the following correctly describe the yeast *Rhodotorula rubra?*
    A. It has been isolated from soil and water, but not from dairy products.
    B. It is the most common fungal cause of diaper rash.
    C. It has been identified as a nosocomial pathogen.
    D. It produces white colonies on Sabouraud's dextrose agar (SDA) and has been found as a contaminant or commensal in specimens of urine, sputum, and feces.

27. A 21-year-old male member of a university track team presents to student health services with a light brown circular lesion on his upper back. The agent most likely responsible for this condition is
    A. *Candida albicans*
    B. *Fusarium* spp.
    C. *Geotrichum candidum*
    D. *Malassezia furfur*

28. Which of the following is likely to be found in clinical specimens as normal microbiota and as clinically significant isolates?
    A. *Aspergillus niger*
    B. *Paracoccidioides brasiliensis*
    C. *Talaromyces marneffei*
    D. *Candida albicans*

29. A 4-year-old child's hair is falling out in patches. The hair fluoresces when subjected to the UV light from a Wood's lamp. When the hair is cultured, a white cottony mold grows at 25°C on potato dextrose agar. Microscopically, rare microconidia, septate hyphae, and terminal chlamydospores are seen. Macroconidia are absent. The mold fails to grow on polished rice grains. The causative agent is
    A. *Microsporum audouinii*
    B. *Microsporum gypseum*
    C. *Trichophyton mentagrophytes*
    D. *Trichophyton rubrum*

30. In tissues infected with *Histoplasma capsulatum*
    A. The hyphae usually invade blood vessels
    B. Encapsulated yeast cells are typical
    C. Tuberculate macroconidia are typical
    D. The fungus is usually intracellular

31. An increased incidence of blastomycosis is most commonly associated with which environment?
    A. Lower Sonoran Life Zone
    B. Mississippi and Ohio River basins
    C. Pigeon roosts
    D. Bat roosts

32. Coccidioidomycosis also known as Valley Fever is more commonly found in this/these geographic region(s).
    A. Lower Sonoran Life Zone
    B. Mississippi and Ohio River basins
    C. North and Central America
    D. Northern United States

33. Even though it can affect other body sites, the organs most commonly affected by infection with *Cryptococcus* are the lungs and the central nervous system. *Cryptococcus* is commonly found in
    A. Rose bushes
    B. Cats and dogs
    C. Pigeon roosts
    D. Bat roosts

34. Exposure to aerosols containing many spores of *Histoplasma* has been associated with a number of "common source" outbreaks of histoplasmosis. *Histoplasma* grows best in soil that contains
    A. Sand
    B. Bird and bat droppings
    C. Decaying vegetation and leaves
    D. Other fungi including mushrooms

35. Sporotrichosis is commonly associated with contact with
    A. Sphagnum moss
    B. Starling roosts
    C. Stagnant fresh water
    D. Colorado River Valley soil

36. White piedra is characterized by soft, white to light brown nodules around and in the hair shaft. The causative agent of white piedra is
    A. *Hortaea werneckii*
    B. *Trichosporon* sp.
    C. *Microsporum* sp.
    D. *Fonsecaea compacta*

37. Black piedra is caused by a fungi, which produces brown to black, gritty nodules on the outside and under the cuticle of the hair shaft. The cause of black piedra is
    A. *Hortaea werneckii*
    B. *Trichosporon* sp.
    C. *Piedraia hortae*
    D. *Fonsecaea compacta*

38. The pigmented, painless lesion, which usually occurs on the palms or fingers when someone has tinea nigra may be mistaken for melanoma. The causative agent of tinea nigra is
    A. *Hortaea werneckii*
    B. *Microsporum audouinii*
    C. *Piedraia hortae*
    D. *Trichophyton mentagrophytes*

39. The cause of tinea versicolor is
    A. *Microsporum canis*
    B. *Malassesia furfur*
    C. *Microsporum gypseum*
    D. *Geotrichum*

40. A example of a keratinophilic saprophyte is
    A. *Malassesia furfur*
    B. *Coccidioides immitis*
    C. *Microsporum gypseum*
    D. *Geotrichum*

41. Otomycosis, an infection of the ear canal, is most frequently caused by
    A. *Aspergillus niger*
    B. *Talaromyces marneffei*
    C. *Microsporum canis*
    D. *Fonsecaea pedrosoi*

The incomplete statements below describe the appearance of growth of yeast or yeastlike fungi on morphology agar, such as rice agar or cornmeal agar with Tween 80, a finding helpful in the presumptive identification of these organisms. For each numbered description, match it to the letter options of the most appropriate species.

---

42. True hyphae and arthroconidia only
43. True hyphae, arthroconidia, and blastoconidia
44. Pseudohyphae, blastoconidia, and chlamydospores
45. Pseudohyphae and blastospores only
46. Blastospores only, without hyphae or pseudohyphae
    A. *Candida albicans*
    B. *Geotrichum*
    C. *Trichosporon*
    D. *Candida tropicalis*
    E. *Cryptococcus neoformans*

Select the letter of the most appropriate specimen source for isolation of each numbered species description.

---

47. *Cryptococcus neoformans*
48. *Histoplasma capsulatum*
49. *Pseudallescheria boydii*
50. *Trichophyton mentagrophytes*
    A. Bone marrow
    B. Cerebrospinal fluid
    C. Chronic draining sinus tract of foot
    D. Chronic interdigital lesion of foot

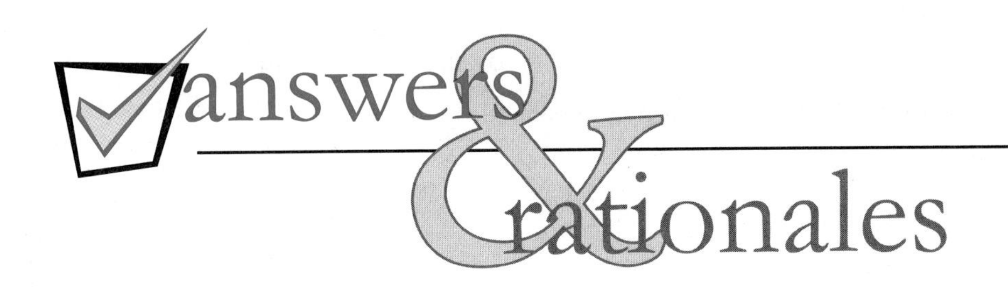

1.

C. Areas of the San Joaquin Valley are highly endemic for *C. immitis*, and infectious arthroconidia of this fungus can be distributed in dust aerosols produced by construction and other disturbances. Symptomatic pulmonary disease patterns vary, but the signs and symptoms given are found in many cases. The fungus grows more rapidly than do other systemic fungal pathogens, and the aerial mycelium will typically produce the characteristic barrel-shaped arthrospores.

2.

D. The distribution of *H. capsulatum* is probably worldwide, but most clinical disease occurs in the western hemisphere. Most cases in the United States occur in the Ohio and Mississippi River valleys. This organism is found in areas contaminated by large amounts of bird excrement, such as starling and blackbird roosts. Inhalation of the spores results in a respiratory illness usually with clinical symptoms within 2 weeks of exposure. Disease ranges from a mild influenzalike illness to acute fulminant lung infection resembling tuberculosis.

3.

D. *S. schenckii* is the agent of sporotrichosis. It usually enters the skin by traumatic implantation. This fungus grows *in vitro* as small yeasts at 35°C and as a mold at room temperature (22–30°C) with delicate hyphae and conidia.

4.

C. All species listed may be urease positive, but *C. terreus* does not grow at 35°C and may assimilate nitrate. *C. krusei* is inositol negative. *C. krusei* and *T. beigelii* produce hyphae on morphology agar. *C. neoformans* typically does not produce hyphae, is nitrate negative, is inositol, urease positive, and grows at 37°C.

5.

D. Infections due to *Talaromyces marneffei* seem to originate in eastern and southeastern Asia. This fungus was first isolated in 1959 from a hepatic lesion from a bamboo rat, a rodent found throughout Southeast Asia. Clinical disease includes fever, weight loss, anemia, and death if untreated. Skin lesions may be present and may drain pus. Diagnosis is made via culture or histopathologic exam of lesions of skin, bone, or liver. The yeastlike cells of *T. marneffei* are oval (3–8 μm) and scattered throughout tissue. Elongated, sausage-shaped cells often contain cross-walls. At 22–30°C, structures typical of the genus *Penicillium* develop. At 35–37°C, round or oval yeastlike cells are seen.

6.

C. Diagnostic features of *H. capsulatum* include large, 8- to 14-μm macroconidia with tuberculate projections. Tuberculate and smooth macroconidia may be seen in the same colony. Microconidia are also produced.

7.

B. Neonatal oral candidiasis is most commonly associated with mothers having vaginal *Candida*, and the newborn acquires the organism from the mother. Diaper rash due to *C. albicans* usually follows oral and perianal candidiasis of the infant. The other three infections are associated with physiologic changes in the host that permit proliferation of *C. albicans* already present in the host's microflora.

8.

A. KOH wet mounts should be used routinely for direct examination of nails, skin, or hair for fungal elements. KOH digests the keratinous tissue and facilitates observation of any fungi present. *E. floccosum* and *Trichophyton* spp. invade nails. *E. floccosum* typically is found as chains of arthroconidia in nail tissue.

9.

A. At 25–30°C, *B. dermatitidis* forms septate hyphae with delicate conidiophores of various lengths that bear round or oval conidia. It is important not to confuse the mold phase of *B. dermatitidis* with either *S. apiospermum* or *Chrysosporium* sp. *S. apiospermum* appears as septate hyphae with simple conidiophores of various lengths that bear oval conidia singly or in groups. *S. apiospermum* is the causative agent of mycetoma and can infect brain, bones, eyes, lungs, etc. *Chrysosporium* sp. appears as septate hyphae with simple to branched conidiophores that bear oval conidia. *Chrysosporium* sp. is commonly considered a contaminant.

10.

B. Conidiophores of *Aspergillus* arise from a foot cell and terminate in a vesicle. The vesicle produces phialides; the phialides then produce the conidia. Before the culture is mature, the presence of a young conidiophore with a foot cell and vesicle is a good clue to the identity of the fungus.

11.

D. Although generally found as laboratory contaminants, the zygomycetes can be clinically significant. Zygomycosis (mucormycosis) is an acute disease that often results in death within a few days in acidotic patients. Fungal agents of mucormycosis include *Rhizopus, Mucor*, and *Absidia*, which are common fungi found in the environment.

12.

D. When speciation of *T. mentagrophytes* or *T. rubrum* is not certain on morphology alone, the *in vitro* hair perforation test is useful; *T. mentagrophytes* is positive and *T. rubrum* is negative. Urease production by *T. mentagrophytes* is less reliable. Neither species produces endothrix infection, and *T. rubrum* rarely infects hair.

13.

D. *Rhizopus* and other fungal agents of mucormycosis are characterized by having coenocytic (nonseptate) hyphae. The finding of broad, nonseptate hyphal elements in sterile body fluids or tissue can provide rapid confirmation of a clinical diagnosis of mucormycosis. The other molds listed have septate hyphae.

14.

D. *E. floccosum* infects skin and nails. This dermatophyte produces thin-walled macroconidia, usually in clusters, but no microconidia. *Microsporum* spp. produce infections in hair and skin. *Trichophyton* spp. may produce infection of the nails, hair, and skin.

15.

D. Essentially all strains of *C. albicans* produce germ tubes within 2 hours of incubation at 37°C in serum. Chlamydospores are produced by most strains of *C. albicans* after 24–48 hours at 22–26°C on cornmeal Tween 80 agar or a similar substrate. Use of EMB medium to screen for *C. albicans* may require 24–48 hours of incubation.

16.

D. The dimorphic pathogenic fungi include the species listed. The tissue phase of *P. brasiliensis* produces large, multiple-budding yeasts, 20–60 µm long. The saprophytic or mycelial phase colonies resemble *B. dermatitidis*, but all cultures produce intercalary chlamydoconidia and coiled hyphae, and conidia development is delayed or absent. Clinical types of paracoccidioidomycosis include relatively benign primary pulmonary infection; progressive pulmonary disease; disseminated disease; or an acute, fulminant, juvenile infection. The disease is endemic in certain areas of Central and South America.

17.

C. The calcofluor white stain requires the use of a fluorescence microscope. It is a rapidly staining method, requiring only 1 minute to complete. Stain binds to chitin in the cell wall of fungi.

18.

A. Barrel-shaped arthroconidia, alternating with empty cells, are typical of the mature mycelial phase of *C. immitis*. Species of *Geotrichum* produce chains of hyaline arthroconidia, and *Trichosporon* is characterized by production of hyaline arthroconidia, blastoconidia, hyphae, and pseudohyphae. Sporothrix is the sole member of the list that does not produce arthroconidia. *Coccidioides* is the only dimorphic fungi in the list.

19.

B. Phenol oxidase breaks down the substrate found in niger seeds producing melanin. This result is characteristic of *C. neoformans*. *C. neoformans* is urease positive, but that reaction is not detected on this medium.

answers & rationales

20.

A. *Absidia* and *Mucor* can cause the uncommon disease mucormycosis in debilitated patients. *Aspergillus* are ubiquitous and opportunistic and cause a variety of human infections (e.g., rhinocerebral syndrome). *Coccidioides* and *Histoplasma* are considered true pathogens that can infect healthy people.

21.

A. Observation of dark-pigmented hyphae in a culture is evidence that the fungus is in one of the dematiaceous genera. Typically, the reverse of a plate will be black. *Alternaria* is a common dematiaceous contaminant.

22.

C. Mycotic keratitis due to *Fusarium* has been reported following injury or cortisone treatment. An ulcerative lesion develops on the cornea. Corneal scrapings may be received for direct exam and culture.

23.

B. *P. jirovecii* produces cysts and trophozoites that can be found in respiratory tract specimens. The fungus primarily infects the lungs, so specimens from the lower respiratory tract are most productive (e.g., brochoalveolar lavage). Specimens can be stained with a silver stain or Giemsa stain.

24.

A. Fungi with only an asexual stage of reproduction are referred to as the imperfect fungi. Fungi able to reproduce sexually are called the perfect fungi. "Septate" and "aseptate" refer to the presence or absence (respectively) of cross-walls in hyphae.

25.

A. Diagnostic features of *Fusarium* spp. include hyaline septate hyphae and sickle- or boat- or banana-shaped macroconidia. Macroconidia are multiseptate with long- or short-branched or unbranched conidiophores. Microconidia (one or two celled) are also produced.

26.

C. *R. rubra* colonies are coral pink on SDA. *R. rubra* has been isolated from soil and water, from a number of food sources (especially dairy products), and as a contaminant of skin, lung, urine, or feces. *Rhodotorula* fungemia has been caused by contaminated catheters, intravenous solutions, and dialysis machines. *C. albicans* is a more common cause of diaper rash.

27.

D. *M. furfur* is the causative agent of tinea or pityriasis versicolor—a superficial skin infection that occurs commonly on the upper back, chest, shoulders, upper arms, and abdomen. Initially, lesions are discrete but in time may coalesce. Lesions may be hyper- or hypopigmented. *M. furfur* is part of the normal skin microbiota of over 90% of adults. There may be an association between the disease and excessive sweating and oily skin. The disease is more common in tropical and subtropical areas.

28.

D. *C. albicans* is an endogenous species (part of normal biota) causing a variety of opportunistic infections. Infection is usually secondary to a predisposing debility. *Aspergillus* spp. are common saprophytic contaminants. *P. brasiliensis* and *T. marneffei* are dimorphic fungi that cause systemic mycoses.

29.

A. *M. audouinii* most commonly affects children. Only rarely are adults infected. Colonies are flat, downy to silky, and gray to white in color. Colony reverse is salmon to brown with a reddish-brown center. Microscopic examination reveals septate hyphae, terminal chlamydoconidia, and occasional microconidia (borne singly). Macroconidia are very rare or absent. Infected hair fluoresces. Growth on polished rice grains aids in differentiating *M. audouinii* from other *Microsporum* species that grow well on rice grains.

30.

D. *H. capsulatum* is found primarily within histiocytes and in macrophages or monocytes in specimens from bone marrow aspirates, biopsies, or the buffy coat of centrifuged blood. Unstained cell wall of the tissue (yeast) form of *H. capsulatum* may be mistaken for a capsular halo in stained preparations. Only the mold phase would exhibit hyphae and macroconidia.

31.

B. *B. dermatitidis* is rarely found in the environment, and there is no reliable skin test for screening for past or subclinical blastomycosis. Outbreaks occur most frequently following exposures to moist environments like streams and rivers. The incidence of clinical cases in the United States is highest in the Mississippi and Ohio River basins, and part of the Missouri River drainage. *Histoplasma* mainly lives in soil in the central and eastern states, particularly areas around the Ohio and Mississippi River Valleys, but it can likely live in other parts of the United States as well.

32.

A. The most highly endemic regions of coccidioidomycosis are semiarid, with dry, hot seasons and wetter, cooler seasons above freezing. The areas of the southwestern United States and northern Mexico with this typical Lower Sonoran Life Zone climate have the highest incidence of coccidioidomycosis. The peak endemic period is fall, when the fungus becomes airborne from the desert surface.

33.

C. Although *C. neoformans* does not appear to infect pigeons, it apparently passes unharmed through their gut. It has been found in large numbers, even as the predominant microorganism, from the debris of old pigeon roosts. Viable, virulent, desiccated cells, small enough to be inhaled into the alveoli, can be present in the dust of these roosts.

34.

B. *Histoplasma* grows best in soil that contains bird or bat droppings. Bats can get histoplasmosis and spread the fungus in their droppings. The most highly endemic areas of histoplasmosis (Missouri, Kentucky, southern Illinois, Indiana, and Ohio) also have the most starlings, whose flocks produce large accumulations of guano. *H. capsulatum* has been found growing in almost pure culture in accumulated starling guano.

35.

A. In temperate countries, including the United States, sporotrichosis is an occupational hazard of gardeners and nursery workers and is frequently associated with contact with sphagnum moss. In Mexico, it has been associated with working with grass, and a well-known epidemic in South Africa involved gold mine workers in contact with untreated mine poles. *Sporothrix schenckii* produces subcutaneous infections that begin at the site of traumatic implantation.

36.

B. White piedra is frequently caused by *Trichosporon ovoides* and *Trichosporon inkin. Trichosporon beigelii* was the name formerly used for the species infecting humans, but use of the name should be avoided. The nodules around and in the hair shaft are composed of hyphae, yeastlike arthroconidia, and sometimes blastoconidia. The beard and body hair are more often affected than scalp hair.

37.

C. Black piedra is caused by *P. hortae*, which produces the characteristic brown to black, nodules on the hair shaft. Scalp hair is the site most often involved. Direct microscopic examination of portions of these nodules in KOH wet mounts can show septate dematiaceous hyphae and ascospores.

38.

A. Tinea nigra is a superficial skin infection caused by *H. werneckii.* Accurate laboratory findings in a KOH preparation of a skin scraping are important in preventing surgical intervention of the patient (if mistaken for melanoma). Microscopic examination of skin scrapings from tinea nigra shows dematiaceous, septate hyphae and budding cells.

39.

B. Tinea versicolor is a chronic, mild, superficial skin infection caused by *M. furfur*, which may also be found on normal skin. Despite the name "tinea versicolor," the causative fungus is not a dermatophyte. Skin scrapings from the lesions demonstrate characteristic yeastlike cells and hyphae ("spaghetti and meatballs").

40.

C. *M. gypseum* is a keratinophilic fungus (dermatophyte). It is a geophilic species that has been isolated from human infections. It is a moderately rapid grower, producing numerous thick-walled rough macroconidia.

41.

A. *A. niger* causes approximately 90% of the otomycoses and external ear infections due to fungi. *Aspergillus fumigatus* also causes otomycosis. Other fungi, far less often involved, include *Scopulariopsis, Penicillium, Rhizomucor, Candida*, and other species of *Aspergillus.*

42.

B. *Geotrichum* spp. typically produce numerous hyphae and arthroconidia. Germinating arthroconidia of *Geotrichum*, however, may be mistaken for blastoconidia production. This may cause confusion between *Geotrichum* and *Trichosporon.*

43.

C. *Trichosporon* spp. produce hyphae and arthroconidia. They may also produce blastoconidia, although these may be rare. If present, blastoconidia can differentiate *Trichosporon* from *Geotrichum.*

44.

A. *C. albicans* and *Candida dubliniensis* both produce pseudohyphae and are germ tube positive. Both are capable of producing chlamydospores and blastoconidia. These two species are difficult to differentiate.

45.

D. *C. tropicalis* typically produces long-branched pseudohyphae. Blastoconidia are produced singly or in short chains. *C. tropicalis* does not produce chlamydospores. The carbon assimilation pattern of *C. tropicalis* resembles that of *C. albicans*, and some strains of *C. tropicalis* may produce a positive germ tube test if incubated more than 3 hours.

46.

E. *C. neoformans* produces only blastoconidia when growing on morphology agar (e.g., cornmeal agar with Tween 80). This species is usually identified by its encapsulated cells, production of urease, failure to assimilate nitrate, and production of brown pigment on bird seed agar. Cryptococcosis can lead to systemic infections in patients who are immunocompromised.

47.

B. The most frequently diagnosed form of cryptococcosis is central nervous system infection. Few or many organisms may be in the cerebrospinal fluid, but a clinical diagnosis of meningitis can often be confirmed by the cryptococcal antigen test. In the past, the use of a microscopic examination of a spun specimen with India ink has been used. The cryptococcal antigen test is much more sensitive and is the recommended test.

48.

A. *H. capsulatum* is found in the mononuclear phagocyte system (reticuloendothelial system) and is seldom extracellular. Specimens such as sternal bone marrow, lymph node, liver and spleen biopsies, or buffy coat of blood should be stained with Giemsa or Wright's stain and examined for small, intracellular yeast cells.

49.

C. *P. boydii* is the most common cause of eumycotic mycetoma in the United States. Mycetoma is a clinical syndrome of localized abscesses, granulomas, and draining sinuses that develops over months or years. It usually occurs on the foot or hand after traumatic implantation of soil organisms.

50.

D. *T. mentagrophytes* is a common cause of intertriginous tinea pedis or athlete's foot. This is a chronic dermatitis most often affecting the areas between the fourth and fifth and third and fourth toes. The acute inflammation often subsides, but recurrences are common.

REFERENCES

Carroll, K. C., et al. (2019). *Manual of Clinical Microbiology*, 12th ed. Washington, DC: American Society for Microbiology Press.

Mahon, C. R., and Lehman, D. C. (2019). *Textbook of Diagnostic Microbiology*, 6th ed. St. Louis: Saunders Elsevier.

Forbes, B. A., Sahm, D. F., and Weissfeld, A. S. (2018). *Bailey and Scott's Diagnostic Microbiology*, 14th ed. Philadelphia: Mosby.

Larone, D. H. (218). *Medically Important Fungi: A Guide to Identification*, 6th ed. Washington, DC: American Society for Microbiology Press.

Gibas, C. F. C., and Wiederhold, N. P. Medically significant fungi. In Mahon, C. R., and Lehman, D. C. (2019). *Textbook of Diagnostic Microbiology*, 6th ed. St. Louis: Saunders Elsevier.

CHAPTER

8 Parasitology

contents

I. INTRODUCTION

A. Parasitic Disease Risk Factors

1. Unsanitary food handling/preparation (i.e., contaminated meats and vegetables)
2. Fecally contaminated water for drinking or recreational use
3. Immunocompromised conditions resulting from disease states or poor nutrition
4. Blood transfusion and organ transplantation
5. Foreign travel to endemic regions of the world

B. Parasitic Disease Characteristics

1. In gastrointestinal tract infections, **diarrhea** is the most frequent symptom, along with abdominal cramping, seen.
2. **Other symptoms** depend on the parasite and the site of infection.
   a. Intestinal obstruction, weight loss, and bloating
   b. Organ involvement with ulcers, lesions, and abscesses
   c. Blood and tissue parasites can cause anemia, fever, chills, bleeding, encephalitis, and meningitis.

C. Specimen Collection and Processing

1. Diagnosis of parasite infections often depends on observing parasite forms that include protozoan cysts or trophozoites, ova, larva, or adult forms.
2. Specimens include stools (most common), tissue, urine, sputum, and blood.
   a. Stool samples should be free of antimicrobial agents or other substances that inhibit parasite growth. Barium (from enemas) can obscure parasites during microscopic examination.
      1) At least **3 grams of fecal sample** on three consecutive days are required for most parasite analyses.
      2) Stool should be free of urine because urea and acidic pH inhibit some parasites and distort their morphology.
      3) **Liquid stools** are best to detect trophozoites, whereas **formed stools** are best to detect ova and cysts.
   b. Stool preservatives
      1) Generally, stool specimens should **not** be frozen, and **unpreserved** specimens should not be stored at room temperature longer than several hours.
      2) Fresh and frozen stool specimens are typically preferred for antigen detection and nucleic acid amplification testing. Fixation is test dependent and the manufacturer's protocol must be followed.
      3) **Formalin** (5 or 10%) is an all-purpose preservative to preserve stool specimens for concentration procedures.
      4) **Polyvinyl alcohol (PVA)** is a mercury-containing preservative for preparing permanent stained smears.
      5) **Sodium acetate formalin (SAF)** is a mercury-free preservative that can be used to preserve stool samples for both concentration and permanent stained smears.

6) Less toxic preservatives generally substitute **zinc sulfate** for mercury. Compared to PVA, these preservatives do not provide the quality of preservation of intestinal protozoa.

c. Optimal microscopic detection of parasites often requires concentration of a fecal specimen.
   1) Gross examination of stool may detect adult forms, particularly helminths (worms).
   2) Fecal concentration procedures remove debris that could obscure parasites. Barium is not removed during concentration procedures.
   3) Fecal concentration methods
      a) **Formalin-ethyl acetate sedimentation:** Approximately 3–4 grams of stool are suspended in 5 or 10% formalin. The suspension is filtered through gauze into a 15 mL centrifuge tube. Either 0.85% NaCl or 5 or 10% formalin is added to fill the tube almost completely. The tube is centrifuged at 500 × *g* for 10 minutes. After centrifugation, the supernatant is discarded. The wash step is usually repeated until the supernatant is clear. After the last wash step, the sediment is resuspended in about 9 mL of formalin. A 4- to 5-mL aliquot of ethyl acetate is added; the tube is shaken vigorously for at least 30 seconds. The cap is loosened slightly to release the pressure in the tube. The tube is centrifuged again, and four layers should be visible (from top to bottom): ethyl acetate, plug of fecal debris, formalin, and fecal sediment. The plug is loosened from the side of the tube with an applicator stick, and the top three layers are poured off. The sediment is resuspended in formalin and used for wet mounts.
      b) **Zinc sulfate flotation:** Approximately 3–4 grams of stool are suspended in 5 or 10% formalin. The suspension is filtered through gauze into a 15 mL centrifuge tube. The tube is centrifuged at 500 × *g* for 10 minutes. After centrifugation, the supernatant is discarded. The wash step is usually repeated until the supernatant is clear. After the last wash step, the sediment is resuspended in about 3 mL of 33% aqueous solution of zinc sulfate. The specific gravity of the zinc sulfate should be adjusted to 1.20 for formalin fixed stools or to 1.18 for fresh (nonformalinized) stools. After resuspending the fecal material, the tube is filled to within 3–4 mm of the top. The tube is centrifuged for 2 minutes at 500 × *g*. Two layers will result: a small amount of sediment and a layer of zinc sulfate. One or two drops of the surface film should be removed with a bacteriological loop before removing the tube from the centrifuge. This liquid is examined for parasites.
      c) **Sheather sugar flotation:** This procedure is similar to the zinc sulfate procedure, except sucrose is used in place of zinc. The sucrose solution has a specific gravity of 1.25–1.27. The Sheather sugar flotation procedure was previously recommended for *Cryptosporidium* and some

ova, but now a modified acid-fast stain on a fecal smear or immunologic procedures is recommended for *Cryptosporidium.*

4) Blood concentration methods

a) The **Knott method** uses low-speed centrifugation to concentrate blood samples suspected of containing minimal numbers of microfilariae.

b) **Buffy coat** slides are used for *Leishmania* or *Trypanosoma* detection.

3. Various stains are used for microscopic detection of stool, tissue, and blood parasites.

a. **Saline wet mounts** made directly from a liquid stool are quick and easy to perform and will allow trophozoite motility and helminth ova and larvae to be seen.

b. **Iodine wet mounts** of fecal concentrates are useful for the detection of larvae, ova, and protozoan cysts in stool samples.

c. Permanent stained smears are used to enhance protozoan morphology and to allow for future study. Stained fecal smears are important in the identification of *Entamoeba histolytica.*

1) **Iron hematoxylin stain** of fecal smears is used when enhanced detail is needed; however, it is difficult to obtain consistent staining results.

2) **Trichome stain (Wheatley or Gomori)** is the most commonly used stain for fecal parasite study.

3) **Modified acid-fast stain** is used to detect ***Cryptosporidium, Cyclospora***, and ***Cystoisospora***.

4) **Modified trichrome stains** for microsporidia: The microsporidia are not easily stained; therefore, the concentration of the stain and the staining time is increased. Alternatively, a hot stain can be used. In the **Weber green stain,** microsporidia stain as 1–3 μm pink ovals, and the background is green. With the **Ryan blue stain**, the microsporidia also stain pink, but the background is blue.

4. Other collection methods

a. The **cellophane (Scotch) tape** method is used to collect ***Enterobius vermicularis*** (pinworm) eggs from the perirectal area.

b. The **EnteroTest®** (string test) or duodenal aspirate is used to obtain duodenal contents for parasitic examination.

c. Sigmoidoscopy is used to collect colon material.

5. Sample types and associated parasites

a. **Feces:** *Giardia, Cryptosporidium, Entamoeba, Ascaris, Enterobius*, etc.

b. **Blood:** *Plasmodium, Trypanosoma*, and microfilariae. *Leishmania* may be found in the bone marrow

c. **Skin:** *Onchocerca*

d. **Vaginal or urethral:** *Trichomonas*

e. **Eye scrapings:** *Acanthamoeba*

f. **Tissue:** *Acanthamoeba* and *Leishmania*

g. **Cerebrospinal fluid:** *Naegleria* and *Balamuthia*

h. **Urine:** *Schistosoma* and *Trichomonas*
i. **Sputum:** *Ascaris* and *Strongyloides* (rarely *Paragonimus westermani*)

D. Diagnostic Test Methods

1. Direct fluorescent antibody: Used to identify *Giardia lamblia, Cryptosporidium, Trichomonas vaginalis*
2. Agglutination test: Used to diagnose leishmaniasis and Chagas disease
3. EIA: Used to identify antigens or antibodies for organisms such as *Giardia duodenalis, Cryptosporidium, Entamoeba histolytica*
4. DNA probes and polymerase chain reactions are used to diagnose selected parasite infections.

E. Terminology

1. **Carrier:** An asymptomatic host that harbors a parasite and is capable of transmitting it to others
2. **Cestode:** Tapeworm
3. **Ciliate:** Protozoa motile by means of cilia
4. **Commensalism:** Symbiotic relationship beneficial to one member and harmless to another
5. **Cyst:** Thick-walled stage of protozoa resistant to adverse conditions
6. **Definitive host:** Host supporting the adult or sexual phase of a parasitic life cycle
7. **Ectoparasite:** Parasite found on the surface of a host
8. **Endoparasite:** Parasite found inside a host
9. **Filariae:** Blood or tissue roundworms
10. **Flagellate:** Protozoa motile by means of flagella
11. **Gravid:** Containing ova
12. **Helminths:** Worms that include nematodes (roundworms), cestodes (tapeworms), and trematodes (flukes)
13. **Hermaphroditic:** Organism capable of self-fertilization
14. **Host:** Living organism that harbors another organism
15. **Hydatid cyst:** Larval stage of *Echinococcus granulosus*
16. **Intermediate host:** Host containing the asexual phase of a parasite
17. **Larva:** Juvenile stage of a parasite
18. **Schizont**
    a. **Immature schizont:** Early stage of asexual sporozoa trophozoite
    b. **Mature schizont:** Developed stage of asexual sporozoa trophozoite
19. **Mutualism:** Symbiotic relationship beneficial to both species
20. **Nematode:** Roundworm
21. **Oocyst:** Infectious cyst-like structure containing the zygote
22. **Parasite:** An organism that obtains its nutrients from another organism (the host) while harming the host
23. **Parasitism:** Symbiotic relationship in which one member benefits at the expense of another member (the host)

24. **Symbiosis:** An association between two or more organisms of different species
25. **Trematode:** Fluke
26. **Trophozoite:** Developmental stage of protozoa
27. **Zoonosis:** An animal infection or disease that humans accidentally acquire

II. INTESTINAL PROTOZOA

A. General Characteristics

1. **Pseudopods** are extensions of cytoplasm providing motility unique to the amebae.
2. **Trophozoite** and **cyst** stages are part of the amebic life cycle and some flagellate life cycles.
3. Most amebic infections are spread to humans through ingestion of fecally contaminated water (sometimes food).
4. Cyst is the **infective stage**, whereas the trophozoite is the active reproduction stage destroyed by stomach acid.
5. **Laboratory identification:** Microscopic identification of cysts (in formed stools) and trophozoites (in liquid stools) is based on size, nuclear characteristics, and inclusions
6. Size is one of the most important criteria for identification.
7. Morphologic terms associated with protozoa
   a. **Karyosome:** Area of chromatin within the nucleus
   b. **Peripheral chromatin:** Nucleic acid combined with protein found along the nuclear membrane
   c. **Excystation:** Development of a cyst into a trophozoite
   d. **Encystation:** Development of a trophozoite into a cyst
   e. **Chromatoid bar:** Rod-shaped, RNA-containing structure characteristic of some species and usually found in the cytoplasm of the cyst

B. Intestinal Amebae

1. ***Entamoeba histolytica***
   a. The only ameba pathogenic for the gastrointestinal tract
      1) **Amebic colitis** is characterized by abdominal cramping, anorexia, fatigue, and diarrhea. Amebic colitis can also cause ulcers and amebic dysentery (often with bloody stools).
      2) Extraintestinal amebiasis primarily involves infections of the **liver**, but it is a rare complication.
      3) Additional extraintestinal conditions include infections of the spleen, brain, and lungs.
   b. **Life cycle:** Cysts are infective when ingested. Excystation occurs in the small intestines Trophozoites live in the large intestine. Infective cysts are passed in stools and are resistant to environmental stress.
   c. **Morphology**
      1) **Cyst characteristics**
         a) Cysts are spherical and range in size from 8 to 22 μm. See Figure 8-1■.

b) *E. histolytica* contains **one to four nuclei**; peripheral chromatin is fine and uniformly distributed.
c) The **karyosome** is small and centrally located.
d) **Cytoplasm** is finely granular. When present, chromatoid bars have parallel sides and round ends.

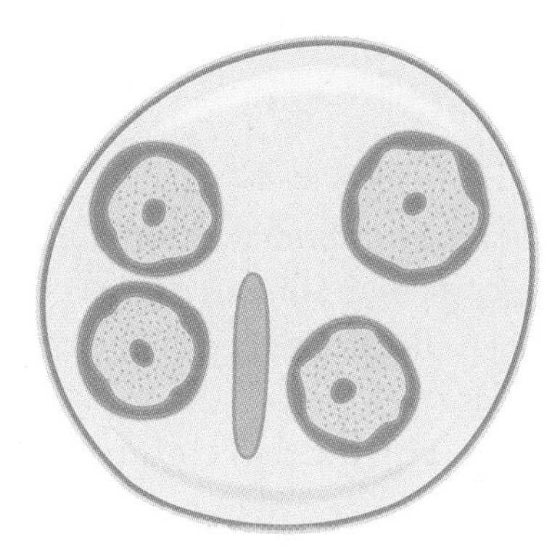

FIGURE 8-1 ■ *Entamoeba histolytica* cyst

2) **Trophozoite characteristics**
   a) Trophozoites range in size from 5 to 70 μm, and they are motile by means of pseudopods. See Figure 8-2■.
   b) *E. histolytica* trophozoites contain one nucleus, and it resembles those found in the cyst.
   c) **Cytoplasm** is finely granular and may contain red blood cell (RBC) inclusions. The presence of intracellular RBCs in intestinal amebae is considered diagnostic of *E. histolytica*.

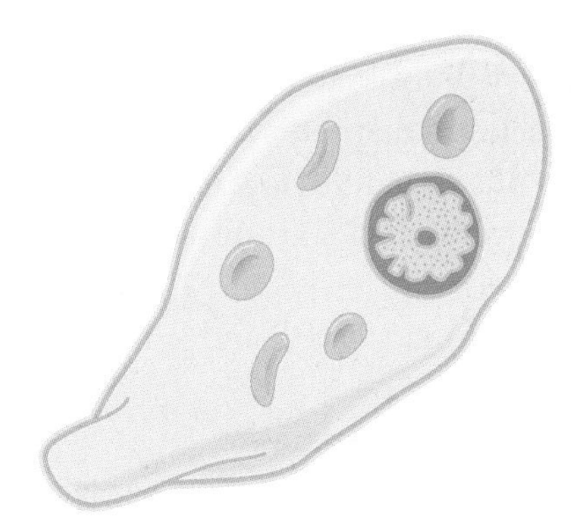

FIGURE 8-2 ■ *Entamoeba histolytica* trophozoite

3) Morphologically, *E. histolytica* is identical to the nonpathogen *E. dispar*. These two species can be differentiated by immunologic assays detecting surface antigens.

2. ***Entamoeba coli***
   a. *E. coli* is generally nonpathogenic but may cause intestinal problems in patients who are immunocompromised.
   b. If found in a stool specimen, *E. coli* can indicate the presence of pathogenic organisms.
   c. Needs to be differentiated from *E. histolytica* for purposes of treatment
   d. **Morphology**
      1) **Cyst characteristics**
         a) Cysts are spherical and range in size from 8 to 40 μm.
         b) *E. coli* contains one to eight nuclei; the peripheral chromatin is coarse and unevenly distributed. Young cysts may contain a large central glycogen mass pushing two nuclei to the periphery of the cell.
         c) The **karyosome** is eccentric and large.
         d) The **cytoplasm** is coarse. When present, the thin chromatoid bars have pointed ends.
      2) **Trophozoite characteristics**
         a) Trophozoites range in size from 10 to 60 μm, and they are motile by means of short/blunt pseudopods.
         b) *E. coli* trophozoites contain a single nucleus with coarse, unevenly distributed chromatin, and resemble those found in the cyst.
         c) The **cytoplasm** is coarse and vacuolated, with bacterial inclusions.
3. ***Blastocystis hominis***
   a. *B. hominis* was classified as an ameba, but rRNA analysis indicates that it is related to algae and water molds.
   b. Associated with diarrhea and abdominal pain in some individuals; others demonstrate no symptoms
   c. Transmission is through contaminated food and water.
   d. **Diagnosis:** Microscopic examination of stool sample
   e. **Morphology:** The **classic form** varies in diameter from 4 to 60 μm and contains a **large central body** that fills about 90% of the cell volume. There is an outer ring of cytoplasm with several nuclei around the central body.
4. Other intestinal tractamebae
   a. ***Entamoeba gingivalis*:** Causes asymptomatic mouth and genital tract infections
   b. ***Iodamoeba bütschlii*:** Nonpathogenic intestinal parasite
      1) **Cyst characteristics:** round to oval; 5–20 μm; nucleus has large karyosome with no peripheral chromatin; large well-defined glycogen vacuole present that may stain red-brown in an iodine wet mount.
      2) **Trophozoite characteristics:** 8–20 μm; single large karyosome often surrounded by achromatic granules; cytoplasm vacuolated
   c. ***Endolimax nana*:** Nonpathogenic intestinal parasite
      1) **Cyst characteristics:** round to oval; 5–10 μm; up to four nuclei with large karyosomes and no peripheral chromatin

2) **Trophozoite characteristics:** 6–12 μm; single nucleus with large irregular karyosome and no peripheral chromatin; vacuolated cytoplasm. Trophozoites of *E. nana* and *I. butschlii* may be difficult to distinguish.

d. ***Entamoeba hartmanni:*** Nonpathogenic intestinal parasite, resembles that of *E. histolytica*

1) **Cyst characteristics:** round, 5–10 μm; up to four nuclei with small central karyosome and even peripheral chromatin. Rounded-end chromatoidal bars may be present.

2) **Trophozoite characteristics:** 5–15 μm; single nucleus with small central karyosome and even peripheral chromatin; granular cytoplasm.

C. Flagellates

1. General characteristics

a. Flagellates are a subclass of protozoa that have one or more flagellum that provide motility.

b. All flagellates have a trophozoite stage, but several lack the cyst stage.

c. Many flagellates live in the small intestines.

d. ***Giardia duodenalis*** is the only pathogenic flagellate. It causes mild to moderate diarrhea. Severe and chronic infections can lead to malabsorption.

e. **Diagnosis** is by microscopic examination of stool for trophozoites or cysts.

f. Morphologic terms associated with flagellates

1) **Axostyle:** Rodlike structure that functions in cellular support

2) **Axoneme:** The intracellular portion of the flagellum

3) **Undulating membrane:** Flagellum finlike structure that generates a wave-like motion

4) **Cytostome:** A rudimentary oral cavity

2. ***Giardia duodenalis***

a. **Taxonomy: *G. lamblia* and *G. intestinalis*** are synonyms.

b. *G. duodenalis* causes giardiasis (a form of **traveler's diarrhea**) characterized by acute diarrhea with gassy, fatty, light-colored stools, abdominal pain, and weight loss. Self-limiting infections last 10–15 days, following a 10- to 35-day incubation period.

c. Infection is due to exposure to contaminated water and food (mostly from wild animal stool). Campers and hunters are prone to infection after drinking untreated fresh water from streams and lakes. Infections have also been reported in day care settings.

1) Cysts are the infective stage.

2) Cysts pass through the stomach and excyst in the duodenum.

3) Trophozoites attach to the duodenal mucosa via ventral disks (suckers).

4) **Encystation** occurs in the large intestines, and cysts will pass in the stool.

d. **Diagnosis**
   1) Microscopic examination of stool samples for trophozoites and cysts
   2) Other diagnostic tests include antigen detection by immunologic assays (e.g., EIA) or fluorescent monoclonal antibody tests. Rarely, a duodenal aspirate or the EnteroTest® will be used to obtain specimens for examination.

e. **Morphology**
   1) **Cyst characteristics**
      a) *Giardia* cysts are oval shaped, and the average size ranges from 12 μm long to 8 μm wide. See Figure 8-3■.
      b) Cysts contain **four nuclei** with large karyosomes and no peripheral chromatin.
      c) **Cytoplasm** is often retracted from the cyst wall and may contain two to four comma-shaped or curved, median bodies.

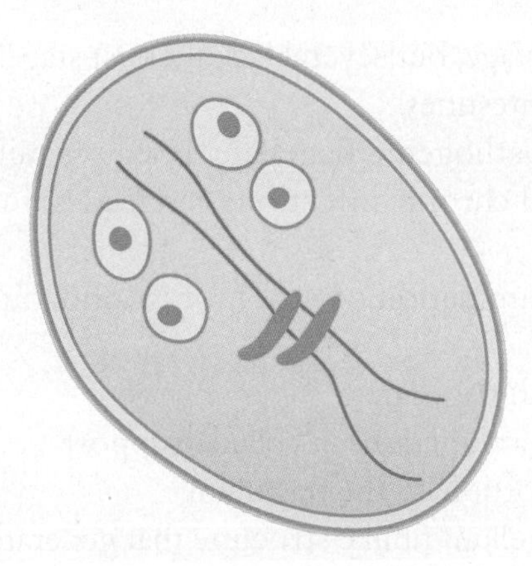

Size Range: 8–17 μm by 6–10 μm
Average Length: 10–12 μm

FIGURE 8-3 ■ *Giardia lamblia* cyst

   2) **Trophozoite characteristics**
      a) *G. duodenalis* trophozoites have an average size of 15 μm long to 10 μm wide. They are motile and pear shaped, with bilateral symmetry and **two large oval-shaped nuclei** on each side of a central **axostyle.** See Figure 8-4■.
      b) The **nuclei** contain a large karyosome and lack peripheral chromatin.
      c) Trophozoites possess four pair of **flagella.**
      d) Two median bodies, two axonemes, and a ventral sucking disk are present.
   3) ***Chilomastix mesnili***
      a) Generally nonpathogenic but has been associated with disease in patients who are immunocompromised

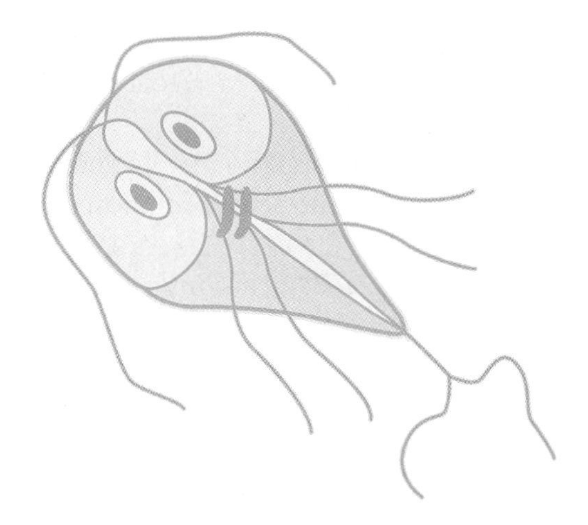

Size Range: 8–20 μm by 5–16 μm
Average Length: 10–15 μm

FIGURE 8-4 ■ *Giardia lamblia* trophozoite

b) Infection is acquired from contaminated food or water containing the infective cyst stage.
c) Diagnosis is by microscopic examination of stool samples.
d) **Cyst characteristics**
   1) The cyst ranges in size from 5 to 10 μm in length and is oval- to lemon shaped with a small hyaline knob at one end.
   2) *C. mesnili* contains a single nucleus without peripheral chromatin.
   3) The **karyosome** is large and centrally located.
   4) The **cytostome** is well defined and has a curved fibril.
e) **Trophozoite characteristics**
   1) Size ranges from 5 to 25 μm in length and 5 to 10 μm in width; they are pear shaped and motile.
   2) Single nucleus without peripheral chromatin
   3) **Karyosome:** Eccentric and small
   4) **Flagella:** Three anterior and one posterior
   5) **Cytostome** is very large, and a spiral groove is present in the cytoplasm toward the posterior end of the organism.

4. ***Dientamoeba fragilis***
   a. Can cause diarrhea and abdominal pain
   b. Many cases of diarrhea caused by *D. fragilis* occur in individuals living in close quarters, such as inmates, college students, and military recruits.
   c. *D. fragilis* infects the mucosal lining of the large intestines. There is no cyst stage, and the life cycle is not well defined; however, it is believed that the trophozoite is infective.
   d. Diagnosis is made from microscopic examination of trophozoites in the stool. Multiple samples are frequently required. The parasite is very delicate and stains poorly.

e. **Trophozoite characteristics**
   1) Size ranges from 5 to 19 μm; they are motile by means of hyaline pseudopods and are round shaped.
   2) Most cells contain two nuclei although up to 20% may be uninucleated. There is no peripheral chromatin and the nucleus is composed of four to eight clumps of nuclear chromatin.
   3) The **cytoplasm** is vacuolated with bacterial inclusions.

D. Ciliates

1. General characteristics
   a. Motile by cilia
   b. Trophozoites and cysts are part of the life cycle.
2. ***Balantidium coli***
   a. The only species pathogenic for humans
   b. Causes balantidiasis, characterized by diarrhea and infrequently dysentery
   c. Transmission of the infective cyst is through ingestion of fecally contaminated water or food.
   d. **Diagnosis**: Microscopic examination of stool for cysts or trophozoites
   e. **Morphology**
      1) **Cyst characteristics**
         a) Round and ranges in size from 43 to 65 μm (Figure 8-5■)
         b) *B. coli* contains two nuclei; the macronucleus, is kidney shaped and very large. The micronucleus is round and much smaller; it is rarely seen.
         c) Has a double cyst cell wall with numerous cilia between the two cell walls

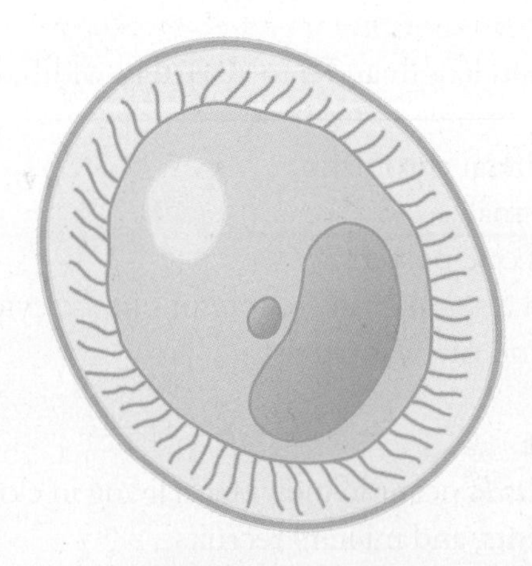

FIGURE 8-5 ■ *Balantidium coli* cyst

      2) **Trophozoite characteristics**
         a) Trophozoites range in size up to 100 μm in length and 70 μm in width. Cilia are present around the cell. See Figure 8-6■.

b) Like the cyst, trophozoites contain two nuclei.
c) Has a prominent cytostome and one or two contractile vacuoles.

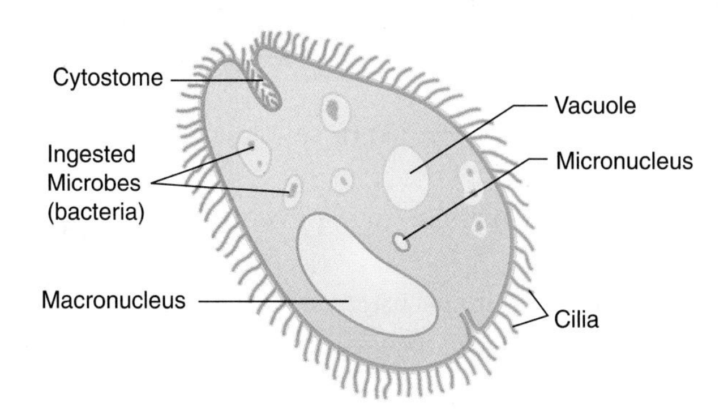

FIGURE 8-6 ■ *Balantidium coli* trophozoite

E. Intestinal Sporozoa

1. ***Cryptosporidium* spp. (*C. parvum and C. hominis*)**
   a. Cause cryptosporidiosis, which is characterized by moderate to severe diarrhea in individuals who are immunocompetent.
   b. In patients with acquired immunodeficiency syndrome (AIDS), *Cryptosporidium* infections are an important cause of death due to dehydration.
   c. In patients who are immunocompromised, the parasite causes a wide range of debilitating problems, including malabsorption and stomach, liver, and respiratory disorders.
   d. Transmission of the infected oocyst is through contaminated food or water (rodent, cow, pig, or chicken feces). Human-to-human transmission has been documented. Humans serve as both intermediate and definitive host.
   e. **Diagnosis**: Microscopic detection of **acid-fast oocysts** in stool or small bowel mucosal epithelial cells. Direct fluorescent monoclonal antibody tests for detection of the oocyst in stools and antigen detection via EIA are also used.
   f. **Oocyst characteristics**
      1) The round oocyst ranges in size from 4 to 6 μm. In an acid-fast stain, the color ranges from light pink to dark red.
      2) Oocysts contain four sporozoites enclosed within a thick cell wall; however, these are rarely visible
      3) The cytoplasm may contain several dark granules.
2. ***Cyclospora cayetanensis***
   a. Humans are the only host for *C. cayetanensis.*
   b. Nonbloody diarrhea is the most common symptom, although infections can be asymptomatic.
   c. **Diagnosis** can be made by examination of a fecal concentrate by light microscopy, or by examination of acid-fast-stained fecal smears. The **oocysts**

will stain with the **modified Kinyoun's acid-fast stain** and are 8–10 μm in diameter. The oocysts may be unstained, light pink, or dark purplish and may appear distorted. The organism will autofluoresce blue at a wavelength of 330–365 nm when UV fluorescent microscopy is used.

3. ***Cystoisospora belli***
   a. Causes cystoisosporiasis, which is characterized by mild diarrhea to severe dysentery
   b. Transmission is by ingestion of the infective oocyst in contaminated food and water.
   c. Humans are the definitive host; there are no intermediate hosts.
   d. **Diagnosis:** Microscopic examination of stool for oocysts by wet mounts and/or acid-fast or auromine-rhodamine stains
   e. **Oocyst characteristics**
      1) The oval oocyst ranges in size from 25 to 40 μm in length.
      2) The cytoplasm is granular. The mature oocyst contains two sporoblasts that contain four sporozoites each. The immature oocyst will demonstrate a single sporoblast.

III. EXTRAINTESTINAL PROTOZOA

A. *Plasmodium*

1. Causative agents of human malaria: *P. vivax, P. falciparium, P. malariae*, and *P. ovale*
2. *Plasmodium* spp. have two life cycle phases.
   a. **Sporogony:** Sexual phase that occurs within the intestinal tract of mosquitoes
   b. **Schizogony:** Asexual phase that occurs in the human host
3. **Transmission**
   a. Occurs with the bite of a **female *Anopheles* mosquito** that harbors the infective **sporozoites** in the salivary gland
   b. Other forms of transmission include contaminated blood products, contaminated needles, and congenital malaria.
4. Diagnosis is made by clinical symptoms and **microscopic examination of blood smears. A direct antigen detection test is also available.**
   a. Because of the rapid progression of *P. falciparum* infections, examination of blood smears for malaria should be considered a **STAT procedure.**
   b. Ideally, blood should be collected by finger stick and blood smears made immediately. Alternatively, **EDTA** (ethylenediaminetetraacetic acid) can be used as an anticoagulant in a venipuncture. Heparin can cause distortion of the parasites.
   c. **Thick smears:** A large drop of blood is placed on a slide and allowed to air dry. The RBCs are lysed in distilled water, and the material is stained with Giemsa stain.
   d. **Thin smears:** A drop of blood is placed on a glass microscope slide, and the blood is spread out on the slide using another slide. The smear is fixed in methanol to prevent RBC lysis and then stained.

e. Both thick and thin smears are thoroughly examined microscopically. The thick smear allows examination of about 20 times more blood volume than the thin smear, so it is much more **sensitive.** However, because the RBCs are intact, it is easier to identify the species of parasites in thin smears, which makes them more **specific.**

f. **The direct antigen test** (rapid diagnostic test) is an immunochromatographic test that detects specific enzymes or antigens from the parasites and is especially useful in detecting infection with *P. falciparum*. The test detects histidine-rich protein II (HRP II) antigen from *P. falciparum* as well as a pan-malarial antigen common to all malarial species infecting humans.

5. ***Plasmodium*** **morphology**
   a. **Trophozoites** or **ring forms**
      1) Erythrocytic intracellular ringlike appearance
      2) Giemsa or Wright's stain will show a blue cytoplasmic ring with a red **chromatin dot.**
      3) Mature trophozoites will lose the ring appearance as the cytoplasm increases but will still contain the chromatin mass.
   b. **Schizonts**
      1) Chromatin masses divide and increase in number within the cytoplasm.
      2) Pigment granules will remain and may be clustered.
      3) Mature schizonts contain **merozoites (a single chromatin mass encased in a small amount of cytoplasm)**; the number and arrangement depend on the species.
   c. **Gametocytes**
      1) Characterized by a chromatin mass staining pink to purple.
      2) The gametocytes of most species are round to oval in shape. *P. falciparium* gametocytes are "banana shaped."
      3) Pigmentation varies by species.
6. Diagnosis is primarily made by microscopic examination of Giemsa (stain of choice) or Wright's stained smears.
7. **Life cycle**
   a. The **sporozoite** is the infective stage transmitted to humans by *Anopheles* mosquitoes.
   b. The sporozoites infect hepatic cells and begin the **exoerythrocytic cycle.** *Plasmodium* spp. undergo **schizogony**, an asexual form of reproduction.
   c. Following schizogony, **merozoites** are produced that invade erythrocytes.
   d. A dormant form of *P. vivax* and *P. ovale,* called **hypnozoites**, can remain in the liver. Reactivation of the hypnozoites results in a **recurrence** (true relapse).
   e. Merozoites released from the liver infect RBCs and initiate the **erythrocytic cycle.** Merozoites develop into ring forms and reproduce by schizogony.
   f. Instead of undergoing schizogony, some merozoites develop into **microgametocytes** or **macrogametocytes.** These stages are transmitted

to the mosquito during human blood meal for completion of the life cycle (sexual phase).

g. The RBC form of the parasites can be nearly eliminated by treatment or an immune response, and the patient may become asymptomatic. However, after several weeks, the parasites can increase in number and the symptoms will return; this is referred to as **recrudescence.** All four *Plasmodium* spp. can cause a recrudescence.

8. ***Plasmodium vivax***
   a. Infected erythrocytes appear enlarged and pale with prominent pale-pink **Schüffner's dots.** Only reticulocytes are infected, thus limiting the parasitemia to 2–5%. Table 8-1■ compares the important characteristics of the *Plasmodium* spp.
   b. **Trophozoite:** Ring stage is one-third the size of an RBC; mature trophozoites fill the entire RBC.
   c. **Schizont** contains 12 to 24 merozoites.
   d. **Gametocyte:** Round to oval with a large chromatin mass that almost fills the RBC
   e. **Fever cycle** lasts 48 hours.
   f. *P. vivax* causes benign tertian malaria following a 10- to 17-day incubation period. It is the most common cause of malaria.

TABLE 8-1 CHARACTERISTICS OF HUMAN *PLASMODIUM* SPP.

Characteristic	*P. vivax*	*P. falciparum*	*P. malariae*	*P. ovale*
Persistence of exoerythrocytic cycle	Yes	No	No	Yes
Length of replication cycle (hours)	44–48	36–48	72	48
Shüffner's dots	Usually present in all infected RBCs except with early ring forms	Absent	Absent	Usually present in all infected RBCs
Number of merozoites in mature schizont	16 (12–24)	Schizonts not seen in peripheral blood	8 (6–12)	8 (8–12)
Important criteria for identification	Infected RBCs enlarged, trophozoites irregular shaped, Shüffner's dots	Multiple ring forms seen in single RBC, crescent-shaped gametes and ring-shaped young trophozoites are only forms seen	Infected RBCs normal size and color, trophozoites compact and band forms may be seen, merozoites often appear in daisy petal arrangement	Infected RBCs enlarged and often oval shaped with fimbriated edges, trophozoites irregular shaped, Shüffner's dots

9. ***Plasmodium falciparum***
   a. Infected erythrocytes appear normal in size, and all ages of RBCs can be infected, which can result in a large number of infected cells (parasitemia).
   b. **Trophozoite:** Ring stage is one-fifth the size of the RBC, and multiple ring forms are found in a single RBC. Some trophozoites will have two chromatin dots in one ring form.
   c. **Schizonts** are rarely seen in peripheral blood smears.
   d. Crescent- or banana-shaped **gametocytes** are diagnostic of *P. falciparium.*
   e. Miscellaneous characteristics: The interval between **paroxysms** (intense fever and chills) is irregular and may be as short as 24 hours. Patients have a high ratio of infected RBCs to uninfected RBCs compared to other *Plasmodium* spp.
   f. *P. falciparum* causes malignant tertian malaria **(blackwater fever)** following a 7- to 10-day incubation period. The organism may also cause cerebral malaria.
10. ***Plasmodium malariae***
   a. Infected erythrocytes appear normal in size without dots; *P. malariae* prefers to infect older RBCs.
   b. **Trophozoites** appear similar to *P. vivax* but stain a more intense blue. Mature trophozoites can produce **band forms**, which spread across the diameter of the RBC.
   c. **Schizonts** average 8 to 12 merozoites arranged in rosettes or daisy-petal arrangement
   d. **Gametocyte morphology** resembles *P. vivax.*
   e. Fever cycle is 72 hours.
   f. *P. malariae* causes quartan or malarial malaria following an 18- to 40-day incubation period.
11. ***Plasmodium ovale***
   a. Infected RBCs appear enlarged with thicker ring forms and contain Schüffner's dots. Infected RBCs resemble those infected with *P. vivax*; however, *P. ovale*-infected RBCs are often oval shaped and have irregularly shaped membranes with projections (fimbriations). Like *P. vivax,* reticulocytes are most commonly infected.
   b. **Trophozoites** maintain their ring appearance as they develop.
   c. **Schizont:** Averages four to eight merozoites arranged in rosettes
   d. **Gametocyte** resembles *P. vivax* but slightly smaller.
   e. *P. ovale* causes benign tertian or ovale malaria following a 10- to 20-day incubation period.

B. *Babesia microti*

1. ***B. microti*** is an intraerythrocytic parasite that causes babesiosis. *B. microti* can cause hemolytic anemia and may invade the spleen, liver, and kidneys.
2. Babesiosis is a self-limiting infection; death is an uncommon outcome.
3. The infective sporozoite is transmitted to humans by a tick bite (*Ixodes scapularis*). Infection may also occur via blood transfusions containing infected RBCs or congenitally.

4. Diagnosis is made by blood smear examination and serologic testing. It is difficult to differentiate *Babesia* spp. from *P. falciparum*.
5. **Ring-form characteristics**
   a. Size ranges from 3 to 5 μm.
   b. Cytoplasm: Minimal with two or more chromatin dots
   c. Two to four rings per RBC are often seen, sometimes appearing like a "**Maltese cross.**"

C. *Toxoplasma gondii*

1. **Toxoplasmosis** is characterized by a broad spectrum of symptoms depending on the individual's state of health. *T. gondii* has a predilection for **central nervous system** (CNS) infections.
   a. In healthy individuals, toxoplasmosis often resembles infectious mononucleosis and produces fatigue, swollen lymph glands, fever, and myalgia. The disease can become chronic and affect the heart and liver.
   b. **Congenital toxoplasmosis** occurs in premature or antibody-deficient infants, where symptoms include splenomegaly, jaundice, and fever. CNS infections can lead to developmental complications, including vision and hearing problems, hydrocephalus, and intellectual disability.
   c. In patients with immunosuppression, such as AIDS, the parasite becomes localized in the CNS with symptoms of encephalitis and brain lesions, often resulting in death.
2. **Transmission to humans**
   a. The sexual stage of reproduction occurs in the intestinal tract of **cats.** The infective form **(oocysts)** of the parasite is passed in the stool, and the **ingestion of cat feces** via contaminated food and water can produce infection.
   b. **Ingestion** of undercooked meat **(lamb and pork)** containing viable tissue cysts
   c. **Transplacental** transmission from an infected mother to the fetus
3. **Diagnosis:** Serologic testing for *Toxoplasma* antibody (IgM and/or IgG)
4. Because both life cycle forms—**tachyzoites** and **bradyzoites**—are small and no single organ is typically involved, it is difficult to diagnose infection by microscopic examination of tissue samples. Cerebrospinal fluid (CSF) specimens are sometimes useful.
5. Molecular assays of amniotic fluid can help diagnose *in utero* infections.
6. Tachyzoites (trophozoites) range in size from 1 to 3 μm and are crescent to round in shape.
7. Cysts contain many bradyzoites.

D. *Naegleri fowleri*

1. Causes primary amebic meningoencephalitis, which is often fatal within 3–6 days

2. *N. fowleri* is a free-living ameboflagellate found in lakes, ponds, and swimming pools where the water is warm.
3. **Life cycle:** Trophozoites are the infective stage. *N. fowleri* does not need a host to survive and can be free living, spending its entire life cycle in the external environment.
4. The amebae are contracted from contaminated water, where trophozoites enter the body through the nasal mucosa and migrate along the olfactory nerve to the brain.
5. Diagnosis is made by finding the trophozoite in CSF or brain biopsies. Only the trophozoite is found in humans.
6. **Morphology**
   a. **Cyst characteristics**
      1) The round cyst ranges in size from 10 to 13 μm.
      2) *N. fowleri* cysts contain a single nucleus, without peripheral chromatin.
      3) The **karyosome** is centrally located and large.
   b. **Trophozoite characteristics**
      1) Size ranges from 10 to 23 μm, and they are motile by means of blunt pseudopods.
      2) Trophozoites contain a single nucleus with a large karyosome without peripheral chromatin.
      3) The **cytoplasm** is granular and vacuolated.
   c. **Flagellate characteristics**
      1) Flagellates range in size from 7 to 15 μm and are pear shaped. They are motile by means of two flagella. They are a transient life cycle stage seen in the environment.
      2) The single nucleus is indented.
      3) **Karyosome** is centrally located and large.
      4) The **cytoplasm** is granular and vacuolated.

E. *Acanthamoeba*

1. Causes amebic encephalitis and amebic keratitis (cornea infection). May cause chronic skin lesions in individuals who are immunocompromised.
2. The life cycle is not well characterized.
   a. The eye is directly invaded by trophozoites, producing keratitis.
   b. Skin, respiratory tract, and CNS infections are caused by the cyst or trophozoite stage.
3. **Diagnosis** is made by finding the cyst or trophozoite stages in corneal scrapings, skin, brain biopsy, or other tissue.
4. **Morphology**
   a. **Cyst characteristics**
      1) Size ranges from 8 to 25 μm with a double wall and a round shape. Exterior wall is wrinkled; interior cyst wall may be star shaped.
      2) Single nucleus without peripheral chromatin
      3) The **karyosome** is centrally located and large.

4) The **cytoplasm** is granular and vacuolated.

b. **Trophozoite characteristics**

1) Size ranges from 15 to 45 μm; motility is by spinelike pseudopods.
2) Contains a single nucleus without peripheral chromatin
3) The **karyosome** is centrally located and large.
4) The **cytoplasm** is granular and vacuolated.

F. *Trichomonas vaginalis*

1. Causes **vaginitis** in women, whereas men are generally asymptomatic carriers
2. *T. vaginalis* is a sexually transmitted disease and can infect neonates (aspiration pneumonia) during delivery.
3. Trophozoites are the infective stage and infect the epithelial or mucosal lining of the vagina, urethra, and prostate gland. *T. vaginalis* does not have a cyst stage.
4. **Diagnosis:** Trophozoites are usually detected during a microscopic urinalysis examination or vaginal wet prep
5. **Trophozoite characteristics**

a. Trophozoites are pear shaped and average about 30 μm in length, with anterior flagella, and an **undulating membrane,**. They move with a jerky motility. See Figure 8-7■.

b. Single prominent nucleus

c. **Flagella:** Three to five anterior and one posterior

d. Large axostyle with cytoplasmic granules

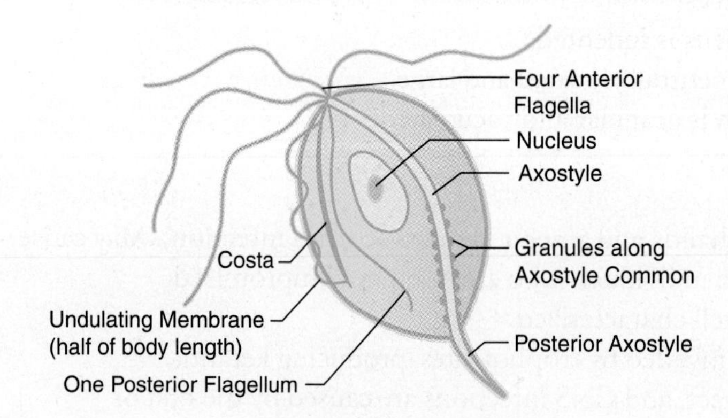

FIGURE 8-7 ■ *Trichomonas vaginalis* trophozoite

G. Hemoflagellates

1. General characteristics

a. Hemoflagellates inhabit the blood and tissues of humans.

b. Four stages of development: amastigote, promastigote, epimastigote, and trypomastigote

1) **Amastigote:** Nonflagellated, oval, intracellular form found in tissue

2) **Promastigote:** Flagellated stage found in the vector, rarely seen in the blood stream
3) **Epimastigote:** Long, slender flagellated form found in arthropod vectors
4) **Trypomastigote:** Has an undulating membrane running the length of the body and an anterior flagellum; found both in the vector and bloodstream of humans. See Figure 8-8■.

c. Transmission to humans is by arthropod bites. With *T. cruzi,* the infective stage is transmitted in the insect's feces.

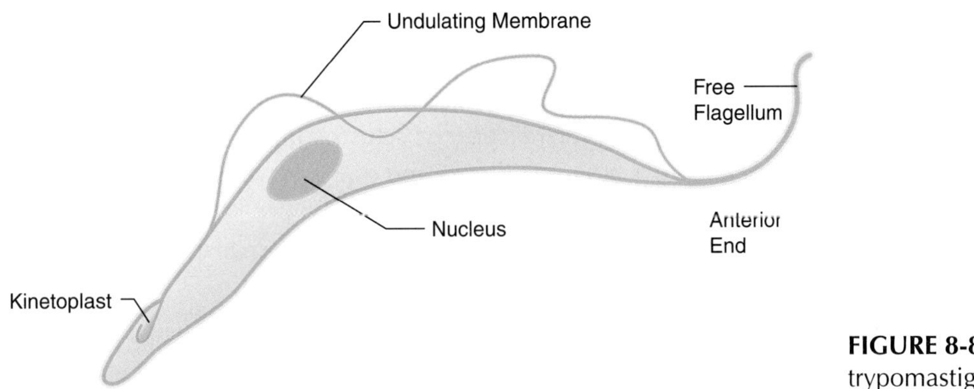

FIGURE 8-8 ■ *Trypanosoma* trypomastigote

2. ***Trypanosoma***
   a. Diagnosis is made by microscopic examination of blood and/or CSF to detect presence of the trypomastigote. Serologic testing may be used to detect antibody to the organism.
   b. Trypanosomiasis occurs mainly in Africa and South America.
   c. Pathogenic species
      1) ***Trypanosoma brucei***
         a) *T. brucei* causes **African trypanosomiasis** or **sleeping sickness**, and infection affects the lymphatic system and CNS. Swollen lymph nodes at the posterior base of the neck (Winterbottom's sign) are sometimes present in the early stage of the disease.
         b) Subspecies ***gambiense*** and ***rhodesiense*** are morplogically identical and named according to their geographic location (*T.b. gambiense*—East Africa; *T.b.rhodesiense*—West Africa)
      2) ***Trypanosoma cruzi***
         a) Causes **Chagas disease** or **American trypanosomiasis**, which is characterized by lesion formation **(chagoma)**, conjunctivitis, edema of the face and legs, and heart muscle involvement leading to myocarditis.
         b) Mostly found in South America
         c) May also be transmitted via blood transfusion or congenitally.
      3) ***Leishmania***
         a) Human leishmaniasis

1) **Cutaneous leishmaniasis** is characterized by skin and mucous membrane ulcers.
2) **Disseminated (visceral) leishmaniasis:** Liver, spleen, and reticuloendothelial (mononuclear phagocyte system) involvement

b) **Diagnosis:** Finding the amastigote in biopsy of tissue or organs or in bone marrow preparations and serologic testing.

c) Mainly a disease of Africa, Eastern Europe, and South/Central America

IV. TREMATODES

A. General Characteristics

1. Trematodes **(flukes)** are a class of helminths pathogenic to humans.
2. Trematodes are flat, hermaphroditic (except the schistosomes), and have at least two suckers: one opens into the digestive tract and one is for attachment.
3. Morphologic terms associated with trematodes
   a. **Cercaria:** Final larval stage of development occurring in snails; motile by means of a tail.
   b. **Metacercaria:** Encysted form occurring in the second intermediate host (fish or crayfish) or on water vegetation
   c. **Miracidium:** First larval stage that emerges from the egg in fresh water
   d. **Sporocyst:** Emerges from the miracidium as a saclike structure containing the larva
   e. **Redia:** Intermediate larval stage occurring in the sporocyst
   f. **Schistosomulum:** Schistosoma stage—resulting from when the cercaria penetrates human skin and loses its tail
4. Life cycle
   a. **Eggs** are usually passed with feces into the water where they hatch and release the free-swimming miracidium.
   b. Miracidia are then ingested by snails (the intermediate host).
   c. **Sporocytes** (schistosomes) or **redia** (trematodes) develop in the snail, resulting in the replication of hundreds of cercariae, which are released into water.
   d. **Cercariae** are infective to second intermediate host. In host tissue, they become metacercaria, which are then ingested by humans. With schistosomes, the cercaria directly penetrate the skin of humans who are swimming in infested water.
   e. **Diagnosis:** Examination of feces for adult forms or ova or, in the case of schistosomes, feces and urine examination for ova.
   f. Tremotodes can infect many organs, especially the intestines, liver, and lungs. However, most are organ specific.

B. *Schistosoma*

1. Species pathogenic for humans include ***S. mansoni, S. haematobium, S. japonicum***, and less frequently *S. mekongi* and *S. intercalatum.*
2. *Schistosoma* spp. cause schistosomiasis, which is characterized by abdominal pain bloody diarrhea, and hepatosplenomegaly. *S. mansoni* and *S. japonicum* adults reside in mesenteric veins surrounding the intestines. The eggs progressively make their way into the intestinal lumen. ***S. haematobium*** adults reside in the blood vessels around the **bladder.** The eggs penetrate the bladder and are passed in the urine. Patients often present with **hematuria.**
3. Prevalent in Africa but also seen in Puerto Rico and South America
4. Humans acquire the infective cercariae from contaminated water when the parasite penetrates the skin.
5. **Diagnosis** is made by microscopic examination of feces or urine for eggs. Adult forms are rarely seen in human blood samples.
6. **Morphology:** Eggs of different species are diagnostic.
   a. *S. haematobium*: Large terminal spine (Figure 8-9■)

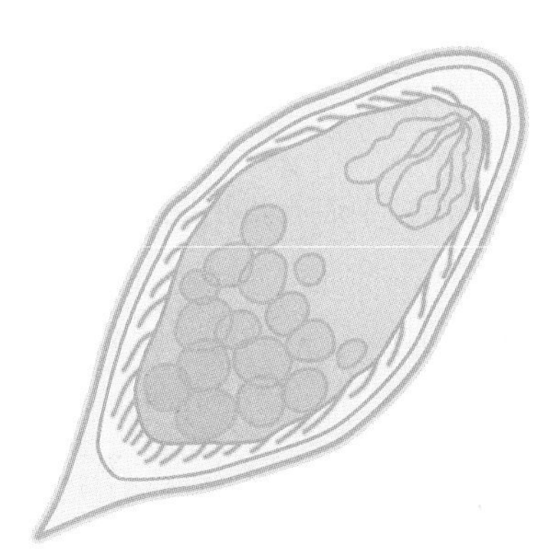

Size Range: 110–170 μm by 38–70 μm **FIGURE 8-9** ■ *Schistomosoma haematobium* egg

   b. *S. mansoni*: Large lateral spine (Figure 8-10■)

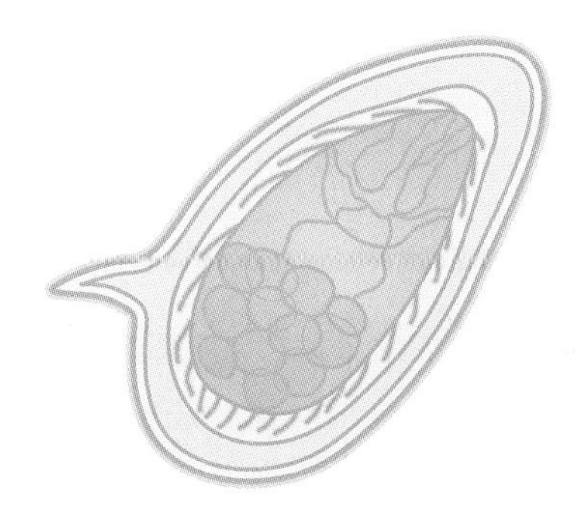

Size Range: 112–182 μm by 40–75 μm **FIGURE 8-10** ■ *Schistosoma mansoni* egg

c. *S. japonicum*: Small inconspicuous lateral spine (Figure 8-11■)

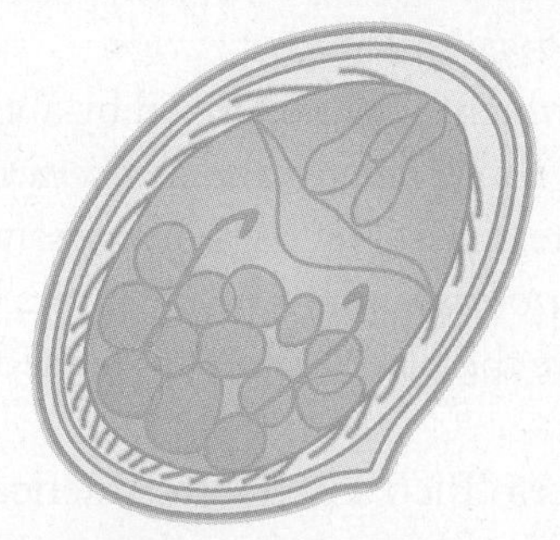

Size Range: 50–85 μm by 38–60 μm **FIGURE 8-11** ■ *Shistosoma japonicum* egg

C. *Paragonimus westermani* (lung fluke)

1. *P. westermani* causes pulmonary infections characterized by chest pain, cough, bronchitis, and sputum with blood.
2. Humans acquire infection by ingesting metacercariae in undercooked crabs and crayfish. Adult forms develop in human lung tissue.
3. Most infections occur in Africa, India, and South America.
4. **Diagnosis:** Microscopic examination of feces for eggs. Eggs may occasionally be found in sputum.
5. **Morphology:** Eggs range in size from 72 to 130 μm in length with an operculum on the flattened end. See Figure 8-12■.

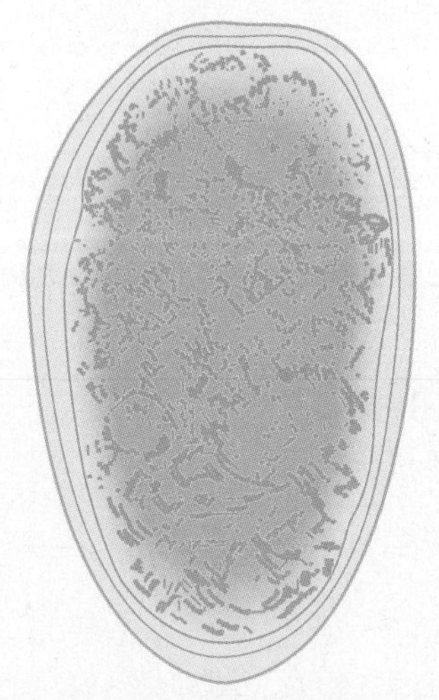

Size Range: 72–130 μm by 48–60 μm **FIGURE 8-12** ■ *Paragonimus westermani* egg

D. *Clonorchis sinensis* (Chinese or oriental liver fluke)

1. Causes liver problems characterized by fever, abdominal pain, and diarrhea
2. Found mainly in China and the Far East
3. Humans acquire the disease by eating undercooked fish containing encysted metacercariae.

4. **Diagnosis:** Egg detection in stool sample
5. **Morphology:** Egg contains miracidium with small knob (abopercular knob) opposite the prominent dome-shaped operculum. See Figure 8-13■.

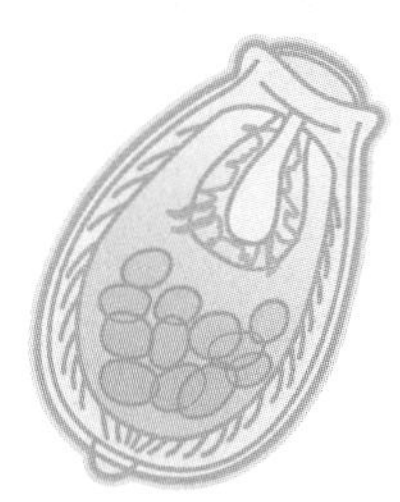

Average Size: 30 μm by 15 μm **FIGURE 8-13** ■ *Clonorchis sinensis* egg

E. *Fasciolopsis buski* (intestinal flukes)
   1. Causes intestinal problems, including diarrhea and ulceration of the intestines and possibly the stomach
   2. Found in China and the Far East
   3. Humans acquire infections by ingesting metacercariae on water plants (e.g., water chestnuts and bamboo).
   4. **Diagnosis:** Egg detection in stool sample
   5. **Morphology:** Eggs are large, oblong (130–140 μm by 80–85 μm) and contain an operculum on the narrow end. See Figure 8-14■. Can be indistinguishable from eggs of *Fasciola hepatica.*

F. *Fasciola hepatic* (liver fluke)
   1. Primarily a zoonosis of sheep affecting the liver
   2. Found in South America and the Mediterranean area
   3. Humans acquire infections by ingesting metacercariae on water plants (e.g., watercress).
   4. **Diagnosis:** Egg detection in stool sample
   5. **Morphology:** Eggs are large, oblong (130–150 μm by 63–90 μm) with an inconspicuous operculum. See Figure 8-14■.

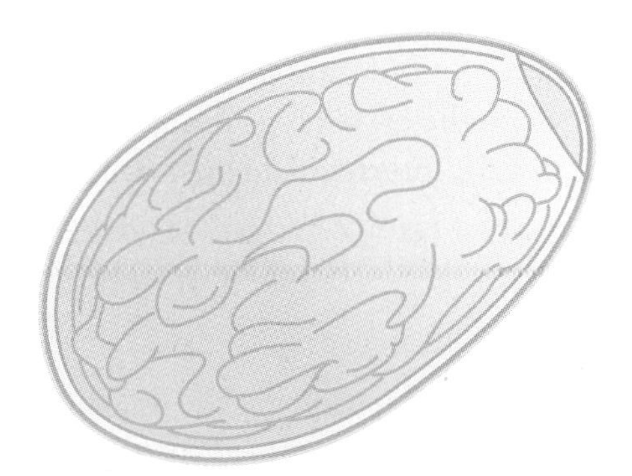

Fasciolopsis Size Range: 128–140 μm by 78–85 μm
Fasciola Size Range: 128–150 μm by 60–90 μm

FIGURE 8-14 ■ *Fasciola hepatica* egg

G. *Heterophyes heterophyes*

1. Besides humans, definitive hosts include cats, dogs, foxes, wolves, and pelicans
2. Found in a number of countries including Egypt, Sudan, Israel, India, and Russia
3. Acquired by ingesting encysted metacercariae on fish
4. Generally mild symptoms but can present with intestinal pain and diarrhea
5. **Diagnosis:** Ova in stool that resemble *C. sinensis*

H. *Metagonimus yokagawa*

1. Besides humans, fish eating animals such as cats, dogs, and birds can be infected.
2. Found primarily in the Far East
3. Acquired by ingesting metacercariae on undercooked fish
4. Typically, symptoms range from asymptomatic to ocassional abdominal pain and diarrhea.
5. **Diagnosis:** Ova in stool that resemble *C. sinensis* and *H. heterophyes*

V. CESTODES

A. General Characteristics

1. Cestodes are a subclass of helminths comprising true **tapeworms.**
2. **Morphology**
   a. The **scolex** is the anterior portion of the body containing suckers and sometimes hooklets responsible for attachment to the host. The "crown" of the scolex is called the **rostellum.**
   b. **Proglottids** are the individual segments that make up the major portion of the tapeworm; they contain male and female reproductive structures.
   c. The **neck region** is located directly behind the scolex and is the site of new proglottid production.
   d. **Strobila** is the entire length of the tapeworm except for the scolex and neck.
3. Cestodes have three **life cycle stages**: egg, larval stage(s), and the adult worm. The cysticercus is the larval stage infective for humans. Eggs are infective for the intermediate host. In all but one species, the egg contains a six-hooked embryo (hexacanth embryo).
4. Cestodes have several intermediate hosts.
5. **Diagnosis:** Microscopic examination of stool samples for eggs or proglottids
6. **Transmission** to humans occurs when the cysticercus is ingested in raw/undercooked meat. Eggs are infective for intermediate host (with *T. solium* eggs may also be infective for humans).

B. Cestodes Pathogenic for Humans

1. ***Taenia saginata*** **and** ***Taenia solium***
   a. *T. saginata* and *T. solium* cause infections that are typically mild and characterized by abdominal pain and mild diarrhea.
   b. Infection is by the ingestion of undercooked **beef** (*T. saginata*) or **pork** (*T. solium*) that contains the **cysticercus larvae.**

c. In rare cases, humans are the **intermediate host** following the ingestion of *T. solium* ova. This causes a larval form of extraintestinal disease called **cysticercosis**, which causes lesions in the cerebral cortex and other body sites that can be fatal.
d. **Diagnosis** is made by microscopic examination of stool specimens for ova. The eggs of the two species are identical. Species identification relies on proglottid or scolex analysis.
e. **Egg morphology**
   1) Range in size from 30 to 40 μm
   2) Hexacanth embryo containing three pairs of hooklets
   3) Thick shell with radial striations

2. ***Diphyllobothrium latum*** (fish tapeworm)
   a. Infection is acquired by eating raw or undercooked fish containing the **pleurocercoid** larva
   b. *D. latum* infection causes intestinal pain, diarrhea, and sometimes vitamin B_{12} deficiency. Individuals may develop a megaloblastic anemia.
   c. Infections occur in populations that eat raw fish, such as northern Europe and Japan.
   d. **Diagnosis:** Egg detected in stool samples; occasionally proglottids may be present.
   e. **Egg morphology**
      1) Range in size from 50 to 80 μm in length and are oblong in shape (Figure 8-15■)
      2) The shell is smooth and color is yellow to brown.
      3) Small terminal abopercular knob is located at the end opposite the operculum.

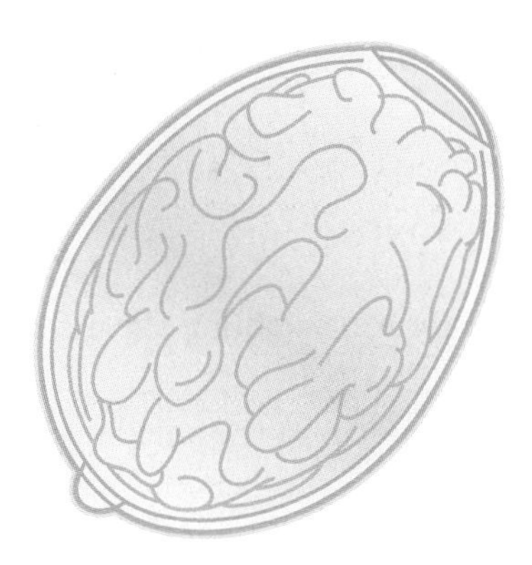

FIGURE 8-15 ■ *Diphyllobothrium latum* egg

3. ***Hymenolepis nana*** (dwarf tapeworm)
   a. Causes abdominal pain and diarrhea
   b. Humans usually acquire the infection by ingestion of **ova** found in mice or human **feces.**

c. Most common tapeworm in the United States
d. **Diagnosis:** Egg detection in stool samples
e. **Egg morphology**
1) The average size is 40 μm, and ova are round.
2) Contains three pairs of hooklets
3) Polar thickening of the shell is common with polar filaments extending into the space between inner and outer shells.

4. ***Hymenolepis diminuta*** (mouse and rat tapeworm)
a. Causes abdominal pain and diarrhea
b. Humans acquire the infection from the ingestion of **insects** containing the **cysticercoids.**
c. **Diagnosis:** Egg detection in stool samples
d. **Egg morphology**
1) Average size of the round egg is 75 μm.
2) Contains three pairs of hooklets
3) No polar filaments and rare polar thickening seen

5. ***Echinococcus granulosus*** (dog tapeworm)
a. Human infection results in the development of a **hydatid cyst** in many body sites (hydatid cyst disease or echinococcosis). As the cyst grows, surrounding tissue is destroyed. Depending on cyst location, death can occur. The release of hydatid cyst fluid may cause anaphylactic shock.
b. Infections are most common where **sheep** (intermediate host) are raised, including England, South America, and Australia. Some cases have been reported in Alaska.
c. Humans, the intermediate host, acquire the infection by ingesting ova in dog feces. The dog acquires the parasite by consuming infected sheep meat.
d. **Diagnosis:** Analysis of hydatid cyst fluid containing cysts and other parasite components, and serologic testing
e. The cyst contains fluid, daughter cysts, brood capsules, and hydatid sand (scoleces of the tapeworm).

6. *Dipylidium caninum*
a. Dogs and cats are reservoirs, and humans typically acquire the infection by ingesting the cysticercoid in infected fleas.
b. The cysticercoid develops into an adult tapeworm in the small intestine.
c. Most infections are aymptomatic.
d. The gravid proglottids detach from the tapeworm and migrate to the anus or are passed in the stool.

VI. NEMATODES

A. General Characteristics

1. Nematodes (roundworms) are a class of helminths.
2. Adult nematodes have a tapered, cylindric body with an esophagus and longitudinal muscles. For most species a male and female exist.

3. **Diagnosis** is based on adult, larvae, or egg morphology.
4. Nematode life cycles vary as to species and can be quite complex.
   a. Some nematodes are transmitted through the ingestion of eggs.
   b. Other nematode infections are transmitted by larvae, which must gain entry through the skin on their way to the intestines.
   c. A few of the tissue nematodes may require intermediate hosts.
5. Nematodes cause diseases associated with the intestines and the skin, including diarrhea, vomiting, and skin lesions.
6. Nematodes are placed into one of two groups: the **intestinal nematodes** and the **intestinal-tissue nematodes.**
   a. Intestinal nematodes
      1) *Enterobius vermicularis*
      2) *Trichuris trichiura*
      3) *Ascaris lumbricoides*
      4) *Strongyloides stercoralis*
      5) *Necator americanus*
      6) *Ancylostoma duodenale*
   b. Intestinal-tissue nematodes
      1) *Trichinella spiralis*
      2) *Dracunculus medinenis*

B. *Enterobius vermicularis*

1. *E. vermicularis,* **pinworm**, causes infections **(enterobiasis)** that are usually self-limiting and characterized by itching and inflammation of the anus. Enterobiasis can be asymptomatic.
2. Pinworm infections are common in the United States, especially in school-age children.
3. **Life cycle**
   a. Infective **eggs** are ingested, and larvae are released in the **small intestines.**
   b. Larvae develop into adult worms in the colon.
   c. Gravid females migrate to the **perianal region** to deposit ova.
   d. The eggs are infective following a 6-hour incubation period.
   e. Itching results from the irritation caused by the deposition of eggs. Eggs are spread from the perianal region by scratching.
   f. The eggs will be infective for several weeks and can be found in dust, clothing, etc.
4. **Diagnosis**
   a. Because eggs are deposited in the perianal area, a routine stool specimen is unlikely to reveal their presence. Instead, ova are detected from a tape preparation in which the sticky side of tape is pressed to the perianal skin and then placed on a microscope slide
   b. Because the gravid female deposits eggs in the perianal folds during the late evening hours, yield is best in children if the specimen is collected in the morning.

5. **Egg morphology**
   a. Eggs range in size from 50 to 60 μm in length and 30 μm in width. They have a thin shell, are oval in shape, and have one side flattened. See Figure 8-16■.
   b. The ovum contains a developing larva (often C-shaped).

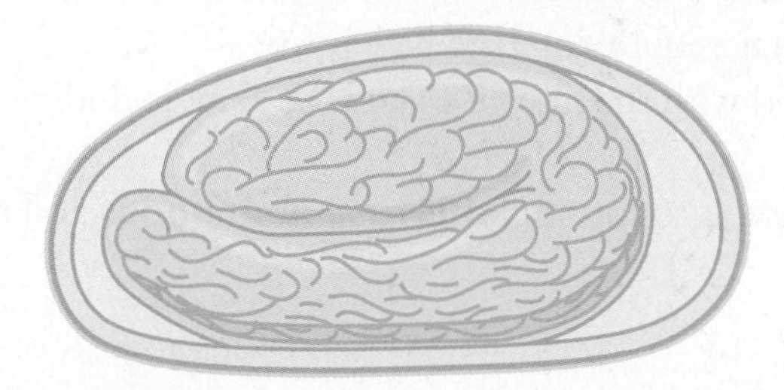

Size Range: 48–60 μm long by 20–35 μm wide

FIGURE 8-16 ■ *Enterobius vermicularis* egg

C. *Trichuris trichiura*
1. *T. trichiura* **(whipworm)** causes infection that in children, presents as colitis and dysentery in heavy infection. Symptoms in adults may include abdominal pain and bloody diarrhea.
2. Most infections occur in Africa and South America, but infections also occur in the deep south of the United States.
3. Eggs from human feces are infective. After ingestion of the ova, the larvae develop into adults in the intestines.
4. **Diagnosis:** Detection of eggs in stool samples
5. **Egg morphology**
   a. The eggs range in size from 50 to 60 μm in length and 25 μm in width and are football shaped with clear plugs at each end.
   b. The shell is thick, smooth, and yellow to brown.
   c. The egg contains a developing embryo.
6. **Adult morphology**
   a. The female adult measures 35–50 mm long, and the male is 30–45 mm long. Adults are rarely found in the stool.
   b. The posterior end is thick and resembles a whip handle.
   c. The anterior end is thin, elongated and resembles a whip.

D. *Ascaris lumbricoides*
1. *A. lumbricoides* is known as the giant intestinal roundworm and causes ascariasis, resulting in intestinal tissue destruction and bowel obstruction that can be fatal. The worms can also migrate to the lungs, where they cause pulmonary disorders, and to other body sites. As part of the life cycle, larva migrate through the lungs, and repeated exposure may cause a pneumonitis-like reaction.
2. Worldwide, *A. lumbricoides* affects over 1 billion people per year; however, infection is rare in the United States.
3. Eggs (the infective stage) are passed in human feces.

4. **Diagnosis:** Examination of stool for eggs and adult forms
5. **Egg morphology**
   a. Infertile ova are oval and measure up to 90 μm in length. See Figure 8-17■.
   b. Fertile eggs are round and range in size up to 75 μm in length and 50 μm in width. The shell is thick, has a bumpy albuminous covering, and contains a single-cell developing embryo. See Figure 8-18■.

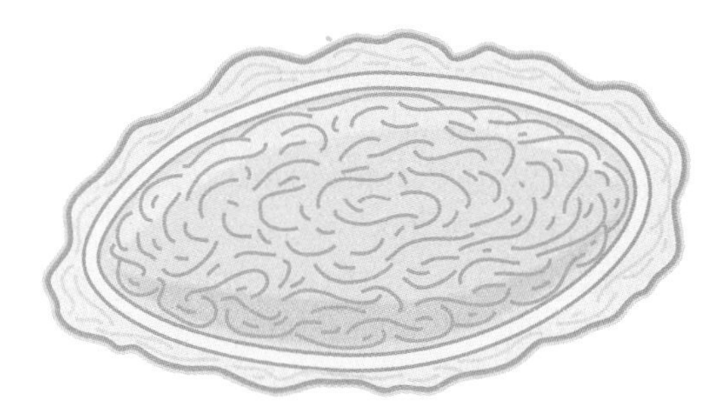

Size Range: 85–95 μm by 38–45 μm

FIGURE 8-17 ■ *Ascaris lumbricoides* infertile egg

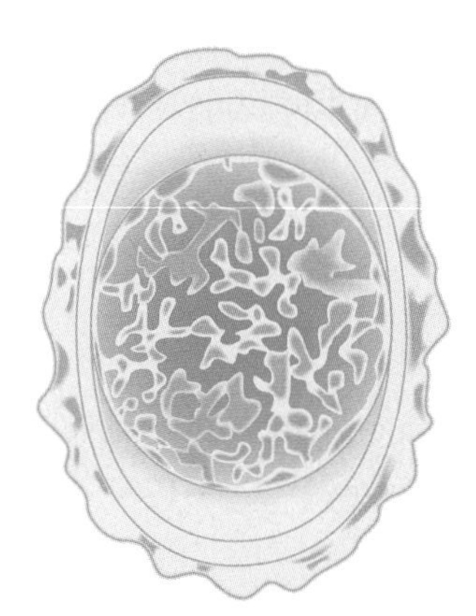

FIGURE 8-18 ■ *Ascaris lumbricoides* fertile egg

6. **Adult morphology**
   a. Females are 20–30 cm long.
   b. Males are 15–31 cm long with a curved posterior end.

E. *Strongyloides stercoralis*
   1. Causes threadworm infections, characterized by diarrhea and abdominal pain
   2. Most infections occur in the tropics.
   3. Skin contact with contaminated soil **(filariform larvae)** is the transmission route for humans. After penetration, larvae migrate through the skin and into the small intestine. Females produce eggs by parthenogenesis, form of asexual reproduction in which an egg can develop into an embryo without being fertilized by a sperm. Eggs usually hatch in the intestine and release a first-stage larva (rhabditiform) into the stool.

4. **Diagnosis:** Because eggs are rarely passed, the rhabditiform larvae are the primary diagnostic stage.
5. **Morphology of rhabditiform larvae**
   a. Larvae range in size up to 700 μm in length. Average is 200–300 um.
   b. Short buccal cavity
   c. Prominent, elongated genital primordium

F. *Necator americanus* and *Ancylostoma duodenale*

1. *N. americanus* (New World hookworm) and *A. duodenale* (Old World hookworm) cause human hookworm infections. Depending on the infected body site, symptoms can include coughing (lung infection) and headaches. Heavy, prolonged infections may cause microcytic, hypochromic anemia.
2. Hookworms are common worldwide, including in North America.
3. Humans acquire the **filariform larvae** through skin penetration. The larvae migrate to the lungs, are coughed up, swallowed, and reach the intestines.
4. **Diagnosis:** Identification of ova or rhabditiform larvae from stool specimens
5. **Egg morphology**
   a. Eggs of the two species are identical.
   b. The eggs are oval and measure 56–75 μm long by 36–40 μm wide.
   c. Eggs are thin shelled, and a developing embryo can sometimes be seen inside.
6. **Rhabditiform larva** morphology
   a. long buccal capsule
   b. inconspicuous genital primordium
   c. 200–300 μm long
7. **Morphology of adult worms**
   a. Adult worms firmly attach to the intestinal mucosa and are rarely seen.
   b. Adults range in size from 7 to 11 mm in length; *Anclyostoma* worms tend to be slightly larger than *Necator* worms.
   c. The buccal cavity of *N. americanus* contains a pair of cutting plates, whereas *A. duodenale* has teeth.

G. *Trichinella spiralis*

1. *T. spiralis* causes trichinosis with symptoms including diarrhea, blurred vision, muscle edema (mostly **striated muscle**), and coughing. Periorbital edema is often present. Infections can be fatal.
2. The parasite is found worldwide; **pigs** are important reservoirs.
3. Humans acquire the infection by eating **undercooked pork** containing encysted larvae.
4. **Diagnosis** can be made by examining muscle tissue for encysted larvae. Laboratory tests reveal high eosinophil count (40–80%), leukocytosis, and increased creatine kinase and lactate dehydrogenase. Antibody tests are available.
5. **Morphology**
   a. Larvae range in size up to 125 μm in length and 7 μm in width. Many encysted forms are found in striated muscle tissue.
   b. Adults range up to 1 mm in length and reside in the intestinal tract.

H. *Dracunculus medinensis*

1. Causes guinea worm infection; symptoms include allergic reactions and painful ulcers
2. Most infections occur in Africa, India, and Asia.
3. Humans acquire the infection by the ingestion of infected **copepods** (water fleas) carrying the larvae.
4. **Diagnosis**: Observing worms emerging from ulcerated areas of the body
5. **Morphology of adults**
   a. Adult females range in size up to 1 m in length and 2 mm in width.
   b. Males are about 2 cm in length.

VII. FILARIAE

A. General Characteristics of the Filarial Parasites

1. Filarial parasites are an order of nematodes consisting of adult threadlike worms.
2. Filariae inhabit the circulatory and lymphatic system and are also found in muscle, connective tissue, and serous cavities.
3. Four primary species cause disease in humans: *Wuchereria bancrofti, Brugia malayi, Loa loa*, and *Onchocerca volvulus.*
4. **Transmission** of the filariae parasites occurs during the bite of mosquitoes or other arthropods.
5. **Diagnosis** is by microscopic examination of blood or tissue for microfilariae. Some species migrate in the daytime (diurnal periodicity), whereas others migrate at night (nocturnal periodicity). It is therefore important to draw blood in the morning (between 10 A.M. and noon) and in the evening (between 10 P.M. and midnight). Characteristics used for identification include the arrangement of nuclei and presence/absence of a sheath (remnant of egg membrane) surrounding the filaria.
6. Most filarial disease occurs in Africa and South America.

B. Filariae Pathogenic for Humans

1. ***Loa loa***
   a. Causes subcutaneous tissue infections and infections of the conjunctival lining of the eye
   b. Most infections occur in Africa.
   c. Transmission of the parasite is through the bite of the *Chrysops* (deer) fly.
   d. **Diagnosis:** Blood smear examination for microfilariae. Adults may be extracted from the skin or eye.
   e. **Microfilariae characteristics**
      1) Size ranges from 250 to 300 μm in length
      2) Contains a row of **nuclei** that extends to the tip of the tail
      3) A **sheath** is present.
2. ***Brugia malayi***
   a. *B. malayi* causes Malayan filariasis, a condition that produces lesions in the lymphatics, and **elephantiasis** may result.
   b. Most infections occur in the Far East, Japan, and China.

c. *B. malayi* is transmitted by the *Anopheles* or *Aedes mosquito.*
d. **Diagnosis** is by microscopic examination of blood smears for microfilariae. Samples collected at night offer the largest yield.
e. **Microfilariae characteristics**
 1) Size ranges from 200 to 300 μm in length.
 2) Two **nuclei** are located in the tail, with a short space between them.
 3) A **sheath** is present.

3. ***Wuchereria bancrofti***
 a. *W. bancrofti* causes Bancroftian filariasis, a condition that produces lesions in the lymphatics. **Elephantiasis** may result.
 b. Disease occurs in the tropics and subtropics.
 c. Vectors for the disease are the *Culex, Aedes*, and *Anopheles* mosquitoes.
 d. **Diagnosis:** Examination of blood smears for microfilariae
 e. **Microfilariae characteristics**
  1) Ranges in size from 250 to 300 μm in length
  2) **No nuclei** are found in the tip of the tail.
  3) A **sheath** is present.

4. ***Onchocerca volvulus***
 a. *O. volvulus* causes **river blindness;** eye infections may lead to blindness.
 b. Most infections occur in Africa, South America, and Mexico.
 c. Transmission of the infective microfilariae is by the bite of the *Simulium* (blackfly).
 d. **Diagnosis:** Tissue (skin snip) or ophthalmologic analysis for microfilariae. Adults maybe found coiled in a subcutaneous nodule.
 e. **Microfilariae characteristics**
  1) Size ranges from 150 to 360 μm in length.
  2) **No nuclei** are located in the tail.
  3) No **sheath** is present.

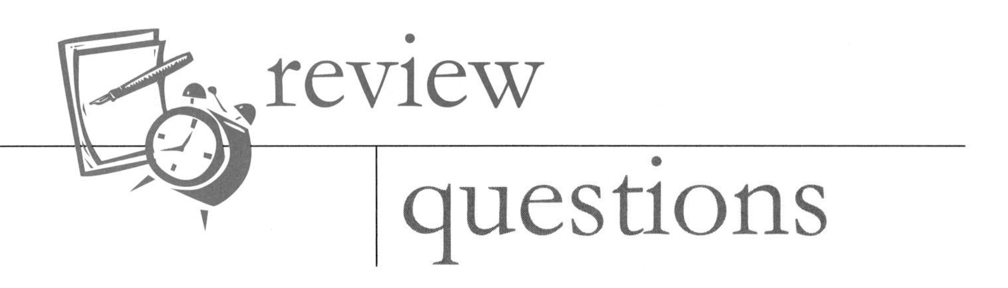

review questions

INSTRUCTIONS Each of the questions or incomplete statements that follows is comprised of four suggested responses. Select the *best* answer or completion statement in each case.

1. *Enterobius vermicularis* infection is usually diagnosed by finding
   A. Eggs in perianal specimens
   B. Larvae in a stool specimen
   C. Adults in feces
   D. Eggs in the feces
2. Which organism infects humans by larval penetration?
   A. *Enterobius vermicularis*
   B. *Ascaris lumbricoides*
   C. *Necator americanus*
   D. *Trichuris trichiura*
3. Which statement is correct for specimen collection and processing?
   A. Stool samples can contain urine.
   B. Stools can be frozen without affecting parasitic structure.
   C. Liquid stools are best for detecting ameba and flagellate trophozoites.
   D. Unpreserved stools can remain at room temperature for up to 72 hours.
4. For which organism is the trophozoite the infective stage for humans?
   A. *Endolimax nana*
   B. *Dientamoeba fragilis*
   C. *Entamoeba coli*
   D. *Giardia duodenalis*
5. The primary diagnostic specimen for detecting infection with *Naegleria fowleri* is a:
   A. Thick blood smear
   B. Corneal scraping
   C. Cerebrospinal fluid sediment
   D. Skin biopsy
6. The host in which sexual reproduction takes place is called the
   A. Commensal
   B. Definitive host
   C. Intermediate host
   D. Vector

7. The presence of ingested red blood cells may be seen in the trophozoite of which organism?
   A. *Giardia duodenalis*
   B. *Entamoeba coli*
   C. *Dientamoeba fragilis*
   D. *Entamoeba histolytica*

8. Which of the following is a characteristic used in identification of *Iodamoeba bütschlii* cysts?
   A. A well-defined glycogen mass
   B. Blunt chromatoidal bars
   C. Four nuclei with large karyosomes
   D. Many ingested bacteria

9. Which of the following is the most important feature in differentiating cysts of *Entamoeba histolytica* from *Entamoeba dispar?*
   A. Number of nuclei
   B. Size of the cyst
   C. Shape and location of the karyosome and peripheral chromatin
   D. Distinguishing surface antigens by immunologic assays

10. An egg was found in an iodine wet mount of a fecal concentrate. The egg was oval, thin shelled, and approximately 55 μm in length. The interior showed an embryo in the four-cell stage of development. The most likely identification is:
    A. *Strongyloides stercoralis*
    B. *Trichuris trichiura*
    C. Hookworm
    D. *Enterobius vermicularis*

11. A 48-year-old male developed fever and weakness 16 days after a safari in northwest Tanzania. After about 8 days, the patient had a temperature of 38.9°C (102°F), and right-sid, anterior cervical lymphadenopathy. Cerebrospinal fluid contained 12 red blood cells and 18 mononuclear cells/μL and a normal protein level (32 mg/dL). Laboratory tests of peripheral blood revealed a hemoglobin level of 12.7 g/dL, a white cell count of $2.4 \times 10^9/L$, and a platelet count of $75 \times 10^9/L$. The peripheral blood smear demonstrated an extra-erythrocytic, flagellated organism about 18 um long with a prominent nucleus, and faintly staining undulating membrane. Which of the following is the most probable etiologic agent of this infection?
    A. *Leishmania donovani*
    B. *Trypanosoma brucei*
    C. *Trypanosoma cruzi*
    D. *Brugia malayi*

12. Which species of malaria parasite usually has ameboid trophozoites and produces small reddish dots in the red blood cell cytoplasm?
    A. *Plasmodium knowlesi*
    B. *Plasmodium falciparum*
    C. *Plasmodium malariae*
    D. *Plasmodium vivax*

13. Which of the following procedures should be used for the accurate, specific diagnosis of an intestinal amebic infection?
    A. Direct saline wet mount
    B. Iodine wet mount of concentrated sediment
    C. Permanently stained smear
    D. Formalin-ethyl acetate sedimentation technique

14. In an examination of stained blood films, *Babesia* spp. are likely to resemble
    A. *Leishmania donovani*
    B. *Plasmodium falciparum*
    C. *Toxoplasma gondii*
    D. *Trypanosoma cruzi*
15. Which of the following is a mercury-containing fixative used to preserve parasites in stool specimens?
    A. Formalin
    B. Sodium acetate
    C. Buffered glycerol
    D. Polyvinyl alcohol
16. Examination of a fecal smear following acid fast staining reveals round acid-fast-positive structures 8–10 μm in diameter. You should suspect what organism?
    A. *Cryptosporidium*
    B. *Cyclospora*
    C. *Cystoisospora*
    D. Microsporidia
17. A 22-year-old male presents to his family physician complaining of fatigue, muscle pain, periorbital edema, and fever. The complete blood count revealed a slightly elevated white blood count, and 45% eosinophilia on the differential. Which of the following conditions should be considered part of the differential diagnosis?
    A. Hydatid cyst disease
    B. Chaga's disease
    C. Trichinosis
    D. Cysticercosis
18. An egg measuring 110 μm with a large lateral projection was observed in an iodine wet mount of a stool specimen. What is the most likely identification?
    A. *Schistosoma haematobium*
    B. *Fasciolopsis buski*
    C. *Chistosoma mansoni*
    D. *Paragonimus westermani*
19. Elephantiasis is a complication associated with which of the following?
    A. Cysticercosis
    B. Guinea worm infection
    C. Hydatid cyst disease
    D. Filariasis
20. A patient with history of human immunodeficiency virus infection presents with an 8-day history of diarrhea and weight loss. A series of stool specimens is collected and examined for the presence of ova and parasites. An acid-fast stain on direct smear reveals pink-stained round structures approximately 4 μm in diameter. The most likely pathogen is
    A. *Blastocystis hominis*
    B. *Cryptosporidium* sp.
    C. *Cyclospora* sp.
    D. Microsporidium
21. A 55-year-old female presents to her physician complaining of a fever that "comes and goes" and fatigue. A complete blood count reveals decreased red blood cell count and hemoglobin. There are small, delicate intracellular ring forms seen on the peripheral blood smear. History reveals no travel outside the United States. She had been backpacking along the Appalachian Trail and into the Northeast. You should suspect what condition?
    A. Trypanosomiasis
    B. Babesiosis
    C. Malaria
    D. Filariasis
22. Keratitis is often caused by which of these organisms?
    A. *Naegleria fowleri*
    B. *Acanthamoeba* sp.
    C. *Loa loa*
    D. *Onchocera volvulus*

23. Which of the following would describe the appearance of microsporidia in a modified trichrome stain?
    A. Purple spheres, 10–15 μm in diameter
    B. Pink ovals, 1–3 μm in diameter
    C. Blue ovals, 4–6 μm in diameter
    D. Fluorescent spheres, 8–12 μm in diameter

24. An iodine wet mount from a formalin concentrate of a stool would most likely demonstrate which of the following?
    A. Mature cyst of *E. coli*
    B. Immature cyst of *Dientamoeba fragilis*
    C. Trophozoite stage of *Endolimax nana*
    D. Oocyst of *Cryptosporidium* sp.

25. Serologic testing is the primary method of diagnosing infection with which organism?
    A. *Schistosoma japonicum*
    B. *Cyclospora cayetanensis*
    C. *Naegleria fowleri*
    D. *Toxoplasma gondii*

26. Pneumonia-like complications due to larval migration through the lungs is most likely associated with infection by which organism?
    A. Hookworm
    B. *Schistosoma japonicum*
    C. *Strongyloides stercoralis*
    D. *Ascaris lumbricoides*

27. Infection with which organism may result in vitamin B_{12} deficiency and megaloblastic anemia?
    A. *Diphyllobothrium latum*
    B. Hookworm
    C. *Hymenolepis diminuta*
    D. *Taenia saginata*

28. Knowledge of nocturnal or diurnal periodicity is especially important in the diagnosis of infections caused by:
    A. *Babesia*
    B. *Plasmodium*
    C. Microfilariae
    D. Trypanosomes

29. Humans develop cysticercosis by:
    A. Ingesting eggs of *Taenia solium*
    B. Eating raw meat containing oocysts of *Toxoplasma gondii*
    C. Skin penetration by larva of *Strongyloides stercoralis*
    D. Ingesting metacercaria of *Fasciola hepatica*

30. Which of the following organisms produces an elongated, barrel-shaped egg (50×22 μm) with a colorless polar plug at each end?
    A. *Ascaris lumbricoides*
    B. *Hymenolepis nana*
    C. *Necator americanus*
    D. *Trichuris trichiura*

31. Which of the following *Plasmodium* spp, is associated with the presence of an intracellular crescent-shaped gametocyte?
    A. *P. falciparum*
    B. *P. malariae*
    C. *P. ovale*
    D. *P. vivax*

32. Which organism below would routinely be considered a nonpathogen?
    A. *Endolimax nana*
    B. *Entamoeba histolytica*
    C. *Giardia duodenalis*
    D. *Dientamoeba fragilis*

33. Which of these organisms is characterized by a uninuclear trophozoite?
    A. *Balantidium coli*
    B. *Giardia duodenalis*
    C. *Dientamoeba fragilis*
    D. *Chilomastix mesnili*

34. A physician suspects that a 10-year-old boy has contracted primary amebic meningo-encephalitis. What clinical history would support this diagnosis?
    A. Swimming in warm stagnant water
    B. Leukemia with chemotherapy
    C. Hiking in the desert of Southwest United States
    D. Visits to Massachusetts and the North-east

35. Which of these diseases would least likely to be associated with poor sanitation and transmission by fecally contaminated water or food?
    A. Amebiasis
    B. Ascariasis
    C. Filariasis
    D. Giardiasis

36. Which stage of *Taenia saginata* is usually infective for humans?
    A. Cysticercus larva
    B. Embryonated egg
    C. Filariform larva
    D. Rhabditiform larva

37. An amebic cyst was seen in an iodine wet mount. It is round, approximately 12–15 μm and has three visible nuclei with fine uniform granules of peripheral chromatin and small, central karyosomes. Name the most likely organism.
    A. *Endolimax nana*
    B. *Entamoeba coli*
    C. *Giardia duodenalis*
    D. *Entamoeba histolytica*

38. Which stage of *Trichuris trichiura* is infective for humans?
    A. Proglottid
    B. Filariform larva
    C. Rhabditiform larva
    D. Embryonated egg

39. An iodine-stained fecal wet mount demonstrates a round structure that is 25 μm in diameter with a homogenously stained central body surrounded by a thin ring of cytoplasm containing a number of nuclei. This best describes which organism?
    A. *Blastocystis hominis*
    B. *Endolimax nana*
    C. *Entamoeba dispar*
    D. *Iodamoeba bütschlii*

40. An egg 38 μm in diameter with a thick shell containing radial striations and several hooklets is seen in a wet mount of a fecal specimen. What is the most likely identification of the egg?
    A. *Hymenolepis nana*
    B. *Taenia* sp.
    C. *Schistosoma japonicum*
    D. *Hymenolepis diminuta*

41. Which of the following descriptions would be associated with a life cycle stage of *Plasmodium malariae*?
    A. Banana-shaped organism in a normal size red blood cell
    B. Compact organism with dark pigment in an enlarged, red blood cell with fimbriated edges
    C. 18 merozoites in an enlarged red blood cell with pink dots in the cytoplasm
    D. 6 merozoites in a daisy petal arrangement in a normal-sized red blood cell

42. Which of the following nuclear characteristics are associated with *Entamoeba coli*?
    A. No peripheral chromatin; large karyosome
    B. No peripheral chromatin; irregular clump of four to eight chromatin granules
    C. Coarse, uneven peripheral chromatin; large eccentric karyosome
    D. Fine, even peripheral chromatin; small central karyosome

43. What is the primary diagnostic stage for *Strongyloides stercoralis*?
    A. Adult female in duodenal aspirate
    B. Egg in stool specimen
    C. Rhabditiform larva in stool specimen feces
    D. Filariform larva in stool specimen or sputum

44. Which species of *Plasmodium* is characterized by a trophozoite, with dark coarse pigment, stretching across a normal-sized infected red blood cell?
    A. *P. falciparum*
    B. *P. ovale*
    C. *P. malariae*
    D. *P. cynomolgi*

45. A Giemsa-stained thin blood film showed many small, delicate intracellular ring forms, and a number of the rings had double chromatin dots. These findings are characteristic of:
    A. *Plasmodium falciparum*
    B. *Plasmodium vivax*
    C. *Plasmodium malariae*
    D. *Plasmodium ovale*

46. Unembryonated eggs with an inconspicuous operculum, small knob on the end opposite the operculum and a size ranging from 65 to 75 μm were seen in the stool of a patient who had extensive travel overseas and often ate raw fish. What is the most likely identification?
    A. *Fasciola hepatica*
    B. *Diphyllobothrium latum*
    C. *Paragonimus westermani*
    D. *Clonorchis sinensis*

47. Which of the following pairs of helminths *cannot* be reliably differentiated by the appearance of their eggs?
    A. *Ascaris lumbricoides* and *Fasciola hepatica*
    B. *Hymenolepis nana* and *H. diminuta*
    C. *Necator americanus* and *Ancylostoma duodenale*
    D. *Diphyllobothrium latum* and *Paragonimus westermani*

48. Oval eggs with a thin shell, flattened side, and containing a curved larva were found in a first-morning urine from a 6-year-old child. They measured approximately 52 μm in length. What is the most likely identification?
    A. Hookworm
    B. *Enterobius vermicularis*
    C. *Schistosoma haematobium*
    D. Infertile Ascaris *lumbricoides*

49. Hematuria is a typical sign associated with infection by:
    A. *Trypanosoma cruzi*
    B. *Trichinella spiralis*
    C. *Trichomonas vaginalis*
    D. *Schistosoma haematobium*

50. Which of the following is the vector for *Babesia?*
    A. Fleas
    B. Lice
    C. Ticks
    D. Mosquitoes

51. An 8-year-old child from Guatemala was seen in the public health clinic. The mother said he was always tired and had difficulty breathing when playing. He had low hemoglobin, and examination of a peripheral blood smear showed the presence of an extracellular organism about 18 μm long with an anterior flagellum and prominent nucleus. The organism seen is most likely:
    A. *Trypanosoma brucei*
    B. *Trypanosoma cruzi*
    C. *Leishmania braziliensis*
    D. *Dracunculus medinensis*

52. Which of the following is the preferred anticoagulant for preparing blood smears for diagnosing malaria?
    A. EDTA
    B. Heparin
    C. Sodium citrate
    D. Sodium fluoride

53. Refer to Color Plate 36■. This is a photomicrograph of a peripheral blood smear from an individual who had recently traveled to Africa. She complained of recurring fevers and chills; magnification is 1000×. What is the most likely identification?
    A. *Plasmodium malariae*
    B. *Plasmodium ovale*
    C. *Plasmodium knowlesi*
    D. *Plasmodium vivax*

54. Refer to Color Plate 37■. This is a photomicrograph of an iodine wet prep made from a stool sample; magnification is 400×. The ovum is about 70 × 50 μm. What is the identification of the parasite?
    A. Hookworm
    B. *Enterobius vermicularis*
    C. *Trichuris trichiura*
    D. *Ascaris lumbricoides*

55. Refer to Color Plate 38■. This is a photomicrograph of a trichrome stain from a fecal smear. The magnification is 1000×. The parasite is approximately 20 μm long and 15 μm wide. This is most likely the trophozoite of what organism?
    A. *Chilomastix mesnili*
    B. *Giardia duodenalis*
    C. *Trichomonas hominis*
    D. *Dientamoeba fragilis*

56. Refer to Color Plate 39■. This is a photomicrograph of a trichrome stain from a fecal smear. The magnification is 1000×. The parasite is approximately 12 μm in diameter. What is the identification of this parasite?
    A. *Iodamoeba butschlii*
    B. *Entamoeba hartmani*
    C. *Dientamoeba fragilis*
    D. *Endolimax nana*

57. Refer to Color Plate 40■. This is a photomicrograph of an iodine wet-mount from a fecal sample. The magnification is 1000×. The parasite is approximately 25 μm in diameter. What is the identification of this cyst?
    A. *Entamoeba histolytica*
    B. *Entamoeba hartmanni*
    C. *Entamoeba coli*
    D. *Entamoeba dispar*

58. Refer to Color Plate 41■. This is a photomicrograph of a trichrome stained fecal smear. The magnification is 1000×. The organism is approximately 11 × 9 μm. What is the identification of this parasite?
    A. *Giardia duodenalis* cyst
    B. *Dientamoeba fragilis* trophozoite
    C. *Endolimax nana* cyst
    D. *Entamoeba hartmanni* cyst

59. Refer to Color Plate 42■. This is a photomicrograph of a trichrome stain from a fecal smear. The magnification is 1000×. The parasite is approximately 15 μm in diameter. What is the identification of this parasite?
    A. *Entamoeba hartmanni*
    B. *Dientamoeba fragilis*
    C. *Iodamoeba bütschlii*
    D. *Blastocystis hominis*

60. Refer to Color Plate 43■. This is a photomicrograph of a blood smear stained with Wright's stain. Identify the parasite.
    A. *Babesia* sp.
    B. *Plasmodium malariae*
    C. *Plasmodium falciparum*
    D. *Plasmodium vivax*

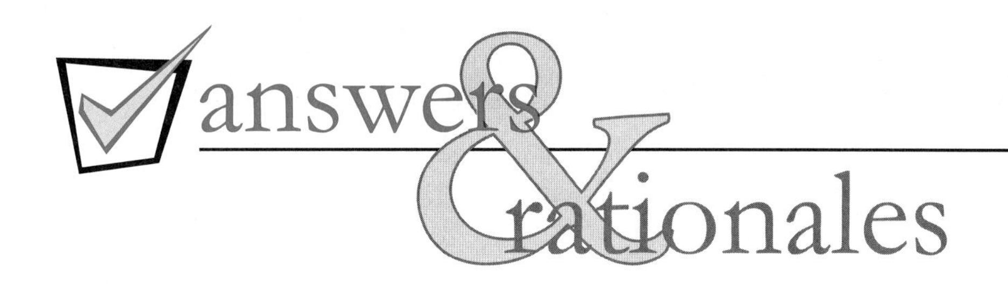

1.

A. Because the eggs of *E. vermicularis* are usually deposited on the perianal area, cellulose tape slides (or sticky paddles) are recommended for collecting the eggs. Recovery is best if specimens are collected late in the evening or before bathing or defecating in the morning. The gravid female worms usually migrate at night to the perianal region to deposit eggs. Because their migration is sporadic, several consecutive collections may be necessary to detect the infection.

2.

C. Humans becomes infected with *Ascaris lumbricoides, Enterobius vermicularis*, and *Trichuris trichiura* by ingesting the egg. *Necator americanus* (hookworm) infects humans when the skin is penetrated by the filariform larva. The larva migrates through the blood stream and eventually matures into an adult in the intestine.

3.

C. Fresh liquid stools are more likely to contain motile protozoan trophozoites that can be detected in saline wet mounts. Urine in stool specimens can damage parasite morphology, as does freezing. Unpreserved stool specimens should only be left at room temperature up to a couple of hours before examining or placing into a preservative.

4.

B. Cysts are the infective stage of most intestinal protozoa. However, *D. fragilis* does not have a cyst stage, and the trophozoite is considered the infective stage.

5.

C. *N. fowleri* is the causative agent of primary amebic meningoencephalitis. Therefore, the cerebrospinal fluid sediment would be the primary specimen used to look for the trophozoite. Corneal scrapings and skin biopsy may be used for diagnosing infection with *Acanthamoeba* sp. Blood smears would be used for stages of organisms such as those causing malaria.

6.

B. In parasites with a sexual and asexual stage of development, the definitive host is the host in which the sexual stage of the parasite occurs. The intermediate host is the host in which the asexual stage of the parasite is found. Vectors are arthropods, like mosquitoes and ticks that transmit infectious agents. A commensal is an organism that benefits from an existence with a host but does not damage the host.

7.

D. *E. histolytica* is a pathogenic organism characterized by its ability to ingest red blood cells. No other intestinal amoebae or flagellates shares this characteristic. *Giardia* and *Dientamoeba* are also considered pathogens; *Entamoeba coli* is considered a nonpathogen.

8.

A. Mature cysts of *I. bütschlii* are usually ovoid, with a single nucleus with a large eccentric karyosome. The cytoplasm contains a compact mass of glycogen, which appears as a clear, well-defined area in unstained or permanently stained preparations but stains dark brown with iodine. Chromatoidal bars are not present. Ingested bacteria are often seen in the cytoplasm of trophozoites.

9.

D. *E. histolytica* and *E. dispar* cannot be morphologically differentiated. The cyst stage of both organisms has four nuclei with a centrally located karyosome and fine, evenly distributed peripheral chromatin. *E. histolytica* is a well-recognized intestinal parasite, whereas *E. dispar* is considered nonpathogenic. Immunologic assays to detect antigens or molecular biology assays are necessary to differentiate these two species.

10.

C. The characteristics describe an egg of hookworm. Although *E. vermicularis* also has a thin shell, it is flattened on one side and usually contains a C-shaped larva. Eggs of *Strongyloides* may resemble those of hookworm; however, they are not routinely found in the feces. *T. trichiura* eggs are barrel shaped with polar plugs.

11.

B. The symptoms and history for this patient are compatible with trypanosomiasis (African sleeping sickness) caused by *T. brucei*. The trypomastigote form of the parasite was found in peripheral blood smears from this patient. Another key clinical sign is the presence of swollen lymph nodes at the posterior base of the neck, known as Winterbottom's sign. *T. cruzi* is the cause of American trypanosomiasis. *B. malayi* infection would demonstrate presence of a microfilaria in the blood. *Leishmania* spp. would be seen as intracellular amastigotes in skin or other organs.

12.

D. The trophozoites of *P. vivax* are described as ameboid and may have large vacuoles; infected red blood cells (RBCs) contain small pink dots called Shüffner's dots. *P. malariae* cytoplasm is much more compact, and infected RBCs lack Shüffner's dots. *P. ovale* resembles *P. vivax*. Shüffner's dots are generally found in *P. vivax* and *P. ovale*-infected RBCs; however, *P. ovale*-infected RBCs have fimbriated edges. Growing trophozoites of *P. falciparum* seen in the peripheral blood remain in the ring form, and infected RBCs lack malarial pigment. *P. knowlesi* is rarely a human pathogen.

13.

C. The permanently stained smear is especially recommended for identification of trophozoites, for confirmation of species, and for keeping a permanent record of the organisms found. Species identification of amebic trophozoites can rarely be made from a single feature; permanent stains enable one to observe the cytoplasm, cytoplasmic inclusions, and the nuclear morphologic features of many cells. Iron hematoxylin and trichrome are commonly used stains.

14.

B. *Babesia* spp. are sporozoan parasites of RBCs that have been recognized as causing febrile illness in humans. *B. microti* has caused a number of tick-borne infections in the United States. The parasites often appear as small rings within infected RBCs, resembling *P. falciparum* trophozoites. The pathognomic form of *Babesia* is the "Maltese cross," four ring forms inside a single RBC. *T. cruzi* has a trypomastigote as the diagnostic stage. *T. gondii* has intracellular forms found in tissue.

15.

D. Polyvinyl alcohol (PVA) is a commonly used fixative for stool specimens. This preservative contains mercury and is used to fix fecal samples for making permanently stained smears. Formalin is commonly used to preserve stool samples in preparation for concentration procedures. Sodium acetate is used with formalin to preserve fecal specimens, but it does not contain mercury and is, therefore, less toxic. Buffered glycerol is sometimes used as a transport medium for stool samples when performing a bacterial culture.

16.

B. Although all the organisms listed have some degree of acid-fast positivity, only *Cyclospora* forms oocysts in the size range of 8–10 μm. The oocysts of *Cryptosporidium* are generally 4–6 μm in diameter and are generally strongly acid-fast positive. Oocysts of *Cystoisospora* are much larger, approximately 25 × 18 μm. Microsporidia are acid-fast variable, and this stain is not recommended for detecting microsporidia. The spores of microsporidia are generally 1–3 μm in diameter.

17.

C. The presence of muscle pain and periorbital edema (swelling around the eyes) in this patient is suggestive of trichinosis. The highly elevated eosinophil count is also characteristic of parasitic infection in the tissues.

18.

C. Ova of *Schistosoma* spp. contain a spine. *S. haematobium* ova have a prominent spine on one end. *S. mansoni* eggs have a prominent lateral spine, whereas the spine of *S. japonicum* is small and inconspicuous. *S. mekongi* is a rare human pathogen.

19.

D. Adult filarial helminths typically inhabit the lymph vessels. They produce inflammation and swelling of the lymph vessels, often in the legs and sometimes the scrotum. This condition is referred to as elephantiasis. The larvae are highly motile and migrate through the body.

20.

B. Although all these organisms are potential pathogens of patients who are immunocompromised, only *Cryptosporidium* produces acid-fast-positive oocysts about 4–6 μm in diameter. The oocysts of *Cyclospora* measure approximately 8–10 μm. The spores of microsporidia are generally 1–3 μm in diameter. Most hospitals today use antigen detection methods to diagnose *Cryptosporidium* infection.

21.

B. The ring forms of *P. falciparum* and *Babesia* sp. are similar. In this case the lack of travel out of the country and travel to the Northeast where *Babesia* infections are endemic suggest babesiosis. Both organisms may cause hemolysis of the RBC leading to a decreased hemoglobin. Trypomastigotes and microfilaria are large, extracellular organisms in the blood.

22.

B. *Acanthamoeba* is a free-living ameba rarely causing human infections. This organism has been associated with granulomatous infections of the skin and lung, as well as meningoencephalitis. However, the most common presentation is keratitis (infection of the cornea), associated with contact lenses. *L. loa* and *O. volvulus* are microfilarial infections. Although *L. loa* adults may be found migrating across the eye, they are not commonly associated with keratitis.

23.

B. The small size and variable staining of the microsporidia make their detection difficult. Tissue examination by electron microscopy is the most specific diagnostic method. In the modified trichrome stain, one of the stains (chromotrope 2R) is used at 10 times the normal concentration. In addition, the staining time is increased to 90 minutes. Alternatively, 15 minutes in heated stain can be used. Under these staining conditions, the spores of microsporidia stain as pinkish ovals, 1–3 μm.

24.

A. A wet mount of a fecal concentrate will not demonstrate trophozoites as they are generally destroyed during processing. *D. fragilis* exists only in trophozoite form and requires a permanently stained smear to demonstrate its presence. *Cryptosporidium* sp. oocysts are small (4-6 um) and frequently require an acid-fast stain to demonstrate their presence.

25.

D. *T. gondii* is a protozoan parasite of humans that generally exists in multiple tissues as a cyst-like form. In humans, there are no forms excreted from the body. Therefore, serologic testing for either IgM antibodies (acute infection) or IgG antibodies (past infection) is the method of choice for detecting infection. The other organisms have life cycle forms that can be detected in stools (*S. japonicum* and *C. cayetanensis*) or cerebrospinal fluid (*N. fowleri*).

26.

D. All of the listed organisms have a larval stage that migrates through the blood stream. However, the larval forms of *A. lumbricoides* are known to cause a pneumonitis-like reaction, especially after repeated exposures.

27.

A. *D. latum* is a tapeworm that has been linked to vitamin B_{12} deficiencies in individuals of Scandinavian descent. *T. saginata* and *H. diminuta* are tapeworms that infect the gastrointestinal tract of humans but have not been linked to vitamin B_{12} deficiencies. Hookworm infections have been associated with a microcytic, hypochromic anemia.

28.

C. Transmission of filariasis depends on the presence of microfilariae in the bloodstream at the time the vector bites, and the periodicity of microfilariae in the peripheral blood varies with the species and sometimes with the geographic area. Nocturnal periodicity is marked in *W. bancrofti* in Africa, Asia, and the western hemisphere, and thick blood films for detection of these microfilariae should be made between 10 P.M. and midnight. The other choices do not exhibit nocturnal periodicity.

29.

A. Ingestion of *T. solium* eggs by humans results in individuals becoming the intermediate host in the life cycle. This host is characterized by the presence of the cysticerci in tissue. Eating raw meat would result in ingesting the cysticerci and becoming a host to the adult tapeworm. Metacercaria and other larva are not stages in the life cycle of the pork tapeworm.

30.

D. Typical eggs of *T. trichiura* are yellow to brown, with colorless polar plugs. They are shaped like a football or a barrel, and they are in the cellular, or unsegmented stage, when passed in the feces. The usual egg range is 49–65 × 35–45 μm. *Necator* eggs have a thin shell with a four- to eight-cell stage embryo. *Ascaris* eggs are characterized by a thick mammilated shell. *H. nana* has a double wall with the presence of polar filaments.

31.

A. The gametocytes of *P. vivax, P. malariae*, and *P. ovale* are round and somewhat similar in appearance. Those of *P. falciparum* have a typical crescent or banana shape. The gametocytes of *P. falciparum* may remain in the peripheral blood a month or more and are often found with the ring stages.

32.

A. *E. nana* is considered a nonpathogenic ameba. *E. histolytica* is a known pathogen associated with amebic dysentery. *Giardia* and *D. fragilis* are also considered pathogens. *Giardia* may cause malabsorption. *Dientamoeba* is considered a mildly pathogenic organism that causes diarrhea, especially in children.

33.

D. *C. mesnili* is the only trophozoite which always has a single nucleus. *B. coli* has a kidney bean–shaped macronucleus and a small round micronucleus (rarely seen). *Giardia* has two large nuclei and *Dientamoeba* is usually binucleated although there are some uninucleated forms.

34.

A. *N. fowleri* is found in warm freshwater ponds and lakes, especially those with disturbed or suspended soil. It has caused a number of cases of primary amebic meningoencephalitis in children and adults who have swum in these bodies of water. Diagnosis is difficult as the symptoms resemble those of bacterial meningitis and identification of the organism in spinal fluid is difficult.

35.

C. Infectious cysts of amebae and *G. duodenalis* and eggs of *A. lumbricoides* may all be ingested in fecally contaminated water or food. These infections are most prevalent in areas lacking good public sanitation, that is, sanitary disposal of human waste and adequately treated and protected drinking water. Filariasis is transmitted by blood-feeding insects (vectors).

36.

A. Humans are infected with *T. saginata* by eating beef containing live cysticerci, the infectious larval stage of this parasite. Cattle become infected by ingesting viable eggs from human feces. Unlike *T. solium*, if humans ingest *T. saginata* ova, infection with the cysticercus does not develop.

37.

D. Cysts of *E. histolytica* are round and range from 10 to 20 μm with characteristic nuclei (small central karyosome and even peripheral chromatin). Although *E. hartmanni* has morphologically identical nuclei, its size range is 5–10 μm, *Giardia* nuclei lack peripheral chromatin and have large prominent karyosomes. *E. coli* may have up to eight nuclei with uneven peripheral chromatin and large, eccentric karyosomes.

38.

D. The fertilized ova of *T. trichiura* are unembryonated when released, and embryonic development occurs outside of the host. In moist, warm, shaded soil, the first-stage larva develops within the egg in about 2 weeks. This fully embryonated egg is infective when ingested by a susceptible host, and it hatches in the small intestine. During development from larva to adult, the worm usually passes to the cecum, where it embeds its slender anterior portion in the intestinal mucosa.

39.

A. The most common form of *B. hominis* seen in human feces is called the "classic form." This form contains a central body that was previously thought to be a vacuole. The central body can take up to 90% of the volume of the cell, displacing the nuclei to the outer edge of the cell. The other organisms will show nuclei distributed throughout the cytoplasm.

40.

B. *Taenia* sp. eggs are characteristically round with a thick shell with radial striations. *H. nana* and *H. diminuta* also have a hexacanth embryo but the shells are thin and *H. nana* will have polar filaments present. *D. latum* lacks a hexacanth embryo. *S. japonicum* will have a thin shell with a small curved inconspicuous spine.

41.

D. The description fits that of a schizont of *P. malariae*. *P. vivax* will have between 12 and 24 merozoites in an enlarged RBC. *P. ovale* trophozoites are compact and in an enlarged, oval RBC that will show fimbriated edges. *P. falciparum* demonstrates a banana-shaped gametocyte.

42.

C. The nuclear description fits that of *E. coli*. *E. nana* lacks peripheral chromatin around the karyosome. *D. fragilis* nuclei also lack peripheral chromatin and have a clump of chromatin granules forming the karyosome. *E. histolytica* nuclei will have even peripheral chromatin and a small central karyosome.

43.

C. The rhabditiform larvae of *S. stercoralis* are the diagnostic stage typically passed in the feces of infected persons. The larvae measure up to 380 μm long $\times$ 20 μm wide. They have a short buccal cavity and a prominent, ovoid, genital primordium midway along the ventral wall of the body. The infective stage is the filariform larva, which differs from the hookworm filariform larva by having a notched tail tip and a long esophagus.

44.

C. *P. malariae* is characterized by the band form trophozoite. Pigment is often dark brown to black and is large and coarse. Infected RBCs are not enlarged. Cells infected with *P. ovale* are enlarged and oval and have fimbriated edges. *P. falciparum* has small delicate ring-form trophozoites. *P. cynomolgi* is found in primates.

45.

A. *P. falciparum* infections tend to produce a large number of rings that frequently have double chromatin, which is only occasionally found in other species. *P. falciparum* differs from other plasmodia of humans in that only early trophozoites (ring forms) and gametocytes are found in peripheral blood except in severe cases. Sex differentiation of the gametes, when present, is difficult.

46.

B. The description fits that of eggs of *D. latum*. This is also supported by the patient's history of travel and ingesting raw fish. Eggs of *F. hepatica* have an inconspicuous operculum but are much larger in size. *P. westermani* has a flattened, shouldered operculum and lacks the knob. *C. sinensis* does have a knob opposite the operculum but the operculum is domed and the egg is much smaller.

47.

C. *N. americanus* and *A. duodenale* are two species of hookworms infecting humans. Their eggs are so similar when found in stool specimens that they are reported as "hookworm ova." The two hookworms can be differentiated by the morphologic characteristics of the adult worms, which are intestinal parasites.

48.

B. The description matches that of *E. vermicularis* eggs. Because the eggs are laid in the perianal area at night, it is possible to find some that may have dropped off the body in a first-morning urine. *S. haematobium* eggs are found in urine but they are larger and have a terminal spine. Hookworm eggs also have a thin shell but have a four- to eight-cell embryo and are found in feces. Eggs of *A. lumbricoides* are larger and have a brown bumpy (mamillated) coating.

49.

D. A common sign of *S. haematobium* infection is the presence of blood in the urine. This is due to the damage caused when the eggs break out of the blood vessels of the vesicular plexus into the bladder. Falciparum malaria may also cause severe hemoglobinuria or "blackwater fever."

50.

C. *B. microti* is a sporozoan parasite commonly found in voles and field mice. The vector is the tick *Ixodes*, normally a parasite of deer. Humans are accidental hosts when bitten by an infected tick. Many *B. microti* infections within the United States occur in the Northeast. It is important to differentiate this parasite from *Plasmodium* in a stained blood film. Antimalarial drugs are not effective in babesiosis.

51.

B. Chagas disease is found throughout the American continents. The infectious agent, *T. cruzi*, is transmitted to humans by reduviid bugs, primarily the triatomids. Chagas disease can be acute or chronic. The trypomastigote is found in blood during the acute phase. *T. brucei* is associated with African sleeping sickness.

52.

A. Collection of blood by finger stick is preferred for preparing blood smears for the detection of malaria. When a venipuncture is performed, the preferred anticoagulant for malarial blood smears is EDTA (ethylenediaminetetraacetic acid). Heparin can be used, but it may cause distortion of some parasite forms.

53.

D. The trophozoite, seen in Color Plate 36■, is that of *P. vivax*. The shape is ameboid; the infected RBC is enlarged. There are faint Schüffners dots. *P. malariae* would show compact trophozoites in normal-sized RBCs. *P. ovale* would demonstrate a compact trophozoite and the infected RBC would be enlarged and oval and possibly have fimbriated edges. *P. knowlesi* is considered a primate malaria but may infect humans. Trophozoites of *P. knowlesi* are morphologically similar to those of *P. falciparum*.

54.

D. Color Plate 37■ demonstrates a fertilized egg of *A. lumbricoides*. Eggs measure 45–75 × 35–50 μm. The thick, brown, mamillated coating is typical of *Ascaris*. Although the size range of all eggs overlap, hookworm eggs and the eggs of *E. vermicularis* have thin shells. *T. trichiura* has a barrel shape, thick shell, and polar plugs.

55.

B. Color Plate 38■ demonstrates a *G. duodenalis* trophozoite; notice the two prominent nuclei. Trophozoites of *C. mesnili* are approximately 6–24 μm in length but have a single nucleus, whereas *G. duodenalis* trophozoites have two nuclei. Trophozoites of *Trichomonas* are about the same size as *G. duodenalis*, but they are rounder than the pear-shaped trophozoites of *G. duodenalis* and *C. mesnili*. *Trichomonas* spp. have a single nucleus. *D. fragilis* would demonstrate an ameboid shape and have two nuclei that are composed of four to eight chromatin granules.

answers & rationales

56.

C. Color Plate 39■ demonstrates a *D. fragilis* trophozoite. Although this organism lacks a flagellum and morphologically resembles the ameba, based on its ultrastructure and molecular biology studies, it is classified as a flagellate. Like the trichomonads, *D. fragilis* does not have a cyst stage. Most trophozoites of *D. fragilis* have two nuclei; none of the other organisms are binucleated. *E. hartmanni* would demonstrate peripheral chromatin on the nuclear membrane. Both *I. butschlii* and *E. nana* have large karyosomes with no peripheral chromatin.

57.

C. Color Plate 40■ demonstrates an *E. coli* cyst. These cysts may resemble *E. histolytica* and *E. dispar*. The key distinguishing feature is that *E. coli* cysts contain up to eight nuclei, whereas *E. histolytica* and *E. dispar* have up to four nuclei. *E. coli* cysts are larger than those of *E. histolytica* and *E. dispar*. Although nuclear detail is difficult to determine in an iodine prep, the presence of eccentric karyosomes and irregular coarse peripheral chromatin may be seen in several nuclei. It is often necessary to use the fine adjustment to see all the nuclei. In this image, six nuclei can be seen.

58.

A. Color Plate 41■ demonstrates a cyst of *G. duodenalis*. The oval shape, large karyosomes, and presence of curved median bodies are keys to identification. *D. fragilis* lacks a cyst form, and trophozoites frequently demonstrate two nuclei with four to eight chromatin granules inside the nuclear membrane. Both *E. nana* and *E. hartmanni* cysts would have up to four nuclei; those of *E. hartmanni* would demonstrate peripheral chromatin. Cysts of *E. nana* would show large karyosomes but no median bodies would be present.

59.

D. Color Plate 42■ demonstrates the "classic form" of *B. hominis*., rRNA studies indicate it is related to algae and water molds. The classic form usually seen in human feces varies in size from 6 to 40 μm in diameter. It contains a large central body, resembling a vacuole that pushes several nuclei to the periphery of the cell.

60.

A. Color Plate 43■ demonstrates multiple RBCs infected with *Babesia* sp. There are small single ring forms in several RBCs of normal size. There is also a "Maltese cross" form present which helps to distinguish it from *P. falciparum*. There is no pigment present. A trophozoite stretching across the infected RBC, called a band form would be characteristic of *P. malariae*. Trophozoites of *P. vivax* would be ameboid and the infected RBCs would be enlarged.

REFERENCES

Tille, P. (2018). *Bailey and Scott's Diagnostic Microbiology*, 14th ed. Philadelphia: Mosby.

Garcia, L. S. (2016). *Diagnostic Medical Parasitology*, 6th ed. Washington, DC: American Society for Microbiology Press.

Mahon, C. R., and Lehman, D. C. (2018). *Textbook of Diagnostic Microbiology*, 6th ed. St. Louis: Saunders Elsevier.

Carroll, K. C., et. al. (Eds.) (2019). *Manual of Clinical Microbiology*, 12th ed. Washington, DC: American Society for Microbiology Press.

Soares, R., and Tasca, T. Giardiasis: an update review on sensitivity and specificity of methods for laboratorial diagnosis. *Journal of Microbiol Methods* 2016. 129:98-102.

CHAPTER

9 Virology

contents

I. INTRODUCTION

A. General Characteristics of Viruses

1. Viruses are acellular, **obligate intracellular parasites unable to self-replicate.** Once inside living cells, viruses induce the host cell to synthesize virus particles. For these reasons, they are generally considered nonliving.
2. With rare exceptions, the genome is either **DNA or RNA** (single or double stranded).
3. Viruses do not have a system to produce ATP.
4. Viruses range in size from 25 to 270 nm.
5. The classification of viruses is based on nucleic acid type, size and shape of virion, and presence or absence of an envelope.
6. Chemotherapeutic agents active against bacteria have no effect on viruses. Therapy is centered around destruction of viral-infected host cells.

B. Viral Structure

1. **Virion** is the entire viral particle.
2. **Capsid** is the protein coat that encloses the genetic material.
3. **Capsomer** is the protein subunit that makes up the capsid.
4. **Nucleocapsid** is composed of the capsid and genetic material.
5. The **envelope** is the outer coating composed of a **phospholipid bilayer** derived from a host cell's membrane, and containing viral-encoded glycoproteins and sometimes viral-encoded matrix proteins. Some viruses use the plasma membrane, whereas others use endoplasmic reticulum, Golgi, or nuclear membranes. **Naked nucleocapsids** are viruses with no envelopes.

C. Replication

1. **Adsorption** is attachment of the virus to a specific receptor on the host cell.
2. **Penetration** is entry of the virus into the host cell.
3. **Uncoating** occurs when there is either the separation of the capsid from the genome or rearrangement of the capsid proteins exposing the genome for transcription and replication.
4. The **eclipse period** is the stage when the genetic material is replicated but intact virions are not yet detectable.
   a. Viral DNA or RNA serves as the template for mRNA production.
   b. mRNA codes for viral protein and enzymes necessary for nucleic acid synthesis.
5. **Assembly (maturation):** Genetic material is assembled into a protein coat (capsid).
6. Viruses are then released from the host cell.
   a. **Cell lysis:** Naked viruses lyse host cell and leave through a hole in the plasma membrane.

b. **Budding:** Intact virion pushes outward from a host's membrane. The membrane wraps around the virion; the membrane is cleaved and then resealed around the virion, thus becoming the viral envelope.

D. Specimen Processing for Diagnosing Viral Diseases

1. Viruses are in highest concentrations during the first several days following onset of symptoms. Therefore, samples should be collected early in the disease course.
2. While bacterial contamination typically will not impact nonculture viral detection, specimens should be obtained aseptically whenever possible.
3. Swabs generally do not collect sufficient material. If swabs are used, FLOQSwabs™ (Copan, Brescia, Italy) should be used.
4. Samples should generally come from the infected site.
   a. **Skin infections:** Rash site and, depending on the virus, serum and urine
   b. **Respiratory infections:** Sputum, nasal swabs, nasal washings, or throat swabs; aspirates and washes generally better than swabs
   c. **Central nervous system** (e.g., meningitis and encephalitis): For diagnosis of meningitis, cerebrospinal fluid (CSF) and serum, as well as stool or throat swabs, can be collected because viruses are sometimes shed into these sites. In cases of encephalitis, brain biopsy material and sometimes serum are used.
   d. **Blood (venipuncture) and bone marrow aspirate:** Specimens should be collected in the anticoagulants ethylenediaminetetraacetic acid (EDTA) or acid-citrate-dextrose.
   e. **Urogenital infections:** Needle aspirates, and endocervical and urethral swabs
   f. **Gastrointestinal tract:** Stool samples and rectal swabs
   g. **Eye infections:** Eye swabs and corneal scrapings

E. Sample Transport

1. Samples for viral culture must be placed into a **viral transport medium** (VTM).
2. VTM contains the following:
   a. Buffered saline
   b. Protein stabilizers
   c. Antimicrobials that inhibit bacterial and fungal growth
3. Samples for viral cultures can be refrigerated in VTM for about 24 to 48 hours, but they should never be frozen at −20°C. Samples can be stored at −70°C; however, infectivity will be diminished.
4. Samples received after extensive delay in collecting or not in VTM should be rejected after consultation with the primary care provider.

F. Prions

1. **Pro**teinaceous **in**fectious particles
2. They cause progressive relentless degeneration of the central nervous system conditions referred to as transmissible spongiform encephalopathies. The disease in humans is called Creutzfeldt-Jakob disease.

II. SAMPLE SITES AND ASSOCIATED VIRAL AGENTS

A. Respiratory System

1. **Upper respiratory tract** infections are commonly caused by viruses, including rhinovirus, influenza virus, parainfluenza virus, respiratory syncytial virus (RSV), Epstein-Barr virus (EBV), metapneumovirus, and coronavirus.
2. **Croup and bronchitis** can be caused by influenza virus, parainfluenza virus, RSV, and adenovirus.
3. **Pneumonia in children** can be caused by **RSV,** parainfluenza virus, adenovirus, metapneumovirus, and varicella-zoster virus (VZV).
4. **Pneumonia in adults** can be caused by influenza virus, VZV, cytomegalovirus (CMV), metapneumovirus, coronavirus, and RSV.

B. Viral Meningitis

1. Caused by enterovirus, echovirus, herpes simplex virus type 1 (HSV-1), HSV-2, and VZV
2. Viral meningitis is often less severe than bacterial meningitis. **Aseptic meningitis** is an older term referring to meningitis not caused by easily cultured bacteria. The term has become synonymous with viral meningitis.

C. Encephalitis

1. Encephalitis typically has a viral etiology. Infections are caused by HSV, VZV, and **arboviruses.** Arboviruses are genetically unrelated viruses transmitted by arthropods (e.g., mosquitoes); they include the families *Togaviridae* (eastern and western equine viruses) and *Flaviviridae* (West Nile virus and St. Louis encephalitis virus). A number of animals, including birds and horses, serve as reservoirs for these viruses. Rabies virus is also an uncommon cause of encephalitis.
2. Encephalitis is an infection of the brain or spinal cord and is much more severe than viral meningitis.

D. Cutaneous Infections

1. Caused by HSV-1, HSV-2, VZV, echovirus, measles virus, rubella virus, enterovirus, molluscum contagiosum virus, and parvovirus B-19
2. Cutaneous infections often result in a rash that, depending on the virus, can have a variety of presentations.

E. Genital Infections (Urethritis, Cervicitis, etc.)

1. Frequently caused by HSV-2 and human papillomavirus
2. Genital tract infections are typically sexually transmitted.

F. Gastroenteritis

1. Caused by a number of viruses, including **rotaviruses, Norwalk viruses,** noroviruses adenoviruses, and calciviruses

2. The symptoms can range from mild self-limiting diarrhea to severe diarrhea with dehydration, particularly with **rotavirus** infections in young children.

G. Eye Infections

1. Caused by HSV, adenovirus, and VZV
2. Viruses can cause conjunctivitis and severe cases of keratitis, resulting in blindness.

H. Neonatal Infections

1. Neonatal infections are acquired *in utero,* during childbirth, or soon after childbirth (perinatally).
2. The infections can be caused by HSV, CMV, and rubella virus.

III. VIRAL IDENTIFICATION

A. Histology and Cytology

1. Cellular inclusions are diagnostic for many viruses. Visible changes in cells due to virus are referred to as **cytopathic effect** (CPE).
2. Because most **DNA viruses** replicate in the nucleus, they often produce nuclear inclusions. However, some DNA viruses are assembled elsewhere in the cell.
3. **RNA viruses** produce cytoplasmic inclusions (assembled in the cytoplasm).
4. HSV and VZV cause intranuclear inclusions. CMV induces enlarged (cytomegalic) cells with a basophilic intranuclear inclusion referred to as **"owl eye" inclusion.**
5. Microscopic examination of tissue is not a sensitive method of diagnosing viral infections and is therefore not commonly performed. One exception is Pap smears, cervical samples collected for detecting cervical cancer and human papillomavirus infection.

B. Viral Isolation

1. **Cell culture**
   a. Because of the expense, expertise required, and time for results, cell culture is no longer an important means of diagnosing viral infections. Clinical specimens are processed and added to cell cultures. Viruses have an affinity for specific cell types (e.g., respiratory epithelium, neurons, etc.). Propagation of viruses is therefore dependent upon providing suitable host cells. Some viruses have not yet been grown *in vitro.*
   b. **Primary cell cultures** are derived directly from tissue. These cells have a normal number of chromosomes (diploid) and are permissive for a number of viruses, but they can only be maintained for a short time in the laboratory. An example of a primary cell line is primary monkey kidney cells. Transferring cells from one container (e.g., test tube or flask) to another is called **"splitting"**

or **"passaging."** Primary cell lines can only be passaged a few times. They are used to grow influenza virus, parainfluenza virus, enteroviruses, and adenoviruses.

c. **Established cell lines,** also referred to as low passage or finite cell lines, are also diploid. They can be maintained longer than primary cell lines, but they are not as permissive. Examples of established cell lines include WI-38, MRC-5, and IMR-90.

d. **Continuous cell lines** are altered cells that can be maintained indefinitely. These cells are **heteroploid,** having an abnormal karyotype from the original parent cell. HeLa, HEp-2, A549, and Vero cells are examples of continuous cell lines. They can be used to grow HSV, VZV, CMV, adenovirus, and rhinoviruses.

e. Slides are made from infected cell cultures and examined for CPE, including clumping, vacuoles, inclusions, granules, cell fusion (i.e., **syncytium**—multinucleated cell development), and cellular destruction. However, many viruses replicate without producing CPE.

2. Embryonated eggs are sometimes used for growth of viruses. Eggs are not typically used for diagnosis of viral infection but to cultivate viruses for research studies and vaccine preparation, as in the case of influenza virus.
3. Animal models are sometimes used in research studies.

C. Electron Microscopy

1. Due to size, most individual virions can only be seen by electron microscopy. However, the poxviruses are about the size of some small bacteria.
2. Electron microscopy is expensive, requires expertise, and is usually insensitive. For these reasons, electron microscopy is not commonly used.

D. Other Methods for Identification

1. Detection of host antibodies directed against specific viruses is useful in many cases and is the method generally used for screening.
2. Direct detection of viral antigens in clinical specimens is commonly used. These assays provide accurate results quickly and are less expensive than nucleic acid amplification tests (NAATs).
3. Viral gene probes and NAATs (e.g., polymerase chain reaction [PCR]) have become the preferred method for diagnosing viral infections. These assays are typically highly sensitive and specific and rapid. Assays from many viruses are available for several manufacturers.

IV. MEDICALLY IMPORTANT DNA VIRUSES

A. Herpesviruses

1. **General characteristics**

a. Herpesviruses capsids are icosahedral shaped, have an envelope, and range in size from 90 to 100 nm. Table 9-1■ lists some medically important DNA viruses.

TABLE 9-1 FAMILIES OF DNA VIRUSES

Family	Important Human Viruses
Poxviridae	Variola virus, molluscum contagiosum virus
Herpesviridae	Herpes simplex viruses types 1 and 2, varicella-zoster virus, Epstein-Barr virus, cytomegalovirus, human herpesviruses 6, 7, and 8
Adenoviridae	Adenovirus
Hepadnaviridae	Hepatitis B virus
Papillomaviridae	Papillomavirus
Polyomaviridae	JC and BK viruses
Parvoviridae	Parvovirus B19

b. They are members of the family ***Herpesviridae.***
c. Except for neonates, infections are generally more severe in adults than in children.
d. All herpesviruses produce **latent infections.** Viral genome will persist in host cell chromosomes, and viral replication can occur at a later time.
e. Sites of latency include **leukocytes** and **peripheral nerves.**
f. **Reactivation** may result from physiological stress. The symptoms are milder than primary infection. The exception is shingles, which is a reactivation of VZV.
g. Herpesviruses include VZV, HSV-1 and HSV-2, CMV, EBV, and human herpes viruses 6, 7, and 8 (HHV-6, HHV-7, and HHV-8). Table 9-2■ lists important clinical manifestations associated with the herpesviruses.

2. **Herpes simplex virus type 1**
   a. HSV-1 causes mouth lesions and **fever blisters** (i.e., cold sores). Most cases are very mild, and symptoms may include mild fever and general malaise. Infections can also be asymptomatic.
   b. **Diagnosis** is by clinical symptoms, immunologic assays that detect viral antigens, and viral isolation.
3. **Herpes simplex virus type 2**
   a. HSV-2 is a causative agent of genital herpes, a common sexually transmitted disease (STD). HSV-1 causes about 20% of genital herpes cases.
   b. Lesions appear on the penis, cervix, and vagina.
   c. Infant infection acquired during childbirth can cause severe eye infections and central nervous system (CNS) damage.
   d. **Diagnosis** is by clinical signs and symptoms, NAATs, immunologic assays that detect viral antigens, and sometimes viral isolation and serology.
4. **Varicella-zoster virus**
   a. **Chickenpox**
      1) Before routine use of a vaccine, chickenpox was a common childhood disease. Symptoms are more severe in adults than children.

TABLE 9-2 MAJOR CLINICAL SYNDROMES OF HUMAN HERPESVIRUSES

Virus	Major Clinical Syndrome	Site of Latent Infection
Herpes simplex virus Type 1	Gingivostomatitis in children and young adults, recurrent oral-labial infection (cold sores), infection of the cornea (keratitis), herpes encephalitis	Trigeminal nerve root ganglion and autonomic ganglia of superior cervical and vagus nerves
Type 2	Genital herpes, neonatal herpes	Sacral nerve root ganglia
Varicella-zoster	Chickenpox (primary infection), shingles or zoster (reactivation)	Thoracic, cervical or lumbar nerve root ganglia
Cytomegalovirus	Asymptomatic infection, heterophile-negative mononucleosis, fever hepatitis syndrome in neonates and patients undergoing transplants, interstitial pneumonia in patients who are immunocompromised	Leukocytes (neutrophils and lymphocytes)
Epstein-Barr virus	Heterophile-positive mononucleosis	B lymphocytes
Human herpesvirus 6	Roseola (sixth disease)	Peripheral blood mononuclear cells
Human herpesvirus 7	Roseola and febrile disease in children	Peripheral blood mononuclear cells
Human herpesvirus 8	Kaposi's sarcoma	Peripheral blood mononuclear cells

2) Viruses are spread by respiratory aerosol from vesicular skin lesions of individuals with infection.
3) The incubation period is from 1 to 2 weeks.
4) Symptoms include a rash and fever.
5) Individuals are contagious 48 hours before the rash and will remain contagious until scabbing of all lesions.

b. **Shingles**

1) **Reactivation** of VZV in the peripheral or cranial nerves leads to shingles and occurs mainly in the elderly.
2) Characterized by skin vesicles, often on one side of the body, and severe pain around the skin lesions
3) Complications include CNS disorders, eye problems, and facial paralysis.
4) **Diagnosis** is often based on clinical signs and symptoms.
5) A vaccine recommended for individuals over the age of 50 years is effective in preventing reactivation of the virus.

5. **Cytomegalovirus**

a. CMV infections are typically **asymptomatic.** Severe infections can occur in patients who are immunocompromised and can include pneumonia and encephalitis. Severe infections are sometimes seen in patients with acquired immunodeficiency syndrome (AIDS).

b. Congenital infections are severe and cause developmental problems for the newborn.
c. The virus is transmitted through contact with saliva or blood.
d. CMV results in persistent infections in humans, including endothelial cells and leukocytes. The tubular cells of the human kidney shed CMV for prolonged periods into the urine.
e. **Diagnosis** is by serologic testing and the absence of antibodies to EBV, which can produce a similar clinical syndrome. Viral isolation from blood, respiratory secretions, or urine samples can be attempted in complicated cases.

6. **Epstein-Barr virus**
   a. EBV causes **infectious mononucleosis,** a common but relatively mild disease. It is also associated with **Burkitt lymphoma, nasopharyngeal carcinoma,** and Hodgkin disease and other lymphomas.
   b. The virus is transmitted in **saliva.** The incubation period is 1–2 months.
   c. **Signs** include fever, enlarged lymph nodes, and swollen tonsils.
   d. **Diagnosis**
      1) Signs and symptoms
      2) Hematologic abnormalities include lymphocytosis and the presence of reactive (atypical) lymphocytes.
      3) Serology
         a) **Heterophile antibodies:** Individuals with EBV infection produce antibodies that will agglutinate sheep and horse red blood cells. These assays are effective in diagnosing about 85% of infectious mononucleosis cases.
         b) Viral-specific antibody assays may be necessary in the roughly 15% of the patients with infectious mononucleosis who do not produce heterophile antibodies. Tests for antibodies to EBV antigens include EA (early antigen), VCA (viral core antigen), and EBNA-1 (Epstein-Barr nucleic antigen-1). Anti-VCA IgM is the most useful marker for diagnosis.
7. **Human herpesvirus 6**
   a. HHV-6 is a very common virus and is acquired by respiratory secretions.
   b. HHV-6 infects T lymphocytes.
   c. Infections are generally mild or subclinical in patients who are immunocompetent. HHV-6 causes exanthem subitum, also known as **roseola** or **sixth disease.**
   d. Sixth disease is a childhood disease characterized by fever, rash, and sore throat; neurologic involvement is rare.
8. **Human herpesvirus 7**
   a. HHV-7 is also a very common virus, with serologic prevalence rates in healthy adults of about 90%.
   b. The virus is mostly transmitted via saliva and infects lymphocytes.

c. In individuals who are immunocompetent, infections are mild or asymptomatic. HHV-7 causes about 5% of all cases of roseola; neurologic involvement is rare.

9. **Human herpesvirus 8**
   a. HHV-8 is associated with Kaposi sarcoma in patients who are immunocompromised (e.g., AIDS) and is also known as Kaposi sarcoma herpes virus (KSHV).
   b. The virus is probably transmitted via oral secretions.
   c. Little is known about primary HHV-8 infections. In latent infections, viral DNA has been found in B cells and peripheral blood mononuclear cells.
   d. Serologic assays are the best method to diagnose infection.

B. Human Papillomavirus (HPV)

1. HPV has an icosahedral-shaped, enveloped virion. The viruses range in size from 40 to 55 nm.
2. Member of the family *Papillomaviridae*
3. HPV causes plantar warts, genital warts, and flat warts. Some HPVs are **associated with cervical cancer.** Genital warts are the most common STD in the United States, and HPV is the most common cause of cervical cancer.
4. Most accurate diagnosis is DNA hybridization.
5. A **vaccine** is approved for use in males and females. The vaccine contains the strains of HPV most often associated with genital warts and those associated with cervical cancer. It is recommended for children 11 or 12 years of age.

C. Poxviruses

1. Identifying characteristics
   a. Poxviruses are large, ranging in size from 220 to 450 nm.
   b. Virions also contain a DNA polymerase for DNA replication and an RNA polymerase system for transcription of viral genes. Poxviruses replicate entirely within the cytoplasm.
   c. Poxviruses belong to the family *Poxviridae.*
2. **Variola virus**
   a. **Variola major** caused a severe disease known as smallpox that had a fatality rate of about 30%. **Variola minor** strains produced milder infections with a fatality rate of less than 1%.
   b. Due to a worldwide vaccination program, the World Health Organization was able to declare the world smallpox free in 1979. The **vaccinia virus** is an attenuated vaccine that prevents variola infection.
   c. Variola virus is considered a potential **bioterrorism agent.**
3. Other poxviruses
   a. **Molluscipoxvirus** causes **molluscum contagiosum,** a skin infection that occurs worldwide.

b. **Monkeypox virus** causes a **zoonosis** found primarily in Africa. An outbreak occurred in the United States in 2003. Infections were traced back to rodents imported from Africa that transmitted the virus to prairie dogs.

D. Adenoviruses

1. Identifying characteristics
   a. Adenoviruses are naked icosahedral virions. They range in size from 70 to 90 nm.
   b. Adenoviruses belong to the family *Adenoviridae* and have been isolated from humans and animals.
2. **Infections**
   a. **Respiratory tract infections,** especially in young children
   b. **Urinary tract** and **gastrointestinal infections,** and pharyngitis
   c. **Eye infections** in newborns, patients who are immunocompromised, and military recruits (because of close living conditions) are common. Adenoviruses have been associated with epidemics of keratoconjunctivitis.
3. **Sample collection:** Throat swabs, eye samples, and stool

E. *Parvoviridae*

1. Parvoviruses are small single-stranded DNA viruses.
2. The main human pathogen in the family, parvovirus B19, belongs to the genus *Erythrovirus.* Parvovirus B19 causes a common, mild childhood disease called erythema infectiosum or fifth disease. It is characterized by a rash, fever, headache, and runny nose.
3. Diagnosis is often made clinically based on the appearance of a "slapped cheek" rash on the patient's face. Serologic assays can be performed for confirmation.

F. *Polyomaviridae*

1. Polyomaviruses are naked double-stranded DNA viruses with a circular genome. They infect mammals and birds. Approximately 13 species are known to infect humans.
2. The main human pathogens in the family are the BK and JC viruses. Both viruses are ubiquitous with an estimated 80% of the population having antibodies by 15 years of age. Cases are usually asymptomatic. BK virus has been associated with cystitis and pyelonephritis in patients undergoing transplants. JC virus causes progressive multifocal leukoencephalopathy in patients with AIDS.
3. Viruses can be detected in urine and other body fluids including blood and CSF using probes, PCR, or direct antigen detection. In addition, the viruses will cause hemagglutination of urine.

V. MEDICALLY IMPORTANT RNA VIRUSES

A. Retroviruses

1. The retroviruses have an icosahedral-shaped, enveloped virion. They range in size from 80 to 130 nm. Some medically important RNA viruses are listed in Table 9-3■.
2. Retroviruses contain an RNA-dependent DNA polymerase (**reverse transcriptase**) for replication. Reverse transcriptase uses viral RNA as a template to make double-stranded DNA that then moves into the nucleus where it is integrated into the host chromosome. This stage is referred to as a **provirus.** The genome is transcribed into mRNA by host RNA polymerase.
3. **Lentiviruses**
   a. The **human immunodeficiency virus** 1 (HIV-1) and HIV-2 are members of the genus *Lentivirus.*
   b. **HIV** is the causative agent of **AIDS.** HIV-1 causes a more severe infection and is much more prevalent than HIV-2.
   c. **Spread of the virus** is by sexual contact with individuals who are infected: (homosexual or heterosexual), intravenous drug use, congenital transmission, or contaminated blood products.
   d. The virus initially infects macrophages and dendritic cells, then the host's **CD4-positive T cells.** These cells are key to both humoral-mediated and

TABLE 9-3 FAMILIES OF RNA VIRUSES

Family	Important Human Viruses
Paramyxoviridae	Measles, mumps, respiratory syncytial, parainfluenza, and metapneumo viruses
Orthomyxoviridae	Influenza A, B, and C viruses
Coronaviridae	Coronavirus
Arenaviridae	Lymphocytic choriomeningitis and Lassa fever viruses
Rhabdoviridae	Rabies virus
Filoviridae	Marburg and Ebola viruses
Phenuiviridae	Rift Valley fever virus
Hantaviridae	Hantaan and Sin Nombre viruses
Nairoviridae	Crimean-Congo viruses
Retroviridae	Human T-lymphotropic and human immunodeficiency viruses
Reoviridae	Rotavirus and reovirus
Picornaviridae	Rhinovirus, poliovirus, enterovirus, ECHO virus, coxsackievirus, hepatitis A virus
Togaviridae	Rubella virus and western, eastern, and Venezuelan equine encephalitis viruses
Flaviviridae	Yellow fever, dengue, St. Louis encephalitis, hepatitis C, and West Nile viruses
Caliciviridae	Norwalk and Sapporo viruses

cell-mediated immune responses. As more T cells are destroyed, immune function deteriorates. CD4 is the primary receptor for the virus; important coreceptors include CXCR4 and CCR5.

e. **Acute infection** (acute retroviral syndrome) is often mild and can resemble infectious mononucleosis. This stage of HIV infection occurs 3 to 6 weeks after infection, and antibodies are generally undetectable. The virus exhibits high level of replication. Viral RNA in serum can sometimes be detected in amplification assays as can p24. Acute HIV infections are rarely diagnosed.
f. Virus replication occurs at a high rate in lymphoid tissue, but the patient remains asymptomatic for many years. The host is able to replace infected T cells as fast as they are destroyed. This condition is referred to as **"clinical latency." However, some viruses remain latent in resting CD4+ T cells.**
g. Eventually, the virus begins to destroy T cells faster than they can be replaced. As immune function is compromised, the patient presents with chronic and recurrent infections, including *Pneumocystis* pneumonia, CMV infections, mycobacteriosis, cryptosporidosis, candidiasis, and toxoplasmosis. This stage is sometimes referred to as **AIDS-related complex.**
h. As immune function continues to deteriorate, the opportunistic infections become more severe and life threatening (Table 9-4■). This stage is referred to as AIDS or full-blown AIDS. CD4+ T cell counts and presence of a variety of opportunistic infections are used to stage the severity of the disease.
i. HIV has also been associated with malignant conditions such as **Kaposi sarcoma** and B-cell lymphomas.
j. **Diagnosis** is by clinical history, serology, and detection of viral antigens or RNA. p24 is present before antibodies can be detected.

TABLE 9-4 AIDS DEFINING CONDITIONS*
Candidiasis of esophagus, bronchi, trachea, or lungs
Cervical cancer, invasive
Coccidioidomycosis, disseminated or extrapulmonary
Cryptococcosis, extrapulmonary
CMV disease (other than liver, spleen, or nodes), onset at age >1 month
HSV: chronic ulcers (>1 month's duration) or bronchitis, pneumonitis, or esophagitis (onset at age >1 month)
Histoplasmosis, disseminated or extrapulmonary
Kaposi sarcoma
Lymphoma, primary, of brain
Mycobacterium avium complex or *Mycobacterium kansasii*, disseminated or extrapulmonary
Pneumocystis jirovecii pneumonia
Progressive multifocal leukoencephalopathy
Toxoplasmosis of brain, onset at age >1 month

*This is a partial list defined by the Centers for Disease Control and Prevention.

i. The Centers for Disease Control and Prevention (CDC) recommends that patients be screened with an HIV-1/HIV-2 antibody p24 antigen combination test. Reactive samples should be tested with an assay that differentiates HIV-1 antibodies from HIV-2 antibodies. Samples that are reactive should be considered positive for HIV antibodies, and a diagnosis of HIV infection can be made. Samples that are negative or indeterminate in the differentiating tests should be tested with an FDA-approved HIV-1 NAAT.

ii. Commercial assays are available that can detect HIV RNA and DNA in clinical specimens, primarily peripheral blood mononuclear cells.

4. Human T-cell lymphotropic virus (HTLV)
   a. This group of viruses includes HTLV-1 and HTLV-2.
   b. These viruses are transmitted via sexual contact, mother to child by breast feeding, and parenteral drug use.
   c. HTLV-1 has been linked to **adult T-cell leukemia** and **HTLV-1-associated myelopathy/tropical spastic paraparesis** (HAM/TSP).
   d. Although HTLV-2 has not been associated with malignancies, it has been linked to a neurologic disease resembling HAM/TSP.

B. Orthomyxoviruses

1. Orthomyxovirus virions contain a segmented RNA genome and have a helical-shaped virion with an envelope. They range in size from 75 to 125 nm.
2. The **influenza viruses,** A, B, and C, are the only members of the family *Orthomyxoviridae.* Influenza A and B viruses are most clinically significant.
3. Orthomyxoviruses have **hemagglutinin** (HA) and **neuraminidase** (NA) on their surface. These molecules are immunogenic, and antibodies to these molecules confer protection. HA allow the viruses to attach to the surface of respiratory epithelial cells and also agglutinate red blood cells. NA has enzymatic activity, cleaving budding viruses from infected cells.
4. **Antigenic drift** develops when point mutations occur in the viral genes encoding the HA and NA spikes. Antigenic drift can occur within any of the three influenza viruses.
5. **Antigenic shift** occurs following a major change (reassortment) of the RNA genome when a single host cell is infected with two different influenza viruses. Among the influenza viruses, antigenic shift only occurs in influenza A viruses. Antigenic shift results in a new combination of viral surface glycoproteins (e.g., from H1N1 to H2N1). Influenza A can infect other animals, including birds and pigs. In these animals, the virus often undergoes recombination events, resulting in new strains. Epidemics and pandemics are generally due to antigenic shifts. Other viruses, such as HIV, can also undergo antigenic shift.
6. **Influenza trivalent and quadrivalent vaccines** are available; each year the formulation of the seasonal influenza vaccine can vary as the CDC tries to predict which influenza strains will predominate in the upcoming flu season.

7. **Diagnosis** is based on clinical signs and symptoms, serology, direct antigen detection, and viral isolation. A number of rapid diagnostic influenza tests are commercially available. Results are available in about 15 minutes. The assays utilize an upper respiratory sample like a nasopharyngeal swab or throat swab and are based on direct antigen detection. NAATs are also available and take 1 to 8 hours.

C. Paramyxoviruses

1. Paramyxoviruses have helical-shaped enveloped virions. They range in size from 150 to 300 nm.
2. The family *Paramyxoviridae* contains paramyxoviruses, morbilliviruses, pneumoviruses, and megamyxoviruses.
3. **Parainfluenza viruses** cause childhood **croup,** which is a respiratory infection characterized by fever and a hoarse cough. There are four human parainfluenza viruses: 1–4. Diagnosis is based on clinical symptoms and confirmed by direct antigen detection of NAATs.
4. **Mumps,** caused by the **mumps virus,** is an infection of the **parotid glands,** causing swelling and difficulty in swallowing. Mumps is rare in developed countries because of widespread use of a vaccine. Diagnosis is generally made clinically.
5. **Morbillivirus** causes **rubeola** or **measles,** typically a childhood illness. Necrotic vesicles with a white center surrounded by erythema on the oral mucosa, referred to as **Koplik spots,** are a characteristic of measles. Vaccination programs have nearly eliminated measles in developed countries. However, in 2019, a measles outbreak began in the United States, and measles is still relatively common in some developing countries, particularly in Africa and Asia.
6. **Respiratory syncytial virus** (RSV) is a member of the genus *Pneumovirus.*
   a. RSV causes respiratory and ear infections that are most common in newborns and young children. Worldwide, it is the most common cause of bronchitis and pneumonia in infants and children.
   b. RSV is characterized by the formation of giant multinucleated cells, **syncytia** as infected cells' membranes fuse with adjacent cells. Diagnosis is best made with real-time reverse transcriptase-PCR. Direct antigen detection is highly sensitive in children but not in adults.

D. Picornaviruses

1. The picornaviruses have a naked virion ranging in size from 20 to 30 nm.
2. The family *Picornaviridae* includes a number of viruses such as the enteroviruses, hepatitis A virus, and the rhinoviruses.
3. **Enteroviruses**
   a. Members of the genus *Enterovirus* (e.g., poliovirus, coxsackie viruses, and echoviruses) are a common cause of a variety of human infections worldwide. They most commonly produce an acute nonspecific febrile syndrome. Enteroviruses also cause infections of the respiratory and gastrointestinal tracts.

b. **Diagnosis** is generally made by NAATs of clinical specimens: serum, CSF, throat swabs, rectal swabs, etc.

4. **Poliovirus**

a. Poliovirus is transmitted by the **fecal-oral route.** The virus initially infects the gastrointestinal tract but spreads to the CNS. Most infections are mild but can result in meningitis or **paralytic polio.**

b. **Vaccines**

1) The **Salk vaccine** is a formalin-inactivated vaccine.
2) The **Sabin vaccine** is an attenuated vaccine.
3) Because of vaccination programs, the current risk for polio is extremely small. The Sabin vaccine produces a stronger immune response. However, because the attenuated virus can sometimes produce severe infection, most countries now routinely use the Salk vaccine.

5. **Coxsackie virus**

a. Coxsackie A viruses cause **hand, foot, and mouth disease of humans;** this is not the same disease as foot and mouth disease of animals. Coxsackie A virus is also associated with conjunctivitis.

b. Coxsackie B viruses cause about one-third of all cases of **myocarditis.** They are also associated with meningitis.

6. **Rhinoviruses**

a. Rhinoviruses are a frequent cause of the **common cold.** Other viruses, including coronaviruses, are also associated with colds. The rhinoviruses grow better at temperatures just below core body temperature (e.g., 33°C). This is near the typical temperature of the nasal passage.

b. Over 100 serotypes are known, and immunity to one does not provide immunity to the others. This is why colds are so common.

c. Infection prevention includes handwashing and avoiding hand-to-nose contact.

E. Rotaviruses

1. Rotaviruses have a double-stranded RNA genome. The virion is about 70 nm in diameter and has a **wheel-like (spokes) appearance.** Rotaviruses belong to the family *Reoviridae.*
2. Rotaviruses are the most important cause of gastrointestinal infections in children less than 2 years of age. Severe diarrhea and dehydration are common in this age group. Two oral vaccines are available and recommended beginning at 2 months of age.
3. **Diagnosis:** Antigen detection via latex agglutination or ELISA and, less commonly, immunoelectron microscopy

F. *Coronaviridae*

1. The coronaviruses cause colds, lower respiratory tract infections, and gastrointestinal tract infections in humans and other animals.

2. In 2003, a coronavirus (CoV) was linked to the global outbreak of severe acute respiratory syndrome (SARS), a lower respiratory tract infection with a significant mortality rate. No SARS cases have been reported since 2004.
3. Middle East respiratory syndrome (MERS) was first reported in 2012 and shown to be caused by a coronavirus. This lower respiratory tract infection also has a significant mortality rate. Currently, all cases of MERS have been linked to residence in or travel to countries in and near the Arabian Peninsula.
4. Diagnosis is generally made by detecting antibodies in serum.

G. *Caliciviridae*

1. The family *Caliciviridae* contains four genera: *Norovirus, Sapovirus, Lagovirus,* and *Vesivirus*. They are small, naked viruses.
2. The noroviruses and Norwalk viruses (members of the genus *Norovirus*) are highly contagious and are important causes of gastroenteritis.

H. *Togaviridae*

1. The virions are about 70 nm in diameter and contain an envelope.
2. The family *Togaviridae* contains two genera.
   a. *Rubivirus:* **Rubella virus** is the only member of this genus. The virus causes a mild infection. However, it can produce severe **congenital infections** if women are infected in the early stage of pregnancy; therefore, pregnant women and women of childbearing age are often tested for immunity. Rubella is rare in developed countries because of an effective vaccine.
   b. *Alphavirus:* This genus contains about 25 viruses, all of which are transmitted by arthropods. Alphaviruses can produce generalized symptoms of fever, malaise, headache, and/or symptoms of encephalitis. Examples include eastern equine encephalitis, western equine encephalitis, and Venezuelan equine encephalitis.

I. *Flaviviridae*

1. Many viruses belonging to the family *Flaviviridae* are arboviruses. Important members of this family include West Nile virus (WNV), St. Louis encephalitis virus, yellow fever virus, dengue virus, and Zika virus.
2. **West Nile virus**
   a. First reported in the United States in 1999 in New York
   b. Birds are the primary reservoir for WNV, and mosquitoes are the vectors.
   c. WNV typically produces mild or asymptomatic infections in many individuals who are otherwise healthy. However, the most serious complication of WNV infection is fatal encephalitis (inflammation of the brain). People over the age of 60 years are most susceptible to encephalitis.
   d. Laboratory diagnosis of WNV infection can be made by detecting antibodies to the virus in serum or CSF. ELISA antigen capture and RT-PCR assays are also available.

3. **Dengue virus**
   a. Four serologically distinct dengue viruses cause the tropical disease dengue. An estimated 400 million people are infected yearly. Mosquitoes are the vectors.
   b. The signs and symptoms of dengue are variable but generally include a high fever along with other symptoms such as severe headache, joint pain, muscle and/or bone pain, low white blood cell count, and mild bleeding problems. A severe form is known as dengue hemorrhagic fever.
   c. Diagnosis is based on travel history, clinical presentation, serologic assays, and molecular tests.
4. **Yellow fever virus**
   a. Yellow fever is another tropical disease transmitted by mosquitoes. The disease is rare in the United States. A vaccine is available.
   b. Most people infected with yellow fever virus are asymptomatic or have mild symptoms. Early symptoms include sudden onset of fever, chills, severe headache, back pain, general body aches, nausea, and vomiting, fatigue, and weakness. Approximately 15% of cases progress to a more severe disease.
   c. Diagnosis is made on travel and vaccine history and clinical presentation. Laboratory testing includes testing serum for virus-specific IgM and IgG antibodies.
5. **Zika virus**
   a. Zika virus has been reported in Africa, Central and South America, and the southern United States.
   b. Zika virus is transmitted by mosquitoes, sexual contact, and to a fetus during pregnancy. Most Zika virus infections are asymptomatic. However, infections acquired *in utero* can result in microcephaly and other severe fetal brain defects.
   c. Travel history is important in diagnosing Zika virus infection. Laboratory diagnosis is based on RT-PCR on serum or urine and detection of antibodies. RT-PCR can be performed following an amniocentesis to diagnose in utero infections.

J. *Phenuiviridae*

1. This family includes the Rift Valley fever virus. The disease is common among domestic animals, such as cattle, buffalo, sheep, goats, and camels. The disease is primarily found in Africa. Recently, outbreaks were reported in Saudi Arabia and Yemen.
2. The virus is transmitted among hosts by mosquitoes. In humans, most infections are asymptomatic or produce a mild illness associated with fever and liver abnormalities. Patients with symptoms often experience fever, generalized weakness, back pain, and dizziness. A small percentage of those infected progress to more serious infection that can include ocular disease, encephalitis, or hemorrhagic fever.

3. In the early stage of infection, the virus can be identified using antigen-detection ELISA and RT-PCR. Antibody testing using ELISA can be used to confirm the presence of IgM antibodies, which appear early.

K. *Arenaviridae*

1. This family includes the Lassa virus, which causes a disease called Lassa fever or Lassa hemorrhagic fever. Most infected people are asymptomatic, but symptoms can range from mild to severe and life threatening. Rats are reservoirs and infection is acquired by contact with these animals. The disease is relatively common in West Africa.
2. The lymphocytic choriomeningitis virus (LCMV) is also a member of this family. It generally causes asymptomatic or mild infection, although neurologic symptoms are present in some individuals. The mortality rate is less than 1%. Mice are reservoirs, and it is estimated that 5% of house mice in the United States carry LCMV.
3. Laboratory diagnosis is usually made by detecting antibodies in the serum or CSF. During the acute stage, virus can be detected by PCR or virus isolation in the CSF.

L. *Hantaviridae*

1. The hantaviruses are found worldwide, and rodents are important reservoirs. Contact with rodent feces, urine, or saliva can lead to human infections. In humans, the viruses can cause severe, life-threatening infections referred to as hantavirus pulmonary syndrome (HPS) and hemorrhagic fever with renal syndrome.
2. In the United States, the Sin Nombre virus produced a multistate outbreak in the southwest United States in 1993. Human-to-human transmission has not been documented in the United States. The disease is relatively uncommon in the United States but has a mortality rate of 36%.
3. HPS diagnosis can be suspected clinically and confirmation requires detecting antibodies in serum.

M. Rhabdovirus

1. Rhabdoviruses have a bullet-shaped, enveloped capsid ranging in size from 150 to 350 nm.
2. Rabies virus, a member of the family *Rhabdoviridae* and the genus *Lyssavirus,* causes **rabies.**
3. The rabies virus gains entry into humans by animal (e.g., cat, dog, or raccoon) bites, as well as contact with bats. The virus first infects the muscle tissue but preferentially infects neurons. The virus migrates along the peripheral nerves to the **CNS.** The disease progresses to produce convulsions, coma, and fatal encephalitis.
4. **Diagnosis** is through medical history of animal bites and a positive direct fluorescent-antibody test. Detection of **Negri bodies** in infected brain cells has a low sensitivity and is not recommended. Negri bodies are virus inclusions inside infected cells.

5. A rabies **vaccine** is available to prevent infection. It is only administered to those at risk for exposure to the rabies virus.
6. Post-exposure treatment is effective if administered within 72 hours. Without rapid treatment, the infection is essentially 100% fatal.

N. *Filoviridae*

1. Virions range in size from 800 to 1000 nm.
2. The family *Filoviridae* includes the **Marburg** and **Ebola** viruses.
3. Bats are thought to be the reservoir, but the mode of transmission is unclear.
4. Infection by these viruses produces **hemorrhagic fever** with high fatality rates.
5. Most cases occur in Africa.
6. Antigen capture by ELISA, RT-PCR, and detection of IgM antibodies can diagnose Ebola virus infection a few days after onset of symptoms.

VI. HEPATITIS VIRUSES

A. Hepatitis A Virus (HAV)

1. **Identifying characteristics**
   a. HAV contains RNA, and the naked virion has an icosahedral shape. HAV ranges in size from 24 to 30 nm.
   b. It is a member of the family ***Picornaviridae*** and the genus ***Hepatovirus.*** Table 9-5■ summarizes other important causes of hepatitis.
2. **Infections**
   a. Infections are spread by the **fecal-oral route** and are generally due to poor sanitation and hygiene. Food handling transmission is common.
   b. Humans can also acquire the infection from contaminated shellfish, including shrimp, oysters, scallops, etc.
   c. **Vaccines are available.**

TABLE 9-5 IMPORTANT HUMAN HEPATITIS VIRUSES

	Hepatitis A	Hepatitis B	Hepatitis C	Hepatitis D	Hepatitis E
Family	*Picornaviridae*	*Hepadnaviridae*	*Flaviviridae*	Unclassified	*Hepeviridae*
Genome	RNA	DNA	RNA	RNA	RNA
Transmission	Fecal-oral	Parenteral, blood, sexually, needles, perinatal	Parenteral, blood, needles, perinatal	Parenteral, blood, sexually, needles, perinatal	Fecal-oral
Comments	No chronic liver disease, rarely fatal, severity increases with age	5–10% chronic hepatitis, associated with hepatocellular cancer	Chronic infections are common	Coinfection/ superinfection in patients infected with HBV	Wide range of clinical outcomes, high mortality rate in pregnant women

3. **Clinical characteristics**
   a. The incubation period is 15–40 days.
   b. Liver involvement (jaundice), nausea, anorexia, and malaise
   c. Mortality rate is less than 1%.
4. **Diagnosis**
   a. Clinical symptoms and liver enzymes, particularly alanine aminotransferase, are elevated.
   b. Serology
5. **Serologic indicators**
   a. Anti-HAV IgM is positive in acute infections.
   b. Anti-HAV IgG (positive) and anti-HAV IgM (negative) indicate a past HAV infection.
   c. General serology testing also includes ruling out hepatitis B and C viruses.

B. Hepatitis B Virus (HBV)

1. **Identifying characteristics**
   a. HBV contains partially double-stranded DNA. The complete virion has an envelope, ranges in size between 42 and 47 nm, and is sometimes referred to as **Dane particles.**
   b. The virus is unusual in that an RNA intermediate is required for replication of the genome. The virus needs a viral-encoded reverse transcriptase for replication.
   c. Member of the family ***Hepadnaviridae***
2. **Infections**
   a. Infections are spread by contaminated body fluids, including blood. HBV can be sexually transmitted.
   b. Infections are associated with contaminated blood products, needle sticks, tattoos, body piercing, intravenous drug abuse, and hemodialysis.
   c. Recombinant HBV vaccines are available and are recommended for newborns and all healthcare workers. The vaccine contains hepatitis B surface antigen (HBsAg).
3. **Clinical characteristics**
   a. The incubation period is 50–180 days.
   b. **Acute infections** produce symptoms resembling HAV infections.
   c. **Chronic infections** are common and can result in **cirrhosis** and **hepatocellular carcinoma.**
4. **Diagnosis**
   a. Clinical symptoms and elevated liver enzymes
   b. Serology
5. **Serologic indicators**
   a. HBsAg is the first marker to be detected, but it will become negative as the patient produces antibody to HBsAg and recovers. In **chronic infections,** HBsAg will remain positive. Presence of this marker indicates that the patient is infectious.

b. **Antibody to HBsAg** (anti-HBs) indicates **recovery or immunity** after HBV vaccination. The antibody is generally present for life.
c. **IgM antibody to HB core antigen** (anti-HBc IgM) indicates **acute infection.** As anti-HBs is forming, the level of HBsAg is decreasing. During this transition, there is a point when both markers are undetectable. At this time, the only indicator of HBV infection is anti-HBc IgM; this time period is called the **"core window."**
d. Antibody to HBcAg is positive in acute infection stages. It indicates current or past infections but does not indicate recovery or immunity.
e. **HBeAg** is positive in acute and chronic stages of infection. Presence of this marker also indicates that the patient is infectious.
f. **Anti-HBe** is associated with a good prognosis.

C. Hepatitis D Virus (HDV)

1. HDV contains RNA, and the naked viruses range in size from 35 to 37 nm.
2. HDV is also called the **delta virus.** HDV requires but does not encode for HBsAg; therefore, it only replicates in cells also infected with HBV. Because of this dependency on HBV, it is sometimes referred to as a subvirus.
3. **Coinfection** occurs when an individual acquires both HDV and HBV at the same time. A **superinfection** is when a patient with an HBV infection is exposed to HDV. Superinfections are more severe than coinfections.
4. **Diagnosis**
   a. Detection of anti-HDV and HDV RNA
   b. Serologic markers for HBV will also be positive; in particular, HBsAg.

D. Hepatitis C Virus (HCV)

1. **Identifying characteristics**
   a. HCV contains RNA and has a lipid envelope.
   b. The virus is a member of the family *Flaviviridae* and the genus *Hepacivirus.*
2. **Infections**
   a. HCV is a common cause of hepatitis worldwide and the primary factor requiring a liver transplant.
   b. Spread through contaminated blood products, organ transplants, hemodialysis, and intravenous drug abuse
   c. No vaccine currently exists for HCV.
3. **Clinical characteristics**
   a. The incubation period is 2–25 weeks.
   b. **Acute** HCV infection is often mild or asymptomatic and is rarely diagnosed in this phase. HCV is more likely to cause **chronic hepatitis,** resulting in cirrhosis, than HBV. HCV infection is one of the most common reasons for liver transplant in the United States.

4. **Diagnosis**
   a. Elevated liver enzymes
   b. **Serologic indicators** (anti-HCV and HCV antigen) and **NAATs**
   c. The virus has not been grown in cell cultures.

E. Other Human Hepatitis Viruses

1. **Hepatitis E virus (HEV)**
   a. HEV contains RNA, and virions range in size from 32 to 34 nm.
   b. HEV is spread by the **fecal-oral route,** often in contaminated water. It is the most common cause of hepatitis in some countries with poor sanitation.
   c. Diagnosis: Serology
2. **Hepatitis G virus (HGV)**
   a. HGV contains RNA and has an envelope.
   b. It is in the same family, *Flaviviridae,* as HCV.
   c. Although HGV is most commonly transmitted by contact with blood, it can also be sexually transmitted and transmitted from mother to children. Infection seems to be relatively common worldwide, but HGV is believed to be nonpathogenic.

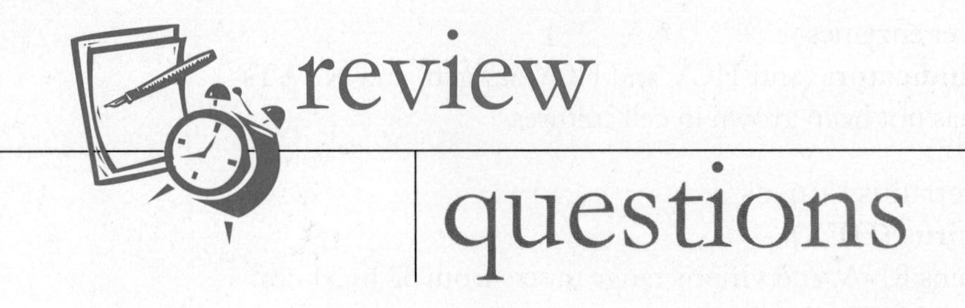

INSTRUCTIONS Each of the questions or incomplete statements that follows is comprised of four suggested responses. Select the *best* answer or completion statement in each case.

1. The retrovirus responsible for causing acquired immune deficiency syndrome is a member of which of the following families?
   A. *Orthomyxoviridae*
   B. *Paramyxoviridae*
   C. *Retroviridae*
   D. *Flaviviridae*

2. A nasopharyngeal swab in bacterial transport medium is received in the laboratory at 8 A.M. The physician has requested a direct antigen test for influenza. The sample was collected at 6 P.M. the previous evening from a patient admitted to the hospital through the emergency department. You should perform which of the following step?
   A. Process the sample according to the package insert for the kit.
   B. Freeze the sample at −20°C for processing later that day.
   C. Place the swab into sterile saline and refrigerate until processed that day.
   D. Contact the physician and request another specimen.

3. Which of the following RNA viruses causes hepatitis and has a high incidence in countries with poor sanitation in handling human feces?
   A. Polyomavirus
   B. Hepatitis A virus
   C. Hepatitis B virus
   D. Hepatitis C virus

4. Which of the following has been declared eradicated by the World Health Organization?
   A. Smallpox
   B. Human T-cell lymphotropic virus
   C. Hepatitis G virus
   D. Eastern equine encephalitis

5. Rotavirus is the most common etiologic agent of which of the following?
   A. Acute nonbacterial encephalitis in children
   B. Acute nonbacterial gastroenteritis in infants and young children
   C. Chronic nonbacterial pharyngitis in children and young adults
   D. Chronic nonbacterial retinitis in children

6. Kaposi sarcoma is associated with infection by which of the following?
   A. Adenovirus
   B. Cytomegalovirus
   C. Hepatitis E virus
   D. Human herpes virus 8
7. Which of the following is the molecular receptor for the virus causing acquired immune deficiency syndrome?
   A. CD 4
   B. CD 8
   C. Fc receptor
   D. Complement receptor
8. Which of the following is the most clinically relevant disease associated with Zika virus?
   A. Pneumonia in the elderly
   B. Severe diarrhea in infants
   C. Neurologic disease in newborns
   D. Cancer in patients who are immuno-compromised
9. Which of the following viruses is predominantly associated with respiratory disease and epidemics of keratoconjunctivitis?
   A. Adenovirus
   B. Molluscum contagiosum virus
   C. Norwalk virus
   D. Rotavirus
10. A 50-year-old male presents to the emergency department of a hospital in Arizona in severe respiratory distress. He states that he has fatigue, headache, muscle aches and pain, and fever before he developed difficulty in breathing. He reports that he recently cleaned the loft of his barn and noted a large amount of rodent feces. He is most likely suffering from which of the following disease?
    A. Hantavirus pulmonary syndrome
    B. Rabies
    C. West Nile fever
    D. Yellow fever
11. The Sabin polio vaccine uses which of the following?
    A. Formalin-inactivated viruses
    B. Attenuated viruses
    C. Recombinant viral antigens
    D. DNA
12. Which of the following is caused by a herpes virus?
    A. Cold sores
    B. Hemorrhagic fever
    C. Polio
    D. Rabies
13. Which of the following is a general characteristic of a virus?
    A. Genome is immediately surrounded by a lipid membrane.
    B. Does not produce ATP
    C. Each virion contains both DNA and RNA.
    D. Can self-replicate in the appropriate host cell
14. The viral disease shingles, which causes extreme tenderness along the dorsal nerve roots and a vesicular eruption, has the same etiologic agent as which of the following?
    A. Rubeola
    B. Vaccinia
    C. Varicella
    D. Variola
15. The etiologic agents of many common colds are RNA viruses that grow better at 33°C than at 37°C. These viruses include which of the following?
    A. Adenoviruses
    B. Orthomyxoviruses
    C. Lassa viruses
    D. Rhinoviruses

16. Influenza A virus undergoes recombination events that produce new strains; this is referred to as which of the following?
    A. Antigenic drift
    B. Antigenic shift
    C. Reactivation
    D. Viral latency

17. The rapid diagnosis of rabies is best made by which of the following?
    A. Detecting Negri bodies in brain tissue
    B. Direct fluorescent antibody test of brain tissue
    C. Detecting antibody to the virus in serum
    D. Detecting antibody to the virus in cerebrospinal fluid

18. Which of the following is a mild childhood disease caused by parvovirus B19?
    A. Measles
    B. Rubeola
    C. Rubella
    D. Erythema infectiousum

19. A clinical specimen is received in viral transport medium for viral isolation. The specimen cannot be processed for 72 hours. At what temperature should it be stored?
    A. −80°C
    B. −20°C
    C. 4°C
    D. 22°C

20. Which of the following is a characteristic of arboviruses?
    A. Only infect humans
    B. Often cause hepatitis
    C. Typically infect lymphocytes
    D. Are transmitted by arthropods

21. Mumps is characterized by an infection of which of the following?
    A. Central nervous system
    B. Parotid glands
    C. Pancreas
    D. Thymus

22. Following a diagnosis of human immunodeficiency virus infection, the disease is staged based on which of the following?
    A. CD4+ cell count and opportunistic infections
    B. CD4+:CD8+ cell ratio and p24 concentration
    C. Anti-gp120 antibody titer and CD4+ cell count
    D. Anti-gp41 antibody titer and CD4+:CD8+ cell ratio

23. Which of the following is the greatest risk factor for severe West Nile virus infection?
    A. Exposure to rodents
    B. Exposure to bats
    C. Age, over 60 years old
    D. Concurrent enterovirus infection

24. The "core window" refers to the time
    A. During hepatitis B virus infection when anti-HBc IgM is the only serologic marker
    B. During hepatitis B virus infection when HBc is the only serologic marker
    C. During hepatitis A virus infection when HAc is the only serologic marker
    D. During hepatitis C virus infection when the virus is latent

25. Which of the following childhood diseases is associated with human herpesviruses 6 and 7?
    A. Chickenpox
    B. Measles
    C. Roseola
    D. Zoster

26. A baby was admitted to the hospital in February for dehydration due to severe diarrhea. Cultures for bacterial pathogens revealed normal fecal biota at 24 hours. Which of the following additional tests would be most appropriate given the case history?
    A. Heterophile antibody test
    B. Rotavirus antigen assay of stool specimen
    C. Hepatitis virus screening tests
    D. Urine microscopic analysis for presence of CMV cellular inclusion bodies

27. Rhabdovirus is most noted for causing infections of which of the following?
    A. Central nervous system
    B. Gastrointestinal tract
    C. Lower respiratory tract
    D. Upper respiratory tract

28. Jaundice is a common clinical symptom of which of the following viral diseases?
    A. Hepatitis A
    B. Infectious mononucleosis
    C. Rabies
    D. Varicella

29. An 18-year-old male presents to his family physician complaining of sore throat and fatigue. The patient is found to have a fever and swollen cervical lymph nodes. A complete blood count and differential reveal lymphocytosis and many reactive lymphocytes. The physician should suspect an infection caused by which of the following viruses?
    A. Adenoviruses
    B. Epstein-Barr virus
    C. Parainfluenza virus
    D. Varicella-zoster virus

30. The poliovirus, an RNA virus, is a(n)
    A. Adenovirus
    B. Coxsackie virus
    C. Enterovirus
    D. Rhinovirus

31. The virus that causes hepatitis B is characterized as a
    A. Defective DNA virus requiring delta virus to complete its replication cycle
    B. DNA virus utilizing reverse transcriptase
    C. Nonenveloped DNA virus
    D. Single-stranded RNA virus

32. Hepatitis C virus infections
    A. Are commonly diagnosed during the acute stage
    B. Are uncommon in the United States.
    C. Are most often acquired by contact with blood
    D. Seldom results in chronic infection

33. Which of the following animals is the primary reservoir for the lymphocytic choriomeningitis virus?
    A. Dogs
    B. Rodents
    C. House cats
    D. Poultry

34. Which of the following viruses is associated with warts?
    A. Flavivirus
    B. Morbillivirus
    C. Mumps virus
    D. Papillomavirus

35. RNA-dependent DNA polymerase is also called
    A. Gyrase
    B. Ligase
    C. Reverse transcriptase
    D. Transaminase

36. Coxsackie viruses are associated with which of the following diseases?
    A. Gastrointestinal disease
    B. Hepatitis
    C. Myocarditis
    D. The common cold

37. The tubular cells of the human kidney shed which of the following viruses for prolonged periods?
    A. Adenovirus
    B. Cytomegalovirus
    C. Epstein-Barr virus
    D. Rubella virus

38. Which of the following togaviruses is known to produce fetal defects?
    A. Influenza
    B. Rotavirus
    C. Rubella
    D. Varicella

39. An 8-week-old infant was admitted to the hospital with symptoms of low birth weight, jaundice, and neurologic defects. Intranuclear inclusions were found in epithelial cells from the urine. The most likely diagnosis in this case would be infection by which of the following viruses?
    A. Cytomegalovirus
    B. Epstein-Barr virus
    C. Herpes simplex virus
    D. Rubella virus

40. Which of the following viruses is the most common cause of cervical cancer?
    A. Cytomegalovirus
    B. Enterovirus
    C. Polyomavirus
    D. Papillomavirus

41. Select the statement that is correct concerning the influenza A viruses.
    A. Humans are the only animal hosts for influenza A viruses.
    B. Pandemics are characteristically produced by influenza A.
    C. The incidence of infection peaks in the summer months.
    D. They are DNA viruses.

42. Which of the following is an example of a virus associated with latent infections?
    A. Influenza
    B. Rotavirus
    C. Rubella
    D. Varicella-zoster

43. After receiving the hepatitis B vaccine, immunity is indicated by the presence of which of the following?
    A. Hepatitis B surface antigen
    B. Anti-hepatitis B surface antigen antibody
    C. Anti-hepatitis Be antigen antibody
    D. Anti-hepatitis B core antigen antibody

44. Which of the following is associated with the rubella virus?
    A. It is a DNA virus.
    B. It is a member of the same taxonomic family as measles virus.
    C. It is known to produce defects in fetuses during the early stages of pregnancy.
    D. It is transmitted by an arthropod vector.

45. Acute retroviral syndrome is characterized by which of the following?
    A. Chronic recurrent infection
    B. Slow rate of virus replication
    C. High titer of autoantibodies
    D. Lack of detectable antiviral antibody

46. Which of the following is an acquired immunodeficiency syndrome defining condition?
    A. *Pneumocystis* pneumonia
    B. Chronic infectious mononucleosis
    C. Severe acute respiratory syndrome
    D. Malaria

47. Although there have been no natural cases of this serious disease in about 40 years, which of the following is considered a potential bioterrorism disease?
    A. Dengue fever
    B. Ebola hemorrhagic fever
    C. Shingles
    D. Smallpox

48. Poliovirus is a member of which of the following families?
    A. *Flaviviridae*
    B. *Paramyxoviridae*
    C. *Picornaviridae*
    D. *Reoviridae*

49. A primary care provider suspects an 18-year-old patient has infectious mononucleosis. However, the serologic markers for the test are all negative. Which of the following is the most likely explanation?
    A. Varicella-zoster virus infection
    B. Cytomegalovirus infection
    C. Blood sample was taken too early in the course of the infection.
    D. False negative results due to the presence of heterophile antibody

50. What is the most accurate test for identifying the presence of human papillomavirus?
    A. DNA hybridization
    B. Enzyme immunoassay
    C. Cell culture
    D. Serology

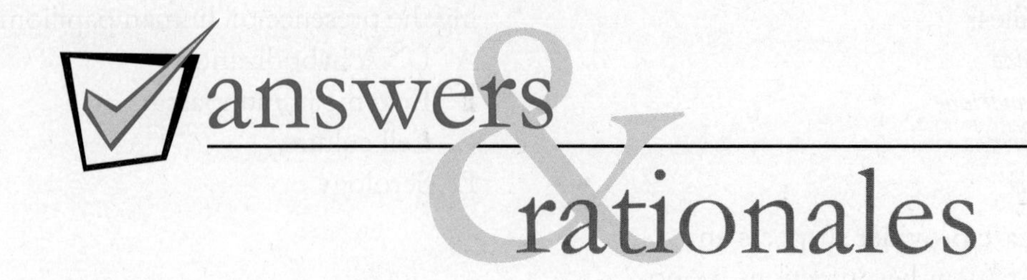

1.

C. Retroviruses are RNA viruses that replicate by means of DNA intermediates produced by the viral enzyme reverse transcriptase. The viruses associated with acquired immune deficiency syndrome are human immunodeficiency viruses (HIVs). These viruses belong to the family *Retroviridae.*

2.

D. Specimens for viral detection should be placed into viral transport medium and taken to the laboratory immediately after collection. If there will be delay, the specimen can be stored at 4°C for up to 24 hours. Because this specimen was in bacterial transport medium for several hours, a new specimen should be requested.

3.

B. Hepatitis A virus is a naked virus spread via the fecal-oral pathway. It is therefore seen more frequently in countries with poor sanitation. The virus rarely causes chronic infections and has a very low mortality rate.

4.

A. The last natural case of smallpox was in 1977, and the World Health Organization declared the world smallpox free in 1979. Elimination of the virus was due to a worldwide vaccination program. Because of the highly contagious nature of variola virus, the cause of smallpox, the ability of the virus to produce severe infections, and the termination of routine vaccinations, the virus is considered a potential bioterrorism agent.

5.

B. One of the major viral agents associated with cases of acute gastroenteritis in children is rotavirus. In particular, this agent is the cause of epidemic nonbacterial gastroenteritis in infants and young children that occurs most commonly during the winter months. Rotavirus has a fecal-oral route of transmission and has been documented as a nosocomial pathogen in pediatric areas of hospitals.

6.

D. During acquired immune deficiency syndrome (AIDS), as the immune system becomes weakened, the patient presents with chronic and recurrent infections and various neoplasms. Kaposi sarcoma, a relatively common cancer in patients with AIDS, has been linked to human herpes virus 8. Viral genome has been found in the cancerous growths in these patients.

7.

A. HIV causes AIDS. The major target of the virus is the CD+ positive T-helper cell, which functions to control disease. Other coreceptors are also important for attachment.

8.

C. With Zika virus infection, most individuals who are otherwise healthy are asymptomatic or have mild symptoms. The greatest concern is when a pregnant woman acquires the infection. The virus can infect the fetus and produce severe neurologic disease such as microencephaly.

9.

A. Adenoviruses are well known as respiratory pathogens and have been the cause of acute respiratory disease among military recruit populations. Also associated with adenoviral infection is the severe ocular disease keratoconjunctivitis, which typically occurs in epidemic form. Adenoviruses may remain in tissues, lymphoid structures, and adenoids and become reactivated.

10.

A. In the southwestern United States, hantavirus pulmonary syndrome is caused by Sin Nombre virus. It is associated with inhalation of rodent excrement. The overall mortality rate is about 36%.

11.

B. The Salk vaccine utilizes a formalin-inactivated poliovirus. The Sabin polio vaccine uses an attenuated virus; therefore, the virus is still able to infect cells and cause an asymptomatic infection. The Sabin vaccine provides a stronger immune response than the Salk vaccine.

12.

A. Members of the herpes virus group are responsible for a number of diseases, including cold sores. Hemorrhagic fevers are caused by a number of tropical viruses, such as Ebola and dengue. Polio is caused by a picornavirus, and rabies is caused by the rhabdovirus.

13.

B. Viruses are obligate intracellular parasites that cannot self-replicate. They cannot produce ATP, and their genome is surrounded by a protein capsid. Most viruses contain either DNA or RNA; however, some large DNA viruses do contain viral mRNA and microRNAs.

14.

C. Zoster or shingles occurs predominantly in adults, whereas varicella occurs more commonly in children. The varicella-zoster virus, following the primary infection known as chicken pox, remains latent in the sensory ganglia. Reactivation of this virus, which occurs years later, is usually associated with a slightly immunocompromised state.

15.

D. Rhinoviruses, members of the picornavirus group, are a common cause of the respiratory disease known as the common cold. Hand transmission, not aerosols, appears to be the primary means of transmission. In contrast to other picornaviruses, the optimum temperature for rhinoviruses is 33°C.

16.

B. Influenza A virus undergoes recombination events that produce significant changes in the RNA genome of the virus. These changes lead to alteration of surface antigens. This process is referred to as antigenic shift. Antigenic drift is a slight change in a gene, usually a point mutation. Influenza A, B, and C viruses can undergo antigenic drift.

17.

B. Rabies is a neurotropic virus that causes extensive destruction in the brain. Negri bodies are seen in the cytoplasm of large ganglion cells and are demonstrated by Seller's stain. Rabies in humans or lower animals can be diagnosed by demonstration of these characteristic inclusions. However, the more sensitive direct fluorescent antibody test is more commonly used.

18.

D. Parvoviruses are small single-stranded DNA viruses. Erythema infectiosum, or fifth disease, is caused by parvovirus B19. This common childhood disease is generally diagnosed clinically based on a characteristic rash resembling a "slapped face."

19.

A. Prolonged storage of clinical specimens for viral isolation requires −80°C. Specimens can be stored at 4°C for approximately 48 hours without appreciable loss of viability. Specimens should not be stored at −20°C for any length of time.

20.

D. Arbovirus is short for arthropod-borne virus. These genetically diverse viruses share a common feature: they are transmitted by arthropods (e.g., mosquitoes and ticks). Arboviruses include West Nile virus and western equine encephalitis virus.

21.

B. The mumps virus infects the parotid glands. Infection results in swelling of the neck. Without routine vaccination programs, mumps is primarily a childhood infection, and swelling of the parotid glands is diagnostic.

22.

A. HIV infections are staged based on the absolute CD4+ cell count and the presence and severity of opportunistic infections. As the HIV infection persists, CD4+ T cells are destroyed faster than they can be replaced. CD4+:CD8+ ratio is also used to aid the prognosis but is not involved in staging the infection.

23.

C. West Nile virus, the cause of West Nile fever, is transmitted by mosquitoes. Individuals over the age of 60 years are more likely to develop encephalitis or meningitis. About 1 in 150 people infected develops a severe illness affecting the central nervous system.

24.

A. During the course of acute hepatitis B virus infection, hepatitis B surface antigen (HBsAg) is the first marker detected. The host will ultimately begin to produce antibody (anti-HBs) to the antigen. As the antibody titer increases, there is a corresponding decrease in the antigen. However, there is a time period when neither of these markers is detectable. During this time period the only serologic marker is antibody to the hepatitis B core antigen (anti-HBc). This period is called the core window.

25.

C. Human herpes viruses (HHVs) 6 and 7 cause the childhood disease roseola, also called sixth disease. The disease is characterized by fever, rash, and sore throat. More cases are caused by HHV 6 than HHV 7.

26.

B. Rotavirus is the cause of diarrheal disease in at least half of all infants and young children admitted to the hospital with dehydration requiring fluid replacement therapy. Because rotaviruses are difficult to propagate in cell culture, the method of choice for the detection of rotavirus infection is the direct examination of stool for the presence of viral antigen. Commonly used rotavirus antigen assay tests include latex agglutination and enzyme immunoassay.

27.

A. Rhabdovirus causes rabies, an infection of the central nervous system. The virus is transmitted in the saliva of an infected animal during a bite. At the bite site, the virus initially infects muscle tissue but will move to the peripheral nerves. The virus then migrates along the peripheral nerves to the central nervous system.

28.

A. Hepatitis A is one of several infectious diseases characterized by liver damage and icterus (jaundice). The appearance of jaundice, in the icteric phase, is correlated by liver biopsy with extensive parenchymal destruction. Convalescence is usually accompanied by subsequent complete regeneration of the diseased organ.

29.

B. The Epstein-Barr virus, which is associated with Burkitt lymphoma and nasopharyngeal carcinoma, is the etiologic agent of infectious mononucleosis. Infectious mononucleosis is an acute disease most commonly affecting young adults. The virus is thought to be transmitted by intimate contact and produces a condition called the "kissing disease." The patient's blood demonstrates a leukocytosis with a marked increase in T lymphocytes, and serologically the disease is characterized by a positive heterophile antibody and antibodies to various viral antigens.

30.

C. Poliovirus, an enterovirus, is shed by both respiratory and fecal routes. Laboratory identification relies on isolation (especially from feces) and subsequent virus neutralization in tissue culture. Spread of the disease is associated with poor sanitary conditions and crowding.

31.

B. The hepatitis B virus is an enveloped, partially double-stranded DNA virus. During viral replication, full-length RNA transcripts of the viral genome are inserted into maturing virus particles. The viral enzyme reverse transcriptase then transcribes these RNA transcripts to a full-length DNA strand but only partially completes synthesis of the complementary DNA strand—hence a partially double-stranded DNA genome.

32.

C. Hepatitis C virus infections, unlike hepatitis A or hepatitis B infections, do not commonly produce jaundice. There are tens of thousands of individuals in the United States chronically infected with hepatitis C; chronic infection appears to be the rule rather than the exception. Transmission of the virus at present occurs mainly through needle sharing. Cases also occur among healthcare workers who contact infected blood.

33.

B. The lymphocytic choriomeningitis virus is carried by about 5% of mice in the United States. Most people infected with this virus are asymptomatic. However, neurologic symptoms can be present.

34.

D. The etiologic agents for the numerous benign cutaneous and mucosal lesions known as warts are the human papillomaviruses (HPVs). The diagnosis of lesions caused by these agents is based on clinical appearance and histopathology, because there are no *in vitro* systems available for isolation. Some HPV types are strongly associated with squamous cell carcinoma of the cervix and anus.

35.

C. RNA-dependent DNA polymerase is also known as reverse transcriptase. The enzyme uses an RNA template to synthesize the complementary DNA strand. The retroviruses and hepatitis B virus require this enzyme for replication.

36.

C. The coxsackieviruses are enteroviruses named after the town of Coxsackie, New York, where they were first isolated. The viruses are divided into groups A and B based on viral and antigenic differences. The group B coxsackieviruses are strongly associated with myocarditis that may cause sufficient damage to require heart transplantation. The group A coxsackieviruses are associated with various diseases, characterized by vesicular lesions, such as herpangina. Neither group of coxsackieviruses is associated with gastrointestinal disease.

37.

B. Cytomegalovirus infections may be asymptomatic for normal healthy hosts. Infections tend to be more severe in patients who are immunosuppressed or in neonates infected perinatally. Cytomegalovirus is readily isolated from urine because it is shed by the tubular cells of infected hosts.

38.

C. The rubella virus is a member of the family *Togaviridae*. In adults and children, rubella infections are generally a mild contagious rash disease. When a pregnant woman becomes infected, the consequences are more serious. If the fetus is infected during the first trimester of pregnancy, a variety of congenital defects can result. Anatomic abnormalities produced by this agent include cataracts, deafness, and cardiac problems.

39.

A. Infants usually acquire cytomegalovirus infections before birth or at the time of childbirth. These infections may lead to death during the first month of life or may result in residual neurologic impairment. The virus can be detected in several different body fluids, with urine being the most commonly examined.

40.

D. Papillomaviruses are responsible for warts, including genital warts. Some serotypes of papillomavirus are associated with cervical cancer. A vaccine providing protection against these serotypes is available for women.

41.

B. Influenza viruses are RNA viruses able to infect humans and other animals, such as birds and pigs. Influenza viruses are associated with epidemic and pandemic disease. There are two main types of influenza viruses (A and B), which differ antigenically and in epidemic periodicity. All recorded pandemics have been caused by influenza A viruses. The incidence of respiratory disease caused by these agents peaks during the winter months.

42.

D. Herpes simplex viruses, cytomegalovirus, and varicella-zoster viruses (VZV) produce latent infections. The genomes of these viruses can remain dormant in host cells for decades. Shingles (zoster) represents reactivation of latent VZV.

43.

B. The vaccine for hepatitis B virus infection is recombinant hepatitis B surface antigen. Successful immunization is indicated by the presence of anti-hepatitis B surface antigen antibody. This antibody also indicates immunity after infection with hepatitis B virus.

44.

C. The rubella virus causes an exanthematous disease resembling a milder form of measles in children. This single-stranded RNA virus, transmitted from person to person, is of medical importance to females of childbearing years because of the teratogenic effects it has on the fetus. Congenital rubella, resulting from an intrauterine fetal infection, is most severe when contracted during the first trimester of gestation.

45.

D. Acute retroviral syndrome is the name given to the acute phase of HIV infection. The stage is characterized by mild symptoms resembling infectious mononucleosis: malaise, swollen cervical lymph nodes, sore throat, and low grade fever. This stage occurs before the development of detectable antibodies to HIV. The virus exhibits high level of replication.

46.

A. As HIV progresses, the T-helper cell count drops gradually leading to severe immunosuppression. At this point, the individual presents with chronic, recurrent, progressively more severe infections and cancers with an infectious etiology. Common infections include disseminated candidiasis, encephalitis due to HIV or cytomegalovirus, cryptosporidiosis, and *Pneumocystis* pneumonia, among several others (Table 9-5■).

47.

D. Although smallpox has not caused a natural infection since 1977, it is regarded as a potential bioterrorism agent. Routine vaccination against smallpox is no longer in effect, so the majority of the world's population is again susceptible. The United States has stockpiles of vaccine available to vaccinate everyone in the country in case of an attack.

48.

C. Poliovirus is a member of the family *Picornaviridae*. These are small RNA viruses lacking an envelope. Other members of the family include coxsackieviruses, echoviruses, enteroviruses, and rhinoviruses. Many are spread by the fecal-oral pathway.

49.

B. Epstein-Barr virus is the cause of infectious mononucleosis. The disease can often be diagnosed in a young adult by the symptoms pharyngitis, fever, swollen cervical lymph nodes, and malaise. Historically, the heterophile test was used to diagnose this condition. Today, it is generally recommended that viral-specific serologic tests be performed. If these tests are negative in patients with symptoms compatible with infectious mononucleosis, then another etiology, such as cytomegalovirus, should be suspected.

50.

A. HPV is the greatest risk factor for cervical cancer. The Pap smear is commonly used to screen cervical specimens for abnormal cells that could develop into cancer. A DNA hybridization test is the most accurate means of diagnosing HPV infection. However, a positive test does not mean the patient has cervical cancer.

REFERENCES

Tille, P. (2018). *Bailey and Scott's Diagnostic Microbiology*, 14th ed. Philadelphia: Mosby.

Mahon, C. R., and Lehman, D. C. (2018). *Textbook of Diagnostic Microbiology*, 6th ed. St. Louis: Elsevier.

Carroll, K. C., et al. (Eds.) (2019). *Manual of Clinical Microbiology*, 12th ed. Washington, DC: American Society for Microbiology Press.

CHAPTER

10 Molecular Diagnostics

contents

I. INTRODUCTION

A. Genetic Information

1. Genetic information in procaryotic and eucaryotic cells is contained in **deoxyribonucleic acid** (DNA) sequences, which are arranged as genes and packaged into chromosomes.
2. The human genome (all DNA in human chromosomes) is **3 billion base pairs** in size.
3. Based on computer analysis of the human genome, the estimated number of protein-coding genes in the human genome is less than 25,000.
4. Genetic information is transferred from parent to daughter cells by DNA copying or **replication.**

B. Central Dogma

1. Central dogma describes the transfer of genetic information within a cell. DNA is used as a template for **ribonucleic acid** (RNA) synthesis, and the RNA sequence determines the protein amino acid sequence: **DNA → RNA → Protein.**
2. The process of **DNA → RNA** is termed **transcription.** One strand of DNA is copied into messenger RNA (mRNA) by RNA polymerase in procaryotes and by RNA polymerase II in eucaryotes.
3. The process of **RNA → Protein** is termed **translation.** A molecule of mRNA is read by ribosomal machinery, resulting in the production of proteins that perform cellular functions.
4. Nucleotide sequence is translated to amino acid sequence through the **genetic code,** which assigns three-base RNA sequences (codons) to amino acids.

II. NUCLEIC ACIDS

A. Basic Structure of Nucleic Acids

1. Nucleic acid is a linear polymer of nucleotides. Nucleotides have three components: nitrogenous bases, five-carbon sugars, and phosphate groups.
   a. The **nitrogenous heterocyclic base** (purine or pyrimidine) is attached to the 1′ carbon atom of the sugar by an N-glycosidic bond.
      1) **Purines** have a double ring and include adenine (A) and guanine (G).
      2) **Pyrimidines** have a single ring and include cytosine (C), thymine (T), and uracil (U).
      3) Both DNA and RNA contain A, G, and C. T is only found in DNA, and U is only found in RNA.
   b. Cyclic five-carbon sugar residue
      1) RNA contains a ribose sugar, which has OH groups bound to its 2′ and 5′ carbons.
      2) DNA contains a deoxyribose sugar. Deoxyribose is identical to ribose except that the OH group at the 2′ position has been replaced with a hydrogen atom (H).

c. A phosphate group is attached to the 5′ carbon of the sugar by a phosphoester bond, and it is responsible for the strong **negative charge** of both nucleotides and nucleic acids.

2. The nucleotides are joined to one another by a **phosphodiester** bond between the 5′ phosphate of one nucleotide and the 3′ OH group of the adjacent nucleotide.

B. Physical and Chemical Structure of DNA

1. **Base pairing**
   a. Base composition of DNA varies from organism to organism; however, A always pairs with T (or U in RNA) and G always pairs with C. This is termed **complementary base pairing.**
   b. **In a double-stranded DNA molecule, the concentration of purines always equals the concentrations of pyrimidines** (Chargaff's rule).
2. **Structure**
   a. Watson and Crick (1953) described DNA as two polynucleotide strands coiled about one another to form a **double-stranded helix.**
   b. **Sugar–phosphate backbones** of each strand form the outer edge of the molecule, and bases are in the central core.
   c. Each base in one strand is hydrogen bonded to a complementary base in the other strand, which forms the purine-pyrimidine base pair (bp) (e.g., AT and GC). Two hydrogen bonds form between A and T, whereas three hydrogen bonds form between G and C.
   d. At physiological temperatures, the DNA base pairs are stable; however, they can break and reform rapidly.
   e. A DNA helix has two external grooves: the **major groove** and the **minor groove,** where various proteins and other molecules bind to DNA.
3. **Complementary strands**
   a. Due to base pairing rules, the two strands are complementary. For example, if one strand has the sequence 5′ GATACC 3′, the other strand's sequence is its complement: 3′ CTATGG 5′. See the following:

      5′ G-C 3′
      A-T
      T-A
      A-T
      C-G
      3′ C-G 5′

   b. The two strands of the DNA double helix are **antiparallel;** their chemical orientations run in opposite directions.
      i. As diagrammed above, one strand runs in the 5′ to 3′ direction, whereas the complementary strand goes from 3′ to 5′. The 3′ OH end of one strand is opposite the 5′ P end of the other.
      ii. By convention, a base sequence is usually written with the 5′ P terminal end on the left.

4. **Eucaryote chromosomes**
   a. **Eucaryotes** have multiple chromosomes.
   b. Helical human DNA is compacted into chromosomes and bound to basic proteins called histones as well as nonhistone proteins.
      i. DNA wrapped around a complex of eight histone proteins is called a **nucleosome.**
      ii. DNA and its associated histone and nonhistone proteins is **chromatin.**
   c. The chromosomes are contained within the nucleus surrounded by a nuclear membrane.
   d. The human nucleus contains **46 chromosomes.**
      i. Humans have two copies of each chromosome and therefore are **diploid.** There are two types of chromosomes: somatic and sex.
      ii. There are 22 pairs of **somatic chromosomes,** numbered 1 to 22, according to size, with 1 being the largest.
      iii. There are two **sex chromosomes,** X and Y, females have two X chromosomes (XX) and males have one X and one Y chromosome (XY).
5. **Eucaryotic Genes**
   a. Unlike procaryotic genes, eucaryotic genes are discontinuous.
   b. Protein coding parts of a gene are called **exons** (**ex**pressed sequences). They contain codons and are well conserved; the nucleotide sequence does not vary significantly among individuals of the same species.
   c. Noncoding regions of a gene are called **introns** (**in**tervening sequences). They do not contain codons, but they can contain regulatory/transcriptional elements and have other functions.
   d. Approximately 25% of all human genes have multiple allelic forms called **polymorphisms.**
      i. **Allele** refers to a different version or form of a gene or noncoding region. For example, the human leukocyte antigen (**HLA**) locus, which codes for peptides that establish self-identity of the immune system, is highly polymorphic.
      ii. **Loci** (singular locus) are the physical locations or positions of a gene or noncoding region on a chromosome.
6. **Mitochondrial DNA (mtDNA)**
   a. Eucaryotic cells have a second genome located in the mitochondria. There are thousands of mitochondria per cell. Each mitochondrion has 1–10 circular genomes of about 16,500 bp.
   b. Mitochondrial DNA (mtDNA) contains 22 tRNA genes, 3 rRNA genes, and 12 genes coding for oxidation-phosphorylation components. Mutations in these genes are responsible for neuropathies and myopathies.
   c. Mitochondrial DNA contains two noncoding regions (610 bp): hypervariable regions I (342 bp) and II (268 bp). Single nucleotide polymorphisms in these regions are sequenced for forensic studies.

7. **Procaryotic chromosomes**
   a. Procaryotic cells have a single chromosome.
   b. Procaryotes lack a nucleus and nuclear membrane.
   c. The procaryotic chromosome is generally circular DNA with groups of related genes arranged in a linear fashion as **operons.**
   d. Approximately 95% of the procaryotic chromosome contains coding sequences and 5% is noncoding sequences.
8. **Plasmids**
   a. Plasmids are extrachromosomal DNA containing nonessential genetic information found in procaryotes and lower eucaryotes. In certain situations, plasmids give organisms a growth advantage.
   b. Resistance (R) plasmids contain genes that confer antimicrobial resistance in a bacterium.
   c. Fertility (F) plasmids confer the ability to transfer genetic information between bacteria by **conjugation.**
   d. High copy number plasmids (500–700 plasmids/cell) replicate independently of the chromosome in cells, while low copy number plasmids may be dependent on host replication factors and therefore are synchronized to host replication.
   e. Plasmids enter cells by the process of **transfection.**
9. **Viruses and bacteriophage**
   a. Viruses are tiny particles that can only replicate with the aid of a host cell. They may be the most abundant of biological forms.
   b. Viruses are comprised of nucleic acid (DNA or RNA) and a protein, glycoprotein or lipid coat.
   c. Viruses invade cells and use the host replication machinery to synthesize viral proteins and nucleic acids ultimately bursting the host cell, and releasing the replicated virus particles.
   d. Some viruses can integrate their genome into the host cell DNA where they can remain latent, and the cell can survive until the viral DNA is activated to produce virus particles.
   e. Bacteriophages are viruses that infect bacteria.
   f. Bacteriophage also use host replication machinery to make more viruses.
   g. Bacteriophage can carry genetic information from cell to cell through the process of **transduction.**

C. Secondary Structure of DNA and RNA

1. The native conformation of DNA is double stranded (ds); whereas the disrupted form, known as **denatured** (or melted) DNA, is single stranded (ss).
   a. Denaturation can be accomplished through **heating** or **chemicals.**
   b. Although denaturing temperatures for DNA vary by species, assays requiring denaturation of human DNA are conducted at about 94°C.

2. **Renaturation,** or **annealing,** is the association of denatured DNA to native dsDNA through hydrogen bonds between complementary bases.
   a. Many molecular biology techniques are based on the reassociation of complementary base sequences (i.e., **hybridization**) and can be used to:
      i. determine whether certain sequences occur more than once in DNA of a particular organism.
      ii. locate specific base sequences in a DNA molecule.
      iii. detect a particular type or structure of RNA.
   b. The two requirements for annealing are as follows:
      i. Salt concentration must be high enough to overcome electrostatic repulsion between negatively charged phosphate groups in two strands.
      ii. Temperature must be high enough to disrupt the random, nonspecific intrastrand hydrogen bonds. Depending on base content, annealing of human DNA will occur around 52°C. Sequences with more G:C base pairs will have a higher annealing temperature than sequences with more A:T base pairs.

D. DNA Replication

1. DNA replication is a process in which genetic information is copied and transferred from parent to daughter cells. It requires energy to unwind the helix and disrupt H-bonds.
2. **Proofreading and repair systems** minimize replication errors; however, mistakes do sometimes occur and on occasion can be expressed as altered phenotypes.
   a. Base changes occur resulting in **mutations;** mutations found frequently in a population generally do not have an adverse phenotypic effect, and are classified as **polymorphisms.**
   b. Often mutations have detrimental effects. However, some mutations result in a selective advantage for the organism that is the basis for evolution.
   c. Changes in the DNA sequence from a reference sequence are indicated by the nucleotide location, followed by the reference base(s), an arrow, and the replacement base. For example, a change from G to A at nucleotide position 315 is indicated as g.315G>A. The "g" indicates a genomic reference sequence (containing introns). A "c" would indicate only exon sequences as would be found in cDNA made from spliced RNA. A "p" is used for the corresponding change in the protein amino acid sequence, for instance, if the change replaces a threonine with a leucine at position 105, then the protein change would be p.Thr105Leu or p.T105L using the single letter amino acid code. Note the different formats for nucleotide versus amino acid sequence.
3. The synthesis of each nucleotide chain of a double helix occurs in the 5′ → 3′ direction. In order to accommodate unidirectional copying of the antiparallel strands of DNA, one strand is synthesized continuously, whereas the other strand

is synthesized discontinuously, resulting in **Okazaki fragments** that must be ligated together by the enzyme ligase.

4. Each parental DNA strand serves as a template to create a complementary daughter strand.
   a. As replication proceeds, the parental double helix unwinds by the action of helicase enzymes.
   b. Polymerization of DNA is catalyzed by **DNA polymerase** enzymes.
   c. As a new strand is formed, it is hydrogen bonded to its parental template. Each new double helix consists of one parental strand and one newly formed daughter strand.

E. RNA Overview

1. Most RNA molecules are **single stranded;** however, RNA readily forms secondary structures required for its many functions.
2. Generally, RNA is environmentally labile and easily degraded by ubiquitous RNA nucleases.
3. **Types of RNA**
   a. **Ribosomal RNA (rRNA)** makes up 80–90% of total RNA in a cell; it is part of ribosomes and is involved in translation of mRNA into proteins.
   b. **Messenger RNA (mRNA)** makes up 1–5% of total RNA in a cell; it is an intermediate between the genetic code in DNA and the protein product.
      i. mRNA is read by ribosomes to produce proteins.
      ii. In eucaryotes, transcription of DNA forms a pre-mRNA molecule with both introns (noncoding) and exons (coding regions). This molecule is referred to as **heteronuclear RNA** (hnRNA). The introns are removed, and the exons are joined together by **splicing.**
      iii. Processing into mature mRNA also includes addition of a 5′ methylguanine cap and polyadenylate (poly A) tail of up to 200 adenylate nucleotides at the 3′-OH terminus of the RNA.
   c. **Transfer RNA (tRNA)** reads mRNA triplets and brings the appropriate amino acid to the ribosome for polypeptide (i.e., protein) synthesis. There is at least one tRNA for each amino acid.
   d. Other RNAs: **Small nuclear RNA** (snRNA) is involved in removal of introns and **small and micro RNAs** (including siRNA, stRNA, miRNA, snoRNA) are involved in regulation of transcription and translation of RNA into protein. A related class of **long noncoding RNAs** (eRNA, lincRNA, lncRNA, pseudogene transcripts) 200 to over 100,000 bases in length also regulates gene expression.

III. NUCLEASES AND RESTRICTION ENZYMES

A. Definitions

1. A variety of enzymes called **nucleases** break phosphodiester bonds in nucleic acids (they usually exhibit chemical specificity).

2. **DNases:** Deoxyribonucleases
   a. Many act on either ss or dsDNA.
   b. Some act on both ss and dsDNA.
3. **RNases:** Ribonucleases
   a. RNases are tiny ubiquitous proteins that are difficult to permanently inactivate.
   b. RNases can survive a wide range of temperatures: below −20 to >100°C.
   c. Humans secrete RNases, possibly as a defense mechanism against RNA viruses; thus, it is necessary to wear gloves when working with RNA.
4. **Exonucleases** cut only at the **end** of a nucleic acid, removing a single nucleotide at a time. **Endonucleases** cut within the nucleic acid strand.

B. Restriction enzymes

1. **Restriction enzyme/endonucleases** are enzymes produced by bacteria to ward off invasion by external DNA.
   a. Bacteria have a restriction/modification system that uses enzymes to methylate their own DNA, so that restriction enzymes can distinguish any incoming nonbacterial DNA from their own.
   b. Restriction enzymes are traditionally classified into four types (Types I–IV) on the basis of methylation capability, how they separate DNA and cofactor requirements. Sequence analysis has revealed a great deal of variety in the four enzyme types.
2. Some restriction enzymes cut only methylated DNA, others only nonmethylated DNA, and some enzymes can cut both.
   a. Restriction enzymes recognize a specific base sequence in a DNA molecule and cut near or within the sequence. These enzymes make two cuts, one in each strand, generating a 3′-OH and a 5′-P terminus.
   b. **Star activity** refers to nonspecific cleaving by the enzyme when incubation conditions are not optimal.
   c. **Type II restriction enzymes** make cuts at predictable sites within or near the recognition sequence; they have the greatest utility in recombinant DNA experiments.
      i. Sequences recognized by most type II enzymes are known as **palindromes,** due to the **bilateral symmetry** of the enzyme.
      ii. A double-stranded palindromic sequence reads the same from the 5′ to 3′ direction on both strands.
      iii. The enzyme binds the specific sequence and cleaves the DNA directly at the binding site.

      For example, the enzyme *Eco*RI recognizes the sequence 5′ GAATTC 3′ and cuts between the G and A. On the complementary strand, the sequence reads 3′ CTTAAG 5′ and is cut between A and G.
3. A particular restriction enzyme generates a unique set of fragments for a particular DNA molecule. A different enzyme generates a different number and size of fragments from the same DNA molecule.

4. In human DNA, occurrence of restriction enzyme sites is polymorphic, so that the pattern of DNA fragments produced by a particular restriction enzyme digest may differ from person to person.
   a. Analysis of **restriction fragment length polymorphisms** (RFLPs) had been used to screen and diagnose hereditary diseases and in forensic science but is rarely used today.
   b. Southern blot analysis using probes to detect fragments at hypervariable loci produces a characteristic RFLP pattern for each individual and thus produces a unique "genetic fingerprint."

IV. LABORATORY TECHNIQUES IN MOLECULAR DIAGNOSTICS

A. Nucleic Acid Isolation

1. **Sources**
   a. A variety of clinical specimens can be used: body and lavage fluids, saliva, buccal cells, stool filtrate, bone marrow, and whole blood.
      i. **Nucleated cells** (e.g., white blood cells) are the classic source for DNA isolation.
      ii. Clinical tests have been developed requiring isolation of **cell-free DNA** from blood plasma or urine. **Cell-free RNA** can also be isolated but is not yet part of clinical testing.
   b. Nucleic acid is also commonly isolated from fresh, frozen, or formalin-fixed paraffin-embedded (FFPE) tissue.
   c. FFPE tissue may be dewaxed with xylene or other agents and then rehydrated before isolation.
   d. **Mitochondrial DNA** is most often obtained from hair follicles.
      i. Due to its small circular structure and natural amplification, mitochondrial DNA is more resistant to degradation than chromosomal DNA.
      ii. Mitochondrial DNA is also isolated from muscle tissue to assess mutations associated with nerve and movement disorders.
   e. A diploid cell contains approximately 6.6 pg of DNA and 10–30 pg of RNA.
      i. Most (80%) of the RNA in a cell is rRNA.
      ii. The actual amount of RNA will depend on the cell type and the metabolic state of the cell.
   f. **Microorganisms:** Nucleic acid can be isolated directly from samples (tissues, body fluids) or from cultures.
      i. Gram-negative bacteria are treated with detergents to release nucleic acids.
      ii. Gram-positive bacteria and fungi are treated chemically with enzymes or physically by sonication or shaking with beads to disrupt cell walls.
      iii. Viral nucleic acid is isolated from tissue, plasma, or from cultures.
2. **Special considerations for RNA isolation** to avoid degradation of RNA are as follows:
   a. Because hands have high concentration of RNase, gloves should always be worn when working with RNA.

b. Use equipment designated as RNase free for RNA testing.
c. RNase-free reagents must also be used.
d. Reserve areas in the laboratory specifically for storage of reagents and RNA work.
e. Use disposable items certified as nuclease-free by the manufacturer.
f. Avoid reusable glassware or bake 4–6 hours at >270°C to inactivate RNase.
g. Lyse cells using detergent, or phenol, in presence of high salt or **RNase inhibitors** (e.g., guanidine isothiocyanate) and a strong reducing agent, such as 2-beta-mercaptoethanol.

3. **Nucleic acid isolation methods**
   a. **Organic isolation**
      i. Organic isolation is performed with a mixture of phenol and chloroform to remove contaminating proteins, lipids, carbohydrates, and cellular debris (for RNA isolation, use acidic phenol pH 4–5).
      ii. This mixture forms an emulsion that separates into two phases. DNA and RNA collect in the aqueous phase.
      iii. DNA or RNA from the aqueous phase is precipitated using **ethanol** or **isopropanol** in high salt concentration and recovered as pellet by centrifugation.
      iv. The pellet is rinsed with 70% ethanol and the DNA resuspended in 10 mM Tris, 1 mM EDTA (TE), or sterile DNase-free water and RNA in RNase-free buffer/water.
   b. **Inorganic isolation**
      i. Most manual laboratory DNA isolations are performed by inorganic methods.
      ii. Low pH and high salt concentration are used to precipitate protein leaving DNA in solution.
      iii. DNA is precipitated using isopropanol and resuspended as previously noted.
   c. **Solid phase isolation**
      i. Solid phase isolation is the basis for most automated nucleic acid isolation systems.
      ii. Silica-based beads or columns bind DNA or RNA in high salt solution.
      iii. The column is washed to remove impurities, and the nucleic acids are eluted with low-salt buffer.
   d. **Chelex extraction**
      i. Chelex is a cation-chelating resin used in forensic applications.
      ii. A solution of 10% Chelex is mixed with the specimen. The mixture is boiled. The contaminating substances will bind to resin and are removed by centrifugation.
      iii. DNA will be in the supernatant.
   e. **Isolation of poly-(A)-enriched RNA (i.e., mRNA)**
      i. The poly-A tail of mRNA binds to oligomers of poly-T or poly-U immobilized to a **matrix** (i.e., beads or column).

ii. Total RNA lysate is poured over the matrix. Poly-A RNA binds poly-T or poly-U; the matrix is rinsed and then mRNA is eluted.
iii. Generally, 1 μg total RNA yields 30–40 ng poly-(A)-enriched RNA.

4. **Measurement of quality and quantity of isolated nucleic acids**
   a. **Electrophoresis:** DNA and RNA are anionic (negatively charged).
      i. Intact **genomic DNA** has a high molecular weight and will, therefore, migrate very slowly during electrophoresis.
      ii. RNA is electrophoresed in the presence of **chaotropic agents** to inhibit secondary structure. A chaotropic agent, or chaotrope, is a substance that disrupts the three-dimensional structure of macromolecules.
      iii. In total RNA preparation, intact 28S and 16S rRNA bands should be present at about 4.8 and 1.7 kilobases.
      iv. Semiquantitative estimates of nucleic acid are made by comparison to ethidium bromide stained standards.
   b. **Spectrophotometry**
      i. Absorptivity maximum for nucleic acids is near 260 nm.
      ii. One Absorbance (Abs) unit equals 50 μg/mL dsDNA. Therefore, the concentration of dsDNA can be determined by multiplying the absorbance reading by 50.
      iii. One Abs unit equals 40 μg/mL RNA or ssDNA. Therefore, the concentration of RNA or ssDNA can be determined by multiplying the absorbance reading by 40.
      iv. Absorptivity maximum of phenol is 270 nm; therefore, phenol contamination can give falsely high readings.
      v. Absorptivity maximum of protein is 280 nm.
      vi. **Quality estimates** are determined from the ratio of Abs 260 nm:Abs 280 nm:
         For high-quality DNA, the ratio will be 1.6–2.0.
         For high-quality RNA, the ratio will be 2.0–2.3.
   c. **Fluorometry** is a more accurate measurement of intact dsDNA than spectrophotometry.
      i. For dsDNA, Hoechst 33258 dye binds minor groove of A-T base pairs; thus, the DNA must be intact (spectrophotometry measures natural absorbance from nitrogen bases).
      ii. Fluorometry requires internal standards with each measurement.

B. Nucleic Acid Sequence Detection by Hybridization

1. A particular gene or base sequence is called the **target sequence.**
2. The target sequence is detected by hybridization (hydrogen bonding) with a **probe** containing the complementary (i.e., **homologous**) sequence or part thereof.
   a. A double-stranded target sequence must be denatured (converted to single stranded) prior to hybridization.
   b. The probe must be single stranded and labeled, and attached to a molecule that produces a color, light, or fluorescent signal.

3. Probe hybridization has applications in microbiology, immunology, forensics, oncology, and genetics.
4. There are two types of hybridization methods: in solution and solid membrane support.
   a. With solution methods, both target and probe sequences are in a liquid state.
   b. In immobilized methods, target sequences (i.e., DNA, RNA, or proteins) in samples are bound onto solid membranes made of nitrocellulose, nylon, or polyvinyldifluoride.
      i. **Southern blot:** Template molecules are DNA fragments produced by restriction enzyme digestion separated by gel electrophoresis, chemically denatured, and transferred to the membrane.
      ii. **Northern blot:** After electrophoresis, total RNA or mRNA is transferred to a membrane.
      iii. **Western blot:** Proteins are separated by sodium dodecyl sulfate-polyacrylamide gel electrophoresis (SDS-PAGE) and then transferred to a membrane.
5. **Transfer** of macromolecular template (i.e., DNA, RNA, or proteins) onto solid matrix can be accomplished by capillary action, electrical current, pressure, or vacuum.
6. **Probes** are single-stranded DNA, or RNA complementary to the target sequences.
   a. dsDNA probes must be denatured, or made single stranded, by heating at 95°C or heating in formamide.
   b. The probe will detect the target sequence within a large amount of other nucleic acid sequences.
      i. Short probes (<500) bases are less specific but good for mutation analysis.
      ii. Probes of 500–5000 bases have greater specificity and are less affected by mutations.
      iii. Because of secondary structure formation, high GC content in the probe decreases efficiency of binding to target.
   c. Probes are covalently attached to radioisotopes (e.g., ^{32}P), enzymes (e.g., alkaline phosphatase or horseradish peroxidase), fluorochromes, or chemiluminescent compounds to produce a measurable signal.
      i. Multiple fluorescent dyes can be used concurrently to detect different targets in the same reaction mixture.
      ii. Labels are incorporated through labeled primers or a labeled deoxynucleotide triphosphate (dNTP) in a DNA synthesis reaction.
   d. Detection methods include fluorescent microscopy, or measurement by a fluorometer, colorimeter, spectrophotometer, or luminometer.
7. Labeled probes of known sequence are incubated in liquid hybridization buffer with the immobilized target sequences to hybridize with DNA or RNA sequences on the blot that are complementary to the labeled probe.

8. Factors that influence hybridization conditions (**stringency**) for probe binding (annealing) and removal of probe (washing) include temperature and salt and/or denaturant concentration in buffer.
   a. **Temperature**
      i. **Melting temperature** (T_m) is the temperature required to separate hybridized strands of complementary nucleotide sequences. At the T_m, half of the double-stranded structure has dissociated into single strands.
      ii. The **annealing temperature** optimal for specific probe:target hybridization is estimated to be ($T_m - 5°C$).
      iii. With high stringency, specificity of probe binding is increased, but sensitivity (ability of the probe to bind) may be decreased.
      iv. With low stringency, the probe can bind robustly (high sensitivity); however, the specificity is compromised by binding to other than exact complementary sequences.
   b. The salt concentration of the hybridization buffer also affects stringency.
      i. Hybridizing single strands are electrostatically repelled by their negative charges in a buffer with low salt concentration. Distilled water is a highly stringent liquid.
      ii. A buffer solution with high salt concentration excludes the nucleic acids, so that they are pushed together and can more easily form hydrogen bonds (low stringency).
   c. The presence of a denaturant, such as formamide, in the hybridization buffer can increase stringency by interfering with hydrogen bonding.
9. For **dot blots and slot blots,** total cellular DNA or RNA is denatured and spotted onto a membrane and hybridized in a single labeled probe solution.
   a. Dot blots allow probe hybridization to multiple samples on the same blot.
   b. Dot blots require highly specific probe–target recognition.
   c. Elongated, rather than circular, spots (slot blots) facilitate densitometry tracings for quantification of target sequences (e.g., RNA expression).
10. In **macroarray** and **microarray** analyses, often termed **reverse hybridization,** known sequences (unlabeled probes) are spotted onto a solid support.
    a. The support can be a membrane, a glass slide, or microelectrode.
    b. Nucleic acids from patient samples are labeled with a fluorescent dye in solution (using polymerase chain [PCR] technology) and incubated with the bound probes.
    c. Cellular DNA or RNA will bind to the complementary probes and produce fluorescence in those spots.
       i. Target and/or probe sequences can be DNA, RNA, protein, complementary DNA (cDNA), PCR products, or synthesized oligonucleotides.
       ii. Multiple genes, gene sequences, mutations, and polymorphisms can be simultaneously analyzed by this method.
       iii. Starting with RNA, cDNA, or protein products obtained from patient samples allows gene expression analysis.

11. **Chromosomal structure and mutations**
   1. The complete set of chromosomes in a cell is displayed in a **karyotype**.
      a. Cells are stimulated to divide in culture with phytohemagglutinin and then arrested at metaphase with colchicine.
      b. Cells are lysed with hypotonic buffer to produce a chromosome spread.
      c. The released metaphase chromosomes are then fixed and stained with dyes to better assess chromosome structures.
         i. Giemsa stain produces reproducible banding patterns on the chromosomes (G-banding).
         ii. Quinacrine dyes were originally used to produce a fluorescent banding pattern (Q-banding).
         iii. Heat denaturation before Giemsa staining reverses the G-banding pattern (R-banding).
      d. The chromosomes are numbered and arranged in order from the largest to smallest in size.
      e. Karyotyping can detect translocations, deletions, insertions, and copy number abnormalities.
   2. **Fluorescence *in situ* hybridization (FISH)**
      a. Interphase nuclei are hybridized to a probe complementary to genomic regions of interest.
      b. The probe is a 60- to 200-kb fragment of DNA specific for a chromosomal region and covalently attached to a fluorescent molecule.
      c. An advantage of interphase FISH over karyotyping is that it does not require culturing of cells.
      d. Interphase FISH detects chromosomal copy number, translocations, deletions, and amplified chromosomal regions in cells in interphase.
   3. **Metaphase FISH** uses chromosomes in metaphase and probes that bind to part of or the whole chromosome (chromosome painting).
      a. Metaphase FISH allows detection of complex abnormalities involving the "painted" chromosome.
      b. More complex changes are detected using **spectral karyotyping** in which each chromosome has a different fluorescent color.

C. Amplification Methods

1. Amplification of specific regions of DNA (or RNA) provides sufficient material for further analysis. These methods also increase the sensitivity of detection of specific nucleic acid targets by making more copies of the target, or probe, or attaching more signal producing molecules onto the target.
2. The three basic approaches to amplification are as follows:
   a. Target amplification is produced by PCR, reverse transcriptase PCR (RT-PCR), quantitative PCR, and transcription-mediated amplification (TMA).
   b. Probe amplification methods include ligase chain reaction (LCR), strand displacement amplification (SDA), and Qβ replicase.

c. Signal amplification is performed using branched chain DNA (bDNA) amplification, hybrid capture assay (HCA), and cleavage-based amplification.

3. PCR is the prototype method used to exponentially increase the amount of target DNA found in a sample, making detection more sensitive and providing sufficient DNA for further analyses.
   a. The PCR takes place in a **reaction mix** consisting of template DNA with target sequences, synthetic primers complementary to sequences flanking the target sequence, nucleotide triphosphates, and DNA polymerase in a buffer containing monovalent and divalent cations.
   b. The reaction mix is then subjected to an **amplification program** comprised of 30–50 cycles. Standard PCR amplification programs use a conventional three-step cycle.
      i. The first step of the first cycle is **denaturation** of the target by heating to **94–96°C** for 20–60 seconds.
      ii. The second step of the first cycle is **annealing** where the primers hybridize to the template at **50–70°C** for 20–90 seconds.
      iii. The third step of the first cycle is extension where DNA polymerase extends or adds nucleotides to the 3′ ends of the primers, copying both strands of the template.
   c. At the end of the first cycle, there are two double-stranded copies (amplicons) per double-stranded starting target sequence. After a second three-step cycle, there will be four copies. The number of copies per starting copy will be approximately 2^n, where n = the number of PCR cycles completed. The yield is not exactly 2^n because the efficiency of amplification is not always 100%.
   d. Thermostable DNA polymerases isolated from thermophilic bacteria such as *Thermus aquaticus* (*Taq* polymerase) are used for PCR to withstand the denaturation temperatures. A variety of polymerases have been applied to different PCR methods.
   e. The amplification process is performed in a **thermal cycler,** which automatically changes temperatures for the appropriate times.
   f. **Repeat the cycle** 20–30 times to produce detectable levels of amplicons.
   g. Unlabeled products can be detected by gel electrophoresis or labels can be introduced into the product using labeled primers or dNTP. Alternatively, labeled probes or antibodies that recognize products that emit colorimetric, fluorescent, or chemiluminescent signals can be used.
   h. Controls in PCR testing
      i. A **positive control** for PCR is a known sample containing the target sequence. The positive control ensures that the DNA polymerase enzyme is active, buffer is optimal, primers are recognizing the intended target, and that the thermal cycler is working properly.
      ii. The **blank control or reagent blank** is a reaction mix without DNA added to ensure that reagent mix is not contaminated with template or previously amplified PCR products.

iii. The **negative template control** is a DNA sample known to lack target to ensure that primers do not anneal to unintended sequences.

iv. The **internal control** or **amplification control** is a second primer set for a sequence unrelated to target sequence of interest but present in all samples tested. This control confirms true negative results for the target sequence. It can be performed in the same tube or can be run as a duplicate sample.

4. Quantitative Real-Time PCR (qPCR)
   a. In addition to amplification, qPCR estimates the amount of starting template (e.g., copy number/mL).
   b. Fluorescent signal increases as target copy number increases during the amplification process.
   c. The amount of fluorescence generated is directly proportional to amount of starting template; however, the time to its accumulation (the point when it crosses a predetermined amount of fluorescence or threshold) is inversely proportional, such that large amounts of target cross the threshold early.
   d. The cycle number at which fluorescence crosses a threshold is designated **C_T (threshold cycle).** C_T is inversely proportional to the amount of starting target. Thus, detection of a large amount of target is indicated by a lower C_T value.
   e. Applications of qPCR include viral load, tumor load, and treatment monitoring.
   f. **SYBR green** is a fluorescent dye that binds double-stranded DNA and monitors accumulation of PCR products as they are made (i.e., in real time). SYBR green lacks specificity in reactions where mispriming and/or primer dimers can generate fluorescence.
   g. Probe systems increase specificity as they produce fluorescence only when hybridized to target sequences. Several types of qPCR probes exist including the following.

i. **TaqMan probe** is a ssDNA oligomer complementary to a specific sequence in the targeted region of the PCR template. The intact probe has a fluorescent reporter dye covalently attached to its 5′ end and a quencher dye covalently attached to its 3′ end. As PCR product is amplified, the probe is displaced and hydrolyzed by the polymerase, releasing the quencher and producing fluorescence.

ii. Fluorescence resonance energy transfer probes are two oligomers that hybridize close to one another on the target sequence. One oligomer has a reporter dye and the other has a donor dye required for fluorescence from the reporter. Signal is detected only when probes are bound next to each other on the target sequence. Signal is detected in the annealing step of the qPCR program.

iii. **Molecular beacons** also measure accumulation of product at the annealing step in the PCR cycle. At one end of the probe is a reporter dye and at the other end is a quencher dye. In the absence of target sequence, the probe forms a loop structure with a few base pairs of complementarity between the two ends of the 20–30 base probe. The proximity of the reporter and quencher prevents the production of signal. In the presence of target sequence, the hairpin is opened when hybridization of the probe overcomes the hydrogen bonds holding the ends together, separating the quencher and reporter. Signal is then detected only when probes are bound to template before displacement by polymerase.

iv. **Scorpion primer/probes** are tailed with hairpin molecular beacons structures. In the presence of template, primer/probe is extended moving reporter molecule away from quencher molecule, which generates fluorescence. An advantage of scorpion probes is that the signal is covalently attached to the PCR product, which can be useful for further analyses such as size measurement by capillary electrophoresis.

5. **Reverse transcription PCR (RT-PCR)**, or reverse transcriptase PCR, starts with an RNA template.
   a. The RNA template is converted to a DNA copy (**cDNA**) by RNA-dependent DNA polymerase, also known as **reverse transcriptase.**
   b. The cDNA product then serves as a template to make millions of dsDNA copies of the target RNA sequence.
   c. RT-qPCR is used to detect and/or quantify RNA in microbiology and oncology applications.
6. RNA is also the target for transcription-based amplification systems such as TMA, nucleic acid sequence–based amplification (NASBA), and self-sustaining sequence replication. Transcription-based amplification systems are target amplification methods.
   a. RNA is the target and primary product.
   b. Reactions are isothermal.
   c. Applications include direct detection of RNA viruses and RNA from other infectious agents, as well as transcribed gene sequences.
7. Probe amplification methods do not amplify the entire target sequence; rather, the synthetic primers/probes complementary to target nucleic acid are amplified.
   a. The **ligase chain reaction** uses four oligomers designed from the target sequence. Two oligomers are unlabeled primers and the other pair of oligomers are probes holding a capture molecule on one oligomer and a signal molecule on the other. It is no longer used much today in clinical laboratories.
   b. In **SDA**, the major amplification products are the probes/primers.
      i. SDA is an isothermal two-stage process of target generation followed by an exponential amplification phase.
      ii. In the first stage of target generation, two primers bind on each strand of the target sequence, one displacing the product of the other. The probes thus generated have a restriction enzyme recognition site introduced by the primers extended to generate them.
      iii. A second set of complementary primers then copies the displaced (probe) sequences. The probes are the target DNA for the next stage of the process.

iv. In the second stage (exponential probe/target amplification), the probes generated in the first stage are nicked by the restriction enzyme.
v. The nick in the DNA is extended, and the opposite strand is simultaneously displaced. The displaced strand is copied by the primers.
vi. The process takes place at 52°C without temperature cycling and produces millions of copies of the initial sequence.

c. **Qβ replicase** is an RNA-dependent RNA polymerase from the bacteriophage Qβ. The target can be either denatured DNA or RNA.
i. Template-bound probe is amplified by mixing with Qβ replicase, which can generate a billion RNA molecules/probes in less than 15 minutes.
ii. This method is used for identification of infectious agents, such as *Mycobacterium tuberculosis.*

8. Signal amplification methods include bDNA amplification, HCA, and cleavage-based amplification.
a. In signal amplification systems, the number of target sequences does not change; instead, large amounts of signal are bound to the target sequences present in the sample, making detection more sensitive. These systems carry less risk of target contamination.
b. **bDNA** is frequently used for quantification of target sequences in clinical samples, especially **viral load** determinations.
i. A series of immobilized capture probes hybridize to target nucleic acids. The capture probes are attached to the wells of a microplate.
ii. Additional probes bind target nucleic acids to attach the branched DNA molecules (amplifiers), which will bind multiple reporter molecules.
iii. Binding of target at multiple sequence locations increases the specificity of the procedure.
iv. The reporter molecules, which bind the branched amplifier DNA, are labeled with alkaline phosphatase. Dioxetane is added as substrate for alkaline phosphatase, and multiple chemiluminescent signals are emitted from each target molecule.
c. HCA is based on the formation of DNA:RNA hybrids.
i. Target DNA released from cells binds to ssRNA probes to form DNA/RNA hybrid molecules.
ii. A DNA/RNA hybrid forms a unique structure, which can be bound by antibodies on the surface of a microtiter well.
iii. Captured hybrids are detected by binding alkaline phosphatase-conjugated anti-DNA/RNA hybrid antibodies in a typical "sandwich" assay.
iv. Substrate is added, and signal is measured. The signal is amplified by multiple antibody conjugates binding to each captured target.
d. Cleavage-based amplification is based on the activity of the cleavase enzyme.
i. Detects target nucleic acid by two probes that bind to the target sequence and overlap forming a triplex DNA structure

ii. **Cleavase** recognizes overlapping sequence of DNA and cuts the end off of the longer sequence-specific probe. Triplex formation and cleavage will only occur if the target and probe are complementary. If not, no cleavage will occur.
iii. The cleaved end of the probe then forms another triplex structure with a fluorescent signal probe. Cleavage of the triplex structure releases a reporter molecule resulting in a fluorescent signal. The fluorescent signal will only occur when the first sequence-specific probe is complementary to the target sequence.
iv. Cleavase assays are used in genetics, hemostasis (e.g., factor V Leiden mutation detection), and infectious disease.

9. Contamination must be avoided in amplification methods.
   a. Physical separation of areas for preparation of sample, reagent mixes, and amplification and post-amplification procedures is the best way to assure post-amplification products do not contaminate pre-amplification materials.
      i. Positive air pressure in the preparation area and negative air pressure in post-amplification areas prevent air-borne contamination.
      ii. Work areas should be decontaminated with bleach or alcohol.
      iii. Ultraviolet (UV) light breaks up DNA; however, the effectiveness of UV light depends on the wavelength, strength, and distance of the light energy from the target.
      iv. Unidirectional organization of workflow is recommended such that work and equipment never goes from post-amplification area to preparation areas.
   b. The uracil triphosphate-uracil-N-glycosylase (**dUTP-UNG**) system chemically removes contamination from PCR and qPCR.
      i. The system uses PCR mixtures with dUTP rather than dTTP, producing amplicons containing uracil rather than thymidine residues.
      ii. Uracil-N-glycosylase (UNG) is added to the reaction mixture before amplification.
      iii. The mixture is incubated at 50°C for 2–10 minutes to allow digestion of any uracil-containing DNA from previous amplifications. Native DNA lacks uracil and is immune from degradation.
      iv. During the first denaturation step of the PCR cycle, UNG enzyme is destroyed and amplification occurs only if target sequence is found in sample.

D. Sequencing methods determine the order or sequence of nucleotides in a DNA (or RNA) molecule.

Applications in the clinical laboratory include genotyping of microorganisms, detecting mutations, identifying human haplotypes, and determining polymorphisms.

1. Classic (Sanger) sequencing utilizes **dideoxynucleotides (ddNTPs)** in a DNA replication reaction. The ddNTP lack the 3′OH group required for formation of a phosphodiester bond.

a. Addition of ddNTPs to a DNA synthesis reaction terminates the DNA chain growth.
b. Manual sequencing requires a single-stranded sequencing template and one labeled primer to visualize the products of the reaction. Alternatively, a labeled nucleotide is used. The label is radioactive, ^{32}P or ^{14}C or other isotopes.
c. In manual sequencing, four separate reaction mixes were prepared, each containing template, primer, and all four dNTPs and a different ddNTP: ddATP, ddCTP, ddGTP, or ddTTP.
d. Upon addition of DNA polymerase, the template was copied into fragments all ending with a ddNTP.
e. The resulting product from all four reactions was a **DNA ladder,** a series of products ending at each nucleotide in the template sequence.
f. The DNA ladder was resolved by gel electrophoresis. The band pattern can be read according to the size of the DNA products, revealing the DNA sequence.

2. Automated sequencing methods have replaced manual methods. Advances in sequencing technology from manual automated dye terminator sequencing were made in the course of sequencing the 3 billion base pair human genome in the Human Genome Project.
   a. Manual Sanger sequencing run on heat blocks followed by gel electrophoresis has been replaced by automated dye terminator methods performed in a thermal cycler and capillary electrophoresis.
   b. A single reaction mix is prepared containing all four dNTPs and ddNTPs. The ddNTPs carry fluorescent labels, each a different "color": ddATP-green, ddCTP-blue, ddGTP-black (or yellow), and ddTTP-red.
   c. All four reactions take place in the same solution in a thermal cycler (**cycle sequencing**).
   d. Cycle sequencing is performed on a double-stranded template, but since only one primer is used, each sequence reaction represents a single strand.
   e. The fluorescently labeled DNA ladder is then resolved by capillary electrophoresis producing an **electropherogram.**
   f. Instrument software provides a textual sequence read by the order of colors of fragments as they travel through the capillary passing by the detector.
3. **Pyrosequencing** is an alternative method to Sanger sequencing used for **resequencing** to test small regions of DNA.
   a. Pyrosequencing requires a single-stranded template. Newer instrument models generate the template on board the instrument.
   b. Neither primer nor nucleotides are labeled in the sequencing reaction.
   c. The instrument will introduce nucleotide triphosphates into the reaction mix in a predetermined order.
      i. If the nucleotide is complementary to the template, DNA polymerase will form a phosphodiester bond, releasing pyrophosphate.
      ii. The pyrophosphate will go through a cascade of enzymatic reactions to produce a light signal detected by the pyrosequencer.

iii. If the nucleotide is not complementary to the template, no phosphodiester bond will be formed and no signal will occur.

d. The results of the pyrosequencing reaction is a **pyrogram** of peaks of light units (chemiluminescence).

e. In comparison to Sanger or dideoxy sequencing, pyrosequencing produces shorter reads of 150 bp or less.

4. Next generation sequencing (NGS) offers the ability to sequence many genes, regions, or even whole genomes in a single sequencing run.
   a. Whole genome sequencing is not done as a clinical laboratory test. Whole exome (the part of the genome consisting of exons) sequencing is used in special applications such as with congenital abnormalities of unknown cause. Most clinical laboratory testing involves gene panels ranging from a few to over a thousand genes.
   b. Currently, the two major platforms for NGS in the clinical laboratory are as follows:
      i. Ion conductance sequencing, which detects sequence by release of a hydrogen atom with the introduction of a complementary nucleotide.
      ii. Reversible dye terminator sequencing, which produces a fluorescent signal from fluorescently labeled nucleotides.
   c. A third platform, long-read single molecule sequencing is used in research applications. Although this method has the advantage of long reads (median >30,0000 bases) and high accuracy, most clinical applications are not aimed at de novo sequencing where such long reads would be useful.
   d. Ion conductance and reversible dye terminator sequencing start with the preparation of a sequencing **library.** The library is a collection of fragments less than 500 bp in length that will be the sequencing template.
      i. Libraries for whole genome sequencing are enzymatically fragmented genomic DNA.
      ii. Libraries for whole exome sequencing utilize bead bound probes or primers to select exome regions to be sequenced.
      iii. Fragments for targeted libraries are selected by primer sets or probes complementary to regions to be sequenced. Libraries can be designed to sequence genes associated with particular disease states, organs, or types of mutations such as single nucleotide variants, translocations, or copy number variants.
      iv. Libraries are prepared for sequencing by the ligation of adaptors, or short sequences with primer binding sites or other recognition sites. The selected fragments are then amplified.
      v. The amplified products are then "bar-coded" by introduction of patient-specific sequences usually on the 5′ end of primers used for an additional amplification step.
   e. The bar-coded libraries can then be sequenced together in the same sequencing reaction.
   f. The instrument software provides an initial sequence quality assessment and variant (DNA base change) detection.

g. Further filtering of the variants, based on confidence of detection, predicted effect on the protein sequence, and previous observations of the variant in other studies, is used to generate the final report. The complexity of this bioinformatic analysis depends on the size of the initial library, with a few genes being relatively straightforward.

5. Other sequencing methods are applied to specific applications as follows:
   a. RNA sequencing is accomplished by converting RNA to cDNA and sequencing the cDNA by Sanger, pyrosequencing, or NGS. This method can also provide gene expression data.
   b. Bisulfite sequencing is performed to detect DNA methylation.
      i. DNA methylation in vertebrates occurs mostly by the addition of a methyl ($-CH3$) group on the 5 position of the cytosine pyrimidine ring.
      ii. When cytosines in DNA, followed by guanines (CG), in genes are methylated, transcription of that gene is inhibited.
      iii. When methylated DNA is treated with sodium bisulfite, cytosines are converted to uracil while methylated cytosines are unaffected.
      iv. Sequencing of the DNA by Sanger, pyrosequencing, or NGS reveals the methylated cytosines as those not converted to uracil when compared to the unconverted sequence.
   c. A variety of other specialized sequencing technologies are being developed but are not yet used routinely in the clinical laboratory.

E. **DNA polymorphisms** are base changes in DNA compared to a reference sequence that are present in at least 1–2% of a particular population. Polymorphisms and mutations differ only by their frequency of occurrence, with mutations usually being more rare.

1. All humans have a unique set of DNA sequences with a variety of polymorphisms.
2. The major histocompatibility locus on chromosome 6 is the most polymorphic area of human DNA.
   a. This locus encodes human leukocyte antigens (HLAs) that recognize self versus non-self molecules.
   b. HLA testing is performed before organ and tissue transplants to find the best "match" of HLAs. The closer the match between the recipient and the transplanted organ, the higher likelihood that the transplant will be successful.
      i. HLAs can be tested serologically with known antibodies using flow cytometry.
      ii. Higher resolution testing of HLAs is achieved by PCR analysis.
      iii. Sanger or NGS is used to perform sequence-based typing, which yields the highest resolution HLA typing.
3. Other highly polymorphic regions of DNA include the mitochondrial genome, centromeric regions, and repeated sequences in DNA.

4. A certain degree of polymorphism occurs throughout the genome. Four types of polymorphic sequences used in clinical applications are: restriction fragment length polymorphisms (RFLPs), variable number tandem repeats (VNTRs), short tandem repeats (STRs), and single nucleotide polymorphisms (SNPs).
   a. RFLP were the first polymorphic structures to be used for DNA sequence analysis.
      i. The first human DNA fingerprinting was developed with RFLP.
      ii. RFLP can also be performed in conjunction with PCR by amplifying regions containing polymorphic bases in restriction enzyme recognition sites. The method is frequently used to find mutations as well.
      iii. Genomic RFLP require the use of Southern blots to detect a large range of fragment sizes. This requirement limited its use in DNA fingerprinting as input DNA had to be in sufficient amounts and quality required for Southern blotting.
   b. STR and VNTR are similar structures in DNA, tandem repeats of base pairs. The repeat units in STR are less than 10 bp, while the repeat units in VNTR are more than 10 bp up to over 100 bp in length. For technical ease of use, most methods utilize STR.
      i. Every STR (and VNTR) can differ (are polymorphic) in the number of repeat units.
      ii. Different individuals will have different numbers of repeat units at STR loci throughout the genome. The number of repeat units is an allele or version of an STR.
      iii. No two people (except identical twins) have the same number of STRs repeat units at all STR loci. In this way, humans can be positively identified by the number of repeat units in their STRs.
      iv. STRs are identified by PCR using primers that flank the STR. Amplicons are resolved by gel or capillary electrophoresis. The size of the PCR product reflects the number of repeats in the amplified locus.
      v. By having one of each of the primer pairs labeled with a fluorescent molecule, the PCR product can be analyzed in fluorescent detection systems (e.g., capillary electrophoresis). The number of loci that can be resolved on a single run has been increased by the use of multicolor dye labels.
      vi. STR typing in forensics uses tetranucleotide (four bp) and pentanucleotide (five bp) repeat units.
      vii. The Combined DNA Indexing system (**CODIS**) now uses 20 "core" polymorphic loci and the nonpolymorphic amelogenin locus on the X and Y chromosomes for positive legal identification.
      viii. The amelogenin gene (not an STR) is a gender-specific locus. Two different sized amelogenin PCR products are seen in males (XY), whereas only one size amelogenin product is seen in females (XX).
      ix. STR match is made by comparing alleles at the 20 loci and calculating probability statistics as indicator of relatedness.

c. SNPs are the most informative of polymorphic DNA structures. A SNP is the presence of a different base at the same location in a DNA sequence among different individuals.
   i. Mutations can be SNPs as well as HLA types and mitochondrial DNA polymorphisms. A SNP is considered a polymorphism, rather than a mutation, if the different base is present in more than 1–2% of a given population.
   ii. The Human Genome Project revealed that SNPs occur about every 1000 bases, making them more informative in identifying DNA from different individuals.
   iii. The International HapMap Project aimed to map all SNPs in the human genome in genetically linked groups or haplotypes.
   iv. Despite the superior level of informativity of SNPs, their use in forensics and clinical analysis is limited by the highly complex methods required to identify the single bp changes. Advances in sequencing technology have facilitated identification of SNPs.

5. Despite numerous polymorphisms, any two people are 99.9% identical at the DNA sequence level. A 0.1% difference accounts for disease susceptibility and other variations among "normal" human traits. In addition, about 80% of the 0.1% will be SNPs.
6. Polymorphisms be used for genetic mapping, disease prediction, disease associations, and human identification.

V. CLINICAL LABORATORY APPLICATIONS

A. *In vitro* diagnostic (IVD) devices are used in the analysis of human samples. This designation includes commercial test products and instruments used in testing.

1. There are four IVD classes.
   a. Class I low risk, for example, nonsterile enzymes or tissue processor
   b. Class II moderate risk, for example, reagents for viral screening of blood units
   c. Class III high risk, for example, reagents used to test for human immunodeficiency virus (HIV) or tuberculosis
   d. Laboratory-Developed Test (LDT) is a class of IVD test that is developed within a single laboratory. It is also called "home-brew test."
2. The three types of test components are as follows:
   a. Analyte specific reagents have a particular diagnostic purpose, for example, antibodies.
   b. "Research Use Only" or "Investigational Use Only" reagents have not been approved, cleared, or licensed by FDA.
   c. Companion diagnostic reagents are developed with intended use for treatment guidance. They are FDA-reviewed.
3. Federal regulations from the FDA require validation of the performance of clinical test methods and reagents in accurately detecting or measuring analytes prior to use in human testing.

a. Validation establishes test performance, limits of detection, and sample type.
b. FDA-approved tests require demonstration of expected performance but not full validation unless the test is modified by the testing laboratory.

B. Detection, identification, and quantification of microorganisms have been greatly facilitated by molecular testing.

1. Methods: HCA, NASBA, TMA, PCR, bDNA, RT-PCR, qPCR, SDA, and DNA sequencing
2. Targets: 16S and 23S rRNA, rDNA, housekeeping genes, toxin genes, antimicrobial resistance genes, interspersed repetitive elements, strain-specific sequences, and internal transcribed spacer elements
3. Molecular epidemiology typing during outbreaks, genotyping, and drug resistance screening
   a. Genotypic methods are highly reproducible and can discriminate between closely related organisms.
   b. Chromosomal RFLP analysis by pulsed-field gel electrophoresis can be used for trace back studies during outbreaks of infectious diseases.
   c. Mass spectrometry matrix-assisted laser desorption ionization-time of flight, (MALDI-TOF) has been applied to identification, hierarchal clustering, and epidemiology of bacteria and fungi.
      i. Peptide profiles generated from mass spectrometry are compared to reference databases of profiles of known organisms.
      ii. The analysis mainly uses peaks consistently appearing in moderate-to-high amounts in a genus or species.
4. Viral load (quantitative) testing is performed using bDNA, NASBA, RT-PCR, and qPCR; especially for HIV, hepatitis C virus, hepatitis B virus, and cytomegalovirus
5. Infectious disease testing of blood donor units: Units of blood are screened for a number of blood-borne infectious agents using NAATs (e.g., PCR).
6. Bacteria frequently identified by molecular techniques include the following:
   a. Respiratory pathogens: *Mycoplasma pneumoniae*, *Chlamydophila pneumoniae*, *Legionella pneumophila*, *Bordetella pertussis*, *Streptococcus pneumoniae*, and *Mycobacterium tuberculosis*
   b. Urogenital pathogens: *Chlamydia trachomatis*, *Neisseria gonorrhoeae*, *Treponema pallidum*, *Mycoplasma genitalium*, *Mycoplasma hominis*, and *Haemophilus ducreyi* Can be Individually identified by multiplex qPCR.

C. Molecular Detection of Inherited Diseases

1. Chromosomal abnormalities can be differences in chromosome number or structure.
   a. Determine abnormalities in chromosome number and structure using karyotype and Giemsa staining

b. Determine specific abnormalities by FISH
   i. Centromeric probes detect changes in chromosome number in interphase.
   ii. Interphase FISH with gene specific probes detect changes in number (amplification or deletion) of specific genes. Gene specific probes can also detect translocations.
   iii. Metaphase FISH (chromosome painting, spectral karyotyping) can detect complex changes in chromosome structure.

c. Comparative genomic hybridization (microarray) provides high-resolution detection of deletions and insertions.

2. **Single gene disorders**
   a. DNA sequencing, PCR-RFLP, linkage analysis, Southern blot, LCR, and capillary electrophoresis are used to detect DNA changes causing disease phenotypes.
      i. Single base changes, such as the factor V Leiden mutation, a G to A change (c.1523G>A), results in substitution of the arginine (R) at position 506 by glutamine (Q), R506Q.
      ii. The base change results in loss of the recognition site for the *Mnl*I restriction enzyme. An amplicon containing this site will not cut with *Mnl*I if the mutation is present (PCR-RFLP).
      iii. The single base change can also be detected by sequence-specific primer PCR (SSP-PCR). One of the primer pair is sequence-specific, that is, the 3′ base is complementary to either the mutant or normal base. A product will only occur if the template has the base complementary to the sequence-specific primer.
   b. The cystic fibrosis transmembrane conductance regulator (CFTR) gene codes for a chloride channel membrane protein, and its loss of function causes cystic fibrosis.
      i. There are about 1700 CFTR mutations, with c.1523T>G (Phe508del or F508del) being the most common.
      ii. Each of 23 CFTR gene mutations and four polymorphisms are detected simultaneously by multiplex PCR and bead array.
      iii. Other methods include RFLP, PCR-RFLP, heteroduplex analysis, temporal temperature gradient gel electrophoresis, SSP-PCR, bead array, and direct sequencing.

3. Trinucleotide repeat expansion disorders are caused by a subset of STRs with three bp repeating units that expand in length over generations.
   a. Fragile X syndrome is due to expanding copies of the CGG codon in the gene *FMR-1* located on the X chromosome. It results in neurological symptoms in males and females.
      i. Normally, there are less than 55 CGG repeats 5′ to the *FMR*1 gene. Expansion up to 200 repeats results in a premutation state with variable severity of symptoms.
      ii. The full mutation introduces thousands of repeat units that become methylated, inhibiting expression of the *FMR*1 gene.
      iii. Since the expansion is on the X chromosome, females are more likely to be carriers, passing the mutation to their sons.

iv. The premutation can be detected by PCR and gel or capillary electrophoresis. The full mutation is detected using Southern blot or PCR and capillary electrophoresis.

b. Huntington disease (HD) is due to CAG expansion at 4p16.3 inside the *HTT* gene that codes for the gene product, huntingtin.
   i. Normally, there are 6 to 35 CAG repeats in the *HTT* gene. Expansion to 36–39 repeats increases the risk for HD. Over 40 CAG repeats will result in the disease phenotype.
   ii. HD repeat expansion is detectable by PCR and gel or capillary electrophoresis.

c. Myotonic Dystrophy type 1 (DM1) results from repeat expansions of (CTG) of the *DMPK* gene.
   i. The diagnosis of DM1 is based on characteristic muscle weakness and molecular testing for repeat expansions 5′ to the DMPK gene.
   ii. More than 34 CTG repeats is abnormal.
   iii. DM1 repeat expansion is detectable by PCR and gel or capillary electrophoresis.

d. Triplet repeat expansion diseases display anticipation, that is, expanding repeat sizes and increased severity of symptoms with each generation of an affected family.

D. Molecular biology is especially useful in oncology testing as cancer is caused by gene mutations.

1. Genes mutated in cancer are those that affect cell growth and survival, tumor suppressor genes that negatively regulate growth and survival, and oncogenes that drive growth and survival.

   a. Oncogenes promote growth by movement throughout the cell cycle and inhibition of apoptosis (cell death). Oncogene mutations in cancer are gain of function mutations and are usually dominant.

   b. Tumor suppressor genes arrest movement through the cell cycle and promote apoptosis. Tumor suppressor gene mutations in cancer are loss of function mutations and a usually recessive.

   c. Inherited tumor suppressor gene mutations increase the risk of cancer. This is the Knudson or "two-hit" hypothesis. With two copies of every gene, both alleles have to be damaged to manifest the cancer phenotype. The first "hit" could be the inheritance of an allele that increases one's risk for cancer, a so-called "susceptibility gene." If that individual later acquired damage to the same gene on the second chromosome, that cell could become cancerous.

   d. Gene and chromosomal mutations in solid tumors can be detected by SSP-PCR, single-strand conformation polymorphism analysis, direct sequencing, immunohistochemical staining, and FISH.

e. Translocations in hematologic malignancies are frequently used to quantify tumor load.
    i. Since only tumor cells carry the translocation, qPCR amplifying the translocated DNA can be used to monitor tumor load similar to how viral load is monitored.
    ii. Translocations used for monitoring are present in acute lymphoblastic and chronic myelogenous leukemia (t(9;22)), promyelocytic leukemia (t(15;17)), and follicular lymphoma, t(14;18).
    iii. Other detection methods such as karyotype FISH, Southern blot, slab gel and capillary gel electrophoresis may be used for rare breakpoints not recognized by the consensus primers or where the size of the product is informative.

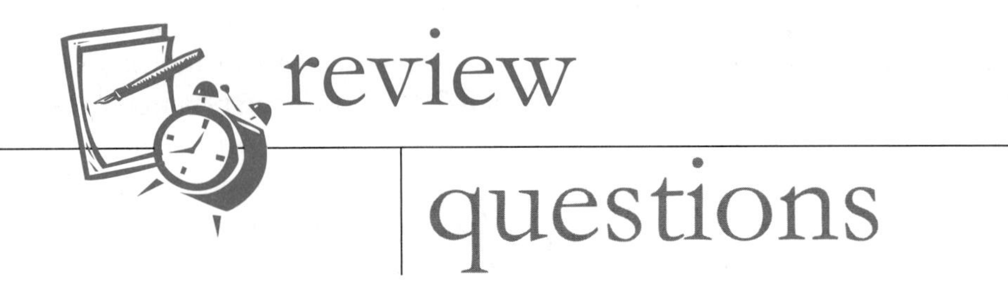

INSTRUCTIONS Each of the questions or incomplete statements that follows is comprised of four suggested responses. Select the *best* answer or completion statement in each case.

1. If 20% of the nucleotides in an organism are adenine, predict the percentage of nucleotides that are guanine.
   A. 20%
   B. 30%
   C. 40%
   D. 60%
2. Which of the following is *not* required for DNA replication by PCR?
   A. Oligonucleotide primers
   B. DNA polymerase
   C. DNA ligase
   D. Deoxynucleotides
3. In naming restriction endonucleases, the first letter of the name comes from which of the following?
   A. Bacterial genus
   B. Bacterial species
   C. Scientist who discovered it
   D. Geographic location of its discovery
4. A restriction enzyme recognizes the sequence, 5′ CT^ATAG 3′, and cuts as indicated. Predict the ends that would result on the *complementary* DNA strand.
   A. 3′ G 5′ 3′ ATATC 5′
   B. 3′ GA 5′ 3′ TATC 5′
   C. 3′ GATA 5′ 3′ TC 5′
   D. 3′ GATAT 5′ 3′ C 5′
5. The absorbance of a 1:100 dilution of isolated dsDNA solution, measured at 260 nm, is 0.062. What is a reasonable estimate for the dsDNA concentration of the sample, expressed in μg/mL?
   A. 3.1
   B. 6.2
   C. 310
   D. 5000
6. In the isolation of RNA, guanidine isothiocyanate (GITC) is used to
   A. Inhibit RNase
   B. Lyse the cells
   C. Precipitate the DNA
   D. Remove buffer salts

7. Total RNA isolated from white blood cells contains which of the following?
   A. 25% mRNA
   B. 80% rRNA
   C. 50% DNA
   D. 10% rRNA

8. After performance of DNA electrophoresis, the isolated bands appear too close together. Which of the following can be done with the next run to improve the appearance/separation of the bands in the samples?
   A. Increase the percent agarose concentration of the matrix
   B. Increase the running time of the electrophoresis assay
   C. Increase the sample volume applied to the gel
   D. Decrease the sample volume applied to the gel

9. Which of the following classes of DNA isolation is used in automated isolation systems?
   A. Solid phase
   B. Organic
   C. Inorganic
   D. Chelex

10. In forensic testing, DNA fingerprinting can identify individuals with high accuracy because
    A. Human genes are highly conserved
    B. Only a small amount of sample is needed
    C. Human gene loci are polymorphic
    D. DNA is stable and not easily contaminated

11. The technique that makes ssDNA from an RNA template is called
    A. Strand displacement amplification
    B. Translation
    C. Ligase chain reaction
    D. Reverse transcription

12. A 5850-base plasmid possesses *Eco*RI restriction enzyme cleavage sites at the following base pair locations: 36, 1652, and 2702. Following plasmid digestion, the sample is electrophoresed in a 2% agarose gel. A DNA ladder marker, labeled M in Color Plate 54■, is included in the first lane, with base pair sizes indicated. Which of the following lanes represents the sample pattern that is most likely the digested plasmid?
    A. A
    B. B
    C. C
    D. D

13. Which of the following is characteristic of DNA chips (i.e., DNA microarrays)?
    A. Allow detection and discrimination of multiple genetic sequences at the same time
    B. Thousands of oligonucleotide probes are labeled and placed on glass or silicon surfaces.
    C. Unlabeled target sequences within the patient sample are detected by hybridization to labeled probes.
    D. All of the above

14. The most useful feature of the molecules streptavidin and biotin is that they bind
    A. Specifically to nucleic acids
    B. Only in neutral pH conditions
    C. To each other with very high affinity
    D. Directly to DNA immobilized on nitrocellulose

15. What is the theoretical estimation of the number of DNA target sequences present (per original dsDNA in solution) following 15 cycles of PCR?
    A. 30
    B. 2^{10} (i.e., 1024)
    C. 2^{15} (i.e., 32,768)
    D. 2^{20} (i.e., 1,048,576)

16. "Star activity" for a restriction enzyme refers to which of the following?
    A. An ability to cleave DNA at sequences different from their defined recognition sites
    B. The enzyme's specificity for sites of methylation within the nucleotide sequence
    C. The temperature and pH conditions at which the enzyme will function optimally
    D. The percent increased accuracy of the enzyme when placed in ideal conditions of pH

17. Which of the following enzymes recognizes and cuts triplex DNA sequences formed between mutant or normal probes and target sequences within samples?
    A. Restriction endonuclease
    B. DNA ligase
    C. Cleavase
    D. RNase H

18. If a DNA probe is added to nitrocellulose after the transfer step but before the blocking step, which of the following will occur?
    A. The probe will nonspecifically bind to its DNA target.
    B. Unoccupied spaces on the nitrocellulose will bind the probe.
    C. The DNA target on the nitrocellulose will be unable to bind the probe.
    D. Bound probe will be washed away in the next wash step.

19. Which of the following is considered a "high stringency" condition for DNA probe protocols?
    A. Using wash buffer with highly acidic pH
    B. Washing the matrix with high salt buffer
    C. Radiolabeling the probe with ^{35}S rather than ^{32}P
    D. Washing the transfer membrane (e.g., nitrocellulose or nylon) at high temperature

20. When compared to Southern blot hybridization testing, PCR
    A. Is less sensitive to DNA degradation than Southern blot
    B. Includes transfer of DNA onto a nylon membrane
    C. Requires no specialized equipment
    D. Is more labor intensive

21. Which of the following specimen types is *not* acceptable as a source material for molecular genetic tests?
    A. Whole blood
    B. Reticulocytes
    C. Amniocytes
    D. Feces

22. In the presence of salt, DNA is precipitated from solution by which of the following?
    A. 10 mM Tris, 1 mM EDTA
    B. 0.1% sodium dodecyl sulfate (SDS)
    C. Alkaline buffers, such as 0.2 N NaOH
    D. Alcohols, such as 95% ethanol or isopropanol

23. TaqMan probes used to increase specificity of real-time PCR assays generate a fluorescent signal
    A. At the beginning of each cycle during the denaturation step
    B. When the probes bind to the template (i.e., during annealing)
    C. When the probe is digested by $5' \rightarrow 3'$ exonuclease activity during extension of primers (i.e., DNA synthesis)
    D. When the reporter fluorophore on the probe is separated from the quencher molecule by a restriction enzyme

24. For the purpose of diagnosing genetic diseases, which of the following components of whole blood is used for the extraction of DNA?
    A. Leukocytes
    B. Plasma
    C. Platelets
    D. Red blood cells

25. Which of the following statements best describes characteristics of RNase?
    A. It degrades mRNA but not rRNA.
    B. It is found in large concentrations on hands.
    C. Its activity can be eliminated by autoclaving.
    D. Its activity occurs in a limited temperature range between 25 and 65°C.

26. Which of the following is the *least* likely inhibitor of PCR?
    A. Heme
    B. Sodium heparin
    C. Diethylpyrocarbonate (DEPC)
    D. Ethylenediaminetetraacetic acid (EDTA)

27. Frequently, DNA probes are used to detect target sequences in Northern or Southern blots. Hybridization occurs between DNA probe and RNA or DNA on the blot, respectively. To ensure that only exactly matched complementary sequences have bound together, the blot is washed under stringent conditions. Stringency of the wash steps to remove unbound and mismatched probe can be increased by which of the following?
    A. High temperature, high NaCl concentration, and high detergent (i.e., SDS) solution
    B. High temperature, low NaCl concentration, and high detergent (i.e., SDS) solution
    C. High temperature, high NaCl concentration, and low detergent (i.e., SDS) solution
    D. Low temperature, high NaCl concentration, and high detergent (i.e., SDS) solution

28. In RNA, which of the following nucleotide bases replaces thymine of DNA?
    A. Adenine
    B. Cytosine
    C. Guanine
    D. Uracil

29. The component parts of a dNTP include a purine or pyrimidine base, a
    A. Ribose sugar, and one phosphate group
    B. Deoxyribose sugar, and three phosphate groups
    C. Ribose sugar, and two phosphate groups
    D. Deoxyribose sugar, and two phosphate groups

30. When comparing two dsDNA sequences of equal length, the strand that has a higher
    A. G + C content has a higher melting temperature (T_m)
    B. A + T content has a higher T_m
    C. A + T content has more purines than pyrimidines along its length
    D. G + C content has more purines than pyrimidines along its length

31. Molecular typing of bacterial strains can be based on restriction fragment length polymorphisms (RFLPs) produced by digesting bacterial chromosomal DNA with restriction endonucleases. Which of the following techniques is used to separate the large DNA fragments generated?
    A. Ribotyping
    B. DNA sequencing
    C. Pulsed-field gel electrophoresis
    D. Capillary electrophoresis

32. Which of the following amplification methods does *not* employ isothermal conditions?
    A. Nucleic acid sequence–based amplification (NASBA)
    B. Polymerase chain reaction (PCR)
    C. Strand displacement amplification (SDA)
    D. Transcription-mediated amplification (TMA)

33. The coding region of a human gene is called
    A. Exon
    B. Intron
    C. SNP
    D. VNTR

34. Central dogma is that DNA is used to make RNA, which is then used to make protein. In this scheme, the two processes that are involved (i.e., DNA to RNA and RNA to protein) are termed
    A. Replication and transcription
    B. Synthesis and encryption
    C. Transcription and translation
    D. Initiation and elongation

35. How many chromosomes are contained in a normal human somatic cell?
    A. 22
    B. 23
    C. 44
    D. 46

36. An ordered sequence of events makes up the cell cycle. Which of the following describes the correct sequence of events starting at G1?
    A. G1, G2, S, M
    B. G1, S, G2, M
    C. G1, M, G2, S
    D. G1, S, M, G2

37. Purified DNA remains stable indefinitely when stored as
    A. Small aliquots at 4°C
    B. Large aliquots at 25°C
    C. Small aliquots at −70°C
    D. Large aliquots at −20°C

38. In Color Plate 55■, the procedure of Southern blotting is diagrammed. In the upper panel, restricted genomic DNA fragments have been separated by electrophoresis in an agarose gel. In lane 1 is a molecular weight marker, in lanes 2–4 are three patient samples, and in lane 5 is a positive control DNA sequence for the probe used. After electrophoresis, DNA was transferred from the gel onto a nylon membrane and then hybridized with a fluorescence-labeled probe that recognizes the CGG trinucleotide repeat. In individuals with fragile X syndrome, expansions of the trinucleotide repeat within the fragile X gene increase to greater than 200 repeats. The bottom panel shows the resultant autoradiogram after a series of high-stringency washes. The three patient samples (lanes 2–4) are DNA from individuals of a single family, one of them suffering from fragile X syndrome. In which lane is the sample from the patient who has an intellectual disability?
    A. Lane 2
    B. Lane 3
    C. Lane 4
    D. Cannot be determined by the results given

39. An advantage of amplification technologies for clinical laboratories is that
    A. They require inexpensive test reagents.
    B. They lend themselves to automated methods.
    C. Each target molecule sought requires a unique set of primers.
    D. Contamination is not a concern when performing these assays.

40. The assay method that detects the expression of a gene rather than the mere presence or structure of a gene is termed
   A. RT-PCR
   B. TMA
   C. Multiplex PCR
   D. Ribotyping

41. Which of the following assays *cannot* be accomplished using PCR methods employing only *Taq* polymerase?
   A. Diagnosis of *Chlamydia trachomatis* and *Neisseria gonorrhoeae* infection
   B. Detection of single base pair gene mutations, such as in cystic fibrosis
   C. Detection of HLA-A, B, and DR genotypes
   D. Determination of viral load for hepatitis C virus (HCV)

42. One method to prevent "false-positive" PCR results includes the use of dUTP in the reaction mix, resulting in amplicons containing U in place of T. The enzyme used to decrease contamination is
   A. Uracil-*N*-glycosylase
   B. *Taq* polymerase
   C. S1 nuclease
   D. DNase

For questions 43-45, refer to Color Plates 56a and b.

43. Which of the following temperatures is best for use in Step 1 in a PCR?
   A. 35°C
   B. 55°C
   C. 75°C
   D. 95°C

44. Which of the following temperature ranges is most appropriate for Step 2 in a PCR?
   A. 25–35°C
   B. 55–65°C
   C. 70–80°C
   D. 90–100°C

45. Which of the following substances within the PCR mix influences the accuracy of cDNA?
   A. Oligonucleotide primers
   B. Monovalent cation K^+
   C. Divalent cation Mg^{2+}
   D. Deoxyribonucleotide triphosphate molecules

46. The following question refers to Color Plate 57■. Factor V Leiden mutation causes increased risk of thrombosis. It is caused by a single base mutation in which guanine (G) is substituted for adenine (A) with a subsequent loss of a restriction site for the enzyme *Mnl*I. Primers used in this example generate a 223 bp PCR product from patient DNA. After resulting PCR products are digested with *Mnl*I, normal patients produce the following DNA fragments: 104 bp, 82 bp, and 37 bp. In Color Plate 57■, the 37 bp fragment is not seen in all lanes because it is sometimes below detectable levels. Lane identities are as follows: M (molecular weight marker), 1–5 (patient 1 to patient 5, respectively), + (positive control showing 104, 82, and 37 bp fragments), and Neg (sterile water used in place of sample DNA). Which of the following patients is heterozygous for the factor V Leiden mutation?
   A. Patient 1
   B. Patient 2
   C. Patient 3
   D. Patient 4

47. The translocation resulting in the Philadelphia chromosome is detected by
    A. Southern blot analysis only
    B. Cytogenetic analysis (e.g., karyotyping) only
    C. PCR, Southern blot, and cytogenetic analysis
    D. RT-PCR, Southern blot, and cytogenetic analysis

48. Which of the following samples in Color Plate 58■ contains the largest amount of cytomegalovirus?
    A. Sample 4
    B. Sample 5
    C. Sample 11
    D. Only qualitative results can be determined in this assay.

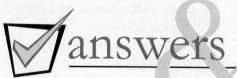

answers & rationales

1.

B. Because of the base pairing property within DNA, the presence of 20% adenine (A) means there must also be 20% thymine (T) in the organism. This means 40% of the DNA is A or T, leaving 60% of the DNA to be cytosine (C) or guanine (G). Because there must be an equal amount of each base type within the base pair, 60% divided by 2 gives 30% each of cytosine and guanine.

2.

C. DNA ligase is an enzyme that catalyzes the reaction between the 5′-phosphate end of one DNA fragment and the 3′-hydroxyl end of the next. This "nick sealing" requires energy from ATP hydrolysis, thus remaking the broken phosphodiester bond between the adjacent nucleotides. Ligase is a very important enzyme in DNA repair, but it is not used in a polymerase chain reaction (PCR). PCR does require a DNA template, two primers to anneal to nucleotide sequences flanking the desired amplification sequence, deoxynucleotide triphosphates (dNTPs) to be used as building blocks for the growing DNA chain, DNA polymerase, and magnesium chloride as an essential cofactor for DNA polymerase activity.

3.

A. The first letter of a restriction endonuclease's name comes from the bacterial genus from which it originated. The second and third letters derive from the bacterial species. The last letter indicates the subspecies or strain from which the enzyme was obtained. The last Roman numeral represents the numerical place the enzyme has among those which have been isolated from that bacterial genus/species/strain. For example, *Eco*RI is the first restriction endonuclease isolated from the bacterium *Escherichia coli*, strain R, whereas *Eco*RV is the fifth such enzyme to be discovered.

4.

C. The complementary strand for this DNA sequence would be, read left to right, 3′ GATATC 5′. Restriction endonucleases require dsDNA, because they use as their substrate palindromic molecules, meaning a molecule that will "read" the same left to right and right to left. In this instance, the complementary strand, read 5′ to 3′ (right to left), reads the same as the sense strand, read 3′ to 5′. If the enzyme cuts the sense strand as indicated, between the thymine and adenine, it will cut the complementary strand identically. This will leave, on the sense strand, the two sequences 5′ CT 3′ and 5′ ATAG 3′. The complementary strand will show 3′ GATA 5′ and 3′ TC 5′.

5.

C. The concentration of dsDNA can be estimated by taking its absorbance reading at 260 nm and multiplying that absorbance by a factor of 50, because one absorbance unit at 260 nm equals approximately 50 μg/mL. To solve this problem: 100 (dilution factor) × 0.062 (sample Abs. at 260 nm) × 50 μg/mL (conversion factor for dsDNA) = 310 μg/mL.

6.

A. In the isolation of RNA, it is very important to remove all RNase activity. Such enzymes are considered ubiquitous, so precautions must always be taken. GITC, diethylpyrocarbonate, or diethyl oxydiformate, will inactivate RNase, thus protecting RNA from degradation. It is used in solution at 0.1–0.2% (w/v) concentration.

7.

B. The amount of RNA in a cell depends on the type of cell and its developmental stage. In most cells, ribosomal RNA (rRNA) is the predominant form of RNA. In white blood cells about 80% of the RNA is rRNA. mRNA accounts for only 1–5% of the total cellular RNA.

8.

B. The rate of electrophoretic separation when using polyacrylamide or agarose gels is affected by time, current, and the percent matrix used. Sample volume will not affect rate of separation but only makes the resulting bands more visible when stained. Achieving increased separation can be accomplished by increasing the time or current used. It can also be achieved by decreasing the percent matrix, because the "pores" present in a 1% agarose gel will be larger than those in a 5% gel. This larger size pore will allow easier molecular passage of DNA molecules during electrophoresis. Conversely, achieving a tighter band pattern (i.e., higher resolution of smaller DNA molecules) can be accomplished by decreasing time or current, or increasing percent matrix used.

9.

A. Solid phase isolation is used for most automated nucleic acid isolation systems. Silica-based beads or columns bind DNA or RNA in high-salt solution. The column is washed to remove impurities, and the nucleic acids are eluted with low-salt buffer.

10.

C. Although human genes are highly conserved in gene coding regions, human gene loci are polymorphic, which means many forms of the gene can exist at a given locus, making each person "unique." Only identical twins are not "unique." Short tandem repeats (STRs) account for the many polymorphisms used in DNA fingerprinting. STRs are short, repetitive sequences of 3–7 base pairs and are abundant in the human genome. This testing does not require large quantities or high-quality DNA for successful results. It uses PCR, which is highly sensitive; however, this characteristic also makes the PCR method prone to contamination.

11.

D. The process whereby a strand of RNA is synthesized from template DNA is called transcription. The enzyme involved is RNA polymerase. It is possible, however, as retroviruses have shown to produce DNA using template RNA. This reversal of the nucleic acid central dogma is called "reverse transcription," and the enzyme that performs this is called reverse transcriptase. After synthesizing a single-stranded DNA molecule from RNA, a different enzyme (DNA polymerase) then synthesizes a complementary strand to produce a DNA double helix.

12.

C. To solve this problem, it is necessary to recognize that plasmid DNA exists as a closed circle. This means that base pair #1 is adjacent to base pair #5850. If the enzyme cleaves the plasmid at positions 36, 1652, and 2702, this will result in three pieces of DNA. One piece will contain base pairs (bps) 37 through 1652 (with a size of 1616 bp), a second will contain bp 1653 through 2702 (with a size of 1050 bp), and the third will span the sequence from bp 2703 through 5850 and from 1 to 36 (with a size of 3184 bp). Note that to determine the size of each piece, subtract the numbers corresponding to each adjacent cut site (e.g., 1652 − 36 = 1616 and 2702 − 1652 = 1050). For the third piece, subtract the highest numbered cut site (i.e., 2702) from the total size of the plasmid (i.e., 5850), and add the size of the piece beginning at bp #1 through bp #36. Use the DNA ladder marker (lane M) in Color Plate 54■ to predict the placement of these pieces (3184 bp, 1616 bp, and 1050 bp) of DNA on the final electrophoresis pattern.

13.

A. DNA chips (i.e., DNA microarrays) allow detection and discrimination of multiple genetic sequences at the same time. DNA chips have thousands of oligonucleotide probes arranged on glass or silicon surfaces in an ordered manner. Target sequences within the patient sample are fluorescently labeled in solution. The labeled sequences in solution are then incubated with the DNA chips containing the oligonucleotide probes attached to the silicon or glass surface. Hybridization will occur between labeled complementary sequences within the patient samples and their corresponding probe on the chip. The DNA chip is placed in an instrument that scans the surface with a laser beam. The intensity of the signal and its location are analyzed by computer and provide a quantitative description of the genes present. Because placement of the oligonucleotides is known, identification of the gene or organism may be determined.

14.

C. Biotin is a vitamin involved physiologically in single carbon transfers. Streptavidin is a protein derived from *Streptomyces avidinii*, consisting of four subunits, each of which can bind one biotin molecule. This bond formation is rapid and essentially irreversible. The interaction between streptavidin and biotin is the strongest known noncovalent biologic interaction between a protein and its ligand. *In vitro* assays take advantage of this strong and specific binding by covalently attaching streptavidin to a reporter molecule (e.g., a primary antibody) and then incubating this with a secondary fluorescent-labeled antibody conjugated to biotin. Each streptavidin molecule will bind four biotin-conjugated molecules, thereby increasing fourfold the signal generated.

15.

C. Assuming 100% efficiency, each cycle of the PCR doubles the number of DNA molecules present in the solution. Starting with one DNA template molecule, there would be $2^2 = 4$ DNA molecules present after two cycles. After five cycles, this would result in $2^5 = 32$. Based on a starting single molecule of double-stranded DNA, after 15 cycles there would theoretically be 2^{15} molecules (32,768). Actual yield is somewhat less than theoretical yield because PCR products created in the first two PCR cycles are slightly longer than the target amplicon. Thus, yield may be better calculated as $2^{(n-2)}$. Actual yield may be decreased by a plateau effect that may occur in later PCR cycles when some components of the PCR become reaction limiting.

16.

A. Restriction enzymes will show specificity for a target nucleotide sequence when used under optimal conditions of temperature and glycerol, salt, and substrate concentrations. If these conditions are not optimal, some enzymes will lose their specificity and begin to cleave randomly. This undesirable, nonoptimal digestion is called "star activity." Such activity is evident when the following parameters are altered in the reaction environment: more than 100 units of enzyme per microgram of DNA, more than 5% glycerol content, less than 25 mM salt concentrations, pH >8.0, presence of dimethyl sulfoxide (DMSO), ethanol, or other organic solvents.

17.

C. Cleavase is an enzyme isolated from bacteria that is likely important in DNA repair *in vivo.* The enzyme recognizes overlapping sequences of DNA and cleaves in the overlapping sequence and is the basis of the Invader® system (Hologic, Marlborough, MA). Target nucleic acid is mixed with Invader and signal probes. When the Invader and signal probes bind the target, the 5′ end of the signal overlaps with the Invader probe, and cleavase cleaves the signal probe. In the next step, the cleaved signal probe binds a fluorescent-labeled reporter probe containing complementary sequences and a quencher molecule, thus forming an overlapping structure. This molecule is subsequently cut by cleavase, which removes the reporter molecule from the quencher. The signal generated is directly related to the amount of target sequences in the original sample. Restriction endonucleases are also bacterial enzymes that recognize specific sequences within DNA and cut DNA near or within the recognized sequence. DNA ligase catalyzes the formation of a phosphodiester bond between adjacent 3′ hydroxyl and 5′ phosphate groups of adjacent nucleotides. RNaseH hydrolyzes RNA strands of a RNA:DNA hybrid molecule.

18.

B. After DNA is transferred to a nitrocellulose or nylon membrane, many sites on the membrane will not be occupied. Adding a probe at this point will not only allow for specific binding of the probe to the target DNA sequence but also the nonspecific binding of the probe to the available binding sites on the membrane. This will cause nonspecific signal generation throughout the matrix. To prevent this, the membrane must first be treated with blocking agents. Denhardt solution and denatured nonhomologous DNA (e.g., salmon sperm DNA) are often used to bind up all the available sites on the matrix and allow for specific binding of the probe in the next step.

19.

D. In Southern blots, hybrids can form between molecules with similar but not necessarily identical sequences. The washing conditions used after adding the labeled probe can be varied so that hybrids with differing mismatch frequencies are controlled. The higher the wash temperature or the lower the salt concentration in the wash buffer, the higher the stringency. Increasing the stringency will decrease the number of mismatches that form between the probe and the target DNA.

20.

A. Standard Southern blot techniques recommend the use of 10 μg of high-quality genomic DNA when studying single-copy genes. In a subsequent step, the genomic DNA is restricted (i.e., cut into small fragments of predictable size). The resulting fragments of the gene of interest generally range in size from 1.0 to 10.0 kilobases. In contrast, the gene sequence of interest to be amplified in a routine PCR targets a smaller portion of the gene (generally 150–500 bases in length). Because the target is a smaller size, partially degraded DNA (i.e., genomic DNA samples of lesser quality) can be amplified successfully. Long-range PCR methods are available that extend the range of PCR products synthesized from 5 to 35 kilobases. Because PCR targets are usually a few hundred bases in length, high-molecular-weight DNA is not necessary for successful PCR. It requires a thermocycler to take the reaction through the cycles of three temperatures needed for denaturation, hybridization, and elongation steps. Turn-around time is also an advantage of PCR because results can be completed in less than 4 hours, whereas Southern blotting takes up to 1 week to complete because of multiple steps required for this procedure.

21.

D. Many frequently used protocols in molecular biology involve PCR. Several substances can inhibit this reaction. For example, because of the nature of fecal material, it is not routinely used, and materials in swabs have also been reported to inhibit PCR. Therefore, a more appropriate specimen that could be used for PCR would be a stool filtrate. Nucleated cells are necessary for isolation of DNA. Whole blood is an acceptable specimen. White blood cells are the source of DNA in this type of specimen and must be separated from red blood cells as soon as possible because hemoglobin will inhibit PCR. For diagnosis of blood parasites, such as *Babesia* and *Plasmodium*, a hemolyzed and washed red blood cell sample is preferred for recovery of the DNA from the parasites. Amniocytes are used for molecular cytogenetic testing to prenatally screen for genetic diseases. Noninvasive collection of cells for genetic and forensic testing can be obtained from the buccal (oral) mucosa.

22.

D. Alcohol precipitation of nucleic acids is a standard method in molecular biology. Sterile water, 10 mM Tris, 1 mM EDTA, or 0.1% SDS can be used to rehydrate DNA; 1 mM EDTA and 0.1% SDS are included in these mixes to inhibit DNases. Alkaline solutions, such as 0.2 N NaOH, are used to denature nucleic acids.

23.

C. Real-time PCR or quantitative PCR (qPCR) is a modification of PCR that allows quantification of input target sequences without addition of competitor templates or multiple internal controls. qPCR is used to measure copy numbers of diseased human genes and viral and tumor load and to monitor treatment effectiveness. The accumulation of double-stranded PCR products during PCR as they are generated can be measured by adding fluorescent dyes that are dsDNA-specific to the reaction mix, such as SYBR green. However, misprimed products or primer dimers will also generate fluorescence and give falsely elevated readings. Thus, more specific systems utilizing probes to generate signal, such as the TaqMan probes, Molecular Beacons, and Scorpion-type primers, have been developed. In the TaqMan probe-based system, specific primers are present to prime the DNA synthesis reaction catalyzed by *Taq* polymerase, thus forming the cDNA product. The TaqMan probe binds to a smaller region within the target sequence. The TaqMan probe has a 5′ reporter fluorophore and 3′ quencher molecule. During extension of the primers by *Taq* polymerase to form cDNA product (i.e., DNA synthesis), the 5′ → 3′ exonuclease activity of *Taq* polymerase digests the TaqMan probe separating the reporter molecule from the quencher to generate a fluorescent signal. Molecular Beacon probes form hairpin structures due to short inverted repeat sequences at each end. The probe has a reporter dye at its 5′ end and a quencher dye at its 3′ end. In the unbound state, fluorescence is suppressed because reporter and quencher dyes are bound closely together by the short inverted repeat sequences. In qPCR assays, fluorescence occurs when molecular beacon probe binds the denatured template during the annealing step because reporter dye is separated from the quencher molecule. Scorpion primers, which contain a fluorophore and a quencher, are covalently linked to the probe. In the absence of the target, the quencher absorbs fluorescence emitted by the fluorophore. During the PCR reaction, in the presence of the target, the fluorophore and the quencher of the Scorpion primers separate, resulting in an increase in the fluorescence emitted. All of these systems require excess concentrations of the labeled probe/primer, so fluorescence emitted is directly proportional to the amount of template available for binding.

24.

A. Leukocytes are routinely used for extraction of DNA from human blood. Mature red blood cells and platelets have no nuclei. Plasma or serum can be used for detection of viremia, but it is not used for analysis of genetic diseases.

25.

B. The highest concentration of RNase is found on hands; thus, it is imperative that gloves be worn when working with RNA. RNases are ubiquitous and can act at temperatures below freezing (−20°C) and above boiling. For long-term storage, purified RNA is best stored at −70°C or below. Autoclaving does not eliminate RNase activity. To remove RNases, glassware must be pretreated with an RNase inhibitor, such as DEPC, followed by autoclaving; alternatively, baking glassware in a >250°C oven for 4 hours will destroy RNase. To prevent RNA degradation, isolation of RNA should be done using chaotropic agents e.g., guanidine isothiocyanate, (GITC) that inhibit RNase activity. When analyzing RNA in a gel, formaldehyde or other agents that denature RNases must be included in the gel. High-quality (i.e., undergraded) RNA will appear as a long smear with two or three distinct areas that correspond to the rRNA subunits: 28S (~4800 bases), 18S (~1800 bases), and 5.8S (~160 bases), whereas degraded RNA will appear as a smear at the bottom of the gel.

26.

D. EDTA and ACD (acid citrate dextrose) are the preferred anticoagulants for specimens that will undergo PCR. These reactions can be inhibited by a variety of substances. PCR inhibitors are concentration dependent; inhibition can often be overcome by simply diluting the DNA sample. Heme and sodium heparin can inhibit PCR. However, laboratory methods can be used to remove these inhibitors, if necessary. DEPC is a substance used to inhibit RNases; it can also inhibit PCR.

27.

B. Stringency of hybridization is accomplished at two steps in the blotting technique. The first step is hybridization conditions of the labeled probe in solution with the transferred RNA or DNA targets on the membrane. The second step occurs when the membrane is washed to remove unbound probe. In the hybridization reaction, formamide and temperature can be used to increase stringency. During wash steps, increasing temperature and increasing detergent concentration (e.g., 1% SDS) will increase stringency; whereas lowering NaCl concentration also increases stringency. At the end of the highest stringency wash, only specific hybrids of interest should remain on the blot.

28.

D. The four nucleotide bases found in RNA are adenine (A), guanine (G), cytosine (C), and uracil (U). The purines A and G are the same as in DNA. C is present in both DNA and RNA; however, in RNA, the DNA nucleotide base thymine (T) is replaced by uracil (U). RNA is usually single stranded, although double-stranded areas (hairpin loops) can occur. A pairs with U, and C pairs with G.

29.

B. dNTP stands for deoxyribonucleotide triphosphate. Nucleotides are the building blocks of nucleic acids. They are composed of phosphate groups, a five-sided sugar molecule, and a nitrogenous base. Nitrogenous bases are either purines (A, G) or pyrimidines (C, T, or U, an RNA-specific base). The sugar molecules are either ribose (in RNA) or deoxyribose (in DNA), with the only difference in structure being the lack of a hydroxyl group at position 2′ in the deoxyribose molecule. When the sugar is bound to a base without the phosphate group, the molecule is called a nucleoside. A nucleotide can have 1, 2, or 3 phosphate groups, which are termed monophosphate, diphosphate, and triphosphate, respectively.

30.

A. DNA is composed of two strands of polynucleotides coiled in a double helix. The outside backbone is composed of sugar–phosphate moieties, whereas the purine and pyrimidine bases are stacked inside the helix. The size and stability of the DNA molecule is such that only specific bases can hydrogen bond to each other to hold the two strands together (A-T and C-G). This is referred to as complementary base pairing. An A-T base pair is less stable than a C-G base pair, because three hydrogen bonds form between C and G and only two hydrogen bonds form between A and T. The increased stability between C-G causes the melting temperature (T_m) to be greater in a dsDNA segment with more C-G pairs than a segment with more A-T pairs. In all dsDNA molecules, the number of purines (A + G) equals the number of pyrimidines (C + T).

31.

C. Pulsed-field gel electrophoresis (PFGE) is used to separate extremely large DNA molecules by placing them in an electric field that is charged periodically in alternating directions, forcing the molecule to reorient before moving through the gel. Larger molecules take more time to reorient; thus, they move more slowly. Bacterial DNA is digested by restriction enzymes in agarose plugs. The PFGE of the digested fragments provides a distinctive pattern of 5 to 20 bands ranging from 10 to 800 kilobases. DNA sequencing determines the exact nucleotide sequence base by base of any organism; however, it is too laborious for epidemiologic purposes. Ribotyping is a Southern blot type of analysis using rRNA probes to detect ribosomal operons (i.e., sequences coding for 16S rRNA, 25S rRNA, and one or more tRNAs) of individual bacterial species. Its discriminatory power is less than PFGE. Reverse transcription-PCR (RT-PCR) is a method that determines whether a gene is being expressed. The starting material for RT-PCR is ssRNA.

32.

B. PCR requires a thermocycler because cycling at three different temperatures is required for this technique. First, template DNA (i.e., which may contain the target sequence) is denatured at 94°C. Next, the temperature is lowered to allow specific primers to anneal to the single-stranded target, generally at temperatures near 55°C. In the third portion of the cycle, primers are extended using dNTP molecules to form a complementary copy of DNA under the direction of a thermostable DNA polymerase enzyme, such as *Taq* polymerase. The optimal temperature at which *Taq* polymerase acts to extend the primers is 72°C. Cycles are generally repeated about 30 times to theoretically yield 2^{30} DNA molecules. The three steps of each cycle are termed denaturation (94°C), annealing of primers (~55°C), and extension of primers (72°C). The other methods listed, nucleic acid sequence–based amplification, strand displacement amplification, and transcription-mediated amplification, are also amplification methods; however, they have been modified so all reactions take place at a single temperature (isothermal).

33.

A. The coding regions of eucaryote genes are called exons. The noncoding intervening regions are called introns. In eucaryotes, the introns and exons are transcribed into mRNA; however, before mRNA is translated, the introns are removed and the exons are spliced together. SNP is an abbreviation for single nucleotide polymorphism, and VNTR refers to variable number tandem repeats.

34.

C. Central dogma describes the flow of genetic information from DNA to RNA to protein. Individual DNA molecules serve as templates for either complementary DNA strands during replication or complementary RNA molecules during transcription. In turn, RNA molecules serve as templates for ordering of amino acids by ribosomes to form polypeptides during protein synthesis, also known as translation.

35.

D. DNA in human somatic cells is compartmentalized into 22 pairs of chromosomes, referred to as autosomes. They are numbered 1 through 22. In addition, humans have two sex chromosomes, X and Y (in males) or two X chromosomes (in females). Thus, the total number of chromosomes is 46 in a normal diploid cell. The genetic information of one set of chromosomes comes from the mother of the individual and the other set from the father. Gametes (i.e., ova and spermatozoa) are haploid and contain only one set of chromosomes (23 chromosomes in human gametes), so that upon fertilization, a diploid zygote is formed.

36.

B. Most of the lifetime of a cell is spent in G1 phase, during which the cells can produce their specialized proteins and accomplish their essential functions. However, when the signal is received for cell division, the cell enters S phase. In S phase, the DNA in all chromosomes is duplicated. At the end of S phase, the duplicated chromosomes remain attached at the centromere. A time delay, G2, separates events of the actual separation of individual chromosomes from their duplicated pairs. Next, the M phase or mitosis is when the two members of each pair of chromosomes go to opposite ends of the original cell. This separates 46 chromosomes into two sets of 23 in each cell. Finally, a cleavage furrow is formed and separates the original cell into two daughter cells. Each cell contains a copy of all the genetic information from each parent.

37.

C. Purified DNA is relatively stable provided it is reconstituted in buffer that does not contain DNases. Therefore, high-quality reagents and type I sterile water should be used in preparing buffers for this purpose. Experiments have shown that purified DNA is stable for as long as 3 years at refrigerated temperature (4°C). However, long-term storage of purified DNA is best accomplished at −20 to −70°C in a freezer that is not frost free to avoid freeze-thaw cycles that may damage DNA and by dividing the original DNA sample into multiple small aliquots for storage.

38.

C. Refer to Color Plate 55■. Given that the probe used will recognize the trinucleotide repeat found in the fragile X gene, *FMR-1*, the location of positive signals will give information about the size of the repeat sequence within each person's DNA. The normal allele for *FMR-1* has 6–50 trinucleotide repeats, the premutation for *FMR-1* contains 50–200 trinucleotide repeats (found in unaffected individuals), and the disease allele (found in affected individuals) has >200 repeats. Because electrophoresis separates DNA by size such that the larger fragments travel shorter distances than smaller fragments, then the larger fragment in the affected individual caused by the expansion of the trinucleotide repeat would be represented in Color Plate 55■ by lane 4 of the diagram.

39.

B. Amplification methods can be automated and standardized, which is proven by the variety of test systems presently on the market. Amplification methods are very sensitive and theoretically can detect one target DNA molecule in a sample. However, increased sensitivity raises the likelihood of false positive results due to contamination of testing areas with PCR amplicons. In addition, most amplification methods can be completed within 4–6 hours and can detect microorganisms that do not grow readily by standard culture techniques. At this time, test reagents are still expensive, although if decreased turn-around time would translate into shorter hospital stays, then resultant healthcare costs could be reduced by use of these methods in the clinical laboratory. A disadvantage of amplification technologies is that they require a unique set of primers for each target DNA being sought. Thus, amplification techniques may be replaced by use of DNA microarrays because thousands of genes can be assessed at one time, rather than a limited number of molecules of interest being assayed.

40.

A. RT-PCR is used to detect gene expression; genes are expressed by transcription into mRNA. The starting material for RT-PCR is mRNA. The only method listed whose target sequence is found in mRNA is RT-PCR. Transcription-mediated amplification targets are usually rRNA. In ribotyping, rRNA probes detect rRNA genes present in total bacterial DNA; bacteria can be grouped on the basis of resulting banding patterns. Multiplex PCR describes a method in which DNA is the target or template, and several different primer sets are included in the reaction mix.

41.

D. Hepatitis C virus (HCV) has an RNA genome, and thus a reverse transcription step is needed to convert RNA into complementary DNA for use in the subsequent PCR that makes multiple copies of the target sequence. RT-PCR is both highly specific and sensitive. Viral load testing also requires that the methodology be quantitative. Quantification can be accomplished by qPCR techniques or by inclusion of a known amount of a synthetic nucleic acid, a quantification standard (QS), in the sample. The QS binds the same primers as the viral target, and so the kinetics of amplification for both may be assumed to be approximately equal. The viral target and QS are coamplified in the same reaction, and the raw data are manipulated mathematically to determine the viral load present in the specimen. To detect genetic sequences specific for the human leukocyte antigen loci, bacteria, and gene mutations, the starting material is usually DNA; therefore, PCR methods, rather than RT-PCR, would be employed.

42.

A. The sensitivity of amplification techniques can be viewed as a double-edged sword. On one hand, the techniques have allowed detection of genetic sequences that are found in limited numbers within a sample. However, because the method creates large amounts of target sequence, the areas within the laboratory can become contaminated with amplicons. Amplicon contamination produces false positive results. The use of dUTP in the reaction mix results in PCR products (i.e., amplicons) containing uracil in place of thymidine. The enzyme used to decrease contamination of previously generated dU-containing amplicons is uracil-N-glycosylase (UNG). Samples are pretreated with this enzyme before their use in subsequent PCR reactions to remove contaminating dU-containing amplicons if present. Pretreatment with UNG has no effect on sample DNA containing thymidine residues. Other procedures necessary to avoid contamination include dedicated areas for reagent preparation, impeccable technique, amplification and post-amplification analysis, and use of aerosol-barrier pipette tips. Treatment of work surfaces, equipment, and pipettors with UV light can also be used to prevent contamination.

answers & rationales

43–45.

(45:D, 46:B, 47:C)
Questions 45–47 are associated with Color Plates 56a■ and b■. A PCR is depicted in Color Plates 56a■ and b■. It is the prototype of target amplification methods. Traditional PCR is the *in vitro* equivalent of DNA replication *in vivo.* The components of PCR are a DNA template (containing target sequence of interest), a set of oligonucleotide primers (that flank the region of interest), building blocks of deoxynucleotide triphosphates (dATP, dCTP, dGTP, TTP, collectively referred to as dNTPs), and a heat-stable DNA polymerase (e.g., *Taq* polymerase) and buffer providing optimal conditions for primer annealing and DNA synthesis. Optimal salt concentrations (e.g., KCl) are needed for annealing of primers. In addition, optimal concentrations of the divalent cation Mg^{2+}, a cofactor for *Taq* polymerase that determines the fidelity of DNA replication *in vitro*, are essential. PCR consists of cycles of three steps: (1) denaturation of doubl stranded oligonucleotide primers to complementary sequence in denatured template, and (3) DNA synthesis catalyzed by *Taq* polymerase. During synthesis, primers are extended in the 5′ → 3′ direction, adding adenine, guanine, cytosine, and thymidine nucleotide bases into the growing chain according to the complementary sequence to which it is bound. The steps generally occur at the following temperatures and duration: denaturation ≥94°C (20–60 seconds); annealing (dependent on base sequences of primers) between 55 and 65°C (20–90 seconds); and DNA synthesis at 72°C, the optimal temperature for *Taq* polymerase (10–60 seconds). The resulting cDNA products are called amplicons. Starting with one dsDNA molecule (1A:1B) containing a target sequence, denaturation separates the dsDNA template into two ssDNA strands (1A and 1B). Next, the temperature is lowered to a point where specific hybridization of each primer to its complementary sequence in the denatured strands occurs. Then, the temperature is increased to 72°C, and extension of the primers ensues. At the end of cycle #1, two dsDNA parent (1) daughter (2) hybrid molecules result (i.e., 1A:2B and 1B:2A). At the end of cycle #2, four dsDNA products are produced. Intermediate-length products, larger than the target sequence of interest (4A and 4B length) but smaller than the original DNA template (1A:1B), are present. In subsequent cycles, the precise length target sequence is amplified most efficiently and becomes the preferred target for amplification. At each cycle, the number of copies doubles such that after *N* doublings, 2^{N-2}, copies of target are produced. For example, after 30 cycles, 2^{28} amplicons = 2.68×10^8 (over a billion) copies are made.

46.

C. Refer to Color Plate 57■. Factor V Leiden mutation (A506G) causes activated protein C resistance that results in increased risk of hypercoagulability. The mutation destroys a *Mnl*I restriction enzyme site in an amplified 223 bp PCR product from patient DNA. From the electrophoretic pattern, wild-type or normal factor V will show three bands after *Mnl*I digestion (104 bp, 82 bp, and 37 bp), as in patients 1, 4, and 5. The pattern seen with patient 2 is that of a homozygous mutant with two bands (141 bp and 82 bp). In the heterozygous patient 3, one allele is normal and the other is mutant. Thus, the banding pattern results in four bands (141 bp, 104 bp, 82 bp, and 37 bp). Sometimes, the 37 bp fragment band is not seen because it is below detectable levels.

47.

D. The translocation resulting in the Philadelphia (Ph) chromosome can be detected by RT-PCR, Southern blot, and cytogenetic analysis. The presence of a Ph chromosome confirms the diagnosis of chronic myelogenous leukemia. The Ph chromosome is a shortened chromosome 22 that arises from a reciprocal translocation involving the long arms of chromosomes 9 and 22. This translocation involves the proto-oncogene c-*ABL*, normally present on chromosome 9q34, and the *BCR* gene on chromosome 22q11. The juxtaposition of *ABL* with *BCR* results in the formation of a *BCR-ABL* fusion gene, which is subsequently transcribed into a chimeric BCR-ABL mRNA that is ultimately translated into a chimeric BCR-ABL protein product. Traditionally, this rearrangement can be seen cytogenetically by visualization of the patient's karyotype (i.e., metaphase spread of patient's chromosomes). Techniques have been developed in which fluorescent-labeled probes for this gene rearrangement can be used to probe the patient's metaphase or interphase spread, called fluorescence *in situ* hybridization. Molecular methods to check for this gene rearrangement include Southern blotting and RT-PCR. PCR cannot be used for this particular gene rearrangement because BCR/*abl* breakpoints span large segments of DNA, which prevents direct PCR testing. Instead, RT-PCR is used. The BCR/*abl* chimeric mRNA is used as a template because primer annealing sites in the breakpoint region of the mRNA are of a smaller size, suitable for amplification.

48.

B. Color Plate 58■ is graphic display of a real-time PCR (i.e., qPCR) for cytomegalovirus (CMV). Real-time PCR assays can measure the amount of starting target sequence (i.e., template in sample) accurately. Rather than measuring PCR product generated at the stationary or endpoint of the PCR assay, qPCR analysis is done as PCR products are formed (i.e., during the exponential phase) where time needed to detect fluorescence is inversely proportional to the amount of starting template (i.e., the shorter the time to accumulate signal, the more starting material). Optimal threshold level is based on the background or baseline fluorescence and the peak fluorescence in the reaction and is automatically determined by the instrument. Using 10-fold dilutions of known positive standards, a standard curve can be made. The qPCR cycle at which sample fluorescence crosses the threshold is the threshold cycle (C_T). Using the standard curve based on DNA of known concentration, the starting amount of target sequence in each sample can be determined by its C_T. Fluorescence versus C_T is an inverse relationship. The more starting material, the fewer cycles it takes to reach the fluorescence threshold (i.e., large amounts of fluorescence accumulate in a short time). The C_T for sample 5 is 21, sample 4 is 25, and sample 11 is 38; therefore, sample 5 has more CMV copies than sample 4, which has more CMV copies than all the other samples with C_T values indicated, including sample 11 with the least CMV. The samples below the threshold fluorescence of 30 are negative for CMV.

REFERENCES

Alberts, B., et al. (Ed.) (2017). *Essential Cell Biology*, 3rd ed. St. Louis: Elsevier.

Buckingham, L. (2007). *Molecular Diagnostics: Fundamentals, Methods, & Clinical Applications*, 3rd ed. Philadelphia: F. A. Davis.

Coleman, W., and Tsongalis, G. (Eds.) (2012). *Molecular Diagnostics for the Clinical Laboratorian*, 2nd ed. Totowa, NJ: Humana Press.

Rifai, N., et al. (2018) *Principles and Applications of Molecular Diagnostics*. St. Louis: Elsevier.

CHAPTER

11 Urinalysis and Body Fluids

contents

I. INTRODUCTION TO URINALYSIS

A. Introduction

1. Urinalysis is the practice of examining urine for diagnostic purposes; it aids in following the course or treatment of disease.

B. Importance of Urine

1. Urine **contains** most of the body's water-soluble **waste products.**
2. Urine chemical changes are directly related to pathologic conditions.
3. A complete urinalysis is composed of multiple tests, including **physical, chemical**, and **microscopic** analysis.
4. Urinalysis is used for disease diagnosis, disease monitoring, drug screening, and initial diagnosis of inborn errors of metabolism.

C. Urine Composition

1. Urine contains **mostly water** and various amounts of dissolved organic/inorganic compounds.
2. Composition varies according to diet, physical activity, metabolism, and disease processes. Composition is directly related to the amount and type of waste material that is to be excreted.
3. Urine **organic** substances
   a. **Urea** accounts for roughly 50% of all dissolved solutes in the urine.
   b. Other organic substances in relatively large amounts include **creatinine** and **uric acid.**
   c. Organic substances in small amounts include **glucose, protein, hormones, vitamins**, and **metabolized medications.**
4. Urine **inorganic** substances (listed in order of highest to lowest average concentration)
   a. **Chloride, sodium**, and **potassium**
   b. Other inorganic substances in small amounts include **sulfate, phosphate, ammonium, calcium**, and **magnesium.**
5. Nondissolved formed elements may include **bacteria, crystals, casts, mucus**, and **various types of cells.**

II. THE KIDNEY AND URINE FORMATION

A. Renal Anatomy

1. The **kidneys** are two bean-shaped organs located under the diaphragm on either side of the aorta in the posterior, upper abdominal region.
2. The **ureter** is a muscular tube that connects the pelvis of the kidney to the bladder.
3. Urine is stored in the **bladder** until excretion through the **urethra.**
4. The **renal pelvis** is a cavity area within the kidney that is an expansion of the ureter. The pelvis functions to collect urine from the calyces for transport from the kidney to the ureter.

5. The kidneys consist of two regions, the **cortex** (outer layer) and the **medulla** (inner layer). The cortex comprises the renal corpuscles and the proximal and distal convoluted tubules of the nephron. The medulla comprises the loops of Henle and the collecting ducts.
6. The **abdominal aorta** supplies blood to the **renal artery**, which in turn provides blood to the kidney, and the **renal vein** functions to return blood to the **inferior vena cava.**
7. Microscopically, the functional unit of the kidney is the **nephron**, which is responsible for **urine formation.** It comprises a renal corpuscle and a tubular system. These areas are further delineated with the **renal corpuscle** consisting of the glomerulus and Bowman's capsule and the **tubular system** consisting of the proximal convoluted tubule, loop of Henle, distal convoluted tubule, and collecting duct. More than a million nephrons may be found in each kidney.
   a. The **glomerulus** is a tuft of capillaries that lie in a tubular depression called Bowman's capsule. The **afferent arteriole** ("a" = "arrives") carries blood into the glomerulus, and the **efferent arteriole** ("e" = "exits") carries blood away. The **peritubular capillaries**, which arise from the efferent arteriole, aid in the tubular reabsorption process by surrounding the various segments of the renal tubule. The main function of the glomerulus is to filter the blood.
   b. The **proximal convoluted tubule** is located in the cortex.
   c. The **loop of Henle** begins in the cortex, with the descending limb of the loop extending into the medulla where the bend of the loop is formed that then becomes the ascending limb, which ends in the cortex.
   d. The **distal convoluted tubule** (DCT) is located in the cortex, and DCTs from multiple nephrons direct the urine flow into a collecting duct.
   e. The **collecting duct** joins with other collecting ducts, forming a papillary duct to carry urine into a calyx of the **renal pelvis.**

B. Renal Physiology

1. In order to form and excrete urine, three processes function together: glomerular filtration, tubular reabsorption, and tubular secretion.
   a. The glomerulus functions as a semipermeable membrane to make an **ultrafiltrate** of plasma that is protein free.
      1) Large molecules (proteins, cells) remain in the arterioles, whereas smaller molecules (glucose, urea, sodium, chloride, potassium, bicarbonate, calcium, etc.) pass through the glomerular capillary walls to become part of the filtrate.
      2) These smaller molecules and ions flow into the proximal convoluted tubule.
      3) The **glomerular filtration rate (GFR)** is about 115–125 mL of filtrate formed per minute by the glomeruli. The **renal tubules** will **reabsorb** all but 1 mL of the filtrate, which will be passed in the urine.

b. **Reabsorption** is the process by which filtered water, ions, and molecules leave the tubules for return to the blood via the peritubular capillaries.
c. **Secretion** is the process by which a substance from the peritubular capillary blood is transported across the wall of the tubule into the filtrate.

2. Function of the nephron
   a. **The proximal convoluted tubule**
      1) Responsible for most of the reabsorption (approximately 65%) and secretion that occurs in the tubules
      2) For some analytes, there is a limitation as to how much solute can be reabsorbed. This is defined as the "**renal threshold.**"
      3) **Reabsorbs** water, Na^+, Cl^-, K^+, urea, glucose (up to renal threshold of 160–180 mg/dL), amino acids, etc.
      4) **Secretes** hydrogen ions and medications
   b. **Loop of Henle**
      1) **Descending limb** reabsorbs water; therefore, it is referred to as the diluting segment.
      2) **Ascending limb** reabsorbs Na^+ and Cl^-; therefore, it is referred to as the concentrating segment.
      3) **Filtrate leaves the loop of Henle** and moves into the distal convoluted tubule.
      4) Approximately 85% of tubular reabsorption of water and salt is complete before the filtrate passes into the distal convoluted tubule.
   c. **Distal convoluted tubule**
      1) Reabsorbs Na^+
      2) Reabsorption of water is controlled by **antidiuretic hormone** (ADH).
      3) Secretion of H^+ and K^+
      4) **Aldosterone** controls the reabsorption of sodium and secretion of potassium and hydrogen into the filtrate. It influences the reabsorption of water, secondary to the reabsorption of sodium.
   d. **Collecting duct**
      1) Final site for water reabsorption to make urine more dilute or concentrated
      2) Na^+ Cl^- reabsorption is controlled by **aldosterone.**
      3) Water reabsorption occurs by osmosis as well as in response to **ADH.**

C. Endocrine Functions

1. **Renin-angiotensin-aldosterone axis**
   a. **Renin** is secreted by the juxtaglomerular apparatus of the **kidneys** and catalyzes the conversion of angiotensinogen to **angiotensin I** (a hormone in the inactive form).
   b. Angiotensin I stimulates the production in the lungs of **angiotensin II** (a hormone in the active form).
   c. **Angiotensin II** regulates renal blood by causes:
      1) **Constriction** of arterioles in the kidney and throughout the body, causing an increase in blood pressure.
      2) **Secretion** of **aldosterone** from the adrenal glands to facilitate retention of sodium by the DCT and CT.

2. **Aldosterone**, made in the cortex of the adrenal glands, acts on the kidneys by promoting the reabsorption of Na^+ from the filtrate into the blood and the secretion of K^+ from the blood into the filtrate. Water will be reabsorbed along with the Na^+.
3. **Antidiuretic hormone** (ADH, vasopressin), secreted by the posterior pituitary gland, promotes water reabsorption from the filtrate into the blood. ADH primarily affects the reabsorption of water from the distal convoluted tubule and the collecting duct.
4. **Parathyroid hormone** (PTH), made in the parathyroid glands, promotes Ca^{2+} reabsorption from the filtrate into the blood and excretion of phosphate ions from the blood into the filtrate.
5. Erythropoietin is an alpha-globulin produced by the peritubular fibroblasts in the kidneys to stimulate red blood cell production in response to lowered oxygen levels.

III. RENAL PATHOLOGY AND RENAL FUNCTION TESTS

A. Renal Pathology

1. **Acute glomerulonephritis**: Inflammation of the glomerulus seen in children and adults; can follow a Group A Streptococcus respiratory infection; characterized by **hematuria, proteinuria, WBCs**, and **casts** (RBC, granular and hyaline)
2. **Rapidly progressive glomerulonephritis**: A more serious condition than acute glomerulonephritis that may result in renal failure; urinalysis results would be similar to acute glomerulonephritis
3. **Acute interstitial nephritis**: Inflammation of the renal interstitium that may be caused by an allergic reaction to medication; characterized by **hematuria, proteinuria, WBCs** (especially eosinophils), and **WBC casts**
4. **Membranous glomerulonephritis**: Caused by immune IgG complexes. Thickening of the glomerular capillary walls and basement membrane; characterized by **hematuria** and **proteinuria**
5. **Nephrotic syndrome**: May be caused by renal blood pressure irregularities; characterized by **proteinuria (>3.5 g/24 hr), hematuria, lipiduria, oval fat bodies, renal tubular epithelial cells**, and **epithelial, fatty, and waxy casts**
6. **Focal segmental glomerulosclerosis**: Affects a specific number of glomeruli, not the entire glomerulus; often seen in African-American patients; characterized by **hematuria** and **proteinuria**
7. **Chronic glomerulonephritis**: Results in a long-term progressive loss of renal function; characterized by **hematuria, proteinuria, glucosuria,** and presence **of casts, including broad casts. Berger disease, an IgA nephropathy, can lead to chronic glomerulonephritis**
8. **Acute pyelonephritis**: An infection of the renal tubules caused by a urinary tract infection; characterized by **hematuria, proteinuria, WBC's, bacteria,** and **WBC and bacterial casts**

9. **Chronic pyelonephritis**: Chronic infection of the tubules and interstitial tissue that may progress to renal failure; characterized by **hematuria, proteinuria, WBCs, bacteria**, and **WBC, bacterial, granular, waxy, and broad casts**
10. **Renal failure**: Tubular necrosis caused by nephrotoxic agents and other disease processes, resulting in a **failure of the kidneys to filter blood**

B. Renal Function Tests

1. **Renal tubular reabsorption tests** (also known as **concentration tests**) are used to detect early renal disease. Examples of these tests include:
   a. **Osmolality** measures the **amount of solute dissolved** in a solution.
   b. **Specific gravity** depends on the **solute dissolved** in a solution **and** the **density** of this solute. **Osmolality and specific gravity** evaluate renal concentrating ability, monitor the course of renal disease, and monitor fluid and electrolyte therapy.
2. Secretion test
   a. **Tubular secretion or renal blood flow test** uses ***p*-aminohippuric acid** (PAH), a substance that is infused into the patient.
   b. PAH is completely removed from the blood by functional renal tissue. If renal problems exist, the PAH will not be removed completely.
3. **Glomerular tests** are used to assess renal **waste removal** and solute **reabsorbing abilities.** A decreased clearance test indicates compromised kidney function. ***Note:*** Urea is not normally used in clearance testing because of tubular reabsorption, diet, and urine flow rate.
   a. **Creatinine clearance** is used to **assess glomerular filtration rate.**
      1) Creatinine levels are not changed by diet (normal) or rate of urine flow. Creatinine is not reabsorbed by renal tubules. **P**: plasma creatinine mg/dL, **U**: urine creatinine mg/dL, **V**: urine flow in mL/min, and **SA**: body surface area. Average body surface area is $1.73\ m^2$.
      2) **Creatinine clearance formula**:

$$C\ (mL/min) = \frac{U \times V}{P} \times \frac{1.73\ m^2}{SA}$$

      3) **24-hour timed urine** is the specimen of choice.
      4) **Reference ranges** differ according to age and sex; values decrease with age.

$$\text{Males: } 105 \pm 20\ mL/min/1.73\ m^2$$

$$\text{Females: } 95 \pm 20\ mL/min/1.73\ m^2$$

   b. **Estimated glomerular filtration rate (eGFR)** uses a **serum creatinine** or serum cystatin C within a formula:
      1) **MDRD** (Modification of Diet in Renal Disease)
         a) Correction for gender, age, and ethnicity required
         b) Results only reported as a number if $<60\ mL/min/1.73\ m^2$

2) **CKD-EPI** (Chronic Kidney Disease Epidemiology Collaboration)
   a) Correction for gender, age and ethnicity required
   b) Results in excess of 90 mL/min/1.73 m^2 can be reported
3) **Schwartz** equation for children
   a) Estimates GFR in children
   b) [0.55 × length (in centimeters)] divided by plasma creatinine
4) The National Kidney Foundation recommends using the CKD-EPI Creatinine Equation (2009) to estimate GFR.

IV. URINE VOLUME AND SAMPLE HANDLING

A. Volume of Urine

1. Determined by the body's state of hydration; normal range of urine output 600–2000 mL/24 hr, with **1200–1500 mL/24 hr** being the **normal adult output**
2. **Factors that affect urine volume**
   a. Fluid intake and fluid loss related to **nonrenal** functions
   b. Diuretic and antidiuretic **hormone** levels
   c. Excretion of dissolved solutes, including **glucose** and **salts**
3. Urine volume terminology
   a. **Oliguria: Decrease** in **urine output** because of dehydration (e.g., vomiting, diarrhea, perspiration, and burns)
   b. **Anuria: No urine output** because of kidney damage or renal failure
   c. **Nocturia: Increased urine output at night**
      1) Caused by a reduction in bladder capacity resulting from pregnancy, stones, or prostate enlargement
      2) Increased fluid intake at night
   d. **Polyuria: Increased daily output**, may exceed 2 L/day
      1) Usually **caused by** such diseases as **diabetes mellitus** and **diabetes insipidus**
      2) May also be caused by **ingestion of diuretics** (medications that block water reabsorption), **caffeine**, and **alcohol** (suppresses secretion of antidiuretic hormone)

B. Specimen Collection and Handling

1. Urine must be treated as a biohazardous material, thus warranting that **standard precautions** be followed.
2. Use clean, dry cups with lids.
3. Label container with name, identification number, and the date and time of urine collection. Note that labeling only the lid is insufficient.
4. Analyze within **2 hours** or preserve.
5. **Preserve** urine
   a. Refrigeration will **decrease** bacterial growth but will cause precipitation of amorphous phosphates/urates.
   b. **Before testing,** urine must be brought to **room temperature.**

c. **Chemical preservatives** can be bactericidal, but they will preserve formed elements and will not, generally, interfere with chemical testing. If the chemical preservative alters the pH, it can interfere with the pH (and possibly the protein) tests on the strips.
d. Changes in unpreserved urine may include:
   1) **Increased** pH, nitrites, bacteria, and turbidity
   2) **Decreased** urobilinogen, glucose, ketones, and bilirubin
   3) Formed element destruction
   4) Change in color

6. Urine specimen types and collection times
   a. **First morning**: Concentrated specimen used for routine screening, pregnancy tests, and for detecting orthostatic proteinuria
   b. **Random midstream clean-catch**: Used for routine screening and microalbuminuria determination; time of collection not a consideration; patient cleans the external urinary meatus, urinates a small volume into the toilet, and then collects the rest of the voided sample.
   c. **Fasting**: Used for glucose monitoring; usually the second voided specimen of the morning following a fasting period
   d. **2-Hour postprandial**: Void 2 hours after eating; used to monitor glucose content
   e. **24-Hour**: Collected over a period of 24 hours for **creatinine clearance** or for quantifying other analytes, including Na^+ and K^+; at time zero, empty bladder into toilet, then collect all urinations in the 24 hours, including the one at 24 hours itself. All collected urine must be delivered to the lab professionals.
   f. **Catheterized**: Collected from a tube placed through the urethra into the bladder; used for bacterial culture and routine screening
   g. **Midstream clean-catch**: Genital area cleansed with a detergent and urine collected in the middle of urination; used for bacterial culture
   h. **Suprapubic aspiration**: Needle inserted into the bladder through the abdominal wall; used for bacterial culture and cytologic testing
   i. **Pediatric collection**: Use small, clear plastic bags with adhesive to adhere to the genital area

V. PHYSICAL EXAMINATION OF URINE

A. Color, Appearance, and Odor

1. **Urine color** varies from colorless to any color shade (black, red, green, etc.). Changes in color can be due to normal metabolism, disease, diet, and physical activity.
   a. The normal color of urine (yellow) is derived from **urochrome**, which is a pigmented substance excreted at a constant rate, which colors both plasma and urine yellow. Variation in shade is a crude indicator of urine concentration.
   b. **Urobilin**, formed from the oxidation of urobilinogen as urine stands, adds minimally to the normal yellow color. As urine sits unpreserved, the color deepens to orange-brown.

c. **Uroerythrin** adds a **slight pink** pigment, mostly apparent following refrigeration, when the pigment attaches to precipitated amorphous urates.
d. **Pale yellow** (straw) samples are generally **dilute**, whereas **dark yellow** samples are usually **concentrated.**

2. **Abnormal urine color**
   a. **Colorless/pale yellow**
      1) Random specimen
      2) Diabetes insipidus or diabetes mellitus with increased urine excretion
   b. **Dark yellow**
      1) Concentrated specimen: First morning or following strenuous exercise
      2) Caused by dehydration from fever, burns, etc.
      3) Concentrated urine will also exhibit high specific gravity.
   c. **Intense yellow/amber/orange**
      1) **Pyridium** (phenazopyridine): This pain medication is prescribed for **urinary tract infections (UTIs)**; resulting **thick orange urine** will mask chemical and microscopic analysis.
      2) **Bilirubin: Bilirubinemia** occurs from liver problems, such as hepatitis, biliary obstruction, etc. With an increase of conjugated, water-soluble bilirubin in the blood, bilirubinuria occurs; **yellow foam** forms when **urine** is **shaken** due to the presence of this **bilirubin.** Note that unconjugated, lipid-soluble bilirubin will never be in the urine, even when increased in the blood.
   d. **Red/pink**
      1) Blood: Glomerular bleeding can also produce brown/black urine.
      2) Hemoglobin, erythrocytes
      3) Myoglobin (muscle trauma)
      4) Porphyrins
   e. **Green/blue**
      1) Medications and dyes such as amitriptyline, indican, and phenols
      2) Infections caused by *Pseudomonas* species
   f. **Brown/black**
      1) Denatured hemoglobin, melanin, or homogentisic acid

   Note: Many abnormal colors are nonpathogenic in nature and are the result of food, drugs, or vitamins.

3. **Appearance of urine** (clarity): The visual inspection of urine uses the following terminology: clear, hazy, slightly cloudy, cloudy, turbid, milky, and bloody.
   a. **Clear**: Indicates the absence of significant numbers of formed elements
   b. **Hazy/slightly cloudy**: May be due to the presence of low numbers of formed elements
   c. **Cloudy**: In acid urine, may be due to amorphous urates showing a slight pink color, calcium oxalate crystals, or uric acid crystals; in alkaline urine, if the sample is white, may be due to amorphous phosphates and carbonates
   d. **Turbid**: May be due to the presence of large numbers of formed elements

4. **Urine odor** is not generally a part of the routine urinalysis but may provide useful information to the physician.
   a. Aromatic odor: Normal
   b. Ammonia odor: Urea metabolized by bacteria into ammonia
   c. Strong odor: Bacterial infection
   d. Sweet or fruity odor: Ketone bodies (diabetic ketosis)
   e. Maple syrup odor: Maple syrup urine disease
   f. Various odors: Different foods

B. Specific Gravity

1. Specific gravity determines the **kidney's ability to reabsorb** essential chemicals and water from the glomerular filtrate. **Reabsorption** is the first renal function to become impaired. Specific gravity also detects dehydration and antidiuretic hormone abnormalities.
2. Specific gravity is the density of a substance compared with the density of a similar volume of deionized water at a similar temperature and is influenced by the number of solutes dissolved and by their size.
3. **Specific gravity instrument: Refractometer** measures a refractive index, by comparing the **velocity of light in air to the velocity of light in a solution.** Method uses a small volume of urine and does not require temperature corrections.
4. **Specific gravity (SG) values: Plasma filtrate** entering the glomerulus has a **SG of 1.010.**
   a. **Normal** random urine **ranges** from **1.003 to 1.035**, with the average SG falling between 1.015 and 1.025.
   b. **Isosthenuric** urine: **1.010** (**fixed SG** indicates loss of concentrating and diluting ability)
   c. **Hyposthenuric** urine: **Less than 1.010**
   d. **Hypersthenuric** urine: **Greater than 1.010**
5. Conditions associated with specific gravity value
   a. **Low specific gravity** may indicate **loss** of the kidney's **ability to concentrate** urine or presence of **disease,** such as diabetes insipidus, glomerulonephritis, and pyelonephritis. It can also be found normally if the person has a large fluid intake.
   b. **High specific gravity** may result from adrenal insufficiency, diabetes mellitus, hepatic disease, congestive heart failure, and dehydration due to vomiting, diarrhea, low fluid intake, or strenuous exercise.
   c. **Interference** from **X-ray contrast media** excretion may result in **SG >1.035.**

VI. CHEMICAL EXAMINATION OF URINE

A. Reagent Strips

1. Reagent strips are used for the following **tests**: pH, protein, glucose, ketones, blood, bilirubin, urobilinogen, nitrite, leukocytes, creatinine, and specific gravity. Reagent strips are the method of choice for the chemical analysis of urine.
2. **Basic use**: Reagent strips are **chemical-containing absorbent pads** that react with urine, producing a chemical reaction that results in a color change. The color is characteristic of positive reactions for various substances. Color intensity is **semiquantitative** for these substances. Confirmatory tests are then performed for some analytes.
3. **Sources of error** in reagent strip use include excess time in the urine, runover between chemicals, not following specific reaction times to read results, and not testing samples at room temperature.
4. Reagent strips should be assessed for accuracy by the use of "normal" and "abnormal" urine controls, run on at least a daily basis.
5. Chemistry testing results can be described as being "accurate" if the result matches what is present in the actual patient; "precise" if repeated measurements of a sample yield the same result. "Sensitivity" of a method is the lowest analyte concentration that can be distinguished from zero. Specificity describes whether the reaction measures what it is meant to measure.

B. Chemical Tests and Clinical Significance

1. **pH**
   a. The **acid-base balance** of the body is primarily **regulated by** the **lungs** and the **kidneys.** The kidneys provide regulation through **secretion of hydrogen ions** via ammonium ions, hydrogen phosphate, and organic weak acids. The kidneys also facilitate the **reabsorption of bicarbonate** from the convoluted tubules.
   b. The **pH** of urine ranges from **4.5 to 8.0** for random urines and from **5.0 to 6.0** for the first morning void. The following urine pHs may indicate various diseases and conditions:
      1) **Acidic pH** (**<6.0**): High-protein diets, after normal sleep, respiratory/metabolic acidosis, uncontrolled diabetes mellitus
      2) **Alkaline pH** (**>7.0**): Excreted after meals in response to gastric HCl, vomiting, increased consumption of vegetables, renal tubular acidosis, respiratory/metabolic alkalosis, and UTIs. Note that urine may also be alkaline as a result of delay in testing due to the action of bacteria on urea to form ammonia.
   c. For **pH**, the **reagent strip** uses **methyl red and bromthymol blue** to detect changes in pH. At pH 5.0 the pad is orange; as the pH increases, the pad will go from orange to yellow to green, and finally to blue at pH 9.0.

2. **Protein**
   a. The reagent strip uses **tetrabromphenol blue** to detect protein.
      1) Principle ("protein error of indicators"): The indicator is yellow in the absence of protein and the pad changes to **shades of green to blue** when **abnormal** amounts of protein (albumin) are present.
      2) **Reaction interference**
         a) **False positives**: Urine pH >9, resulting from alkaline medicine and keeping the reagent strip in urine too long
         b) **False negatives**: Dilute urine; proteins other than albumin present
   b. Normal urine will contain **less than 10 mg/dL** of protein or **100 mg/24 hr.** Protein types include **albumin, microglobulins**, and **uromodulin** (Tamm-Horsfall).
   c. Urine protein is diagnostic for renal disease and many indicate tubular reabsorption problems, increased low-molecular-weight proteins, and glomerular membrane damage caused by toxic agents, lupus, or *streptococcal glomerulonephritis.*
   d. Protein can come from **nonrenal sources**, such as prostate, seminal, and vaginal secretions. However, these other sources of protein will not usually be detectable by the reagent strip method, which is selective for albumin.
   e. **Bence Jones protein** is produced due to a **proliferative disorder of plasma cells** as seen in **multiple myeloma**. Bence Jones proteins are **light chain monoclonal immunoglobulins.**
   f. **Benign proteinuria** can occur in cold temperatures and as a result of exercise, fever, dehydration, late pregnancy, and orthostatic/postural proteinuria in young adults (going from supine to upright).
   g. **Microalbumin** evaluation is useful for patients with **renal complications of diabetes mellitus.** The protein levels found may be less than that detectable by routine protein reagent strip tests. Performed on random urines, microalbumin analysis always requires the simultaneous analysis of creatinine, and it is reported as an Alb/Cr ratio. **Abnormal** values (microalbuminuria) will be **30–299 mg albumin/g creatinine.**
3. **Creatinine**
   a. **Creatinine** testing in a random urine is performed only for **comparison with** the **protein** level to **rule out microalbuminuria.**
   b. Creatinine provides an assurance that the **water volume** of the sample is **not** influencing the protein concentration.
   c. **Methodology of creatinine testing**
      1) **Creatinine** in the urine sample forms a **complex with copper reagent** in the reagent strip pad. This complex has **pseudoperoxidase** activity that **catalyzes** the **oxidation of a chromagen** to a colored end product.
      2) The final concentration from the **creatinine** pad is **matched in a grid** with the concentration from the **protein** pad. The intersection of the two test results will indicate if the protein result is normal or abnormal.

   3) Reagent strips with the creatinine pad will commonly lack a urobilinogen pad.
   4) **Sensitivity** of the **creatinine** method is **10 mg/dL,** which will be **interpreted** as a specimen that is **too dilute to use for analysis.**
      a) **False positives**: None
      b) **False negatives**: Ascorbic acid

4. **Glucose**
   a. **Glucose** testing is most commonly used to detect and monitor **diabetes mellitus.** It may also be important in monitoring the use of medications which purposely place glucose into the urine by interfering with the sodium-glucose cotransporters (SGTR2) which are involved in glucose reabsorption by the proximal convoluted tubules (e.g., Invokana® and Farxiga®).
   b. **Glucosuria** is the presence of **urine glucose** and is seen in the following conditions: diabetes mellitus (either from glycosemia itself or as a therapeutic way of decreasing blood glucose levels), impaired tubular reabsorption seen in Fanconi syndrome, advanced tubular renal disease, central nervous system (CNS) damage, thyroid disorders, and pregnancy.
   c. **Methodology of glucose testing**
      1) **Reagent strip**: Glucose + oxygen are catalyzed by **glucose oxidase** to form gluconic acid and H_2O_2. The H_2O_2 + chromogen are catalyzed by **peroxidase** to form an oxidized colored chromogen + water.
         a) **False positives**: Strong oxidizing agents (e.g., bleach)
         b) **False negatives**: Ascorbic acid; alkaline pH and high specific gravity
      2) **Copper reduction test** (Benedict's, Clinitest tablet): Method utilizes a reduction reaction, in which **glucose** (or other reducing substances) **reduces copper sulfate** (blue) **to cuprous oxide** (various shades of yellow to green). Currently, this test is not used for confirming the presence of glucose, because it is much less sensitive to glucose than the strip test. Instead, this test is mainly used to detect the presence of galactose in urine for pediatric patients with galactosemia.
         a) **False positives**: Antibiotics, ascorbic acid, and other reducing sugars
         b) **False negatives**: None

5. **Ketones**
   a. Include three intermediate **products of fatty acid metabolism: acetone, acetoacetic acid**, and **beta-hydroxybutyric acid**
   b. **Normal** urine contains **no ketones** when metabolized fat is broken down completely, but when fat reserves are needed for energy, ketones will show up in the urine.
   c. **Ketonuria**: The presence of ketones in the urine
   d. **Clinical significance**: Uncontrolled diabetes mellitus, insulin dosage monitoring, electrolyte imbalance, and dehydration due to excessive carbohydrate loss such as vomiting, starvation, exercise, and rapid weight loss

e. **Methodology of ketone testing**

1) Reagent strips use **sodium nitroprusside** (nitroferricyanide) to measure **acetoacetic acid.** The addition of **glycine** permits the measurement of **acetone and acetoacetic acid.**

a) **False positives**: Pigmented urine, dyes, phenylketones

b) **False negatives**: Bacterial breakdown of acetoacetic acid, or if the volatile ketones are released when the sample container is opened.

2) **Acetest** is a **nitroprusside** and **glycine** tablet used to detect ketones; gives an enhanced color reaction and permits serial dilutions to be done. Reaction interference parallels the reagent strip method; may also be used with blood.

3) The **enzymatic method** uses beta-hydroxybutyrate dehydrogenase to detect the presence of beta-hydroxybutyric acid.

6. **Blood**

a. Reagent strip test detects **hematuria** and **hemoglobinuria.**

b. Types of blood/hemoglobin in the urine

1) **Hematuria** (**intact RBCs** in the urine)

a) Caused by renal calculi, glomerulonephritis, pyelonephritis, tumors, trauma, toxins, exercise, menstruation, and pregnancy

2) **Hemoglobinuria** (**hemoglobin** in the urine)

a) Caused by transfusion reactions, hemolytic anemia, severe burns, infections, and exercise

3) **Myoglobin** (hemoglobin-like protein found in **muscle tissue**)

a) The presence of **myoglobin** will cause a **positive reaction** on the reagent strip pad **for blood.** Myoglobin can be detected in muscle trauma, coma, convulsions, muscle-wasting diseases, and extensive exercise.

b) To **screen for myoglobin**, use **ammonium sulfate** to **precipitate hemoglobin** out of the urine; the **urine supernatant** is then filtered and **tested** with a reagent strip. **Positive reaction: myoglobin;** negative reaction: hemoglobin

c. **Reagent strip methodology**

1) Detects the **pseudoperoxidase** activity of **hemoglobin or myoglobin;** H_2O_2 plus chromogen reacts with hemoglobin peroxidase-like activity to form oxidized chromogen and water. The chromogen is **tetramethylbenzidine**, which forms a green-blue color when oxidized.

2) A **speckled pattern** on the reagent strip pad occurs when low numbers of **intact RBCs** lyse upon touching the reagent strip pad, releasing hemoglobin. **Free hemoglobin** or high numbers of red blood cells in the urine will form a **uniform color** on the pad.

d. **Reaction interferences**

1) **False positives**: Vegetable peroxidase and *Escherichia coli* peroxidase

2) **False negatives**: High levels of ascorbic acid and nitrites, formalin preservatives, captopril (hypertension medication)

7. **Bilirubin**
   a. Detects **bilirubinuria**, a degradation product of hemoglobin
   b. Bilirubin is a pigmented yellow compound.
   c. Hemoglobin is metabolized into iron, protein, and **protoporphyrin.** The protoporphyrin is **converted to bilirubin** by reticuloendothelial system cells; bilirubin binds to albumin for transport to the liver as unconjugated bilirubin.
   d. In the liver, **bilirubin** is **conjugated** with **glucuronic acid** to form **bilirubin diglucuronide**, which goes to the intestines and is reduced to **urobilinogen** via bacterial action and excreted in the feces as **urobilin.** Urobilin gives feces its brown color. A small amount of urobilinogen reaches the kidney via the bloodstream and is excreted in the urine.
   e. **Bilirubinuria** may result from hepatitis, cirrhosis, biliary obstruction, and early liver disease when conjugated bilirubin enters the circulation.
      1) **Conjugated bilirubin** is **water soluble** and excreted in urine.
      2) **Unconjugated bilirubin** is ***not*** water soluble and cannot be excreted in urine.
   f. **Bile duct obstruction** is positive for urine bilirubin (conjugated form increased in plasma) but normal for urine urobilinogen.
   g. In **hemolytic disease**, urine urobilinogen is positive and urine bilirubin (unconjugated form increased in plasma) is negative.
   h. **Reagent strip** uses **diazonium salt** reaction (bilirubin → azobilirubin) methodology. The **Ictotest®** tablet is a diazo confirmatory test for bilirubin that is more sensitive and less subject to interference.
   i. **Reaction interferences**
      1) **False positives**: Pigmented urine (i.e., medications, indican, and Lodine)
      2) **False negatives**: Specimen too old, excessive exposure to light (bilirubin exposed to light is converted to biliverdin, which does not react with diazonium salts), ascorbic acid, and nitrite
8. **Urobilinogen**
   a. Formed from hemoglobin metabolism; produced from the reduction of bilirubin by bacteria in the small intestine
   b. Increased urobilinogen in the urine can indicate early liver disease, hepatitis, and hemolytic diseases.
   c. Reagent strip uses **Ehrlich's reagent** (paradimethylaminobenzaldehyde) or a **diazo dye** to detect urobilinogen. Note that it is not possible to detect the absence of urobilinogen by the reagent strip.
   d. **Reaction interferences**
      1) **False positives**: Pigmented urine
      2) **False decrease**: Improper storage, high levels of nitrite
9. **Nitrite**
   a. Rapid test for **UTIs**
   b. A **positive nitrite** can indicate cystitis (bladder infection) and pyelonephritis.
   c. Used for evaluation of UTI antibiotic therapy

d. **Reagent strip** detects the ability of **certain bacteria** to **reduce nitrate** (found in urine normally) **to nitrite** (abnormal in urine). In the reagent strip method, nitrite reacts with an aromatic amine to form a diazonium salt, which then reacts with a dye to produce a pink product.
e. **Reaction interferences**
   1) **False positives**: Old urine samples containing bacteria and pigmented urine
   2) **False negatives**: Ascorbic acid, antibiotics, bacteria that do not reduce nitrate, diet low in nitrates, inadequate time in bladder for reduction of nitrate to nitrite, and heavy concentration of bacteria that reduces nitrate all the way to nitrogen, which does not react

10. **Leukocytes**
   a. Indicate possible **urinary tract infection, inflammation** of urinary tract
   b. Reagent strip method does not quantify the number of WBCs.
   c. The strip method **detects lysed leukocytes** that would not be found under the microscope.
   d. **Reagent strip reaction**: Intact leukocytes lyse on contact with the pad. An acid ester reacts with **leukocyte esterase** to form an aromatic compound that reacts with a diazonium salt, forming a purple color.
   e. **Reaction interferences**
      1) **False positives**: Pigmented urine, strong oxidizing agents
      2) **False negatives**: Increased glucose, protein, and ascorbic acid; yellow-pigmented substances; high specific gravity (prevents release of leukocyte esterases); lymphocytes (do not contain leukocyte esterase); selected antibiotics like gentamicin and tetracycline

11. **Specific gravity**
   a. Gives an approximate specific gravity value in increments of 0.005
   b. **Clinical significance**: Monitors hydration and dehydration, loss of renal tubular concentrating ability, and diabetes insipidus
   c. **Reagent strip reaction**: The **ionization of a polyelectrolyte** in an alkaline solution (due to change in dissociation constant) **produces hydrogen ions** proportionally to the ions present in the solution. This causes a **change in pH** that is detected as a decrease in pH, thus causing a **color change of bromthymol blue**, which is an indicator able to measure pH changes. SG = 1.000, pad color is blue in alkaline solution; SG = 1.030, pad color is yellow in acid solution. Note that the pad is sensitive only to ions in the urine. Cells and nonionized solutes like glucose will not cause a reaction.
   d. **Reaction interferences**
      1) **False positives**: Elevated protein or ketone levels increase the specific gravity.
      2) **False negatives**: If urine pH >6.5, add 0.005 to the reading.

VII. MICROSCOPIC EXAMINATION OF URINE

A. Microscopic Examination of Urine

1. Must be done to identify insoluble substances from the blood, kidney, lower urogenital tract, and external contaminants
2. **Formed elements**: Erythrocytes, leukocytes, epithelial cells, bacteria, yeast, fungal elements, parasites, mucus, sperm, crystals, and artifacts
3. Standard rules for microscopic analysis of urine.
   a. Examine urine while **fresh** or when **properly preserved.**
   b. 10–12 mL of urine are centrifuged leaving 0.5–1.0 mL of sediment for viewing.
   c. Report all cell types (RBC, WBC, epithelials, sperm, yeast) using high-power magnification (i.e., high-power field [hpf]); report casts and crystals using low-power magnification (i.e., low-power field [lpf]).
   d. All formed elements must be identified and quantified.
   e. Microscopic methods include brightfield, phase contrast, and polarized.

B. Normal Urines: Contain 0–2 RBCs (hpf), 0–5 WBCs (hpf), 0–2 hyaline casts (lpf), several epithelial cells (hpf), some types of crystals, and mucus. Note that the reference ranges for these will vary by the method and volume used.

C. Urine Formed Elements

1. **Erythrocytes (7 microns)**
   a. Number of cells counted is related to extent of renal damage, glomerular membrane damage, or urogenital tract vascular damage.
   b. RBCs are associated with infections, toxins, cancer, circulatory problems, renal calculi, menstrual contamination, trauma, and exercise.
   c. **RBCs** in normal urine **appear as colorless disks**; in concentrated urine they **shrink** and appear **crenated**; in dilute or alkaline urine, RBCs **swell** and **lyse** with release of hemoglobin, leaving an **empty cell**, which appears as a **ghost cell.**
   d. RBCs can be confused with yeast cells or oil droplets (highly refractile). Dilute **acetic acid** can be used to **lyse RBCs,** leaving only yeast, oil droplets, and WBCs.
2. **Leukocytes (10–15 microns)**
   a. **Pyuria** is **increased WBCs** in the urine and may indicate **infection** in the urogenital tract. Leukocytes in the urine may indicate the following:
      1) **Bacterial** infections, pyelonephritis, cystitis, prostatitis, and urethritis
      2) **Nonbacterial** pyuria resulting from glomerulonephritis, lupus, and tumors
   b. **Neutrophils** are the **predominant WBC** appearing in the urine with cytoplasmic granules and multilobed nuclei.
      1) **WBCs swell** in dilute alkaline urine (hypotonic), producing **glitter cells**, which have a sparkling appearance due to the Brownian movement of the granules.
      2) **Eosinophils** in the urine may indicate a drug-induced nephritis or renal transplant rejection. If suspected to be present, special staining will be needed to visualize these cells.

3. **Epithelial cells**
   a. **Squamous epithelial (30–50 microns)**: These cells are very common in the urine and usually not clinically significant. Squamous epithelial cells **line the lower urethra and vagina in women and the urethra of males.** They are the **largest** of the cells found in sediment with **abundant, irregular cytoplasm** and a **central nucleus** the size of a RBC. Excessive numbers of these cells may suggest the sample has not been collected properly by the clean-catch method. In the presence of a vaginal infection, **clue cells** may appear; clue cells are squamous epithelial cells covered with *Gardnerella vaginalis* (coccobacillus).
   b. **Transitional epithelial (20–40 microns)**: These cells **line the renal pelvis, ureters, bladder, and upper urethra in males. Smaller** than squamous epithelial cells, transitional cells are **spherical/polyhedral/caudate** and have a **central nucleus.** There is no associated pathology, except in large numbers, with abnormal morphology, including vacuoles and irregular nuclei, which may indicate renal carcinoma or viral infection. Increased number of cells may be present after catheterization due to the invasiveness of the procedure.
   c. **Renal tubular epithelial (RTE) (12–60 microns, depending on the tubule location)**: The RTE cell is the **most significant** epithelial cell in the urine. It has a **small eccentric nucleus.** Cell **size and shape vary** from rectangular, larger cells in the proximal convoluted tubule (PCT) to cells slightly larger than a WBC-shaped cuboidal or columnar originating from the collecting duct (CD). **Cytoplasm varies**, with the PCT being coarsely granulated and the CD being very finely granulated. **Tubular injury** is suggested when **>5/hpf are present.** Can indicate renal cancer, renal tubular damage, pyelonephritis, toxic and allergic reactions, and viral infection. Types of renal tubular cells include:
      1) **Bubble cells** are RTE cells that contain large, nonlipid-filled vacuoles. These cells can be seen in **renal tubular necrosis.** Their presence is associated with dilation of endoplasmic reticulum before the death of injured cells.
      2) **Oval fat bodies** are renal tubular epithelial cells that have absorbed lipids that are highly refractile and stain with Sudan III or oil red O. They may indicate nephrotic syndrome.
   d. **Miscellaneous cells: Histiocytes** in the urine may indicate lipid-storage disease. These cells are filled with fat and are larger than oval fat bodies.
4. **Casts**
   a. Of all the formed elements in the urine, only casts are **unique** to the kidney.
      1) Different casts represent different clinical conditions.
      2) **Cylindruria** is the term for casts in the urine.
      3) Casts are **formed** within the **lumen of the distal convoluted tubule** and **collecting duct**, taking on a shape similar to the tubular lumen. Their formation is favored when there is urinary stasis, acid pH, and increased solute concentration.

4) Casts may have **formed elements** (such as bacteria, WBCs, RBCs, etc.) contained **within** them **or attached** to their surface.
5) **Uromodulin** (Tamm-Horsfall glycoprotein) is the **major constituent of casts** and is poorly detected by reagent strip methods. Uromodulin is made by the **renal tubular epithelial cells** that line the DCT and upper CD. Casts also consist of some albumin and immunoglobulins.

5. **Types of casts**
   a. **Hyaline cast: Most commonly seen** cast, 0–5/lpf normal
      1) Increased hyaline casts normally follow exercise, dehydration, heat, and emotional stress.
      2) **Disease association**: Acute glomerulonephritis, pyelonephritis, chronic renal disease, and congestive heart failure
      3) **Appearance**: Colorless, with varied morphology
   b. **RBC cast**: Cellular casts containing erythrocytes
      1) **Disease association**: Bleeding within the nephron, damage to the glomerulus or renal capillaries as found in poststreptococcal infections
      2) Seen following strenuous contact sports
      3) **Appearance**: Orange to red color, contains hemoglobin and intact erythrocytes
   c. **WBC cast**: A cellular cast containing WBCs
      1) **Disease association**: Infection (pyelonephritis) or inflammation within the nephron (acute interstitial nephritis)
      2) **Appearance**: Primarily contain neutrophils, thus appearing granular with multilobed nuclei
   d. **Bacterial cast:**
      1) **Disease association**: Pyelonephritis
      2) **Appearance**: Bacilli contained within the cast and bound to the surface; mixed cast containing bacteria and WBCs may occur
   e. **Epithelial cell cast:**
      1) **Disease association**: Advanced renal tubular damage; seen in heavy metal, chemical, or drug toxicity, viral infections, and allograft rejection
      2) **Appearance**: Contain renal tubular epithelial cells
   f. **Granular cast:**
      1) **Disease association**: The granular appearance results from degeneration of a cellular cast's encased cells since there has been a slowing of the urine flow, thus keeping the cast in the tubule for a longer time.
      2) Seen with hyaline casts following stress and exercise
      3) **Appearance**: Granular casts can be coarsely or finely granular (differentiation holds no clinical significance). **Finely granular casts** appear gray or pale yellow. **Coarsely granular casts** contain larger granules that may appear black.

g. **Waxy cast**: Contains surface protein, granules adhere to the cast matrix; formed from degeneration of granular casts
   1) **Disease association**: Chronic renal failure with significant urine stasis
   2) **Appearance**: High refractive index, colorless to yellow with a smooth appearance; can have cracks or fissures on the sides
h. **Fatty cast**: Seen with oval fat bodies in disease states that result in lipiduria
   1) **Disease association**: Nephrotic syndrome, toxic tubular necrosis, diabetes mellitus
   2) **Appearance**: Highly refractile, contains yellow-brown fat droplets
   3) Positive identification of fatty casts is by Sudan III stain or polarized light, which shows a characteristic **Maltese cross formation.**
i. **Broad cast**: Formed in the DCT and CD due to **anuria**
   1) **Disease association**: Suggests renal failure
   2) **Appearance**: All types of casts can occur in the broad form, with the most common being granular and waxy.

6. **Bacteria**: Not present in normal sterile urine
   a. **Disease association**: Lower and upper UTI
   b. Bacteria can be distinguished from amorphous crystals by their motility (tumbling or directional movement).
7. **Yeast:**
   a. **Disease association**: UTI, vaginal infections, diabetes mellitus, and in individuals who are immunocompromised
   b. Yeast can be confused with erythrocytes; look for budding yeast forms or the presence of pseudohyphae.
8. **Parasites**: The most common parasite in the urine is ***Trichomonas vaginalis.*** Another parasite sometimes found in the urine is **pinworm ova** from *Enterobius vermicularis*, which is usually due to fecal contamination. A rarer urine parasite is *Schistosoma haematobium*, a significant public health problem in Africa and the Middle East.
9. **Sperm**: Seen in urine following intercourse or nocturnal emissions; no clinical significance except in forensic cases, male infertility, and retrograde ejaculation
10. **Mucus**: Glycoprotein substance produced by the RTE cells and the urogenital glands; not considered clinically significant
    a. **Appearance**: Threadlike structures with low refractive index, view under reduced light; can be confused with hyaline casts
11. **Crystals:**
    a. Crystals are formed by the **precipitation** of urine salts, organic compounds, and medications. Crystal formation can be altered by temperature, pH, and urine concentration. Crystals will appear more frequently if urine stands at room temperature for prolonged time periods or if it is refrigerated. Urine **pH is important** in determining the **type of crystal formation.**
    b. **Crystal formation**: The glomerular ultrafiltrate passes through the renal tubules; then the solutes in the ultrafilrate are concentrated. If an increased

amount of a solute is present, the **ultrafiltrate** becomes **saturated**, leading to the solute precipitating into a characteristic crystal form. Crystal formation is enhanced when **urine flow** through the renal tubules is **inhibited.** The reduced flow allows time for concentration of the solutes in the ultrafiltrate.

c. **Crystal identification**: Crystals differ in their solubility. **All clinically significant crystals are in acidic and neutral urine.**

12. **Types of acidic urine crystals:**

a. **Amorphous urates**
   1) Formed from the urate salts of Na^+, K^+, Mg^+, and Ca^{2+}
   2) No clinical significance
   3) Small, **yellow-to-brown granules** usually in large amounts; may make other urine elements difficult to see
   4) **Refrigerated** samples will produce more **amorphous urates** and may appear as **pink sediment** because of the **presence of uroerythrin** on the surface of the granules.
   5) Amorphous urates will **dissolve at alkaline pH** or by heating above 60°C.

b. **Uric acid**
   1) Seen in **gout**, with chemotherapy for leukemia, and in Lesch-Nyhan syndrome
   2) Appear **yellow to orange/brown** but can be colorless
   3) **Pleomorphic** (many) shapes include four-sided flat plates, rhombic plates, wedges, and rosettes

c. **Calcium oxalate**
   1) Most urine oxalate is from oxalic acid, which is found in such foods as tomatoes, asparagus, spinach, berries, and oranges. In addition, oxalic acid is a metabolite of ascorbic acid.
   2) Colorless, **dihydrate** form appears as **octahedral envelope** or two pyramids joined at their bases; **monohydrate** form appears as **dumbbell or oval** shaped.
   3) These crystals are **associated with renal calculi formation.** Monohydrate form is seen in poison centers where children have ingested ethylene glycol (antifreeze).

d. **Bilirubin**
   1) **Abnormal crystal**: These crystals are formed when urine bilirubin exceeds its solubility, and they appear as **fine needles or granules** that are **yellow to brown** in color.
   2) These crystals are most often seen in **liver disease.** Casts may contain bilirubin crystals in cases of viral hepatitis when there is renal tubular damage.

e. **Tyrosine**
   1) **Abnormal crystal**: Fine delicate **needles, colorless to yellow** found in clumps or rosettes
   2) Associated with **severe liver disease** and in **inherited diseases** that affect amino acid metabolism
   3) May be seen with leucine crystals in urine that tests positive for bilirubin

f. **Leucine**
   1) **Abnormal crystal: Yellow to brown,** oily looking spheres with concentric circles and radial striations; may be found with tyrosine crystals
   2) Associated with **severe liver disease** and in **inherited diseases** that affect amino acid metabolism

g. **Cystine**
   1) **Abnormal crystal: Colorless, hexagonal plates**
   2) These crystals result from a **congenital disorder** that inhibits renal tubular reabsorption of cystine, hence cystinuria. Note that lysine, arginine, and ornithine will also be present but they are more soluble than cysteine so not visible.
   3) Associated with **renal calculi formation**

h. **Cholesterol**
   1) **Abnormal crystal: Clear, flat, rectangular plates** with a **notch in one or more corners**; more commonly seen following refrigeration; seen with fatty casts and oval fat bodies
   2) Associated with **nephrotic syndrome** and other disorders that produce lipiduria

i. **Crystals from medications**
   1) Medications are excreted by the kidneys; any buildup can result in renal damage.
      a) **Ampicillin** crystals appear **colorless** in the form of **needles**, which may form bundles.
      b) **Sulfonamide** crystals appear **colorless to yellow-brown** in the form of needles, sheaves of wheat, fan formations, or rosettes.

j. **Radiographic dyes**
   1) Resemble cholesterol
   2) Correlate with increased specific gravity (>1.050)

13. **Alkaline urine crystals:**

a. **Amorphous phosphate**
   1) Identical in appearance to amorphous urates and generally **colorless; refrigerated** samples appear as a **white sediment**
   2) Amorphous phosphates are **soluble in acetic acid** (amorphous urates are insoluble in acetic acid) and will not dissolve when heated above 60°C.
   3) Not clinically significant

b. **Triple phosphate (ammonium magnesium phosphate)**
   1) **Colorless, three- to six-sided prism** often resembling a **coffin lid**
   2) Not clinically significant; may be associated with **UTI, prostatitis**

c. **Calcium phosphate**
   1) **Colorless**, thin prisms or rectangular plates
   2) Not clinically significant; may be associated with **renal calculi formation**

d. **Ammonium biurate**
   1) Normal crystal commonly seen in old urine samples; converts to uric acid crystals if acetic acid added and dissolves at 60°C
   2) **Yellow to brown** spheres with striation on the surface, also can show irregular, **thorny projections** (thorn apple)

e. **Calcium carbonate**
   1) Appear as small, **colorless** crystals having **dumbbell** or spherical shapes
   2) Not clinically significant

VIII. SPECIAL URINE SCREENING TESTS (USUALLY PERFORMED IN SPECIAL CHEMISTRY)

A. Phenylketonuria (PKU)

1. The presence of phenylalanine in the urine indicates defective metabolic conversion of phenylalanine to tyrosine, which is caused by a gene failure to produce **phenylalanine hydroxylase.**
2. Occurs in 1:10,000 births and, if undetected, will result in **severe intellectual disability.**
3. **PKU screening tests** are required in all 50 states for newborns (at least 24 hours old).
4. The urine gives off a **mousy odor** associated with phenylpyruvate because of the increased ketones.
5. When the PKU test is positive, the diet is changed to eliminate all phenylalanine from the diet.
6. As the child grows, an alternative phenylalanine pathway develops and dietary restrictions are eased.
7. **Types of PKU testing** (all positive screening tests are **confirmed by high-performance liquid chromatography**)
   a. **Guthrie** bacterial inhibition test uses blood from a heel stick. Blood is placed on filter paper disks on culture media streaked with *Bacillus subtilis.* If phenylalanine is present in the blood sample, beta-2-thienylalanine in the media, which is an inhibitor of *B. subtilis,* will be counteracted, resulting in *B. subtilis* growth around the disks (positive PKU).
   b. Urine test for phenylpyruvic acid uses **ferric chloride** (tube or reagent strip); a positive test is blue-green.
      1) **Microfluorometric assay** directly measures phenylalanine in dried blood filter disks.
      2) It is a quantitative test (Guthrie is semiquantitative).
      3) It is not affected by antibiotics.
      4) A pretreated (trichloroacetic acid) patient sample extract is reacted in a microtiter plate containing ninhydrin, succinate, leucylalanine, and copper tartrate.
      5) The sample is measured at 360 nm and 530 nm.

B. Miscellaneous Special Urine Screening Tests

1. **Tyrosinosis**
   a. Excess **tyrosine** (tyrosinuria) or its by-products (*p*-hydroxyphenylpyruvic acid or *p*-hydroxyphenyllactic acid) in the urine
   b. Inherited or metabolic defects
   c. **Metabolic disease states** include transitory tyrosinemia, premature infants with an underdeveloped liver, and acquired severe liver disease. All of these conditions will produce **tyrosine and leucine crystals. Hereditary defects** are usually **fatal**, presenting with liver and renal diseases.
   d. The **nitrosonaphthol** test is used as a **screening** test, whereas **chromatography** is used as a **confirmatory** test.
2. **Alkaptonuria**
   a. This is a **genetic defect** resulting in failure to produce homogentisic acid oxidase, which causes **accumulation of homogentisic acid** in blood and urine.
   b. This condition produces brown pigment deposits in body tissue that can lead to arthritis, liver, and cardiac problems.
   c. **Screening tests** include:
      1) Ferric chloride tube test (blue color)
      2) Benedict's test (yellow color)
      3) Alkalization of fresh urine (urine darkens)
3. **Melanuria**
   a. **Increased melanin** in urine is produced from **tyrosine**; urine darkens upon standing and exposed to air.
   b. Indicates **malignant melanoma**
   c. Screening tests include **ferric chloride** (gray/black precipitate) and **sodium nitroprusside** (red color).
4. **Maple syrup urine disease**
   a. Characteristic of this disorder is **maple syrup smell** of the urine, breath, and skin.
   b. Caused by low levels of **branched-chained keto acid decarboxylase**; inhibits metabolism of leucine, isoleucine, and valine
   c. If **untreated**, the disease causes **severe intellectual disability**, convulsions, acidosis, and hypoglycemia. Death occurs during the first year.
   d. Screening test uses **2,4-dinitrophenylhydrazine** (DNPH) to form yellow turbidity or precipitate.
5. Argentaffinoma
   a. Arise from enterochromaffin cells of the gastrointestinal tract
   b. Produce increased blood serotonin, whose major urinary excretion product is 5-hydroxyindoleacetic acid (5-HIAA)
   c. Detected using 1-nitroso-2-naphthol to yield a purple color
   d. Patient must be on diet free of bananas, pineapples, and tomatoes, which contain significant amounts of serotonin.

IX. BODY FLUIDS AND FECAL ANALYSIS

A. Cerebrospinal Fluid (CSF): (Most CSF analysis is performed in chemistry, hematology, and microbiology.)

1. **CSF** is made by the brain's third choroid plexus as an ultrafiltrate of plasma. It supplies nutrients to nervous tissue, removes wastes, and cushions the brain and spinal cord against trauma. A total volume of 20 mL of CSF is produced each hour. Total adult volume is 140–170 mL, and neonate volume is 10–60 mL.
2. **Specimen collection** is by lumbar puncture, which is performed by a physician between the 3–4 or 4–5 lumbar vertebrae. The samples are collected into sterile, numbered, screw-capped tubes. The **order of draw** is:
   a. Tube #1: Chemistry and serology (glucose, protein, antibodies); note that hematology will also receive this tube initially to compare with tube #3 for determining possibility of traumatic tap
   b. Tube #2: Microbiology (culture and sensitivity)
   c. Tube #3: Hematology (red and white blood cell counts)
3. **Cerebrospinal fluid appearance**
   a. **Clear and colorless**: Normal
   b. **Cloudy**: Indicates WBCs, RBCs, protein, or bacteria; seen in meningitis, hemorrhage, disorders of the blood-brain barrier, etc.
   c. **Bloody**: This may be due to subarachnoid hemorrhage or traumatic tap. Differentiation between the two is made by noting the difference in appearance between tubes #1 and #3. If there is hemorrhage, all tubes will appear bloody. If traumatic tap, there will be less blood in tube #3 than in tube #1.
   d. **Xanthochromic** (yellow): Increased hemoglobin, bilirubin, protein, immature liver in premature infants; note that this term is reserved for CSF.
4. **Chemistry testing**
   a. CSF **glucose**: 60–70% of the patient's plasma glucose
   b. CSF **total protein**: Assayed using trichloroacetic acid precipitation method or Coomassie brilliant blue
5. **Hematology testing**
   a. **Cerebrospinal fluid microscopic**: Normal CSF contains 0–5 WBC/μL; lymphocytes and monocytes predominate
   b. **Lymphocytes**: Seen in normal fluids; **increased in viral and fungal meningitis**
   c. **PMNs: Bacterial meningitis** (cerebral abscess)
   d. **Early cell forms**: Acute leukemia
   e. **Plasma cells**: Multiple sclerosis or lymphocytic reactions
6. **Microbiology testing**
   a. **India ink**: Used to detect *Cryptococcus neoformans*, possible complication of AIDS
   b. **Gram stain and culture**: Used to detect bacteria

B. Seminal Fluid (Semen)

1. Used to evaluate infertility, postvasectomy, and forensic medicine cases
2. **Specimen collection**
   a. Collect in sterile containers after a 3-day period of no sexual activity for infertility studies; **postvasectomy** requires no waiting period
   b. Plastic containers will inhibit motility
   c. No condom collection (may contain spermicidal agents)
   d. Keep at room temperature; transport to the lab professionals within 1 hour.
3. **Semen analysis**
   a. **Volume**: 2–5 mL
   b. **Viscosity**: Normal is no clumps or strings; must have specimen that is completely liquefied, which takes about 30–60 minutes.
   c. **Appearance**: Normal is a **translucent, gray-white color.**
   d. **pH**: 7.2–8.0 is normal (>8.0 could indicate infection).
   e. **Sperm count**: Normal is 20–160 million/mL, borderline is 10–20 million/mL, and sterile is less than 10 million/mL.
   f. **Motility**: Based on the percentage of movement, 50–60% or greater with a motility grade of 2 is normal (0—immotile; 4—motile with strong forward progression).
   g. **Morphology: Oval-shaped head** with a **long, flagellar tail** is **normal. Abnormal** forms include double head, giant head, amorphous head, pinhead, double tail, and coiled tail.
   h. **Cells other than sperm present**: The presence of red blood cells or white blood cells would be significant.

C. Synovial Fluid

1. Synovial fluid is a **plasma ultrafiltrate** and is often called **joint fluid.**
2. Synovial fluid functions as a **lubricant** and **nutrient transport** to articular cartilage.
3. Different joint disorders change the chemical and structural composition of synovial fluid, including inflammation, infection, bleeding, and crystal-associated disorders.
4. Normal **color** of synovial fluid is **clear to straw** colored.
5. **Laboratory analysis** (nonchemistry) includes color, differential count, Gram stain with culture, and crystal identification with a polarizing microscope.
   a. In addition, the presence of hyaluronic acid gives synovial fluid a unique viscosity, which, if absent, can suggest the presence of bacteria secreting hyaluronidase.
   b. Most **crystals** found in synovial fluid are associated with **gout (uric acid)** or **calcium phosphate deposits.**

D. Gastric Fluid: Gastric fluid collection is performed by nasal or oral intubation. Analysis involves physical appearance, volume, titratable acidity, and pH. Most uses of gastric analysis are for toxicology and for the diagnosis of Zollinger-Ellison syndrome.

E. Amniotic Fluid
1. **Protective fluid** surrounding the fetus; needle aspiration termed "**amniocentesis**"
2. Amniotic fluid is mostly used for genetic studies but may be used to check for bilirubin, fetal bleeding, infection, fetal lung maturity, or **meconium** (dark green fetal intestinal secretions) content that in large amounts is associated with meconium aspiration syndrome.
3. Differentiation of the presence of blood versus bilirubin can be achieved by measuring for increased absorbance at 410 nm (absorbance maximum for bilirubin) and 450 nm (absorbance maximum for hemoglobin).
4. Levels of phospholipids (phosphatidyl choline [lecithin], phosphatidyl glycerol) will increase as the fetus's lungs mature.
5. Lamellar bodies are packets of surfactant whose number can predict fetal lung maturity. Counting is usually done on an automated counter, with values greater than 50,000/μL suggesting the lungs are mature.

F. Peritoneal Fluid
1. **Clear to pale yellow** fluid contained between the parietal and visceral membranes in the **peritoneum** (serous membrane that covers the walls of the abdomen and pelvis); also called **ascites fluid**
2. Aspiration is termed "**peritoneocentesis.**"
3. **Laboratory analysis** includes cell counts, Gram stains, gross color examination, and specific gravity.

G. Pleural and Pericardial Fluids
1. Pleural and pericardial fluids are found between the visceral and parietal pleural (around the lungs) and pericardial (around the heart) membranes, respectively. Both fluids are **clear to pale yellow.**
2. Aspiration of pleural/pericardial fluids is termed "**thoracentesis**" and "**pericardiocentesis**," respectively.
3. **Laboratory analysis** includes cell counts, Gram stains, and gross color examination.

H. Fluid Effusions
1. Increases in volume in peritoneal, pleural, or pericardial fluids are called **effusions.**
2. If the mechanism is **noninflammatory**, it is called a **transudate** and will have **fewer than 1000 cells/μL and less than 3 g/dL protein.**
3. **Inflammatory** effusions are called **exudates** and will have **higher than 1000 cells/μL and more than 3 g/dL protein.**

I. Fecal Analysis

1. Used in the detection of gastrointestinal (GI) bleeding, liver and biliary duct disorders, malabsorption syndromes, and infections
2. Types of fecal analysis
   a. **Color and consistency**
      1) **Black (tarry) stool**: Upper GI bleeding; iron therapy
      2) **Red stool**: Lower GI bleeding
      3) **Steatorrhea**: Fat malabsorption
      4) **Diarrhea**: Watery fecal material
      5) **Ribbon-like stools**: Bowel obstruction
      6) **Mucus**: Inflammation of the intestinal wall (colitis)
      7) **Clay-colored, pale**: Bile-duct obstruction/obstructive jaundice
   b. **Fecal leukocytes**: Determine cause of diarrhea
      1) **Neutrophils**: Bacterial intestinal wall infections or ulcerative colitis, abscesses
      2) **No neutrophils**: Toxin-producing bacteria, viruses, and parasites
   c. **Qualitative fecal fat**: Detects fat malabsorption disorders by staining fecal fats with **Sudan III or oil red O**; increased fecal fat (>60 droplets/hpf) suggestive of **steatorrhea**
   d. **Muscle fibers**: Look for undigested striated muscle fibers, which may indicate **pancreatic insufficiency** seen in cystic fibrosis.
   e. **Occult blood**: Used for early detection of **colorectal cancer**; old name, guaiac test
      1) Occult blood most frequently performed fecal analysis
      2) Several chemicals used that vary in sensitivity
         a) **Ortho-toluidine**: Pseudoperoxidase activity of hemoglobin (Hb) reacts with H_2O_2 to oxidize a colorless reagent to a colored product.

$$\text{Hb} \rightarrow H_2O_2 \rightarrow \text{ortho-toluidine} \rightarrow \text{blue oxidized indicator}$$

         b) **Gum guaiac**: Least sensitive, most common
         c) Immunological: Use of an anti-hemoglobin to react with the patient's hemoglobin has the advantage of not requiring any special diet before sample collection. There is the possibility, however, of hemoglobin degradation (and nondetection by antibody), if the gastrointestinal bleed is in the upper intestine.
   f. **DNA test** detects **K-ras mutation**, which is associated with colorectal cancer.

X. AUTOMATION

A. Physical Analysis

1. Physical components of urinalysis are color, clarity, and specific gravity.
2. White light and light scatter analysis in an automated flow cell measures color and clarity, respectively. An aliquot of the urine sample may have specific gravity measured using a refractometer.

B. Chemical Analysis

1. Reflectance colorimetry of the individual reagent strip pads
   a. A wavelength of light is first directed toward a white calibration area on the strip platform, establishing what is 100% reflectance.
   b. Light is then directed toward a pad on the strip, and the intensity of the color developed will affect the amount of light reflected.
   c. Comparison of that amount of reflectance to reflectance stored in memory will determine the concentration displayed for that analyte.

C. Microscopic Analysis

1. Sample is added to a sheathing fluid, making the formed elements travel single file in the flow cytometer.
2. Formed elements pass a flashing strobe light and are captured by a digital camera.
3. Each element is analyzed for size, contrast, shape, and texture.
4. Algorithms classify each element into a category and estimate concentration.
5. Images are visualized by category in a monitor collage for confirmation/reclassification.

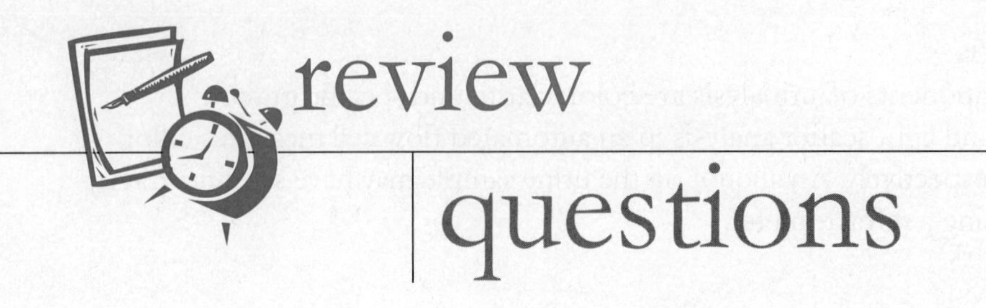

INSTRUCTIONS Each of the questions or incomplete statements that follows comprises four suggested responses. Select the *best* answer or completion statement in each case.

1. Why is the first-voided morning urine specimen the most desirable specimen for routine urinalysis?
   A. It is the most dilute specimen of the day and, therefore, any chemical compounds present will not exceed the detectability limits of the reagent strips
   B. It is the specimen least likely to be contaminated with microorganisms because the bladder is a sterile environment
   C. It is the specimen most likely to contain protein because the patient has been in the orthostatic position during the night
   D. It is the most concentrated specimen of the day and, therefore, it is more likely that abnormalities will be detected

2. The physical characteristic of color is assessed when a routine urinalysis is performed. Which of the following will affect that color significantly?
   A. Bilirubin
   B. Glucose
   C. Albumin
   D. Ketones

3. In which disorder will a urine turn black if the sample's pH becomes alkaline upon standing?
   A. Malignant melanoma
   B. Hemolytic anemia
   C. Alkaptonuria
   D. Hepatitis

4. What is the expected pH range of a freshly voided urine specimen?
   A. 3.5–8.0
   B. 3.5–9.0
   C. 4.0–8.5
   D. 4.5–8.0

5. Urine specimens should be analyzed as soon as possible after collection. If urine specimens are allowed to stand at room temperature for an excessive amount of time, the urine pH will become alkaline because of bacterial decomposition of
   A. Protein
   B. Urea
   C. Creatinine
   D. Ketones

6. Which term is defined as a urine specific gravity which is 1.035?
   A. Anuria
   B. Oliguria
   C. Polyuria
   D. Hypersthenuria

7. The reagent test strips used for the detection of protein in urine are most reactive to
   A. Albumin
   B. Hemoglobin
   C. Alpha-globulins
   D. Beta-globulins

8. A urine specimen that exhibits white foam on being shaken should be suspected of having an increased concentration of
   A. Protein
   B. Hemoglobin
   C. Bilirubin
   D. Nitrite

9. How should controls be run to ensure the precision and accuracy of the reagent test strips used for the chemical analysis of urine?
   A. Positive controls should be run on a daily basis and negative controls when opening a new bottle of test strips.
   B. Positive and negative controls should be run when the test strips' expiration date is passed.
   C. Positive and negative controls should be run on a daily basis.
   D. Positive controls should be run on a daily basis and negative controls on a weekly basis.

10. The colorimetric reagent strip test for protein is able to detect as little as 5–20 mg of protein per deciliter. What may cause a false-positive urine protein reading?
    A. Uric acid concentration is greater than 0.5 g/day.
    B. Vitamin C concentration is greater than 0.5 g/day.
    C. Glucose concentration is greater than 130 mg/day.
    D. pH is greater than 8.0.

11. "Isosthenuria" is a term applied to a series of urine specimens from the same patient that exhibit a
    A. Specific gravity of exactly 1.000
    B. Specific gravity less than 1.007
    C. Specific gravity greater than 1.020
    D. Fixed specific gravity of approximately 1.010

12. A urine specimen is tested by a reagent strip test and the sulfosalicylic acid (SSA) test to determine whether protein is present. The former yields a negative protein, whereas the latter results in a reading of 2+ protein. Which of the following statements best explains this difference?
    A. The urine contained an excessive amount of amorphous urates or phosphates that caused the turbidity seen with the sulfosalicylic acid test.
    B. The urine pH was greater than 8, exceeding the buffering capacity of the reagent strip, thus causing a false-negative reaction.
    C. A protein other than albumin must be present in the urine.
    D. The reading time of the reagent strip test was exceeded (the reading being taken at 2 minutes), causing a false-negative reaction to be detected.

13. Which solute is a major component of a 24-hour urine sample?
    A. Sodium
    B. Mucus
    C. Erythrocytes
    D. Urea

14. Each of the following is included in the quality assurance program for a urinalysis laboratory. Which one represents a preanalytical component of testing?
    A. Setting collection guidelines for 24-hour urines
    B. Setting a maintenance schedule for microscopes
    C. Reporting units to be used for crystals
    D. Requiring acceptable results for control specimens before any patient results are reported out

15. A urine sample arrives in your laboratory from the pediatric unit of your hospital. Routine microscopic urinalysis shows many perfectly shaped six-sided crystals. The first diagnosis you think for this pediatric patient is:
    A. Upper urinary tract infection
    B. Maple syrup urine disease
    C. Cystinuria
    D. Glomerulonephritis

16. Which urinalysis test result is *diagnostic* for glomerulonephritis?
    A. Oval fat bodies
    B. Hyaline casts
    C. Cholesterol crystals
    D. Red blood cell casts

17. A patient whose samples have come to your lab before always have a large concentration of triple phosphate salts in the urine, but today you do not see any triple phosphate crystals microscopically. Which reason could explain this?
    A. You need phase contrast to see this.
    B. The urine pH must be acidic.
    C. You need polarized microscopy to see this.
    D. Concentration of the salt is too high for crystals to form.

18. If a specimen has bacteria in it, what will be the indication that the bacteria were put there at the time of collection rather than from a UTI?
    A. Positive nitrite
    B. Squamous epithelial cells present
    C. Transitional cells present
    D. Renal epithelial cells present

19. Uromodulin protein can be found in urine:
    A. Only from patients with glomerular damage
    B. Mainly from those with urinary tract infection
    C. Without any pathological process happening
    D. Significantly when some patients stand up

20. Which of the following casts represents the **most advanced and pathological** formation?
    A. Hyaline
    B. Granular
    C. Cellular
    D. Waxy

21. Which of the following, in significantly increased numbers, would be a part of the urine microscopy result pattern for a patient who had a catheter inserted into and then removed from his urethra and bladder?
    A. Squamous epithelial cells
    B. Transitional epithelial cells
    C. Renal epithelial cells
    D. Ammonium biurate crystals

22. Which of the following can cause a urine sample to be reddish in color?
    A. Malignant melanoma
    B. Multiple myeloma
    C. Fanconi syndrome
    D. Muscular dystrophy

23. A patient with diabetes mellitus starts taking megadoses of vitamin C for her cold. Her true urine glucose is 250 mg/dL and her urine level of vitamin C is 500 mg/dL. How will the addition of vitamin C change her urinalysis result pattern when the tests are done using reagent strips?
    A. Specific gravity = falsely low
    B. Glucose = falsely low
    C. Protein = falsely high
    D. pH = falsely high

24. The best indicator that the reagent strip is inappropriate to use for testing when you take it out of the bottle is
    A. An obvious odor associated with the strip
    B. A discoloration of any of the pads
    C. The confirmatory test result does not agree with the stix result
    D. Unnecessary since strips are too stable to ever become unsuitable for testing

25. The reagent pad with the longest manual wait time (2 minutes) to read the result is the leukocyte test. Color on this pad that develops only after the 2-minute timer ends should be
    A. Used to determine the final result
    B. Compared to a different color chart than the one on the stix bottle
    C. Repeated with a new reagent strip
    D. Ignored

26. The interference by vitamin C on certain reagent strip test pads is an example of which characteristic of the test method?
    A. Sensitivity
    B. Specificity
    C. Accuracy
    D. Precision

27. A patient's first morning urine albumin is measured as 109 mg/dL, and her creatinine from the same sample is 410 mg/dL. Which value will be reported as her albumin:creatinine ratio?
    A. 0.26 mg/g
    B. 3.76 mg/g
    C. 26.6 mg/g
    D. 266 mg/g

28. If the blood pad on a reagent stix appears "speckled," which of the following may be true?
    A. There are around 5-10 red blood cells/hpf present.
    B. Myoglobin may be present.
    C. Vitamin C is causing a falsely increased result.
    D. White blood cells are interfering with the reaction.

29. A patient's urine sample shows a blood result of "small" on the reagent stix. For which situation could this result happen even when the person is **truly healthy**?
    A. Crash dieting for a weekend event
    B. Going from laying down to standing/walking
    C. Menstruation
    D. Hemorrhoids

30. An infant's urine contains 500 mg/dL galactose and no glucose. Which of the following two test results (glucose pad on the stix and the Clinitest) would be obtained for this patient?
    A. Negative on stix, trace Clinitest
    B. Negative on stix, 500 mg/dL Clinitest
    C. 500 mg/dL on stix, trace Clinitest
    D. 500 mg/dL on stix, 500 mg/dL on Clinitest

31. Which of the following cell types predominate in CSF during a classic case of viral meningitis?
    A. Lymphocytes
    B. Macrophages
    C. Monocytes
    D. Neutrophils

32. The presence of xanthochromia in all three tubes of spinal fluid collected from a patient is highly suggestive of which of the following?
    A. Bloody tap during collection
    B. Hemorrhage in the central nervous system
    C. Presence of bacterial meningitis
    D. Presence of viral meningitis

33. Which tests are the *least* reliable for indicating a patient has a bacterial UTI since they could be found in a *completely healthy* individual?
    A. Alkaline pH, cloudiness = 2+
    B. Positive nitrite, 10–15 WBC clumps/hpf
    C. 25–50 squamous epithelial cells/hpf, moderate bilirubin
    D. Large ketones, 250 mg/dL glucose

34. Why are occult blood tests using anti-hemoglobin unable to detect bleeding happening in the esophagus?
    A. The hemoglobin is degraded by the time of excretion and is not recognized by the antibody.
    B. The K-ras gene will be degraded by bacteria.
    C. The dye used in the test cannot detect intact red blood cells.
    D. Urobilinogen and bilirubin in the intestines will interfere with the test.

35. Which of the following would characterize a serous effusion received in your lab as an *exudate* rather than a *transudate*?
    A. Total protein: 6.5 g/dL
    B. Color: pale yellow
    C. Leukocyte count: 8 cells/μL
    D. Glucose: 70 mg/dL

36. Which of the following correlates with having crenated red blood cells in urine?
    A. Polyuria
    B. Galactosuria
    C. Hyposthenuria
    D. Hypersthenuria
    E. glycosuria

37. A patient's urine shows pH 5.0, many uric acid crystals, 20–50 RBC/hpf. Which disease pattern does this suggest?
    A. Gout
    B. Urinary tract infection
    C. Kidney stones
    D. Leukemia

38. A patient has a negative blood result on the stix but you see over 20 RBC/hpf. Which of the following could be a possible explanation?
    A. Large amounts of ascorbic acid present
    B. Presence of myoglobin in the urine
    C. Diagnosis of hemolytic anemia
    D. Specific gravity = 1.003

39. A patient with painful urination provides a first morning urine specimen (after an 8-hour sleep) for testing. It has been correctly collected as a clean-catch, midstream sample and analyzed within 0.5 hours of collection. While there appears to be a significant number of bacteria microscopically, the nitrite result is negative. Which of the following could be an explanation for these results?
    A. Insufficient incubation time
    B. Bacteria have nitrate reductase.
    C. Patient does not eat green leafy vegetables.
    D. White blood cells are not neutrophils.

40. A routine urinalysis is performed on a young child suffering from diarrhea. The reagent test strip is negative for glucose but positive for ketones. These results may be explained by which of the following statements?
    A. The child has type 1 diabetes mellitus.
    B. The child is suffering from lactic acidosis, and the lactic acid has falsely reacted with the impregnated reagent area for ketones.
    C. The child is suffering from increased catabolism of fat because of decreased intestinal absorption.
    D. The reagent area for ketones was read after the maximum reading time allowed.

41. Which of the following will contribute to a specimen's specific gravity if it is present in a person's urine?
    A. 50–100 RBC/hpf
    B. 85 mg/dL glucose
    C. 3+ amorphous phosphates
    D. Moderate bacteria

42. With infections of the urinary system, white blood cells are frequently seen in the urine sediment. What type of white blood cell is seen the most frequently in urine sediment?
    A. Eosinophil
    B. Lymphocyte
    C. Monocyte
    D. Neutrophil

43. To detect more easily the presence of casts in urine sediments, which microscopic method can be used?
    A. Fluorescent microscopy
    B. Phase-contrast microscopy
    C. Polarized microscopy
    D. Brightfield microscopy

44. Which of the following found in urinary sediment is more easily distinguished by use of polarized microscopy?
    A. Oval fat bodies Lipids
    B. Casts
    C. Red blood cells
    D. Ketone bodies

45. "Glitter cell" is a term used to describe a specific type of:
    A. Ketone body
    B. Oval fat body
    C. Fatty droplet
    D. Neutrophil

46. A 40-year-old female with a history of kidney infection is seen by her physician because she has felt lethargic for a few weeks. She has decreased frequency of urination and a bloated feeling. Physical examination shows periorbital swelling and general edema, including a swollen abdomen. Significant urinalysis results show the following: color = yellow; appearance = cloudy/frothy; specific gravity = 1.022; pH = 7.0; protein = 4+; 0–3 WBC/hpf; 0–1 RBC/hpf; 0–2 renal epithelial cells/hpf; 10–20 hyaline casts/lpf; 0–1 granular casts/lpf; 0–1 fatty casts/lpf; occasional oval fat bodies. Her serum chemistries show significantly decreased albumin, increased urea nitrogen, and increased creatinine. These findings suggest which condition?
    A. Multiple myeloma
    B. Glomerulonephritis
    C. Nephrotic syndrome
    D. Chronic renal failure

47. A 47-year-old female patient with controlled type 2 diabetes mellitus complains of urinary frequency and burning. She provides a first-morning, clean-catch specimen. Results show color = yellow; appearance = cloudy; pH = 6.5; a representative microscopic high-power field is shown in Color Plate 46■. Which of the following is *true* for this patient?
    A. The number of bacteria seen would result in a positive nitrite.
    B. The major formed elements are white blood cells and yeast.
    C. The type and number of epithelial cells suggest incorrect sample collection.
    D. The red blood cells would be sufficient to give a positive blood result on the reagent strip.

48. A 22-year-old female clinical laboratory student performs a urinalysis on her own urine as part of a lab class. Significant results include: color = yellow; appearance = cloudy; pH = 7.5; nitrite = positive; leukocyte esterase = 2+; 25–40 WBC/hpf; 0–3 RBC/hpf; 2–5 squamous epithelial cells/hpf; moderate bacteria. All other chemistries and microscopic results were normal. These findings suggest
    A. Glomerulonephritis
    B. Upper urinary tract infection
    C. Lower urinary tract infection
    D. Nephrolithiasis

49. If a fasting plasma glucose level of 100 mg/dL is obtained on an individual, what is the expected fasting cerebrospinal fluid (CSF) glucose level in mg/dL?
    A. 25
    B. 50
    C. 65
    D. 100

50. A 67-year-old male has routine testing done and shows an estimated glomerular filtration rate (eGFR) of 42 mL/min/1.73 m^2. Which of the following is *true* for this patient?
    A. This test requires a 24-hour urine collection.
    B. The patient does not have chronic kidney damage, based on these results.
    C. The test result is invalid because body surface area was not calculated.
    D. The result is significantly low and should be followed up.

51. Which is *true* about the formed element shown in Color Plate 47■?
    A. May be found in normal alkaline urine
    B. Associated with renal pathology
    C. Characteristic of glomerulonephritis
    D. Associated with lung pathology

52. The major formed element in the high-power field shown in Color Plate 48■ is most likely a:
    A. Granular cast
    B. Hyaline cast
    C. Waxy cast
    D. Fiber artifact

53. The formed element shown in Color Plate 49■ would usually be found in the patient's urine along with which soluble biochemicals?
    A. Phenylalanine and tyrosine
    B. Ornithine and arginine
    C. Isoleucine and leucine
    D. Acetoacetic acid and β-hydroxybutyric acid

54. A 13-year-old ice skater is having her routine physical before the school year. Her first morning urinalysis results include color = straw; appearance = hazy; pH = 6.0; protein = trace; a representative microscopic high-power field is shown in Color Plate 50■. All other chemical results were normal. The major formed elements are ____ and suggest ____.
    A. hyaline casts and waxy casts; nephrotic syndrome
    B. mucus and fibers; no pathology
    C. granular casts and red blood cells; glomerulonephritis
    D. hyaline casts and mucus; normal sediment

55. What condition is suggested by the number of the formed element that predominates in the high-power field of Color Plate 51■?
    A. Glomerulonephritis
    B. Improperly collected specimen
    C. Pyelonephritis
    D. Normal sample

56. Xanthochromia of cerebrospinal fluid (CSF) samples may be due to increased levels of which of the following?
    A. Chloride
    B. Protein
    C. Glucose
    D. Magnesium

57. Which of the following will be characterized by an increased number of the urinary component seen in Color Plate 52■?
    A. Acute glomerulonephritis
    B. Biliary tract obstruction
    C. Contamination from vaginal discharge
    D. Nephrotic syndrome

58. Patients with diabetes insipidus tend to produce urine in ____ volume with ____ specific gravity.
    A. increased; decreased
    B. increased; increased
    C. decreased; decreased
    D. decreased; increased

59. Which of the following characteristics is *true* of the primary urinary components shown in Color Plate 53■?
    A. Consist of uromodulin protein
    B. Presence always indicates a disease process
    C. Can be observed with polarized microscopy
    D. Appear yellowish in brightfield microscopy

60. A characteristic of substances normally found dissolved in the urine is that they are all:
    A. Water soluble
    B. Inorganic
    C. Organic
    D. Waste products

61. Which of the following characteristics is *true* for the urinary components shown in Color Plate 54■?
    A. Never should appear in a freshly collected sample
    B. Can also resemble cysteine crystals
    C. Appear insoluble in alkaline urine
    D. Presence indicates an inborn error of metabolism

62. A patient sends the following question to an online consumer health Web site: "I am a 22-year-old female who experienced increasing headaches, thirst, and decreasing energy. I was studying in the library when I felt lightheaded and passed out. I was taken to a hospital emergency department and they told me that my serum Acetest® was 40 mg/dL and urine glucose was 500 mg/dL. What does this mean?" How would you reply?
    A. Your lab results pattern suggests diabetes mellitus.
    B. You probably have been crash dieting recently.
    C. The two results do not fit any disease pattern.
    D. The tests need to be repeated because they could not possibly occur together.

63. Which urinalysis reagent strip test will never be reported out as "negative"?
    A. Protein
    B. Urobilinogen
    C. Bilirubin
    D. Nitrite

64. The following urinalysis results were obtained on a 40-year-old Caucasian male whose skin appeared yellowish during the clinical examination. Color and clarity—dark brown, clear; protein—negative; glucose—negative; blood—negative; ketones—negative; bilirubin— moderate; urobilinogen—0.2 mg/dL. These results are clinically significant in which of the following conditions?
    A. Bile duct obstruction
    B. Cirrhosis
    C. Hepatitis
    D. Hemolytic anemia

65. Which condition is characterized by increased levels of immunoglobulins in the cerebrospinal fluid, originating from within the central nervous system and not from the general blood circulation?
    A. Gout
    B. Erythroblastosis fetalis
    C. Multiple myeloma
    D. Multiple sclerosis

66. Which of the following statements pertains to screening methods used to determine pregnancy?
    A. Immunoassays will use reagent anti-hCG to react with patient hCG.
    B. A random urine specimen is the preferred specimen for pregnancy screening tests.
    C. Internal controls provided within the kit will assess if the patient's specimen was collected correctly.
    D. External quality control is not needed with these methods.

67. Which of the following is a *true* statement?
    A. Renal tubular cells originate from the renal pelvis.
    B. Red blood cells in acid urine (pH 4.5) will usually be crenated because of the acidity.
    C. Bacteria introduced into a urine specimen at the time of the collection will have no immediate effect on the level of nitrite in the specimen.
    D. Pilocarpine iontophoresis is the method of choice for the collection of pericardial fluid.

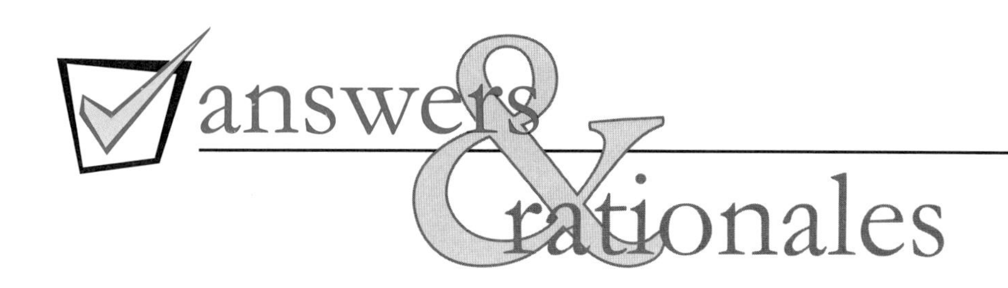

1.

D. The first-voided morning urine specimen is the most desirable for chemical and microscopic analysis because it is the most concentrated specimen of the day. Protein and nitrite testing is better performed on a concentrated specimen, as are the specific gravity determination and the examination of urinary sediment. However, because of the lack of food and fluid intake during the night, glucose metabolism may be better assessed on the basis of a postprandial specimen.

2.

A. Bilirubin is a pigmented waste product of heme metabolism. Its presence in urine will darken the yellow color to shades of amber, based on its concentration.

3.

C. Homogentisic acid, an intermediate in the metabolism of tyrosine, will increase in urine from patients with alkaptonuria, and impart a brown/black color if the urine becomes alkaline. Melanin needs to be exposed to air and oxidized for such a color change to happen.

4.

D. pH is a representative symbol for the hydrogen ion concentration. The kidney plays an important role in the maintenance of the acid-base balance of body fluids by either excreting or retaining hydrogen ions. A normally functioning kidney will excrete urine with a pH between 4.5 and 8.0, depending on the overall acid-base needs of the body.

5.

B. At room temperature, the amount of bacteria present in a urine sample will increase. The bacteria are capable of metabolizing the urinary urea to ammonia. The ammonia formed through this process will cause an alkalinization of the urine.

6.

D. On the average, a normal adult excretes 1200–1500 mL of urine daily. "Polyuria" is a term used to describe the excretion of a urine volume in excess of 2000 mL/day. In oliguria, the daily urine excretion is less than 500 mL, and in anuria the urine formation is completely suppressed. Hypersthenuria refers to urines of any volume containing increased levels of dissolved solute.

7.

A. In healthy individuals, the amount of protein excreted in the urine should not exceed 150 mg/24 hr. When protein is present in the urine, the colorimetric reagent test strips change color, indicating a semiquantification of the amount of protein present. Serum proteins are classified as being albumin or globulin in nature, and the type of protein excreted in the urine is dependent on the disorder present. Although the strip test is a rapid screening method for the detection of urinary protein, it must be noted that this method is more sensitive to the presence of albumin in the specimen than to the presence of globulin, Bence Jones protein, or mucoprotein.

8.

A. Normal urine does not foam on being shaken. If urine contains bilirubin, it will exhibit yellow foaming when the specimen is shaken. In fact, the foam test was actually the first test for bilirubin, before the development of the chemical tests. However, the shaken specimen shows a white foam when increased urine protein is present.

9.

C. For quality control of reagent test strips, it is recommended that both positive and negative controls be used daily. It is necessary that any deterioration of the strips be detected in order to avoid false-positive or false-negative results. The use of positive and negative controls will act as a check on the reagents, on the technique employed, and on the interpretive ability of the person or instrument performing the test.

10.

D. The principle of the reagent strip method for the detection of protein in urine is based on a color change in an indicator system, such as tetrabromophenol blue, that is buffered to pH 3. The buffering capacity of the strip is sufficient provided that the urine pH does not exceed 8.0. Within the normal urine pH range of 4.5–8.0, a change in color in the reagent strip is an indication of the presence of protein in the urine. With a urine pH greater than 8, the buffering capacity of the strip may be exceeded, and a false-positive color change in the impregnated area will reflect the pH of the urine rather than the presence of protein. The presence of vitamin C, uric acid, or glucose in urine will not affect the test for protein.

11.

D. "Isosthenuria" is a term applied to a series of urine specimens that exhibit a fixed specific gravity of approximately 1.010. In isosthenuria, there is little, if any, variation of the specific gravity between urine specimens from the same patient. This condition is abnormal and denotes the presence of severe renal damage in which both the diluting ability and the concentrating ability of the kidneys have been severely affected.

12.

C. When globulin, mucoprotein, or Bence Jones protein is present in a urine specimen, the reagent strip test may give a negative result because the strip is more sensitive to the presence of albumin than to the presence of other proteins in urine. However, the sulfosalicylic acid (SSA) test is able to detect not only albumin but also globulin, mucoprotein, and Bence Jones protein in a specimen. Therefore, it can be seen that a negative reagent strip test result for protein but a positive sulfosalicylic acid test result is possible when the protein present is some protein other than albumin. For this reason, the sulfosalicylic acid test is run as a test for urinary protein if the presence of abnormal proteins is suspected.

13.

D. Although sodium is the major inorganic molecule found in urine, urea is the major organic molecule excreted. Urea is a waste product of protein/amino acid metabolism. Its level in a normal 24-hour urine with a glomerular filtration rate of 125 mL/min would be 400 mmol/day. Glucose excretion will average less than 1 mmol/day. The excretion of the inorganic molecules sodium and potassium would be 130 and 70 mmol/day, respectively.

14.

A. Preanalytical components of laboratory testing include all variables that can affect the integrity or acceptability of the patient specimen prior to analysis, such as correct collection technique. Analytical factors affect the actual analysis of the specimen (temperature, condition of equipment, timing, and presence of interfering substances). Postanalytical factors affect the final handling of the results generated (reporting units, critical values, and acceptability of quality control).

15.

C. Six-sided crystals from a pediatric patient suggests cysteine is present. If observed for the first time, it requires immediate confirmation and notification of the clinician. Since uric acid can resemble cysteine, positive confirmation includes formation of a purple color with the addition of nitroprusside.

16.

D. While patients with glomerulonephritis may exhibit oval fat bodies and hyaline casts in their urine, increased numbers of red blood cells and RBC casts would be most diagnostic. Cholesterol would suggest nephrotic syndrome. Although a positive result on a urine test for ketones is most commonly associated with increased urinary glucose levels, as in diabetes mellitus, other conditions may cause the urine ketone test to show positive results while the urine glucose test shows negative results. In young children, a negative glucose reaction accompanied by a positive ketone reaction is sometimes seen. Ketones in the urine may be seen when a child is suffering from an acute febrile disease or toxic condition that is accompanied by vomiting or diarrhea. In these cases, because of either decreased food intake or decreased intestinal absorption, fat catabolism is increased to such an extent that the intermediary products, known as ketone bodies, are formed and excreted in the urine.

17.

B. Triple phosphate is insoluble in alkaline conditions, becoming easily visible as "coffin-lid" classical shapes in regular light microscopy. The salt will dissolve in acid pH. As with all salts which form crystals, the solute concentration must be high enough to favor crystal formation.

18.

B. If a urine sample is not collected using the midstream clean-catch method, there is a greater possibility of urethral squamous epithelial cells and contaminating bacteria being added to the urine. Transitional and renal cells are from the bladder and kidney, respectively, and would not be present as a result of poor collection technique. Conversion of nitrate to nitrite needs >100,000 bacteria per mL and 4 hours of incubation, neither of which would be conditions present with bacteria introduced at the time of collection.

19.

C. Uromodulin (formerly called Tamm-Horsfall protein) is made by the renal tubular cells and is a normal component of urine. In some patients, urine albumin concentration will increase upon standing due to changes in renal venous pressure and glomerular filtration. It is considered benign functional proteinuria (postural proteinuria).

20.

D. Evolution of cast formation begins with (1) hyaline casts, which can pick up cells during their formation to become (2) cellular casts. With decreased urine flow, the cells will degenerate to form granules, becoming (3) granular casts), which at lowest urine flow rate will degenerate further into (4) waxy casts. These are associated with renal failure.

21.

B. Transitional epithelial cells line the urethra and bladder, so any surface rubbing against those linings may result in sloughing of these cells. Squamous cells would come from the lower urethra and external meatus, while renal cells would originate from the kidney. Ammonium biurate crystals are most often found in urines after prolonged storage.

22.

D. The muscle atrophy in muscular dystrophy may result in the release of myoglobin, which will be filtered into the urine and give a reddish color. Melanin from malignant melanoma will oxidize and cause urine to turn brown/black if exposed to air. Neither multiple myeloma not Fanconi syndrome result in urine color changes.

23.

B. Vitamin C will negatively affect any reaction involving peroxidase. Only glucose, blood, and creatinine reagent strip tests will be affected. Vitamin C will positively affect the Clinitest since it is a reducing substance, similar to glucose and galactose.

24.

B. Even with a desiccator present in the bottle of reagent strips, moisture from repeatedly opening the bottle may still affect the pads, causing them to deteriorate. The first pads on which such subsequent discoloration will be seen are the nitrite and leukocyte pads.

25.

D. Each reagent strip test has a colorimetric reaction whose result should be considered "end-point" rather than "kinetic." Any color development after the end-point time is reached should be ignored.

26.

B. Specificity describes whether the reaction measures what it is meant to measure. Sensitivity is the smallest analyte concentration that can be distinguished from zero. A method is accurate if the result obtained matches the actual concentration in the sample (and in the patient), while precision occurs when repeated measurements of the sample yield the same result.

27.

D. The results are reported as "milligrams of albumin per gram of creatinine." Since 1000 mg = 1 g, this can be calculated by setting up a ratio-and-proportion as follows: UACR (mg/g) = U Albumin (mg/dL)/U Creatinine (g/dL); therefore,

UACR (mg/g) = 109 mg/dL/.41 g/dL
UACR = 266 mg/g

(NOTE: 410 mg/dL of creatinine = .41 g/dL of creatinine).

28.

A. The blood test is based on hemoglobin's peroxidase-like activity on the pad. This means the red blood cells must lyse on contact with the pad. When the number of RBCs is low, it is possible to see the actual localized reaction of the RBC's hemoglobin and the pad reagents, giving a speckled appearance. When the RBCs are higher in number, it is no longer possible to visibly distinguish among the individual RBCs lysing on the pad, giving a homogenous color change on the pad. Since myoglobin is soluble, its presence will always give a homogeneous appearance. If vitamin C is present, it will cause negative interference. The method is not affected by white blood cell presence.

29.

C. Menstruation is a healthy process which can place red blood cells into a woman's urine. Hemorrhoids are never "healthy." Crash dieting may increase urine ketones, while some healthy patients may experience increased albumin in urine as benign postural proteinuria.

30.

B. Galactose is a reducing sugar which can negatively interfere with the glucose reagent stix reaction and give a positive result with Clinitest. Since there is no glucose present, only the Clinitest result will be positive.

31.

A. Viral meningitis will be characterized by increased numbers of lymphocytes. If this were bacterial meningitis, neutrophils would predominate. Monocytes (macrophages) will be present in either case.

32.

B. Xanthochromia is a pink/orange/yellow coloration of CSF if either hemoglobin, bilirubin, or protein (>100 mg/dL) are present. If present in all three tubes, xanthochromia suggests that they have been present in the original CSF itself and not from a bloody tap. Meningitis would be characterized by a cloudiness from increased white blood cell numbers.

33.

A. Both alkaline pH and increased cloudiness may result from diet and the presence of amorphous material or crystals. All of the other choices suggest either inappropriate collection (squamous) or pathology (B = urinary tract infection, C = obstructive jaundice, D = diabetic ketoacidosis).

34.

A Use of anti-hemoglobin relies on finding intact hemoglobin as a sign of the presence of fecal occult blood. Hemoglobin released from the esophagus will have been digested to amino acids by the time it arrives in a fecal sample, leaving nothing to bind with the reagent antibody.

35.

A. Characteristics of an exudate include total protein >3 g/dL, cell counts >1000 cells/microliter, specific gravity >1.015, and a cloudy appearance from the increased cell count.

36.

D. Crenation of red blood cells will occur when the urine sample is hypertonic, making the cytoplasmic water leave the cell. This condition is associated with high specific gravity which is hypersthenuria. In low specific gravity conditions (hyposthenuria), red blood cells will lyse due to movement of water into the cells.

37.

C. An acidic urine with increased uric acid crystals may suggest gout, but this condition does not usually place red blood cells into the specimen. If, however, those crystals are forming aggregates (stones) within the renal tract, this could lead to bleeding.

38.

A. Choices B, C, and D could all result in a positive blood reaction on the pad and no red blood cells seen microscopically. Only ascorbic acid will negatively interfere with the peroxidase reaction on the blood pad, giving a false-negative result.

39.

C. The reaction of nitrate to nitrite requires four conditions to be present at the same time: (1) sufficient nitrate in the urine, usually through a diet of green leafy vegetables, (2) at least 100,000 bacteria per milliliter, (3) bacteria with nitrate reductase, and (4) at least 4 hours of incubation. The only condition not met in this case is that the diet does not provide the source of the required urine nitrate to be used as the substrate.

40.

C. Although a positive result on a urine test for ketones is most commonly associated with increased urinary glucose levels, as in diabetes mellitus, other conditions may cause the urine ketone test to show positive results while the urine glucose test shows negative results. In young children, a negative glucose reaction accompanied by a positive ketone reaction is sometimes seen. Ketones in the urine may be seen when a child is suffering from an acute febrile disease or toxic condition that is accompanied by vomiting or diarrhea. In these cases, because of either decreased food intake or decreased intestinal absorption, fat catabolism is increased to such an extent that the intermediary products, known as ketone bodies, are formed and excreted in the urine.

41.

B. Only dissolved solutes affect specific gravity (e.g., glucose). Cells, mucus, crystals, or any other formed elements will have no effect, regardless of concentration. If the reagent strip method is used, it should be noted that only dissolved ions will contribute to specific gravity results. Thus, glucose would not affect reagent strip results at any concentration. In such instances as diabetes mellitus, with urine glucose levels over 2 g/dL, there may be a discrepancy between specific gravity results obtained with a reagent strip method versus using a refractometer, because such glucose levels are known to increase refractometer results, thus requiring correction. It should also be noted, however, that glucose will not be detected by the reagent strip pad which only detects ions.

42.

D. The majority of renal and urinary tract diseases are characterized by an increased number of neutrophilic leukocytes in the urine. To identify correctly any white blood cells present in a urine specimen, it is necessary to examine the specimen as soon as possible after collection. This is necessary because leukocytes tend to lyse easily when exposed to either hypotonic or alkaline urine.

43.

B. To better diagnose renal and urinary tract diseases, it is necessary to examine urinary sediment carefully by the most appropriate microscopic method available. Formed elements in the urine, such as cells and casts, are more easily differentiated by the use of phase-contrast microscopy. This is especially true for the identification of the more translucent elements such as the hyaline casts. Phase microscopy tends to enhance the outline of the formed elements, allowing them to stand out and be more easily distinguished.

44.

A. Fatty materials in urinary sediment may be identified by means of staining techniques using Sudan III and oil red O or by means of polarized microscopy. Polarized microscopy is especially useful when the composition of fatty casts, fatty droplets, or oval fat bodies is primarily cholesterol. When cholesterol molecules are exposed to polarized microscopy, the effect is such that a Maltese cross formation becomes visible, simplifying the identification process. Casts and red blood cells may be better visualized using phase-contrast microscopy. Ketone bodies will be soluble and, therefore, not seen in a urine sediment.

45.

D. When neutrophils are exposed to hypotonic urine, their physical appearance becomes altered. Under hypotonic conditions, the neutrophils tend to swell and the cytoplasmic granules contained within the cells exhibit Brownian movement. This Brownian movement of the granules causes the neutrophilic contents to refract in such a way that the cells appear to glitter—thus the name "glitter cells."

46.

C. Nephrotic syndrome is suggested by the increased urine protein (with serum albumin significantly decreased), the hyaline and fatty casts, and the presence of oval fat bodies. The patient's symptoms of periorbital swelling and edema reflect the loss of oncotic pressure because of the excretion of albumin. Its loss from the vascular compartment will induce plasma water movement into the tissue spaces. Glomerulonephritis will have many more red blood cells, including red blood cell casts. Multiple myeloma will not show increased urine albumin but rather immunoglobulin light chains. Chronic renal failure will have multiple types of casts present (hyaline, granular, cellular, waxy, and fatty).

47.

B. There are minimal bacteria present in Color Plate 46■. Both budding yeast and white blood cells predominate this microscopic field. Patients with diabetes mellitus are prone to such yeast infections because of the increased glucose in their urine. The epithelial cells visualized in this field are transitional and not squamous. They can be distinguished by their size (about 15–20 μm), less cytoplasm than a squamous cell would have, and their central nucleus. Increased squamous epithelial cells would suggest improper collection, whereas transitional cells, if greater than five cells/hpf, would indicate pathology. There are fewer than five red blood cells in this field, and that would be below the sensitivity of the blood pad on the reagent strip.

48.

C. This student has a lower urinary tract infection (UTI), also known as cystitis. The major distinguishing features between upper and lower UTI include the presence of protein and casts in an upper UTI and not in a lower UTI. This is because both urine protein excretion and cast formation reflect what is happening within the kidney itself. The most common source of either upper or lower UTIs is contamination by enteric gram-negative bacteria. Their presence will not be found in glomerulonephritis or with urinary stones (nephro= "kidney"+ lith = "stone").

49.

C. Cerebrospinal fluid (CSF) is a clear, colorless liquid that may be described as a modified ultrafiltrate of blood. Both active transport and passive diffusion are involved in the passage of glucose from the blood into the CSF. Normally, fasting CSF glucose levels range between 50 and 80 mg/dL, representing approximately 60–70% of the blood glucose level. In hyperglycemia with plasma glucose levels of 300 mg/dL, the active transport mechanism reaches a point of maximum response, so that CSF glucose levels reflect approximately 30% of the plasma glucose level. Decreased CSF glucose levels are associated with hypoglycemia, a faulty active transport mechanism, and excess utilization of glucose by microorganisms, red or white blood cells, or the central nervous system.

50.

D. eGFR calculation is based on the "CKD-EPI Creatinine Equation (2009)" formula recommended by the American Kidney Foundation. It does not use a urine sample at all, but instead requires only a serum creatinine or serum Cystatin C and the patient's age, gender, and ethnicity. Values less than 60 mL/min/1.73 m^2 are considered abnormal and need to be followed up. This patient's value places him in stage 3 kidney damage (35–59 mL/min/1.73 m^2).

51.

A. Normal alkaline (or neutral) urine may contain triple phosphate crystals, as seen in Color Plate 47■. These crystals can be identified by the characteristic "coffin lid" appearance. They usually do not indicate any pathology.

52.

D. Refer to Color Plate 48■. The fringed appearance at the one end of the major formed element strongly suggests that this is a fiber artifact, most likely placed in the sample at the time of collection. Casts, taking the shape of the tubule within which they are formed, will not have such a fringed end.

53.

B. The presence of cystine crystals in a patient sample is always a cause for immediate notification of the physician. Cystinuria is an autosomal recessive disorder characterized by the inability to reabsorb the amino acids cystine, lysine, arginine, and ornithine in either the renal tubules or the intestine. Cystine will crystallize in acid pH more readily than the other amino acids. Tyrosine forms needle-shaped crystals whereas leucine will appear round and oily with concentric rings. Isoleucine and phenylalanine will not form crystals in the urine. Acetoacetate and β-hydroxybutyric acid are two ketone bodies that will be soluble in the sample and give a positive reaction with nitroprusside.

54.

D. The major formed elements in Color Plate 50 ■ are hyaline casts and mucus fibers, which are normal in the numbers shown in this field. Waxy casts will appear yellowish with characteristic serrated edges. There are no obvious granules in the casts shown, and red blood cells are not present.

55.

D. Color Plate 51■ demonstrates sperm and calcium oxalate crystals. Both formed elements are found in correctly collected normal urines from either gender. Calcium oxalate seen here is the dehydrate form. The monohydrate form will appear oval or dumbbell shaped. Neither formed element is usually associated with pathology.

56.

B. Xanthrochromia literally means "yellow color." It is a term used exclusively with cerebrospinal fluid, which is normally colorless. Yellowish color is most frequently associated with erythrocyte hemolysis from a subarachnoid hemorrhage and is therefore used to discriminate this from a traumatic tap. Other causes for xanthochromia are systemic jaundice and conditions associated with increased CSF protein.

57.

A. Refer to Color Plate 52■. Erythrocytes or red blood cells (RBCs) occur in small numbers (0–2/hpf) in a normal urine. Using brightfield microscopy, unstained RBCs appear as colorless discs with an average size of 7 μm in diameter. Increased or large numbers of RBCs are commonly seen with acute glomerulonephritis, renal calculi, acute infections, and menstrual contamination. The nephrotic syndrome is characterized by heavy proteinuria, oval fat bodies, renal tubular epithelial cells, casts, and waxy and fatty casts. Biliary tract obstruction will show pale-colored stools, whereas vaginal discharge contamination may introduce increased numbers of white blood cells.

58.

A. Diabetes insipidus is caused by a deficiency in antidiuretic hormone. Such deficiencies will result in the kidney's inability to reabsorb water at the distal and collecting tubules. This affects only water reabsorption and not the reabsorption of other urinary solutes. Excreted solute amounts will be the same, but the water volume into which they are excreted will be larger. This results in high urine volumes and low final solute concentrations. The low solute will lead to low specific gravities in these patients' specimens.

59.

A. As seen in Color Plate 53■, hyaline casts are the most commonly observed cast, and they consist completely of uromodulin (Tamm-Horsfall) protein. A reference urine may contain 0–2 hyaline casts per low-power field. Hyaline casts appear translucent using brightfield microscopy because they have a refractive index similar to urine. Phase-contrast microscopy may be used to visualize the casts better.

60.

A. To be found in urine, a solute must be water soluble. Solutes can be inorganic (e.g., sodium) or organic (e.g., urea). Excreted waste products, meaning end products of metabolism, are creatinine, urea, and uric acid. Some excreted solutes, however, are not present as waste but as overload, such as glucose or sodium.

61.

B. Uric acid crystals, as seen in Color Plate 54■, are commonly encountered in normal acidic urine but may be observed in neutral urine and rarely in an alkaline urine, because uric acid is soluble at alkaline pH. Using brightfield microscopy, uric acid crystals appear as diamonds, cubes, barrels, rosettes, and may even have six sides and be confused with cysteine. Because they are a reflection of the excretion of purine waste products, they may be pathologically increased in cases of gout and after chemotherapy. They show birefringence (multiple colors) under plane polarized light.

62.

A. A positive urine glucose plus a positive serum ketone strongly suggest uncontrolled diabetes mellitus. There is an increased rate of fatty acid oxidation occurring in light of the inaccessibility of the glucose, especially to skeletal muscle. If the patient had only been dieting, the glucose would be negative.

63.

B. The sensitivity of a method is the lowest concentration of the analyte that will result in a detectable reaction signal. The protein, bilirubin, and nitrite readout color scales each has a color associated with analyte concentrations less than the method's sensitivity, called "negative." Urobilinogen's readout color scale begins with its lowest reportable value, but there is no pad associated with concentrations less than this.

64.

A. In the hepatic phase of bilirubin metabolism, bilirubin is conjugated with glucuronic acid to form water-soluble conjugated bilirubin. The conjugated bilirubin passes into the bile duct and on to the intestinal tract. In the intestine, it is reduced by intestinal bacteria to form urobilinogen. Bile duct obstruction is characterized by an obstruction of the flow of conjugated bilirubin into the intestinal tract to complete its metabolism. The conjugated bilirubin, which is water soluble, will be excreted by the kidney. Because bilirubin is not entering the intestines, the normal production of urobilinogen is decreased. Therefore, the urine biochemical test will indicate a positive reagent strip test for bilirubin, positive Ictotest, and "normal" (0.2 mg/dL) urobilinogen (because there is no reagent strip pad for "negative" urobilinogen).

65.

D. In multiple sclerosis, the immune system attacks the myelin sheath surrounding nerves. The antibodies causing this destruction have a unique pattern on electrophoresis, called "oligoclonal banding," which can be useful in confirming the diagnosis. In contrast, the antibodies produced in excess in multiple myeloma come from clone(s) of cancerous plasma cells and will be found in the plasma and urine.

66.

A. Many simplified yet immunologically sophisticated methods exist currently for determining pregnancy. All are based on the reaction between patient human chorionic gonadotropin (hCG) and anti-hCG. Most kits will use an antibody recognizing one subunit of hCG (alpha or beta), whereas other kits may use both anti-α-hCG and anti-β-hCG. Internal controls in these kits will only check if the procedural steps were performed correctly. They cannot detect problems with any preanalytical variables, like specimen handling or appropriateness. In addition, internal quality control cannot be used to assess the kit's accuracy in distinguishing "positive" from "negative" specimens. Only the use of external quality control specimens can accomplish this. Because the first morning specimen is the most concentrated of the day, it is the preferred specimen for such screenings. Use of a random urine may be too dilute to detect low levels of patient hCG, thus giving a false negative.

67.

C. Renal tubular cells originate from the renal medulla or cortex. Red blood cell crenation is a phenomenon reflecting increased solute concentration (hyperosmolality) and is not caused by urine pH. Red cells will, however, lyse at high alkaline pH. The nitrite reaction requires (a) a sufficient dietary source of nitrate, (b) sufficient numbers of bacteria present in the urine, and (c) sufficient incubation time (>4 hours). Bacteria introduced at collection, even in sufficient number, will not have had sufficient incubation time to convert urine nitrate to nitrite. Pilocarpine iontophoresis is the collection method for sweat.

REFERENCES

Beers, M. H. (Ed.) (2006). *The Merck Manual of Diagnosis and Therapy*, 18th ed. Whitehouse Station, NJ: Merck Research Laboratories.

Brunzel, N. A. (2018). *Fundamentals of Urine and Body Fluid Analysis*, 4th ed. St. Louis MO: Elsevier, Inc.

McPherson, R. A., and Pincus, M. R. (2007). *Henry's Clinical Diagnosis and Management by Laboratory Methods*, 21st ed. Philadelphia: Elsevier.

Mundt, L., and Shanahan, K. (2016). *Graff's Textbook of Urinalysis and Body Fluids*, 3rd ed. Philadelphia: Wolters Kluwer.

Strasinger, S. K., and DiLorenzo, M. S. (2014). *Urinalysis and Body Fluids*, 6th ed. Philadelphia: F. A. Davis Co.

CHAPTER

12 Laboratory Calculations

contents

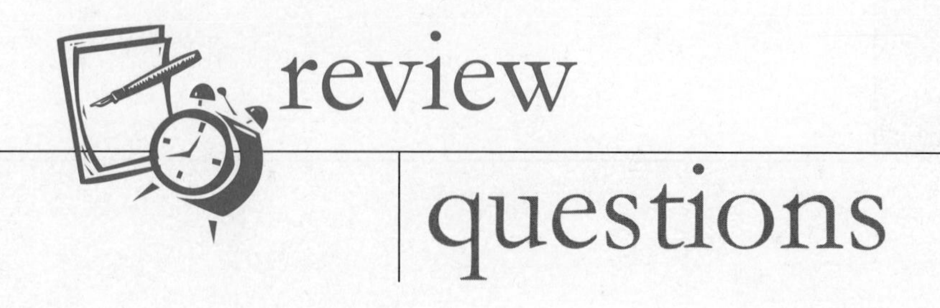

INSTRUCTIONS Each of the questions or incomplete statements that follows is comprised of four suggested responses. Select the *best* answer or completion statement in each case.[1]

1. What is the molarity of a solution that contains 18.7 g of KCl in 500 mL (MW 74.5)?
   A. 0.1
   B. 0.5
   C. 1.0
   D. 5.0
2. A calcium standard solution contains 10 mg/dL of calcium. What is its concentration in millimoles per liter? (MW 40)
   A. 2.5 mmol/L
   B. 5.0 mmol/L
   C. 7.5 mmol/L
   D. 10.0 mmol/L
3. How much solid stock NaCl is needed to prepare 100 mL of a standard solution of concentration 135 mmol/L of Na? (MW sodium 23, NaCl 58.5)
   A. 0.31 g
   B. 0.79 g
   C. 1.2 g
   D. 1.8 g
4. How much 95% v/v alcohol is required to prepare 5 L of 70% v/v alcohol?
   A. 2.4 L
   B. 3.5 L
   C. 3.7 L
   D. 4.4 L
5. You need 80 mL of 2.5% w/v ferric sulfate, and you have solid anhydrous salt to make the solution. How much solid salt is needed? (MW 152)
   A. 0.100
   B. 0.112
   C. 0.113
   D. 1.125

[1]Note: A periodic table of the elements is located on p. 967.

6. You need 80 mL of 2.5% w/v ferric sulfate, and you have a stock bottle labeled "40% w/v ferric sulfate" on your reagent shelf. How much stock is needed to make the desired solution? (MW 152)
   A. 5.0
   B. 9.20
   C. 27.5
   D. 54.4
7. You need 80 mL of 2.5% w/v ferric sulfate, and you have a stock bottle labeled "ferric sulfate trihydrate" on your reagent shelf. How much solid stock is needed to make the desired solution? (MW anhydrous 399.9)
   A. 0.03 g
   B. 1.79 g
   C. 2.24 g
   D. 224 g
8. What is the osmolality of a solution containing 5.85 g NaCl and 18 g glucose in 1 kg water? (MW NaCl 58.5, glucose 180)
   A. 0.2
   B. 0.3
   C. 0.6
   D. 0.9
9. Physiologic saline solution is 0.85% w/v NaCl. What is its osmolarity in osmol/L? (MW 58.5)
   A. 0.15
   B. 0.29
   C. 0.85
   D. 8.5
10. Needed: 400 mL of 100 mEq/L $Zn_3(PO4)_2$ using 10 mol/L stock solution. How much stock is required? (MW 358)
    A. 0.7 mL
    B. 4.0 mL
    C. 667 mL
    D. 4000 mL
11. A 5 N solution is diluted 1:4. The resulting solution is diluted 4:15. What is the concentration in normality of the final solution?
    A. 0.25
    B. 0.33
    C. 2.5
    D. 3.0
12. A colorimetric method calls for the use of 0.1 mL of serum, 5 mL of reagent, and 4.9 mL of water. What is the dilution of the serum in the final solution?
    A. 1 to 5
    B. 1 to 10
    C. 1 to 50
    D. 1 to 100
13. Needed: make 250 mL of 200 mmol/L sodium standard using 6 mol/L Na_2CO_3. How much stock is needed?
    A. 0.42 mL
    B. 4.2 mL
    C. 13.3 mL
    D. 667 mL
14. You need 500 mL of a lithium standard containing 10 mmol/L Li^{+1}. How much solid Li_2SO_4, in grams, should be weighed out to make this solution? (MW salt 110, Li 7)
    A. 0.005 g salt
    B. 0.01 g salt
    C. 0.275 g salt
    D. 0.55 g salt
15. A stock standard solution contains 10 mg/mL of urea nitrogen. How much stock (in milliliters) is needed to prepare 200 mL of a working standard containing 20 mg/dL of urea nitrogen?
    A. 1
    B. 2
    C. 4
    D. 8

16. How many milliliters of a 50% v/v acetic acid solution are required to prepare 1 L of 5% v/v acetic acid?
A. 0.01
B. 0.10
C. 10
D. 100

17. How many grams of sulfosalicylic acid (mol wt = 254) are required to prepare 1 L of a 3% w/v solution?
A. 3.0
B. 7.6
C. 30
D. 254

18. A quantitative protein analysis is performed on an aliquot of a 24-hour urine specimen. The test indicates the presence of 120 mg/dL protein. If a total urine volume of 2.155 L is collected, how many grams of protein are excreted in the 24-hour specimen?
A. 0.056
B. 2.6
C. 25.9
D. 258.6

19. Prepare one deciliter of a nitrate ion standard containing 900 mg/dL nitrate ion using a stock solution containing 10 mol/L $Ca(NO_3)_2$. (MW salt 164, nitrate 62)
A. 0.73 mL stock
B. 7.3 mL stock
C. 13.7 mL stock
D. 137 mL stock

20. How many grams of NaOH are required to prepare 4 L of a 2 Eq/L solution?
A. 40
B. 80
C. 160
D. 320

21. How many milliliters of glacial acetic acid (mol wt = 60; assay = 99.7% w/w) are required to prepare 2 L of a 5% v/v solution?
A. 6
B. 10
C. 50
D. 100

22. Prepare 2 liters of 60 mEq/L H_3PO_4 using concentrated acid (70% w/w purity, 1.64 g/mL, 98 MW).
A. 1.7 mL stock acid
B. 2.4 mL stock acid
C. 3.4 mL stock acid
D. 5.6 mL stock acid

23. Prepare 4.5 liters of 270 mmol/L glacial acetic acid using concentrated acid (67% purity, 1.82 g/mL, 60 MW).
A. 13 mL stock acid
B. 40 mL stock acid
C. 60 mL stock acid
D. 109 mL stock acid

24. An isotonic saline solution contains 0.85% w/v NaCl. How many grams of NaCl are needed to prepare 5 L of this solution? (MW 58.5)
A. 4.25
B. 8.5
C. 42.5
D. 170

25. You have 10 μL of patient spinal fluid. You need to make a 1:5 dilution. What is the maximum total volume which can be made?
A. 0.5 μL
B. 2 μL
C. 5 μL
D. 50 μL

26. How much serum is needed to prepare 50 mL of 1:20 dilution of the sample?
A. 0.4 mL
B. 2.5 mL
C. 5.0 mL
D. 10.0 mL

27. A serum chloride concentration is 369 mg/dL. What is the concentration in millimoles per liter? (MW chloride 35.5)
    A. 5
    B. 10
    C. 36
    D. 104

28. A serum calcium level is 8.6 mg/dL. What is the concentration in millimoles per liter? (MW 40)
    A. 2.2
    B. 2.5
    C. 4.3
    D. 8.6

29. A sample diluted 1:3 gives a total protein result of 4.9g/dL. What is the total protein concentration in the **original** specimen?
    A. 1.6 g/dL
    B. 5.3 g/dL
    C. 14.7 g/dL
    D. 22. g/dL

30. What dilution of a stock standard which contains 46 g of sodium per liter is needed to prepare a working standard whose concentration must be 200 mmol of sodium per liter? Na = 23 MW
    A. 1:10
    B. 1:20
    C. 1:100
    D. 1:200

31. How many moles per liter of nitrate ions (MW 62) are present in a solution containing 96 mol/L calcium nitrate (MW 164)?
    A. 49 mmol/L
    B. 192 mmol/L
    C. 215 mmol/L
    D. 254 mmol/L

32. How many milliliters of a stock solution of 20% w/v NaOH are required to prepare 800 mL of a 2.5% w/v solution?
    A. 20
    B. 50
    C. 100
    D. 125

33. You need 2.6 liters of 0.33 mol/L potassium bicarbonate (MW 100). You only have hydrated solid salt $KHCO_3*3H_2O$ (MW 154) available. How much hydrated salt needs to be weighed out to make this solution?
    A. 33 g
    B. 51 g
    C. 86 g
    D. 132 g

34. How many grams of sodium sulfate (mol wt = 142) are required to prepare 750 mL of a 23% w/v solution?
    A. 17.25 g
    B. 172.5 g
    C. 1725 g
    D. 17250 g

35. You need 5.0 mL of 40% v/v ethanol (MW 47). What amount of stock 75% v/v ethanol is needed?
    A. 1.3 mL
    B. 2.7 mL
    C. 4.8 mL
    D. 9.4 mL

36. You need 350 mL of a solution containing 200 mmol/L sodium ions. Your available stock contains 10 mol/L sodium sulfate. How much stock is needed to make this solution? MW of sodium is 23; MW of sodium sulfate is 142.
    A. 1.8 mL
    B. 3.5 mL
    C. 8.8 mL
    D. 17.5 mL

37. How many milliliters of a 5 Eq/L H_2SO_4 solution are required to prepare 4 L of 10% w/v HCl?
A. 0.82 mL
B. 816 mL
C. 1632 mL
D. 3264 mL

38. After preparing a 1:20 dilution of a patient's cerebrospinal fluid, you perform a protein assay on the diluted sample. This diluted sample has 16.6 mg/dL protein. What is the concentration of the protein in the undiluted, original spinal fluid?
A. 0.83 mg/dL
B. 84 mg/dL
C. 116 mg/dL
D. 332 mg/dL

39. An analysis for sodium is performed on an aliquot of a 24-hour urine specimen. A sodium value of 122.5 mmol/L is read from the instrument. What is the amount of sodium in mmol/L in the 24-hour urine specimen if 1540 mL of urine are collected?
A. 80
B. 189
C. 1887
D. 18,865

40. What is the molarity of a 5% (w/v) solution of urea (MW 60)?
A. 0.08
B. 0.4
C. 0.8
D. 1.2

41. The pleural fluid sample you are testing has too many red blood cells to count accurately using a manual method. You make a 1:200 dilution of the sample, and count a total of 473 rbc/µL. What is the cell count, in cells/µL?
A. 4730
B. 9400
C. 47,300
D. 94,000

42. You add 200 mL methanol (100% v/v, MW 32) to 800 mL water. What is the final methanol concentration in % v/v?
A. 10%
B. 20%
C. 25%
D. 60%

43. Your reagent buffer comes to you from the manufacturer as a 10x solution. The directions state that it must be diluted to 1x before use. For this month's assays, you estimate you will need 2000 mL of the working buffer. What is the amount of stock 10x buffer which needs to be diluted to make the needed working buffer?
A. 100 mL
B. 200 mL
C. 500 mL
D. 1000 mL

44. An enzyme assay is performed at 37°C, and absorbance readings are taken each minute for a total of four minutes. Given the following information, what is the enzyme activity in units per liter at 37°C?

Absorbance Readings	Method Information
0.204 at 1 minute	Reagent volume = 3.0 mL
0.406 at 2 minutes	Sample volume = 200 µL
0.610 at 3 minutes	Light path = 1 cm
0.813 at 4 minutes	ε_{340nm} of NADH = 6.22×10^3

A. 490
B. 522
C. 525
D. 1307

45. Your pregnant patients in their third trimester have serum hCG levels that are usually ~30,000 IU/L. Your hCG method's measured signal is linear only up to 6000 IU/L, so you choose to dilute all samples before running the tests. What dilution will you program your instrument to make of each sample so that the final signal falls within the linear range at that dilution?
   A. 1:2
   B. 1:4
   C. 1:5
   D. 1:10

46. What is the molar concentration of calcium in a solution labeled "5 mol/L calcium phosphate"?
   A. 5 mol/L
   B. 10 mol/L
   C. 15 mol/L
   D. 20 mol/L

47. 0.25 Eq/L $CaCl_2$ is equal to how many mmol/L? (MW 110)
   A. 0.125
   B. 0.250
   C. 125
   D. 250

48. 1800 mmol/L $Fe_2(SO_4)_3$ is equal to how many mg/dL? (MW 304)
   A. 54.72
   B. 180
   C. 54,720
   D. 547,200

49. Morphine has a $T_{½} = 6$ hours. If the initial single dose serum level was 10 μg/mL, how much morphine would be left in the serum after 24 hours?
   A. 5.0 μg/mL
   B. 2.5 μg/mL
   C. 1.2 μg/mL
   D. 0.6 μg/mL

50. What is the relationship between equivalents per liter and moles per liter?
   A. Equivalents per liter will always be the same as or less than the moles per liter value
   B. Equivalents per liter will always be the same as or more than the moles per liter value
   C. Equivalents per liter will never be the same as the moles per liter value
   D. Equivalents per liter will always be less than the moles per liter value

51. What is the relative centrifugal force (× *g*) of a centrifuge operating at 2500 rpm with a radius of 10 cm?
   A. 625
   B. 699
   C. 1250
   D. 6988

52. A 10-mL class A volumetric flask has an accuracy of ±0.2%. Express the ±0.2% tolerance in terms of milliliters.
   A. ±0.002
   B. ±0.01
   C. ±0.02
   D. ±0.04

53. A sample of deionized water is found to contain a lead concentration of 0.01 ppm. What is the equivalent concentration expressed as milligrams per deciliter?
   A. 0.01
   B. 0.001
   C. 0.0001
   D. 0.00001

54. Because of a malfunction, a spectrophotometer can show only the percent transmittance (%*T*) readings on its digital display. Convert 68.0 %*T* to its corresponding absorbance.
   A. 0.109
   B. 0.168
   C. 0.320
   D. 0.495

55. Over the past month, your total protein method's low control shows a standard deviation of 0.22 g/dL with the mean = 3.2 g/dL. What is the coefficient of variation?
A. 3.7%
B. 6.5%
C. 14.5%
D. 70.4%

56. The prefix which means 10^{-9} is
A. Micro
B. Milli
C. Nano
D. Pico

57. A "5 normal" (also can be listed as 5N) solution is the same thing as which concentration unit?
A. 5 mol/L
B. 5% w/v
C. 5 Eq/L
D. 5% v/v

58. Which of the following weighs the least?
A. 0.1 ng
B. 0.01 g
C. 1.0 mg
D. 1000 pg

59. "% (w/v)" means the same thing as
A. 100 g solute per 100 mL
B. Number of grams of solute per deciliter
C. Number of grams of solute per liter
D. Number of milliliters of stock solution per 100 mL final solution

60. How many moles per liter of hydroxyl ions (MW 17) are present in a solution containing 96 mol/L calcium hydroxide (MW 74)?
A. 48
B. 96
C. 192
D. 288

PERIODIC TABLE OF THE ELEMENTS

Main groups (1A–2A); Transition metals (3B–2B); Main groups (3A–8A)

	1A[a] 1	2A 2	3B 3	4B 4	5B 5	6B 6	7B 7	8B 8	8B 9	8B 10	1B 11	2B 12	3A 13	4A 14	5A 15	6A 16	7A 17	8A 18
1	1 **H** 1.00794																	2 **He** 4.002602
2	3 **Li** 6.941	4 **Be** 9.012182											5 **B** 10.811	6 **C** 12.0107	7 **N** 14.00674	8 **O** 15.9994	9 **F** 18.998403	10 **Ne** 20.1797
3	11 **Na** 22.989770	12 **Mg** 24.3050											13 **Al** 26.981538	14 **Si** 28.0855	15 **P** 30.973762	16 **S** 32.066	17 **Cl** 35.4527	18 **Ar** 39.948
4	19 **K** 39.0983	20 **Ca** 40.078	21 **Sc** 44.95591	22 **Ti** 47.867	23 **V** 50.9415	24 **Cr** 51.9961	25 **Mn** 54.938049	26 **Fe** 55.845	27 **Co** 58.933200	28 **Ni** 58.6934	29 **Cu** 63.546	30 **Zn** 65.39	31 **Ga** 69.723	32 **Ge** 72.61	33 **As** 74.92160	34 **Se** 78.96	35 **Br** 79.904	36 **Kr** 83.80
5	37 **Rb** 85.4678	38 **Sr** 87.62	39 **Y** 88.90585	40 **Zr** 91.224	41 **Nb** 92.90638	42 **Mo** 95.94	43 **Tc** [98]	44 **Ru** 101.07	45 **Rh** 102.90550	46 **Pd** 106.42	47 **Ag** 107.8682	48 **Cd** 112.411	49 **In** 114.818	50 **Sn** 118.710	51 **Sb** 121.760	52 **Te** 127.60	53 **I** 126.90447	54 **Xe** 131.29
6	55 **Cs** 132.90545	56 **Ba** 137.327	57 ***La** 138.9055	72 **Hf** 178.49	73 **Ta** 180.9479	74 **W** 183.84	75 **Re** 186.207	76 **Os** 190.23	77 **Ir** 192.217	78 **Pt** 195.078	79 **Au** 196.96655	80 **Hg** 200.59	81 **Tl** 204.3833	82 **Pb** 207.2	83 **Bi** 208.98038	84 **Po** [210]	85 **At** [210]	86 **Rn** [222]
7	87 **Fr** [223]	88 **Ra** [226]	89 **†Ac** [227]	104 **Rf** [261]	105 **Db** [262]	106 **Sg** [266]	107 **Bh** [264]	108 **Hs** [265]	109 **Mt** [268]	110 [269]	111 [272]	112 [277]	113	114 [285]	115	116 [289]	117	118 [293]

*Lanthanide series	58 **Ce** 140.116	59 **Pr** 140.90765	60 **Nd** 144.24	61 **Pm** [145]	62 **Sm** 150.36	63 **Eu** 151.964	64 **Gd** 157.25	65 **Tb** 158.92534	66 **Dy** 162.50	67 **Ho** 164.93032	68 **Er** 167.26	69 **Tm** 168.93421	70 **Yb** 173.04	71 **Lu** 174.967
†Actinide series	90 **Th** 232.0381	91 **Pa** 231.03588	92 **U** 238.0289	93 **Np** [237]	94 **Pu** [244]	95 **Am** [243]	96 **Cm** [247]	97 **Bk** [247]	98 **Cf** [251]	99 **Es** [252]	100 **Fm** [257]	101 **Md** [258]	102 **No** [259]	103 **Lr** [262]

[a] The labels on top (1A, 2A, etc.) are common American usage. The labels below these (1, 2, etc.) are those recommended by the International Union of Pure and Applied Chemistry.

The names and symbols for elements 110 and above have not yet been decided.

Atomic weights in brackets are the masses of the longest-lived or most important isotope of radioactive elements.

Further information is available at http://www.shef.ac.uk/chemistry/web-elements/

The production of elements 116 and 118 was reported in May 1999 by scientists at Lawrence Berkeley National Laboratory.

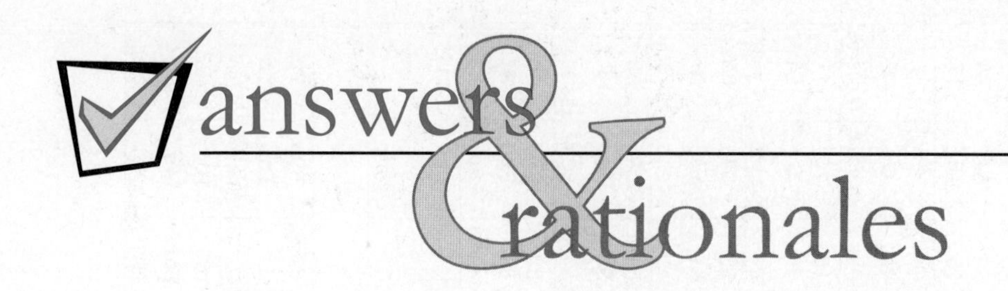

In general, reagent or calibration solution calculations utilize three types of stocks: solid, liquid, and concentrated acids/bases. Each type of stock has its own unique thought process for doing the calculations. Each thought process identifies the desired concentration and needed volume, and then uses factors to arrive at the final needed units (grams or milliliters of stock):

Solid stock: ***use if desired solution is in mol/L or Eq/L; A = anhydrous, H = hydrate***

mol or Eq desired	Volume desired (unit should match first terms to cancel)	→ Eq mole	Moles A→H or vice versa	moles of ions → moles of salt or vice versa	→ mole grams
Volume					

Solid stock: ***use if desired solution is in % (w/v), which equals "grams per deciliter"; A = anhydrous, H = hydrate***

grams desired (A or H)	Volume needed (units matched to dL, mL or L)	MW A or H For what is desired... must be used with denominator below
dL <u>or</u> 100 mL <u>or</u> 0.1 L		MW H or A to cancel first term

Liquid stock:

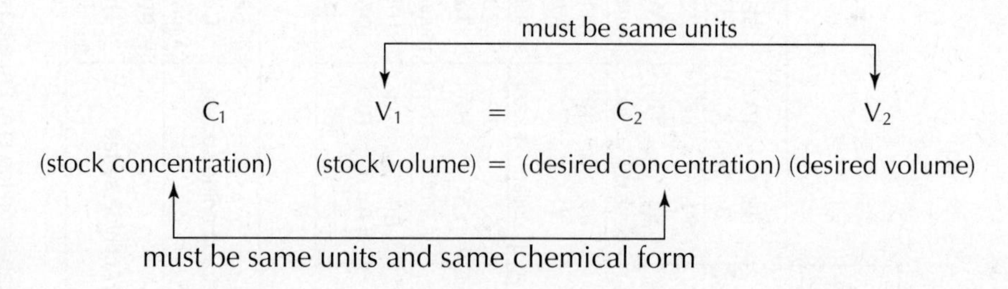

Concentrated acid/base stock:

Eq or moles desired	Volume needed (to match L)	Eq → mole	MW Pure grams	100 g []	mL[]
L			mole	Grams pure	g[]

Note that g [] in the final term is the specific gravity of the acid/base, as provided on the original container, such that "1.037" would mean each milliliter of the concentrated acid weighs 1.037 grams. This weight contains both pure acid/base plus any impurities. "Grams pure" is the percent purity (% assay) of the acid/base, such that "assay = 57%" would mean each 100 grams of the acid/base would contain 57 grams of pure acid. Note that this means this "percent" solution is unique since it is weight to weight (w/w) rather than weight to volume (w/v) or volume to volume (v/v). It is *essential* that you label each term so that they correctly cancel in the final calculation.

These thought processes will be used throughout the explanations, with unique nuances explained, as needed.

1.

B. Recognize a simple conversion, needing grams to moles and mL to L. Put what you know *first*, then the needed conversion factors:

$$\frac{18.7\,\text{g}}{500\ \text{mL}} \left| \frac{1000\,\text{mL}}{\text{L}} \right| \frac{\text{mole}}{74.5\ \text{g}} = 0.5\,\text{mol/L}$$

2.

A. Recognize a simple conversion, needing milligrams to grams and dL to L. Put what you know *first*, then the needed conversion factors:

$$\frac{10\,\text{mg}}{\text{dL}} \left| \frac{10\,\text{dL}}{\text{L}} \right| \frac{\text{mmol}}{40\ \text{mg}} = 2.5\,\text{mmol/L}$$

3.

B. Recognize that (1) stock is solid, so you need the "solid" process above, (2) conversions of mL to L, mmol to mol, ion to salt, and moles to grams are needed. Put what you desire *first*, then the needed conversion factors. Make sure you are changing only *one* unit at a time:

$$\frac{135\,\text{mmol ion}}{\text{L}} \left| \frac{100\,\text{mL}}{} \right| \frac{\text{L}}{10^3\ \text{mL}} \left| \frac{\text{mol ion}}{10^3\,\text{mmol ion}} \right| \frac{\text{mol salt}}{\text{mol ion}} \left| \frac{58.5\,\text{g salt}}{\text{mol salt}} \right. = 0.79\,\text{g salt}$$

4.

C. Recognize that stock is liquid, so you need the "V1C1" process above. Place the *stock* information on the left and the *desired* information on the right, notice that the concentration units are the same on both sides and your final answer will be in liters:

$$(V1)\,(C1) = (V2)\,(C2)$$

$$(x\text{L})\,(95\%) = (5\text{L})\,(70\%)$$

$$V1 = 3.7\,\text{L, which would be } 3700\ \text{mL}$$

5.

C. Recognize that (1) stock is solid, so you need the "solid" process above, (2) conversion of dL to mL is the only one needed, and you do *not* need molecular weight here. Put what you desire *first*, then the needed conversion factors:

$$\frac{2.5\,\text{g}}{\text{dL}} \left| \frac{80\,\text{mL}}{} \right| \frac{\text{dL}}{100\ \text{mL}} = 0.79\,\text{g salt}$$

6.

A. Recognize that stock is liquid, so you need the "V1C1" process above. Place the *stock* information on the left and the *desired* information on the right, notice that the concentration and volume units are the same on both sides, so no conversions needed:

$$(V1)\quad(C1) = (V2)\quad(C2)$$

$$(x\text{mL})\,(40\%) = (80\,\text{mL})\,(2.5\%)$$

$$V1 = 5.0\,\text{mL}$$

answers & rationales

7.

C. Recognize that (1) the stock is a solid, so you need the "solid" process above, (2) conversions of dL to mL, grams anhydrous to grams hydrate, and you *do* need molecular weight here. Put what you desire *first*, then the needed conversion factors. It is *essential* that you write units so you make sure they cancel:

2.5 g anhydrous	80 mL	dL	447.9 g hydrate
dL		100 mL	399.9 g anhydrous

= 2.24 g hydrated salt stock

8.

B. *Given*: weights of NaCl and glucose dissolved in 1 kg of water

Want: osmolality of solution

Relation: osmolality = moles per kilogram of solvent times the number of particles into which solute molecules dissociate

Calculation: express the amount of each solute in terms of moles (grams per molecular weight)

$$5.85\,\text{g NaCl} = \frac{5.85\,\text{g}}{58.5\,\text{g/mol}} = 0.1\,\text{mol NaCl}$$

$$18\,\text{g glucose} = \frac{18\,\text{g}}{180\,\text{g/mol}} = 0.1\,\text{mol glucose}$$

Consider the dissociation of each solute.

$$0.1\,\text{mol NaCl} \rightarrow 0.1\,\text{mol Na}^+ + 0.1\,\text{mol Cl}^-$$

Glucose does not dissociate appreciably.

$$\text{Number of Osmols} = 0.1 \times 2 = 0.2\,\text{osmol NaCl}$$

$$+\ \underline{0.1}\ \text{osmol glucose}$$

$$\text{Total } 0.3\,\text{osmol in } 1\,\text{kg } H_2O$$

$$= 0.3\,\text{osmol}$$

9.

B. *Given*: concentration in grams per deciliter:

0.85% NaCl = 0.85 g/dL

Want: concentration in osmolarity

Relation: osmolarity = moles per liter times the number of particles into which the solute dissociates

Calculation: molecular weight of

$$\text{NaCl} = 23 + 35.5 = 58.5\,\text{g/mol}$$

In dilute solution, NaCl is assumed to be fully dissociated; therefore, each molecule of NaCl will produce two particles, a sodium ion and a chloride ion.

$$\text{Osmolarity} = \text{mol/L} \times \text{No. of particles/dissociate molecule}$$

$$= \frac{\text{g}}{\text{mol wt}}/\text{L} \times \text{No. of particles/dissociate molecule}$$

Convert to grams per liter:

$$0.85\,\text{g/dL} \times 10\,\text{dL/L} = 8.5\,\text{g/L}$$

$$\text{Osmolarity} = \frac{8.5\,\text{g/L}}{58.5\,\text{g/mol}} \times 2 = 0.29\,\text{osmol/L}$$

10.

A. Recognize that the stock is a liquid, so you need the "V1C1" process above. Place the *stock* information on the left and the *desired* information on the right, notice that the concentration units are *not* the same on both sides, so conversion of C1 from mol to Eq and Eq to milliEq is needed:

$$(\text{V1})\quad(\text{C1}) = (\text{V2})\quad(\text{C2})$$

$$(x\,\text{mL})\,(10\,\text{mol/L}) = (400\,\text{mL})\,(100\,\text{mEq/L})$$

Conversion of C1:

10 mol	6 Eq	10^3 mEq
L	1 mol	Eq

= 60,000 mEq/L for the stock, put back into equation

$$\text{V1} = 0.7\,\text{mL}$$

11.

B. When more than one dilution is carried out on a sample, the final concentration is the initial concentration multiplied by each dilution expressed as a fraction. If a 5N solution is diluted 1:4 and then further 4:15, the final concentration is:

$$5\text{N} \times \frac{1}{4} \times \frac{4}{15} = 0.33\text{N}$$

The same principle applies in testing a specimen that is too concentrated to fall within the range of the test procedure. The specimen is diluted, the test repeated, and the result multiplied by the reciprocal of the dilution. Thus, if the specimen had to be diluted 1:10 (1/10) to fall within the range of the test procedure, the result would be multiplied by 10 (10/1) to give the correct value.

12.

D. To find the dilution of serum in a mixture, calculate the total volume. The total volume equals 0.1 mL serum + 5 mL reagents + 4.9 mL water = 10 mL. Therefore, the dilution of serum is 0.1 mL to 10 mL, or 0.1:10. Because dilutions are usually expressed as 1 to some number, multiply both the serum volume (0.1) and the total volume (10) by a common factor of 10. Thus, the 0.1:10 serum dilution may be expressed as 1:100.

13.

B. Recognize that the stock is a liquid, so you need the "V1C1" process above. Place the *stock* information on the left and the *desired* information on the right, notice that the concentration units are *not* the same on both sides on both sides, so conversion of C1 from mmol to mol and ion to salt are needed:

$$(\text{V1})\ (\text{C1}) = (\text{V2})\ (\text{C2})$$

$$(\text{x mL})\ (6\,\text{mol/L salt}) = (400\,\text{mL})\ (200\,\text{mmol/L ion})$$

Conversion of C1:

$$\frac{6\,\text{mol salt} \mid 10^3\,\text{mmol salt} \mid 2\,\text{mmol ion}}{\text{L} \mid 1\,\text{mol salt} \mid 1\,\text{mmol salt}} =$$

12,000 mmol/L ion, put back into equation

$$\text{V1} = 4.2\,\text{mL}$$

14.

C. Recognize that (1) stock is solid, so you need the "solid" process above, (2) conversion of L to mL, millimoles to moles, moles ion to moles salt, and moles salt to grams salt, and you *do* need salt molecular weight here. Put what you desire *first*, then the needed conversion factors:

$$\frac{10\,\text{mmol ion} \mid 500\,\text{mL} \mid \text{L} \mid \text{mole ion} \mid 1\,\text{mole salt} \mid 110\,\text{g salt}}{\text{L} \mid \quad \mid 10^3\,\text{mL} \mid 10^3\,\text{mmol ion} \mid 2\,\text{mole ion} \mid \text{mole salt}} = 0.275\,\text{g salt}$$

15.

C. Recognize that the stock is a liquid, so you need the "V1C1" process above. Place the *stock* information on the left and the *desired* information on the right, notice that the concentration units are *not* the same on both sides, so conversion of C1 from mg/mL to mg/dL is needed:

$$(\text{V1})\ (\text{C1}) = (\text{V2})\ (\text{C2})$$

$$(\text{x mL})\ (10\,\text{mg/mL}) = (200\,\text{mL})\ (20\,\text{mg/dL})$$

Conversion of C1:

$$\frac{10\,\text{mg} \mid 100\,\text{mL}}{\text{mL} \mid \text{dL}} = 1000\,\text{mg/dL}$$

for the stock, put back into equation

$$\text{V1} = 4\,\text{mL}$$

16.

D. Recognize that the stock is a liquid, so you need the "V1C1" process above. Place the *stock* information on the left and the *desired* information on the right; notice that the volume units are *not* the same on both sides, so conversion of V2 from L to mL is needed:

$$(\text{V1})\ (\text{C1}) = (\text{V2})\ (\text{C2})$$

$$(\text{x mL})\ (50\%) = (1\,\text{L})\ (5\%)$$

Conversion of V2:

$$\frac{1\,\text{L} \mid 10^3\,\text{dL}}{\mid \text{L}} = 1000\,\text{mL}$$ for V2, put back into equation

$$\text{V1} = 100\,\text{mL}$$

17.

C. Recognize that (1) the stock is a solid, so you need the "solid" process above, (2) conversion of L to dL, and you *do not* need salt molecular weight here. Put what you desire *first*, then the needed conversion factors:

$$\frac{3g \mid 1L \mid 10\,dL}{dL \mid \quad \mid L} = 30\,g \text{ salt}$$

18.

C. The urine sample contained 120 mg/dL % protein, which is equivalent to 120 mg of protein per deciliter. Because the total urine volume is given in milliliters, it is necessary to express the volume in deciliters so that the units of measurement correspond. This may be done by dividing the 24-hour volume in milliliters by 100, because there are 100 mL in each deciliter. The amount of protein excreted in the 24-hour urine specimen may now be calculated. Make sure you do *not* divide by the "24" in the denominator. It may be less likely to make that mistake if you write "day" instead.

$$\frac{\begin{matrix}\text{Protein conc.} & & \text{urine volume} \\ \text{in g/dL} & \times & \text{in mL/24 hr}\end{matrix}}{100\,mL/dL} = g/24\,hr$$

$$\frac{1.2\,g/dL \times 2155\,mL/24\,hr}{100\,mL/dL} = 25.9\,g/24\,hr$$

19.

A. Recognize that the stock is a liquid, so you need the "V1C1" process above. Place the *stock* information on the left and the *desired* information on the right, notice that the concentration and volume units are *not* the same on both sides, so conversion of C1 from mol salt to mmol salt, mmol salt to mmol ion, mmol ion to mg ion, and L to dL are all needed. V2 needs conversion of dL to mL:

$$(V1)\ (C1) = (V2)\ (C2)$$

$$(x\,mL)\,(10\,mol/L\,salt) = (1\,dL)\,(900\,mg/dL\,ion)$$

Conversion of C1:

$$\frac{10\,mol\,salt \mid 10^3\,mmol\,salt \mid 2\,mmol\,ion \mid 62\,mg\ ion \mid L}{L \mid 1\,mol\,salt \mid mmol\,salt \mid mmol\,ion \mid 10\,dL}$$

$$= 124{,}000\ mg/dL \text{ ion stock}$$

Conversion of V2:

$$\frac{1\,dL \mid 100\,mL}{\quad \mid dL} = 100\,mL$$

Put new C1 and V2 back into formula and solve for V1: 0.73 mL stock

20.

D. Recognize that (1) the stock is a solid, so you need the "solid" process above, (2) Eq to moles, moles to grams, and you *do* need molecular weight here. Put what you desire *first*, then the needed conversion factors. Note that here 1 Eq = 1 mole since the valence x number of sodium ions = 1:

$$\frac{2\,Eq \mid 4L \mid mole \mid 40\,g}{L \mid \quad \mid Eq \mid mole} = 320\,g\ NaOH$$

21.

D. "Percent solution" refers to a specific number of *parts per hundred.* For a volume per volume solution, measure the volume of liquid solute required in milliliters and add solvent to a final volume of 100 mL of solution. Preparation of a 5% v/v CH_3COOH solution may be done as follows: 5% glacial acetic acid = 5 mL of stock concentrated acid per deciliter (remember, 100 mL is equivalent to 1 dL). Thus, to find the number of milliliters needed to prepare 2 L of 5% CH_3COOH, multiply by the required volume in deciliters as follows: $5\,mL/dL \times 10\,dL/L \times 2\,L = 100\,mL$. Thus to prepare 2 L of a 5% acetic acid solution, add 100 mL of glacial acetic acid to deionized water (remember—always add acid to water) and dilute using a volumetric flask to a final volume of 2 L. Note that you do not need to use the MW or the % assay to solve this since the desired solution was in % v/v. If it had been in mol/L or Eq/L, you would have used the long formula found on page **xxx** and which will be used in questions #22 and 23.

22.

C. Concentrated acids require certain unique handling realities: (1) for safety, you will always add acid to water to reduce the chance of splatter, (2) concentrated acids are never 100% pure so you must account for that in the math by using the % assay value listed on the acid bottle; (3) you will never weigh out concentrated acid, so you must convert grams of acid into milliliters of acid, using the specific gravity value listed on the acid bottle. A very easy way of accounting for these realities is the formula on page **xxx**, which looks like the solid stock formula, but will account for both % assay and specific gravity conversions, leaving you with milliliters of stock acid needed to make the solution. As always, start with what you need and then use the required conversions, cancelling one unit at a time, in *this* order, and labeling everything clearly:

60 mEq	2L	Eq	mol	98 g pure	100 g []	mL []
L		10^3 mEq	3Eq	mole	70 g pure	1.64 g []

= 3.4 mL stock acid

23.

C. Concentrated acids require certain unique handling: (1) for safety, you will always add acid to water to reduce the chance of splatter, (2) concentrated acids are never 100% pure so you must account for that in the math by using the % assay value listed on the acid bottle; (3) you will never weigh out concentrated acid, so you must convert grams of acid into milliliters of acid, using the specific gravity value listed on the acid bottle. A very easy way of accounting for these realities is the formula on page **xxx**, which looks like the solid stock formula, but will account for both % assay and specific gravity conversions leaving you will milliliters of stock acid needed to make the solution. As always, start with what you need and then use the required conversions, cancelling one unit at a time, in *this* order, and label everything clearly:

270 mmol	4.5 L	mol	60 g pure	100 g []	mL []
L		10^3 mmol	mole	67 g pure	1.82 g[]

= 60 mL stock acid

24.

C. Recognize that (1) the stock is a solid, so you need the "solid" process above, (2) conversion of L to mL is the only one needed, and you *do not* need molecular weight here. Put what you desire *first*, then the needed conversion factors:

$$\frac{0.85\,g \mid 5\,L \mid 10^3\,mL}{100\,mL \mid \quad \mid L} = 42.5\,g$$

25.

D. Dilutions are always relationships between sample volume (SV) and total volume (TV), with SV always in the numerator and TV in the denominator. The skill in solving dilution problems is in recognizing who the players are. Here, the "1:5" means out of every 5 total volumes, 1 is the sample volume. "Patient" is always considered the "sample volume," so that is the 10 μL. This leaves the total volume to be calculated, based on the relationship between SV and TV being 1:5:

$$\frac{SV}{TV} = \frac{1}{5} = \frac{10\,\mu L}{x\,\mu L}$$

Solving for x = 50 uL as the maximum TV that can be made. One thing to note, however, is that this TV will use up *all* of your sample volume, which is never a good idea when dealing with spinal fluid. The additional reality will be in knowing what TV your testing method requires, which is not a part of this question but definitely has to be a part of the spinal fluid handling process.

26.

B. Dilutions are always relationships between sample volume (SV) and total volume (TV), with SV always in the numerator and TV in the denominator. The skill in solving dilution problems is in recognizing who the players are. Here, the "1:20" means that, out of every 20 *total* volumes, 1 is the *sample* volume. "Serum" is always considered the "sample volume," and that is the unknown here, and the 50 mL is the TV:

$$\frac{SV}{TV} = \frac{1}{20} = \frac{x\,mL}{50\,mL}$$

Solving for x = 2.5 mL as the serum volume needed. One thing to note is that the volume of diluent volume required is never directly calculated in these problems but is definitely assumed to be included in the TV, since that equals SV plus diluent volume. Here, the diluent volume would be 50 mL minus 2.5 mL serum = 47.5 mL diluent.

27.

D. Recognize a simple conversion, needing dL to L and milligrams to millimoles. Put what you know *first*, then the needed conversion factors:

$$\frac{369\,mg \mid 10\,dL \mid mmol}{dL \mid \quad \mid 35.5\,g} = 104\ mol/L$$

28.

A. Recognize a simple conversion, needing milligrams to millimoles and dL to L. Put what you know *first*, then the needed conversion factors:

$$\frac{8.6\,mg \mid 10\,dL \mid mmol}{dL \mid L \mid 40\,mg} = 2.15, \text{which rounded}$$

$$= 2.2\ mmol/L$$

29.

C. Any question indicating a dilution is involved and providing at least one concentration means you can use the formula FC = OC × dilution. "FC" is "final concentration," meaning the one determined *after* the dilution is made. "OC" is "Original concentration," meaning the one *before* the dilution is made. "Dilution" is always "sample volume" in the numerator and "total volume" in the denominator. Therefore, most problems will provide three of these four terms, and the skill is figuring out who the players are!

$$FC = OC \times \frac{SV}{TV}$$

$$4.9\,g/dL = OC \times \frac{1}{3}$$

$$OC = 4.9 \times 3$$

$$= 14.7\,g/dL$$

Note that when you know the diluted concentration and the dilution used, you can always "correct for dilution" by multiplying the FC by the reciprocal of the dilution.

30.

A. Any question indicating a dilution is involved and providing at least one concentration means you can use the formula **FC = OC × dilution**. "FC" is "final concentration," meaning the one determined *after* the dilution is made (so here it would be 200 mmol ion/L). "OC" is "original concentration," meaning the one *before* the dilution is made (so here it would be 46 g ion/L). "Dilution" is always "sample volume" in the numerator and "total volume" in the denominator. Therefore, most problems will provide three of these four terms, and the skill is figuring out who the players are! Note that dilutions are given in lowest terms, so the numerator, representing the "sample volume" will usually be a "1" if the denominator is a whole number.

$$FC = OC \times \frac{SV}{TV}$$

$$200\,\text{mmol ion/L} = 46\,\text{g ion/L} \times \frac{SV}{TV}$$

For this problem, you are given the FC and OC but not the dilution. In addition, the units for the FC are not the same as the OC, so you must make them the same by conversion math before solving for the dilution. Also note that even though sodium **ions** are mentioned, there is no ion to salt conversion needed since "ion" is in both FC and OC. In fact, the salt used to place the sodium ions into the solution is irrelevant!

Conversion of grams ion to mmol ion:

$$\frac{46\,\text{g ion}}{\text{L}} \left| \frac{\text{mole}}{23\,\text{g}} \right| \frac{10^3\,\text{mmol}}{\text{mole}} = \frac{2000\,\text{mmol ion}}{\text{L}},$$

which gets placed back into the formula

$$200\,\text{mmol ion/L} = 2000\,\text{mmol/L} \times \frac{SV}{TV}$$

$$\frac{SV}{TV} = \frac{200\,\text{mmol ion/L}}{2000\,\text{mmol ion/L}} = \frac{1}{10}$$

31.

B. Recognize a simple conversion, needing moles of salt to moles on ions. Note that MW is *not* needed here. Every mole of $Ca(NO_3)_2$ places 2 moles of nitrate into solution. Put what you know *first*, then the needed conversion factors:

$$\frac{96\,\text{mol salt}}{\text{L}} \left| \frac{2\,\text{moles of ion}}{1\,\text{mole salt}} \right. = 192\,\text{mol/L nitrate ions}$$

32.

C. Recognize that the stock is a liquid, so you need the "V1C1" process above. Place the *stock* information on the left and the *desired* information on the right, notice that the concentration and volume units are the same on both sides, so no conversions are needed:

$$(V1)\ (C1) = (V2)\ (C2)$$

$$(x\,\text{mL})\,(20\%) = (800\,\text{mL})\,(2.5\%)$$

$$V1: 100\,\text{mL stock}$$

33.

D. Recognize that (1) the stock is a solid, so you need the "solid" process above, (2) conversion of moles anhydrous to moles hydrate, and moles hydrate to grams hydrate, and you *do* need only the hydrate molecular weight here. Note that the molarity of the anhydrous will *always* be the same as the molarity of the hydrate, regardless of how many waters are associated with the salt. Put what you desire *first*, then the needed conversion factors:

$$\frac{0.33\,\text{mol anhydrous}}{\text{L}} \left| \frac{2.6\,\text{L}}{} \right| \frac{\text{mole hydrate}}{\text{mole anhydrous}} \left| \frac{154\,\text{g hydrate}}{\text{mole hydrate}} \right. = 132\,\text{g hydrate}$$

34.

B. Recognize that (1) the stock is a solid, so you need the "solid" process above, (2) conversion of dL to mL is the *only* one needed, and you *do not* need molecular weight here. Put what you desire *first*, then the needed conversion factors:

$$\frac{23\text{ g} \mid 750\text{ mL} \mid \text{dL}}{\text{dL} \mid \quad \mid 100\text{ mL}} = 172.5\text{ g salt}$$

35.

B. Recognize that the stock is a liquid, so you need the "V1C1" process above. Place the *stock* information on the left and the *desired* information on the right, notice that the concentration and volume units are the same on both sides, so no conversion is needed:

$$(V1)\ (C1) = (V2)\ (C2)$$
$$(x\text{ mL})(75\%) = (5.0\text{ mL})(40\%)$$
$$V1 = 2.7\text{ mL}$$

36.

B. Recognize that the stock is a liquid, so you need the "V1C1" process above. Place the *stock* information on the left and the *desired* information on the right, notice that the concentration units are *not* the same on both sides, so conversion of C1 from mol salt to mmol salt, and mmol salt to mmol ion are needed:

$$(V1)\ (C1) = (V2)\ (C2)$$
$$(x\text{ mL})(10\text{ mol/L salt}) = (350\text{ mL})(200\text{ mmol/L ion})$$

Conversion of C1:

$$\frac{10\text{ mol salt} \mid 10^3\text{ mmol salt} \mid 2\text{ mmol ion}}{\text{L} \mid 1\text{ mol salt} \mid \text{mmol salt}} =$$

20,000 mmol/L ion, put back into formula

$$V1 = 3.5\text{ mL}$$

37.

C. Recognize that the stock is a liquid, so you need the "V1C1" process above. Place the *stock* information on the left and the *desired* information on the right, notice that the concentration and volume units are *not* the same on both sides. For this set of different units, it is easier to change both to mol/L. So conversion of C1 from Eq to mole and C2 from g/dL to mol/L are needed. V2 needs conversion of L to mL:

$$(V1)\ (C1) = (V2)\ (C2)$$
$$(x\text{ mL})(10\text{ mol/L salt}) = (1\text{ dL})(900\text{ mg/dL ion})$$

Conversion of C1:

$$\frac{5\text{ Eg} \mid \text{mol}}{\text{L} \mid 2\text{ Eq}} = 2.5\text{ mol/L stock}$$

Conversion of C2:

$$\frac{10\text{ g} \mid 10\text{ dL} \mid \text{mol}}{\text{dL} \mid \text{L} \mid 98\text{ g}} = 1.02\text{ mol/L desired}$$

Conversion of V2:

$$\frac{4\text{ L} \mid 1000\text{ mL}}{\quad \mid \text{L}} = 4000\text{ mL}$$

Put new C1, C2 and V2 back into formula and solve for V1: 1632 mL stock

38.

D. Any question indicating a dilution is involved and providing at least one concentration means you can use the formula FC = OC × dilution. "FC" is "final concentration," meaning the one determined *after* the dilution is made. "OC" is "Original concentration," meaning the one *before* the dilution is made. "Dilution" is always "sample volume" in the numerator and "total volume" in the denominator. Therefore, most problems will provide three of these four terms, and the skill is figuring out who the players are!

$$FC = OC \times \frac{SV}{TV}$$

$$16.6\ mg/dL = OC \times \frac{1}{20}$$

$$OC = 16.6 \times 20$$

$$= 332\ mg/dL$$

Note that when you know the diluted concentration and the dilution used, you can always "correct for dilution" by multiplying the FC by the reciprocal of the dilution.

39.

B. The urine sample contained 122.5 mmol/L of sodium. Because the total urine volume is given in milliliters, it is necessary to express the volume in liters so that the units of measurement correspond. This may be done by dividing the 24-hour volume in milliliters by 1000, because each liter has 1000 mL. The amount of sodium excreted in the 24-hour urine specimen may now be calculated.

$$\frac{\underset{mmol/L}{Sodium} \times \underset{mL/24\ hr}{urine\ volume}}{1000\ mL/L} = mmol/24\ hr$$

$$\frac{122.5\ mmol/L \times 1540\ mL/24\ hr}{1000\ mL/L} = 188.6\ mmol/24\ hr$$

40.

C. Recognize a simple conversion, needing dL to L and grams to moles. Put what you know *first*, then the needed conversion factors:

$$\frac{5g}{dL}\bigg|\frac{10\ dL}{L}\bigg|\frac{mol}{60\ g} = 0.8\ g\ mol/L$$

41.

C. Any question indicating a dilution is involved and providing at least one concentration means you can use the formula FC = OC × dilution. "FC" is "final concentration," meaning the one determined *after* the dilution is made. "OC" is "Original concentration," meaning the one *before* the dilution is made. "Dilution" is always "sample volume" in the numerator and "total volume" in the denominator. Therefore, most problems will provide three of these four terms, and the skill is figuring out who the players are!

$$FC = OC \times \frac{SV}{TV}$$

$$473\ rbc/\mu L = OC \times \frac{1}{100}$$

$$OC = 473 \times 100$$

$$= 47{,}300\ rbc/\mu L$$

Note that when you know the diluted concentration and the dilution used, you can always "correct for dilution" by multiplying the FC by the reciprocal of the dilution.

42.

B. Any question indicating a dilution is involved and providing at least one concentration means you can use the formula FC = OC × dilution. "FC" is "final concentration," meaning the one determined *after* the dilution is made. "OC" is "Original concentration," meaning the one *before* the dilution is made. "Dilution" is always "sample volume" in the numerator and "total volume" in the denominator. Therefore, most problems will provide three of these four terms, and the skill is figuring out who the players are!

$$\text{FC} = \text{OC} \times \frac{\text{SV}}{\text{TV}}$$

$$\text{FC} = 100\%\ \text{v/v} \times \frac{200\,\text{mL}}{200 + 800\,\text{mL}}$$

$$\text{FC} = 100\%\ \text{v/v} \times \frac{1}{5}$$

$$= 20\%\ \text{v/v}$$

43.

B. Any question indicating a dilution is involved and providing at least one concentration means you can use the formula FC = OC × dilution. "FC" is "final concentration," meaning the one determined *after* the dilution is made. "OC" is "Original concentration," meaning the one *before* the dilution is made. "Dilution" is always "sample volume" in the numerator and "total volume" in the denominator. Therefore, most problems will provide three of these four terms, and the skill is figuring out who the players are!

$$\text{FC} = \text{OC} \times \frac{\text{SV}}{\text{TV}}$$

$$1\text{X} = 10\text{X} \times \frac{\text{SV}}{2000\,\text{mL}}$$

$$\frac{1\text{X}}{10\text{X}} = \frac{1}{10} = \frac{\text{SV}}{2000\ \text{mL}}$$

Solving for SV = 200 mL of stock is needed. Note that when you know the FC and OC, you automatically know the ratio of SV to TV needed since it must equal the ratio of FC to OC.

44.

B. The International Unit is defined as the amount of enzyme activity that converts 1 μmol of substrate in 1 minute under standard conditions. The following formula is used to calculate enzyme activity.

$$\frac{\Delta A/\text{min} \times 1000 \times TV \times 1000 \times Tf}{6.22 \times 10^3 \times LP \times SV} = \text{U/L}$$

where ΔA/min is the average absorbance change per minute and 1000 converts milliliters to liters; *TV* is the total reaction volume and 1000 converts millimoles to micromoles; *Tf* is the temperature factor (1.0 at 37°C); 6.22×10^3 is the molar absorptivity of reduced nicotinamide-adenine dinucleotide (NADH) at 340 nm; *LP* is the light path in centimeters and *SV* is the sample volume. For the problem presented, determine the average ΔA/min and then substitute the given information into the equation.

Absorbance (*A*) Readings	Δ *A*/min	Average Δ *A*/min
0.204 *A* at 1 min		
	0.202	
0.406 *A* at 2 min		
	0.204	0.203
0.610 *A* at 3 min		
	0.203	
0.813 *A* at 4 min		

$$\frac{0.203\,\Delta A/\text{min} \times 1000 \times 3.2\,\text{mL} \times 1000 \times 1}{6.22 \times 10^3 \times 1.0 \times 0.2\,\text{mL}} = 522\,\text{U/L}$$

45.

D. Any question indicating a dilution is involved and providing at least one concentration means you can use the formula FC = OC × dilution. "FC" is "final concentration," meaning the one determined *after* the dilution is made. "OC" is "original concentration," meaning the one *before* the dilution is made. "Dilution" is always "sample volume" in the numerator and "total volume" in the denominator. Therefore, most problems will provide three of these four terms, and the skill is figuring out who the players are!

$$FC = OC \times \frac{SV}{TV}$$

$$6000\,IU/L = 30000\,IU/L \times \frac{SV}{TV}$$

$$\frac{6000}{30000} = \frac{SV}{TV} = \frac{1}{5}$$

Therefore, a 1:5 dilution will bring most patient sample hCG levels into the linear range. However, note that "6000 IU/L" is at the *top* of that range. It would be better to make the dilution place most samples in the mid-linear range, so 3000:30000 = 1:10 dilution would be better. You would not want to dilute much more than that since it would place diluted values too low in the linear range. Mid-range is best!

46.

C. Recognize a simple conversion, where the skill is in writing the salt formula correctly as $Ca_3(PO_4)_2$, which tells you every mole of the salt puts three calcium ions into solution. This one needs only moles of salt converted to moles of ion. It is critical to label everything! Put what you know *first*, then the needed conversion factors:

$$\frac{5\text{ mole salt}}{L} \times \frac{3\text{ mole ion}}{1\text{ mole salt}} = 15\text{ mol/L calcium ions}$$

47.

C. Recognize a simple conversion, needing Eq to moles, and moles to millimoles. There are 2 Eq in a mole of $CaCl_2$ since the calcium valence times number of ions = 2. You do *not* need MW here. Put what you know *first*, then the needed conversion factors:

$$\frac{0.25\text{ Eq}}{L} \times \frac{\text{mole}}{2\text{ Eq}} \times \frac{10^3\text{ mmol}}{\text{mol}} = 125\text{ mmol/L}$$

48.

C. Recognize a simple conversion, needing L to dL and millimole to milligram. You *do* need MW for this one. Put what you know *first*, then the needed conversion factors:

$$\frac{1800\text{ mmol}}{L} \times \frac{L}{10\text{ dL}} \times \frac{304\text{ mg}}{\text{mmol}} = 54{,}720\text{ mg/dL}$$

49.

A. The term "half-life" ($T_{1/2}$) is the time in which the serum level of an analyte will decrease by half. For drugs that are given in a single dose, the decrease will be due mainly to clearance (usually by liver or kidney) and metabolism of the drug into a form that the method does not detect or which is no longer active. For this problem, it has already been established that the $T_{1/2}$ is 6 hours ($T_{1/2}$). So the time course for the drug-level change in the blood would be:

Time of drug-level measurement	0 hr	6 hr	12 hr	18 hr	24 hr
[drug]	10 μg/mL	5 μg/mL	2.5 μg/mL	1.25 μg/mL	0.6 μg/mL

Since the question asks what would be the drug level at the 24-hour blood draw, the answer is 0.6 μg/mL. Note that this math is relevant for a drug given in a *single* dose. The math becomes more complicated (and not shown here) if *multiple* doses over time are given.

50.

B. The Eq/L value will always be the *same as* or *greater than* the mol/L value. Conversion of Eq/L to mol/L uses an easy factor of charge and the number of positive ions. You must know how the molecule dissociates to get these factors. For example, 3 Eq/L NaCl = 3 mol/L, since sodium has a +1 charge and there is only one sodium in the molecule, so the factor is 1, and 3/1 = 3. For 3 Eq/L Na_2SO_4, the molarity would be 1.5 mol/L since sodium has a +1 charge and there are two sodiums in the molecule, so the factor is 2, and 3/2 = 1.5. For 3 Eq/L Na_3PO_4, the molarity would be 1 mol/L since sodium has a +1 charge and there are three sodiums in the molecule, so the factor is 3, and 3/3 = 1.

For a more complex molecule example, 12 Eq/L of $Ca_3(PO_4)_2$ would equal 2 mol/L since calcium has a +2 charge and there are three calciums in the molecule, so the factor is 6, and 12/6 = 2.

51.

B. By use of centrifugal force, a centrifuge effects the separation of substances of different densities. The most common use of a centrifuge in the clinical laboratory is the separation of serum or plasma from the blood cells. The use of the proper amount of centrifugal force with serum separator tubes is especially important. In order for a thixotropic, silicone gel to form a barrier between the serum and the cell clot, it is critical that the tube be centrifuged for a specified time and with the specified centrifugal force. The following formula is used to calculate the relative centrifugal force (RCF) in terms of gravities (*g*), where 1.118×10^{-5} represents a constant, r represents the rotating radius in centimeters, and rpm represents the rotating speed in revolutions per minute:

$$\begin{aligned} \text{RCF} &= 1.118 \times 10^{-5} \times r \times (\text{rpm})^2 \\ &= 1.118 \times 10^{-5} \times 10 \times (2500)^2 \\ &= 698.75 \\ \text{RCF} &= 699 \times g \end{aligned}$$

52.

C. Class A volumetric flasks are calibrated at 20°C. Glassware that is designated as class A must meet the requirements of the National Institute of Standards and Technology. The College of American Pathologists (CAP) requires that CAP-approved clinical laboratories use only class A glassware. A 10 mL class A volumetric flask that is accurate to ±0.2% has a tolerance of ±0.02 mL; 10 mL × 0.2% = 0.02 mL = ±0.02 mL. Thus, the capacity of a 10 mL flask is within the range of 9.98 to 10.02 mL.

53.

B. The term "parts per million" (ppm) is a unit of concentration that describes the number of parts of a substance that are contained in 1 million parts of the solution. "Parts per million" refers to the number of grams of a substance in 1 million grams of solution. To convert from parts per million to concentration, the following formula is used:

$$\frac{\text{g}}{X\text{mL}} \times 1{,}000{,}000 = \text{ppm}$$

In referring to parts per million, it is important to remember that the unit of measure may vary (e.g., milligrams, micrograms, and nanograms), provided that the relationship of some number of parts in 1 million parts is maintained. Therefore, it follows that to convert 0.01 ppm to mg/dL:

$$\frac{\text{mg}}{X\text{mL}} \times 1000 = \text{ppm}$$

$$\frac{\text{mg}}{100} \times 1000 = 0.01$$

$$\text{mg} = \frac{0.01}{1000} \times 100$$

$$\text{mg} = 0.001$$

Thus, 0.01 ppm of lead is equivalent to 0.001 mg/dL or 0.001 mg/100 mL.

54.

B. To convert 68.0 $\%T$ to absorbance (A), use the following formula:

$$A = -\log T = \log\frac{1}{T} = \log\frac{100\%}{\%T}$$

$$A = \log 100 - \log \%T$$

$$A = 2 - \log \%T$$

$$A = 2 - \log 68$$

$$A = 2 - 1.832 = 0.168$$

After determining absorbance values, they may be used in the Beer's law equation, $A = abc$, to determine concentration values. Absorbance and percent transmittance values may both be used to construct standard curves to determine concentration values of unknown samples.

55.

B. Coefficient of variation is calculated by dividing the standard deviation by the mean of the population and multiplying by 100 to express the CV in percent. In clinical quality control practice, a CV over 5% should be investigated since it suggests there is greater variability within the method than is acceptable. In this problem, 0.22 g/dL divided by 3.2 g/dL times 100 = 6.5%, which would not be considered acceptable and should be investigated.

56.

C. In decreasing multiples of 1000, the unit modifiers most commonly used in the clinical laboratory are micro (10^{-3}), milli (10^{-6}), nano (10^{-9}), pico (10^{-12}), femto (10^{-15}), and atto (10^{-18}).

57.

C. A "Normal" solution is the same as "Eq/L." This latter term is more useful since it provides a unit of volume which can be used when needing to cancel units in lab math problems. "% w/v" and "% v/v" mean grams per deciliter and milliliters per deciliter, respectively.

58.

A. To solve this problem, all the values must be converted to a common unit. In metric measurement, the gram is the primary unit for weight. The value 0.1 ng is equal to 1×10^{-10} g, which is the lightest weight given. The gram relationships for the other values stated are 0.01 g $= 1 \times 10^{-2}$ g, 1.0 mg $= 1 \times 10^{-3}$ g, and 1000 pg $= 1 \times 10^{-9}$ g.

59.

B. "% w/v" means grams per deciliter. Therefore, a solution labeled "25% w/v glucose" would contain 25 grams of glucose in every 100 mL. Note that answer D would define "% v/v."

60.

C. You must be able to determine the dissociation of the molecule to do this math. Since every molecule of calcium hydroxide places into solution **one** ion of calcium and **two** hydroxyl ions, those numbers become factors in determining their individual ion concentrations:

$$Ca(OH)_2 \longrightarrow 1Ca^{+2} + 2OH^{-1}$$

$$96\,mol/L \qquad 96\,mol/L \qquad 192\,mol/L$$

Make sure that you recognize that the "2" in the dissociation refers to the entire hydroxyl (OH) ion, and not just to the oxygen.

REFERENCES

Burtis, C. A., and Bruns, D. E. (Eds.) (2015). *Tietz Fundamentals of Clinical Chemistry and Molecular Diagnostics*, 7th ed. Philadelphia: Saunders.

Campbell, J. B., and Campbell, J. M. (1997). *Laboratory Mathematics Medical and Biological Applications*, 5th ed. St. Louis: Mosby-Year Book.

Doucette, L. J. (2015). *Mathematics for the Clinical Laboratory*, 3rd ed. Philadelphia: Saunders.

CHAPTER

13 General Laboratory Principles, Quality Assessment, and Safety

contents

I. GENERAL LABORATORY PRINCIPLES

A. Chemicals and Related Substances

1. **Chemicals**
   a. **Analytic reagent** (AR) **grade** chemicals meet the specifications established by the **American Chemical Society** (ACS) and are used in most analytical laboratory procedures.
   b. **Ultrapure** reagents have undergone additional processing that makes them suitable for special procedures such as atomic absorption, chromatography, molecular diagnostics, or other techniques that require extremely pure chemicals.
2. Laboratory requirements generally call for **reagent grade water.** Reagent grade water meets the specifications of **Clinical Laboratory Reagent Water (CLRW),** the standards for which were established by the Clinical and Laboratory Standards Institute (CLSI). **Reagent grade water (CLRW)** is of the highest quality and is used in test methodologies where minimum interference and maximum precision and accuracy are needed. Resistivity of greater than or equal to 10 MΩ•cm at 25°C is required. Other specifications address microbiological content, silicate, particulate matter, and organics.
   a. Processes required in preparation of reagent grade water (CLRW) are as follows:
      1) **Prefilters** are glass or cotton microfibers that remove 98% of the particulate matter from municipal water supplies.
      2) **Activated carbon** removes organic matter and chlorine.
      3) **A submicron filter** removes all particles or microorganisms larger than the membrane pore size.
      4) **Reverse osmosis** is a process that removes 95–99% of bacteria and organic and other particulate matter.
      5) **Ion exchange** is a system of resin cartridges or tanks connected in series that remove cations and anions to make deionized water.
   b. **Distilled water** is water that has been purified to remove almost all organic materials, using distillation (boiling and condensation). Water may be boiled more than once with each distillation cycle removing more impurities.
   c. **Deionized water** is purified water (prefiltered or distilled) that has had some or all of its ions removed using an anion or cation exchange resin followed by the replacement of removed ions with hydroxyl or hydrogen ions.
   d. Other types of water used in the clinical laboratory are categorized by the **intended purpose** of their use and include the following:
      1) **Special reagent water (SRW):** May require different preparation than CLRW according to intended use, such as sterility specification for tissue or organ culture, nucleic acid content for DNA testing, metal content for trace metal analysis, etc.
      2) **Instrument feed water:** Used for internal instrument rinsing, making dilutions, etc., and needs to meet manufacturer's specifications.

3) **Water for use as a diluent or reagent supplied by manufacturer:** Label states intended use; do not substitute for CLRW or SRW unless label indicates it is of such quality.
4) **Purified water commercially bottled:** Exercise care because some plastic containers permit microorganism growth due to air permeability.
5) **Water for laboratory dishwashers and autoclaves:** Purified to contain only low levels of organics, inorganics, and particulate matter so it does not leave residue on glassware or contaminate solutions and media in autoclaves.

3. **Standards**
   a. **Primary standards** are highly purified chemicals that are weighed or measured to produce a solution with an exact concentration and purity.
   b. **Secondary standards** are solutions whose values are determined by repeated analyses, using a reference method.
   c. **National Institute of Standards and Technology (NIST)** provides standard reference materials for purchase.
   d. **Standard reference materials (SRMs) and certified reference materials (CRMs)** are produced by the NIST. Values of the materials are determined by high-quality analysis, and the chemical composition is certified.
4. Units of measure:
   Quantitative laboratory results consist of two components, the actual test value and the label identifying the units.
   Système Internationale d'Unités is a system of measurement that is known as **SI units.** SI units may be classified as base, derived, or supplemental units. **Base units** were established for each of the **seven fundamental quantities of measurement.**
   Laboratory results are often reported in terms of substance concentration (e.g., moles) or, more commonly, mass of a substance (e.g., mg/dL, g/dL, and IU). These are referred to as **Traditional or Conventional Units.**
5. **Desiccants** are **drying agents** that absorb water from air or other materials. **Magnesium perchlorate** is one of the most effective desiccants, and **silica gel** is one of the least hygroscopic. **Desiccators** provide a dry environment for chemical materials.

B. Laboratory Supplies and Equipment

1. Laboratory supplies such as pipettes, flasks, etc., used for analytical work must meet specific **tolerances of accuracy** as designated by the NIST. Most laboratory supplies must satisfy certain tolerances of accuracy and must fall into two classes of precision tolerance, **Class A** or **Class B.** Class A supplies are stamped with the letter "A" and are preferred for laboratory applications. Class B glassware has twice the tolerance limits of class A and are often found in student laboratories. Class A and Class B are both given by the **American Society for Testing and Materials (ASTM).**

2. **Types of glass:** Whenever possible, clinical chemistry glassware should consist of high thermal borosilicate or aluminosilicate glass and meet Class A tolerances.
   a. **Flint glass** is made from soda-lime glass. It is inexpensive and used in making some disposable laboratory glassware.
   b. **Borosilicate glass** is commonly used for laboratory glassware because of its properties, including resistance to heat, corrosion, and thermal shock.
   c. **Pyrex** and **Kimax** are glasses that can withstand high temperatures. They are made of borosilicate, which has a low alkali content.
   d. **Corex** is aluminosilicate glass that is six times stronger than borosilicate glass. It is used to make high-temperature thermometers, graduated cylinders, and centrifuge tubes.
   e. **Vycor** glass can be heated to 900°C and is used for extremely high temperatures and resists heat shock.
3. **Types of plasticware**
   a. **Polyolefins** (polyethylene/polypropylene): Chemically inert resins; generally resistant to acids, alkalis, and salt solutions
   b. **Polycarbonate** has a clear appearance and because of its strength may be used for centrifuge tubes. Chemical resistance is less than the polyolefins.
   c. **Fluorocarbon resins** (Teflon): Chemically inert and used for temperatures from −270 to +255°C; provide nonwettable surface; used for stir bars and tubing
4. **Pipettes and calibration**
   a. **Transfer pipettes** are volumetric and Ostwald-Folin.
      1) **Volumetric pipettes** are **"to deliver" (TD)** types that have the bulb closer to the center and accurately deliver a fixed volume of aqueous solution. They drain by gravity and should not be blown out.
      2) **Ostwald-Folin pipettes** are **TD** types that have the bulb closer to the delivery tip because they deliver viscous fluids. These pipettes deliver an accurate volume by being "blown out" using a pipetting bulb. An **etched ring** or a **pair of etched rings** near the top of the pipette indicates the need to **"blow out."**
   b. **Measuring pipettes** are serologic and Mohr.
      1) **Serologic pipettes** are **TD** types that are calibrated to the tip and must be **"blown out"** to deliver entire volume. The need to blow out is indicated by the etched rings at the top of the pipette.
      2) **Mohr pipettes** are **TD** types that are calibrated between marks and cannot be "blown out."
   c. Pipettes labeled **"to contain" (TC)** must be **rinsed out** to deliver the entire contents. Sahli pipettes and some capillary pipettes are in this category.
   d. Semiautomatic and automatic pipettes are handheld and automated, respectively.
      1) **Semiautomatic** are handheld pipettes that use disposable tips, and the laboratorian performs aspiration and dispensing.

2) **Automatic pipettes** are electronic and may not require tips. Many use a glass syringe that aspirates and dispenses through the same tube.

e. Verification of pipette calibration

1) **Gravimetric pipette calibration:** This method verifies the amount of liquid dispensed by a pipette. All equipment and water must be at room temperature before beginning. A specific amount of water is pipetted into a weighed container, and the weight of the water is determined. The weight of the water is proportional to the volume of water pipetted. This is the most desirable method for verifying accuracy and precision of pipettes.

2) **Volumetric pipette calibration:** This method uses a dye of known concentration and water. A specific amount of dye is pipetted into a specific volume of water. Depending on the volume of the pipette, the absorbance of the solution will read a predetermined number. The pipette can then be adjusted and the calibration repeated.

3) Class A pipettes do not need to be recalibrated by the laboratory. Automatic pipetting devices as well as non-Class A materials do need recalibration.

5. **Centrifuges**

a. **Centrifuges** accelerate gravitational separation of substances differing in their masses. **Centrifugal force** is dependent on several parameters, including mass, speed, and radius of rotation. The speed is expressed in revolutions per minute (rpm). The centrifugal force is expressed in terms of relative centrifugal force (RCF) by the following equation:

$$\text{RCF} = 1.118 \times 10^{-5} \times r \times (\text{rpm})^3$$

where 1.118×10^{-5} is a constant,
r is the radius in centimeters (measured from center of axis to the bottom of the test tube shield or bucket.

b. Centrifuges are used to separate blood cells from serum or plasma, separate particulate matter in urine, and separate two liquid phases of different densities.

c. Centrifuge speed should be checked periodically with a **tachometer** for accuracy.

d. Types of centrifuges

1) **Horizontal-head or swinging-bucket centrifuges** allow the tubes to attain a horizontal position in the centrifuge when spinning and a vertical position when the head is not moving.

2) **Fixed-angle or angle-head centrifuges** have angled compartments for the tubes and allow small particles to sediment more rapidly.

3) **Ultracentrifuges** are high-speed centrifuges used to separate layers of different specific gravities. They are commonly used to separate lipoproteins. The chamber is generally refrigerated to counter heat produced through friction.

6. **Balances and weighing**

a. **Mass** is a physical property of matter. A balance compares the mass of an unknown against a known mass.

b. NIST recognizes five types of calibration weights for assessing the accuracy of balances. **Class S weights** are used to check **analytical balances** for proper calibration. **Class M weights** have the quality of a **primary standard** and are used to check the accuracy of other weights.

c. Types of balances

1) **Double-pan balance** has a single beam with arms of equal length. Standard weights are added manually to the pan on the right side to counterbalance the weight of the object on the left-side pan.

2) **Single-pan balance** has arms of unequal length. The object is placed on a pan attached to the shorter arm. A restoring force is applied mechanically to the other arm until the indicator is balanced.

3) **Electronic balance** utilizes electromagnetic force to replace the weights as the counterbalance, with the force being proportional to the weight on the pan.

7. **Thermometers**

a. There are three types of thermometers: **liquid-in-glass** (replaces mercury type), **digital,** and **electronic (thermistor probe).**

b. Thermometers should be **calibrated** against a NIST-certified or NIST-traceable thermometer. NIST provides an **SRM thermometer** with several calibration points, such as 30 and 37°C.

C. Sources and Control of Preanalytical Error

1. **Preanalytical variation** includes the following:

a. **Cyclic variation:** Changes in analyte concentration occur at different times during the day, week, or month.

b. **Diurnal variation:** Variation according to sleeping and waking times

c. **Circadian variation:** Occurs during a 24-hour period

d. **Circannual variation:** Occurs twice a year; related to seasonal changes in climate and diet (elevated in the summer, decreased in the winter)

e. **Physical variables**

1) **Exercise:** May cause alteration of serum potassium, phosphate, creatinine, and protein values

2) **Eating:** Causes increased serum glucose, triglycerides, etc.

3) **Stress:** May cause alteration of serum cortisol (increase), total cholesterol (increase), and even decreased hormone production of pituitary hormones and aldosterone

f. **Blood collection technique errors** in preservatives and/or anticoagulants, specimen type, or drawing technique

1) **Short draws** for coagulation studies are not acceptable.

2) **Proper anticoagulants,** plain red top tubes, or gel separator tubes must be selected based on the testing to be done.

3) **Stasis** caused by tourniquet use and repeated fist clenching, as well as improper drawing techniques, can lead to increased serum potassium, proteins, and metabolic by-products, as well as hemolysis of red blood cells.

4) **Hemolysis** causes false increases in serum levels of lactate dehydrogenase (LD), potassium, and magnesium, as well as a decrease in sodium.
5) **Lipemia** interferes with assays for a number of analytes.
6) **Drawing from a vein receiving intravenous (IV) fluid** dilutes blood analytes but increases the value of analytes present in the IV fluid (e.g., sodium, chloride, or glucose).

g. **Patient identification, sample identification,** and **chain of custody** are major concerns in specimen collection. Proper protocol must always be followed.

h. Although **sample transport** is always important, it is of special concern for accurate analysis of some analytes, such as plasma ammonia, plasma lactate, and blood gases/pH. Specimens for ammonia and lactate analysis should be placed on ice for transport to the laboratory. Blood gas/pH specimens drawn in plastic syringes should be transported immediately to the laboratory for analysis.

i. **Sample processing** involves logging the specimen into a laboratory information system (LIS) and assigning the sample an identification number, sorting and delivering specimens to various departments for testing, centrifuging to separate serum or plasma from red blood cells, and removing serum or plasma from red blood cells (if not in a gel separator tube).

j. **Sample storage**
1) **Separate serum or plasma from red blood cells** as soon as possible, and preferably within 2 hours of blood draw (may need to be sooner for some analytes). Gel separator tubes are commonly used in hospital situations, and they provide a good alternative for off-site collection provided a centrifuge is available (physician offices, clinics).
2) **Serum or plasma** can generally be **stored** at 2–8°C for 2–3 days; for long periods, storage at −20°C is recommended for many analytes.

D. Phlebotomy

1. **Patient and collection preparation**

a. **Introduction:** Phlebotomy personnel should engage professionally, introduce themselves, explain the procedure, be courteous, and act professionally.

b. **Identify the patient.**
1) Ask the patient/client to state his or her name.
2) For an inpatient, compare the patient's name and identification number on the patient's identification band to the laboratory requisition. Electronic scanners may be used to scan patient identification band for confirmation.
3) If the patient is an inpatient and an identification band is not present, the patient's nurse or physician must be asked to identify the patient. The name of the nurse or physician must be recorded on the laboratory requisition.
4) If the patient is an outpatient without an identification band, the patient must provide two unique identifiers (e.g., name and date of birth) for proper identification.

c. **Select the venipuncture site:** The preferred collection site includes the median cubital vein and the cephalic vein; as a last resort, the basilic vein can be used but caution must be taken because of its close proximity to the median nerve and the brachial artery.

d. **Assemble all necessary equipment.**
   1) Gloves, alcohol swabs (betadine for blood cultures and alcohol levels), gauze, tape or band aids, evacuated blood collection tubes, needles, needle holders with safety, and tourniquets (Velcro or latex band; alternative nonlatex, **nitrile** materials should be **used** because of **latex allergies**). Lancets are used for finger sticks.
   2) When selecting blood collection tubes, use tubes with the smallest volume necessary for testing to prevent **iatrogenic anemia.**
   3) Apply the tourniquet and palpate using two fingers to select the most appropriate collection site. The phlebotomist should **never leave** the **tourniquet** on the patient **more than 1 minute.** Patient results will be affected; blood may become more concentrated because of blood flow stasis. If the tourniquet is left on the arm for a prolonged time period, it could also increase the chance of pain and discomfort to the patient and the possible formation of a hematoma.
   4) Needles are available according to gauge including 18, 21, 23, and 25 routinely. The gauge refers to the inner measurement or opening of the needle. The gauge of the needle is inversely related to the size of the needle bore, for example, a **higher number** gauge means that the needle has a **smaller** bore (diameter).
   5) Assemble the needle and needle holder with the evacuated tube, or needle and syringe for blood cultures or collection from fragile veins. Because of small-diameter needles (23 gauge), some phlebotomists prefer using the butterfly (winged collection set) method for difficult draws. It is, however, more difficult to collect large quantities of blood using a butterfly needle.

e. **Perform the venipuncture.**
   1) Needle should enter the site at a 15- to 30-degree angle, with the bevel of the needle facing up.
   2) Advance the evacuated tube onto the needle; change tubes carefully without moving the needle. If the collection tube has an anticoagulant, invert 2–3 times before progressing to the next tube.
   3) Once good blood flow is established or the last tube has been advanced onto the needle, the tourniquet should be removed.

f. **After the blood collection**
   1) Remove the needle, and then immediately apply pressure to the site using a gauze pad.
   2) Engage the safety on the needle immediately and discard needle into sharps container. **Phlebotomists should never recap contaminated needles.**
   3) **Invert tubes** containing anticoagulant several times.

4) If bar coding is not used, label all tubes completely. Although labeling requirements vary among facilities, most require date and time of collection, name or initials of phlebotomist, and patient's name and identification number.
5) Dispose of all contaminated materials appropriately.
6) Thank the patient, remove gloves, and wash hands before leaving the patient's room.

g. **Always maintain patient confidentiality.**

2. **Types of evacuated blood collection tubes**
   a. **Red** stopper tubes contain **no anticoagulant, but do contain silica, which is designed to induce clotting.**
      1) Most commonly used when serum is required for a test
      2) May be used for routine chemistries, therapeutic drug levels, immunohematology, and serology
   b. **Lavender** stopper tubes contain ethylenediaminetetraacetate **(K_3 EDTA), an anticoagulant.**
      1) EDTA ratio is 1.5 mg/1 mL of whole blood. Coagulation is prevented by removing ionized calcium (chelation), which forms an insoluble calcium salt.
      2) Used in hematology for complete blood count, slide preparation, and other routine hematology procedures; also used in immunohematology and for some special chemistry assays.
      3) Alternative formulation of **K_2 EDTA** (**pink** stopper tubes) may be used in immunohematology.
   c. **Light blue** tubes contain **sodium citrate, an anticoagulant.**
      1) Sodium citrate (3.2%) in a 1:10 ratio, 1 part sodium citrate to 9 parts whole blood.
      2) Prevents coagulation by removing ionized calcium (chelation).
      3) Used for **coagulation studies** (e.g., prothrombin time and activated partial thromboplastin time).
   d. **Green** tubes contain **heparin, an anticoagulant.**
      1) Several forms of heparin are available (e.g., lithium heparin and sodium heparin).
      2) Heparin ratio is 0.2 mL/1 mL of whole blood.
      3) Prevents coagulation by inactivating thrombin.
      4) Used for routine and special chemistry and cytogenetic testing.
   e. **Speckled, tiger, or marbled** top **serum** separator tubes (SSTs) contain a **gel separator** and often contain **clot activators.**
      1) The **separator** is a **thixotropic gel** that forms a barrier between the cells and the serum during centrifugation.
      2) These tubes are useful when serum is needed; they are used frequently in clinical chemistry for a number of assays. Serum separator tubes are not recommended for immunohematology or drug levels.

f. **Speckled, tiger, or marbled** top **plasma** separator tubes (PSTs) contain a **gel separator** and an **anticoagulant.** In some cases, the PST stopper color is **green,** which indicates that **lithium heparin** is the anticoagulant.
   1) The **separator** is a **thixotropic gel** that forms a barrier between the cells and the plasma during centrifugation.
   2) These tubes are useful when plasma is needed. Plasma separator tubes reduce the time needed for clot formation and thus speed up the assay process. They are used frequently in clinical chemistry for a number of assays but are not recommended for immunohematology.

g. Gray tubes contain sodium fluoride and may be used to collect samples for glucose analysis. The sodium fluoride will preserve glucose.

3. **Correct order of draw**
   a. To **prevent anticoagulant carryover** and contamination when using a needle and needle holder for blood collection, the following order of draw should be used: **sterile specimen** (blood culture), **light blue** top (sodium citrate; see below), **plain red** top or **SST** serum tubes (with or without clot activator), **green** top (heparin or heparin PST), and **lavender** top or pink top (EDTA), gray (sodium fluoride and sodium or potassium oxalate).
   b. When using the butterfly (winged collection set) to collect a sodium citrate tube, if it is the first tube to be collected, then a discard tube (plain red or another sodium citrate tube) must be collected first to remove the air from the tubing. Sodium citrate tubes must be completely filled to ensure the correct plasma:anticoagulant ratio, or the test results could be compromised.

II. LABORATORY QUALITY ASSESSMENT

A. Definitions

1. **Total quality management (TQM)** is a managerial process that focuses on improvement of the quality of all factors that affect laboratory testing and performance. It consists of five elements: quality laboratory process, quality control, quality assessment, quality improvement, and quality planning.
2. **Quality assessment (QA):** This is a systemic laboratory program, encompassing preanalytical, analytical, and postanalytical factors, that monitors excessive variation in specimen acceptability, test methodologies, instruments, reagents, quality control, and personnel competencies. This process is used to ensure accurate patient test results.
3. **Preanalytical error** occurs during sample collection and transport before sample analysis and can include sample preparation and storage conditions.
4. **Analytical error** occurs during the testing process and includes problems related to reagents, instruments, controls, calibration, performance of personnel, etc.
5. **Postanalytical error** occurs after the test is performed and refers to clerical errors, reporting of results, test interpretation, etc.
6. **Accuracy** is a measure of a laboratory test result's closeness to the true value.
7. **Precision** is realized when repeated laboratory test results yield the same number; reproducibility.

8. **Reliability** refers to the ability of laboratory testing to maintain accuracy and precision over an extended period of time.
9. **Quality control (QC):** A system used to monitor the analytical process to detect and prevent errors that would impact on the accuracy and precision of laboratory test results; includes both statistical and nonstatistical parameters.
   a. **Internal QC** is performed by laboratory personnel using control materials of known values and comparing the control values to established, acceptable ranges. The control material values are assessed using Levey-Jennings control charts and Westgard multirules to detect errors.
   b. **External QC** is performed by laboratory personnel when analyzing specimens sent to the laboratory by an external agency, and the results generated are submitted to the agency for assessment. This type of assessment is known as **proficiency testing.** It is required by federal regulations for all laboratories providing results for human diagnosis and/or treatment.
10. **Linearity check** determines the lowest and highest values that can be accurately measured by a particular method. This is an example of a nonstatistical QC parameter.
11. **Random errors** affect precision, are unable to predict because they have no known pattern, and may alternate between a positive or negative direction.
12. **Systematic errors** are predictable and cause a constant difference in results that are consistently positive or negative or stay the same. Such errors may be due to incorrect calibration, deteriorated reagents, instrument malfunction, etc.
13. **Delta check** assesses the patient's most recent result for a particular test as compared to the patient's previous value; the difference between the test results (delta) is calculated and compared to established limits.
14. **Reference ranges** are determined by each laboratory to fit their particular population. Intervals are generally constructed by adding and subtracting two standard deviations from the mean.
15. **Standard** is material of known concentration (should be traceable to NIST) that is used to calibrate an instrument or develop a standard curve.
16. **Control** is material of known value that is analyzed with patient samples to determine acceptability of results.
   a. **Assayed control:** Values are assigned by the manufacturer.
   b. **Unassayed control:** Values are determined by each individual laboratory for their methods/instruments.
17. **Westgard multirules** are statistical "rules" applied to graphical summaries of numerical quality control data to assess the acceptability of such data.
18. **Six Sigma** is a data-driven, business approach to performance improvement; it is oriented toward process identification and process improvement.
19. **Lean principles** are an improvement trend to make work faster by providing ways to streamline through the removal of waste.
20. **ISO 9000 Standards** were established by the International Organization for Standardization as a series of four standards for quality management.

B. Specimen Quality

1. Test result quality depends on the quality of the sample submitted.
2. Specimen quality depends on the following:
   a. Patient preparation
   b. Labeling procedures
   c. Timing of specimen collection
   d. Special collection instructions
   e. Specimen handling and transport requirements
   f. Criteria for unacceptable specimens.

C. Operating Instructions

1. **Laboratory procedures** should contain the following information: test name, method principle, significance of test, patient preparation, test specimen requirements, equipment and materials needed, reagent preparation, test procedure, calculations, quality control procedures, reference intervals, panic values, limitations of the procedure, and references, including the instrument user manual. Each procedure must be reviewed, signed, and dated annually.
2. Instrument user manuals and instrument maintenance manuals must be available, and all maintenance performed must be documented.

D. Selecting Instruments

1. Selection criteria should include instrument cost, reagent cost, throughput, technical support, personnel training, method linearity, range of methods available, test methodologies, analytical sensitivity and specificity, etc.
2. Instruments are evaluated to determine instrument and method accuracy, precision, systematic error, linearity, and calibration stability.

E. Statistical Analysis

1. **Arithmetic mean** ($\bar{x}$) of a set of numbers is obtained by adding all the numbers in the set and dividing the sum by the number of values in that set.
2. **Median** is the middle value in a set of numbers that are arranged according to their magnitude.
3. **Mode** is the most frequently obtained value in a set of numbers.
4. **Standard deviation (*s*)** reflects the variation of data values around the mean.
5. **Variance (s^2)** reflects dispersion around the mean and is the square of the standard deviation.
6. **Coefficient of variation (CV)** reflects random variation of analytical methods in units that are independent of methodology, because it is a percentage comparison of the standard deviation divided by the mean.
7. **Normal distribution** is a symmetric distribution about the mean, where 95.45% of the values lie within $\pm 2\,s$ and approximately 5% will normally fall outside.

8. The diagnostic **sensitivity** of a test is the percentage of individuals with a specific disease that are correctly identified or predicted by the test as having the disease. It reflects the ability of a test to detect a given disease or condition. Diagnostic sensitivity is calculated as follows:

$$\text{Diagnostic Sensitivity (\%)} = \frac{\text{True Positives}}{\text{True Positives} + \text{False Negatives}}.$$

9. The diagnostic **specificity** of a test is the percentage of individuals without the specific disease that are correctly identified or predicted by the test as not having the disease. It reflects the ability of a test to correctly identify the absence of a given disease or condition. Diagnostic specificity is calculated as follows:

$$\text{Diagnostic Specificity (\%)} = \frac{\text{True Negatives}}{\text{True Negatives} + \text{False Positives}}.$$

10. **Predictive value** of a test utilizes the parameters of test sensitivity and specificity as well as disease prevalence (i.e., incidence of a disease or condition).
    a. **Positive predictive value** is the percentage of people with positive test results who have the disease.
    b. **Negative predictive value** is the percentage of people with negative test results who do not have the disease.

F. Reference Intervals

1. **Reference intervals (ranges)** are calculated for each laboratory's menu of tests. Each laboratory serves a unique population, so the reference intervals must be determined for that population.
2. Use a **minimum of 20 specimens** from "healthy" people to determine analyte values, calculate the mean and standard deviation, and compare to the reference interval suggested by the manufacturer.
3. **Preferably,** analyte values should be determined using a **minimum of 120 specimens** from healthy people in each relevant sex and age category.
4. Calculate the **mean** and **standard deviation.**
5. **Reference intervals** are calculated using the **mean +2 standard deviations** (high value) and the **mean −2 standard deviations** (low value) to include 95% of the "healthy" population.

G. Internal Quality Control

1. **Purpose:** It is a comprehensive program involving statistical analysis of control materials, which are analyzed with a batch of patient samples to determine acceptability of the run.
2. **Control material**
    a. Commercially manufactured **lyophilized or liquid materials** that have the **same matrix** as patient specimens and are used to evaluate the test process.

b. Control materials are handled exactly like patient specimens: Analysis conditions (incubation time, analysis temperature, calculation, etc.) and preanalysis conditions if warranted (precipitation, protein-free filtrate, etc.).
c. Control materials are selected so that values will be at **medically significant** levels. Generally, one control will have a value within the reference interval, and a second control will have an abnormal (elevated) value.
d. It is preferred that the **same lot number** of control material be purchased and used for at least a 1-year period.
e. Lyophilized control material must be **accurately reconstituted** according to the manufacturer's directions to avoid vial-to-vial variability. The stability of the reconstituted material is important.
f. For **qualitative controls,** use materials that will provide **both negative and positive results.**

3. **Data evaluation procedures for control materials**
   a. **Levey-Jennings control chart** is constructed monthly for each control material using the mean ± 3 standard deviations to construct a graph that allows visual detection of shifts and trends. The control value is plotted versus the established range, with the **acceptable control range represented by ± 2 standard deviations.**
      1) Control values that exceed the mean ± 2 standard deviations are generally considered unacceptable and alert personnel to investigate the cause, unless using multirule where a ± 2 standard deviation violation serves as a warning.
      2) **Trend** is a gradual change in the mean that is reflected as either a decrease or increase of consecutive control values (generally the number of consecutive observations signifying a trend is six or more). The change occurs only in one direction.
      3) **Shift** is a sudden change in the mean that is reflected as consecutive control values above or below the mean.
      4) **A loss of precision** is obvious on the chart when control values become more dispersed.
      5) The difference between a test and reference method results in error. There are two types of error, random and systematic.
         a) **Random error** is unpredictable and can be either positive or negative. Random error can be due to instrument, operator, reagent, and environmental variation. It is calculated as the standard deviation of the points about the regression line, also known as S_{y}/x. The higher the S_{y}/x, the wider the scatter, and the higher the random error.
         b) **Systematic error** is predictable and affects data consistently in one direction. There are two types of systematic error: 1) **constant systematic error,** which results in continual difference between test and reference regardless of the concentration, and 2) proportional systematic error where the difference between the test and reference increases with the analyte concentration.

c) Constant systematic error is defined by the y-intercept, and proportional systematic error is defined by the slope. Both slope and y-intercept are part of the linear regression equation: Y = mx + b (b = y-intercept and M = slope). When two methods perfectly agree, the slope is 1.0 and the Y-intercept is 0.

b. **Westgard multirule** is a control procedure that utilizes control rules to assess numerical quality control data; the control rules establish the limits for data rejection in a system with two controls. Other rules apply when three controls are used.

1) $\mathbf{1_{2s}}$—1 control value exceeds the mean ± 2 standard deviations; warning rule that triggers inspection of control values using the other rejection rules that follow; only rule that is not used to reject a run; results are reportable if no other rule violation occurs.
2) $\mathbf{1_{3s}}$—1 control value exceeds the mean ± 3 standard deviations; detects random error.
3) $\mathbf{2_{2s}}$—2 consecutive control values exceed the same 2 standard deviation (*s*) limit (same mean +2 *s* or same mean −2 *s*); detects systematic error.
4) $\mathbf{R_{4s}}$—1 control value in a group exceeds the mean +2 *s* and a second control value exceeds the mean −2 *s*, creating a 4 standard deviation spread; detects random error.
5) $\mathbf{4_{1s}}$—4 consecutive control values are recorded on one side of the mean and exceed either the same mean +1 *s* or the same mean −1 *s*; detects systematic error.
6) $\mathbf{10_x}$—10 consecutive control values are recorded on one side of the mean (either above or below the mean); detects systematic error.

4. **Youden plot** is a graphical technique for analyzing interlaboratory data when each laboratory has made two runs on the same analyte or one run on two different analytes. The plot identifies **within-laboratory** and **between-laboratory** variability.

H. External Quality Control

1. **External quality control** refers to a program where a clinical laboratory contracts with an agency (e.g., College of American Pathologists or American Association of Bioanalysts) to receive and assay samples, the concentration of which is unknown to the participating clinical laboratory. The same samples are sent by the agency to reference laboratories for analysis for the purpose of establishing target values and ranges of acceptability. The results generated by the participating clinical laboratory are sent to the agency for comparison to the values established by the reference laboratories for the purpose of assessing the clinical laboratory's level of performance. This is known as proficiency testing.
2. **Proficiency testing:** An agency sends proficiency samples to a clinical laboratory to analyze, and the results generated are assessed by the agency for accuracy to determine the performance of the laboratory. Assessment reports are sent to participating laboratories to assist with performance analysis and test method and

equipment selection. Federal CLIA '88 (Clinical Laboratory Improvement Amendments '88) requires that all laboratories performing human testing for diagnosis and/or treatment must use proficiency testing for all analytes it reports. Failure to comply can result in sanctions, including a complete closure of the laboratory.

3. **Proficiency samples** have a similar matrix to patient specimens, are generally shipped in a lyophilized form with diluent, and are utilized in proficiency testing programs.
4. **Limitations of external quality control programs**
   a. Some laboratories will **treat proficiency samples differently** than normal patient specimens (i.e., special handling, running controls before and after each proficiency sample, calibrating the assay before running the proficiency sample, special selection of personnel to perform the assay, etc.). Such deviation from routine workload procedures will not reflect the accuracy and precision of the laboratory.
   b. Proficiency samples **do not reflect the preanalytical component** of patient identification, collection, and handling procedures. There could be problems in these areas that an external quality control program is not designed to address.
5. For a clinical laboratory to comply with **CLIA '88,** the laboratory must successfully participate in proficiency testing. In turn, the agencies that provide proficiency testing to clinical laboratories must be approved by the Centers for Medicare and Medicaid Services (CMS).

III. LABORATORY SAFETY

A. Regulatory Oversight

1. **Occupational Safety and Health Administration (OSHA)**
   a. Federal agency charged with the enforcement of safety and health legislation
   b. **Occupational Safety and Health Act of 1970** makes employers responsible for providing a safe and healthy workplace for their employees.
   c. **Hazardous Communication Programs,** also known as the **Right to Know Standard:** The purpose of this standard is to ensure that chemical hazards in the workplace are identified and information concerning these hazards is communicated to employers and employees.
2. **Centers for Disease Control and Prevention (CDC):** Federal agency that publishes numerous safety standards
3. **The Joint Commission:** Issues standards and grants accreditation to improve the safety and quality of care provided to the public through inspections of healthcare facilities.
4. **College of American Pathologists (CAP):** Issues standards and offers accreditation through inspections.

B. Safety Program

1. Accreditation organizations require clinical laboratories to have a formal safety program. The program needs to ensure that the laboratory environment meets approved safety standards.
2. **Safety officer or chair of the safety committee:** Responsibility is to implement and maintain a safety program.

3. **Chemical hygiene officer (CHO):** OSHA requires that laboratories have a designated CHO whose responsibility is to provide technical guidance in the development and implementation of the chemical hygiene plan.
4. **Safety data sheet (SDS)** is a major source of safety information for hazardous materials in the laboratory. The SDS must be provided by the manufacturer and includes the following 16 items:
   a. Section 1: Identification
   b. Section 2: Hazard Identification
   c. Section 3: Ingredients Information
   d. Section 4: First Aid Procedures
   e. Section 5: Fire-Fighting Procedures
   f. Section 6: Accidental-Release Measures
   g. Section 7: Handling and Storage
   h. Section 8: Exposure Controls and Personal Protection
   i. Section 9: Physical and Chemical Properties
   j. Section 10: Stability and Reactivity
   k. Section 11: Toxicology Information
   l. Section 12: Ecological Information
   m. Section 13: Disposal Considerations
   n. Section 14: Transport Information
   o. Section 15: Regulatory Information
   p. Section 16: Other Information, Including Date of Preparation or Last Revision
5. **Safety inspections**
   a. The laboratory should have a safety committee or inspection team periodically inspect the laboratory.
   b. Several federal, state, and private accreditation organizations (e.g., CAP and The Joint Commission) conduct inspections of healthcare facilities. These inspections may be regularly scheduled or unannounced. Inspections may also follow a complaint filed against a facility.

C. Personal Safety
1. **Wash hands** before leaving the laboratory and after taking off gloves.
2. **Do not mouth pipet.**
3. Tie back long hair and avoid loose sleeves/cuffs, rings, bracelets, etc.
4. **Do not apply cosmetics** in the laboratory.
5. **Eating and drinking are forbidden in the laboratory.**
6. **Housekeeping**
   a. Maintain orderly work areas.
   b. Keep aisle-ways clear and free of tripping hazards.
   c. Keep floors dry to avoid slipping; attend to spills immediately.

D. Personal Protective Equipment
1. OSHA requires that employers provide all necessary **personal protective equipment** (PPE) to employees.
2. **Eye protection:** Goggles and face shield

3. **Protective clothing**
   a. The **laboratory coat** is designed to protect the clothing and skin from chemicals that may be spilled or splashed. It should be worn buttoned up and with the sleeves extended to the wearer's wrist.
   b. **Foot protection** is designed to prevent injury from corrosive chemicals or heavy objects. If a corrosive chemical or heavy object were to fall on the floor, the most vulnerable portion of the body would be the feet. For this reason, shoes **that completely cover and protect** the foot are worn in the laboratory.
4. **Hand protection:** Heat-resistant gloves for handling hot or cold objects (e.g., dry ice) and latex or nitrile gloves to prevent exposure to biological hazards must be available. Selection of protective gloves is based on chemical hazard and the tasks involved.

E. Safety Equipment

1. **Individual storage containers**
   a. Selecting the best means of storage for chemical reagents will, to a great extent, depend on that reagent's compatibility with the container. A safety can is an approved container of no more than 5-gallon capacity. It has a spring-closing lid and spout cover and is designed to safely relieve pressure buildup within the container.
   b. **Sharps containers:** Hard containers for the disposal of sharp objects such as used phlebotomy needles, broken contaminated glass, and pipettes.
2. **Eye wash stations** must be inspected and tested periodically for proper function.
3. **Safety showers** provide an effective means of treatment in the event that chemicals are spilled or splashed onto the skin or clothing. They must be inspected and tested periodically for proper function.
4. **Refrigerators**
   a. Standard refrigeration units are **not appropriate for storing flammable materials.**
   b. **Laboratory refrigerators are not appropriate for storing food for consumption.** Each refrigerator and freezer must be labeled, "No food or beverages may be stored in this refrigerator."
   c. Each refrigerator and freezer must be monitored daily to ensure proper functioning.
5. **Alarms** are designed so that endangered personnel are alerted. All individuals should become familiar with the exact location of the fire alarm stations nearest to their laboratory.
6. **Chemical spill kits**
   a. Laboratories are equipped with clean-up kits for various types of spills. Wear the appropriate PPE (i.e., gloves, goggles) when cleaning up spills.
   b. **Acid spills**
      1) Apply neutralizer (or sodium bicarbonate) to perimeter of spill.
      2) Mix thoroughly until fizzing and evolution of gas ceases.
      3) Transfer the mixture to a plastic bag, tie shut, fill out a waste label, and place in a fume hood.
   c. **Solvent spills**
      1) Apply activated charcoal to the perimeter of the spill.
      2) Mix thoroughly until material is dry and no evidence of solvent remains.
      3) Transfer absorbed solvent to a plastic bag, tie shut, and place in fume hood.

7. **Chemical fume hood**
   a. The only safe place to work with some highly toxic and volatile chemicals.
   b. Partially enclosed ventilated work space for volatile chemicals.
   c. Chemical fume hoods are generally ducted and vent air outside the building.
   d. Fume hoods are not to be used for the storage of hazardous chemicals.
8. **Biological safety cabinets**
   a. **Class 1 cabinets** have an open front and are under negative pressure. Air is exhausted into the room after passing through high-efficiency particulate air (HEPA) filters.
   b. **Class 2 cabinets** provide added protection by forcing HEPA-filtered air downward at the front of the cabinet where the laboratorian is working. The air can be exhausted into the room **(Class 2A)** or outside the building **(Class 2B).**
   c. **Class 3 cabinets** are gas-tight. The interior of the cabinet is only accessible through glove ports.
   d. Chemical fume hoods and biological safety cabinets **cannot** be used interchangeably. Fume hoods will not protect workers from infectious agents, and biological safety cabinets may not protect against chemical vapors. In addition, chemicals can damage the HEPA filters in biological safety cabinets.

F. Waste Collection and Disposal

1. Discard all nonsharp biohazardous substances into biohazard bags.
2. Dispose of used tubes in biohazard bags.
3. Dispose of swab wrappings, band aid wrappings, used paper towels, kit boxes, and any other nonbiohazardous waste into regular trash bags.
4. Do not discard nonbiohazardous waste into red biohazard bags.
5. Store chemicals in appropriate chemical can. Chemicals should not be poured down sink drains.

G. Mandated Plans

1. **Chemical hygiene plan**
   a. OSHA requires laboratories to have a chemical hygiene plan.
   b. List of responsibilities of employers and employees
   c. Chemical inventory list
   d. Copies of the SDSs must be readily available.
2. **Exposure control plan**
   a. OSHA requires that all laboratories have an exposure control plan to minimize risk of exposure to **bloodborne pathogens** (BBPs).
   b. Regulates disposal of medical waste
3. **Ergonomic plan**
   a. CAP requires laboratories to have an ergonomic plan to minimize risk of work-related musculoskeletal disorders.
   b. Avoid awkward posture, repetitive motion, and repeated use of force.
   c. Employer must provide training and appropriate equipment, and an assessment and documentation system.

4. **Transportation and shipping of clinical specimens**
   a. Laboratories are responsible for preventing people from being exposed to infectious agents during transport.
   b. The Department of Transportation (DOT), International Air Transport Association (IATA), and the International Civil Aviation Organization (ICAO) developed strict guidelines for the handling and shipping of hazardous materials. Only special approved shipping containers can be used. Only individuals who have received training and have a permit are allowed to ship hazardous material.

H. Laboratory Hazards

1. **The United Nations** (UN) established the following nine classes of hazardous materials:
   a. Class 1—explosives
   b. Class 2—compressed gases
   c. Class 3—flammable liquids
   d. Class 4—flammable solids
   e. Class 5—oxidizer materials
   f. Class 6—toxic materials
   g. Class 7—radioactive materials
   h. Class 8—corrosive materials
   i. Class 9—miscellaneous materials not classified elsewhere.
2. **Warning labels**
   a. The DOT requires all chemicals shipped in the United States have labels based on the UN hazardous material classification.
   b. DOT labels are diamond shaped with the classification number in the bottom corner. The hazard is also identified in words along the horizontal axis of the label.
   c. The DOT label is only on the shipping container. Once received, the laboratory must label each individual container in the shipping container.
   d. Although OSHA mandates the use of labels or appropriate warnings, no single uniform labeling system exists for hazardous materials.
   e. As of June 2015, the Hazard Communication Standard (HCS) requires pictograms on labels to alert users of chemical hazards to which they may be exposed. Each pictogram consists of a symbol (representing a distinct hazard) on a white background framed within a red border. The pictogram on the label is determined by the chemical hazard classification.
   f. The **National Fire Protection Association** (NFPA) developed the **704-M Identification System,** which most laboratories use.
      1) The labels are diamond shaped, and each quadrant has a different color: **blue**—health; **red**—flammability; **yellow**—reactivity; and **white**—special information. The chemical is classified 0–4 (least hazardous to most hazardous) in the areas of health, flammability, and reactivity.
      2) The chemical can be identified as a poison, water reactive, etc., in the white quadrant.

Hazard	Pictogram	Descriptors
Health		Carcinogen Mutagenicity Reproductive Toxicity Respiratory Sensitizer Target Organ Toxicity Aspiration Toxicity
Flame		Flammables Pyrophorics Self-Heating Emits Flammable Gas Self-Reactives Organic Peroxides
Exclamation Mark		Irritant (skin and eye) Skin Sensitizer Acute Toxicity (harmful) Narcotic Effects Respiratory Tract Irritant Hazardous to Ozone Layer (Nonmandatory)
Gas Cylinder		Gases Under Pressure
Corrosion		Skin Corrosion/Burns Eye Damage Corrosive to Metals
Exploding Bomb		Explosives Self-Reactives Organic Peroxides
Flame over Circle		Oxidizers
Environment (Nonmandatory)		Aquatic Toxicity
Skull and Crossbones		Acute Toxicity (fatal or toxic)

3. **Chemical hazards**
   a. Approved spill kits must be nearby.
   b. Concentrated acids must be diluted by adding them to water in the sink.
   c. Label all containers **before** adding the chemical.
   d. Some chemicals can become more hazardous if stored for a prolonged time. **Picric acid** has the potential to form peroxides if stored for a long period of time and not used. The material can become **shock sensitive,** with the potential to explode if bumped.
   e. **Sodium azide,** a carcinogen, is sometimes used as a preservative in laboratory reagents. When disposed of in the sewer, the accumulation of copper and iron salts of azide may occur. These metallic salts are explosive, especially when subjected to mechanical shock.
   f. Working with **carcinogens** requires special precautions such as using a fume hood, wearing rubber gloves and a respirator, and cleaning contaminated glassware with a strong acid or organic solvent.
   g. **Chemical containers** made of glass should be transported in rubber or plastic holders that will protect them from breakage.
4. **Fire hazards**
   a. **Flammability** is a measure of how easily a gas, liquid, or solid will ignite and how quickly the flame, once started, will spread. **Flammable** and **inflammable** both mean "to catch fire easily."
   b. **Flammable liquids themselves are not flammable; rather, the vapors from the liquids are combustible.** There are two physical properties of a material that indicate its flammability: flash point and volatility (boiling point).
      1) The **flash point** of a material is the temperature at which a liquid (or volatile solid) gives off vapor in quantities significant enough to form an ignitable mixture with air.
      2) The **volatility** of a material is an indication of how easily the liquid or solid will pass into the vapor stage. Volatility is measured by the boiling point of the material—the temperature at which the vapor pressure of the material is equal to the atmospheric pressure. Volatile solvents should be stored in small amounts in an explosion-proof refrigerator.
      3) The flash point of **flammables** is designated as less than 100°F, and that of **combustibles** as greater than 100°F.
   c. Xylene, ethanol, methanol, and acetone are flammable chemicals commonly used in clinical laboratories that must be stored in a **flammable liquid safety cabinet.**
   d. Some materials are **pyrophoric,** meaning that they can ignite spontaneously with no external source of ignition. Potassium metal, for example, can react with the moisture in air.
   e. **Storage**
      1) **Flammable materials should never be stored near acids.**
      2) **Storage areas should be cool** enough to prevent ignition in the event that vapors mix with air. Adequate ventilation should be provided to prevent vapor buildup.

3) **Avoid storage of flammable materials in conventional** (non-explosion-proof) **refrigerators.** Sparks generated by internal lights or thermostats may ignite flammable material inside the refrigerator, causing an extremely dangerous explosion hazard.
4) Be aware of **ignition sources** in your laboratory area (heat sources, electrical equipment).

f. **Handling**
1) Use gloves and safety goggles when handling flammable liquids or vapors.
2) Dispensing of flammable or combustible liquids should only be done in a fume hood or in an approved storage room.
3) Do not use water to clean up flammable liquid spills.

g. **Extinguishers**
1) Extinguishers are classified according to a particular fire type and are given the same letter and symbol classification as that of the fire.
    a) **Type A**—combustibles: wood, cloth, paper, rubber, and plastics
    b) **Type B**—flammable liquids: oil, grease, and paint thinners
    c) **Type C**—energized electrical equipment: electrophoresis
    d) **Type D**—combustible metals: magnesium, titanium, sodium, lithium, potassium
2) Type A extinguishers are pressurized water extinguishers effective with Class A fires; Type A, B, and C extinguishers are dry chemical extinguishers effective with Class A, B, and C fires; Type B and C extinguishers are carbon dioxide extinguishers effective with class B and C fires; halogenated hydrocarbon extinguishers are recommended for use with computers, electrical equipment, motors, and switches.
3) **Multipurpose extinguishers** are highly recommended because they are effective against multiple types of fires.
4) Class D fires present specific problems, and extinguishment is left to trained firefighters using special dry chemical extinguishers. When encountering a class D fire, it is recommended that you isolate burning metal from combustible surfaces with either sand or a ceramic carrier material.
5) **Biological hazards**
    a) The National Institutes of Health guidelines describe four levels of biosafety depending on the biological agents isolated or studied. The levels are based on the virulence of the agents and the availability of effective treatments and vaccines.
        1) **Biosafety Level 1** laboratories handle agents that have no known potential for infecting healthy people.
        2) **Biosafety Level 2** laboratories are those laboratories that work with microorganisms associated with human diseases that are rarely serious and for which preventive or therapeutic interventions are often available. Most clinical microbiology laboratories are Level 2.

3) **Biosafety Level 3** is recommended for materials that may contain viruses not normally encountered in a clinical laboratory and for the cultivation of mycobacteria. Clinical laboratories offering these services must have a Level 3 facility. Working with mycobacteria requires the use of **N95 HEPA filter respirators;** surgical masks are not acceptable.
4) **Biosafety Level 4** is required for work with dangerous and exotic agents that pose a high risk of aerosol-transmitted laboratory infections and life-threatening disease for which effective treatments are limited.

b) **Exposure risks**
1) Accidental punctures with needles
2) Spraying (aerosols) or spilling infectious materials onto desktop or floor
3) Cuts or scratches from contaminated object
4) Centrifuge accidents: Aerosols, broken tubes, etc.

c) **Bloodborne pathogens** are transmitted through contact with infected blood and body fluids and include **human immunodeficiency virus, hepatitis B virus** (HBV), and **hepatitis C virus.**

d) Use **standard precautions,** and treat all blood or potentially infectious body fluids as if they are contaminated. Avoid contact whenever possible, and whenever it's not, wear personal protective equipment.

e) All surfaces, tools, equipment, and other objects that come in contact with blood or potentially infectious materials **must be decontaminated** and sterilized as soon as possible. Decontamination is recommended with an approved disinfectant or **5.25% chlorine bleach** (sodium hypochlorite; NaOCl) solution, a 1:10 dilution of household bleach. The diluted bleach solution should be made daily.

f) OSHA requires that employers offer employees **HBV vaccine** if their regular duties present a potential for exposure to the virus.

g) Before leaving the laboratory, laboratorians should wipe the countertop with a disinfectant, wash their hands in an antiseptic soap, and remove their laboratory coat.

h) Microbiology laboratories are engineered to maintain negative air pressure with respect to the administrative areas. This maintains airflow into the laboratory, minimizing the risk of airborne pathogens exiting the laboratory when a door is opened.

6) **Compressed gases**

a) Transportation of compressed gases is regulated by the DOT.
b) NFPA labels should be attached to each cylinder.
c) Gas cylinders should be secured onto a hand truck for transporting.
d) Gas cylinders must be stored in a vertical position chained to a wall.
e) When in use, gas cylinders must be securely fastened to a wall or laboratory bench.

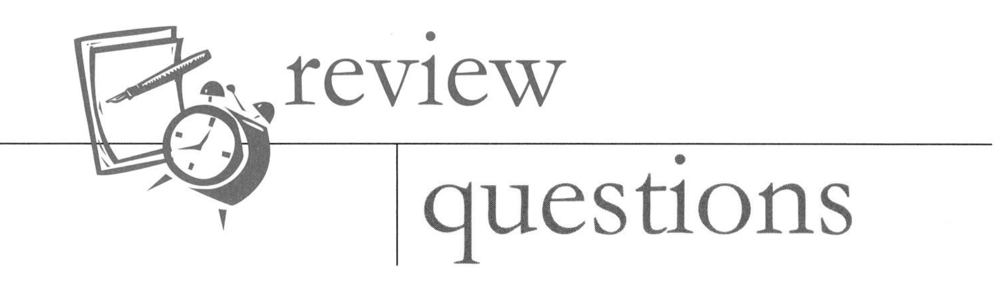

INSTRUCTIONS Each of the questions or incomplete statements that follows is comprised of four suggested responses. Select the *best* answer or completion statement in each case.

General Laboratory Principles

1. Which of the following is an alumina-silicate glass that is at least six times stronger than borosilicate and is resistant to alkaline etching and scratching?
   A. Kimax
   B. Pyrex
   C. Corning boron free
   D. Corex

2. The National Institute of Standards and Technology (NIST) requires that volumetric pipettes and flasks be certified as:
   A. Class A
   B. Class B
   C. Class C
   D. Class D

3. Which of the following types of water is recommended for routine clinical use?
   A. Special reagent water
   B. Instrument feed water
   C. Purified water
   D. Reagent grade

4. Lavender top blood collection tubes are used for complete blood counts. Which of the following anticoagulants is in these tubes?
   A. EDTA
   B. Heparin
   C. Sodium citrate
   D. Sodium oxalate

5. SI units are the designated units employed by the International System of Units. The unit class that encompasses the seven fundamental quantities of measurement is:
   A. Base
   B. Primary
   C. Derived
   D. Elemental

6. Which of the following containers is calibrated to hold only one exact volume of liquid?
   A. Graduated cylinder
   B. Erlenmeyer flask
   C. Volumetric flask
   D. Griffin beaker

7. Which of the following storage temperatures is recommended when storing routine samples 2–3 days?
   A. −80°C
   B. −20°C
   C. 5°C
   D. Room temperature
8. "To deliver" (TD) pipettes are identified by which of the following?
   A. Two etched bands near the top
   B. Self-draining capacity
   C. Dual-purpose pipette labels
   D. Blue graduation levels
9. If a laboratory needs to keep certain chemical materials dry, the apparatus used will be a
   A. Buret
   B. Desiccator
   C. Separatory funnel
   D. Vacuum
10. Which of the following is an advantage of the angle-head centrifuge over the horizontal-head centrifuge?
    A. Less air friction
    B. Smaller increase in sample temperature during centrifugation
    C. Can be operated at a higher speed
    D. All of the above
11. The type of water desired for use in test methods requiring maximum accuracy and precision is
    A. Distilled
    B. Pure grade
    C. Reagent grade
    D. Special reagent water
12. The speed of a centrifuge should be checked at least once every 3 months with a(n)
    A. Tachometer
    B. Wiper
    C. Potentiometer
    D. Ergometer
13. The type of balance that uses an electromagnetic force to counterbalance the load placed on the pan is a(n)
    A. Trip balance
    B. Class A balance
    C. Class S balance
    D. Electronic balance
14. At which of the following angles should a needle be when performing routine venipuncture?
    A. 5°
    B. 20°
    C. 50°
    D. 90°
15. When performing a venipuncture, which of the following is the proper order of draw for evacuated blood collection tubes?
    A. Sterile specimen, light blue top, and plain red top
    B. Light blue top, plain red top, and sterile specimen
    C. Lavender top, light blue top, plain red top
    D. Green top, sterile specimen, and plain red top

Laboratory Quality Assessment

16. Which of the following terms applies to the sum of all the values in a set of numbers divided by the number of values in that set?
    A. Median
    B. Mode
    C. Arithmetic mean
    D. Geometric mean
17. Calculate the coefficient of variation (percent) for a set of data where the mean $(\bar{x}) = 89$ mg/dL and 2 standard deviations $(s) = 14$ mg/dL.
    A. 7.8
    B. 7.9
    C. 15.7
    D. 15.8

18. What does the preparation of a Levey-Jennings quality control chart for any single constituent of serum require?
    A. Analysis of control serum over a period of 20 consecutive days
    B. 20 to 30 analyses of the control serum, on 1 day, in one batch
    C. Analyses consistently performed by one person
    D. Weekly analyses of the control serum for 1 month

19. A batch of test results is out of control. What should you do first?
    A. Report the results to the physician first, and then look for the trouble.
    B. Follow the "out-of-control" procedure specified for the test method.
    C. Repeat the tests with a new lot of standards (calibrators).
    D. Repeat the tests with a new lot of reagents.

20. In addition to utilizing Levey-Jennings charts, what other criteria should be applied to interpret internal quality control data?
    A. Westgard multirule
    B. Cusum
    C. Linear regression
    D. Youden

21. A new standard (calibrator) has been prepared in error at a lower concentration than that required for the test. How would such an error appear on a quality control chart?
    A. Upward trend
    B. Downward trend
    C. Upward shift
    D. Downward shift

22. The ± 2 standard deviation ($\pm 2s$) range of acceptable values for a digoxin control is established as 2.0–2.6 ng/mL. On the average, the expectation that a value will be greater than 2.6 ng/mL is 1 in
    A. 10
    B. 20
    C. 40
    D. 100

23. What is the purpose of a Youden plot?
    A. Compares results on two control specimens, low and high controls, for the same analyte analyzed by several laboratories.
    B. Evaluates the validity of daily results on a single control specimen over a period of 30 days.
    C. Compares results on a single control specimen by two different methods for the same analyte.
    D. Evaluates the validity of daily results of two control specimens within a single laboratory.

24. If the therapeutic range for the gentamicin assay is a trough level of less than 2 μg/mL and a peak level of 5–8 μg/mL, what would be the appropriate mean values for two control levels (in micrograms per milliliter) used to monitor the system?
    A. 1 and 2
    B. 1 and 3
    C. 1.5 and 6
    D. 5 and 6

25. Systematic error can best be described as consisting of:
    A. Random and constant errors
    B. Constant and proportional errors
    C. Total and random errors
    D. Syntax and proportional errors

26. On a quality control chart, when would a statistical out-of-control situation requiring corrective action be suspected?
    A. Six successive plots fall above and below the mean within $\pm 1\ s$.
    B. Six successive plots fall above and below the mean within $\pm 2\ s$.
    C. One plot falls within the area of $\pm 2\ s$ to $3\ s$ within a 20-consecutive-day span.
    D. One plot falls outside the area of $\pm 3\ s$ within a 20-consecutive-day span.

27. Which of the following would result in a sudden shift in daily values on a quality control chart?
    A. Recalibrating the instrument when changing reagent lot numbers during an analytical run
    B. Replacing the instrument's sample aspiration probe
    C. Changing the spectrophotometer lamp in the middle of a sample run
    D. Changing personnel operating the instrument

28. Which of the following terms refers to the measure of scatter of experimental data around the mean of a Gaussian (normal) distribution curve?
    A. Median
    B. Mode
    C. Coefficient of variation
    D. Standard deviation

29. The percentage of individuals without a specific disease who are correctly identified or predicted by the test as not having the disease describes which of the following?
    A. Sensitivity
    B. Specificity
    C. Positive predictive value
    D. Negative predictive value

30. Which of the following terms refers to deviation from the true value caused by indeterminate errors inherent in every laboratory measurement?
    A. Random error
    B. Standard error of the mean
    C. Parametric analysis
    D. Nonparametric analysis

31. Which of the following would result in analytical error?
    A. Sample preparation
    B. Clerical error
    C. Result reporting
    D. Performance of personnel

32. Which of the following terms refers to the closeness with which the measured value agrees with the true value?
    A. Random error
    B. Precision
    C. Accuracy
    D. Variance

33. What percentage of values will fall between $\pm 2s$ in a Gaussian (normal) distribution?
    A. 34.13%
    B. 68.26%
    C. 95.45%
    D. 99.74%

34. Which of the following terms refers to a measure of dispersion or spread of values around a central value?
    A. Range
    B. Validity
    C. Variance
    D. Coefficient of variation

35. Which of the following describes the ability of an analytical method to maintain both accuracy and precision over an extended period of time?
    A. Reliability
    B. Validity
    C. Probability
    D. Sensitivity

36. Which of the following is calculated by the formula $\frac{\sum (x - \bar{x})^2}{n - 1}$?
    A. Coefficient of variation
    B. Variance
    C. Confidence limits
    D. Standard deviation
37. Given the following regression equation, what is the slope?

    $$Y = 2.0 + 1.03X.$$

    A. Y
    B. 2.0
    C. 1.03
    D. X
38. A group of physicians consistently complains that they are not receiving stat patient results quickly enough. The supervisor is likely to refer to which quality assessment variable?
    A. Specimen separation and aliquoting
    B. Test utilization
    C. Analytical methodology
    D. Turnaround time
39. To provide independent validation of internal quality control programs, external surveys have been developed. Which of the following is a representative survey program?
    A. Clinical and Laboratory Standards Institute (CLSI)
    B. American Society for Clinical Laboratory Science (ASCLS)
    C. American Society for Clinical Pathology (ASCP)
    D. College of American Pathologists (CAP)
40. A tech is scheduled to perform a specialized test that she/he is familiar with, but is not *exactly* certain of the steps required. What is the best course of action to take?
    A. Ask another tech to perform the test.
    B. Consult the procedure manual and notify the supervisor.
    C. Run the test as best as possible, being careful to note control values.
    D. Reject the specimen.
41. A tech has completed the first run of morning specimens. She/he notices that the one control being used is outside $\pm 3\ s$. What course of action should be taken?
    A. Release the results.
    B. Repeat the control only, and if it comes in, release results.
    C. Check equipment and reagents to determine source of error; repeat the entire analysis, including the control and patients; if the control value is within $\pm 2\ s$, release results.
    D. Repeat the control; if the same thing happens, attribute the cause to random error; release results.
42. Which of the following describes the Westgard multirule 2_{2s}?
    A. Two control data points are within $\pm 2\ s$.
    B. One control data point falls outside $+2\ s$ and a second point falls outside $-2\ s$.
    C. Two consecutive data points fall outside $+2\ s$ or fall outside $-2\ s$.
    D. Two consecutive data points fall outside $+2\ s$.

43. Which of the following Westgard multirules applies to a situation where one control point exceeds the mean by +2 *s* and a second control point exceeds the mean by −2 *s*?
   A. 1_{2s}
   B. 2_{2s}
   C. 4_{1s}
   D. R_{4s}

44. Upon admission to the hospital, a chemistry profile is performed on a patient. The patient has a total bilirubin of 2.0 mg/dL. The next day a second chemistry profile is done, and the patient's total bilirubin is 6.2 mg/dL. What should be done in regard to these results because the normal and abnormal controls are within acceptable limits?
   A. Immediately call the physician to alert him/her to the second abnormal result.
   B. Immediately send the second result to the patient's floor for charting.
   C. Repeat the entire second run of patient specimens because there must be an error.
   D. Perform a delta check and, if warranted, look for possible sources of error.

45. When comparing a potential new test with a comparative method in order to bring a new method into the laboratory, one observes error that is consistently affecting results in one direction. What is this type of error known as?
   A. Systematic error
   B. Random error
   C. Constant systematic error
   D. Proportional systematic error

46. When establishing a reference interval for a new test being introduced into the laboratory, what is the preferred number of subjects that should participate?
   A. 30
   B. 50
   C. 75
   D. 120

47. A small laboratory has collected blood samples from 20 individuals as part of a reference interval study for a new test being introduced into the laboratory. Of the test results, four are outside the reference interval published by the manufacturer. How should you proceed?
   A. Delete the four results and only use the 16 within the range to establish the lab's reference interval.
   B. Use all 20 results when calculating the ±2 *s* range because outliers are to be expected.
   C. Run four additional samples, and if within the manufacturer's range, add them to the original 16 for statistical analysis.
   D. Obtain an additional 20 samples for testing, and if two or less are outside the suggested range, then the manufacturer's reference interval can be accepted.

48. Given the following regression equation for a comparison between two cholesterol methods, which of the following statements is true?

$$Y = 1.01x + 3.0$$

   A. There is no error.
   B. There is random error.
   C. There is constant systematic error.
   D. There is proportional systematic error.

49. Which of the following must be known in order to determine the sensitivity of a test?
   A. True positives and false negatives
   B. True negatives and false positives
   C. True positives and false positives
   D. True negatives and false negatives

50. A new test to assess for the presence of malignancy has been developed. By testing a group of benign individuals, it is determined that 45 of 50 subjects test negative for the new marker. What is the specificity of this new assay?
    A. 10%
    B. 11%
    C. 90%
    D. 100%
51. Which of the following must be known in order to determine the predictive value of a negative test—that is, the percentage of individuals who test negative and are not diseased?
    A. True negatives and false negatives
    B. True positives and false positives
    C. True positives and false negatives
    D. True negatives and false positives
52. Which of the following statements is *false* about proficiency-testing programs?
    A. Participation is mandated by the Centers for Medicare and Medicaid Services under CLIA '88.
    B. College of American Pathologists and the American Association of Bioanalysts are two major providers of these programs.
    C. Samples of unknown concentrations are periodically sent to labs participating in the program.
    D. Acceptable ranges are provided with the samples so labs can determine if it is necessary to repeat the assay.

Laboratory Safety

53. Which of the following is a reactive chemical that has the potential to become shock sensitive if stored for a prolonged period of time?
    A. Xylene
    B. Picric acid
    C. Chloroform
    D. Phenol
54. A fire extinguisher used in the event of an electrical fire should include which of the following classifications?
    A. Type A
    B. Type B
    C. Type C
    D. Type D
55. In the National Fire Protection Association identification system, four color-coded, diamond-shaped symbols are arranged to form a larger diamond shape. What type of hazard does the blue diamond identify?
    A. Flammable
    B. Health
    C. Reactivity
    D. Contact
56. Xylene, ethanol, methanol, and acetone would be in which of the following hazard classes?
    A. Corrosive
    B. Flammable
    C. Oxidizer
    D. Carcinogen
57. Which of the following organizations is responsible for enforcement of safety and health legislation?
    A. The Joint Commission
    B. College of American Pathologists
    C. Occupational Safety and Health Administration
    D. Centers for Disease Control and Prevention

58. A Biosafety Level 2 (BSL-2) laboratory is designed to work with microorganisms that are:
    A. Not associated with disease in healthy adult humans
    B. Associated with serious or lethal human disease for which preventative or therapeutic interventions may be available
    C. Likely to cause serious or lethal human disease for which preventative or therapeutic interventions are not usually available
    D. Associated with human disease that is rarely serious and for which preventative or therapeutic interventions are often available

59. The flash point of a liquid may be defined as the:
    A. Minimum temperature at which self-sustained ignition will occur
    B. Maximum vapor pressure at which spontaneous ignition will occur
    C. Temperature at which an adequate amount of vapor is produced, forming an ignitable mixture with air at the liquid's surface
    D. Temperature that is 10°C greater than the liquid's boiling point

60. A corrosive material was spilled onto the hand of a laboratorian. After diluting the material under running cold water, what should be done next?
    A. Consult the material safety data sheet.
    B. Wipe up the spill with paper towels.
    C. Dilute the spill with water and remove it in a biohazard bag.
    D. Go to the nearest hospital emergency department.

61. Most clinical microbiology laboratories are categorized at what biosafety level?
    A. 1
    B. 2
    C. 3
    D. 4

62. The maximum chemical exposure allowable for an employee during one 8-hour day is the
    A. Flash point
    B. HEPA standard
    C. Threshold limit value
    D. Limit established by the United Nations

63. Which of the following types of fire extinguishers should be used on electrical fires?
    A. Type A
    B. Type B
    C. Type C
    D. No extinguisher will work on these types of fires; it is recommended you call the fire department

64. The air-handling system for a microbiology laboratory should
    A. Maintain negative pressure with respect to the administrative areas
    B. Maintain positive pressure with respect to the administrative areas
    C. Have no particular requirement
    D. Have a HEPA filter

65. Precautions such as using a chemical fume hood, wearing rubber gloves, donning a respirator, and cleaning glassware with a strong acid or organic solvent are consistent with working with
    A. Corrosives
    B. Carcinogens
    C. Azides
    D. Acids

66. A laboratorian, properly dressed in white pants, laboratory coat, and shoes, prepares to leave the laboratory for lunch. In addition to washing his/her hands, he/she should:
    A. Put on safety goggles
    B. Remove his laboratory coat
    C. Wipe the bench with water
    D. Remove polyvinyl gloves and place them into lab coat pocket for future use

67. Which of the following may be a potentially hazardous biological situation?
    A. Handling specimens collected from patients in isolation according to standard precautions
    B. Keeping the centrifuge lid closed until the system has stopped completely
    C. Discarding sharp objects, including broken glass, in a puncture-proof container
    D. Discarding disposable blood collection needles in the patient's wastebasket

68. Which of the following is associated with proper storage of chemicals?
    A. All chemicals should be stored in alphabetical order for ease of handling.
    B. Flammable chemicals should be stored in a chemical fume hood.
    C. Large containers of liquid chemicals should be stored on a top shelf to allow easy visibility from below.
    D. Volatile solvents should be stored in small amounts in an explosion-proof refrigerator.

69. A laboratorian spills a bottle of concentrated sulfuric acid and slips in the fluid, exposing the lower length of her body to the burning fluid. What would be the most advisable action for a coworker to take?
    A. Call security.
    B. Put the person under the safety shower.
    C. Take the injured person to the nearest hospital emergency department.
    D. Pour concentrated base on the person to neutralize the acid.

70. A stat procedure requiring a corrosive reagent (organic acid) is requested. To transport this reagent to the work area under the chemical fume hood, a laboratorian should:
    A. Employ a rubber carrier with handles
    B. Pour an amount near the storage site and transport it
    C. Pipette the required volume and carry the pipette to the work area
    D. Carry the brown bottle by the loop with one hand under the bottom of the container

71. Which of the following statements pertains to the safe handling of compressed gases?
    A. Large cylinders should be loosely placed on a hand cart when being transported.
    B. Cylinders must be secured to a wall or bench when in use.
    C. Cylinders should be stored along with flammable liquids because both are combustible.
    D. Large cylinders should be ordered to avoid frequent movement in and out of stock.

72. The major job-related disease hazard in clinical laboratories is
    A. Tularemia
    B. Salmonella
    C. Tuberculosis
    D. Hepatitis

73. The responsibility to implement and maintain a safety program in a clinical laboratory belongs to the:
    A. State public health laboratory
    B. Chemical hygiene officer
    C. Laboratory safety officer
    D. Chief pathologist

74. Based on the chemical properties of azides, which of the following factors has motivated laboratories to monitor their use?
    A. The buildup of salts can lead to explosions.
    B. They are corrosive to pipes even when diluted.
    C. They are extremely volatile.
    D. They are flammable and dangerous near an open flame.

75. A biological safety cabinet that forces HEPA-filtered air downward at the front of the cabinet where the laboratorian is working describes a
    A. Class 1 cabinet
    B. Class 2 cabinet
    C. Class 3 cabinet
    D. Class 4 cabinet

76. The phrase "Standard Precautions" refers to a concept of bloodborne disease control that requires all human blood and other potentially infectious materials:
    A. Be treated as if known to be infectious for bloodborne pathogens regardless of the perceived "low risk" of a patient population
    B. Be treated as if it is not infectious unless it is known to be infectious
    C. Must be handled using a respirator for aerosol exposure
    D. Need not be treated with caution unless there is a cut on your hand

77. The biological safety cabinet is the single most useful safety device in the microbiology laboratory. How do Class 2A cabinets differ from Class 2B?
    A. Class 2A exhausts HEPA-filtered air into the room.
    B. Class 2B exhausts HEPA-filtered air into the room.
    C. Class 2B cabinets are larger.
    D. Class 2A cabinets contain gas jets for a Bunsen burner.

78. Chlorine is most often used in the form of sodium hypochlorite (NaOCl), found in household bleach, for a disinfectant. Which of the following dilutions of household bleach is recommended by the Centers for Disease Control and Prevention to clean up blood spills?
    A. 1:1
    B. 1:10
    C. 1:20
    D. 1:100

79. The clinical hematology laboratory just received a new disinfectant to use in place of the one normally used. Never having used this particular disinfectant before, how should the lab professional proceed?
    A. Use it full strength; you can always be sure if you do this.
    B. Read the manufacturer's package insert and prepare the product according to directions.
    C. Make the concentration 10% higher than the manufacturer's recommendations.
    D. Put the new disinfectant under the sink for storage.

80. What written plan of specific measures must laboratories have in place to minimize the risk of exposure to bloodborne pathogens?
    A. Chemical hygiene plan
    B. Exposure control plan
    C. Material safety data sheets
    D. Infection control plan

81. A fire caused by a flammable liquid should be extinguished using which of the following types of extinguishers?
    A. Class B
    B. Halogen
    C. Pressurized
    D. Water Class C

82. Work is being done with *Mycobacterium tuberculosis* in the microbiology laboratory. It is important that you enter this laboratory while work is being done with positive samples. What is the most important personal protective equipment you should don before entering this laboratory?
    A. Carbon cartridge respirator
    B. Mask
    C. Gloves
    D. N95 HEPA filter respirator

83. When working with chemicals, the selection of your gloves depends on
    A. The chemical hazard and the tasks involved
    B. How far you must transport the chemical
    C. Whether or not you use a chemical fume hood
    D. Whatever is available in the laboratory

84. What is the maximum capacity of a chemical storage safety that can be used in the laboratory?
    A. 1 gallon
    B. 5 gallons
    C. 20 gallons
    D. 55 gallons

answers & rationales

General Laboratory Principles

1\.

D. Several types of glassware are commonly used in the laboratory, each having its specific purpose. Corex glass is used in the manufacture of centrifuge tubes and thermometers. Pipettes, beakers, and flasks are generally made from Pyrex or Kimax borosilicate glass.

2\.

A. The National Institute of Standards and Technology (NIST) and the College of American Pathologists (CAP) state that volumetric pipettes and flasks must be of certified accuracy. Class A glassware meets federal guidelines and fulfils the CAP requirements. All non–class A glassware must be recalibrated periodically by an acceptable verification procedure.

3\.

D. Water is the most frequently used reagent in the laboratory; however, tap water is unsuitable for most laboratory applications. The lab, therefore, purifies water through multiple processes to create reagent grade water, the type of water suitable for most routine laboratory purposes.

4\.

A. Lavender top blood collection tubes contain EDTA as an anticoagulant. The EDTA chelates calcium, which is required for the coagulation cascade. Heparin is the anticoagulant in green top tubes, sodium citrate in blue top tubes, and potassium oxalate in gray top tubes.

5\.

A. The Système Internationale d'Unités was established to facilitate a uniform system of measurement. SI units may be classified as base, derived, or supplemental units. Base units were established for each of the seven fundamental quantities of measurement: length (meter), mass (kilogram), time (second), electric current (ampere), amount of substance (mole), temperature (kelvin), catalytic amount (katal), and luminous intensity (candela). Derived units are mathematically calculated from more than one base unit.

6.

C. Flasks, beakers, and graduated cylinders are used to hold solutions. Volumetric and Erlenmeyer flasks are two types of containers in general use in the clinical laboratory. The volumetric flask is calibrated to hold one exact volume of liquid, also known as to contain (TC). Graduate cylinders, Griffin beakers, and Erlenmeyer flasks are calibrated to measure different volumes of liquids and are not as accurate as the volumetric flask.

7.

C. When samples arrive to the laboratory, they are processed and analyzed. Samples should be analyzed within 4 hours and properly capped and kept away from areas of light, airflow, and heat to help maintain the integrity of the sample. The recommended storage temperature for most routine samples is 4–6°C. If the samples are being held longer, storage at −20 and −80°C is appropriate for most analytes.

8.

A. Serologic pipettes are "to deliver" (TD) types and are not rinsed out. These pipettes are not self-draining but must be blown out to deliver their entire contents, as is indicated by the two etched rings at the top of the pipette. "To contain" (TC) pipettes, such as Sahli pipettes, must be rinsed out to deliver their entire contents.

9.

B. Desiccators provide a dry environment for chemical materials. A shelf is placed on top of the desiccant on which the material to be stored can be set. A heavy glass cover closes the system. An airtight seal is provided by placing stopcock grease around the ground glass joints between the desiccator and the lid.

10.

D. In an angle-head centrifuge, the cups are rigidly supported in the head at a fixed angle to the shaft, and they are fully enclosed within the head. In a horizontal-head centrifuge, the cups hang down in a vertical position when the centrifuge is at rest and swing out to a horizontal position when the centrifuge is rotating. Because cups in the angle-head centrifuge are enclosed in a head specifically designed to reduce wind resistance, there is less air friction and, consequently, less of an increase in sample temperature during centrifugation. Because of the reduced wind resistance, angle-head centrifuges can provide a force of over 9000 × *g*, whereas horizontal-head centrifuges provide about 1650 × *g*.

11.

C. Reagent grade water should be used when a high degree of accuracy is desired, as in quantitative chemistry assays and in the preparation of standards and buffers. Reagent grade water requires deionization through acidic and basic ion-exchange columns, removal of organic materials by activated charcoal adsorption, and semipermeable membrane filtration for the removal of microorganisms and other particulate material. Special reagent water is for specific uses and, depending on the use, may need to be sterilized.

12.

A. Centrifugal force may be determined by knowing the mass of the solution and the speed and radius of the centrifuge. With aqueous solutions having a specific gravity near 1.0, the specific mass need not be known. To determine the speed, use either a strobe light, positioned over the revolving centrifuge head, or a tachometer to establish the revolutions per minute (rpm).

13.

D. An electronic balance is a single-pan balance that uses an electromagnetic force to counterbalance the load placed on the pan. These balances are top-loading in design and permit weighings to be made quickly. The Mettler Instrument Corporation makes a representative electronic balance.

14.

B. For phlebotomy procedures performed on most individuals, the recommended angle of insertion is 15–30 degrees with the bevel of the needle facing up.

15.

A. To prevent anticoagulant carryover and contamination when using a needle and needle holder for blood collection, evacuated blood collection tubes should be collected in a proper order. Sterile specimens should be drawn first to minimize risk of contamination for blood cultures. After sterile collections, the following order should be used: light blue top, plain red top or serum separator tube, green top (heparin or heparin PST), and lavender top.

Laboratory Quality Assessment

16.

C. The arithmetic mean of a set of numbers is obtained by adding all the numbers in the set and dividing the sum by the number of values in that set. It is a precise way of expressing what is often called the average. It is not to be confused with the mode, which is the value that occurs most frequently in the set. The geometric mean is the antilogarithm of the sum of the logarithms of all the values divided by the number of values. The median is the middle value in a set of numbers that are arranged according to their magnitude.

17.

B. The coefficient of variation is calculated from the following formula:

$$CV = \frac{s}{\bar{X}} \times 100\%,$$

where CV = coefficient of variation, s = 1 standard deviation, and $\bar{x}$ = mean. Given that the mean = 89 mg/dL and 2 s = 14 mg/dL,

$$CV = \frac{7}{89} \times 100\% = 7.86\%.$$

Because there are only two significant figures in each of the given numbers, there can be only two figures in the answer. Therefore, when rounded to the nearest tenth, the answer is 7.9, not 7.8.

18.

A. Any analytical result has some degree of uncertainty because of unavoidable random errors in the procedure. A Levey-Jennings quality control chart is a graphic representation of the acceptable limits of variation in the results of an analytical method. To prepare such a chart, it is first necessary to obtain a large-enough batch of normal and abnormal pooled serum to last for a minimum of 12 months. Analyses of aliquots of the pools are done in duplicate over a period of 20 days, preferably by all workers who will subsequently be using the controls. The data thus collected are statistically analyzed to determine the mean and standard deviation. Any results falling above or below the mean $\pm 3\,s$ are discarded. The mean and standard deviation are then recalculated. The acceptable range is assigned, usually the mean $\pm 2\,s$. The data thus developed are used to prepare the Levey-Jennings quality control chart. A similar protocol may also be followed when setting up standard deviation parameters for new lots of assayed control materials.

19.

B. The purpose of a quality control chart is to facilitate the identification of analytical problems that are not otherwise apparent. A quality control program must include clearly written instructions for the steps that are to be taken when a control serum value is out of control. These instructions must be used whenever a set of test results is out of the established control limits. Usually the procedures will include a visual inspection of the equipment, reagents, and instruments used, and a check of calculations. The next step might be to rerun the batch of tests with a fresh aliquot of control serum. Additional steps to take include preparing newly reconstituted controls, recalibrating the instrument, and using a fresh bottle of reagent. Out-of-control results should never be reported to the physician.

20.

A. When assessing daily, internal quality control, the Westgard multirule procedure aids in interpretation of control data. A chart similar to the Levey-Jennings chart is constructed with control limits drawn at the mean as well as $\pm 1\,s$, $\pm 2\,s$, $\pm 3\,s$, and even $\pm 4\,s$. The Westgard multirules are then applied to the graphical representation, giving a more structured approach to data interpretation.

21.

C. On a quality control chart, when the control values change abruptly and on several consecutive days are consistently on one side of the mean, although within the $\pm 2\,s$ limits, this is called a shift. An upward shift could be produced by changing to a new standard (calibrator) that was prepared in error at a lower concentration than specified. A downward shift could be caused by the use of too concentrated a standard (calibrator) than what is specified. A gradual change observed over the course of several days is called a trend. It may be upward or downward. Its presence suggests gradual deterioration of one of the reagents or instrument components.

22.

C. If the range of acceptable values for a quality control material is based on the $\pm 2\,s$ intervals on either side of the expected mean value for the control, then about 19 of every 20 values obtained for the control are expected to fall within the acceptable range. Conversely, about 1 of every 20 values obtained are expected to fall outside the $\pm 2\,s$ range with about 1 of every 40 values above the upper acceptable limit and the same number below the acceptable limit. For example, if a digoxin control is established to have an acceptable range from 2.0 to 2.6 ng/mL, about 1 value in 40 would be expected above 2.6 ng/mL.

23.

A. A Youden plot is a type of quality control chart that is used to compare results obtained on a high and low control serum by several different laboratories. It is particularly useful for interlaboratory quality control programs. The Youden plot displays the results of the analyses by plotting the mean values for one specimen on the ordinate and the other specimen on the abscissa. It is desirable for a laboratory to have its point fall at the center of the plot.

24.

C. The choice of appropriate concentrations for control materials is important in implementing a quality control program. The concentrations chosen should be sensitive to assay variability in the clinically significant region of the particular compound being measured. For instance, the therapeutic range for the drug gentamicin in many laboratories is a trough level that is less than 2 μg/mL and a peak level of 5–8 μg/mL. Control levels of 1.5 and 6 μg/mL would appropriately monitor both trough and peak regions of the standard curve. If both controls are above 5 or below 4 μg/mL, only one region of the curve would be monitored.

25.

B. The difference between two methods is known as error. There are two types of error, systematic and random. Random error is unpredictable, is present in all measurements, and can be either positive or negative on both sides of the assigned target value. Systematic error is predictable error and is further broken down into two types, constant and proportional errors.

26.

D. On a quality control chart, the acceptable range generally encompasses the mean ±2 *s*. The control values should occur randomly in this area, falling to both sides of the mean. If more than five successive plots occur at a constant level in one area (e.g., near the ±2 *s* line), an out-of-control situation should be considered. One plot falling outside the mean ±2 *s* in 20 successive days is expected statistically. Although one should be alert to the possibility of a potential problem, it does not necessarily imply an out-of-control situation. However, the occurrence of a value outside the area of ±3 *s* would require corrective action.

27.

C. When a quality control chart shows a sudden shift in daily values, there are several possible causes. Use of a new batch of reagents or reference standards (calibrators) that have been improperly made can cause such a shift. Another cause for a sudden shift in daily values might be a change in one of the components of the instrument, such as a new lamp in a spectrophotometer. Whenever an instrument component is changed, the instrument must be recalibrated. A change in operating personnel should not cause any change in quality control values.

28.

D. The standard deviation reflects how much the data values vary around the mean. The mean is the arithmetic average of the data and is a measure of the location of the distribution. The median describes the middle value; half of the observations are greater than the median, half are less than the median. The mode is the most frequently obtained value. The coefficient of variation expresses random variation of analytical methods in units independent of methodology, because it is a percentage comparison of the standard deviation divided by the mean.

29.

B. Specificity is the percentage of individuals without the specific disease who are correctly identified or predicted by the test as not having the disease. The sensitivity of a test is the percentage of individuals with a specific disease who are correctly identified or predicted by the test as having the disease. The positive predictive value is the percentage of people who tested positive with the test who have the disease, and the negative predictive value is the percentage of people who tested negative with the test who do not have the disease.

30.

A. Random errors are deviations from the true value caused by unavoidable errors inherent in laboratory measurements. The standard error of the mean is a statistical concept reflecting sampling variation. It is the standard deviation of the entire population. Parametric statistics refer to a Gaussian (normal) distribution of data. Nonparametric statistics are more general and require no assumptions.

31.

D. There are three types of variation that exist in the laboratory, preanalytical, analytical, and postanalytical. Preanalytical errors, like the name implies, occurs due to processes before the analysis of the patient sample, such as cyclic variation, diurnal and circadian variation, physical variables (exercise, eating, and strass), and blood collection technique errors. Analytical errors occur during the sample analysis phase of testing and include instrument errors and calibration errors. Postanalytical errors occur after the sample has been analyzed including, interpretation errors, time delay to the physician, etc.

32.

C. The accuracy of an analytical result is the closeness with which the measured value agrees with the true value. Precision is reproducibility. Accuracy and precision are independent, but it is the goal of the clinical laboratory to design methods that are both precise and accurate.

33.

C. The normal distribution is a symmetric distribution about the mean. In a normal distribution, 95.45% of the values will be within an area enclosed by the mean $\pm 2\ s$ and approximately 5% will normally fall outside; 68.26% will lie within $\pm 1\ s$; 99.74% will lie within $\pm 3\ s$. The $\pm 2\ s$ (95.45%) interval forms the basis of statistical quality control in the laboratory.

34.

C. Variance is one way in which members of a group are dispersed about the mean. It is a square of the standard deviation (s^2). Both standard deviation and variance are measures that describe how observed values vary.

35.

A. The reliability of an analytical procedure is its ability to maintain accuracy and precision over an extended period of time during which supplies, equipment, and personnel in the laboratory may change. It is often used interchangeably with the term "consistency." It is the goal of every clinical laboratory to produce reliable results.

36.

B. The variance is the measure of dispersion, which is the square of the standard deviation. To determine the variance, find the difference between each value and the mean, square this difference, add the differences, and divide by one less than the number of values. The variance reflects scattering about the mean.

37.

C. Before introducing a new method/instrument into the clinical laboratory, assurances need to be made regarding the precision and accuracy of the new method compared to the procedure currently in place and measured against allowable error limits set by CLIA'88. One criteria used in the method evaluation process is a comparison of methods study involving a split-sample study of 40–100 clinical specimens. All samples should be assayed by both methods within a 4 hour period of time and over several days. Data analysis involves plotting test method results on the y-axis and the comparative method on the x-axis. One statistical technique used during this study is regression analysis to determine a regression equation with a slope and y-intercept. The regression equation $Y = mx + b$ with m being the slope and b being the y-intercept.

38.

D. Maintaining quality assessment includes control of preanalytical, analytical, and postanalytical factors. One variable to assess is turnaround time. It is the total amount of time required to procure the specimen, prepare the specimen, run the test, and relate the results. The supervisor should refer to the turnaround time of the stated procedure and relate to the techs they need to work within the stated limits.

39.

D. The College of American Pathologists comprehensive survey involves thousands of participating clinical chemistry laboratories. This survey and others have been established to provide independent validation of quality control programs. A CAP survey provides unknown samples for analysis. The program, when properly used, gives valid estimation of the inherent accuracy of a system. CLSI develops laboratory standards to improve the quality of medical care. ASCLS and ASCP are organizations to which medical laboratory personnel may apply for professional membership.

40.

B. Whenever one needs to review the details of a procedure, one should review the procedure manual and notify the supervisor so that guidance can be received. The procedure manual is one way in which a laboratory can document analytical protocols. This leads to consistency in test results regardless of which person is performing the analysis.

41.

C. When checking control results that fall outside acceptable limits, one can apply the Westgard multirule procedure, specifically 1_{3s}. Anytime only one control is used and it exceeds the mean $\pm 3s$, you must reject the test run. You should check the instrument and reagent system to locate the problem, if possible. A new control along with the patient specimens should be analyzed. No results should be reported until the control is within the limits of $\pm 2s$ from the mean.

42.

C. Westgard multirule 2_{2s} describes an out-of-control situation where two consecutive data points fall outside the same mean +2 *s* or fall outside the same mean –2 *s*. This is an example of systematic error. The test run would be rejected, and all samples would need to be retested.

43.

D. When one control point exceeds the mean by +2 *s* and a second control point exceeds the mean by –2 *s*, the R_{4s} multirule will apply. In this case, the out-of-control problem is most likely due to random error. The test run would be rejected, and all samples would need to be retested.

44.

D. When the same test is ordered on a patient more than once, a delta check can be performed to compare consecutive test results. Bilirubin results obtained on two consecutive days on an adult should not vary by more than 50%. If the results vary by greater than 50%, it is most likely that an error has occurred or an acute change has taken place. One of the first things to check is proper identification of the patient's specimen. As part of a quality assessment program, one should also check patient results based on the clinical correlation of laboratory test results.

45.

A. When comparing a potential new test with a comparative method in order to bring a new method into the laboratory, linear regression analysis should be performed using the results of the two methods. By calculating the slope and *y* intercept, the presence of systematic error can be identified. Unlike random error that is due to chance and can occur in either direction, systematic error consistently affects results in only one direction. Specific types of systematic error are termed constant and proportional, but the stated question did not give sufficient information to differentiate between the types.

46.

D. Although some laboratories may use the reference interval recommended by the manufacturer or ranges published in medical books, it is preferred that laboratories establish their own limits. When subjects are not easily available, a laboratory should use at least 20 individuals to verify a published range. Whenever possible, a minimum of 120 subjects with representatives from each age and sex group should be included in the reference interval study.

47.

D. When the population served by a laboratory is similar to that described by a manufacturer, then the reference interval published by the manufacturer can be adopted provided the laboratory successfully completes a small study. Such a study need only include 20 individuals. If two or less subjects tested have test values that fall outside the suggested range, then the manufacturer's reference interval can be used. If three or more subjects have test values that fall outside the range, then an additional 20 subjects need to be tested. Provided that two or less are outside the range on this second attempt, then the manufacturer's reference interval can be accepted. In the event that this second attempt fails, the laboratory should assess what differences there may be between their population and that of the manufacturer. If differences cannot be determined, then a complete reference interval study using 120 subjects should be completed by the laboratory.

48.

A. When performing a method comparison study, a commonly used statistical analysis involves regression analysis to develop a regression equation. The regression line provides an equation that can be used to predict Y from X ($Y = bx + a$). In a perfect relationship between two methods, the slope would be 1.0 and the y-intercept 0. However, that is rarely the case in the clinical laboratory. The slope in this equation is an indicator of proportional error while the y-intercept is an indicator of constant error. In this case, with the regression equation of $Y = 1.01x + 3.0$, there is little to no proportional error as defined by the 1.01 (slope near 1.0). There is constant error present with a y-intercept of 3.0 (ideal is 0).

49.

A. The *sensitivity* of a test is the percentage of individuals with a specific disease that are correctly identified or predicted by the test as having the disease. To determine the sensitivity of an assay, the true positives, represented by the number of individuals correctly identified by the test as having the disease, and the false negatives, represented by the number of diseased individuals not correctly identified by the test, must be established for the assay in question. The formula for determining sensitivity follows, where TP = true positives and FN = false negatives,

$$\text{Sensitivity} = \frac{TP}{TP+FN} \times 100.$$

50.

C. The *specificity* of a test is the percentage of individuals without the specific disease who are correctly identified or predicted by the test as not having the disease. To determine the specificity of an assay, the true negatives, represented by the number of individuals correctly identified by the test as not having the disease, and the false positives, represented by the number of nondiseased individuals not correctly identified by the test, must be established for the assay in question. The formula for determining specificity follows, where TN = true negatives and FP = false positives,

$$\text{Specificity} = \frac{TN}{FP+TN} \times 100$$

$$= \frac{45}{5+45} \times 100$$

$$= \frac{45}{50} \times 100$$

$$= 90\%.$$

51.

A. The predictive value of a test utilizes the parameters of test sensitivity and specificity as well as disease prevalence. The predictive value of a negative test (i.e., the percentage of individuals who test negative and are not diseased) may be determined by knowing the number of true negatives and false negatives. The formula for determining the predictive value of a negative test (PV^-) follows, where TN = true negatives and FN = false negatives,

$$PV^- = \frac{TN}{TN+FN} \times 100.$$

52.

D. A proficiency testing program is part of external quality control that aids a lab in assessing the quality of its testing methods. Samples of unknown concentrations are purchased through a recognized professional agency such as the College of American Pathologists or the American Association of Bioanalysts. Samples are periodically sent to labs participating in the program. Following analysis of the samples, the lab sends its results to the agency for review. If significant problems are detected, the laboratory needs to take corrective action. Participation is mandated by the Centers for Medicare and Medicaid Services under CLIA '88.

Laboratory Safety

53.

B. Picric acid has the potential to form peroxides if stored for a long period of time and not used. If this happens, the bottle can become shock sensitive with the potential to explode if knocked. All other chemicals listed do not pose this risk.

54.

C. A fire extinguisher is classified and labeled for the type of fire on which it should be used. An ABC fire extinguisher is commonly found in laboratories. Type A extinguishers are used on fires of ordinary combustibles such as paper, cloth, wood, rubber, and plastics. Type B extinguishers are used on fires of flammable liquids including oils, gasoline, and solvents. Type C extinguishers are used on electrical equipment fires. Type D extinguishers are used on fires involving combustible metals (e.g., magnesium, sodium).

55.

B. The National Fire Protection Association developed the 704-M Identification System to provide common, recognizable warning signals for chemical hazards. The system consists of four color-coded, diamond-shaped symbols arranged to form a larger diamond shape. The blue diamond symbol located to the left identifies potential health hazards. The diamond symbol located at the top of the larger diamond is color-coded red, indicating a flammability hazard. The yellow diamond symbol to the right represents reactivity-stability hazards. The white diamond symbol located at the bottom provides information on special precautions. Contained within each color-coded diamond is a number ranging from 0 to 4, indicating the severity of the respective hazard (0 = none and 4 = extreme). A number of chemical manufacturers have adopted this warning system for their labels.

56.

B. All hazardous chemicals in the workplace must be identified and clearly marked with a National Fire Protection Association label. All the chemicals listed are flammable. Corrosive chemicals are harmful to mucous membranes, skin, eyes, or tissues.

57.

C. Safety is an important part of requirements for initial and reaccreditation of health care institutions. The Occupational Safety and Health Act (OSHA) was enacted by U.S. congress in 1970. It is the federal body that sets and regulates safety in laboratories.

58.

D. The National Institutes of Health guidelines describe Biosafety Level 2 laboratories as those laboratories that work with microorganisms associated with human disease that is rarely serious and for which preventive or therapeutic interventions are often available. Biosafety Level 1 laboratories handle agents that have no known potential for infecting healthy people. Biosafety Level 3 is recommended for materials that may contain viruses not normally encountered in a clinical laboratory.

59.

C. Both flammable and combustible liquids are commonly used in the laboratory. These two categories are differentiated on the basis of their flash points—that is, the temperature at which a liquid forms an adequate amount of vapor to produce an ignitable mixture with the air at the liquid's surface. The flash point of flammables is designated as less than 100°F and that of combustibles as greater than 100°F.

60.

A. Manufacturers of chemicals, reagents, and kits provide material safety data sheets (SDSs) for all products. These sheets must be available to all laboratorians in case of emergency. When an individual goes to the emergency department, he or she should have the SDS to give to the physician in order to get prompt, correct treatment. A laboratory professional must be confident to report any accident and take appropriate measures to clean it up.

61.

B. Biosafety level 1 laboratories handle agents with no known potential for infection. Biosafety level 2 laboratories are those where employees work with microorganisms associated with human diseases that are rarely serious. Most clinical microbiology labs are biosafety level 2 laboratories. Biosafety level 3 labs are those that may contain viruses not normally encountered in a clinical laboratory and for the cultivation of mycobacteria. Biosafety level 4 labs work with dangerous and exotic agents that pose a high risk of aerosol-transmitted laboratory infections and life-threatening disease for which effective treatments are limited.

62.

C. The threshold limit value (TLV) is the exposure allowable for an employee during one 8-hour day. The TLV will be listed in the material safety data sheet for each chemical. More toxic chemicals will have a smaller TLV.

63.

C. Fire extinguishers are divided into different types corresponding to the types of fires they are recommended to be used with. Class A fires (wood, paper, cloth) should be extinguished using a class A extinguisher. Class B fires (liquids, grease, gasoline, paints, oils) should be extinguished using class B extinguisher, Class C fires (electrical equipment, motors, switches) should be extinguished using a class C extinguisher, and Class D fires should not be extinguished by anyone other than a trained firefighter.

64.

A. Laboratory areas should maintain negative pressure with respect to the administrative areas to prevent toxic or pathogenic materials used in laboratory work areas from escaping and injuring humans or contaminating the environment. The amount of air provided to the negative pressure laboratory should be equal to 85% of the air exhausted from the area. Positive pressure is maintained in the office areas.

65.

B. Some of the precautions that should be followed when working with carcinogenic chemicals include performing the procedure in a chemical fume hood, wearing rubber gloves and proper protective clothing, and wearing a respirator when working with organic vapors and dust-producing materials. If possible, use disposable glassware. All other glassware should be washed with a strong acid before being processed in the general wash cycle.

66.

B. Safe practices in the laboratory are essential to the well-being of all employees. Each laboratorian should disinfect his/her work area daily. Pens and pencils placed on laboratory bench tops may be contaminated and should never be placed near one's mouth. Laboratory coats should never be worn in the cafeteria because they may be contaminated. Laboratory personnel should never smoke, eat, or drink in the laboratory, nor should food be placed in a refrigerator used for storage of reagents or biologic specimens. Cosmetics should not be applied in the laboratory because of potential contamination. Personnel should always wash their hands before leaving the laboratory, discarding their used gloves in a biohazard receptacle.

67.

D. It should be remembered that all body fluids from patients are potentially hazardous to one's health. Specimens collected from infectious patients in isolation should be handled according to standard precautions. Blood specimens need to be centrifuged, and inhalation of aerosols is prevented by never raising centrifuge lids prematurely. All sharp objects, including broken glass and needles, should be disposed of in a puncture-proof container. Blood collection needles should never be discarded in a wastebasket in a patient's room, because housekeeping personnel or others may easily be injured and infected.

68.

D. Chemicals should not be stored in alphabetical order because some chemicals are incompatible with others and will react adversely. Large containers of chemicals should always be stored on a shelf as close to the floor as possible to avoid severe injury in the event of breakage. Flammable chemicals should be stored in a fire-safety cabinet. Although flammables should be used in a chemical fume hood, the hood is not a proper storage area.

69.

B. Emergency showers must be available to anyone working with corrosive materials. The victim should be removed from the area as rapidly as possible and showered with water. No attempt should be made to neutralize the acid on the person's skin.

70.

A. Bottles of chemicals and solutions should be handled carefully. Chemical containers made of glass should be transported in rubber or plastic holders that will protect them from breakage. In the event of breakage, the plastic holders will contain the spill.

71.

B. Compressed gas cylinders should be stored in a vertical position in a ventilated, fire-resistant location. Gas cylinders must never be stored in the same area as flammable liquids, because both are highly combustible. Because of their shape, gas cylinders may easily fall, causing the regulator valve to rupture. To prevent such an occurrence, cylinders must always be fastened when stored, transported, and used in the laboratory.

72.

D. Viral hepatitis is the major job-related disease hazard in all clinical laboratories. All laboratorians who handle blood or body fluids are at risk. The modes of transmission include ingestion and injection. Thus, it is crucial that the laboratorian follows proper safety practices at all times.

73.

C. The responsibility to implement and maintain a safety program belongs to the laboratory safety officer. The responsibility of the chemical hygiene officer is to provide technical guidance in the development and implementation of the chemical hygiene plan. Accreditation agencies typically require laboratories to have both a safety officer and a chemical hygiene officer.

74.

A. Although now considered a carcinogen, sodium azide has been used as a preservative in some laboratory reagents. When disposal of this reagent is made in the sewer, a buildup of copper and iron salts of azide may occur. These metallic salts are explosive, especially when subjected to mechanical shock.

75.

B. The single most useful safety device used in a clinical microbiology laboratory is the Class 2 biological safety cabinet. This engineering device is designed with inward airflow at a velocity to protect personnel. In addition, it is constructed with HEPA-filtered vertical laminar flow for protection of laboratorians.

76.

A. In 1987, the Centers for Disease Control and Prevention (CDC) established guidelines for universal precautions. These guidelines were established to lower the risk of hepatitis B virus and human immunodeficiency virus transmission in clinical laboratories and blood banks. In 1996, the CDC published new guidelines, called standard precautions, for isolation precautions in hospitals. Standard precautions (updated in 2007) synthesize the major features of body substance isolation and universal precautions to prevent transmission of a variety of organisms.

77.

A. Class 2A biological cabinets force HEPA-filtered air downward at the front of the cabinet where the laboratorian is working. This provides a barrier between the worker and the infectious material. Class 2A biological cabinets exhaust HEPA-filtered air into the building, whereas Class 2B cabinets exhaust air out of the building.

78.

B. Halogens, especially chlorine and iodine, are frequently used as disinfectants. Chlorine is most often used in the form of sodium hypochlorite ($NaOCl$), the compound known as household bleach. The Centers for Disease Control and Prevention recommends that counter tops be cleaned following blood spills with a 1:10 dilution of bleach.

79.

B. The most important point to remember when working with biocides or disinfectants is to prepare a working solution of the compound exactly according to the manufacturer's package insert. Many people think they will get a stronger product if they use a more concentrated dilution. The ratio of water to active ingredient may be critical, and if sufficient water is not added, the free chemical for surface disinfection may not be released.

80.

B. Each employer having an employee with occupational exposure to human blood or any other infectious materials including bloodborne pathogens must establish a written exposure control plan designed to eliminate or minimize employee exposure. The plan identifies tasks that are hazardous and promotes employee safety. The plan incorporates education, proper disposal of hazardous waste, engineering controls, use of personal protective equipment, and a post-exposure plan.

81.

A. Class B fires are fires due to flammable liquids, grease, gasoline, paints, and oils. Class B extinguishers should be used to put out flammable liquid fires.

82.

D. *Mycobacterium tuberculosis* is spread by the aerosol route. The risk of inhalation of infectious materials can occur in the laboratory environment and poses a significant potential health hazard to the employees. The proper personal protective equipment is extremely important when working with particular infectious materials. The N95 HEPA filter respirator is a high-energy particulate air filter and is used for microorganisms spread via the aerosol route.

83.

A. Hands are more likely to contact chemicals than any other part of the body. Gloves made of appropriate materials can effectively protect the hands from exposure if they are worn during routine handling of chemicals. Selection of protective gloves is based on chemical hazard and the tasks involved. The glove fabric must have an acceptable slow breakthrough time and permeation rate for the chemical of interest.

84.

B. A safety can is used to store used chemicals until the material is removed from the laboratory. An approved container has a capacity of no more than 5 gallons. A safety can has a spring-closing lid and spout cover, and it is designed to safely relieve pressure buildup within the container.

REFERENCES

Bishop, M. L., Fody, E. P., and Schoeff, L. (Eds.) (2018). *Clinical Chemistry Principles, Techniques, and Correlations*, 8th ed. Philadelphia: Wolters Kluwer.

Burtis, C. A., and Bruns, D. E. (Eds.) (2015). *Tietz Fundamentals of Clinical Chemistry and Molecular Diagnostics*, 7th ed. Philadelphia: Saunders.

American Society for Microbiology, Jorgensen, Pfaller, and Carroll (Eds.) (2015). *Manual of Clinical Microbiology*, 11th ed. Washington, DC: ASM Press.

Murray, P. R., et al. (Eds.) (2007). *Manual of Clinical Microbiology*, 9th ed. (pp. 97–104). Washington, DC: American Society for Microbiology Press.

United States Department of Health and Human Services. (2007). *Biosafety in Microbiological and Biomedical Laboratories*, 5th ed. Washington, DC: U.S. Government Printing Office. Available at: http://www.cdc.gov/od/ohs/biosfty/bmbl5/BMBL_5th_Edition.pdf

Westgard, J. O., Quam, E., and Barry, T. (Eds.) (1998). *Basic QC Practices.* Madison, WI: WesTgard® Quality Corporation.

CHAPTER

14 Laboratory Management

contents

I. NATURE OF MANAGEMENT

A. Information Age: Management has changed from supervision of "factory" workers to coordination of knowledge workers.

B. Organizational Structure

II. MANAGEMENT PROCESSES

A. Managerial Roles and Functions

1. Managerial functions include planning, organizing, directing, decision making/problem solving, coordinating, and communicating.
2. Managerial roles include the following:
    a. Represent the organization
    b. Hold formal authority
    c. Develop and implement strategies to accomplish mission and goals of the organization
    d. Manage personnel
        1) Evaluations
        2) Hiring
        3) Promoting
        4) Mentoring
        5) Empowering
    e. Manage financial responsibilities
        1) Budget
            a) Capital
            b) Operating
        2) Revenue
        3) Expenses
    f. Facilitate communication: Employees, supervisors/team leaders, colleagues (internal and external), and patients
    g. Motivate: Employees, supervisors/team leaders, colleagues, and self
    h. Implement time management strategies
    i. Oversee customer service
    j. Implement innovative ways to expand services, expand or redirect customer base, and fulfill the bottom line
    k. Demonstrate servant leadership

B. Planning

1. **Definition:** Develop strategies/pathway(s) to accomplish the organization's mission and goals using resources and time
2. **In order to plan for the future, one must first determine where the organization stands.** A **SWOT** analysis should be performed to determine both internal and external factors.

a. Internal factors
    1) **S:** Strengths of the organization
    2) **W:** Weaknesses of the organization
b. External factors
    1) **O:** Opportunities available to the organization
    2) **T:** Threats to the organization

3. Once the SWOT analysis is complete, the manager can plan a course of action for the organization to follow that will accomplish its goals and mission.
4. Formulating **goals**
    a. Written goals allow all employees to work toward a common result.
    b. Goals should be broad; objectives are written to achieve specific tasks.
5. Writing **objectives**
    a. Objectives are tasks to achieve goals.
    b. Objectives are focused on achieving one goal.
    c. Each objective deals with one task.
    d. Objectives are very specific.
    e. Objectives are written using action verbs.
    f. Objectives are evaluated against specific and specified numerical criteria.
6. **Types of plans**
    a. **Short range or tactical plans** cover a 1- to 5-year period and focus on tasks that can be completed in this time frame.
    b. **Operational planning** may be for 1 year or one budget period and concerns operations.
    c. **Strategic planning** maps out the course of an organization for approximately 5–10 years. Strategic plans involve tactical and operational plans as well as forming alliances and partnerships with key players (sometimes even competitors). This plan is evaluated and modified yearly.

C. Organizing

1. **Time management**
    a. Laboratorians have their work dictated by the healthcare system—patient admissions, emergency patients, and outpatients. Managers have more flexibility to plan their work because it is dictated by administration (organization).
    b. Managers have more control over their workload and, therefore, they must identify, control, and eliminate or curtail specific situations that rob them of time.
        1) These tasks may require most of a manager's resources. Identify important tasks, and make sure these are accomplished first.
        2) Develop skills necessary to facilitate use of manager's time.
            a) **Managerial skills:** Organized, ability to delegate, knows when to say "no," takes control, effective planning, ability to prioritize, conducts effective meetings, exhibits good listening skills, articulate giving clear and concise instructions, and understands team dynamics

b) **Educated:** Self-study through seminars, management journals, experience, on-line webinars, access to list serves, or formal management course work
c) **Awareness of the work culture:** Knows the organization and/or goals, able to see the "big" picture
d) **Controls interferences:** Avoids lengthy unnecessary phone calls, "drop-in" visitors, reading junk mail, and too much socializing
e) **Decision-making capabilities:** Controls perfectionism, able to make a decision, appropriately detail oriented
f) **Develops resources:** Adequate money in budget, functional and up-to-date equipment, adequate staff, and support from the administration
g) **Self-discipline:** Avoids procrastination, inappropriate socializing, meets deadlines, behavior sets example for employees
h) **Servant leadership:** Focuses on the growth of the employee and the team

2. **Structure**
   a. The manager develops a structure that allows plans to be carried out and objectives accomplished.
   b. The organizational structure is based on authority, responsibility, and accountability.
      1) **Authority**
         a) Formal: Assigned by organization or administration
         b) Informal: Gained informally through competence or leadership qualities that encourage teamwork within the immediate team and across the organization
      2) **Responsibility:** Assigned by administration through delegation
      3) **Accountability** occurs when the person responsible for completing a task is evaluated to determine if the task was completed.
3. **Reengineering**
   a. **Definition:** Reorganizing work processes in an organization
   b. Use of Lean principles and tools including flow diagramming the specific work processes to determine if more effective processes could be implemented
   c. Examples of reengineering
      1) Use of robotics to automate (particularly specimen processing)
      2) Computerization
      3) Pneumatic tube system to transport specimens
   d. **Benchmarking** is a process of measuring a service or process in one organization against those of another considered the best in the industry to identify internal opportunities for improvement.
   e. Examples of benchmarking
      1) Cost per test
      2) Number of tests performed per FTE (full-time equivalent/employees) paid for 2080 hours per year
      3) Number of corrected reports

4. **Inventory management**
   a. Objective of an efficient laboratory is to experience few shortages in testing reagents, supplies, and materials.
   b. Requisitions for contract and purchase orders to obtain necessary quantities of materials, etc., in suitable time frames
   c. Managers are responsible for purchasing laboratory instruments and service contracts to maintain instruments.
   d. Instrument selection includes technical evaluation and cost comparison of instruments from various instrument manufacturers.
   e. Many hospital laboratories contract with outside agencies to provide blood products for patients.
   f. Hospitals contract with outside companies to manage biohazardous waste and/or hazardous waste disposal.

D. Directing

1. **Definition:** Persuading employees to effectively perform the tasks that help the organization accomplish its mission and goals
2. Techniques of directing
   a. **Authoritative** encompasses issuing orders and telling someone what to do. It does not allow employee to decide how best to accomplish task.
   b. **Coaching** allows the instilling of confidence and motivation into an employee about accomplishing a task. The employee has more "say-so" in how to accomplish a task.
   c. **Empowerment** allows an employee to determine what task and how to accomplish the task to help the manager solve a problem or to allow an organization to come closer to accomplishing their mission and goals. Employees are allowed to be creative and innovative to solve problems. Employees are allowed to take risks without fear of admonishment for failing.
3. **Communicating**
   a. Face-to-face **spoken communication**
      1) **Advantages**
         a) Immediate message conveyed
         b) Feedback immediate
         c) Can determine other factors: body language, tone of voice, eye contact, and implied meanings
         d) Encourages buy-in, volunteerism, cross-fertilization of ideas
      2) **Disadvantages**
         a) Cannot save the communication
         b) Receiver interpretation of message may be different from that of speaker's intentions.
         c) Body language, tone of voice, and eye contact may confuse recipient or sender.
         d) Cannot retract spoken words

e) Gender, age groups, ethnicity, professional, emotional state, and other biases exist for effective communication.
f) Perception of favoritism

b. **Written communication**
1) **Advantages**
a) Can save communication encounter
b) Deliver same message to many receivers
c) Can add graphics to explain or clarify message
d) Readers can review, interpret, and thoughtfully respond to initial message.
2) **Disadvantages**
a) Feedback delayed
b) Tone of written message is interpreted by the reader.
c) Can be impersonal
d) Final
e) Memos and e-mail are considered informal communication; letters are considered formal communication.

c. **Listening**
1) Active listening components
a) Privacy
b) Eliminate (reduce) physical barriers
c) Listen to words, but look at behavior, and interpret implied meaning.
2) Restate what you think you have heard to ensure accuracy and capture any implied meanings.
3) Remain objective, but give signals (nod, keep eye contact, say "go on") to show speaker that you are listening.
4) Identify what the sender wants from the listener.
5) Summarize the plan for action and the time when action will be complete.

4. **Motivating**
a. **Definition:** Influencing a person to act in a particular way and to generate initiative within that person
b. **Motivators include the following:**
1) Reward (i.e., bonus)
2) Empowerment
3) Praise
4) Recognition
5) Salary
6) Encouragement
7) Career development opportunities

5. **Delegating**
a. **Definition:** Assigning responsibility, authority, and accountability for a task to an employee

b. **Effective delegation** occurs when the manager selects the right task for the right person, prepares an overview of exactly what must be done, allows time for the task to be completed, and then provides recognition for performing the task.

6. **Coaching**
   a. Create an atmosphere of trust
   b. Allow employees to take risks and not be reprimanded for failures
   c. Make everyone feel that he or she is important
   d. Work through emotions of players
   e. Seek feedback by asking questions

E. Giving Directives and Managing Change

1. Managerial function that enables the manager to get his or her people to do the most and their best
2. Work done through employees with management development of their work skills
3. Good directives
   a. **Reasonable:** An employee is able to, desires to, and has resources to do so
   b. **Understandable:** The employee has clear expectations and can repeat the directive in his/her own words accurately.
   c. **Appropriately worded** and delivered in a nonthreatening tone; presented in the form of a suggestion or recommendation; avoid giving orders
   d. **Important** for getting the job done; requests should not be made for personal gain of supervisor.
   e. **Time limits** should be included in directives and should be of reasonable length.
4. Major techniques for directives
   a. **Autocratic**
      1) Detailed instructions given of exactly how and what is to be done.
      2) The manager's way is the defined expectation, and employees need not think of another way to complete the task.
      3) This inhibits employees from thinking for themselves. They lose interest and initiative. Ambition, creativity, and involvement in daily job will be diminished or lost.
   b. **Consultative**
      1) Also called participative, democratic, permissive, or empowered management
      2) Views employees as eager to do a good job and equipped with the skills to do so
      3) Believes employees will become more motivated if left alone to do their job
      4) Input is sought from employees to help solve a problem or tackle a project. They perform the job and know best the challenges.
      5) Employees are consulted about tackling a project. When in agreement, an employee is assigned to the project and needs to complete it within a specific time frame. The employee decides how the project is to be accomplished.

6) Information must flow back and forth freely between manager and employee. Good ideas need to be explored, no matter who thinks of them.
7) Employees are allowed to think for themselves and make worthwhile contributions to the organization.
8) Atmosphere is created of mutual confidence in which the employee can call on the manager when necessary with no fear of reprisal.
9) It is similar to active learning, which is more effective than passive learning. Employees work out solutions to problems and projects more effectively than management giving them the solutions.

c. **Change and influence**

1) Organizations are constantly changing in leadership positions to capture more market share and to meet technological advancements.
2) The degree and complexity of changes vary among departments in organizations.
3) Change is best accepted by employees if presented in a nonthreatening way. Managers must promote change and keep morale high.
4) Explaining the reasons for change may lead to acceptance by many employees.
5) Reasons people resist change
   a) **Uncertainty:** They do not want to be moved out of their comfort zone, because it will take effort on their part to analyze the change, learn new procedures, or perform additional tasks. There is concern of failure.
   b) **Perception:** Everyone has particular life experiences, values, and perceptions. Each individual has a different perception of the same event.
   c) **Loss:** Within the organization, there exist relationships among all workers that are built upon respect, trust, and expertise. Change can destroy all those relationships and make people lose status or perceived status among peers.
   d) **Self-interests:** Change disturbs the current state of affairs. Even though it may not be perfect, people have arranged their lives so their need satisfaction is stable. Change produces instability and uncertainty.
   e) **Insecurity:** Job security and being able to earn a wage that will allow an individual to pay the bills and maintain a decent standard of life is why people work. Change usually produces insecurity because people see their jobs threatened or taken away from them.
6) Overcoming resistance to change
   a) Managers should allow ample time for the change and not expect to follow a rigid timeline for implementing the change.
   b) Employees deserve to know why changes are being made. Managers should give employees plenty of time to have their questions and concerns answered. The manager should also state the desired effects of the change. Communicate, communicate, communicate at all times.

c) Managers should involve employees in planning and implementing the change. When employees take part in making something happen, they are more likely to take ownership and accept the change more readily.
d) **Change is stressful for everyone.** It is important to include stress management techniques to help decrease the stress of change. Be available to the team.

F. Leadership

1. Essential component of every organization; different from management
2. **Purpose:** Leadership produces change.
   a. **Management** involves planning and budgeting, organizing and staffing, controlling, and problem solving.
   b. **Leadership** involves **establishing direction, aligning, motivating,** and **inspiring people.**
3. Structure of leadership
   a. **Purpose:** To create leadership processes and help produce changes needed to cope with a changing environment
   b. **Content:** Can vary from very focused to very broad
   c. **Assignment:** Roles are assumed or assigned in a more fluid way in businesses that change often.
4. The origin of leadership
   a. Personal characteristics: High drive/energy level, good intelligence and thinking skills, articulate, good mental and emotional health, and integrity
   b. Career experiences
      1) **Promote leadership:** Challenging assignments early in a career, visible leadership role models who are very good or very bad, assignments that broaden a person's experience
      2) **Inhibit leadership:** A long series of narrow and tactical jobs, vertical career movement, rapid promotions, measurements and rewards based on short-term results only
5. The following steps can assist a leader in producing meaningful change in an organization:
   a. **Establish direction:** A vision of the future of the organization is established, and strategies are developed and implemented to bring the organization closer to that vision.
   b. **Align people:** Communicate the vision and strategies to other people using words and deeds so that the vision and strategies are understood and accepted. Be sensitive to diversity issues.
   c. **Motivate and inspire:** Energize people to implement the vision and strategy changes by satisfying basic needs (achievement, belonging, recognition, self-esteem, and a control of one's life) that may go unmet.
   d. Foster Servant Leadership: A main goal of the leader is to serve.

III. REGULATORY ELEMENTS

A. Definitions

1. **Accreditation:** The approval of an institution, part of an institution, or program, demonstrating that it meets all formal standards as defined by the accrediting body
2. **Certification:** Official acknowledgement of the passing of a qualifying examination
3. **Licensure:** The process by which a competent public authority grants permission to an organization or an individual to engage in a specific professional practice, occupation, or activity
4. The body of laws that govern the practice of laboratory medicine is **the Clinical Laboratory Improvement Amendments of 1988** (CLIA '88), the legislation that mandates the conditions that must be met for laboratories to be certified. All laboratories performing laboratory testing, regardless of where the labs are based, must maintain an active CLIA license and be subject to inspections by their State branch of the federal CLIA agency. The requirements cover quality assurance, quality control, proficiency testing, record retention, complexity of tests (high, moderate, and waived), job categories, and personnel requirements to perform testing, supervise, and direct laboratories.

B. Regulatory Agencies

1. **American Association of Blood Banks** (AABB) is an international association established to promote the highest standards of care in all aspects of blood banking. Blood Bank laboratories that are part of hospitals can be accredited and inspected jointly by AABB and CAP.
2. **American Society for Clinical Pathology** (ASCP) is a professional organization for individuals working in clinical laboratory medicine. The ASCP Board of Certification (BOC) offers examinations for clinical laboratory personnel.
3. CMS, Centers for Medicare & Medicaid Services, oversees many federal health care services, including laboratory medicine, assessing best practices to ensure patient safety.... **College of American Pathologists** (CAP) accredits laboratories under deemed authority from CMS, thus eliminating a CMS inspection. The survey is on a 2-year cycle with interim participation in proficiency testing required to assure ongoing quality of all laboratory test procedures.
4. **Food and Drug Administration** (FDA) reviews and approves new analytical methods prior to marketing by the manufacturer to laboratories. The FDA also inspects all blood banks to assure the ongoing safety of the nation's blood source.
5. **The Joint Commission** evaluates and accredits most of the healthcare organizations in the United States under deemed authority from CMS. If the laboratory is accredited by CAP, the on-site inspection of the facility by the Joint Commission will include only the transfusion service, safety, and employee competency and education. The Joint Commission can accredit laboratory services. NAACLS, National Accrediting Agency for Clinical Laboratory Sciences, is an international agency for accreditation and approval of educational programs in the clinical laboratory sciences and related health professions.

IV. MANAGING FINANCES

A. Principles

1. **Budget statement**
   a. Income statement or **revenue/expense spreadsheet**
      1) Shows revenue generated and expenses incurred over a period of time (month, quarter, year)
      2) Net income = revenue generated − expenses incurred
   b. **Balance sheet**
      1) Shows the financial situation of the organization at a specific point in time
      2) This sheet contains current assets (cash, patient receivables, inventory), current liabilities (accounts payable, accrued salaries), property and equipment (land, building, equipment, and instruments), and long-term obligations (bonds payable, loans).
      3) Equation is: **assets = liabilities + net worth**
   c. **Cash-flow statements**
      1) Show the inflow and outflow of cash for a specific period
      2) These statements show the net cash flow from operations, net flow from investments, and net cash flow from financial activities.
   d. Miscellaneous data needed by managers: Test volumes per laboratory section, supply costs, labor costs, cost per billable test, workload, rejection rates, contamination rates, repeat frequency and productivity
2. **Budgets**
   a. Usually done annually as a plan for spending for the next year
   b. Incorporates workload data, new (or eliminated) programs, test costs, previous year revenues, previous year costs, capital equipment costs, operating expenses, labor costs, and equipment maintenance costs
   c. Most organizations use data from the previous year, then estimate increased costs for the coming year and add this figure to the budget.
   d. Zero-based budgeting involves starting the budget process from a zero figure and justifying and researching every cost that will be incurred before arriving at the final budget.
3. **Revenue**
   a. **Medicare and Medicaid**
      1) The federal government pays healthcare organizations for providing care to beneficiaries using a method called **Prospective Payment System** (PPS).
      2) Healthcare organizations are paid a lump sum for services according to the **Ambulatory Payment Classification** (APC) for **outpatient** services and the **Diagnosis-Related Group** (DRG) for **inpatient** services. **Current Procedural Terminology** (CPT) is a Medicare coding system for reimbursement at the procedural level.

3) The government established a database and derived average costs for many illnesses based on the **International Classification of Disease** (ICD-10). The APC and DRG are based on ICD-10 codes.
4) The government develops a payment schedule, and this is the amount an organization is paid.

b. **Commercial payers**

1) Insurance providers contract with hospitals to provide services for the patients whose lives they are contacted to cover.
2) Capitated contracts—Negotiated between the hospital and the insurance provider for **outpatient** services, the healthcare provider is paid a **set fee** to provide specific services per HMO enrollee. For example, if a plan has 300 enrollees (covered lives), it may contract with the hospital to provide X-ray, laboratory, and physical therapy services for its patients at $100/patient per year.
3) This method is called **capitated reimbursement;** it is based on the number of enrollees at a specific payment amount per enrollee.
4) For **inpatient** services, a specific amount is paid per day (per diem) based on the **admitting ICD-10 code.**

4. Operating Costs

a. **Operating costs** are what it costs to produce test results. This includes direct and indirect costs.
b. **Direct costs** are directly associated with producing test results. These include supplies, quality control materials, and labor.
c. **Indirect costs** indirectly contribute to producing laboratory tests. These include electricity, water, paper towels, soap, bleach, computer software, and the labor that supports these services, as well as supervisory, managerial, and administrative labor.
d. **Fixed costs** remain the same from month to month no matter how many tests are produced—an example is instrument service contracts.
e. **Variable costs** change with the amount of work performed—an example is test reagents.
f. **Capital costs** are related to purchasing equipment or instruments that have a life span of more than 1 year and cost more than a set dollar amount. This figure is determined by the organization and usually ranges from $3000 to $5000. Key to organizational approval of capital expenditure for instrumentation is a return on investment (ROI) document including instrument payback calculation.

B. Cost Management

1. **Definition:** Keeping cost as low as possible without compromising the quality of care delivered to patients
2. Employees become very valuable sources for suggestions to increase efficiency and effectiveness of work patterns.

C. Cost Analysis

1. **Cost per billable test** entails gathering data on wages, collection and handling fees, reagent cost, control and reference materials cost, disposables cost, instrument maintenance, depreciation, miscellaneous costs, and indirect costs.
2. **Cost per billable test calculation**

Cost for testing = instrument cost + administration costs + supplies + labor

Revenue pertest = total revenue ÷ total number of tests

Profit = revenue per test − cost per test

D. Breakeven Analysis

1. **Breakeven analysis = where revenues equal expenses**
2. Calculation

Breakeven (BE) test volume = annual fixed costs ÷ (test price − variable costs per test)

BE minimum price per test = [annual fixed costs + (test volume × variable costs per test)] ÷ test volume

BE minimum revenue = annual fixed costs ÷ [(test price − variable costs per test) ÷ test price]

E. Cost Accounting

1. **Definition:** Systems that study costs associated with performing tests
2. Focuses on internal processes

F. Cost Containment

1. Focuses on ways of first reducing costs, then maintaining quality
2. Centralizing services is one way to control costs.
   a. Centralized purchasing
   b. Centralization of jobs or the location where the test is performed
3. Decreases unnecessary testing
4. Encourages employee retention, retraining, cross training, and flexible wage and benefits programs

V. QUALITY MANAGEMENT

A. Championed by Deming, Juran, Crosby, and Shewhart

B. Quality Programs

1. Components
   a. **Statistical analysis** is especially important in production control. It is used to analyze the quality of results. In the laboratory, statistical analysis includes internal and external quality control.
   b. **Training and education:** Employees need adequate training and education to perform the best possible job. Inadequate training and education leave

an employee unprepared to perform their best. Development plans direct employee corrective actions.

c. **Evaluation:** Quality programs establish goals or targets. The progress toward accomplishing these goals is assessed. If satisfactory progress toward a goal is not achieved, then the process needs to be changed or modified to achieve satisfactory progress toward a goal.

d. **Feedback:** This is a continuous process. Monitoring and evaluation takes place for several indicators.

C. Performance Improvement (PI)

1. Synonyms and processes:
   a. **Total quality improvement** (TQI), **total quality management** (TQM), and continuous quality improvement (CQI): The focus is on looking at the system processes when evaluating errors and determining opportunities for improvements.
   b. Executive management must be committed to performance improvement for it to work.
   c. The data teams generate are vital and important to the process, but the success of PI is dependent upon using this data to improve existing processes.
   d. **Lean thinking** focuses on removing waste and increasing the value of the service. Only do things that add value and eliminate all other activity. Kaizen is an activity that continuously looks for ways to eliminate waste by standardizing processes. Lean processing does not require a lot of mathematical analysis.
   e. **Six Sigma** focuses on reducing the variation in a process to remove error. Six Sigma uses a disciplined methodology that is data driven.
2. The cycle of quality improvement that was developed by Deming:
   a. **P.D.C.A.: Plan → Do → Check → Act**
   b. **Feedback is a crucial step in this cycle.** Without feedback, there is no improvement.
3. Tools used in evaluating quality management opportunities include Pareto charts, flowcharts, cause-and-effect charts, fish-bone diagrams, and value stream analysis.

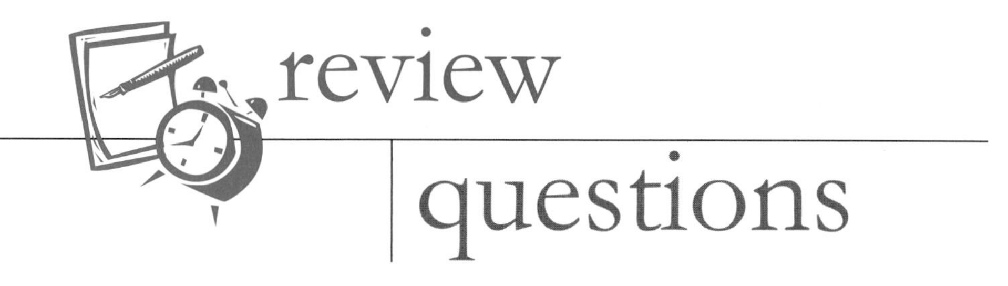

review questions

INSTRUCTIONS Each of the questions or incomplete statements that follows is comprised of four suggested responses. Select the *best* answer or completion statement in each case.

1. Which of the following sections of the clinical laboratory is regulated by the Food and Drug Administration?
   A. Chemistry
   B. Blood bank
   C. Serology
   D. Hematology

2. In order to plan for the future, one must first determine where the organization stands. A SWOT analysis should be performed to determine both internal and external factors. The term "SWOT" stands for which of the following?
   A. Successes, Weaknesses, Opportunities, Threats
   B. Strengths, Weaknesses, Opportunities, Threats
   C. Strengths, Weaknesses, Opportunities, Testing
   D. Successes, Wastes, Opportunities, Threats

3. A number of management styles are used by supervisors in laboratories. Which of the following is a management style that includes the employee in decisions about how to accomplish tasks and encourages creativity?
   A. Autocratic
   B. Persuasive
   C. Empowerment
   D. Democratic

4. What is the meaning of the abbreviation FTE?
   A. Full-time equivalent
   B. Full-time expenditure
   C. Fixed total expenditure
   D. Fixed-timely equivalency

5. Most laboratories have a definite structure that establishes the formal setup of the various departments and levels. Which of the following refers to this structure?
   A. Administration table
   B. Laboratory directory
   C. Report of contact
   D. Organizational chart

6. In a budget, which of the following terminologies is used to describe money spent for a nonexpendable item that has a life expectancy greater than one fiscal year?
   A. Expenditure
   B. Annual cost
   C. Capital expenditure
   D. Depreciable item

7. Which of the following governmental legislations has had the greatest impact on the regulation of the laboratory industry?
   A. Clinical Laboratory Improvement Act
   B. Medicare and Medicaid
   C. Fair Labor Standards Act
   D. Occupational Safety and Health Administration Act

8. Which of the following is the process by which a competent public authority grants permission to an organization or an individual to engage in a specific professional practice, occupation, or activity?
   A. Accreditation
   B. Certification
   C. Licensure
   D. Credentialing

9. Delegation is a responsibility of most laboratory managers. Effective delegation occurs when:
   A. The employee is given the freedom to decide what to do
   B. The employee has a limited time to complete the assignment
   C. The manager assigns responsibility, authority, and accountability to the employee
   D. The manager offers the assignment to the most senior employee

10. A proper understanding of why a laboratory may become liable for the actions of its personnel requires a basic knowledge of the laws involved. This area is known as tort law and involves three types of wrongful conduct. Which of the following is considered wrongful conduct?
    A. Occupational injuries
    B. Negligent acts
    C. Personal leaves
    D. Requesting work reassignment

11. DRG is a commonly used abbreviation. Which of thc following statcmcnts is associated with DRGs?
    A. Capitated contracts for services
    B. Diagnosis and payment
    C. Lean 6 Sigma strategies
    D. Decision-making responsibilities of managers

12. Which of the following is associated with the outpatient PPS system of reimbursement?
    A. DRG
    B. Capitated rate
    C. APC
    D. PPO

13. Which of the following factors is needed for an effective employee performance appraisal?
    A. Employee–supervisor discussion with written evaluation
    B. Organization standards
    C. Current cash flow documentation
    D. Kaizen review

14. Which of the following is associated with benchmarking?
    A. Measurement of labor-hours with worked and paid productivity
    B. Employee safety records
    C. Performance standards
    D. CAP accreditation

15. Which of the following is a part of the budget-making process as related to laboratories?
    A. ICD-10 codes
    B. Performance standards
    C. Organization chart
    D. Projected volume of testing

16. Which of the following areas of questioning in the interview process is inappropriate or illegal?
    A. References
    B. Age
    C. Education
    D. Experience

17. Which of the following should be included in a job description?
    A. Incumbent name
    B. Promotion potential
    C. Qualifications and job duties
    D. Job securities

18. Disciplinary action is a responsibility of supervision. Which of the following characteristics should be included for discipline to be effective and positive?
    A. Public
    B. Casual
    C. Timely
    D. Written

19. Which of the following voluntary agencies develops and implements blood bank practices for the clinical laboratory?
    A. OSHA
    B. FDA
    C. AABB
    D. PPS

20. Which of the following is associated with the goals of a laboratory continuing education program?
    A. Cost-cutting measures
    B. Elimination of promotional opportunity
    C. Staff development
    D. Increased workload

21. Which of the following is considered a line item of the laboratory budget?
    A. Labor union dues
    B. Legal fees
    C. Maintenance and repair of instruments
    D. Electricity

22. Which of the following agencies is generally responsible for the inspection and accreditation of clinical laboratories in the United States?
    A. CAP
    B. NCA
    C. CDC
    D. ASCP

23. What is the strategic process of attracting and maintaining a customer base called?
    A. Marketing
    B. Discretionary factors
    C. Market environment
    D. Product differentiation factors

24. For marketing purposes, which of the following terms best describes the laboratory customer?
    A. Captive market
    B. Patient–physician as partners
    C. Discretionary buyer
    D. Person or organization paying the bill

25. Assume that the chemistry analyzer in the laboratory of a 500-bed hospital yields 60,000 profiles per year made up of 10 results each. The number of quality control (QC) tests performed per year numbers 2400, and the total direct labor cost is $1.50 per test. The cost for a year's supply of QC reagents is $3000. What are the QC direct labor cost per profile and the QC consumable cost per profile, respectively?
    A. $0.05, $0.06
    B. $0.06, $0.05
    C. $0.08, $0.05
    D. $0.60, $1.25

26. Your lab has added a new test. It is important that you determine what the breakeven point is in the number of tests. The revenue per unit has been $10.00, whereas your fixed cost is $400.00 and your variable cost is $2.00. What is the breakeven point, if you expect your net income to be zero (no profit and no loss)?
    A. 45
    B. 48
    C. 50
    D. 52
27. A laboratory has 14,159 total hours paid. Of the total hours paid, 1263 hours are nonproductive hours. Assuming that a full-time employee works 2080 hours annually, what is the total number of FTEs needed to run the laboratory and the number of productive FTEs, respectively?
    A. 6.2, 5.8
    B. 6.8, 6.2
    C. 7.4, 6.8
    D. 11.2, 10.2
28. As a result of fraud and abuse identified by the Office of the Inspector General (OIG), what are laboratories required to develop?
    A. Chemical hygiene plan
    B. Compliance plan
    C. PPE plan
    D. Quality control plan
29. Which of the following refers to the portion (percentage) of the cost of an item or service that the Medicare beneficiary must pay?
    A. Deductible
    B. Balance bill
    C. Coinsurance
    D. Reasonable charges
30. Which of the following established the Equal Employment Opportunity Commission (EEOC)?
    A. Title VII of the Civil Rights Act of 1964
    B. Age Discrimination Employment Act of 1967
    C. Rehabilitation Act of 1973
    D. The Equal Pay Act of 1963
31. Which of the following refers to a program where the overall activities conducted by the institution are directed toward assuring the ongoing quality of the products and services provided?
    A. Quality control
    B. Cost containment
    C. Value stream analysis
    D. Continuous quality improvement
32. Who introduced the use of statistical tools in decision making, in problem solving, and for troubleshooting the production process?
    A. Philip Crosby
    B. Joseph Juran
    C. James Westgard
    D. Edward Deming
33. Your laboratory is considering expansion. You will have to buy land and build a new lab. One of the financial aspects to consider is the annual depreciation of the project. The total cost of the project is $800,000 ($200,000 for the land and $600,000 for the building). At current estimates, the building is expected to be used for 20 years, with a salvage value of $40,000. What is the annual depreciation of the project?
    A. $38,000/year
    B. $30,000/year
    C. $28,000/year
    D. $10,000/year

34. Which of the following processes is designed to measure the value (level of success) of performing diagnostic tests and other services related to the improvement of a patient's disease or condition?
    A. Clinical pathways
    B. Outcomes assessment
    C. Clinical practice guidelines
    D. Quality assurance

35. Which of the following categories of personnel is required in laboratories performing tests using high-complexity methodology?
    A. General supervisor
    B. Clinical consultant
    C. Technical consultant
    D. Director

36. Which of the following is *not* contained in the standard operating procedure manual (SOPM)?
    A. Literature references
    B. Control procedures
    C. Reference ranges
    D. Personnel requirements

37. When a manager does not possess the expertise or knowledge to implement change and the resisters have significant power to impede the efforts, which of the following strategies for change will be used?
    A. Facilitation and support
    B. Participation and involvement
    C. Negotiation and agreement
    D. Manipulation and co-optation

38. The struggle is underway, and the behavior of the participants makes the existence of the conflict apparent to others who are not directly involved. What is this stage of conflict known as?
    A. Perceived
    B. Felt
    C. Manifest
    D. Latent

39. Influence exerted through the control of support services, such as a safety officer or quality assurance coordinator, which provide recommendations to the manager and set policies, is a type of authority known as:
    A. Staff
    B. Line
    C. Formal
    D. Functional

40. What is horizontal communication?
    A. The official communication message generated by the business activities of the organization
    B. The formal messages that are channeled through the hierarchical network of the organization
    C. The activity that occurs during the normal conduct of business among departments, managers, and staff
    D. Live discourse in which all parties exchange ideas and information and receive spontaneous feedback

41. Which of the following agencies develops and monitors engineering and work practice controls?
    A. The Centers for Disease Control and Prevention
    B. Occupational Safety and Health Administration
    C. The Joint Commission
    D. College of American Pathologists

42. Which of the following refers to the continuum of care under one common computerized communication channel that links hospitals, labs, pharmacies, physicians, employers, payers, and medical information systems?
    A. Common Healthcare Integrated Network
    B. Continuum Health Internal Network
    C. Community Health Information Network
    D. Computerized Health Information Network

43. Which of the following budgeting processes attempts to set expenditures on a variable workload volume?
A. Operational
B. Capital
C. Project
D. Flexible

44. In addition to preparing a capital budget for the institution's own use, federal and state regulations require healthcare facilities to submit capital plans on certain projects for approval and to obtain a:
A. Certificate of Approval
B. Certificate of Need
C. Capital Budget Appropriation
D. Capital Need Assessment

45. What will be the payback period be for a new chemistry analyzer that costs $150,000 and produces an annual income of $420,000?
A. 2.3 months
B. 2.8 months
C. 4.3 months
D. 33.6 months

46. Which of the following is *not* a part of the calculation of the total cost per test?
A. Direct and indirect labor
B. Direct and indirect materials
C. Equipment and overhead costs
D. Depreciation

47. Which of the following best describes the role of a team leader?
A. Decision-maker
B. Taking minutes at team meetings
C. Leading, guiding, and teaching
D. Terminating employees

48. What is the primary coding system that is used by the federal government to determine levels of reimbursement at the procedural level for Medicare services?
A. CAP codes
B. CPT codes
C. Modifiers
D. ICD-10 codes

49. Your laboratory wants to buy a new hematology analyzer. In determining the total cost per test analysis, you need to know what the cost will be for equipment per test. The analyzer costs $55,000 and has a useful life of 7 years. After the 1-year warranty expires, the annual maintenance contract will cost $8000. You estimate that you will perform 3500 tests per year on this analyzer. What is the equipment cost for each test performed?
A. $1.38
B. $2.10
C. $2.81
D. $4.20

50. Which of the following styles of directing allows an employee to determine the task and how to accomplish the task in order to help the manager solve a problem?
A. Coaching
B. Autocratic
C. Empowerment
D. Authoritative

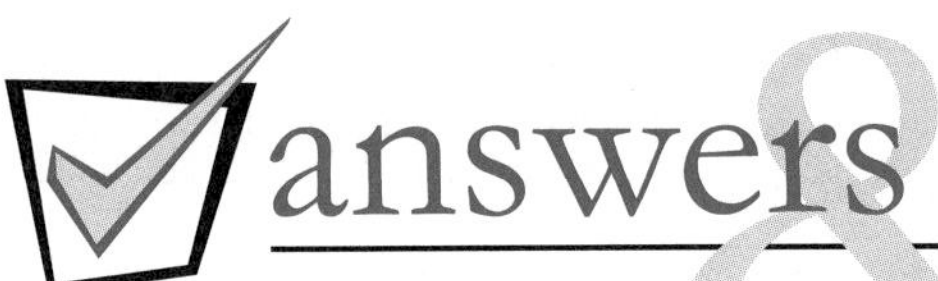

answers & rationales

1.

B. Immunohematology (blood bank) is the only laboratory section that is regulated by the Food and Drug Administration (FDA). The FDA enforces the Food, Drug, and Cosmetic Act. This Act regulates the preparation of blood and blood products as well as the facilities, including hospital laboratories and transfusion services, where preparation occurs.

2.

B. In order to plan for the future, management must first assess where the organization stands. A SWOT analysis should be performed to determine both internal and external factors. Internal factors include strengths and weaknesses of the organization. External factors include opportunities available and threats to the organization.

3.

C. The word "liberal" is not descriptive of the type of leadership style used by laboratory managers. "Autocratic," "consultative," "persuasive," and "democratic" are words that describe the styles routinely used, although rarely as purely one style; instead, a combination of various styles is used generally. Managers who are autocratic hold Theory X philosophies and allow for little input from their staff. Managers who are democratic are Theory Y managers and are participatory in their leadership style. Empowerment is the style that includes the employee in decisions about how to accomplish tasks and encourages creativity.

4.

A. "Full-time equivalent" (FTE) is a term routinely used by every laboratory, particularly during the budget process. An FTE equals 2080 person-hours paid in 1 year's time. An FTE combines productive hours and nonproductive hours (i.e., vacation, holiday, and sick time). The FTE is based on a 40-hour workweek and is more easily used in a discussion of personnel and hours worked. In one FTE, one full-time person or two or more part-time persons may occupy the 40-hour position.

5.

D. The organizational chart shows the lines of supervision, relationships of various staff members, and interrelationships of the various departments. There are generally three types of organizational charts: vertical, horizontal, and circular. Most hospital administrations use the vertical chart, which is a summary or a snapshot of the structure of the organization. It is also used by many levels of laboratory management.

6.

C. The term "capital expenditure" refers to the money spent for nonexpendable items having a life expectancy of more than one fiscal year. Capital expenditures are generally for permanent items of equipment and laboratory improvements in the physical setup of the laboratory. Very often such equipment items are high-cost items and require the approval of the institution's budgetary administration.

7.

A. Although Medicare and Medicaid legislation has had the greatest influence on the health care industry, the Clinical Laboratory Improvement Act has had the greatest impact on the laboratory industry. The CLIA 88 legislation mandates the conditions that must be met for laboratories to be certified. All laboratories performing laboratory testing, regardless of where the labs are based, must maintain an active CLIA license and be subject to inspections by their State branch of the federal CLIA agency. The requirements cover quality assurance, quality control, proficiency testing, record retention, complexity of tests (high, moderate, and waived), job categories, and personnel requirements to perform testing, supervise, and direct laboratories.

8.

C. Requiring a license is the most restrictive form of government regulation of professional practice. Licensure makes it illegal for an unlicensed organization or individual to provide a professional service within a scope of practice that is defined by statute. Licensing is designed to protect the public from inadequate manufacturing practice and incompetent practitioners.

9.

C. Delegation is defined as assigning responsibility, authority, and accountability for a task to an employee. Effective delegation occurs when the manager selects the right task for the right person, prepares an overview of exactly what must be done, allows time for the task to be completed, and then provides recognition for performing the task.

10.

B. Negligent acts are defined as the failure to do something that a reasonable person, guided by the considerations that ordinarily regulate human affairs, would do or not do. Strict liability applies to product liability and to the performance of a service.

11.

B. DRG stands for diagnosis-related group. These groups of diagnoses were developed by the federal government in the 1970s and adopted in the 1980s. The groupings provide a method of determining reimbursement for Medicare patient care by the federal government and have been used by hospital management for budgeting and planning.

12.

C. On August 1, 2000, the Centers for Medicare and Medicaid Services (CMS) and the Office of Inspector General (OIG) instituted the use of an outpatient prospective payment system (PPS) known as Ambulatory Payment Classification (APC). Mandated by the Omnibus Budget Reconciliation Act (OBRA) of 1990, APCs comprise an outpatient PPS that parallels the inpatient DRGs. PPS rates are established for each group of services provided in hospital outpatient departments for the diagnosis and treatment of Medicare beneficiaries. Services are grouped by the APC groups, which categorize services according to similarity of clinical diagnosis and resource use. The capitated rate is a fixed rate of reimbursement for health care organizations to a minimum amount per covered life. This is a process used by managed care organizations and insurers. Under capitation, a payer pays a provider a fixed amount for each member of the plan who is assigned to receive services (laboratory, radiology, cardiology, etc.) during any given month.

13.

A. A good performance appraisal should include a complete job description, performance standards based on the job description, and a regularly scheduled evaluation using the first two factors. The performance appraisal system as a whole should combine the evaluation process with a thorough discussion with the employee once he/she has had time to review the written evaluation. The appraisal should occur on a regular basis, and at a minimum of once a year.

14.

A. Benchmarking is the process whereby the best process in one organization is modified to fit similar processes in another organization. Generally, a business case is developed for making changes that will result in improvements. Examples of benchmarking data utilized in the laboratory environment include cost per test, productivity, tests performed per FTE, number of corrected reports, and capital expenditures.

15.

D. Cost analysis, forecasting, determination of fixed and variable costs, projected volume of testing, and breakeven analysis are all parts of the budget-making process. These tools must be used in the determination of all costs before any intelligent forecast or budget can be made. All have become increasingly important in today's climate of stringent reimbursement methods.

16.

B. Questions regarding race, age, and childcare needs are all inappropriate in an interview; only the applicant's experience is relevant. There are many other areas, such as marital status, arrests, credit history, religious affiliation, and spouse's occupation, that also should not be discussed. Education and past employment experience as well as interests and short- and long-range plans are appropriate areas in which to concentrate.

17.

C. Job descriptions will vary from one institution to another. However, the position title, job responsibilities, necessary qualifications, and job relationships should be part of any job description. Some other aspects that may also be covered include immediate supervisor, limitations or hazards, training, working conditions, skills, shift worked, and section or division assigned.

18.

C. Positive discipline should involve privacy, be timely, and be progressive, although it is not necessary that it be in a written format. Discipline can be informal and oral in the early stages, and it should always be private. Disciplinary action may progress through the following stages: oral, informal talk; oral warning or reprimand; written warning; disciplinary layoff or similar penalty; demotional downgrading; and discharge.

19.

C. The Food and Drug Administration (FDA) is the only compulsory agency that currently develops and implements standards and practices for blood banks. The American Association of Blood Banks (AABB) is also an agency that performs these functions, but it is a voluntary, not compulsory, program. The Occupational Safety and Health Administration addresses safety practices in the laboratory overall but does not develop specific practices for blood banks. The Prospective Payment System has to do with Medicare reimbursement and is not an agency dealing with blood banks.

20.

C. Staff development that generally improves the capabilities of the laboratory worker, improvement of laboratory functioning through in-service programs, and the meeting of accreditation requirements are important goals of a continuing education program. These goals may be accomplished by means of seminars, journal clubs, lectures, workshops, and so forth. Participation in continuing education programs is the responsibility of every laboratory professional and should be maintained throughout the career.

21.

C. Employee salaries, supplies, repair and maintenance of instruments, and fixed expenses are line items in a laboratory budget. Also considered line items are employee benefits, purchased services, allocations, and miscellaneous expenses. The aforementioned items can be further broken down into smaller, more specific components; for example, employee benefits include such items as life and health insurance, vacations, holidays, sick leave, and pensions.

22.

A. The College of American Pathologists (CAP) accredits hospitals and associated laboratories. CAP inspects clinical laboratories every 2 years. The FDA is responsible for the inspection of blood banks, and this is done on an annual basis. In the event a laboratory is not accredited by CAP, the Joint Commission will handle the inspection as part of the overall hospital assessment.

23.

A. Marketing, as a specific function of management, may be defined as the strategic process of attracting and maintaining a customer base. Without success in this area, the very survival of the organization may be placed in jeopardy. Marketing has to do with how the laboratory deals with the new reimbursement and the restructuring of the laboratory delivery system.

24.

C. There is no question that the person toward whom the laboratory directs its professional concerns is the patient. However, the laboratory must also identify the customer—the entity that sends the patient to the laboratory. The discretionary buyer is the entity that decides where a service is performed. The discretionary buyer may be the patient, a physician, a third-party payer, or even another institution. Market research shows that the mother is usually the one who decides where the family receives medical care. For this reason, much of healthcare's promotional focus is on the mother and on women in general and associated family issues.

25.

B. Product costs are an integral part of cost accounting. Labor and consumables are product costs. To calculate the cost per test of a particular assay, you must include quality control (QC) material as part of the total cost to perform a particular assay. When calculating the QC direct labor cost per test, you need to know the total number of QC tests performed each year, the total profiles performed per year, and the total direct labor cost. Therefore, the QC direct labor cost per profile would be as follows:

$$\frac{(2400 \times \$1.50)}{60{,}000} = \$0.06/\text{profile}.$$

To calculate the QC consumable costs, you need to know the cost for a year's supply of QC reagents and the total profiles performed per year. Therefore, the QC consumable cost per profile would be as follows:

$$\frac{\$3000}{60{,}000} = \$0.05/\text{profile}.$$

26.

C. Breakeven analysis is used to determine how many units, or in this case tests, you must run to recoup your costs (both fixed and variable) and make your net income (in this case, zero). A laboratory might use this to see how much a new test would cost them to implement. The formula to calculate the breakeven point is as follows:

$$rx = vx + f + c,$$

where

r = revenue per unit
x = breakeven point
v = variable costs
f = fixed costs
c = net income.

For this particular problem, the values are as follows:

x = breakeven point—this is the unknown that you are trying to determine
r = \$10.00 per test
v = \$2.00
f = \$400.00
c = 0 (net income with no profit and no loss).

So

$$\begin{aligned} 10(x) &= 2(x) + 400 + 0 \\ 10x - 2x &= 400 \\ 8x &= 400 \\ x &= 50. \end{aligned}$$

The laboratory would have to perform a minimum of 50 tests to reach the breakeven point and meet both the fixed and variable costs. Once the lab determines that the test should be included in its menu, the next step might be to determine what net income is necessary to maintain the test.

27.

B. An important concept in salary and wage management is the calculation of full-time equivalents (FTEs), which can be used for setting and measuring budgeting and staffing goals. To calculate FTEs, divide the number of hours (total = productive and nonproductive) by 2080, the number of hours a full-time person works in 1 year (40 hours per week × 52 weeks = 2080). In this example, in order to calculate the total FTE needed, you need to know the total hours paid and the number of hours an FTE works in a year:

$$\frac{14{,}159 \text{ total hours paid}}{2080 \text{ hours/person}} = 6.8 \text{ total FTEs.}$$

To calculate the productive FTE, you need to know the productive hours worked. This is determined by

$$14{,}159 \text{ total hours paid} - 1263 \text{ nonproductive hours} = 12{,}896 \text{ productive hours.}$$

The number of productive FTEs equals:

$$\frac{12{,}896 \text{ productive hours}}{2080 \text{ hours/person}} = 6.2 \text{ productive FTEs.}$$

28.

B. The Office of Inspector General (OIG) and other federal agencies charged with responsibility for enforcement of federal law have emphasized the importance of developing and implementing compliance plans. In recent years, the OIG has been asked to supply guidance as to the elements of a model compliance plan. The purpose of this issuance, therefore, is to respond to those requests by providing some guidance to health care providers that supply clinical laboratory testing services for Medicare and Medicaid beneficiaries.

29.

C. Coinsurance is the portion of the cost of an item or service that the Medicare beneficiary must pay. Currently, the Medicare Part B coinsurance is generally 20% of the reasonable charge for the item or service. Typically, if the Medicare reasonable charge for a Part B item or service is $100, the Medicare beneficiary (who has met the deductible) must pay $20 of the physician's bill and Medicare will pay $80.

30.

A. The Equal Employment Opportunity Commission (EEOC) was established by Title VII of the Civil Rights Act of 1964 and began operating on July 2, 1965. The EEOC enforces the principal federal statutes prohibiting employment discrimination, including Title VII of the Civil Rights Act of 1964, the Age Discrimination in Employment Act of 1967, the Equal Pay Act of 1963, Title I of the Americans with Disabilities Act (ADA) of 1990, and Section 501 of the Rehabilitation Act of 1973.

31.

D. Continuous quality improvement programs assure the ongoing focus on quality of the products and the services provided.

32.

D. Edward Deming is often credited with providing the Japanese with the information and training that brought them to their position as the world's leader in the production of quality products. A statistician who worked with Walter Shewhart introduced the use of statistical tools in decision making, problem solving, and troubleshooting the production process. Deming is also frequently cited as the source of most of the concepts and methods contained in the total quality management (TQM) model.

33.

C. Straight-line depreciation is a method based on the time element. As a product grows older, its value decreases and maintenance costs increase. This method can be used for all capital items, but it is usually used to establish depreciation rates for buildings and other structures with an extended life expectancy (i.e., greater than 10 years). Land is considered to last forever and is never depreciated. Therefore,

$$\text{Annual depreciation} = \frac{\text{cost of project} - \text{salvage value}}{\text{Life expectancy}}$$

$$\text{Annual depreciation} = \frac{\$800{,}000 - (\$200{,}000 + \$40{,}000)}{20\,\text{years}}$$

$$= \frac{\$800{,}000 - \$240{,}000}{20\,\text{years}}$$

$$= \$28{,}000/\text{year}.$$

34.

B. Clinical practice guidelines are published by professional medical groups, insurers, federal agencies and departments, and other groups that recommend when a selected medical procedure, test, or practice should be used. Clinical pathways are developed by hospitals for specific diseases or conditions (e.g., pneumonia, hip replacement) by the medical staff and other healthcare personnel. They may include some of those practice guidelines determining what test, procedure, or practice should be used when treating a patient with that disease or condition so that quality treatment is consistent from patient to patient. Quality assurance is a program in which the overall activities conducted by the hospital are directed toward assuring the quality of the products and services provided. The outcomes assessment is used to measure the value of the clinical practice guidelines, clinical pathways, and quality assurance program that the hospital has decided to put in place.

35.

A. A general supervisor, who must be responsible for day-to-day supervision, is stipulated for laboratories doing high-complexity testing. This is a laboratorian with an associate's degree or higher in medical laboratory technology and 2 years of training and experience in a high-complexity laboratory. The director and technical consultant must be a doctoral-level scientist with an appropriate laboratory specialty or a physician with training or experience in laboratory medicine. A physician or doctoral-level clinical scientist may provide the services of a clinical consultant.

36.

D. Personnel requirements are not required to be part of the Standard Operating Procedure Manual (SOPM). Tests are categorized by waived, moderate complexity, and high complexity. The type of personnel allowed to perform testing is determined by these categories as described by the Clinical Laboratory Improvement Amendments (CLIA) of 1988.

37.

B. Participation and involvement allows subordinates to be part of the planning or implementation of change. It is an excellent method when the manager does not possess the expertise or knowledge to implement change himself /herself, and the resisters have significant power to impede the manager's efforts. Participation often generates commitment by the participants to the change process. This approach can also result in time-consuming compromise that does not fit the organizational needs. It must be carefully handled, because once a decision has been made by the group, it is difficult for the manager to push it aside.

38.

C. Conflict does not usually appear overnight. It often festers without the knowledge of the recipient party. Conflict usually passes through several progressive stages before it manifests itself to others. The parties may be at different stages of the conflict cycle, which complicates management of conflict. The manager must have a keen sensitivity to and understanding of his/her work environment to deal effectively with conflict at all stages.

39.

A. Staff authority is exercised through such positions as the lab safety officer or quality assurance coordinator—those areas that provide supportive services in a more indirect fashion, where ability to implement change depends on the action of the section supervisors. They exercise their influence by making recommendations, providing specific support services, giving assistance and advice in technical areas, facilitating paperwork and other procedures, and developing general lab policies. Line authority is supervisory responsibility assigned through the formal delegation of authority—in the lab this is from administration to department head to supervisor to staff. Functional authority is the power to enforce directives, such as physician's medical orders, within the context and boundaries of a clearly defined specialty and span of control. Formal authority is the official, sanctioned lines of authority assigned by the owners of the organization.

40.

C. Members of organizations receive communications from two sources, formal and informal. Formal comes from two directions in a company—from above or below. Vertical communications take the form of memos and other directives that come down through the bureaucratic hierarchy and the responses and other information that make their way back up through the same network. Horizontal communication occurs in the course of the normal exchange of services, information, and work orders, when managers and staff talk to each other as peers.

41.

B. Engineering and work practice controls involve taking physical steps to isolate or remove any possible pathogen hazards from the workplace. The Occupational Safety and Health Administration (OSHA) requires specific engineering action by employers. Some primary areas where these actions are required include hand-washing facilities, needles and sharps, and procedures that minimize splashing, spraying, and generating aerosols. Although work practice controls are developed by OSHA, the Joint Commission and the College of American Pathologists (CAP) also require that these work practice controls be in place to become accredited. The Centers for Disease Control and Prevention (CDC), just like any other lab, is required to follow the same work practice controls.

42.

C. The Community Health Information Network (CHIN) links all healthcare participants involved in the continuum of care under one computerized communication channel. This channel, or electronic highway, serves as the information's translation medium. It enables members of the healthcare community to talk to one another without leaving their computer terminals, learning another computer language, or buying another computer system. A sophisticated security system allows only authorized users to access information contained in various databases at its members' systems.

43.

D. At a certain patient census, the hospital should have a specific number of employees. When the number of patients increases, more staff is hired; when the census drops, employees are laid off. In practice, this has been difficult to implement because of recruitment and retention problems. Even supplies must be ordered in advance to ensure adequate levels. For this reason, a flexible budget similar to the forecast method is prepared and then closely monitored to ensure that projections are on target.

44.

B. The process of submitting capital plans for governmental approval is required for projects, equipment, or buildings above an established monetary level. Most states have set this limit at $150,000, following federal guidelines. A certificate of need (CON) must also be obtained before new services such as oncology or obstetrics can be offered. This program was established in an attempt to control medical costs and to avoid duplication of services and the overbuilding of hospital beds.

45.

C. Payback period $= P/I$, where $P =$ purchase price of project and $I =$ annual income generated. Many investors and lenders perform this calculation to determine the length of time needed to recover their investment. Businesses use this same formula to assist in determining the affordability of a project. By the nature of the business, laboratory instruments need a relatively shorter payback period because of the rapid technological obsolescence in the field.

$$\text{Payback period} = \frac{\$150{,}000}{\$420{,}000/\text{year}} = 0.36\,\text{year} \times \frac{12\,\text{months}}{1\,\text{year}} = 4.3\,\text{months}.$$

46.

D. Depreciation is not part of the total cost per test but is part of the overall budget. The way depreciation is determined and recorded has a direct impact on the financial status of the company as a whole. The total cost per test can be determined by adding together direct and indirect labor, direct and indirect materials, and equipment and overhead costs. Direct labor cost includes the cost of technical personnel who actually perform the testing. Indirect labor cost represents the cost of all other laboratory support and supervisory personnel. Direct material includes reagents, sample cups, and pipette tips. Indirect material cost encompasses the cost of shared equipment and supplies that cannot be directly allocated to individual tests, such as the cost of the LIS, centrifuge, or refrigerator. Overhead cost includes the hospital's allocation for utilities, housekeeping, administration, and other costs.

47.

C. The team leader, to be successful, must be skilled at leading, guiding, and teaching the team. Basic knowledge of the project area and skills for getting cooperation from multiskilled and multidisciplinary team members are crucial.

48.

B. The CPT is actually Level I of the HCPCS codes. CPT is authored by the American Medical Association and, therefore, most codes are historically identified physician provided procedures. They relate to signs, symptoms, and conditions; their use is important in substantiating procedural orders. Modifiers are attached to CPT codes to further describe a procedure. They can be alpha or numeric in nature. An example used in lab procedures is modifier "91," indicating that the same procedure was performed more than once on the same date of service.

49.

D. Equipment cost is an essential part of determining the total cost per test. In order to determine the equipment cost per test, you need to know the cost of the equipment, the useful life of the equipment, the annual maintenance cost after warranty expiration, and the estimated number of tests to be performed by the equipment you want to purchase.

$$\text{Equipment cost} = \frac{[(E \div L) + M]}{A},$$

where

E = Cost of equipment
L = Useful life of equipment
M = Maintenance costs
A = Annual tests performed.

Equipment cost =

$$\frac{[\$55{,}000 \pm (\$8000 \times 6)]/7}{3500} = \$4.20$$

50.

C. Empowerment allows an employee to determine what task and how to accomplish the task to help the manager solve a problem or to allow an organization to come closer to accomplishing its mission and goals. Employees are allowed to be creative and innovative to solve problems. Employees are allowed to take risks without fear of admonishment for failing.

REFERENCES

Toussaint, J. (2015). *Management on the Mend: The Healthcare Executive Guide to System Transformation.* Theda Care Center for Health Care Value, Appleton, WI.

Optum360. (2017). *Coding and Payment Guide for Laboratory Services.* OptumInsight, Inc., West Valley City, UT.

CHAPTER

15 Medical Laboratory Education and Research

contents

I. FUNDAMENTALS OF EDUCATION

A. Components of Education

1. **Curriculum** is driven by the **body of knowledge** of the profession.
2. **Competencies** are the **skills** that must be mastered by students to become an entry-level medical laboratory professional.
3. **Goals** are general statements of **learning outcomes** that typically apply to a whole course or curriculum.
4. **Objectives** are **measurable** and **observable behaviors** that will enable students to master entry-level competencies. Objectives guide the students to the expectations of content mastery and performance.
5. **Instruction** is the **process of passing knowledge and skills** to students. Learning activities can include lecture, reading, demonstration, assignments, research, and group projects. It includes design of activities and experiences to develop psychomotor skills and behaviors in the affective domain.
6. **Tests** measure the amount of **knowledge** students have **learned.** Tests should be **objective measures** of learning that correlate with the stated objectives and goals.
7. **Evaluation** measures **cognitive, psychomotor**, and **affective learning.** It documents how well students master entry-level competencies.

B. Competency-Based Education (CBE)

1. **Definition:** Program curriculum is based on entry-level competencies as determined by the profession.
2. The competencies are set by the **National Accrediting Agency for Clinical Laboratory Sciences** (NAACLS) in the *Standards for Accredited and Approved Programs.* These competencies are supported by the **certification examination content guidelines** of the **American Society for Clinical Pathology Board of Certification** (ASCP BOC) and the former **National Credentialing Agency for Laboratory Personnel** (NCA).
3. **Objectives** are **action statements** that reflect the **skill (psychomotor domain)**, the **behavior (affective domain)**, and the **knowledge (cognitive domain)** to be mastered by a student. The objectives must be **measurable** so that student progress toward mastery of the objectives can be assessed.
   a. Each objective must contain:
      1) The **doer** (A = Audience)
      2) The **activity** (B = Behavior, the action verb; success is measurable)
      3) The **specified conditions** (C = Conditions, circumstances)
      4) The **standard** (D = Degree that implies mastery)
      5) For example, the *student* (doer) must *classify* the bacteria (the activity) in *5 minutes* (condition) with *100% accuracy* (the standard).
   b. **Objectives benefit students by:**
      1) Clearly stating **expectations** of students
      2) Helping students **capture relevant subject matter**

3) Providing students with **self-direction**
4) Establishing a **lifelong learning** process for students

c. **Objectives benefit instructors by:**
1) Clearly defining **expectations** of students
2) Identifying **important subject matter**
3) Establishing **criteria** for testable material
4) Holding instructors **accountable**
5) Helping instructors **plan** course content, lectures, and laboratory experiences

II. LEARNING DOMAINS

A. Cognitive Domain

1. Consists of progressive levels of difficulty
   a. **Knowledge:** Recall, facts
   b. **Comprehension:** Linking to what you already know
   c. **Application:** Relating new knowledge to a new situation
   d. **Analysis:** Breaking down a situation into its components and determining the interrelation of its parts
   e. **Synthesis:** Taking separate components and bringing them together to produce a meaningful new product
   f. **Evaluation:** Judging the value of information (such as research articles or data) for a specific purpose

B. Affective Domain

1. Consists of progressive levels of commitment, depth, and sophistication
   a. **Receiving:** How students listen; their attitude toward constructive criticism and directions.
   b. **Responding:** How students reply and demonstrate new behaviors as a result of experience.
   c. **Valuing:** Students exhibit involvement and a commitment to learning opportunities, constructive criticism, and directions.
   d. **Organization:** How students integrate a new value into their current set of values, and rank the new value among the current set.
   e. **Characterization:** The inherent personality manifested in behavior that is consistent with the new set of values.

C. Psychomotor Domain

1. Consists of progressive levels of complexity
   a. **Observation:** Watches a procedure or assay being performed
   b. **Preparation:** Organizes work space to perform an assay or procedure
   c. **Manipulation:** Completes the assay or procedure
   d. **Coordination:** Performs many tasks in an efficient manner; multitasks
   e. **Adaptation:** Transfers old skills when performing a new procedure
   f. **Origination:** Develops new manual dexterity to perform tests more easily or efficiently

III. INSTRUCTORS

A. Roles of the Instructor

1. **Expert:** Must be knowledgeable about the subject she/he is teaching; must be capable of using resources.
2. **Authority:** Instructors are given formal authority over students.
   a. Formal authority includes developing course syllabi, policies and procedures, grading structure, course activities, assessment structure, and relevant cognitive, affective, and psychomotor objectives.
   b. Instructors need to be familiar with the institution's policy on academic misconduct and must follow established guidelines. Honesty and integrity are essential in health professions. Establishing a culture where academic integrity is critical prepares students for the professional integrity that is expected and required in the field of medical laboratory science.
   c. Instructors must oversee that students develop entry-level competencies.
3. **Facilitator:** Organize and present knowledge to students in an orderly, understandable manner and guide students through the learning process.
   a. The instructor must take into account different student learning styles and different student learning rates.
   b. The instructor is responsible for helping students to apply what they have learned.
4. **Compliance manager:** Responsible for ensuring students follow the policies and rules of the program and institution.
5. **Responsibilities:**
   a. Compliance with governmental safety regulations
   b. Be prepared for class.
   c. Provide appropriate turnaround time for the grading of assignments, grades, and assessments.
   d. Communicate in a timely manner.

B. Teaching Methods

1. **Lesson plan** is an outline of what should be accomplished using:
   a. Cognitive, affective, and psychomotor objectives
   b. Lecture notes and/or handouts
   c. Digital presentations to share information can incorporate multimedia to appeal to different learning styles; time-consuming to create, may require special equipment to present
   d. PowerPoint presentations are easy to prepare, but sometimes contain too much information
   e. Presentations with images, such as parasites or blood cells, require special equipment and a darkened room to present; fine details may not be visible on screen
   f. Demonstrations
   g. Web-based and application resources

2. **Lecture** is a setting in which an expert talks to a group of people about a particular topic.
   a. Good for disseminating large amounts of information to many students simultaneously
   b. Popular format
   c. Allows little opportunity for discussion
3. **Cooperative learning**
   a. Small group learning topics
   b. Groups use all members as resources, cooperating in a friendly environment to learn.
4. **Problem-based learning** (PBL)
   a. Presentation of a problem/scenario to students
   b. Students work together to find the solution
5. **Electronic-assisted learning** provides software programs and applications for students to use in learning and reviewing topics.
6. **Simulation activities**
   a. Students act out situations
   b. Provides nonthreatening learning environment
   c. Identify solutions to difficult/challenging scenarios
   d. Develop and improve team skills
7. **Online education** utilizes alternative delivery methods to facilitate students' learning.
   a. Lectures delivered at specific outreach sites away from a higher-learning institution.
      1) Via the Internet for online courses
      2) Via video conferencing equipment
8. **Experiential learning** allows the student to practice skills in a learning environment such as a student laboratory or clinical site
   a. Allows the student to learn and practice
   b. Can be expensive and time-consuming to design and facilitate

C. Assessment

1. **Definition:** Means of determining how well students understand, remember, and can apply the subject matter presented to them
2. **Types of evaluation tools**
   a. **Checklist:** Often used in conjunction with a practical examination or experience to assess competency pertaining to a particular task, lists components within a particular task and each component is checked for completion.
   b. **Pretest:** Test given to students to determine what students **already know** about a subject.
   c. **Posttest:** Test given to students to determine what they **have learned**; pretest score compared with posttest score to assess learning.

d. **Norm-referenced test:** A test in which the students are **evaluated** based upon their performance **in relation to** that of their **peers.**
e. **Criterion-referenced test:** A test in which the students are **evaluated** based **upon actual mastery** of the material; **criteria** for scoring are **established prior** to administration of the test (e.g., summative test such as a national certification examination).
f. **Diagnostic examination:** Used to assess the presence/extent of disability and need for accommodations.

3. **Test attributes**
   a. **Reliability:** Refers to how stable and consistent a test is from year to year.
      1) Consistency relates to reviewing the subject matter annually and editing the test appropriately.
      2) Adequate test questions
      3) Objective test questions
   b. **Validity:** When a test asks questions about specific information
   c. **Objectivity:** Questions that **relate back to stated objectives**, fairness, adequate time to complete, good format (sufficient space to answer questions).
4. **Structure and assessment of test questions**
   a. Three levels: **Level I** (Recall), **Level II** (Interpretation), and **Level III** (Problem-solving)
      1) **Level I—Recall:** This is the lowest level question because it asks the student to recite information.
      2) **Level II—Interpretation:** The student is asked to use material learned to tell something about a process, test, or principle.
      3) **Level III—Problem-solving:** The student is presented with a problem and asked a specific question related to that problem.
   b. **Assessing test question responses** using **rubrics**
      1) **Level I questions** are typically objective (i.e., multiple choice, true/false, matching, short answer). These can be challenging to create but are easy to grade.
      2) **Level II questions** may be objective. Other formats include short answer or essay.
      3) **Level III questions** may also be objective, but typically are not. They can be easy to create (i.e., short answer or essay questions to demonstrate the ability to solve/resolve a problem). However, these questions are challenging to grade. A **rubric** is a **list of criteria** or **expectations** established and utilized **to assess a student's mastery** of a written assignment or problem. The rubric should be scaled with varying levels of achievement based upon the expectations of the instructor, and it should be presented to the student prior to completion of the assignment whenever possible.

IV. STUDENTS

A. Learners/Students

1. **Definition:** Students are contracted customers who take classes to earn a degree, diploma, or certification, or to learn specific information. Graduates of a program are products of the educational process.
2. **Responsibilities:**
   a. Know degree requirements from the school
   b. Attend all classes and be on time
   c. Maintain academic integrity
   d. Maintain a professional demeanor
   e. Adhere to institution, department, and course policies and procedures
   f. Notify instructor as soon as possible if absent, tardy from class, or something prevents completion of an activity
   g. Respect the role of the instructor and the right of fellow students to a productive learning environment

V. PROFESSIONAL COMPETENCY

A. Medical Laboratory Science Educational and Professional Organizations

1. **NAACLS** (National Accrediting Agency for Clinical Laboratory Sciences) is an organization that **accredits** medical laboratory science/clinical laboratory scientist and medical laboratory technician/clinical laboratory technician **educational programs.**
   a. Develops the *Standards for Accredited and Approved Educational Programs*
   b. Monitors institutional compliance with the *Standards* to ensure that students have the ability to: meet the entry-level competencies ater successful completion of the program of study.
   c. Requires affiliation agreements between academic institutions and clinical education sites to align responsibilities, expectations, and provide for student safety.
2. **ASCP BOC** (ASCP Board of Certification) is a **credentialing agency** that develops and administers an examination to certify medical laboratory scientists (MLSs) and medical laboratory technicians (MLTs). To maintain the professional credential, laboratory professionals are expected to participate in the Credential Maintenance Program (CMP) through ASCP. The superscript "cm" will appear in the credential listing for individuals participating in the form of MLS(ASCP)^{cm} or MLT(ASCP)^{cm}.
3. **NCA** (National Credentialing Agency for Laboratory Personnel) was a **credentialing agency** that developed and administered certification examinations for clinical laboratory scientists (CLSs) and clinical laboratory technicians (CLTs). NCA merged with the ASCP in 2009.
4. AMT (American Medical Technologists) is an alternative **credentialing agency** that also develops and administers an examination to certify medical technologists

(MTs) and medical laboratory technicians (MLTs). To maintain the professional credential, laboratory professionals are expected to participate in the Certification Continuation Program (CCP) through AMT.

5. **ASCLS** (American Society for Clinical Laboratory Science) is a **professional organization** for clinical laboratory science practitioners that promotes all aspects of the profession and to which an individual can hold membership. ASCLS has state chapters in which clinical laboratory professionals may hold membership.
6. **ASCP** (American Society for Clinical Pathology) is a **professional organization** that promotes the laboratory profession and to which clinical laboratory practitioners can hold membership.

B. Certification versus Licensure

1. **Certification** is the process of recognizing an **individual's qualifications** by a **nongovernmental** organization or agency. It is a voluntary process that involves meeting specific academic requirements and successfully passing an examination. Although certification is voluntary, many institutions require it for employment and/or compensation as an MLS/MLT or CLS/CLT.
2. **Licensure** is the process by which a **governmental** agency (e.g., state) **grants permission to an individual** that she/he is qualified **to work** in a certain field. In the profession of medical laboratory science, this requires meeting specific academic requirements and successful completion of an examination that may be administered by the particular state or an approved credentialing agency.

VI. INTRODUCTION TO RESEARCH METHODS

A. Research Definitions

1. **Theory:** An explanation to a problem, or how variables relate to other variables.
2. **Hypothesis:** A statement regarding supposed relationships among variables; the research conducted will support or not support the hypothesis.
3. **Null hypothesis (H_0):** A hypothesis that attempts to prove no difference between two groups for the variable being investigated.
4. **Statistical significance:** Used to show differences or similarities that support a theory or hypothesis.
5. **Control group:** A group that is untreated or receives no special treatment.
6. **Variables:** Factors influencing data or outcomes; must be accounted for in final statistical analysis.

B. Types of Research

1. **Experimental-comparison design:** Comparing different groups that have been assigned to receive different treatments.
2. **Single-case experimental design:** The same subjects receive different treatments, and comparisons or changes are noted.

3. **Correlational design**
   a. The most common design that is nonexperimental
   b. Two or more variables are measured to determine relationships.
   c. **Example:** Is self-esteem related to grades?
4. **Descriptive research**
   a. A type of nonexperimental quantitative research
   b. Describes a group or set of variables as they exist without external or internal interference
   c. **Example:** New medical laboratory/clinical laboratory science (MLS) employees are compared with experienced MLS employees.
5. Questions related to research design development
   a. Is the problem an important one?
   b. Does the theory regarding the problem make sense?
   c. Does the collected data confirm the hypothesis?
   d. Is the study feasible given the available resources?

VII. RESEARCH METHODS

A. Experimental-Comparison Design

1. Introduction
   a. Answers questions that involve comparison of one treatment or condition with another
2. Random assignment
   a. One of the most important features of the experimental-comparison design is the use of random assignment of subjects to various treatments.
      1) Random assignment solves one of the most critical problems of research design, which is selection bias.
      2) **Example:** The names of 100 hospital laboratories are put into a box, and 50 laboratories are chosen randomly. Personnel from 25 of the chosen laboratories are given in-service training in safety, whereas personnel from the remaining 25 laboratories are not given the safety in-service. Which laboratory's personnel will have the best safety record?
   b. Stratified random assignment
      1) The process of random assignment in the **same category**
      2) **Example:** Random selection of private laboratories

B. Single-Case Experimental Design

1. Introduction
   a. In single-case experiments, one or more subjects are observed over a period of time.
      1) The observations establish a baseline of the variables being observed.
      2) Once the baseline is established, a treatment is started.
      3) The baseline is then analyzed to determine if the treatments have made a difference to the original observations.

C. Nonexperimental Quantitative Design

1. Introduction
   a. This type of design uses a series of observations about a subject or group of subjects in order to determine differences or similarities. No treatment is applied to the observed subjects.
   b. **Example:** Edward Jenner in the 1700s observed dairymaids who had cowpox but did not get smallpox. He determined that people with cowpox would not get smallpox.
   c. Quantitative research is a type of descriptive research in which the researcher is observing a subject in relation to determining differences and similarities.
   d. Types of quantitative (descriptive) research
      1) Survey research
         a) Uses questions to study a population or problem
      2) Assessment research
         a) Typically, uses criterion-referenced tests constructed to measure skills believed to be important.
      3) Historical research
         a) Uses historical documents rather than people
         b) The goal of historical research is to find connections among events in the past rather than among variables in the present.

D. Qualitative Research

1. Introduction
   a. Qualitative research is intended to explore important environmental phenomena by immersing the investigator in the situation for extended periods of time.
   b. Characteristics of qualitative research
      1) Uses the natural setting as the direct source of data and the researcher as the key instrument
      2) Descriptive
      3) Concerned with process rather than simply with outcomes or products
      4) Tends to analyze data inductively
      5) Meaning is of essential concern to the qualitative approach.
   c. Types of qualitative research
      1) **Naturalistic observations** are those when the observer tries not to alter the situation being observed in any way but simply records whatever is seen.
      2) **Open-ended interviews** attempt to let the person being interviewed tell their story in detail without interference by the interviewer.
      3) Data used in qualitative research include:
         a) Field notes
         b) Documents and photographs
         c) Statistics

VIII. MEASURES AND SAMPLING

A. Concepts of Critical Importance

1. **Reliability** refers to the degree to which a measure is consistent in producing the same readings when measuring the same things.
   a. In the case of questionnaires, tests, and observations, the goal is to create measures that will consistently show differences between groups that occur in all situations where those measures are used.
2. **Validity** refers to the degree to which a measure actually measures the concept it is supposed to measure.
   a. Types of validity
      1) **Content validity:** The degree to which the content of a test matches some objective criterion.
      2) **Predictive validity:** The degree to which scores on a scale or test predict later scores.
      3) **Concurrent validity:** The correlation between scores on a scale and scores on another scale that has been established to be valid.
      4) **Construct validity:** The degree to which scores on a scale have a pattern of correlations with other scores or attributes that would be predicted to exist.

B. Types of Measures

1. **Questionnaires** can be developed to assess personality, attitudes, and other noncognitive variables.
   a. Characteristics involved in constructing questionnaire:
      1) Questions should be as short and clear as possible.
      2) Double negative questions should be avoided.
      3) Cover all possibilities if multiple choice questions are used.
      4) Include points of reference or comparison when possible.
      5) Emphasize words that are critical to the meaning of the questions.
      6) Ask only important questions.
2. **Interviews** are used to ask individuals specific questions; however, interview data are more difficult to collect and analyze.
   a. Constructing an interview protocol
      1) Develop questions.
      2) Develop notes that will indicate a course of action in response to certain answers.
      3) Be prepared for clarification of questions and responses.
      4) Have a plan to analyze the collected data.

C. Sampling

1. Introduction to sampling
   a. Sampling is very important in research design; it is designed to assess part of the larger group.

   b. Each member of the population from which the sample is drawn should have an equal and known probability of being selected.
   c. The larger the sample size, the smaller the sampling error.
2. Types of samples
   a. **Cluster samples** include sampling groups rather than individuals.
   b. **Stratified random samples** include random assignment of subjects to one or more groups that will ensure that each group has certain characteristics.
   c. **Samples of convenience** include sampling a small group and making the argument that these findings will apply to the larger group.
3. Sample size
   a. A critical element of research design
   b. If the sample is too small, chances are good that no statistically significant results will be obtained.
   c. The sample size depends on the amount of error accepted, the number of variables being tested, and the type of statistical analysis to be used (Student's *t*-test, chi-square test, ANOVA, etc.). There are statistical programs that can be used to establish the minimal number of samples needed to obtain statistically useful data.
   d. Generally, the larger the sample size, the better chance there will be to observe statistical significance.

IX. PLANNING THE STUDY

A. Criteria for a Research Topic

1. Of interest to you and others
2. Important
3. Build on previous research.
4. Timely
5. Resources (time, money, research tools) available to adequately study the topic.

B. Gather Information

1. Start with a widely focused literature search: Internet searches are a good way to start, along with abstracts, journals, and books.

C. Steps in the Proposal (What You Want to Do and How You Will Do It)

1. **Statement of the problem:** Briefly introduces the questions to be answered and discusses the importance of the problem
2. **Hypothesis:** A statement that summarizes what one expects to find or learn.
3. **Literature review:** A summary of the research relevant to the topic
4. **Procedures** should include the following:
   a. Subjects and sampling plan
   b. Procedures
   c. Measures
   d. Analysis of the collected data
5. **Time frame** for study completion

X. INTRODUCTION TO STATISTICAL TERMS

A. Scales of Measurement

1. **Nominal scale:** Uses numbers as names for certain categories or groups. Nominal scale numbers have no relationship to one another.
2. **Ordinal scale:** Ordinal scale numbers are in a definite order, but without regard to distance among numbers.
3. **Interval scale:** Scores or numbers differ from one another by the same amount, without regard to a zero point.
4. **Ratio scale** is an interval scale with a true zero point.

B. Measures of Central Tendency

1. **Mean:** Average of a set of numbers.
2. **Median:** The middle number of a set.
3. **Mode:** The most frequent number.

C. Measures of Dispersion

1. **Standard deviation** (SD) is the dispersion or scatter of a set of numbers. SD is the square root of the variance.
2. **Variance** is the degree of dispersion or scatter of a set of numbers. The variance is the square of the standard deviation.

D. Statistical Comparisons

1. **Statistical significance:** Two or more statistics are found to be more different than would be expected by random variation.
2. **Student's *t*-test:** Statistics used to determine if means from two different samples are different beyond what would be expected due to sample to sample variation.
3. **Student's *t*-test for comparison of two means from matched groups:** Used to compare the same subjects under two different conditions or at two different times.
4. **Analysis of variance (ANOVA):** Used to compare means of more than two groups.
5. **Analysis of covariance (ANCOVA):** Used to compare two or more group means after **adjustment** for a control variable.
6. **Chi-square test:** Uses frequency count data, such as the number of individuals falling into a particular category.

XI. WRITING A JOURNAL ARTICLE

A. Format and Style of Journal Articles

1. **Abstract:** Brief synopsis (about 150 words) that summarizes the purpose, methods, and study results.
2. **Introduction:** Brief review of the literature supporting the topic, describing the purpose and significance of the study.
3. **Methods:** Description of the procedures and methods used in the study.
4. **Results:** Description of the findings of the study.

5. **Discussion:** Analysis of results and correlation to support the theory and literature discussed in the introduction.
6. **Summary:** One or two paragraphs capturing key results.
7. **References:** Citations of other people's work used in the body of the article; substantiates theory and results.

B. Tips for Getting Published
1. Have several people read your manuscript for accuracy, content, etc.
2. Follow the format, style, and other journal requirements very carefully.
3. If your article is rejected, make editorial adjustments and resubmit.
4. Send rejected articles to another journal for possible publication.

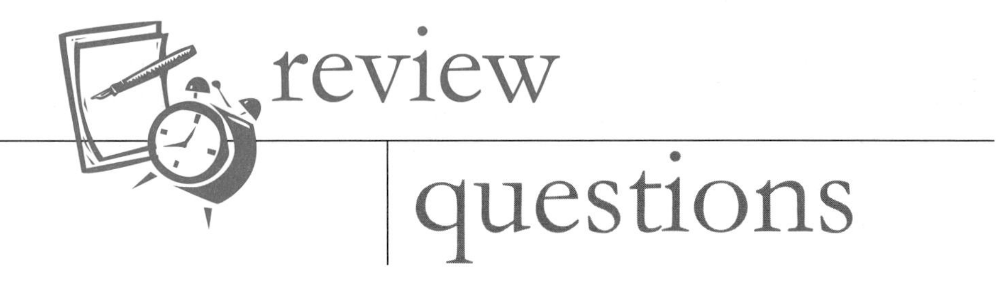

review questions

INSTRUCTIONS Each of the questions or incomplete statements that follow are comprised of four suggested responses. Select the *best* answer or completion statement in each case.

1. The three levels of test questions are:
   A. Recall, synthesis, interpretation
   B. Recall, interpretation, problem-solving
   C. Recall, synthesis, problem-solving
   D. Easy, interpretation, case studies
2. The statement, "The curriculum is designed to prepare graduates to develop procedures for the analysis of biological specimens," is an example of a(n):
   A. Course description
   B. Goal
   C. Task analysis
   D. Objective
3. The statement, "Given a hemocytometer, the student will perform manual red cell counts with 90% accuracy," is an example of a(n):
   A. Course description
   B. Goal
   C. Task analysis
   D. Objective
4. Which of the following represents a non-measurable verb?
   A. Differentiate
   B. Diagram
   C. List
   D. Understand
5. Of the major domains for learning objectives, which domain contains objectives that involve the performing of a task, for example, performing a white blood cell differential?
   A. Affective
   B. Analytical
   C. Cognitive
   D. Psychomotor

6. Which of the taxonomic levels in the cognitive domain is represented by the following objective?
   Objective: When given prothrombin time values and the ISI information, the student will be able to calculate and interpret the INR value.
   A. Knowledge
   B. Comprehension
   C. Application
   D. Analysis

7. What part of the following statement represents the conditions of the objective?
   Objective: Given the appropriate tools and written procedure, the student will perform daily maintenance on the chemistry analyzer without error.
   A. Given the appropriate tools and written procedure
   B. The student will perform daily maintenance on the chemistry analyzer
   C. The student will
   D. Without error

8. A name tag reads: "Jane Smith, MLS(ASCP)^{cm}" What does this tell us about Jane Smith's professional credentials? She is:
   A. Accredited
   B. Certified
   C. Licensed
   D. Registered

9. Which of the following terms refers to the process by which an agency evaluates a medical laboratory science program and recognizes that it has met certain preset standards?
   A. Accreditation
   B. Certification
   C. Licensure
   D. Registration

10. An instructor observes a medical laboratory science student cheating on an examination. What is the best action to take?
    A. Ignore the behavior because the student is hurting only himself/herself.
    B. Stop the examination and collect all the papers.
    C. Document the incident, but do not report it unless it is repeated.
    D. Document the incident and report it to the appropriate authority.

11. Which of the following activities is associated with problem-based learning (PBL)?
    A. Students perform laboratory procedures using a checklist.
    B. Student work independently to solve a problem.
    C. Students work together to identify the resources needed and solve the problem proposed.
    D. The instructor presents a lecture series for each instructional unit.

12. Which of the following is an advantage of the lecture method?
    A. Useful for teaching technical skills
    B. Student is an active participant
    C. Pace is controlled by the learner
    D. Disseminates large amounts of information

13. Which of the following teaching methods involves students working in a team where each student has a role in the efforts to work through a situation?
    A. Lecture
    B. Simulation activities
    C. Online courses
    D. Cooperative learning

14. Which of the following best describes the term "**reliability**" as it relates to assessment?
    A. The test question pertains to a specific learning objective.
    B. The test questions and student performance results are consistent from year to year.
    C. All of the test questions are level 1 questions.
    D. Each student is given a different set of questions to evaluate their knowledge.

15. Simulation is designed to strengthen skills in which educational domain?
    A. Affective
    B. Psychomotor
    C. Aesthetic
    D. Cognitive

16. Which of the following best describes licensure?
    A. A credentialing agency that develops and administers an examination
    B. An organization that sets standards and reviews educational programs for compliance
    C. A process where a governmental agency grants permission for an individual to work in a specific state upon meeting the requirements
    D. The promotion of all aspects of the laboratory profession by an organization

17. Which of the following testing types assesses a student's performance on an examination independent of peer performance?
    A. Norm referenced
    B. Objective referenced
    C. Criterion referenced
    D. Standard referenced

18. The ASCP Board of Certification examination is an example of which of the following types of tests?
    A. Placement
    B. Formative
    C. Summative
    D. Diagnostic

19. What is the level of the following test question: "List the normal range for serum protein levels."
    A. Level I question
    B. Level II question
    C. Level III question
    D. The question level cannot be determined from the information given.

20. The evaluation tool that monitors the performance of each step comprising a technical procedure is called a:
    A. Checklist
    B. Rating scale
    C. List of objectives
    D. Practical exam

21. Which of the following is a type of research design where two or more variables are measured to determine relationships?
    A. Single-case experimental design
    B. Experimental-comparison design
    C. Descriptive research
    D. Correlational design

22. Stratified random assignment is:
    A. Nonrandom assignment in a different category
    B. Nonrandom assignment in the same category
    C. Random assignment in a different category
    D. Random assignment in the same category

23. Quantitative research is a type of descriptive research where the researcher observes a subject:
    A. For bad habits
    B. For characteristic traits
    C. To determine differences
    D. In relation to determining differences and similarities
24. Which of the following refer to the degree to which a measure is consistent in producing the same reading when measuring the same things?
    A. Concurrent reliability
    B. Construct validity
    C. Reliability
    D. Validity
25. The larger the sample size, the smaller the:
    A. Population bias
    B. Sampling error
    C. Reliability error
    D. Random sample
26. Standard deviation is:
    A. Used for frequency count data
    B. The dispersion of a set of numbers
    C. Used to compare more than two samples
    D. The statistic used to determine if means are from two different populations

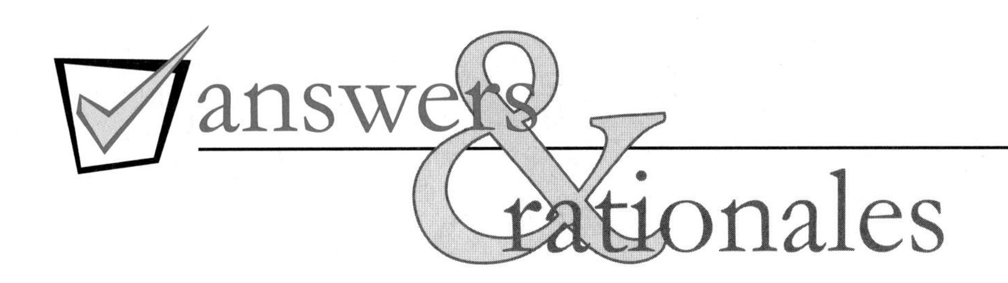

1.

B. The three levels of test questions are recall of the knowledge imparted by the teacher, interpretation or the ability to apply that knowledge to data presented, and problem-solving, in which the student selects the appropriate path to resolve a problem. Problem-solving is the most complex level of the three. Synthesis refers to a student's ability to take parts and create a new "whole." Case studies are typically used in problem-based learning.

2.

B. Goals describe what a student will be able to do and are written in general terms and do not describe behaviors. An objective is a statement that describes what a student will be able to do at the end of a unit of instruction. A task analysis is a description of the knowledge and skills needed for competence in the work setting. Course descriptions differ from objectives in that the former do not describe what the student is expected to achieve but give information about course content.

3.

D. An objective is a statement that describes what a student will be able to do at the end of a unit of instruction. Goals also describe what the student will be able to do; however, they are written in general terms and do not describe behaviors. A task analysis is a description of the knowledge and skills needed for competence in the work setting. Course descriptions differ from objectives in that the former do not describe what the student is expected to achieve but give information about course content.

4.

D. Action verbs describe an activity that is observable and measurable. Nonmeasurable verbs are not observable. Using action verbs in writing objectives clearly conveys the instructor's expectations of students. Verbs that are more general, such as "understand," "know," and "realize" do not describe performances that are measurable; they may be used for goals. Differentiate, diagram, and list are all measureable verbs as an activity or assessment question can be designed to evaluate the student's ability to demonstrate their ability to meet the learning objective.

5.

D. Objectives have been classified into three major domains: cognitive, affective, and psychomotor. The cognitive domain includes those objectives that emphasize the intellect. Cognitive behavior includes the recall of information, the comprehension of that information, and the processes of application, analysis, synthesis, and evaluation. The affective domain includes those objectives that emphasize values and attitudes, such as the importance of maintaining patient confidentiality and the desire to follow laboratory safety procedures. The psychomotor domain deals with those behavior outcomes that require neuromuscular function, such as the actual performance of a laboratory procedure.

6.

D At the analysis level, the student is taking previously learned material and using it to resolve a problem such as a calculation and then interpreting/analyzing that value to evaluate the clinical significance. The student understands the organization of the material and can reorganize the component parts so that they form a new pattern or structure. Knowledge is the lowest level of cognitive learning and involves simply recalling learned material. At the comprehension level, the student grasps the meaning of the material but does not see the fullest implication of that material. Application requires the students to take learned material and use it to solve a problem such as a calculation. For this learning objective, the student needs to recall the INR calculation and then use the data provided to perform the calculation and interpret (analyze) the value obtained.

7.

A. The conditions in an objective, "Given the appropriate tools and written procedure", describe what will be provided or denied to the student in order to accomplish the objective. Other parts of an objective include the terminal behavior required by the learner ("the student will perform daily maintenance on the chemistry analyzer") and the standards of performance ("without error"). The terminal behavior addresses what the learner must be able to do after completing the instructional unit. The standards of performance indicate how well the learner must perform for an acceptable behavior.

8.

B. The initials MLS(ASCP)^{cm} indicate that Jane Smith is certified by the American Society for Clinical Pathology as a medical laboratory scientist Certification is the process by which an individual's qualifications are recognized by a nongovernmental organization or agency. It is a voluntary process and usually involves meeting specific academic requirements and passing an examination. The superscript "cm" indicates that Jane participates in the credential maintenance program (CMP) for the professional certification.

9.

A. The National Accrediting Agency for Clinical Laboratory Sciences (NAACLS) is responsible for the evaluation and recommendation of accreditation of medical laboratory science programs after a review process including a self-study and a site visit. The term "certification" refers to the process by which an individual's competency is recognized by a nongovernmental agency or association. Licensure is the process by which a governmental agency grants an individual the permission to work in a certain field after successful completion of an examination. The term "registration" refers to the process by which individuals are identified by a nongovernmental agency as being certified. The term "registration" has been replaced by "certification."

10.

D. An instructor should be familiar with the institution's procedure for handling academic misconduct which includes cheating and should follow established guidelines when misconduct is detected. Ignoring the problem or assigning a failing grade does not help the student. Ignoring the problem will also damage the morale of the other students, who are often aware when an individual is cheating.

11.

C. Problem-based learning (PBL) is designed for the instructor to serve as a facilitator in the learning process. The goal for students is to resolve problems, develop critical thinking skills, and learn team communication skills while working together. The students determine what information is needed to solve the problems posed and select the appropriate resources. Traditional lecturing is not a characteristic component of PBL.

12.

D. The lecture format is good for disseminating large amounts of information to the learner. It is the most popular learning format and is useful for bringing together information from a variety of sources. It can be limiting, however, because of the lack of involvement of the learner.

13.

B. In simulation or role-playing activities, each student participates in a specific role and works through a situation in that role. Simulation activities allow for a team of students to work through a situation in a nonthreatening, practice environment which helps to further develop team skills. In a lecture, an instructor presents large amounts of information to a group. In online courses, the course content can be to a large audience located in different places through a learning management system. Cooperative learning involves students working in small groups on a given topic.

14.

B. Assessments are reliable when the results of the test are stable and consistent from year to year. Objectivity refers to questions relating back to the specific learning objectives. The level of a question refers to the type of test question being used—recall, interpretation, or problem-solving. If each student is given a different set of test questions, the reliability cannot be determined as it varies student to student and with each offering.

15.

A. Simulation represents a learning format that is specifically designed to promote cooperative problem-solving and communication skills. For these reasons, simulation is useful for developing learning outcomes in the affective domain. Simulation is especially effective when it represents a situation that the student will be likely to encounter in the future.

16.

C. Licensure is a process where a governmental agency sets the requirements for an individual to work in a specific state. The agency may require a specific certification, but having the certification may not equate to licensure. Educational programs can be accredited.

17.

C. Criterion-referenced examinations assess a student's mastery of a skill or body of knowledge with the use of predetermined minimal standards. Unlike a traditional norm-referenced test, in which students compete with one another on test performance, it is possible and even desirable for all students to do well on a criterion-referenced test. Examples of criterion-referenced examinations are the certification examinations of the ASCP Board of Registry (American Society for Clinical Pathology) and the National Credentialing Agency for Laboratory Personnel, Inc. (NCA).

18.

C. The certification examination of the ASCP Board of Certification is an example of a summative test, because it is comprehensive and designed to assess the mastery of a body of material. Placement tests are designed to test for prerequisite skills necessary for a course of study. Formative tests are administered during a course of study and allow the student to assess their knowledge at that time. Diagnostic tests are administered to aid in defining learning disabilities.

19.

A. Level I test questions are recall questions where the student has to recall a fact. Level II questions require the student to use the factual information to interpret or explain more about the problem, test principle, etc. Level III questions require the student to solve a problem using the factual information and applying it to the problem presented. Level III questions are complex and require recall, interpretation, and application.

20.

A. A checklist is a list of statements describing expected student behaviors in performing the steps that comprise a particular task or procedure. The behaviors are checked to indicate whether or not they occurred. A checklist is differentiated from a rating scale by its "all or none" format.

21.

D. Correlational design is where two or more variables are measured to determine relationships. Experimental-comparison design compares different groups that have been assigned to receive different treatments or studies of before and after treatment. Descriptive research is a type of non-experimental quantitative research. Single-case experimental design is where the same subjects receive different treatments, and comparisons or changes are noted.

22.

D. Stratified random assignment is the process of random assignment in the same category. Random assignment of individuals to groups helps overcome sampling errors or bias. Selection bias is one of the most critical problems of research design.

23.

D. Quantitative research is a type of descriptive research where the researcher is observing a subject in relation to determining differences and similarities. Survey research where questions are used to study a population or problem is an example of quantitative research. Historical and assessment research are other examples.

24.

C. Reliability is the degree to which a measure is consistent in producing the same readings when measuring the same things. Validity is the degree to which a measure actually measures the concept it is supposed to measure. Worthwhile research data must have reliable and valid measurement tools.

25.

B. The larger the sample size, the smaller the sampling error. Sample size is an important part of research design. If the sample is too small, chances are good that no statistically significant results will be obtained. However, as the sample size increases, the cost of performing the study increases.

26.

B. The standard deviation (*s* or SD) is the dispersion or scatter of a set of numbers. Standard deviation is the square root of the variance. Along with the mean, a measure of central tendency, the standard deviation is a descriptive statistic used to summarize data in a sample.

REFERENCES

Anderson, L. W., and Krathwohl, D. R. (Eds.) (2001). *A Taxonomy for Learning, Teaching, and Assessing: A Revision of Bloom's Taxonomy of Educational Objectives*. New York, NY: Longman.

Beck, S. J., and LeGrys, V. L. (2007). *Clinical Laboratory Education* (CD ROM). Bethesda, MD: The American Society for Clinical Laboratory Science.

Bishop, M. L., Fody, E. P. and Schoeff, L. E. *Clinical Chemistry: Principles, Techniques, and Correlations*, 8th ed. Philadelphia: Lippincott Williams & Wilkins.

Depoy, E., and Gitlin, L. N. (2016). *Introduction to Research: Understanding and Applying Multiple Strategies*, 5th ed. St. Louis: Elsevier.

Harmening, D. M. (2012). *Laboratory Management Principles and Processes*, 3rd ed. St. Petersburg: D. H. Publishing & Consulting Inc.

McKeachie, W. J., and Svinicki, M. D. (2013). *McKeachie's Teaching Tips: Strategies, Research, and Theory for College and University Teachers*, 14th ed. Belmont: Wadsworth Publishing.

Riegelman, R. K. (2012). *Studying a Study and Testing a Test*, 6th ed. Philadelphia: Lippincott Williams & Wilkins.

Weissman, J. (2008). *Presenting to Win: The Art of Telling Your Story*. Upper Saddle River, NJ: Pearson FT Press.

CHAPTER

16 Computers and Laboratory Information Systems

contents

I. DEFINITIONS

A. A personal computer (PC), also referred to as a microcomputer or desktop computer, is a stand-alone computer that contains a central processing unit (CPU), monitor, hard drive, etc., and can be used for processing data.

B. An operating system is a computer program that controls the basic operation of a computer and allows other software to interact with the computer hardware (e.g., Windows Operating System, UNIX, and Mac OS).

C. A server is a computer with a large amount of memory and storage capacity that stores data accessed by other computers, called clients or workstations. Programs (applications) can also be stored on servers.

D. A mainframe is a large-capacity computer designed to support many users at once with little or no down time. The term can have different meanings, but today it often refers to computers compatible with the IBM System/360 series of computers.

E. Supercomputers are computers that, at the time of their production, are on the forefront of processing speed. They contain hundreds of CPUs.

F. A local area network (LAN) is a collection of hardware, including printers and PCs, or clients connected to at least one server through cables (hardwired) or via a wireless network. The PCs are able to send data and share files with others on the network.

G. An intranet is a network of computers and other hardware that is not accessible to anyone outside that organization or office.

H. A wide area network (WAN) is a computer network over a large geographic area that crosses metropolitan or national boundaries.

I. Computerized provider order entry (CPOE) is a method of digital entry of instructions for the diagnosis and treatment of patients by a medical practitioner.

J. An electronic health record (EHR) is a digital patient record that can include demographics, test results, medical history and examination, images, etc. EHRs can encompass the entire patient history and is designed to be shared with other providers across practices.

K. An electronic medical record is also a digital patient record. However, EMRs differ from EHRs in that EHRs are designed to share information within a single organization.

L. A hospital information system (HIS) is a powerful computer system that includes hardware and software responsible for storing patient, business, and employee data. An HIS is often linked to other digital information systems (e.g., laboratory information system).

M. A community health information network (CHIN) is a network of computers in a community or city that shares information on patients. Hospitals, reference laboratories, physician offices, pharmacies, health insurance companies, etc., can have access to patient information.

N. Malware is malicious software that can damage computers and includes viruses, Trojans, spyware, etc.

O. Informatics is the science of information, the practice of processing information, and the development of information systems.

P. Bluetooth: Wireless technology that is used for short distance connections. Most input devices can use Bluetooth connectivity.

Q. Terminal Server: Hardware that is used to provide a common IP address to many devices. This is most commonly used for laboratories connecting many analyzers or instrumentation using a common IP address.

II. GENERAL COMPUTER INFORMATION

A. Digital Data

1. Computers process and store data using numbers.
2. **Binary (base 2):** Computers use a series of 0s (zeroes) and 1s (ones); 0 is off and 1 is on.
3. **Bit:** A 0 or 1
4. A **Byte** is a series of 8 bits. It takes one byte to represent one character. There are 2^8, or 256, combinations of bytes. Storage capacity is measured in kilobytes (KB), 1024 bytes; megabytes (MB), 1024 kilobytes; or gigabytes (GB), 1024 megabytes.

B. Computer Hardware

1. The **CPU** contains millions of transistors and performs mathematical and logical operations. The speed of the CPU is measured in **clock speed**, or gigahertz (GHz), which is the number of cycles per second. **Cache memory** is the location of data being processed by the CPU and is located on the CPU. Cache memory is the fastest memory on a computer, but it is also the most expensive. Modern computers have dual or quad processors.
2. **Memory modules** are the location where **random access memory** (RAM) is stored. RAM contains data waiting to be processed or that has recently been processed by the CPU. RAM requires continuous electricity to be maintained; any data in RAM is lost when the computer loses power. Modern computers generally have 8–16 GB of RAM.
3. The **motherboard** is a circuit board connecting the other components of the computer. The CPU, memory modules, and other circuit boards are plugged into the motherboard. When the power is turned on, the motherboard distributes power to the integrated circuits and moves data through the components. The electronic pathway for the movement of data is referred to as the **databus.**

4. **Input devices:** A number of devices can input data into a computer.
   a. Keyboard
   b. Pointing device (e.g., mouse and touch-sensitive pad) is used with a **graphical user interface** (GUI).
   c. Bar code reader or scanner reads printed bar codes, a series of parallel lines that represent letters or numbers. Bar codes are used to identify patients and patient samples.
5. **Output devices**
   a. **Monitor**
      1) **Resolution** is measured in the number of **pixels** (**pic**ture **el**ements) and the **dot pitch.** A pixel is the smallest piece of information in an image. It is composed of three dots: red, green, and blue. A monitor with a resolution of 1024 × 768 has 1024 columns and 768 rows of pixels. Dot pitch refers to the distance between dots of light of the same color. The smaller the dot pitch and the greater the number of pixels, the better is the image.
      2) **Liquid crystal display** (LCD) monitors have become the industry standard. They take up less space, are lighter, and use less electricity than the older **cathode ray tube** (CRT) monitors.
      3) Light-emitting diode (LED): Also an industry standard, it uses two semiconductors which emit light when activated. LEDs share the same advantages as LCDs.
   b. **Printers**
      1) **Inkjet printers** spray ink onto paper.
      2) **Laser jet printers** use the precision of a laser to position dots on a drum with magnetized toner. The particles are fixed to the paper with heat. Laser jet printers are faster but more expensive to purchase compared to inkjet printers. Generally, however, the cost per page is less for a laser jet printer.
      3) **Plotters** are vector graphic printing devices that print line art by moving a pen over the surface of paper. They are used for large technical drawings (architecture) and computer-aided designs.
6. **Storage devices**
   a. **Hard drives** use magnetized microscopic particles embedded in a surface. Data are added and retrieved using a read/write head. Hard drives can be internal or external. **Disk arrays** are a series of linked, generally external, hard drives with much larger storage capacity. Hard drives allow **random accessing** of data, meaning the computer can directly read or write to any location on the disk.
   b. **Tape drives**, or streamers, read and write data to a magnetic tape. Data are stored **sequentially**, meaning the data can only be accessed in an ordered sequence. They are generally used to back up large amounts of data and typically have a storage capacity of 4–20 GB. Sequential storage is an effective use of space, but it takes longer to access the data compared to accessing data on a hard drive.
   c. **USB flash drives** contain a universal serial bus (USB) connector and a flash memory chip (circuit). Because of their compact size, large storage capacity, and ease of use, these storage devices are widely used.

d. **Compact discs (CDs)** and **digital versatile discs or digital video discs (DVDs)** are optical storage devices. Data are stored as either "pits" or "grounds" on the disks in thin closely spaced **tracks.** A laser is used to read the data on the disks. DVDs have tracks that are much closer together and, therefore, they have greater storage capacity.
e. Solid state storage (SSD): Storage device that does not rely on moving, mechanical parts, similar to USB drives but faster.

7. **Cables** are used to connect external components **(peripherals)** to the computer via the motherboard.
   a. **Serial cables** move one bit of data at a time. Serial cables are no longer commonly used; they have been replaced by USB cables.
   b. **Parallel cables** move one byte of data at a time. Parallel cables had been used to connect printers and laboratory instruments to a computer. Parallel connections have generally been replaced by USB connections, which are much faster and use thinner cables.
   c. **USB** cables are commonly used to connect peripherals. They allow multiple devices to be connected through a single port; allow plug and play (hot swapping), where a device can be removed without restarting the computer; and provide power to low-consumption devices.
   d. **IEEE 1394** interface (i.e., Firewire, Apple Inc.) is a high-speed serial connection commonly used to connect digital cameras and audio/visual components to a computer.
   e. High Definition Multimedia Interface (HDMI): Interface used between any audio or visual source displaying a higher resolution.

C. Electronic Communication

1. The **Internet** is a worldwide network of computers.
2. **Transmission control protocol** (TCP) is the protocol computers use to exchange data on the Internet. It allows electronic mail (**e-mail**) and the content of Web sites to be sent electronically. TCP divides messages and files into smaller pieces called **segments.**
3. **Internet protocol (IP) address** is a unique address that electronic devices (e.g., computers and printers) use in order to communicate with each other on a computer network.
4. **Bandwidth** refers to the rate data are transferred; it is usually measured in kilobits/second (Kbps). A **broadband** connection is one that transfers a lot of **digital data** at once or when multiple pieces of data are sent simultaneously. Computers need a **network interface card** (NIC) to connect to a broadband cable. Examples of cable connections include:
   a. **Ethernet cable** (1 gigabit+/second)
   b. **Coaxial cable** (10 megabits+/second)
   c. **Fiber-optic cable** (600 megabits+/second)

5. **Wi-Fi**, or "wireless fidelity," allows wireless access to computer networks via radio waves. Although distances vary, with a standard antenna distance is limited to about 100 feet.
6. The **World Wide Web**, or the Web, is a body of information (documents) interlinked and accessed via the Internet. Sir Tim Berners-Lee is credited with creating the Web in 1989.
   a. **Hyperlinks:** A navigational element in one document links to another section of the same document or to a different document
   b. **Hypertext transfer protocol** (HTTP) is a communication protocol for the transfer of information (hypertext) over a computer network.
   c. **File transfer protocol** (FTP) is a network protocol used for uploading documents to a Web server.
   d. **Uniform resource locator** (URL) is a string of characters that provides the address or location of a unique document available over the Internet.
   e. **Hypertext markup language** (HTML) and extensive markup language (XML) are standard languages used for Web pages. Web browsers read the text (i.e., HTML code) and display the information.
7. **Search engines** use **spiders** or **bots** (short for robots) to retrieve information found in Web pages and create a searchable database.
8. **Telemedicine** is the use of technology to send healthcare-related information (e.g., patient test results) for clinical diagnosis and treatment.
9. Virtual Private Network (VPN): Extends a private network over a public network. For example, a hospital private network can be accessed from a remote location through the use of a VPN.

III. LABORATORY INFORMATION SYSTEMS

A. A laboratory information system (LIS) is a computer network of hardware and software for receiving, processing, and storing laboratory data and information. It can interface with laboratory instruments to transfer data into patient records, evaluate quality control data, and store preventive maintenance records. In addition, an LIS can interface with an HIS, pathology information system, and other information systems.

B. Components of an LIS
   1. The LIS software **user interface**, typically a GUI, determines how the user will interact with the system. It will have specific screens for entering data, sending reports, reporting results, etc. The software will have features such as security, access control, file maintenance, etc.
   2. **Request entry:** Requests for laboratory tests to be performed can be entered through clients located in the nursing units or remote primary care practitioner's office. In the case of outpatients, requests can be entered when the patient arrives at the laboratory.

3. **Data (results) entry**
   a. **Electronic data interface (EDI)** connections between an LIS and a clinical instrument allow automatic transfer of patient test results to the LIS.
   b. **Manual data entry:** Laboratory scientist will enter patient result into the LIS. This is usually done when there is no interface (EDI) between an analyzer and an LIS.
   c. **Release patient results:** The results are added to the LIS, but they are not released to clients outside the laboratory until the results and quality control are reviewed and verified. Alternatively, **autoverification** can be used. In this case, the computer uses a set of instructions to determine if the results should be released. Because the results are not held up for manual review, autoverification is quicker. To help with verification, reference ranges and panic values are programmed into the LIS. In most hospitals, autoverification is dependent on quality control being in-range in the LIS in a 24-hour period. Autoverification can be set up to be halted entirely or just by test if a control is out of range. Most LIS systems will also have a way to manually suspend autoverification. When results are released, patient values are **flagged** or marked as being outside the reference range.
   d. **Point of care (POC) testing:** POC testing is performed at the patient's bedside often using portable laboratory instruments, like handheld analyzers, that can connect to an LIS via a wireless connection. Many POC tests are waived tests, meaning that they are low in complexity, low risk for incorrect results, and can be performed by health professionals not educated in laboratory testing.
4. **Data storage**
   a. **Redundant arrays of independent disks (RAID):** LISs are regulated by the Food and Drug Administration and considered a medical device, and they are required to have **mirrored hard drives.** Data are stored on two separate hard drives of the LIS server.
   b. **System backup:** Each day the data are to be copied to an external or other portable storage device and removed from the laboratory.
   c. **Cloud based:** Remote servers that allows for storage and access of information via the Internet.
   d. Node: Any computer or device with a unique IP address.
5. **System security:** Ongoing procedures to ensure the security of patient data and user profiles (usernames and passwords) to prevent unauthorized access must be in place. **Phishing** is an illegal attempt to obtain any sensitive information such as usernames and passwords. Users should have access only to the patient information and LIS functions needed to perform their job (minimum necessary use). The Health Insurance Portability and Accountability Act requires that healthcare providers maintain strict confidentiality of patient medical records. Antiviral software should be installed to protect the system from harmful **malware**, especially for networks with a Windows operating system.

6. **Barcoding** can facilitate processing of clinical specimens.
   a. Bedside Labeling: A feature from either LIS and/or HIS, this involves printing a specimen label at patient bedside or point of collection. A printed label would be accessible with the LIS so no further labeling is required.
7. **Interface:** The LIS can be connected to clinical instruments and other information systems through an EDI. An interface is typically **bidirectional**, meaning information is sent to and from the instruments and the information systems. With a **unidirectional** interface, analyte results from an instrument are sent to the LIS, but the LIS cannot send requests to the instrument. So that instruments and computers used in healthcare can communicate with each other, the **Health Level 7** (HL7) communication standard was adopted. HL7 is an international committee formed in 1987 to formulate data standards, a set of rules that allow healthcare information to be shared and processed in a uniform and consistent way.
8. **Manual procedures:** Also called "downtime" when the computer system goes down; a contingency plan for manual procedures and forms needs to be in place.
9. **System maintenance:** LISs need to be shut down (taken offline) periodically for software upgrades and other maintenance. Occasionally, the system will become nonresponsive (crash).
10. **Disaster recovery:** Every laboratory needs a plan to restore the system after system disruption by a storm, fire, or other hardware damaging situation.
11. **Middleware:** An interface that bridges software between an analyzer and the LIS. It can be used to modify patient results before sending them to the LIS.
12. **Audit Trail:** Important function of any LIS that can track single user activity from specimen accessioning to result verification

C. Information Provided by an LIS

1. **Patient demographics**
2. **Work lists**
3. **Data retrieval (inquiry)**
   a. Generate patient results: Flag critical values, print reports if requested, etc.
   b. Perform **delta checks:** Results of an analyte assay are compared to the most recent previously performed results on the same patient
   c. Patient results can be retrieved electronically at a client or via the Internet with a Web browser.
4. **Reflex testing:** If an initial test result is positive or outside normal parameters, the LIS can automatically order a second appropriate test.
5. **Current procedural terminology (CPT) codes:** The CPT codes describe medical, surgical, and diagnostic services and are designed to communicate information about medical services and procedures among physicians and other healthcare professionals. CPT codes are used for billing purposes and can be programmed into the LIS.

6. **Quality control:** An LIS can analyze quality control entered manually or sent via an interface and prepare charts and reports (e.g., Westgard rules and Levey-Jennings charts).
7. **Quality assurance** can provide reports on turn-around time, documentation of critical result reporting, and corrected reports.
8. **Management reports:** Cost per billable test calculations, test volume, turn-around time, employee hours, workload data, etc.
9. **Encoding systems:** Systemized Nomenclature of Medicine—Clinical Terms **(SNOMED—CT)** is a comprehensive database of standardized terminology for healthcare. Once implemented, it will allow automatic data analysis over a wide range of clinical information systems. Logical observation identifiers names and codes (**LOINC**) is another database of universal standards for healthcare.
10. Turn-around-Time (TAT): An estimated amount of time it takes for the completion of a test. This information can be built into tests in LIS to generate reports or visual monitors.

D. Selecting an LIS

1. The process begins with a laboratory **needs assessment**, where data are collected on the information needs of the laboratory.
2. **Needs are analyzed** to determine feasibility of a system and what is needed to get the job done.
3. Laboratory managers and administrators form a committee and prepare a **request for proposal** (RFP). The RFP contains information about the laboratory facility, lists specific requirements needed in an LIS, and poses questions about LISs. This information may include interface capabilities to hospital information systems and laboratory instruments, remote user access, system requirements, custom features, hardware and software maintenance contracts, training, etc. The RFP is distributed to vendors.
4. Vendors will respond to the RFP describing how their systems will meet the needs of the laboratory and the estimated cost of the systems.
5. The RFP responses will be reviewed by the committee. To prevent information overload and confusion, only a few of the vendors, those that submitted an RFP response that match the needs assessment, should be selected to give demonstrations.
6. **Vendor demonstrations and visits to other laboratories** using the systems help narrow the choices. Vendor demonstrations should be scheduled within a short time frame so that information is fresh in everyone's mind.
7. **Selection** is based on the system that can best meet the laboratory's needs at the lowest cost (i.e., the cost does not outweigh the benefit).

E. Installation

1. The installation process is important and very time-consuming. It is critical to identify any errors early in the process before the system is activated **(goes live).**

2. Vendor representatives will install the server, clients, network connections, and software.
3. **Testing:** A thorough test of individual components **(unit test)** and a test of the system **(integration test)** are performed.
4. **Training** laboratory personnel and other healthcare providers on the LIS is an expensive process. It is important to discuss this with the vendor before accepting a proposal. Management needs to know how many people the vendor will train. It will become the responsibility of the laboratory personnel receiving training to train others. Training will also be needed for healthcare providers outside the laboratory.
5. **Communication:** Before the LIS goes live, it is important to communicate to all members of the healthcare team about the planning and timeline of the process.

F. System Validation

1. Validation of the laboratory information system is an ongoing process of proving the system performs its intended use initially and over time.
2. Validation consists of defining, collecting, maintaining, and reviewing evidence that the system is performing consistently according to specification. It is tedious, difficult, and costly, but it must be done to assure that the system meets the needs of the laboratory.

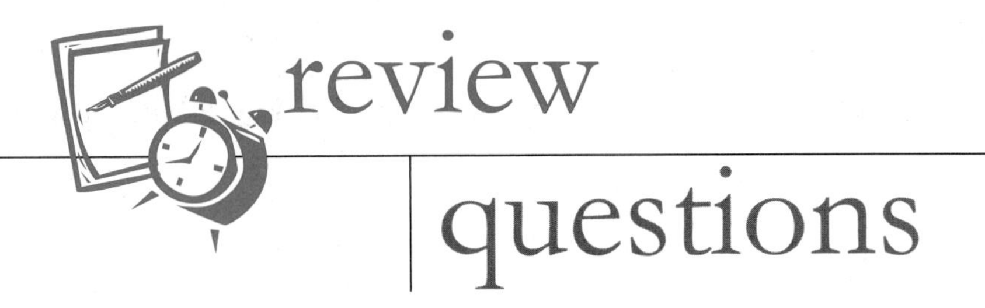

review questions

INSTRUCTIONS Each of the questions or incomplete statements that follows is comprised of four suggested responses. Select the *best* answer or completion statement in each case.

1. You have been asked to chair a committee to recommend the purchase of a laboratory information system (LIS). What is the first step you should take?
   A. Issue a request for proposal (RFP)
   B. Develop a needs assessment
   C. Contact vendors for product demonstrations
   D. Determine the encoding system that will be used
2. What devices usually use Bluetooth connectivity?
   A. Wireless speakers
   B. Monitor
   C. Mouse
   D. Both A and C
3. An electronic data interface (EDI) is used to
   A. Access the Internet
   B. Connect instruments to a laboratory information system
   C. Manually enter patient results into a laboratory information system
   D. Provide security to patient records
4. The fastest type of memory a computer has access to is
   A. Random access
   B. Sequential
   C. Serial
   D. Cache
5. What is an illegal attempt to obtain any sensitive information?
   A. Anti-virus
   B. Malware
   C. Phishing
   D. System security
6. In networked computer systems, what does the term "client" refer to?
   A. Manufacturer of the software
   B. Software that allows the connected hardware to communicate
   C. Computer that provides software to user terminals
   D. Workstation from which the user requests services from the server

7. A worldwide network of computers describes
   A. Hyperlinks
   B. Hypertext markup language
   C. Search engines
   D. The Internet
8. A secure connection from a public network can be established through?
   A. Terminal Server
   B. Virtual Private Network
   C. Ethernet capability
   D. File Transfer Protocol
9. Which of the following is an example of an optical storage device?
   A. Compact disk (CD)
   B. Universal serial bus (USB) drive
   C. Computer tape
   D. Hard drive
10. Computers process and store data using a binary system. This is equivalent to
    A. Base 2
    B. Base 4
    C. Base 8
    D. Base 10
11. Which one of the following may be used as a pointing device with a graphical user interface?
    A. Databus
    B. Internet connection
    C. Keyboard
    D. Mouse
12. Disk arrays are
    A. High-performance printers
    B. Large-capacity storage devices
    C. Broadband Internet connections
    D. Methods used to search a database
13. Patient results from an autoanalyzer are released to the primary care provider without being reviewed is referred to as:
    A. Autoverification
    B. Delta check
    C. Reflexing
    D. Host query
14. Which of the following is *not* an important part of laboratory information systems?
    A. Specimen tracking
    B. Data retrieval
    C. Transportation
    D. Order entry
15. USB drives have a universal serial bus connector and a
    A. Disk drive
    B. Flash memory chip
    C. Parallel connection
    D. Tape drive
16. What device would allow multiple analyzers to share a common Internet protocol (IP) Address?
    A. Wide area network
    B. Graphical user interface
    C. USB drive
    D. Terminal server
17. The speed of Internet access is partly determined by the carrying capacity of the communication line. What is this called?
    A. Bandwidth
    B. Interface
    C. Internet protocol
    D. Uniform resource locator
18. Many laboratory information systems allow users the option to define actions in response to certain patient results, such as performing additional tests or sending test results to public health authorities. What is this feature called?
    A. Flagging
    B. Hot key inquiry
    C. Host query
    D. Reflexing

19. Communication among laboratory information systems in different hospitals is becoming more common. Data transfers can be facilitated if laboratories use which standardized communication interface?
    A. Health level 7
    B. RS-232C
    C. Hypertext transfer protocol
    D. UNIX
20. Search engines use computer programs to collect information found in Web pages. These programs are commonly called
    A. Hyperlinks
    B. Spiders
    C. Malware
    D. Trojans
21. When documents are uploaded to Web servers, special software is used. This software uses a standard protocol called
    A. File transfer protocol (FTP)
    B. Hypertext markup language (HTML)
    C. Hypertext transfer protocol (HTTP)
    D. Uniform resource locator (URL)
22. After a hospital has decided to purchase a laboratory information system, what do laboratory administrators issue to solicit bids from vendors?
    A. Ancillary report
    B. Good manufacturing practice request
    C. Request for proposal
    D. Needs analysis
23. What feature of a laboratory information system compares a patient's test value to a previous value?
    A. Archiving
    B. Delta check
    C. Prompt
    D. System validation
24. Of the following hardware, which one is an input device?
    A. Keyboard
    B. Monitor
    C. Printer
    D. Motherboard
25. A networked computer's unique address is called the
    A. FTP address
    B. Community health network (CHIN) address
    C. IP address
    D. URL
26. The laboratory is requesting an interface that will send information only to the LIS. What type of interface is the laboratory requesting?
    A. Bidirectional
    B. Unidirectional
    C. Unilateral
    D. None of the above

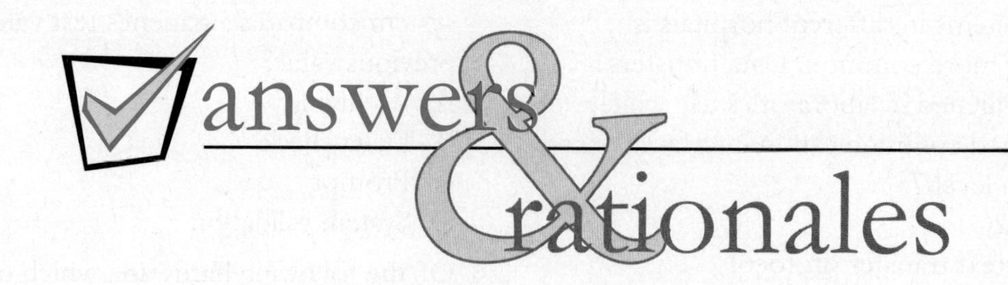

1.

B. The first step in recommending a laboratory information system is determining the informational needs of the laboratory. Needs are analyzed to determine the feasibility of a system and what is needed to get the job done. Once the needs assessment is complete, an RFP is announced. Vendors will read the RFP and submit a proposal to the laboratory.

2.

D. A mouse is an example of an input that can be wireless and connect via Bluetooth. Speaker can also connect wirelessly to a computer by Bluetooth or Wi-Fi. An output device such as a printer can also use Bluetooth connectivity.

3.

B. An electronic data interface connects a laboratory information system (LIS) to clinical instruments. The connection allows data (test results) from the instrument to be automatically added to the LIS. This method of entering results is much faster and more accurate than manual entry.

4.

D. Cache memory is located on the central processing unit and is the fastest memory to which the computer has access. It is also the most expensive type of memory. Increasing cache memory does, however, reach a point of diminishing returns—after a certain point, the addition of more cache memory does not increase computer performance.

5.

C. Phishing is an illegal attempt at obtaining sensitive information. Malware is software that is intended to damage or disable a computer. Usually, anti-virus software, like Windows Defender, is used to prevent malware from being installed to a computer. Hospital information technology teams will have system security in place to prevent phishing attempts.

6.

D. The client is the workstation or terminal requesting data from the server. In other words, the server provides information to the client or user. The client can be a stand-alone desktop computer or a thin client that is only a terminal (monitor and keyboard).

7.

D. The Internet is simply a global collection of computers. The computers providing the information are called servers. Each computer on the Internet has a unique Internet protocol (IP) address or location.

8.

B. VPNs are used to establish a secure connection using a public network to a private network. This establishes an encrypted connection between your computer and the VPN remote server.

9.

A. From the list, only a CD is an optical storage device. The data on the CD are read using a laser. Hard drives are magnetic storage devices, and a USB drive uses a circuit to store data.

10.

A. Computers function on two states: off or on. Data are stored as a series of zeroes and ones. This is equivalent to a base 2 or binary system.

11.

D. Pointer devices control the movement of a movable icon, usually an arrow, on the monitor. A mouse is the most common type of pointing device. Touch-sensitive pads are pointing devices commonly found on laptop computers.

12.

B. Disk arrays are a series of hard drives used for storing digital data. Because mainframe computers need to store a lot of information, they often have disk arrays. Disk arrays can be internal or external.

13.

A. Autoverification is when a computer uses a set of instructions to determine if test results should be released. In most hospitals, autoverification dependents on quality control being in-range in the LIS in a 24-hour period and the patient result is reasonable. Because the results are not held up for manual review, autoverification releases results sooner. Values outside reference ranges will be flagged, marked as such.

14.

C. LISs can increase the efficiency of clinical laboratories by allowing for specimen tracking, data (e.g., patient results) retrieval, and order entry. The LIS does not transport specimens; a robotics system would be necessary to handle this function. Features of LISs vary considerably among the different vendors and can be customized to the needs of individual laboratories.

15.

B. USB drives store data on a flash memory chip (circuit). These storage devices are small, easy to use, and have a high storage capacity. These features have made flash memory drives very popular.

16.

D. Terminal Servers are used especially in places like clinical laboratories to allow multiple analyzers to share a common IP Address. A WAN, or wide area network, extends over a large distance.

17.

A. Bandwidth is measured in bits per second (bps). It is the amount of information that can be transmitted through a channel or communication line at one time. Internet protocols (IPs) are the standards allowing computers to exchange data via the Internet. Uniform resource locators (URLs) are the addresses used to find Web sites.

18.

D. Most LISs allow users to program additional operations to be performed based on specified patient results. If a patient result for a particular test falls within certain parameters, an additional test may be suggested. These reflexes should automatically include billing codes. Flagging is simply marking high or low values and critical (panic) values. Hot key inquiries are keys on the computer keyboard programmed to provide the user with additional information, such as reference ranges during data entry. A host query is a type of bidirectional interface between an instrument and the LIS.

19.

A. Hospitals, health maintenance organizations, and physician offices in an area may want to share patient information. In order for the computer information systems to communicate with each other and to exchange data, they must use a standardized transfer protocol. The most widely used interface for this purpose is Health Level 7 (HL7). The RS-232C is a type of serial interface with 25 pins. Hypertext transfer protocol (HTTP) is the protocol followed for the exchange of information on the Web. UNIX is a text-based operating system for servers.

20.

B. Spiders "crawl" along the Web and are used by Internet search engines to collect information found on Web pages. Malware refers to malicious software that can damage a computer or steal a user's identity. Trojans are an example of malware.

21.

A. In order for computer files to be accurately transferred on the Internet, standard protocols must be used. The protocols for uploading documents to a Web server are called file transfer protocols (FTPs). Hypertext markup language (HTML) is the language used to create Web pages. Hypertext transfer protocol (HTTP) is the protocol followed for the exchange of information on the Worldwide Web, and a uniform resource locator (URL) is a unique address for a Web page.

22.

C. In order to get the best price and solutions to a laboratory's computer needs, a request for proposal (RFP) is issued. The laboratory's needs are described, and companies submit proposals describing how the needs would be addressed and at what cost. Good manufacturing practice is a regulation issued by the Food and Drug Administration. Laboratories would do a needs analysis to help write an RFP.

23.

B. An LIS can be programmed to compare a patient's test value to a previous value for the same assay. This is called a delta check. A prompt is the user interface of a text-based operating system such as UNIX. System validation is a tool within the LIS allowing the user to set up and monitor testing, regulatory compliance, and quality control. Archiving refers to storing patient data that are no longer needed onto a backup system to free storage space on the LIS.

24.

A. Input devices are those that send data to the computer. The keyboard is an input device. The monitor displays information (output); however, touch screen monitors can be an input device. Printers are also output devices.

25.

C. A computer's unique address is called the Internet protocol (IP) address. A uniform resource locator (URL) is a unique address for a Web page. A community health network (CHIN) is a computer network in a community that shares data on patients.

26.

B. A unidirectional interface will send information from the analyzer to the LIS. Bidirectional interfaces will send information from analyzer to LIS (results) and also send information from LIS to analyzer (patient demographics).

REFERENCES

Chou, D. (2009). Laboratory Information Systems. In Kaplan, L. A. and Pesce, A. J. (Eds.), *Clinical Chemistry: Theory, Analysis, Correlation*, 5th ed. St. Louis: Elsevier.

Jackson, B. R., and Harrison, J. H. (2008). Clinical Laboratory Informatics. In Burtis, C. A., Ashwood, E. R. and Bruns, D. E. (Eds.), *Tietz Fundamentals of Clinical Chemistry*, 6th ed. Philadelphia: Elsevier.

PC Encyclopedia. Available at: https://www.pcmag.com/encyclopedia. Accessed May 18, 2018.

Sepulveda, J. L. and Young, D. S. (2013). The Ideal Laboratory Information System. *Archives of Pathology & Laboratory Medicine* 137:1129–1140.

CHAPTER

17 Self-Assessment Test

contents

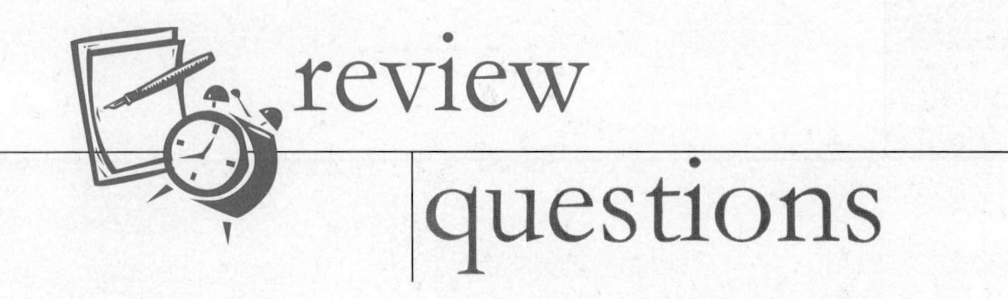

CHAPTER 1: CLINICAL CHEMISTRY

1. Which of the following instruments requires a primary and secondary monochromator?
   A. Spectrophotometer
   B. Atomic absorption spectrophotometer
   C. Fluorometer
   D. Nephelometer
2. There are six known defects associated with the development of congenital adrenal hyperplasia (CAH). Which of the following defects is the most common one seen?
   A. 11-Hydroxylase defect
   B. 11-Dehydrocorticosterone defect
   C. 11-Deoxycortisol defect
   D. 21-Hydroxylase defect
3. Insecticides that are organic phosphorus compounds, such as parathion and tetraethyl pyrophosphate, may cause insecticide poisoning by inhibiting:
   A. Lactate dehydrogenase
   B. Acid phosphatase
   C. Cholinesterase
   D. Glucose-6-phosphate dehydrogenase
4. Which of the following hormones involved in calcium regulation acts by decreasing both calcium and phosphorous?
   A. PTH
   B. Vitamin D
   C. Calcitonin
   D. Estrogen
5. Which of the following is a laboratory assay used for detecting cystic fibrosis?
   A. Serum lipase
   B. Serum amylase
   C. Serum trypsin
   D. Sweat chloride
6. In primary hypothyroidism one would expect the serum FT_4 level to be ________, the thyroid stimulating hormone level to be ________, and the thyroxine-binding globulin level to be ________.
   A. Decreased, increased, slightly increased
   B. Decreased, decreased, slightly increased
   C. Increased, decreased, slightly increased
   D. Decreased, increased, slightly decreased
7. Insulin release will stimulate the cellular uptake of which of the following electrolytes?
   A. Sodium
   B. Potassium
   C. Chloride
   D. Bicarbonate
8. Usually _______ are required after the onset of chest pain before creatine kinase-muscle/brain (CK-MB) or the troponins become elevated in a patient with myocardial infarction?
   A. 1–2 hours
   B. 2–4 hours
   C. 4–6 hours
   D. 6–8 hours

9. A blood specimen is drawn in the morning, and the serum is removed from the clot and left standing at room temperature until late in the afternoon. Which of the following parameters would be most severely affected by delayed analysis?
   A. Urea
   B. Potassium
   C. Alanine aminotransferase
   D. Bilirubin
10. In ketoacidosis, the anion gap would most likely be affected in what way?
    A. Unchanged from normal
    B. Increased
    C. Decreased
    D. Balanced
11. If the aspartate aminotransferase (AST) and the alanine aminotransferase (ALT) serum levels are increased 50-fold over the reference range, what would be the most consistent diagnosis?
    A. Extrahepatic cholestasis
    B. Cirrhosis
    C. Carcinoma of the liver
    D. Viral hepatitis
12. A decreased bicarbonate level in the blood without a change in PCO_2 will result in what acid/base imbalance?
    A. Respiratory acidosis
    B. Respiratory alkalosis
    C. Metabolic acidosis
    D. Metabolic alkalosis
13. Elevated serum levels of urea, creatinine, and uric acid would be suggestive of what disorder?
    A. Gout
    B. Chronic renal failure
    C. Cirrhosis
    D. Malnutrition
14. As part of a gestational diabetes screening test, 1 hour after ingesting 50 grams of glucose the plasma glucose was 152 mg/dL. Based on this result, what interpretation is most correct?
    A. The result indicates normal glucose metabolism
    B. The result indicates gestational diabetes mellitus
    C. The result indicates type 1 diabetes mellitus
    D. The result indicates need for a diagnostic oral glucose tolerance test
15. Which of the following methods may be used to quantify total protein in serum, urine, or cerebrospinal fluid?
    A. Coomassie brilliant blue
    B. Sulfosalicylic acid
    C. Bromcresol green
    D. Ponceau S
16. A patient who received a blood transfusion experienced a hemolytic transfusion reaction. Because of the presence of free hemoglobin in the plasma, which serum protein will exhibit a decreased level?
    A. Ceruloplasmin
    B. Transferrin
    C. α_2-Macroglobulin
    D. Haptoglobin
17. When employing a diazo method to quantify serum bilirubin, which of the following blood constituents when present in an elevated amount will cause a falsely depressed bilirubin result?
    A. Ammonia
    B. Creatinine
    C. Hemoglobin
    D. Uric acid

18. The incorporation of which of the following into a spectrophotometer can sometimes improve the linearity of a chemistry procedure?
A. Flow-through cuvette
B. Wider bandwidth
C. Narrower bandwidth
D. Chopper

19. What hormone plays a primary role in controlling the reabsorption of sodium in the tubules?
A. Cortisol
B. Cortisone
C. Estriol
D. Aldosterone

20. Which of the following is associated with individuals diagnosed with Addison disease?
A. Hypoglycemia
B. Casual plasma glucose ≥200 mg/dL
C. Fasting plasma glucose ≥126 mg/dL
D. 2-Hour post-load glucose ≥200 mg/dL

21. Which of the following tests when used together are helpful in monitoring treatment and identifying recurrence of testicular cancer?
A. Alpha-fetoprotein (AFP) and carcinonoembryonic antigen (CEA)
B. AFP and human chorionic gonadotrophin (hCG)
C. CEA and hCG
D. Cancer antigen (CA) 125 and CA 19-9

22. The main substance used in the production of androgens and estrogens is:
A. Catecholamines
B. Cortisol
C. Cholesterol
D. Progesterone

23. High levels of cholesterol associated with increased risk of coronary artery disease would be associated with which lipoprotein fraction?
A. LDL
B. VLDL
C. HDL
D. Chylomicrons

24. The calculated osmolality given a sodium = 135 meq/L, glucose = 95 mg/dL, and BUN = 10 mg/dL is:
A. 240 mOsm/kg
B. 278 mOsm/kg
C. 375 mOsm/kg
D. 480 mOsm/kg

25. If the ratio of bicarbonate to carbonic acid is 30:1, what would be the blood pH?
A. Increased
B. Decreased
C. Stable
D. Normal

26. Upon what principle is nephelometric measurement based?
A. Fluorescence produced
B. Phosphorescence produced
C. Light transmitted
D. Light scattered

CHAPTER 2: HEMATOLOGY

27. A patient with beta-thalassemia characteristically has a(n):
A. Elevated A2 hemoglobin
B. Low fetal hemoglobin
C. High serum iron
D. Normal red blood cell fragility

28. The main source of thrombopoietin is the:
A. Kidney
B. Lymph node
C. Bone marrow
D. Spleen

29. Red blood cell distribution width is a measurement of the:
   A. Average size of the red blood cells
   B. Hemoglobin content of the red blood cells
   C. Coefficient of variation of the red cell population
   D. Various maturation stages of red blood cells
30. Aminolevulinic acid synthase is an enzyme involved in:
   A. Early stages of heme synthesis in the mitochondria
   B. Intermediate stages of heme synthesis in the cytoplasm
   C. Globin chain synthesis
   D. Embden-Meyerhof pathway
31. Hemoglobin A consists of:
   A. Two alpha-globin and two beta-globin chains
   B. Two alpha-globin and two gamma-globin chains
   C. Four beta-globin chains
   D. Two alpha-globin and two delta-globin chains
32. Increased osmotic fragility test results could be expected in which of the following disorders?
   A. Sickle cell anemia
   B. Iron-deficiency anemia
   C. Beta-thalassemia minor
   D. Hereditary spherocytosis
33. Which of the following conditions would *not* exhibit the red blood cell morphology seen in Color Plate 9■?
   A. Pyruvate kinase deficiency
   B. Sideroblastic anemia
   C. Posttransfusion
   D. Iron-deficiency anemia post-treatment
34. Complement-induced red blood cell lysis and glycosyl phosphatidylinositol–anchored protein deficient peripheral red blood cells are seen in which disorder?
   A. Glucose-6-phosphate dehydrogenase deficiency
   B. Hereditary spherocytosis
   C. Paroxysmal nocturnal hemoglobinuria
   D. Paroxysmal cold hemoglobinuria
35. Which of the following will be increased in polycythemia vera?
   A. Plasma volume
   B. Leukocyte alkaline phosphatase
   C. 2,3-Bisphosphoglyceric acid
   D. Urine bilirubin
36. Which of the following stains is used to visualize reticulocytes?
   A. Wright's
   B. Crystal violet
   C. Prussian blue
   D. New methylene blue
37. The function of the hexose monophosphate shunt is to:
   A. Produce adenosine triphosphate (ATP)
   B. Produce 2,3-bisphosphoglyceric acid
   C. Prevent oxidation of hemoglobin
   D. Participate in heme synthesis
38. Hemoglobin is measured spectrophotometrically at what wavelength?
   A. 410 nm
   B. 472 nm
   C. 540 nm
   D. 610 nm
39. The red blood cells seen in Color Plate 8■ would most likely be associated with:
   A. Sideroblastic anemia or beta-thalassemia major
   B. Hereditary spherocytosis or warm autoimmune hemolytic anemia
   C. Iron-deficiency anemia or beta-thalassemia minor
   D. Aplastic anemia or following chemotherapy

40. Deletional and nondeletional mutations in globin genes that reduce or eliminate synthesis of corresponding globin chain would result in?
A. Hemoglobinopathies
B. Thalassemias
C. Unstable hemoglobins
D. Porphyrias

41. The first leukocyte to migrate, engulf, and destroy a foreign body in the tissue is the:
A. Macrophage
B. Monocyte
C. Neutrophil
D. Lymphocyte

42. What immunoglobulin is increased in plasma cell myeloma?
A. IgA
B. IgE
C. IgG
D. IgM

43. The leukocyte alkaline phosphatase stain is most helpful in the differentiation of:
A. Neutrophilic leukemoid reaction and degenerative left shift
B. Neutrophilic leukemoid reaction and chronic myelogenous leukemia
C. Chronic myelogenous leukemia and acute myelogenous leukemia
D. Acute myelogenous leukemia and acute lymphoblastic leukemia

44. Which cell line is normally the most numerous in the bone marrow?
A. Lymphocytic
B. Megakaryocytic
C. Erythroid
D. Myeloid

45. Which French-American-British (FAB) type of myelodysplastic syndrome presents with less than 1 percent blasts in the peripheral blood, less than 5 percent blasts in the bone marrow, and no ringed sideroblasts?
A. Refractory anemia
B. Chronic myelomonocytic leukemia
C. Refractory anemia with excess blasts
D. Refractory anemia with excess blasts in transformation

46. A 5-year-old girl was recently diagnosed with acute lymphoblastic leukemia. Which of the following is *not* typical of this diagnosis?
A. Using World Health Organization criteria, bone marrow blasts will be $\geq 20\%$.
B. Common acute lymphoblastic leukemia antigen (CD10) positive type has a poor prognosis.
C. Central nervous system involvement is common.
D. Leukemic blast cells show periodic acid Schiff positivity.

47. Antigens expressed by precursor B-cells in B acute lymphoblastic leukemia (B-ALL) include:
A. CD3, CD4, and CD8
B. CD10, CD19, and CD34
C. There are no antigens specific for precursor B-ALL
D. Myeloperoxidase

48. A 59-year-old patient is evaluated for severe anemia, thrombocytopenia, and neutropenia. What test(s) will provide the most useful information?
A. Complete blood count and differential
B. Bone marrow aspirate and biopsy
C. Reticulocyte count and immature reticulocyte fraction
D. Test for heterophile antibodies

49. The Philadelphia chromosome is a consistent finding in patients with what disorder?
    A. Chronic myelogenous leukemia
    B. Acute myelomonocytic leukemia
    C. Myelodysplastic syndrome
    D. Primary myelofibrosis
50. Pelger-Huët anomaly is associated with:
    A. Large Döhle-like bodies and giant platelets
    B. Large azurophilic granules in all types of leukocytes
    C. Defective neutrophilic phagocytosis
    D. Morphologically immature but functionally normal neutrophils
51. Plasma cells are found in large numbers in the bone marrow and occasionally in the peripheral blood of patients with what disorder?
    A. Multiple myeloma
    B. Burkitt lymphoma
    C. Acute lymphoblastic leukemia
    D. Infectious mononucleosis
52. The blood smear shown in Color Plate 12■ is from a 16-year-old male with complaints of extreme fatigue and sore throat. His white blood cell, hemoglobin, and platelet count results are within reference ranges. Based on the clinical and laboratory information, which of the following is the most likely cause of his condition?
    A. Staphylococcal pneumonia
    B. Infectious mononucleosis
    C. Chronic lymphocytic leukemia
    D. Non-Hodgkin lymphoma
53. Which of the following disorders is associated with pancytopenia?
    A. Neutrophilic leukemoid reaction
    B. Acute lymphoblastic leukemia
    C. Chronic myelogenous leukemia
    D. Aplastic anemia
54. Inability to obtain a bone marrow aspirate is frequently encountered in patients with which of the following disorders?
    A. Acute monocytic leukemia and myelodysplastic syndromes
    B. Primary myelofibrosis and hairy cell leukemia
    C. Polycythemia vera and essential thrombocythemia
    D. Erythroleukemia and acute megakaryocytic leukemia
55. The cytoplasmic inclusion present in the cell shown in Color Plate 17■ excludes a diagnosis of:
    A. Acute myelogenous leukemia without maturation (FAB M1)
    B. Acute promyelocytic leukemia (FAB M3)
    C. Acute myelomonocytic leukemia (FAB M4)
    D. Acute lymphoblastic leukemia
56. Which of the following is considered diagnostic for Hodgkin lymphoma?
    A. Sézary cell
    B. Burkitt cell
    C. Reed-Sternberg cell
    D. Reider cell

CHAPTER 3: HEMOSTASIS

57. The test of choice to detect abnormalities in the intrinsic pathway of secondary hemostasis is the:
    A. PFA-100
    B. Thrombin time
    C. Activated partial thromboplastin time
    D. Prothrombin time
58. A 39-year-old male patient shows evidence of poor wound healing and a history of joint bleeding. What protein deficiency is most likely present?
    A. Factor II
    B. Factor V
    C. Factor X
    D. Factor XIII

59. Which of the following describes plasmin?
    A. Enzyme that can digest cross-linked fibrin into D-dimers
    B. Activator of plasminogen
    C. Circulates freely in the plasma ready to digest fibrin clots
    D. Forms a complex with tissue plasminogen activators to digest fibrinogen
60. By what mechanism does aspirin therapy impair platelet function?
    A. Blocks glycoprotein receptors on the surface of the platelet
    B. Decreases thrombopoietin levels and subsequent bone marrow platelet production
    C. Interferes with the ability of platelets to adhere to subendothelial collagen
    D. Decreases thromboxane A_2 formation by inhibiting cyclooxygenase
61. Which of the following describes thrombotic thrombocytopenic purpura?
    A. Occurs only in a chronic form
    B. A platelet autoantibody is responsible for platelet destruction
    C. Develops in the majority of cases after recovery from a bacterial infection
    D. Causes decreased bone marrow synthesis of platelet precursors
62. The most clinically significant naturally occurring inhibitor to clotting is:
    A. Antithrombin
    B. Lupus inhibitor
    C. Protein C
    D. α_2-Antiplasmin
63. Factor XII deficiency is associated with:
    A. Increased risk of thrombus
    B. Severe liver disease
    C. Poor clotting
    D. Bleeding in the spinal cord
64. An 18-year-old male was seen in the emergency department following a motorcycle accident. The patient was not wearing a helmet at the time of the accident. He was comatose and was admitted to the hospital with a diagnosis of severe closed head injury. The next day the patient was noted to have increased bleeding from venipuncture sites. Given the following results, what was the most likely diagnosis for this patient?

Tests	Patient Results	Reference Ranges
PT	25.0 seconds	11.0–13.0 seconds
aPTT	89.0 seconds	22.0–38.0 seconds
Fibrinogen	65 mg/dL	150–400 mg/dL
Thrombin time	45 seconds	15–20 seconds
Platelet count	$32 \times 10^9/L$	$150-450 \times 10^9/L$
FDP test	>20 μg/mL	<5 μg/mL
D-dimer	>1.0 μg/mL	<0.5 μg/mL

    A. Hemophilia A
    B. Primary fibrinogenolysis
    C. Thrombotic thrombocytopenic purpura
    D. Disseminated intravascular coagulation
65. Of the following conditions that cause bleeding, the most common is:
    A. Hemophilia A
    B. Thrombocytopenia
    C. von Willebrand disease
    D. Hemophilia B
66. Thrombocytopenia and loss of high molecular weight von Willebrand factor multimers are features of which of the following conditions?
    A. Type 2B von Willebrand disease
    B. Type 2M von Willebrand disease
    C. Type 1 von Willebrand disease
    D. Type 2A von Willebrand disease

CHAPTER 4: IMMUNOLOGY & SEROLOGY

67. How are individuals with cellular immune deficiencies best identified?
    A. Determining serum complement concentration
    B. Human leukocyte antigen typing
    C. Serum electrophoresis testing
    D. Skin testing
68. Which of the following is characteristic of DiGeorge syndrome?
    A. Defective T lymphocyte production
    B. Depressed B cell development
    C. Suppressed intracellular killing by polymorphonuclear cells
    D. Suppressed complement levels
69. The interaction between antigen-presenting cells and T-helper cells is mediated by surface expressed antigen and:
    A. Interferon gamma
    B. Interleukin 2
    C. Interleukin 3
    D. MHC class II molecules
70. Which of the following cell types is an important mediator of antibody-dependent cellular cytotoxicity reactions?
    A. B cells
    B. Cytotoxic T cells
    C. Natural killer cells
    D. Suppressor T cells
71. What is the portion of an antigen that binds specifically to the binding site of an antibody called?
    A. Epitope
    B. Hapten
    C. Idiotope
    D. Paratope
72. Which of the following is *true* of the alternative complement pathway?
    A. Activated by bacterial polysaccharide
    B. C3 is not involved
    C. C1 initiates activation
    D. Does not form membrane attack complexes
73. Role of T-helper cells in celiac disease:
    A. Release of IgE
    B. Mark host cells for destruction
    C. Secretion of proinflammatory molecules
    D. Inactivate the enzyme transglutaminase 2
74. A substance able to induce an immune response describes which of the following?
    A. Allotype
    B. Antigen
    C. Epitope
    D. Immunogen
75. The B cell surface receptor for antigen is:
    A. CD5
    B. Immunoglobulin
    C. Interleukin 2
    D. MHC I antigen
76. Which of the following frequently functions as an antigen-presenting cell?
    A. Dendritic cell
    B. Cytotoxic T lymphocyte
    C. Natural killer cell
    D. T-helper cell
77. Antibody normally present in the greatest concentration in serum:
    A. IgA
    B. IgE
    C. IgG
    D. IgM
78. The presence of antinuclear antibodies is suggestive of a(n):
    A. Acute glomerulonephritis
    B. Autoimmune disease
    C. Cell-mediated immune deficiency
    D. Humoral-mediated immune deficiency
79. Graves' disease is an autoimmune disease primarily affecting the:
    A. Adrenal gland
    B. Nerve synapses
    C. Pancreas
    D. Thyroid

80. Which of the following markers is found on mature T-helper cells?
A. CD4
B. CD8
C. CD10
D. CD25

81. An immunochromatographic assay for human chorionic gonadotropin (hCG) has a visible color at the *test* and *control lines*. How should you interpret the result?
A. Positive for hCG
B. Negative for hCG
C. Indeterminate
D. Invalid

82. In patients with myasthenia gravis, you would expect to find:
A. CD8 positive T cells reactive to myelin sheath
B. Antibodies to thyroid-stimulating hormone receptor
C. Antibodies to acetylcholine receptors
D. Decreased levels of IgA

83. Which of the following is a nonphagocytic cytotoxic cell able to kill cells rapidly without having been previously exposed to antigens on that cell?
A. Cytotoxic T cell
B. T-helper cell
C. Natural killer cell
D. Suppressor T cell

84. Which of the following is a granulocytic cell with IgE receptors?
A. Cytotoxic T cell
B. Mast cell
C. Natural killer cell
D. Plasma cell

85. Which of the following is an oncofetal antigen whose presence in adult serum is suggestive of carcinoma?
A. **α**-Fetoprotein
B. C-reactive protein
C. Lymphocyte function-associated antigen 1
D. Nuclear antigens

86. An adaptive or specific immune response includes:
A. Antibody synthesis
B. Complement activation
C. Inflammation
D. Phagocytosis

CHAPTER 5: IMMUNOHEMATOLOGY

87. Information obtained from a volunteer blood donor at the time of registration is designed to protect the health of both donor and recipient. Of the following responses, which would cause the donor to be deferred from the collection process?
A. Received his last injection in a vaccine series for hepatitis B 3 weeks ago
B. Had a tooth filled 1 week ago
C. Took aspirin yesterday for a headache
D. Taking Tegison

88. Interpret the following reactions:

	A_1 cells	B cells		Anti-A	Anti-B
Patient serum	$+^w$	4+	Patient cells	3+ mf	0

A. Group A_2 patient with anti-A_1 in his serum
B. Group A patient having rouleaux
C. Group A patient transfused with group O cells
D. Group A patient with acquired B antigen

89. A physician would like to increase the hemoglobin level of a patient before surgery by 3 g/dL. How many units of packed red blood cells will this patient need to meet the minimum criteria?
A. 2 units
B. 3 units
C. 4 units
D. 5 units

90. When testing blood donors for human immunodeficiency virus (HIV), what is the major advantage of nucleic acid amplification test over enzyme immunoassay testing for anti-HIV1?
   A. Simplicity of performance
   B. Less expensive
   C. Requires less "tech time"
   D. Increased specificity
91. What is the expiration date for fresh frozen plasma that is stored at −18°C or colder?
   A. 1 year
   B. 3 years
   C. 5 years
   D. 7 years
92. A 35-year-old male is found to have a factor V deficiency. He should be treated for the deficiency with:
   A. Cryoprecipitated antihemophilic factor
   B. Red blood cells
   C. Fresh frozen plasma
   D. Pooled platelet concentrates
93. Which of the following donors would most likely be allowed to donate autologous blood for elective surgery if all other criteria are acceptable?
   A. 15-year-old girl with a hemoglobin of 12 g/dL
   B. 17-year-old boy with intermittent bacteremia
   C. 30-year-old man with aortic stenosis
   D. 25-year-old woman who had a baby 4 weeks ago
94. A 32-year-old female, pregnant with her fourth child, is seen in the emergency department for childbirth. There are no records of her prenatal care available. She is group AB, D-negative, weak D negative. She gives birth to a group O, D-negative, weak D positive girl. Her husband is group O, D-negative, weak D positive. Which of the following may explain these results?
   A. Nonpaternity
   B. Mother carries the *cis-AB* gene
   C. Father has been mistyped
   D. Child has been switched with another woman's infant
95. A and B blood group antigens are derived when glycosyltransferases add specific sugars to precursor H. What is the terminal sugar for the B antigen?
   A. Fucose
   B. *N*-acetylglucosamine
   C. *N*-acetylgalactosamine
   D. D-Galactose
96. A patient has the Rh phenotype below. What is the most likely Rh genotype?
   D+, C+, c+, E+, e+
   A. R1R1
   B. R1R2
   C. R2r
   D. R2r"
97. Which of the following antigens is the most immunogenic after A, B, and D antigens?
   A. C
   B. E
   C. Fy^a
   D. K
98. What is likely to be found in the serum of a person diagnosed with transfusion related acute lung injury?
   A. Anti-D antibody
   B. Anti-leukocyte antibody
   C. IgA antibody
   D. Red blood cell alloantibody

99. An antibody screen gives the following results. What do the results indicate about the patient?

	SC I	SC II	Auto-control
IS	1+	0	0
37°C LISS	0	1+	0
AHG (monospecific)	0	3+	0
CC	√		√

A. Autoantibody reacting at all phases of testing
B. Alloantibody showing dosage
C. More than one alloantibody
D. Rouleaux reaction

100. In which of the following situations would a DAT (direct antiglobulin test) be of value?
A. Transfusion reaction work-up
B. Alloimmune thrombocytopenia
C. Negative autocontrol
D. Negative antibody screen

101. A "type and screen" established that an infant is group A, D-positive with a negative antibody screening test. Numerous small volume transfusions are predicted. If only group O red blood cells are to be transfused, how often must the infant be crossmatched?
A. Before transfusion and whenever 3 days have elapsed before the next transfusion
B. Before transfusion and whenever 7 days have elapsed before the next transfusion
C. If during the same admission, not until he reaches 2 months of age
D. If during the same admission, not until he reaches 4 months of age

102. What antibody is most likely to cause compatibility issues when O-negative packed cell units are emergency released without being crossmatched?
A. Anti-A
B. Anti-C
C. Anti-c
D. Anti-e

103. Using the chart below, what is(are) the most likely antibody specificity(ies) in this patient's serum?

Cell #	D	C	E	K	Jk^a	Jk^b	AHG	CC
1	+	0	0	+	0	0	2+	
2	+	0	0	0	+	0	0	√
3	+	+	+	0	+	0	0	√
4	0	+	0	+	0	+	4+	
5	0	0	+	0	0	+	1+	

A. Anti-C and anti-Jk^a
B. Anti-K and anti-Jk^b
C. Anti-C showing dosage and anti-E
D. Anti-Jk^b

104. What is the most common cause of anemia leading to transfusion in neonates who are ill?
A. Bleeding from the umbilicus
B. Red blood cell destruction because of hemolytic disease of the newborn
C. Blood drawn for laboratory testing
D. Immature bone marrow response

105. What is the initial step to perform when a patient is suspected of having a transfusion reaction?
A. Perform a DAT on a posttransfusion specimen
B. Compare the pretransfusion and posttransfusion serum for evidence of hemolysis
C. Check identification of the patient and donor blood
D. Stop the transfusion

106. A patient has anti-c. If 80% of donors are c-positive and 68% are C-positive, how many red blood cell units will need to be tested in order to find two compatible units?
A. 5
B. 7
C. 10
D. 15

107. To which organization must the hospital transfusion service laboratory report all cases of transfusion-associated disease?
   A. Blood-collecting facility
   B. Centers for Disease Control and Prevention
   C. Food and Drug Administration
   D. State Health Department

108. To comply with the requirements of AABB *Standards for Blood Banks and Transfusion Services,* which of the following tests must be performed on each unit before blood bank personnel may issue autologous units of blood drawn in their facility?
   A. ABO and Rh typing
   B. HBsAg
   C. Anti-HIV1
   D. DAT

109. The Centers for Disease Control and Prevention recommends that "standard precautions" be exercised by all healthcare workers to prevent transmission of hepatitis B virus, HIV, and other blood-borne pathogens. What do these precautions include?
   A. Wearing protective clothing when testing blood specimens from patients in specific areas
   B. Using special precautionary methods when testing blood specimens with a biohazard label
   C. Handling every patient blood specimen as if it were infectious
   D. Carefully recapping needles before discarding

110. To ensure proper reactivity, how frequently must all blood bank reagents be quality controlled?
   A. With each test
   B. Daily
   C. Each day of use
   D. Weekly

111. What should one do to validate the reaction obtained in the antiglobulin test?
   A. Use antiglobulin reagent
   B. Add IgG-coated red cells to each test tube
   C. Add IgG-coated red cells to each positive reaction
   D. Add IgG-coated red cells to each negative reaction

112. What is the term defining the identification and notification of recipients of blood products who tested positive for transfusion-transmitted disease?
   A. Exclusion
   B. Deferral
   C. Lookback
   D. MSBOS

113. Which of the following antibodies could be identified using a patient specimen collected in a red top tube (plain glass), but may not be identified if a purple top tube (EDTA) was used for the collection?
   A. Anti-M
   B. Anti-E
   C. Anti-Jk^a
   D. Anti-D

114. Which antibody would not be detected by group O screening cells?
   A. Anti-B
   B. Anti-C
   C. Anti-K
   D. Anti-Fya

115. An immediate spin crossmatch or a computer crossmatch (if the computer system is validated for this use) may be used as the sole compatibility test when a patient has a confirmed blood type, a negative antibody screening test, and:
   A. A negative DAT result
   B. No history of unexpected antibody
   C. No record of previous transfusion
   D. The same ABO and Rh type as the donor

116. Within how many hours after pooling must pooled platelet concentrates be transfused?
A. 4
B. 6
C. 8
D. 12

CHAPTER 6: BACTERIOLOGY

117. Pus with a blue-green color was aspirated from an empyema. A Gram stain of the aspirated material showed many white blood cells and numerous gram-negative bacilli. What is the most likely etiologic agent?
A. *Legionella pneumophila*
B. *Pseudomonas aeruginosa*
C. *Morganella morganii*
D. *Serratia marcescens*

118. In the early stages of typhoid fever, *Salmonella* Typhi is most likely to be recovered from which of the following specimen types?
A. Blood
B. Feces
C. Urine
D. Skin lesions

119. Symptoms of gastritis and peptic ulceration are most closely associated with which of the following?
A. *Campylobacter jejuni*
B. Enterotoxigenic *Escherichia coli*
C. *Helicobacter pylori*
D. *Vibrio cholerae*

120. A patient with impaired cell-mediated immunity presents with evidence of a pulmonary abscess and neurologic involvement. A brain abscess was detected by magnetic resonance imaging. Material from the abscess grew an aerobic, filamentous, branching gram-positive organism, which stained weakly acid-fast. What is the most likely etiologic agent?
A. *Cutibacterium (Propionibacterium) acnes*
B. *Nocardia* spp.
C. *Actinobacillus israelii*
D. *Bacillus cereus*

121. The organism *Borrelia recurrentis* is the etiologic agent of:
A. Lyme disease
B. Relapsing fever
C. Undulant fever
D. Weil disease

122. Most cases of legionellosis are acquired from:
A. Environmental water sources
B. Person-to-person transmission
C. Mosquitoes
D. Farm animals

123. What chemical(s) is(are) commonly added to blood culture media as an anticoagulant and to prevent the killing of bacteria by innate cellular and humoral factors?
A. Tween 80
B. Colistin and naladixic acid
C. Cefsulodin, irgasin, and novobiocin
D. Sodium polyanethole sulfonate

124. Which of the following statements is *true* regarding anaerobic infections?
   A. Anaerobic pulmonary infections are rare because lung tissue is well saturated with oxygen.
   B. Because of the inaccessibility of organs such as the liver and brain to indigenous biota, they are seldom infected with anaerobes.
   C. Bacteremia due to anaerobes is benign because anaerobes do not possess endotoxin.
   D. Intra-abdominal abscesses, peritonitis, and wound infections can occur postoperatively when devitalized tissue is contaminated with bowel contents.

125. Foul-smelling pus aspirated from a postsurgical cholecystectomy patient grew a gram-positive bacillus. When cultured on an anaerobically incubated blood agar plate, it grew colonies surrounded by an inner zone of complete red blood cell lysis and an outer zone of incomplete cell lysis. What would be the most likely identification of this isolate?
   A. *Fusobacterium nucleatum*
   B. *Clostridium perfringens*
   C. *Clostridium tetani*
   D. *Bacteroides fragilis*

126. A common cause of mild, primary atypical pneumonia is:
   A. *Bordetella parapertussis*
   B. *Mycoplasma pneumoniae*
   C. *Pseudomonas aeruginosa*
   D. *Streptococcus pneumoniae*

127. Which of the following antimicrobial susceptibility tests would provide the minimal inhibitory concentration?
   A. D-test
   B. Hodge test
   C. Disk diffusion
   D. Gradient diffusion

128. Which of the following is associated with *Streptococcus agalactiae?*
   A. Common cause of pharyngitis in adults
   B. Important cause of neonatal sepsis and meningitis
   C. Is also called viridans *Streptococcus*
   D. Is implicated in dental caries

129. The presence of spirochetes seen in material collected from a chancre is diagnostic for
   A. Chancroid
   B. Lyme disease
   C. Relapsing fever
   D. Syphilis

130. Which of the following is associated with *Vibrio cholerae?*
   A. Sucrose fermentation negative
   B. Requires media with high salt concentration
   C. Is a component of the normal microbiota of the human intestine
   D. Produces a toxin that causes increased secretion of water and electrolytes from the intestines

131. A blood culture grew a small, pleomorphic, anaerobic, gram-negative rod. It grew on kanamycin-vancomycin laked-sheep blood agar, in the presence of 20% bile, and was esculin positive. This organism is most likely:
   A. *Bacteroides fragilis*
   B. *Clostridium perfringens*
   C. *Fusobacterium nucleatum*
   D. *Veillonella* sp.

132. A coagulase-negative *Staphylococcus* was isolated from a urine culture. It was identified as *Staphylococcus saprophyticus* on the basis of it being:
   A. Coagulase negative
   B. Resistant to novobiocin
   C. DNase positive
   D. Mannitol positive

133. In a cefoxitin disk diffusion test, a *Staphylococcus aureus* isolate exhibits a 20 mm zone of inhibition, this indicates:
A. Cefoxitin sensitive
B. Oxacillin resistant
C. Ketolide resistant
D. Chloramphenicol sensitive

134. Refer to Color Plate 26■. The organism seen on this Gram stain was isolated from the cerebrospinal fluid of an infant. It grew on sheep blood agar with faint beta-hemolysis. It was catalase positive. What microorganism should be suspected?
A. *Bacillus subtilis*
B. *Lactobacillus* sp.
C. *Bifidobacterium dentium*
D. *Listeria monocytogenes*

135. You isolate a small, pleomorphic, gram-negative rod from the cerebrospinal fluid of a 9-month-old infant. It fails to grow on sheep blood agar or MacConkey agar, but it grows well on chocolate agar incubated in 5% CO_2. What bacterium should you suspect?
A. *Escherichia coli*
B. *Streptococcus agalactiae*
C. *Haemophilus influenzae*
D. *Listeria monocytogenes*

136. How might MALDI-TOF MS be able to predict resistance to an antimicrobial agent?
A. Detects drug resistant gene
B. Detects protein responsible for drug resistance
C. Identifies bacteriophage carrying drug resistant marker
D. Performs antimicrobial susceptibility test during identification

137. What is the primary risk factor for *Clostridioides (Clostridium) difficile*-associated infection?
A. Age less than 1 year
B. Age greater than 50 years
C. Recent administration of oral antimicrobial agents
D. Immune suppression

138. A stool culture yields moderate growth of clear colonies and pink colonies on a MacConkey agar plate. On a Hektoen-enteric agar plate, moderate growth of clear colonies with black centers is found. A possible pathogen is:
A. *Salmonella* Typhimurium
B. *Shigella sonnei*
C. *Proteus mirabilis*
D. *Edwardsiella tarda*

139. A 60-year-old male presents to the emergency department with fever, chills, and difficulty breathing. He has a productive cough. A stat Gram stain of his pinkish-yellow sputum reveals gram-positive cocci in pairs. You should suspect:
A. *Chlamydophila pneumoniae*
B. *Staphylococcus aureus*
C. *Streptococcus pneumoniae*
D. *Streptococcus mutans*

140. A 45-year-old woman came to the emergency department after being bitten on the hand by her cat. The wound was extremely painful and produced a large amount of pus. The pus was cultured on sheep blood agar (SBA) and MacConkey agar. After 24 hours, growth was observed on the SBA plate as tiny colonies that produced a slight greening on the medium. A Gram stain revealed tiny gram-negative rods. There was no growth on the MacConkey agar. Biochemical tests gave the following reactions:
TSI-A/A
Oxidase positive
Nonmotile
Urease negative
The most likely organism would be:
A. *Pasturella multocida*
B. *Corynebacterium diphtheriae*
C. *Brucella abortus*
D. *Bordetella pertussis*

141. Buffered charcoal yeast extract agar is the primary medium for the isolation of:
A. *Bartonella bacilliformis*
B. *Chlamydia pneumoniae*
C. *Legionella pneumophila*
D. *Mycoplasma pneumoniae*

CHAPTER 7: MYCOLOGY

142. What form of the fungus *Coccidioides immitis* is found in human tissue?
A. Yeast
B. Spherule
C. Hyaline aseptate hyphae
D. Macroconidia with budding yeast

143. Selective medium for the isolation of the dimorphic fungi often contain what agent to inhibit the growth of the saprophytic fungi?
A. Cyclohexamide
B. Chloramphenicol
C. Sulfonamide
D. Gentamicin

144. A yeast or yeast-like fungus is growing on cornmeal agar with Tween 80, and the only structures observed are branched pseudohyphae and blastospores grouped in short chains or alone. Based on that description, what is the most probable species?
A. *Geotrichum* sp.
B. *Candida tropicalis*
C. *Candida albicans*
D. *Trichosporon* sp.

CHAPTER 8: PARASITOLOGY

145. A peripheral blood smear of a patient who had recently been on safari in Africa showed the presence of intracellular organisms. The infected red blood cells were enlarged with a smooth membrane. The organism filled about 1/3 of the cell and was amoeboid in shape. Based on this description what is the most likely identification?
A. *Plasmodium malariae*
B. *P. vivax*
C. *P. knowlesi*
D. *P. ovale*

146. An iodine wet mount of a stool concentrate demonstrates the presence of multiple oval structures about 11 um in length. There appears to be 4 nuclei each with a large karyosome. There are several curved, rod-like inclusions. The most likely identification is a cyst of:
A. *Cyclospora* sp.
B. *Endolimax nana*
C. *Entamoeba histolytica*
D. *Giardia duodenalis*

147. The presence of multiple *ring forms* in a single red blood cell is suggestive of:
A. *Babesia* sp.
B. *Plasmodium malariae*
C. *Plasmodium ovale*
D. *Trypanosoma* sp.

CHAPTER 9: VIROLOGY

148. In what way are hepatitis B virus and human immunodeficiency virus similar?
A. Preferred target cell
B. Have cross-reacting antigens
C. Nucleic acid composition
D. Require RNA-dependent DNA-polymerase for replication

149. A 16-year-old male presents with fever, enlarged cervical lymph nodes, and mild fatigue. A heterophile test is negative. The primary healthcare provider suspects infectious mononucleosis and orders an IgM viral core antigen (VCA) test, which is also negative. You should suspect:
A. Chicken pox
B. Cytomegalovirus infection
C. Epstein-Barr virus infection
D. A false-negative IgM VCA test

150. Other than viral RNA, the first detectable serum marker for human immunodeficiency virus (HIV) infection is:
A. p24
B. gp41
C. Anti-HIV-1 antibodies
D. Anti-HIV-2 antibodies

CHAPTER 10: MOLECULAR DIAGNOSTICS

151. A probe with the sequence 5′AGCGTGAGCT 3′ will bind to which single-stranded product?
A. 5′AGCGTGAGCT 3′
B. 5′TCGAGTGCGA 3′
C. 5′TGCGATCGAG 3′
D. 5′AGCTCACGCT 3′

152. A common activating mutation in the oncogene *KRAS* is reported as G12A. What does G12A denote?
A. Adenine is replaced by guanine in exon 12 of the *KRAS* gene.
B. Adenine is replacing glycine at amino acid position 12 of the *KRAS* gene.
C. Alanine is replacing glycine at amino acid position 12 of the *KRAS* gene.
D. Glycine is replacing alanine at amino acid position 12 of the *KRAS* gene.

153. Southern blot methods were replaced by polymerase chain reaction (PCR) procedures in forensic applications. What is the advantage of PCR?
A. PCR is more informative on high quality DNA.
B. Since PCR does not require an electrophoresis step, it is more rapid than Southern blot.
C. Unlike Southern blot, PCR can amplify DNA from degraded samples and DNA in limited amounts.
D. The PCR process does not require temperature changes.

154. Which of the following is an example of a signal amplification method?
A. Branched DNA
B. Ligase chain reaction
C. Polymerase chain reaction
D. Strand displacement amplification

155. Stringency can be decreased by increasing:
A. Incubation time
B. Incubation temperature
C. Ionic strength (e.g., NaCl)
D. pH

156. A single base change abolishes a restriction enzyme site in a disease gene. Using specific primers that target a portion of the gene, a 282 base pair PCR product is generated. After enzyme digestion of PCR products from normal individuals, fragments of 201 bp and 81 bp are produced. Which of the following restriction fragment patterns represent the results you would see in a patient heterozygous for the single base change?
   A. Two bands—282 bp and 81 bp
   B. Three bands—282 bp, 201 bp, and 81 bp
   C. Two bands—201 bp, and 81 bp
   D. Three bands—365 bp, 201 bp, and 81 bp

157. A PCR test is performed on a male patient with mild learning disabilities. Results from PCR amplification of the 5′ region of the gene *FMR1* followed by capillary electrophoresis produced a series of peaks less than 40 bp.
   A. This result is positive for fragile X syndrome.
   B. This is a negative result for fragile X syndrome.
   C. The patient is a fragile X carrier.
   D. The patient has a premutation for fragile X.

158. In a PCR assay, which control is necessary to distinguish between a true negative result and a false negative result?
   A. Reagent blank (no DNA template) control containing all PCR reagents
   B. Negative template control containing DNA sample known not to contain target sequence
   C. Internal control containing second primer set to sequence found in all samples but unrelated to target sequence
   D. Positive control containing target sequence

159. Which of the following qPCR systems utilizes a probe that contains a short target-specific sequence flanked by a short inverted repeat whose 5′ end is a fluorescent reporter molecule that forms a stem and loop structure with a 3′ end quencher molecule when not bound to the target sequence?
   A. SYBR green detection system
   B. TaqMan probe detection system
   C. Fluorescent resonance energy transfer detection system
   D. Molecular Beacons® detection system

160. Which of the following is(are) output signals for ion conductance sequencing?
   A. Fluorescent signals of four colors
   B. Changes in pH
   C. Chemiluminescence
   D. Absorbance at 260 nm

CHAPTER 11: URINALYSIS AND BODY FLUIDS

161. Which reagent strip test utilizes copper and a peroxidase-link principle as a part of its method?
   A. Glucose
   B. Clinitest
   C. Blood
   D. Creatinine

162. In what area of the nephron does approximately 65% of renal reabsorption occur?
   A. Proximal tubule
   B. Distal tubule
   C. Bowman capsule
   D. Glomerulus

163. What is the renal blood flow for a 70-kg individual?
   A. 12 mL/min
   B. 120 mL/min
   C. 1200 mL/min
   D. 12 L/min

164. Which of the following filtrate glucose concentrations will result in glucose being found in the urine?
A. 98 mg/dL
B. 126 mg/dL
C. Renal threshold 152 mg/dL
D. Blood threshold 173 mg/dL

165. When mixing a patient urine sample, you notice that a stable yellow foam forms at the surface of the urine. Which biochemical test will you expect to see as "positive" when testing is completed?
A. Glucose
B. Bilirubin
C. Protein
D. Blood

166. Given the following data, calculate the creatinine clearance?

Analyte	Result
Serum Creatinine	1.4 mg/dL
Urine Creatinine	118 mg/dL
Urine Volume	1.70 L/day
Surface Area	1.80 m^2

A. 70 mL/min
B. 90 mL/min
C. 100 mL/min
D. 120 mL/min

167. Ascites fluid is derived from which source?
A. Abdominal cavity
B. Knee joints
C. Central nervous system
D. Space around the lungs

168. Which of the following formed elements are present in the high-power field seen in Color Plate 53■?
A. Transitional epithelial cells, oval fat bodies, spermatozoa
B. Renal epithelial cells, mucus, calcium oxalate
C. Red blood cells, squamous epithelial cells, white blood cells
D. Yeast, squamous epithelial cells, mucus

169. Which of the following is *true* about uromodulin (Tamm-Horsfall) protein?
A. Measured using the conventional reagent test strips
B. Appears only in abnormal urine
C. Matrix of hyaline casts but not granular casts
D. Produced by renal tubules in small quantities

170. Which of the following procedures is used to assess the filtration ability of the glomeruli?
A. eGFR
B. Sulfosalicylic acid
C. Nitroprusside
D. Specific gravity

171. With which crystals are urinary cysteine crystals often confused?
A. Calcium pyrophosphate
B. Uric acid
C. Cholesterol
D. Calcium oxalate

172. In what sequence does urine formation occur?
A. Proximal convoluted tubule, loop of Henle, distal convoluted tubule, collecting duct, Bowman's space
B. Glomerulus, Bowman's space, proximal convoluted tubule, loop of Henle, distal convoluted tubule, collecting duct
C. Bowman's space, glomerulus, proximal convoluted tubule, loop of Henle, distal convoluted tubule, collecting duct
D. Bowman's space, glomerulus, distal convoluted tubule, proximal convoluted tubule, collecting duct

173. New glucose control therapy used by those with type 2 diabetes have a mechanism which will ________ but can have the side effect of ________.
   A. increase glucose excretion, high risk of yeast urinary tract infection
   B. increase insulin production, increased ketone production
   C. decease glucose reabsorption, lower urine protein levels
   D. decrease ketone production, higher bilirubin levels
174. Which of the following do the formed elements present in the high-power field in Color Plate 44■ suggest?
   A. Nephrotic syndrome
   B. Pyelonephritis
   C. Excessive exercise
   D. Diabetic nephropathy
175. The formed elements present in the high-power field in Color Plate 50■ can be detected by the appropriate reagent strip pad reacting with their:
   A. Pseudoperoxidase
   B. Esterase
   C. Glucose oxidase
   D. Acetoacetate
176. When using polarized light microscopy, which urinary sediment component exhibits Maltese cross formation?
   A. Red blood cells
   B. White blood cells
   C. Yeasts
   D. Oval fat bodies
177. Which urinary sediment component is frequently confused with the component in Color Plate 46■?
   A. Yeasts
   B. WBCs
   C. Parasites
   D. Casts
178. Which of the following is the component of synovial fluid that provides the cushioning needed for the joint?
   A. Glucose oxidase
   B. B.Hyalurane oxalate
   C. Hyaluronic acid
   D. Hyaluronidase
179. What type of microscopy may also be used to observe the urinary components in Color Plate 48■?
   A. Polarized
   B. Darkfield
   C. Phase contrast
   D. Electron
180. Which of the following urine biochemical result would be obtained in hemolytic anemia?
   A. Negative bilirubin
   B. Negative blood
   C. Positive nitrite
   D. Negative urobilinogen

CHAPTER 12: LABORATORY CALCULATIONS

181. A patient serum was diluted by adding 3.5 mL of buffer to 0.5 mL of the patient sample. The absorbance of a 20.0 mmol/L hormone standard is 0.831. The diluted patient serum has an absorbance of 0.509. What is the value of the unknown which you will report to this patient's physician?
   A. 12.3 mmol/L
   B. 32.7 mmol/L
   C. 85.8 mmol/L
   D. 98.0 mmolL

182. You need 400 mL of a glucose calibrator which must contain 100 mg/dL glucose, and your stock is labeled "80 mmol/L glucose." What volume of stock do you need to add to the diluent to make this calibrator? Mol. wt. of glucose = 180 g/mol
A. 2.8 mL
B. 18 mL
C. 136 mL
D. 500 mL

183. Into a test tube you place 500 μL patient serum, 1 mL of 200 mmol/L sulfuric acid, 2.5 mL of 10% (w/v) sodium tungstate, and 1000 μL distilled water. What's the final serum dilution?
A. 1:3
B. 1:5
C. 1:9
D. 1:10

CHAPTER 13: GENERAL LABORATORY PRINCIPLES

184. Which of the following statements describes standard precautions?
A. Everyone should be careful before entering a patient room.
B. Treat all human blood and other potentially infectious materials as though they contained infectious particles.
C. Treat human blood as infectious only if it is known to be.
D. All human blood and other infectious material must be handled while wearing a respirator.

185. Which of the following is *true* of a volumetric pipette?
A. Blow out the last drop
B. Is labeled "to contain" (TC)
C. Is used for diluting control material
D. Is rinsed out

186. Which type of fire extinguisher should be used to deal with a laboratory fire consisting of ordinary combustibles (e.g., wood and paper)?
A. A
B. B
C. C
D. D

187. When performing a method evaluation, which of the following types of error is measured using a replication study?
A. Random error
B. Constant systematic error
C. Proportional systematic error
D. Total error

188. Which of the following is the range of values described as the mean plus or minus some number of standard deviations, forming the basis of statistical rules for acceptance and rejection of quality control values?
A. Variance
B. Degrees of freedom
C. Coefficient of variation
D. Confidence interval

189. Serum samples are collected from patients over a 2-week period and are split into two aliquots and analyzed for cholesterol by two methods. Each sample was assayed by both methods within 30 minutes of collection by a laborataory scientist familiar with both methods. The reference method is method x (upper reference limit 200 mg/dL). Linear regression analysis was performed and the results are as follows:

Linear regression	Correlation coefficient	Standard error of the estimate
Y = 2.50 + 1.03x	0.998	0.23

Which statement below best characterizes the relationship between the methods?
A. There is a significant amount of proportional error
B. There is no disagreement between the two methods because the correlation coefficient is approaching 1.0
C. There is a significant bias caused by constant error
D. There is a significant amount of random and systematic error

CHAPTER 14: LABORATORY MANAGEMENT

190. Which coding system is a systematized series of numbers corresponding to all diseases, and other medical, surgical, and mental health conditions, published annually by the American Medical Association for the purpose of standardizing and coding for statistical and billing activities in healthcare?
A. CPT
B. HCPCS
C. ICD-10-CM
D. DRG

191. When pricing new tests, a laboratory must use a factor to calculate the allowance for the hospital's cost for utilities, housekeeping, administration, and other services. What are these costs known as?
A. Direct
B. Overhead
C. Depreciation
D. Indirect labor

192. What is the authority relationship from administration to department head to supervisor to staff known as?
A. Line authority
B. Staff authority
C. Formal authority
D. Job-related authority

CHAPTER 15: EDUCATION

193. The verbs "perform" and "analyze" would most likely be used in writing an objective in which of the following domains?
A. Affective
B. Cognitive
C. Psychomotor
D. Technical

194. Classify the following *objective:* "The student will list the substances contained in the dense bodies and alpha granules."
A. Cognitive domain
B. Psychomotor domain
C. Psychosocial domain
D. Affective domain

195. Which of the following best describes criterion-referenced tests?
A. Students are evaluated based on performance compared to their peers.
B. Used to assess students' knowledge of a subject prior to researching a topic.
C. Students are evaluated based on mastery of the specific content where the scoring criterion is established prior to the test administration.
D. Used to assess the presence of a learning disability.

196. Which of the following types of research are used to compare different groups that have been assigned to receive different treatments?

A. Experimental-comparison design
B. Correlational design
C. Descriptive research
D. Single-case experimental design

197. Which of the following types of validity is used to demonstrate the correlation between scores on a scale and scores on another scale that has been validated?

A. Content validity
B. Predictive validity
C. Concurrent validity
D. Construct validity

CHAPTER 16: COMPUTERS

198. What do laboratories need to send results from an auto-analyzer to a laboratory information system?

A. Malware
B. Interface
C. Reflex Testing
D. Audit Trail

199. A contingency plan that takes place when the laboratory information system is unavailable is also nicknamed:

A. Recovery
B. Middleware
C. Back-up
D. Downtime

200. An example of standardized terminology in healthcare where specific codes are given to tests:

A. LOINC
B. Demographic
C. Request for proposal
D. Electronic data interface

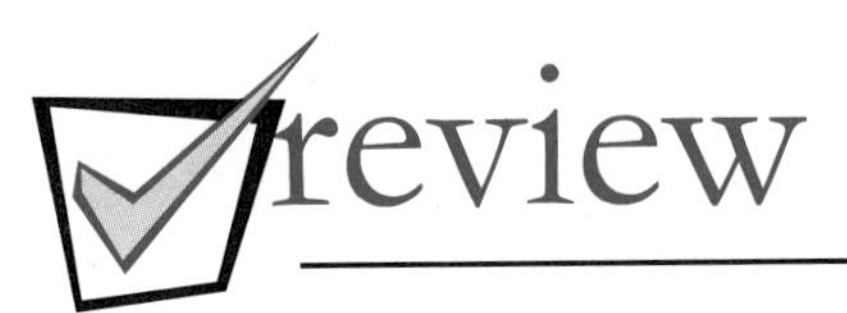

review answers

CHAPTER 1: CLINICAL CHEMISTRY

1. C
2. D
3. C
4. A
5. D
6. A
7. C
8. C
9. D
10. B
11. D
12. C
13. B
14. D
15. A
16. D
17. C
18. C
19. D
20. A
21. B
22. C
23. A
24. B
25. A
26. D

CHAPTER 2: HEMATOLOGY

27. A
28. A
29. C
30. A
31. A
32. D
33. A
34. C
35. B
36. D
37. C
38. C
39. B
40. B
41. C
42. C
43. B
44. D
45. A
46. B
47. C
48. B
49. A
50. D
51. A
52. B
53. D
54. B
55. D
56. C

CHAPTER 3: HEMOSTASIS

57. C
58. D
59. A
60. D
61. B
62. A
63. A
64. D
65. B
66. A

CHAPTER 4: IMMUNOLOGY & SEROLOGY

67. D
68. A
69. D
70. C
71. A
72. A
73. C
74. D
75. B
76. A
77. C
78. B
79. D
80. A
81. A
82. C
83. C
84. B
85. A
86. A

CHAPTER 5: IMMUNOHEMATOLOGY

87. D
88. C
89. B
90. D
91. A
92. A
93. A
94. B
95. D
96. B
97. D
98. B
99. C
100. A
101. D
102. C
103. B
104. C
105. D
106. C
107. A
108. A
109. C
110. C
111. D
112. C
113. C
114. A
115. B
116. A

CHAPTER 6: BACTERIOLOGY

117. B
118. A
119. C
120. B
121. B
122. A
123. D
124. D
125. B
126. B
127. D
128. B
129. D
130. D
131. A
132. B
133. B
134. D
135. C
136. B
137. C
138. A
139. C
140. A
141. C

CHAPTER 7: MYCOLOGY

142. B
143. A
144. B

CHAPTER 8: PARASITOLOGY

145. B
146. D
147. A

CHAPTER 9: VIROLOGY

148. D
149. B
150. A

CHAPTER 10: MOLECULAR DIAGNOSTICS

151. D
152. C
153. C
154. A
155. C
156. B
157. B
158. C
159. D
160. A

CHAPTER 11: URINALYSIS AND BODY FLUIDS

161. D
162. A
163. C
164. D
165. B
166. C
167. A
168. C
169. D
170. A
171. B
172. B
173. A
174. B
175. A
176. D
177. D
178. C
179. C
180. A

CHAPTER 12: LABORATORY CALCULATIONS

181. D
182. A
183. D

CHAPTER 13: GENERAL LABORATORY PRINCIPLES

184. B
185. C
186. A
187. A
188. D
189. C

CHAPTER 14: LABORATORY MANAGEMENT

190. C
191. B
192. A

CHAPTER 15: EDUCATION

193. C
194. A
195. C
196. A
197. C

CHAPTER 16: COMPUTERS

198. B
199. D
200. A

Index

G

H

N

O

P